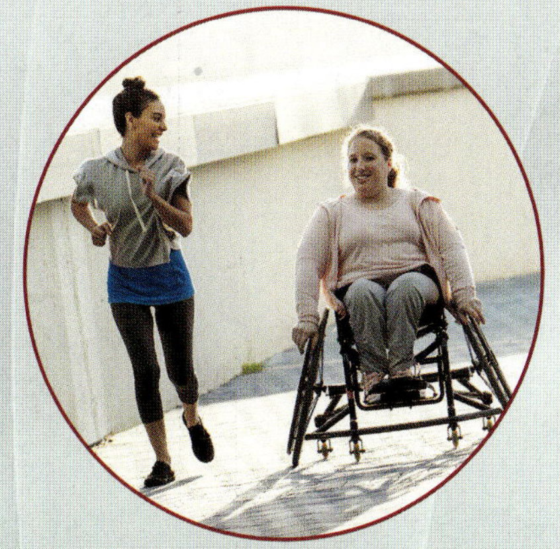
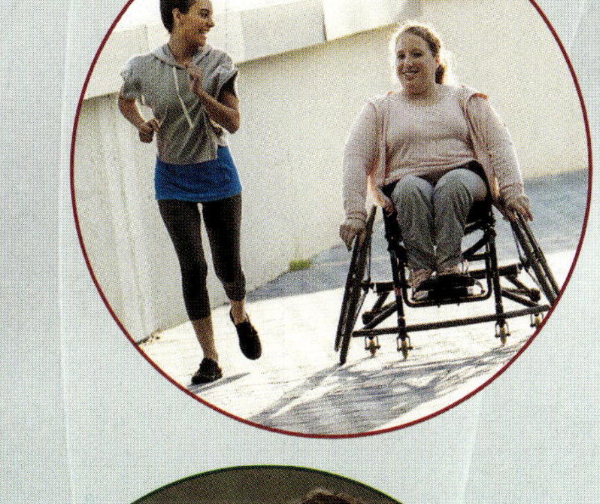
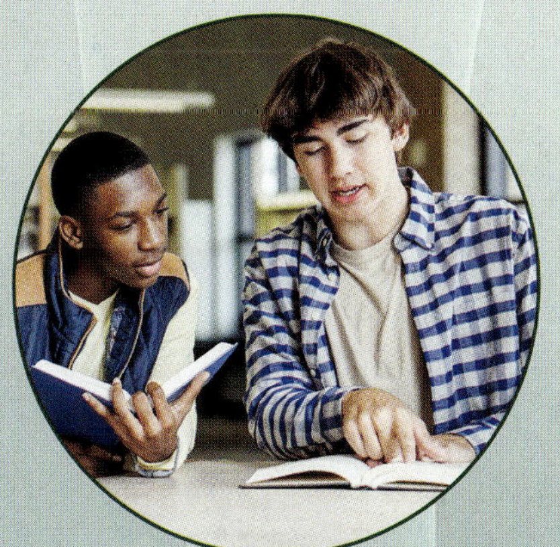
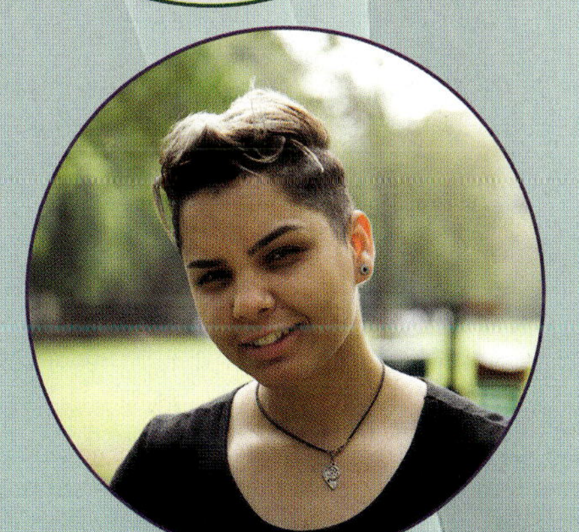
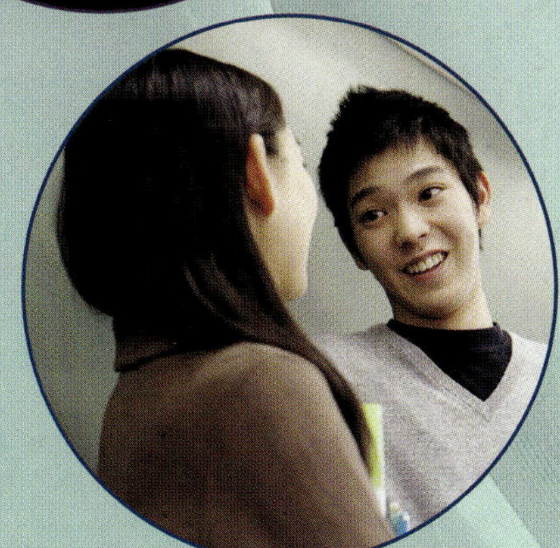

Comprehensive Health Skills

Third Edition

Catherine A. Sanderson, PhD
Professor of Psychology
Amherst College
Amherst, Massachusetts

Mark Zelman, PhD
Professor of Biology
Aurora University
Aurora, Illinois

Pedagogy Developers

Diane Farthing, NBCT
Health Educator
Pleasanton, California

Melanie Lynch, M.Ed.
Health Education Specialist
Pittsburgh, Pennsylvania

Melissa Munsell
Instructional Specialist
Physical Education and Health Department
San Antonio, Texas

Publisher
The Goodheart-Willcox Company, Inc.
Tinley Park, Illinois
www.g-w.com

Previously published as *Comprehensive Health*

Previous editions copyright 2018, 2015

Manufactured in the United States of America.

ISBN 978-1-64564-409-5

1 2 3 4 5 6 7 8 9 — 21 — 25 24 23 22 21 20

Cover images: Left column, top to bottom: kali9/E+/GettyImages, kali9/E+/GettyImages, FG Trade/E+/GettyImages, KPG_Payless/Shutterstock.com; Right image: Shift Drive/Shutterstock.com
Blue background element: ArtFish/Shutterstock.com
Big Ideas icon: Hilch/Shutterstock.com
Health Management Plan icon: IconBunny/Shutterstock.com
Skills icon: Goodheart-Willcox Publisher
Reading and Notetaking icon: Webicon/Shutterstock.com
Setting the Scene icon: Legend_art/Shutterstock.com
Research in Action icon: Lucky Creative/Shutterstock.com
Health in the Media icon: Dacian G/Shutterstock.com
Case Study icon: FishCoolish/Shutterstock.com
Quiz icon: VectorKnight/Shutterstock.com
Local and Global Health icon: Oleh Svetiukha/Shutterstock.com
Spotlight on Health and Wellness Careers icon: Imagine Room/Shutterstock.com
Health Across the Life Span background: Triff/Shutterstock.com

About the Authors

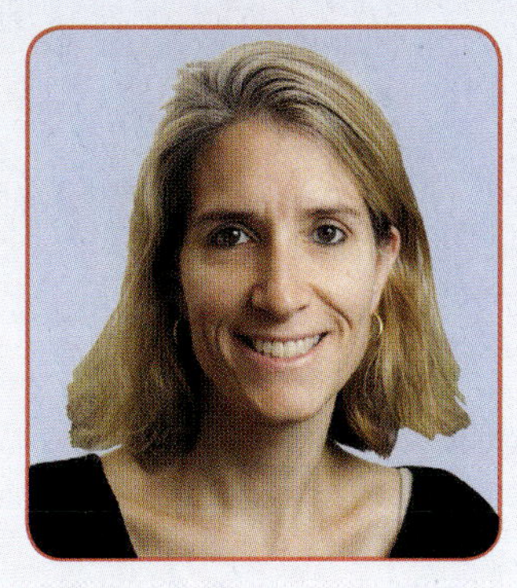

Catherine A. Sanderson is the Manwell Family Professor of Life Sciences (Psychology) at Amherst College. She received a bachelor's degree in psychology, with a specialization in Health and Development, from Stanford University, and received both master's and doctoral degrees in psychology from Princeton University. Professor Sanderson's research examines how personality and social variables influence health-related behaviors, such as safer sex and disordered eating. Her research also examines the development of persuasive messages and interventions to prevent unhealthy behavior and predictors of relationship satisfaction. This research has received grant funding from the National Science Foundation and the National Institutes of Health. Professor Sanderson has published more than 25 journal articles and book chapters; four college textbooks; high school and middle school health textbooks; and a trade book, *The Positive Shift*, which examines how mind-set influences happiness, health, and even how long people live. Her latest book, *Why We Act: Turning Bystanders into Moral Rebels*, examines why good people often stay silent or do nothing in the face of wrongdoing. In 2012, she was named one of the country's top 300 professors by the Princeton Review.

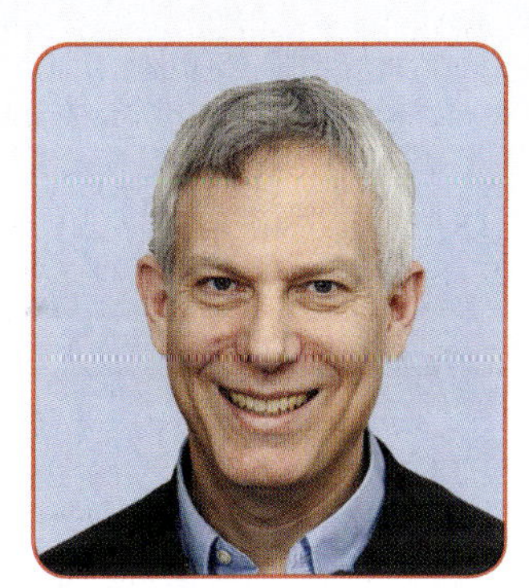

Mark Zelman is a Professor of Biology at Aurora University, Aurora, Illinois. He received a bachelor's degree in biology at Rockford College, with minors in chemistry and psychology. He received a PhD in microbiology and immunology at Loyola University of Chicago, where he studied the molecular and cellular mechanisms of autoimmune disease. During his postdoctoral research at the University of Chicago, he studied aspects of cell physiology pertaining to cell growth and cancer. Dr. Zelman supervises undergraduate research on streptococcal and staphylococcal infections, and mechanisms of antibiotic resistance. He teaches science education courses for high school teachers. He has published articles on microbiology, infectious disease, autoimmune disease, and biotechnology, and he has written two college texts on human diseases and infection control. Dr. Zelman works with the West Africa AIDS Foundation and other public health projects in the US and abroad. He is an officer of the Illinois State Academy of Sciences.

Pedagogy Developers

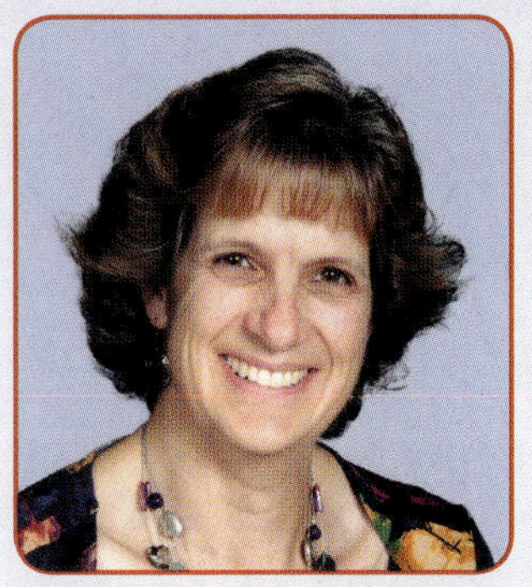

Diane Farthing received her bachelor's degree and teaching credentials from Kent State University in Ohio and has been teaching health education for 37 years. In 2010, she became a National Board Certified Teacher. Diane's teaching career includes 16 years at a continuation high school and five years at the middle school level. Since 2004, she has been teaching health education and anatomy and physiology at Amador Valley High School in Pleasanton. She is a strong believer in the power of collaboration. She spent seven years as part of the Bay Area Physical Education-Health Subject Matter Project leadership team designing and delivering professional development institutes. In 2014, she took on the role of Health Program Director for the Health and Physical Education Collaborative (H-PEC), a nonprofit organization dedicated to helping teachers develop physical and health literacy in their students. Diane was a member of the CDE's Framework and Evaluation Criteria Committee and helped write the Health Education Curriculum Framework for California Public Schools. She is the 2019 California Association for Health, Physical Education, Recreation, and Dance (CAHPERD) Health Teacher of the Year and the 2020 Western District Teacher of the Year.

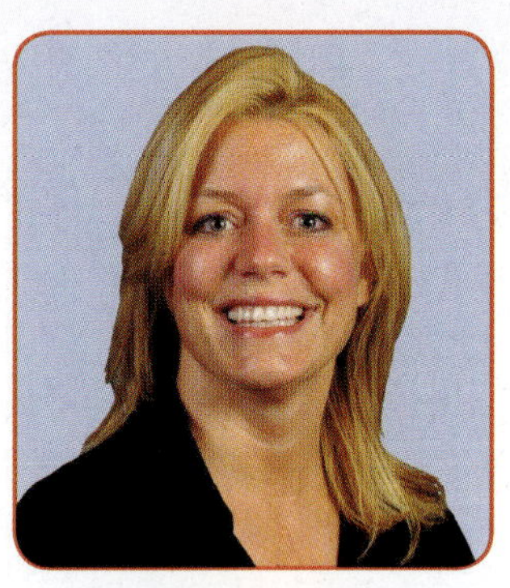

Melanie Lynch is an experienced teacher with more than 25 years in the classroom. She spent the first 21 years of her career specializing in teaching only health education. She now teaches health and physical education in Pittsburgh, Pennsylvania, at North Allegheny Intermediate High School. She has served as Vice President of Health Education for SHAPE Pennsylvania for five years and served as their President in 2016. Also in 2016, SHAPE America named Melanie the National Health Education Teacher of the Year. Melanie's love of working with students and her creative, skills-based lesson ideas have taken her all over the country, where she has spoken to thousands of teachers. Melanie is grateful to work, learn, and grow with so many amazing teachers.

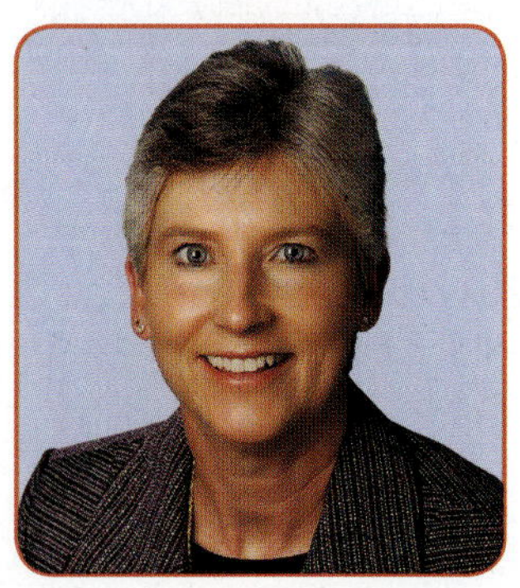

Melissa Munsell has worked as an instructional specialist in the Physical Education and Health Department at North East Independent School District in San Antonio, Texas, and served as the K–12 Health Education Lead for the district. Melissa received a bachelor's degree in kinesiology from The University of Texas at Austin and is certified to teach Physical Education K–12 and Health Education 6–12, among other endorsements, in the state of Texas. She has 26 years of teaching and administrative experience, including six years teaching health education at the high school level. She has also served as vice president of the Health Division and General Division of the Texas Association for Health, Physical Education, Recreation, and Dance (TAHPERD) and presents workshops and lectures on various health topics locally and statewide.

Contributors and Reviewers

Contributors

Goodheart-Willcox Publisher would like to thank the following classroom instructors who contributed to the development of the *Warm-Up*, *Real World Health Skills*, *Health and Wellness Skills*, and *Hands-On Activities*.

Michael A. Cleffi, II
Health and Physical Education Instructor
Bethlehem Area School District
Bethlehem, Pennsylvania

Haillie Moody
Health and Physical Education Instructor
Sierra Sands Unified School District
Ridgecrest, California

Kathryn Smith, MAT
Family and Consumer Sciences Instructor
Issaquah High School
Issaquah, Washington

Advisory Board

Goodheart-Willcox Publisher would like to thank the following advisory board members who provided guidance in the development of the third edition of *Comprehensive Health Skills*.

Carolyn Cleaves
Health Instructor
Alisal High School
Salinas, California

Susan Gabin
Health Educator
Frontier High School
Bakersfield, California

Mary Irilian
Health Instructor
Hart High School
Newhall, California

Kellie A. Johnson
Assistant Athletic Coordinator, Health Instructor
LEE High School
San Antonio, Texas

Beth Kahn
Health Instructor
North Salinas High School
Salinas, California

Janelle Merry
Health and Physical Education Instructor
North County Trade Technical High School
Vista, California

Haillie Moody
Health and Physical Education Instructor
Sierra Sands Unified School District
Ridgecrest, California

Tracey Rudnick
Health Instructor
Bradley Middle School
San Antonio, Texas

Nancy Searle
Health Instructor
McCallum High School
Austin, Texas

Shasta Smith
Health Education Instructor
Sitka High School
Sitka, Alaska

Delia Thibodeaux
Health Instructor
Westside High School
Houston, Texas

Goodheart-Willcox Publisher would also like to thank the members of the **2019 CAHPERD Convention Focus Group**, who shared feedback and insight that influenced the development of this book.

Professional Reviewers

Goodheart-Willcox Publisher would like to thank the following health professionals who reviewed selected chapters and contributed valuable input into the development of *Comprehensive Health Skills*.

Kelsey Banaszynski
Food Scientist, Research & Innovation
Danone North America
Louisville, Colorado

Kathy Barnes, Ed.D.
Educational Consultant
Texas

Jennifer Carroll, MSW
Resource Development Manager
National Eating Disorders Association (NEDA)
New York, New York

Maryann Y. Davis, CATC II
Addiction Counselor and Mental Health Program Technician
The Gooden Center
Pasadena, California

Michael Dorcas
Registered Pharmacist
Apple Valley, Minnesota

Pam Garramone, M.Ed.
Positive Psychology Keynote Speaker
Wholebeing Institute
Quincy, Massachusetts

Shawn V. Giammattei, PhD
Psychologist
Quest Family Therapy
Santa Rosa, California

Heidi Hanna, PhD
CEO, Stress Mastery Academy; Fellow, American Institute of Stress
Stress Mastery Academy
San Diego, California

Deb Kimberlin, PhD, RDN, LDN
Associate Professor
Olivet Nazarene University
Bourbonnais, Illinois

Linnea L. Mavrides, PsyD, CGP
Clinical Psychologist, Adjunct Professor
LIU-Post
Brookville, New York

Merle Wilder
High School Counselor
Belleville East High School
Belleville, Illinois

Instructor Reviewers

Goodheart-Willcox Publisher would like to thank the following health education instructors who reviewed selected chapters and contributed valuable input into the development of *Comprehensive Health Skills*.

Lindsay Armbruster
Health Education Teacher
Burnt Hills-Ballston Lake Central School District
Burnt Hills, New York

Trish Armstrong
Health Educator
Northampton High School
Northampton, Massachusetts

Michael Bargas
Health Education Instructor
Estancia High School
Costa Mesa, California

Kyle Bell
Health/Physical Education Instructor
Canyon High School
Anaheim Hills, California

Cheryl Berude
Dual Credit Instructor/ Health Science Pathway
Boerne-Champion High School
Boerne, Texas

Susie Blucher
Health Instructor
Tejeda Middle School
San Antonio, Texas

Andrew Bonsall
Health Science Instructor and Physical Educator
Marina High School
Huntington Beach, California

Margaret Brown
Health Educator
Deerfield Academy
Deerfield, Massachusetts

Amanda Browning
Health and Physical Education Instructor
Weaver Academy, Guilford County Schools
Greensboro, North Carolina

Dr. Graciela Lea Bryant
Health Educator
Huntsville High School
Huntsville, Alabama

Kim Cherre
Health/Physical Education Department Chair
Cary Academy
Cary, North Carolina

Dominique Clarke
Physical Education Instructor
First Coast High School
Jacksonville, Florida

Bryan Cromer
Instructor, Coach
Panther Creek High School
Cary, North Carolina

Maureen T. Delaney
Assistant Principal
Bowie High School
Bowie, Maryland

Sara Fiorini
Health and Physical Education Instructor
Arlington Public Schools
Arlington, Virginia

Susan Gabin
Health Educator
Frontier High School
Bakersfield, California

Dr. Stacy Germany
Health Science Educator
Westwood High School
Austin, Texas

Kyle Gilmer
Physical Education Upper School Instructor
Greensboro Day School
Greensboro, North Carolina

Dr. Cara D. Grant
Supervisor, PreK–12 Health and Physical Education
Montgomery County Public Schools
Rockville, Maryland

Glenn Hagood
Health and Physical Education Chair
St. John Paul II Catholic High School
Huntsville, Alabama

Lori Hewlett
Chairperson for Health Education
Sachem Central School District
Lake Ronkonkoma, New York

Mary Irilian
Health Instructor
Hart High School
Newhall, California

Kellie A. Johnson
Assistant Athletic Coordinator, Health Instructor
LEE High School
San Antonio, Texas

Beth Kahn
Health Instructor
North Salinas High School
Salinas, California

Katie Laraway
Healthful Living Instructor
Raleigh Charter High School
Raleigh, North Carolina

Rachael McClure
Health Instructor
Pelham High School
Pelham, Alabama

Jolene Meza
Instructor
Cleveland Charter High School
Reseda, California

Haillie Moody
Health and Physical Education Instructor
Sierra Sands Unified School District
Ridgecrest, California

Heather R. Perrigan
Professional Health Educator
Corvallis High School
Corvallis, Oregon

Mary Record
High School Health Instructor
Scarborough High School
Scarborough, Maine

Dr. Chuck Rhoades
Health Instructor
Portsmouth High School
Portsmouth, New Hampshire

Tracey Rudnick
Health Instructor
Bradley Middle School
San Antonio, Texas

Julia Russell
Health Instructor
South Tahoe High School
South Lake Tahoe, California

Nancy H. Searle
Health Instructor
McCallum High School
Austin, Texas

Bill Shandor
Director of Athletics/ Physical Education Instructor
Desert Academy
Santa Fe, New Mexico

Shasta Smith
Health Education Instructor
Sitka High School
Sitka, Alaska

Cynthia Smyser
Science and Health Instructor
University of Illinois Laboratory High School
Urbana, Illinois

Leah Swedberg
Health Instructor
West Fargo High School
West Fargo, North Dakota

Lyle Takeshita
Health Instructor
Temple City High School
Temple City, California

Delia Thibodeaux
Health Instructor
Westside High School
Houston, Texas

James Tulley
Health Education Instructor
Scarsdale High School
Scarsdale, New York

Deb Van Klei
QCOMP Coordinator
Stillwater Area Public Schools
Stillwater, Minnesota

Julie Woodruff
Health Science Technology Instructor
Champion High School
Boerne, Texas

Brief Contents

Contents

Feature Contents

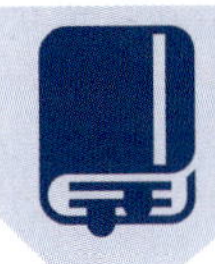

Case Studies

Research in Action

Local and Global Health

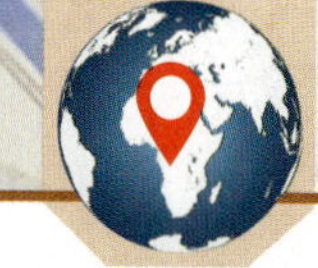

Health in the Media

Skills for Health and Wellness

Health Across the Life Span

Quizzes

Spotlight on Health and Wellness Careers

To the Student

We wrote this exciting textbook for high school health and wellness classes based on our experiences as professors of psychology (Catherine Sanderson) and biology (Mark Zelman), and as the accomplished authors of high school and college-level textbooks. Our backgrounds give us a deep well of knowledge of the most current scientific theory and research to draw from.

Perhaps the most valuable experience we had in preparing us to write this book is our roles as parents to a combined total of seven children, ages 8 through 22. After all, in writing this book, we both reflected frequently on our experiences as parents and our goal of ensuring that our own children maintain excellent physical, mental and emotional, and social health.

This book includes all of the standard topics found in high school health and wellness books—including self-talk, self-compassion, and self-care; body positivity, neutrality, and compassion; health effects of vaping; medication and drug abuse (including opioids); digital citizenship and personal digital footprint; how social media affects physical, mental and emotional, and social health; and healthy relationships. We wanted our book to give high school students the most current health information, presented in an engaging writing style so students would enjoy reading the book. Additionally, we included a focus on practical health skills that young people can use to develop and promote positive health and wellness habits throughout their lives.

As the authors of high school and college-level textbooks, we felt confident in our research and writing abilities, but felt that the pedagogy was better left to health teachers. We would like to thank Diane Farthing, Melanie Lynch, and Melissa Munsell for developing the skills-based questions, activities, and resources that are a vital part of this course. We are delighted with the final product, and wish all readers of this book a lifetime of health.

Catherine A. Sanderson

Mark Zelman

Unit 1

Promoting a Lifetime of Health and Wellness

Big Ideas

- *Health* describes the state of your physical, mental, and social well-being. In contrast, *wellness* is the process of becoming aware of your state of health and taking steps to improve it. Your *well-being* is your satisfaction with life.
- The different dimensions of health—physical, mental and emotional, and social—affect each other and all contribute to overall well-being.
- Health is a continuum. The steps you take to improve your health move you closer to optimal health.
- Different risk and protective factors affect your health and decisions. Some factors you can change. Others you cannot.
- Making healthy decisions is critical to your health. The decision-making process can help you with this. When you are setting goals, be sure they are specific, measurable, achievable, relevant, and timely.
- Reliable health information enables you to make healthy decisions. To find reliable health information, evaluate websites and other sources critically.
- As a minor, you have certain rights to access health services. Knowing how to access these services and get help is important to your health.
- Your community and world affect your health. Fortunately, there are steps you can take to improve your community health and promote health around the world.
- Effective communication is an essential skill for building relationships and setting boundaries. You also need to know how to resolve conflicts in a healthy way and resist negative peer pressure.

Drazen_/E+/Getty Images ▸

Health Management Plan › Skills for Your Future

Over your years of school, you have studied many subjects. Health, unlike many of these subjects, is about *you*. Your health is a critical part of your future. It allows you to set and pursue your goals, make wise decisions, have fun, and live a good life. In this book, you will learn skills for having positive health—now and in the future.

As with any long-term goal, having positive health requires a plan. This plan does not have to be boring or like anyone else's plan. Your plan should address what *you* care about and what you want for your future.

Over the course of this book, you will make this plan as a series of entries about each major topic. Your plan can be physical or digital and can take any form. For example, you could use a journal or spreadsheet. You could also use a blog, video blog, or illustrated book. Title your project "*Your Name's* Health Management Plan."

Once you have chosen the format for your plan, create a first entry, titled "My Health." For this first entry, answer the following questions:

1. What do you think of when you hear the word *health*? What have people told you about health? Do you think these impressions are accurate or not?
2. How good do you feel in your life right now? How do you feel physically? mentally and emotionally? How close are your relationships?
3. What areas of your life would you like to improve? Be specific and honest with yourself. Explain why you want to improve each area.
4. What skills do you think you will need to improve your life in these areas? What skills do you hope to practice as you learn about health?

After answering these questions, save your entry. As you read this unit, revisit your entry and add to your answers. You will return to your plan before and after each unit in this book.

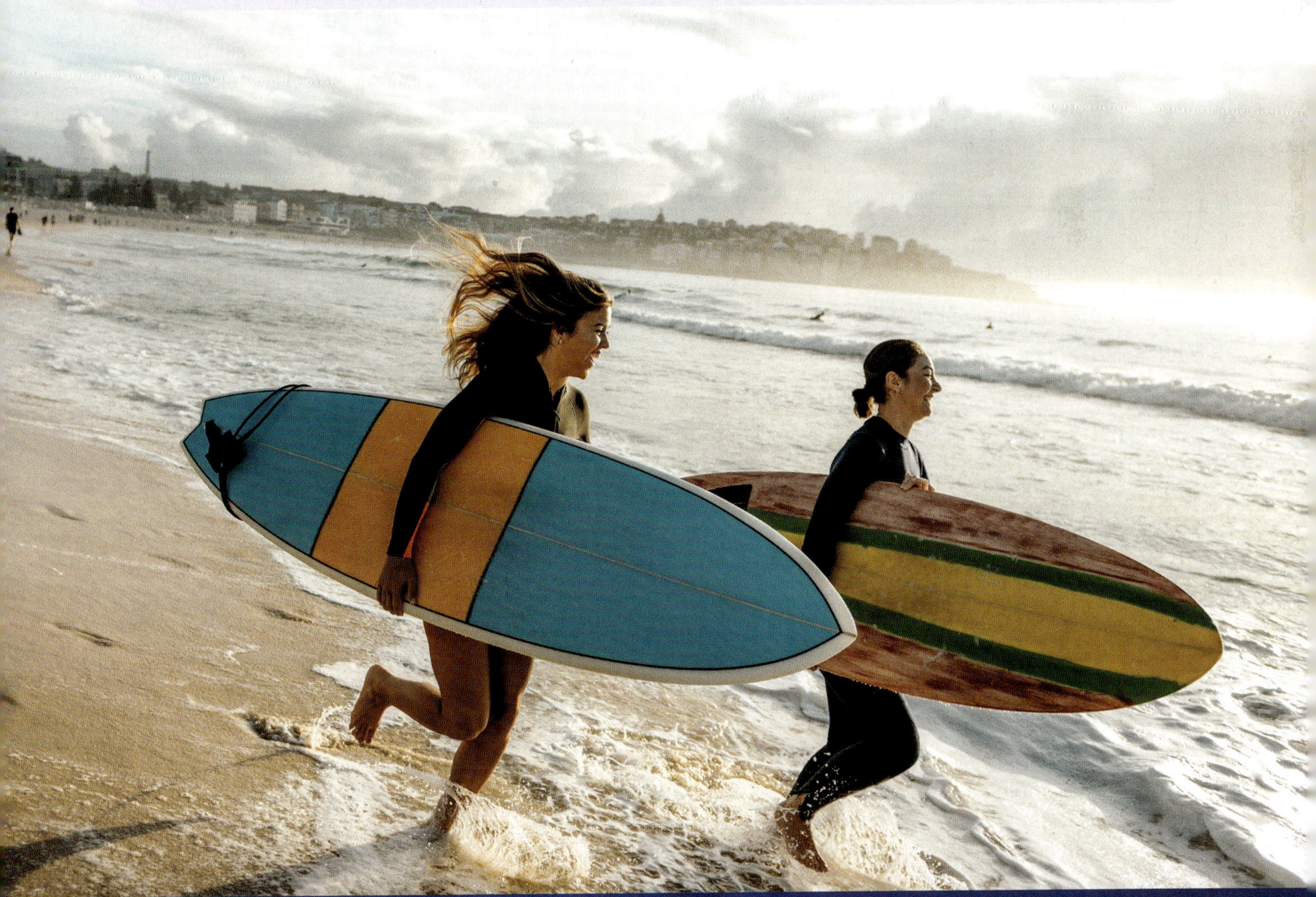

Chapter 1

Health and Wellness Fundamentals

Look for the skills icon throughout this chapter for opportunities to practice your health skills.

Check Your Health and Wellness Skills

In this chapter, you will learn skills for understanding health and wellness and analyzing influences in your life. To understand the skills you currently use, take the following inventory of your behaviors. Indicate how well you think you use each skill. Use a scale of 1–5, *1* meaning you do not use the skill and *5* meaning you feel completely comfortable using it.

Skill	How Well Do You Use Each Skill?
I spend as much time taking care of my mental health as I do my physical health.	
I make time for relationships, even when I'm busy.	
I see setbacks in my health as opportunities for growth.	
I ask questions about my family history of disease.	
I think about the long-term effects of my behaviors now.	
I avoid risky behaviors like drug use and sexual activity.	
I wear a helmet when bicycling.	
I avoid places I know are contaminated with pollutants like lead or asbestos.	
I promote respect and a sense of belonging in my community.	
I think carefully about how the media I'm consuming affects my health.	
I try to do well in school.	
	Total:

Add up your responses to each statement. The higher your score, the more comfortable you feel practicing health skills related to maintaining health and analyzing influences. Which skill do you think is most important for you? Which skill is the most challenging for you? Which skill would you most like to improve? In this chapter, you will learn how to perform these skills better and more often.

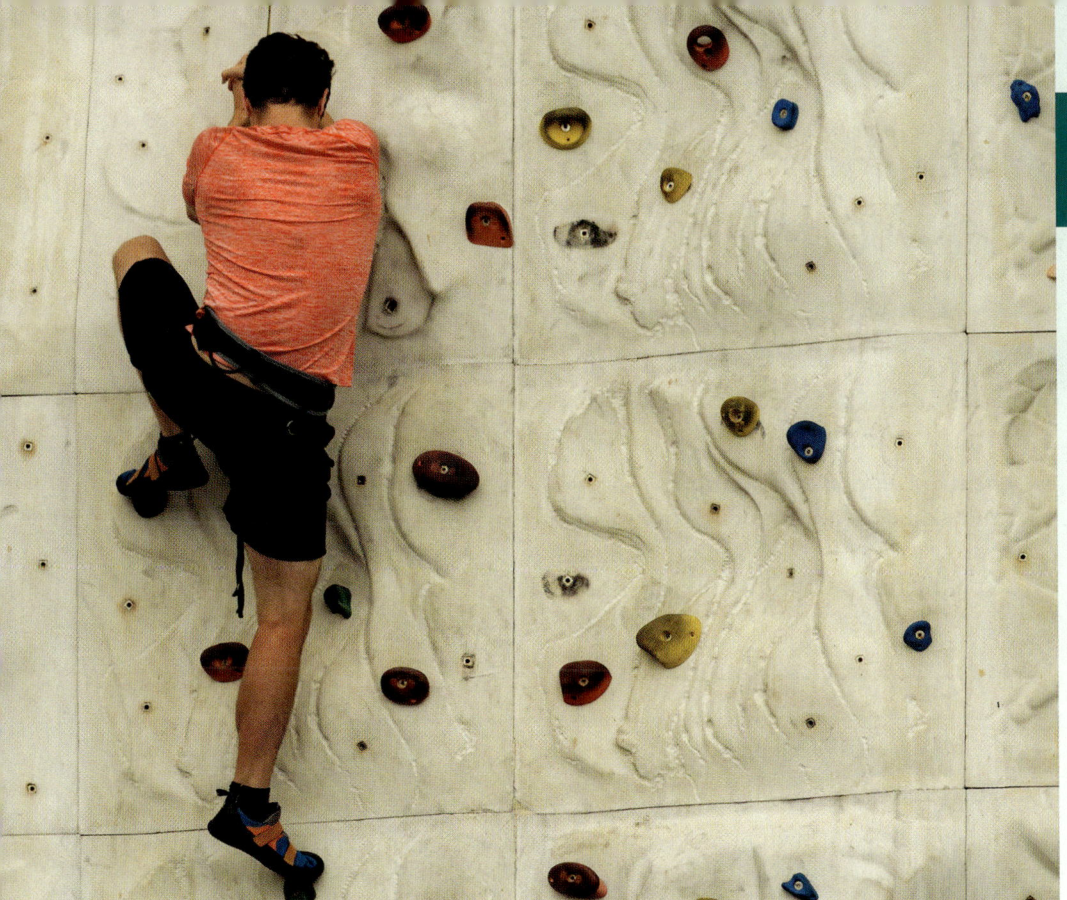

CLS Digital Arts/Shutterstock.com

Reading and Notetaking

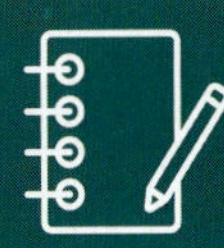

Skim this chapter from top to bottom and from left to right and list all of the headings. Then, identify key terms with which you are unfamiliar and scan through the chapter to find their definitions. Write a "topic sentence" and brief summary for each heading, using the key terms to explain what you think you will learn. After you read this chapter, write a new topic sentence and summary for each section, outlining the main points you learned.

Heading	Topic Sentence and Summary	New Topic Sentence and Summary
	Topic sentence: Summary:	Topic sentence: Summary:

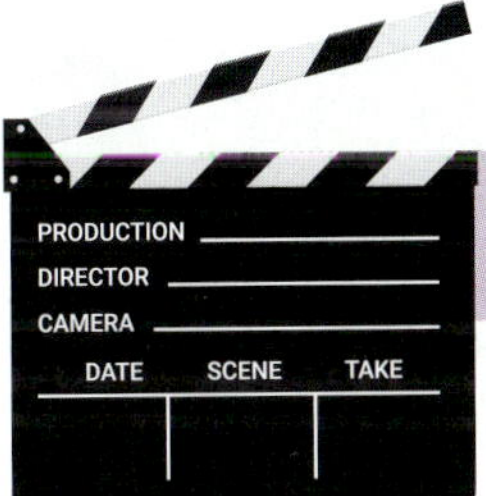

Setting the Scene

Stressed, Sick, and Now What?

When you started this school year, you had lots of energy and felt great after a summer volunteering and seeing friends. Now that you are halfway through the school year, however, you feel stressed out and tired most days.

No matter what you do, it seems like you cannot keep up with studying and all of your homework. You are not getting enough sleep and eat mostly chips, convenience store foods, and fast food on the go. Because you are so busy, you feel irritable and do not enjoy activities with your friends. When you are not with your friends, you stay home and feel sad and overwhelmed. Lately, your grades have been slipping, and you think you might be catching a cold. After school, you talk with the school nurse, who recommends you see a doctor.

Thinking Critically

1. What are the different challenges you are facing in this scenario? List these challenges and create a drawing showing how the different challenges are related to each other.
2. What steps could you take in this situation to begin resolving these challenges? Where would you start? How would resolving one challenge affect challenges in other areas of your health?

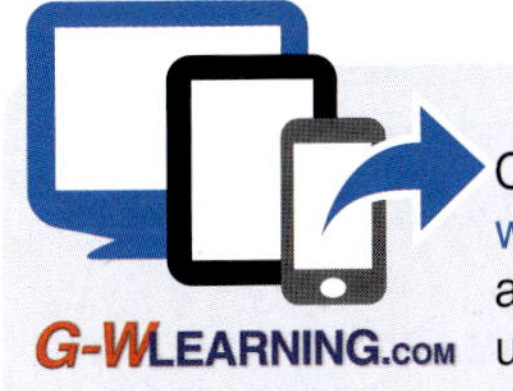

G-WLEARNING.com

Click on the activity icon or visit www.g-wlearning.com/health/4095 to access online vocabulary activities using key terms from the chapter.

Lesson 1.1

What Are Health and Wellness?

Essential Question

What does it mean to have health and wellness?

Learning Outcomes

After studying this lesson, you will be able to

- define *health*, *wellness*, and *well-being*;
- analyze how the physical, mental and emotional, and social dimensions of health are interrelated; and
- explain the status of health as it relates to a continuum.

Key Terms

emotional health
health
illness
life expectancy
life span
mental health
optimal health
physical health
quality of life
social health
well-being
wellness

Warm-Up Activity

Different Dimensions

Comprehend Concepts In this lesson, you will learn about the three dimensions of health: physical health, mental and emotional health, and social health. Given what you already know, give a real-life example you think fits into each dimension. Your examples can be positive or negative. In a few sentences, brainstorm how each example might also affect the other two dimensions of health positively or negatively.

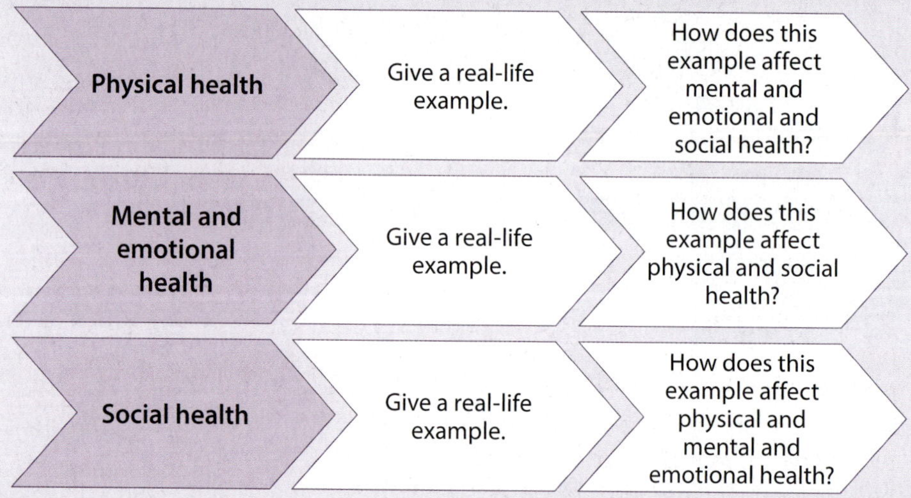

According to her doctor, 16-year-old Janine is the picture of health. She has a healthy weight, rarely gets sick, and gets regular physical activity. When she is under stress—which is often—Janine is so anxious she cannot sleep or focus on her schoolwork. Frequently tired, Janine fights with her friends regularly and eats on the go since her family has little money for groceries. Recently, she stopped running and took up smoking with her partner. Janine avoids making decisions and planning for her future. Instead, she prefers to "go with the flow."

Alex, also 16, was born with a genetic disorder he inherited from his father. This makes running and playing most sports difficult. Alex manages his disorder by following his doctor's instructions and taking the medication prescribed for his condition. He also makes sure to eat well, get plenty of sleep, get a moderate amount of physical activity, and avoid smoking or drinking. His optimistic and upbeat attitude attracts other people to him, so he has many friends and is close with his grandparents who are raising him. Alex sets goals for his future and is confident he will succeed if he works hard.

Who do you think is healthier—Janine or Alex? In the past, many people would say that Janine is healthier. In many Western societies, including the United States, *health* was defined in purely medical terms as the absence of physical illness and disease.

Many public health experts and medical professionals now embrace a broader definition of health and may conclude that Alex is the healthier one. For example, although Janine does not have a health condition, she smokes.

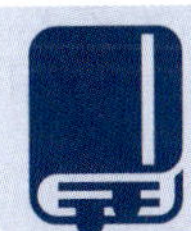

Case Study

The Interactions of Your Health

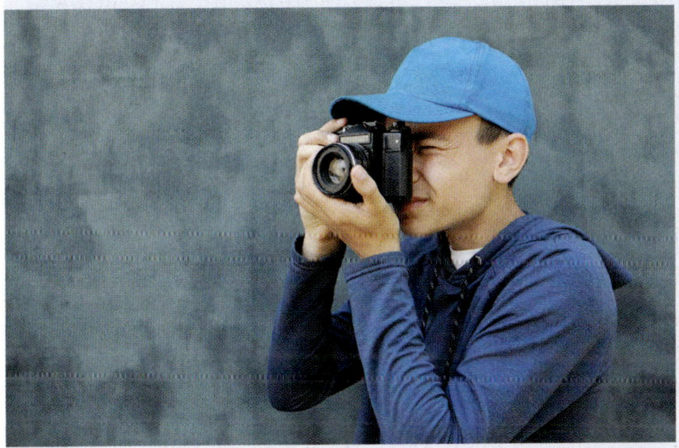

Arthur Linnik/Shutterstock.com

Dexter has experienced anxiety his whole life, but it has gotten especially bad since he started high school. His doctor prescribed medication, but Dexter wanted to do more. He researched different ways to improve his mental health and found that eating healthy foods and getting regular physical activity could help. Dexter started eating more fresh fruit and vegetables and joined the cross country team. After a few weeks of regular running and healthy eating, Dexter notices the symptoms of his anxiety have lessened.

Skye and her brother used to ride bikes and play basketball together. While Skye has remained active, her brother has not. Her brother recently got into a fight with his friends on the basketball team. He stopped playing basketball to avoid his friends and instead hides away in his room after school. He does not even come out to ride bikes with Skye. Skye's brother has been sluggish and short of breath after quitting basketball, while Skye feels energetic and ready for anything.

As a freshman, Malik struggled to find where he belonged at his new school. He felt frustrated with himself for not making new friends. He also often felt sad and lonely. Even though Malik's childhood friends rooted for him, they went to different schools. His friends suggested that Malik join a club to meet new people. He joined the Photography Club and volunteered with a school group for Habitat for Humanity. Through these groups, Malik met his first friends at school and has remained friends with a few throughout high school.

Practice Your Skills

Comprehend Concepts

In groups of three, assign one person to each dimension of health: physical, social, or mental and emotional. On a piece of paper, describe a scenario in which a person experiences either a positive or negative impact to the dimension of health assigned. Within your group of three, trade papers with one another. On your partner's paper, add a second scenario describing how a different dimension of health may be impacted by that situation. Then, trade papers again, and add a third scenario describing how the last area of health might also be impacted. In your group of three, discuss how the dimensions of health are interrelated.

This puts her at risk of someday becoming one of the 480,000 people in the US who die prematurely from a smoking-related disease each year. Janine also does not get the sleep and nutritious foods her body needs. While Alex is confident and optimistic, Janine is often anxious and lacks the skills needed to set goals and make decisions that benefit her health and well-being.

Dimensions of Health and Wellness

health state of complete physical, mental and emotional, and social well-being

well-being person's ability to function positively and overall satisfaction that life's present conditions are good

wellness process of identifying one's state of health and taking steps to improve it

physical health dimension of health that refers to how well the body functions

The *World Health Organization (WHO)*, an international organization that promotes health across the world, defines **health** as not just the absence of disease, but as a state of complete physical, mental and emotional, and social well-being. **Well-being** refers to a person's ability to function positively and overall satisfaction that life's present conditions are good (**Figure 1.1**).

To achieve health, people practice wellness. While often used synonymously with *health*, **wellness** refers to the process of identifying one's state of health and taking steps to improve it. Wellness is different for each individual. Steps that will help you achieve well-being and your full potential may be different from the steps taken by your friends. Wellness is affirming of these differences and is also *holistic*, which means it takes into account the many areas of a person's health. These areas, also identified in the WHO's definition of *health*, include physical health, mental and emotional health, and social health. Only by paying attention to and practicing wellness in *each* area can people achieve well-being and positive health.

Physical Health

Physical health is the area of health that refers to how your body functions. If you have a physically healthy body, your body allows you to participate in the activities of daily life. You can cope with the stresses of disease, injury, and aging and maintain an active lifestyle. In other words, being physically healthy enables you to do more than walk to school or lift a bag of books. With positive physical health, you can recover from a sprained ankle, fight off the flu, and have the energy to cope with daily stresses.

Like all areas of health, physical health exists on a spectrum. Having a disease, for example, does not mean a person cannot be physically healthy in other ways. Someone who has a disease or disability can still maintain physical health by eating nutritious foods, getting plenty of physical activity, and avoiding hazardous substances.

People in a state of well-being...

- have a sense of fulfillment and a positive attitude
- enjoy a long life
- engage in behaviors that promote health
- are socially connected, have relationships, and participate in social activities
- are productive at school, work, and home
- have a sense of purpose
- have access to resources for meeting basic needs such as food, sleep, and physical activity
- have a safe physical and social environment at home, at school and work, and in the community

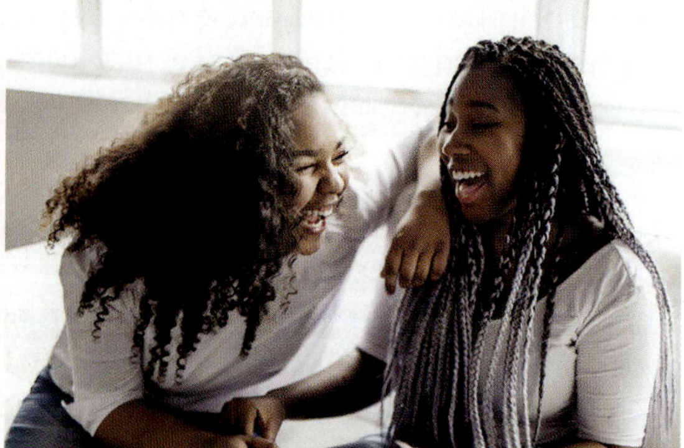

Lopolo/Shutterstock.com

Figure 1.1 These characteristics describe people in a state of well-being, according to research among people of all ages and from many cultures. ***What process do people practice to achieve health?***

Mental and Emotional Health

Mental and emotional health refer to the health of your internal life—the thoughts and feelings that cross your mind and influence your decisions (**Figure 1.2**). Compared to other areas, these areas of health may not be as visible from the outside. Without taking steps to promote your mental and emotional health, however, it is impossible to reach a state of well-being.

Mental health describes how you observe and interpret information. It affects your ability to make decisions, solve problems, and examine situations. For example, a person who is mentally healthy can think clearly, critically, and optimistically, even in challenging circumstances. People who are mentally healthy also enjoy exploring new ideas and excel at learning, adapting, and growing. In contrast, people with mental health conditions might be unable to identify the root of a social problem and may think badly about themselves instead of solving the problem.

mental health dimension of health that describes how a person observes and interprets information to make decisions, solve problems, and examine situations

While similar to mental health, **emotional health** refers to how you express yourself and your thoughts and feelings. Your emotions, mood, feelings about yourself, and way of viewing the world are all parts of your emotional health. People who have positive emotional health express their thoughts and feelings clearly and cope well with stress. They maintain mature relationships by respecting and valuing others and themselves.

emotional health dimension of health that refers to the expression of thoughts and feelings, including emotions, moods, feelings about one's self, and views about the world

Sometimes, people do not realize they are experiencing challenges with mental and emotional health. For example, persistent feelings of sadness or worry are not healthy. Ongoing negative feelings can keep you from doing well in school or participating in your favorite activities. They can also interfere with your sleep, diet, or physical activity and prevent you from forming healthy friendships. The good news is that, like medications and good nutrition can improve your physical health, treatment and skills for maintaining your mental and emotional health can help you feel better.

Social Health

Can you imagine your life with no human interaction? It is unhealthy for humans to live in isolation, without relationships to provide them support. Humans are social animals who must interact and communicate with one another. **Social health** is the dimension of health that refers to how well you get along with other people.

social health dimension of health that refers to how well a person gets along with others

Having positive social health means having enjoyable, supportive, and healthy relationships with family members, friends, dating partners, and people in your community. Healthy relationships make you feel good about yourself and are characterized by trust and honest communication.

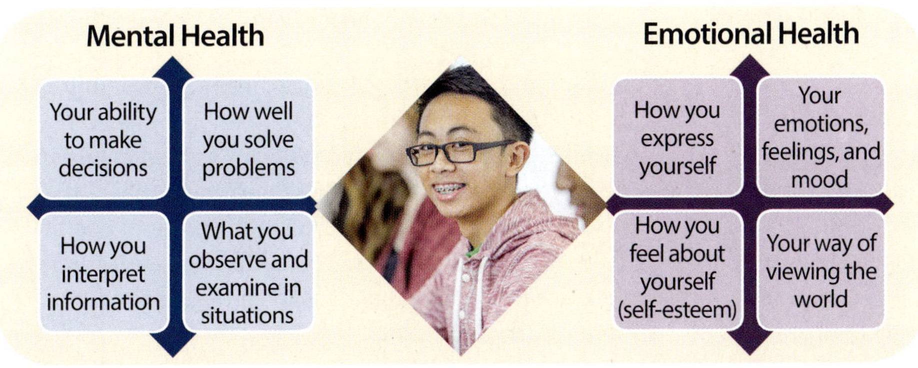

FatCamera/E+/GettyImages

Figure 1.2 While mental health and emotional health are related, they are not exactly the same.

These relationships are among your most valuable resources and give you the support you need to enjoy life and meet its challenges.

Unhealthy relationships make you feel bad about yourself. Any relationship that causes you harm is also unhealthy. You should never be harmed or threatened by friends, dating partners, family members, or any other people in your life. Interpersonal skills can help you build healthy relationships and change, leave, or get help for relationships that are unhealthy.

Interaction of Health Dimensions

The physical, mental and emotional, and social dimensions of health interact with and affect each other. A disturbance in one dimension of health may lead to a disturbance in another. Likewise, an improvement in one dimension may lead to improvements in others.

For example, suppose someone who is physically fit and eats well also has the mental illness known as *major depressive disorder*. When people have major depressive disorder, their emotional health suffers, but the condition also impacts other dimensions of health. People with major depressive disorder may feel less motivated to eat properly (physical health). They may have difficulty concentrating (mental health) and distance themselves from their friends and family members (social health).

Research in Action

The Areas of Health Affect Each Other

Have you ever felt happier after spending time with friends? been better able to concentrate after taking a walk? Scientific studies have confirmed that the physical, mental and emotional, and social dimensions of health are deeply interconnected. Each area affects the others in many ways.

One example of this is the relationship between physical activity and mental and emotional health. A study of young adults found that as people increased their amounts of physical activity, symptoms of depression and anxiety decreased. This was true for light physical activity (walking) and moderately vigorous activity (jogging). The mental health benefits were greater for people who were more active each day.

Social relationships also affect mental health. In a study of immigrants, those with social support systems had fewer mental health conditions such as anxiety and depression. Immigrants were less likely to have mental health conditions if they had a greater sense of belonging and strong social support within their new community.

Social health can also impact physical health. Research about addiction has shown that teens from families with unhealthy or abusive relationships are more likely to use drugs and alcohol, which impacts physical health, and run away from home. To develop effective treatments, researchers also compared individual therapy for substance use with family-based therapy. Family-based therapy taught teens and their family members relationship and communication skills. Teens taking part in family-based therapy abstained from drugs more, remained in therapy longer, and ran away from home less often.

Practice Your Skills

Analyze Influences

Suppose a teen has a healthy body weight, gets plenty of physical activity, and eats nutritious meals. You could say this teen is physically healthy. With a partner, discuss how this teen's physical health influences other areas of health, including mental and emotional health and social health. How might challenges in other areas of health impact physical health? Write a case study in which this teen focuses on physical health to improve other areas of health. Also write a case study in which other areas of health influence this teen's physical health. Trade case studies with another pair and discuss the other pair's case study with your partner.

At the same time, making improvements in one area of health can positively impact other areas of health. For example, if a person with major depressive disorder eats well, engages in physical activity, and seeks professional treatment, this may benefit emotional health.

The Continuum of Health

In Japan, women born today are expected to live to 86 years of age. In Kenya, women are expected to live to 65 years of age. Are women in Japan healthier than women in Kenya? In the US, children die before five years of age at twice the rate of children in Germany. Are children in Germany healthier than children in the US? How long people are expected to live, or **life expectancy**, is just one of many ways to measure health. Other ways of measuring health include **life span**, which is the actual number of years a person lives, and **quality of life**, or the extent to which a person experiences a healthy, happy, and fulfilling life. Quality of life is typically assessed using a *quality of life index*. This gauges each person's ability to fully engage in activities of daily living and level of satisfaction with personal and social life.

When measuring health and well-being, people often think that being healthy and being unhealthy are totally different. In this model, you are either healthy or you are not. This is not an accurate model for describing health. A person's health status normally lies somewhere between the extremes of poor and excellent. This range in health status is called a *continuum* (**Figure 1.3**).

life expectancy length of time a person is expected to live

life span actual number of years a person lives

quality of life extent to which a person experiences a healthy, happy, and fulfilling life

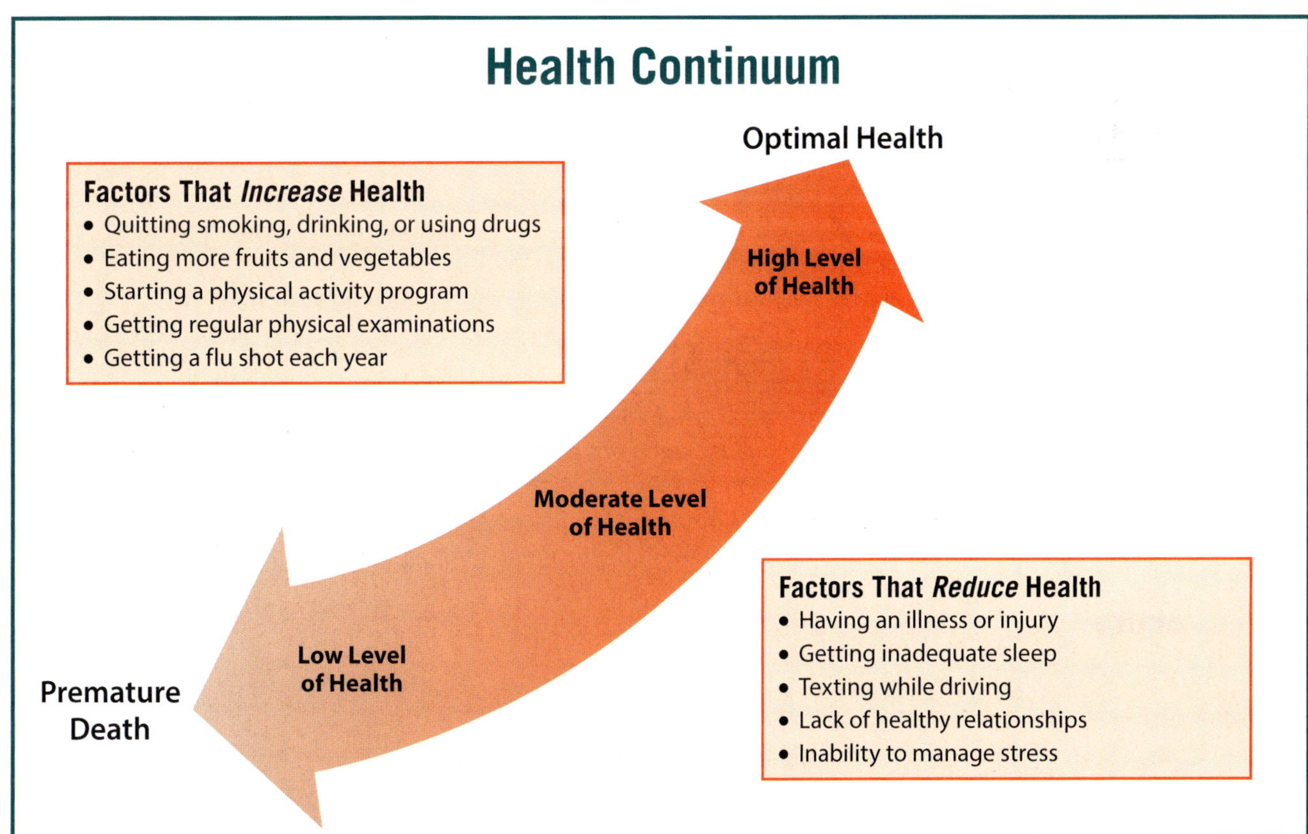

Figure 1.3 Your level of health can be plotted on a continuum. The choices you make largely determine where you are on the continuum. ***Where would you plot your health status on this continuum today? Explain.***

optimal health state of excellent health and wellness, including physical, mental and emotional, and social health

illness poor overall state of health in which a person cannot function normally; caused by factors such as disease, risky behaviors, hazardous substances, and concerns with mental or emotional health

Most people experience one or more factors that put their health status near the center of the health continuum.

At one end of the continuum lies **optimal health**. Optimal health is a state of excellent physical, mental and emotional, and social health. People want their health status to be at or near this end of the continuum. At the other end of the continuum lies illness and premature (early) death. The term **illness** describes an overall poor state of health. Diseases or disorders, risky behaviors, hazardous substances, and poor mental or emotional health can lead to illness.

People can change their place on the health continuum by increasing factors that improve health and decreasing factors that reduce health. Achieving health does not mean eliminating all factors that hinder health. Some factors, like genetic disorders, the environment in which you live, and your family members' decisions, are outside your control. As a teen, however, you have more control over your health decisions than ever before. By taking responsibility for the factors you *do* control and making healthy, informed decisions, you can improve all areas of your health.

Lesson 1.1 Review

Know and Understand

1. Explain the difference between health and wellness.
2. How do you know if you are physically healthy?
3. Which dimension of health refers to how you express thoughts and feelings?
4. What does it mean to have positive social health?
5. With a partner, discuss the following question: Can a person with a physical disability, disease, or mental illness still have positive health?

Think Critically

6. With a partner, discuss the different ways you have heard the word *health* used. How do these definitions compare to the definition used by the WHO?
7. Why do you think many people do not see mental and emotional health as clearly as they see physical health? What are the consequences of this difference?
8. Give one example of a time the dimensions of health have affected each other in your life.

REAL WORLD Health Skills

Make Decisions Draw and label a continuum of health. Make a list of both positive and negative decisions you make that affect your health. Place these decisions or actions onto your health continuum. After labeling your health continuum, circle where you fall. Below your health continuum, list some decisions or actions you can make in the future to improve your health or keep your place near optimal health.

Individual Factors Affecting Health and Wellness

Essential Question?

What genetic and behavioral factors influence health?

Lesson 1.2

Learning Outcomes

After studying this lesson, you will be able to

- explain how risk and protective factors impact health;
- identify genetic factors; and
- describe the impact that behavioral choices and lifestyle have on health and wellness.

Key Terms

behavioral factors
deoxyribonucleic acid (DNA)
genes
genetic disorders
protective factors
risk factors

Warm-Up Activity

Daily Health

Set Goals Outline the schedule of your typical day, including choices you make regarding nutrition, physical activity, and entertainment. List your activities and write one or two sentences about how you think each activity affects your health and risk of injury or illness. Brainstorm two goals you know you could set and act on to improve your health.

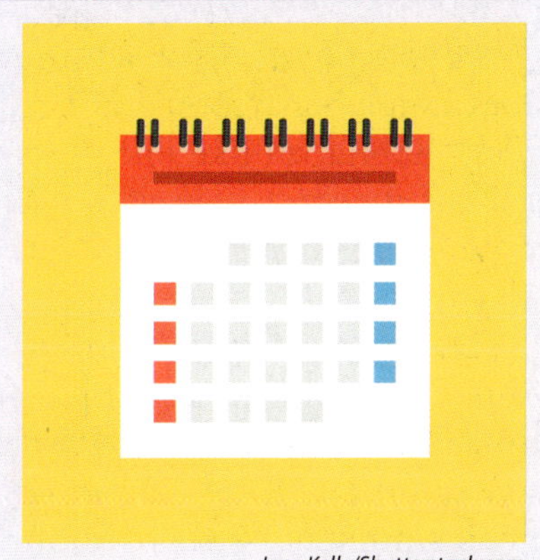

Jane Kelly/Shutterstock.com

As you approach adulthood, you will be faced with more and more choices that will affect your health and wellness now and in the future. Learning about factors that affect health and wellness can help you make decisions that improve your health. **Risk factors** are aspects of people's lives that *increase* the chance of a disease, injury, or decline in health. **Protective factors** are aspects that *reduce* risk. For example, risk factors for Janine from the previous lesson include her family's income, which makes it hard for her to eat well, and her lifestyle choices. Alex faces risk factors related to his genetics since he inherited a genetic disorder. His positive lifestyle choices and family support are protective factors that improve his health.

risk factors aspects of people's lives that increase the chances they will develop a disease or disorder or experience an injury or decline in health

protective factors aspects of people's lives that reduce risk and increase the likelihood of optimal health

The presence of risk and protective factors does not mean that a person is guaranteed to develop a health condition or have positive health. Even if Janine has little money to spend on healthy food, for example, she can still make the healthiest choices possible using what she has. Compared with someone who does not have this risk factor, however, Janine has a greater chance of developing a health condition due to her diet.

Risk and protective factors come in two types—modifiable and nonmodifiable. *Modifiable factors* can be changed. Many behavioral or lifestyle factors are modifiable. For example, Janine can stop smoking and thereby remove that risk factor. *Nonmodifiable factors* cannot be changed. Age and genetic factors are typically nonmodifiable.

Understanding your risk and protective factors can help you make healthy decisions. You can make choices to reduce or eliminate risk factors. If a risk factor cannot be eliminated, you can reduce other risk factors and increase protective factors. For example, if you have a close relative with high blood pressure, you cannot change your genetic risk factor. You can, however, eat nutritious foods and get physical activity to decrease your risk.

Risk and protective factors—both modifiable and nonmodifiable—fall into two basic categories. These categories are *individual factors*, or factors relating to identity and decisions, and environmental factors. In this lesson, you will explore individual factors related to genetics and behaviors.

Genetic Factors

genes DNA segments that contain the blueprint for the structure and function of a person's cells; affect development, personality, and health

deoxyribonucleic acid (DNA) chemical that carries genetic information; found in chromosomes

People physically resemble their biological parents. They may even share some behaviors, abilities, likes, and dislikes. For example, your nose might be shaped like one parent. If your other parent does not like the taste of cheese, you may not either. You may be uncoordinated or allergic to pollen like your parents. These characteristics are partly shaped by your genes.

Genes contain the blueprint for the structure and function of your cells. Your genes direct how you grow and develop and influence your personality and health. Humans have 20,000–25,000 genes, which are composed of **deoxyribonucleic acid (DNA)**. Within a cell's nucleus, genes are bundled in packages called *chromosomes* (**Figure 1.4**). Humans inherit half of their chromosomes from each biological parent. The unique combination of genes from your parents determines many of your characteristics.

Genes can significantly influence your health. For example, if members of your biological family develop a disease such as cancer, you have a *family history* of that disease. This means the genes you inherited from your biological parents might make you more likely to develop cancer.

Genes do not act alone, however. Other factors, such as your environment and lifestyle choices, also impact whether you will develop a health condition. For example, getting regular physical activity and avoiding hazardous substances can reduce your risk for developing cancer. Some examples of how genetic factors affect your risk of developing health conditions follow.

Cell Structure

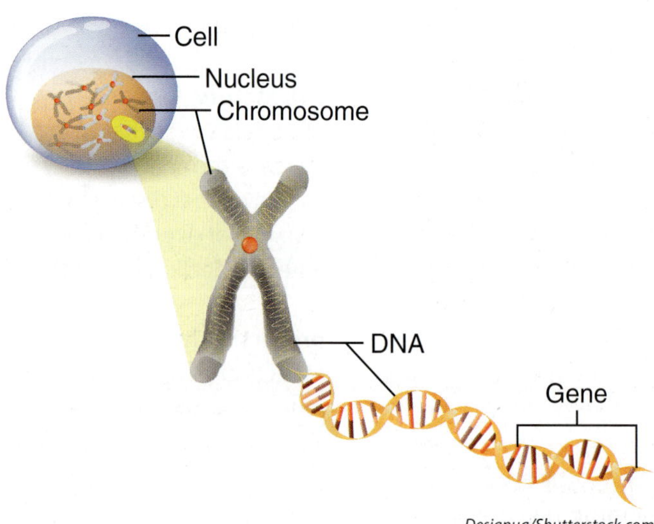

Figure 1.4 Cells contain thousands of chromosomes, which contain hundreds to thousands of genes. These genes contain DNA and form the blueprint for your personality and health.

Weight

Research shows that the tendency to have a certain weight is rooted in genetics. In most cases, multiple genes are responsible. These genes affect a person's ability to burn calories and store and burn fat. Genes also influence a person's appetite and levels of physical activity.

A combination of genetic, behavioral, and environmental factors explains the widespread increase in people with overweight and obesity in the US. These factors include easy access to high-calorie foods and drinks, sedentary lifestyles, and jobs with little physical activity. People with genetic risk factors are exposed to multiple environmental and behavioral risk factors, which increases the chance for experiencing overweight and obesity.

Diseases and Disorders

The role of genes in diseases or disorders varies. For example, *communicable diseases* are caused by microscopic *pathogens* (bacteria, viruses, fungi, and parasites). Genes do not affect whether you encounter pathogens, but they do influence your immune system and resistance to diseases.

On the other hand, genes significantly influence whether you develop a *noncommunicable disease* (**Figure 1.5**). Noncommunicable diseases develop due to changes in health over time, and your genes guide many of these changes. Sometimes, noncommunicable diseases only develop with the presence of additional risk factors. Other times, genetic risk factors can cause noncommunicable diseases without any other risk factors. Disorders that develop in this way are called **genetic disorders**.

genetic disorders health conditions that develop due to a person's genes; do not require the presence of other risk factors

The Role of Genes in Noncommunicable Diseases

Disease	Explanation
Cardiovascular disease	Cardiovascular disease is the leading cause of death in the US, and risk runs in families. Several genes contribute to cardiovascular disease. Having a close relative with this disease suggests a person may have inherited a tendency toward developing it. A genetic disorder called *familial hypercholesterolemia* is also associated with heart disease. People who have this disorder develop extremely high levels of *cholesterol*, a fatty substance that blocks arteries, leading to cardiovascular disease.
Cancer	Genes have an impact on a person's risk of developing cancer. The genes *BRCA1* and *BRCA2* increase a female's risk of developing some types of breast or ovarian cancer. Colon cancer affects many people with *familial polyposis*, a condition that causes the growth of abnormal masses in the colon. While exposure to the sun's ultraviolet radiation is the main cause of skin cancer, genetic factors like having fair skin and light-colored eyes and hair increase a person's risk.
Diabetes mellitus	Type 1 diabetes usually begins in childhood when the body cannot make insulin. Certain genes increase risk for type 1 diabetes, but environmental factors also play a role. In type 2 diabetes mellitus, the hormone insulin does not lower blood sugar. A family history of obesity or type 2 diabetes and an ancestry that is African-American, Hispanic, or Native American increase risk for type 2 diabetes mellitus.
Sickle cell anemia	People who have sickle cell anemia inherit a single mutated gene from each biological parent. These mutated genes cause red blood cells to be shaped abnormally, which reduces the blood's ability to carry oxygen. This reduced ability leads to symptoms such as fatigue and pain.

Figure 1.5 Genes impact your body's likelihood of developing certain diseases. ***How can genes also affect your risk of communicable diseases?***

Mental Health Conditions and Illnesses

Mental health conditions are thoughts and feelings that reduce mental and emotional health. When mental health conditions interfere with daily life for a period of time, they are called *mental illnesses*. Major depressive disorder, anxiety disorders, bipolar disorder, and schizophrenia spectrum disorder are examples of mental illnesses. Studies of families and identical twins have shown that genes influence the development of these conditions. As with many other diseases and disorders, however, genes are only part of the story. A person's environment also influences the risk for developing a mental illness.

Behavioral Factors

Did you know that one in four teens has ridden in a car with a driver who has been drinking alcohol? Driving under normal conditions can be risky, but getting into a car with someone who has been drinking puts you and others at increased risk for injury. Driving under the influence of alcohol or riding with a person who has been drinking is an example of a behavioral risk factor that can harm your health.

behavioral factors
choices and behaviors that affect a person's chance of developing a disease, unhealthy condition, or injury

Behavioral factors, also called *lifestyle factors*, are choices and behaviors that affect a person's chance of developing a disease or health condition. These choices and behaviors are often based on a person's values, habits, and beliefs. These factors are modifiable, and many begin during childhood and adolescence, continue into adulthood, and affect a person's health for years to come.

Some behaviors, like getting into a motor vehicle accident, have an immediate impact on health. Other behaviors have both short- and long-term effects. For example, children with an active lifestyle are more likely to become physically active adults. Physically active adults have a lower risk for developing obesity, high blood pressure, and cardiovascular disease.

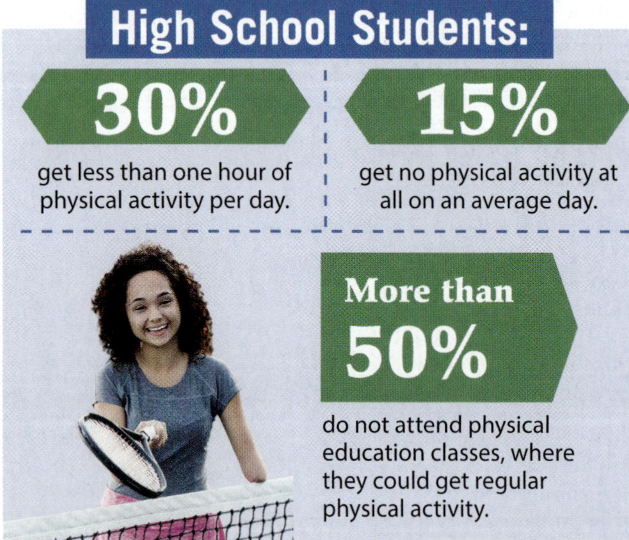

Figure 1.6 Unfortunately, many high school students do not get the physical activity they need. Physical activity is a protective factor against health conditions. ***Why do you think students may be getting so little physical activity?***

Nutrition and Physical Activity

What you eat, how much you eat, and how much physical activity you get all influence your health. Nutritional excesses or deficiencies are risk factors for many health conditions. For example, diets low in fiber and high in red meat increase a person's risk for developing cancer of the colon. Diets high in calories, salt, and fat can lead to cardiovascular disease, high blood pressure, stroke, cancer, and obesity.

Physical activity is also an important factor. Getting enough physical activity is a protective factor for maintaining a healthy weight and heart health. Being physically inactive can lead to short-term health consequences of weakness and weight gain. It can also lead to long-term health conditions such as cardiovascular disease, high blood pressure, cancer, type 2 diabetes mellitus, arthritis, and muscle and bone weakness (**Figure 1.6**).

The dietary and physical activity habits of children and teens tend to persist into adulthood. As behavioral factors, your nutrition and physical activity are modifiable. If you do not have a healthy diet, you can take steps to eat nutritious foods. You can get more physical activity by making time in your schedule and being active with friends.

Sleep

Lack of sleep is a risk factor for poor health. It reduces a person's resistance to disease and impairs motor skills, such as for driving. It also increases the risk for mental health conditions such as depression and anxiety.

Teens need at least eight to 10 hours of sleep each night and sometimes require more. Fewer than one out of three high school students get eight hours of sleep on school nights. The amount of sleep you get is a modifiable factor. Setting a schedule for sleep and avoiding *blue light* from phone, computer, and TV screens before bed can help you get the sleep you need (**Figure 1.7**).

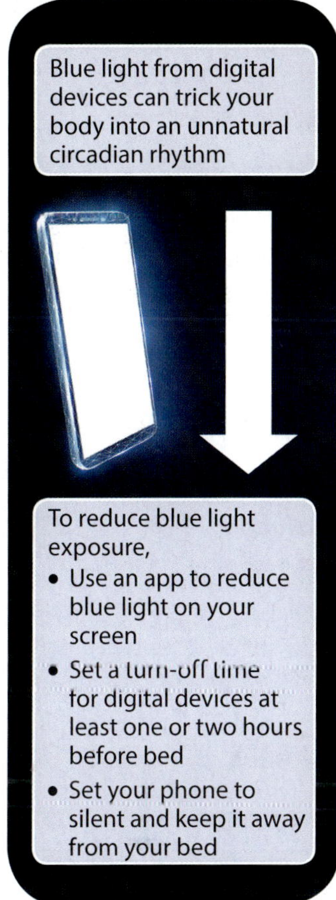

Butusova Elena/Shutterstock.com

Figure 1.7 Blue light from digital devices interferes with how your body produces *melatonin*, the hormone that makes you feel sleepy.

Tobacco, Alcohol, and Drug Use

Using medications properly and following your doctor's directions can improve your health and wellness. Misusing or abusing medications and using tobacco, alcohol, or drugs, however, can cause serious health conditions that will last a lifetime. For example, smoking and vaping can raise your blood pressure, harden your arteries, and greatly increase your chance for a heart attack or stroke. Alcohol use can lead to impaired judgment and brain damage, and the abuse of medications and drugs can cause serious damage and even death. Use of these substances is a modifiable factor because people can choose not to use tobacco, drink alcohol, or abuse medications and drugs.

Sexual Activity

Research shows that sexual activity among teens tends to be fairly risky and have negative health outcomes. Of teens who have sex, many fail to use contraception, leading to significant risks for pregnancy and sexually transmitted infections (STIs), including HIV. In addition, sexual activity among teens, who are still establishing their identities and learning to set goals and build relationships, can be emotionally traumatic. Sexual activity among teens can lead to unhealthy relationships, broken trust, negative feelings, and regret. Sexual activity is a modifiable factor. You have the right and ability to say *no* to sexual activity, no matter the kind of relationship.

Injuries and Accidents

Accidents are the leading cause of death among children and teens in the US and worldwide. Even if they do not cause death, accidents can cause significant injury and sometimes disabilities. You can help prevent injuries from accidents by reducing the risky behaviors that lead to them.

Teen Drivers at Higher Risk for Injury

According to researchers, teen drivers (ages 16–19) are **three times** more likely than adult drivers to be in a fatal motor vehicle accident.

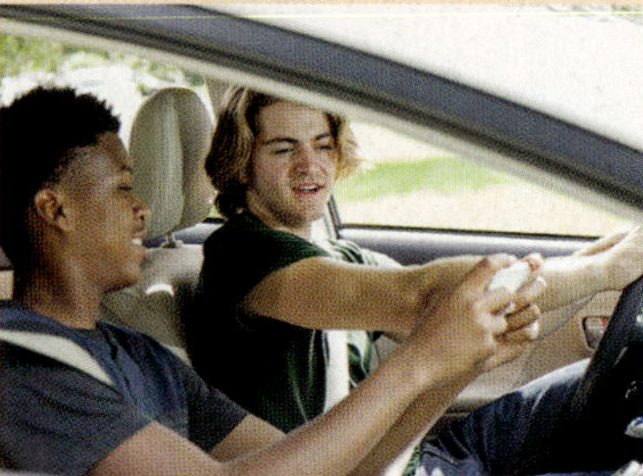

Teen drivers are significantly more likely to engage in behaviors that increase their risk of possibly fatal accidents:

- texting or using phones while driving
- driving with more than one passenger under 18 years of age
- distracted driving
- not using seatbelts

kali9/iStock/Getty Images Plus/GettyImages

Figure 1.8 Risky behaviors, such as texting and driving, are common among teens. These types of actions are behavioral risk factors for accidents and injuries.

Motor vehicle accidents cause most injury-related deaths for teens. Thousands of teens die in motor vehicle accidents each year, and hundreds of thousands are injured (**Figure 1.8**).

Injuries can also arise from other risky behaviors. Head injuries occur more frequently when people do not wear a helmet while bicycling, skateboarding, or snowboarding. Despite this evidence, many teens still make the choice not to wear helmets. Other outdoor activities, such as canoeing, can be risky if people do not take proper safety measures. For example, you can prevent accidental drowning by wearing a personal flotation device while canoeing. If you are caught outdoors during a thunderstorm or other severe weather situation, you can avoid serious injury by simply going inside and taking precautions.

Lesson 1.2 Review

Know and Understand

1. Give one example of a risk factor and one example of a protective factor.
2. What steps can you take to improve health if a risk factor is nonmodifiable?
3. What does it mean to have a family history of a disease?

Think Critically

4. With a partner, discuss why behaviors you adopt today will affect your health into adulthood. Why do these behaviors persist? What does this mean for the decisions you make today?
5. Make a plan for getting enough rest and sleep. How much sleep do you get now? What changes could you make to get more?

REAL WORLD Health Skills

Access Information Using reliable resources, research how many deaths the following behaviors caused in the US in the past year:

- motor vehicle accidents
- alcohol use
- illegal drug use
- medication abuse
- sexual activity (including sexually transmitted infections)
- poor nutrition
- extreme sports

Which behaviors caused the most deaths? How did these deaths occur? Also conduct research to identify precautions that can help prevent these risky behaviors. Share this information with your class.

Environmental Factors Affecting Health and Wellness

Essential Question?

What factors in a person's environment influence health?

Lesson 1.3

Learning Outcomes

After studying this lesson, you will be able to

- summarize how factors in a person's physical environment influence health;
- analyze the importance of social environment;
- assess the impact of media and technology on teens; and
- describe how economic environment affects health.

Key Terms

culture
environment
geography
homelessness
media
pollution

Warm-Up Activity

You and the Environment

Practice Health-Enhancing Behaviors Environmental factors are sometimes modifiable and sometimes not. For example, you can modify many aspects of your social environment, such as the friends you choose. You may not be able to modify where you live or your family's income level. With a partner, discuss the following question: *How much control do I have over my environment?* List aspects of your environment you can and cannot control. Also list aspects you might be able to influence, even if you cannot control them. Brainstorm a few actions you could take to improve aspects of the environment you can control.

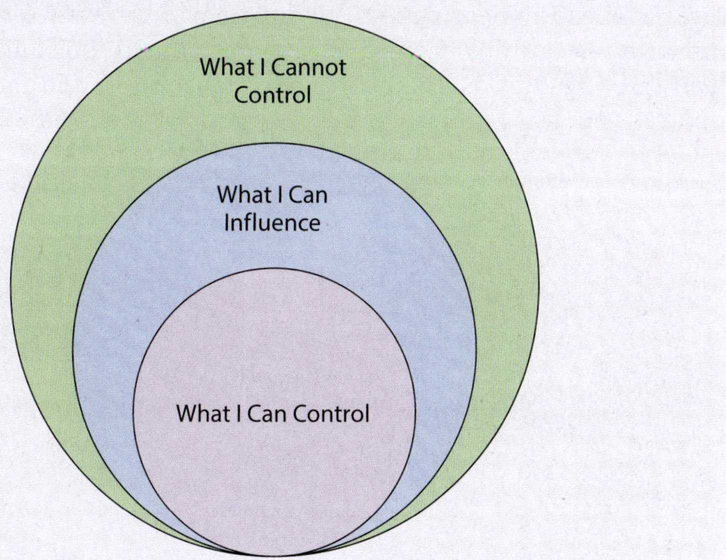

Environmental factors relate to your **environment**, or the circumstances, relationships, or conditions that surround you. Climate, workplace, home, family and peers, culture, media and technology, and community are all part of your environment. Every environment has protective factors that can increase your health and risk factors that can create barriers to positive health practices.

environment
circumstances, objects, or conditions that surround a person in everyday life

Physical Environment

Your *physical environment* includes the places you spend your time—outside, at school, at home, or in the workplace. Factors in all of these areas can influence your chances of developing health conditions. Some aspects of your physical environment are modifiable, while others are not. Eliminating risk factors whenever possible and taking advantage of protective factors in your environment can help you have positive health.

Climate, Geography, and Pollution

geography land features and any bodies of water present in an area

pollution presence of waste in the environment

One environmental factor is your region's *climate*, or overall pattern of weather conditions. Frequent destructive weather events, such as hurricanes or tornados, can increase your risk for injury. Sun exposure can put you at risk for skin cancer. **Geography**, or the features of the land and any bodies of water, can also affect health. Many mountains can provide opportunities for physical activity, but increase your risk for an accident or injury. Unless you move, climate and geography are factors you cannot control. You can, however, take safety precautions to reduce your risk of injury.

Another environmental factor is **pollution**, or the presence of waste in the environment. Each year, diseases related to polluted air, water, and soil cause the deaths of nine million people—about the population of New York City. Air pollution has the largest impact worldwide, accounting for four million deaths per year (**Figure 1.9**).

Home, School, and Work Conditions

Dangerous substances or conditions at home, school, or work increase your risk for injury or disease. For example, exposure to loud noises can lead to hearing loss. Flying debris or power tools can cause injury, and hazardous chemicals can cause burns, poisoning, and respiratory conditions. Exposure to lead, asbestos, and radon gas, even in places you visit regularly, can cause cancer and brain or lung damage.

The WHO estimates
90%
of the world's
population is exposed
to unhealthy air.
Air pollution can cause
• asthma
• cardiovascular disease
• stroke
• cancer
• lung infections
VanderWolf Images/Shutterstock.com

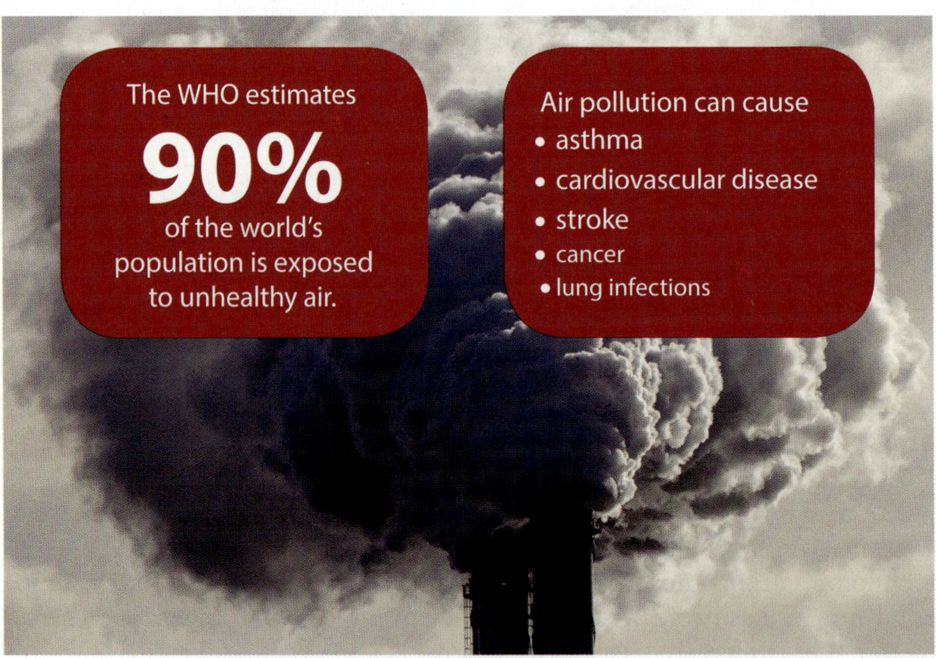

Figure 1.9 Air pollution is widespread and dangerous and can cause many health conditions.

Computer use and time spent sitting also impact health. If you use a computer at home or school, this can cause eye strain and repetitive use injuries. A job that involves continuous computer use might also limit opportunities to engage in physical activity (**Figure 1.10**). Your level of activity at school or work may not be a modifiable factor, but you can control your level of physical activity at home. Simple changes such as waking up early to jog, walk, or bike can increase your level of physical activity.

Another physical environmental factor is **homelessness**, or a lack of stable housing. People who are homeless are more likely to experience health conditions, crime, violence, and assault. Without access to healthcare, even minor health conditions, such as skin or wound infections, can become dangerous. People can become homeless for many reasons, including loss of a job or home, low income, untreated mental illness, or running away from home.

homelessness state of being without regular, consistent housing

Social Environment

Your *social environment* includes the relationships all around you. Relationships with family, peers, and community members all affect health. In some cases, factors in your social environment are nonmodifiable. You cannot make another person behave respectfully, for example. You can, however, build and maintain your own healthy relationships and advocate for a positive community environment.

Family

Family relationships are a key part of social environment. A supportive, safe family environment is a protective factor because it promotes and maintains the health of family members. Family support during childhood and adolescence promotes language and intellectual development. Children and teens with supportive families have fewer health conditions and are more likely to get treatment for existing conditions.

Physical Activity Needs Depend on Lifestyle
Female • 28 years old • 145 pounds
Website Designer
Works mainly at a desk throughout the day.
102 calories per hour
Carpenter
Lifts heavy objects and runs errands.
260 calories per hour
Firefighter
Carries a heavy backpack, works in extreme conditions.
892 calories per hour

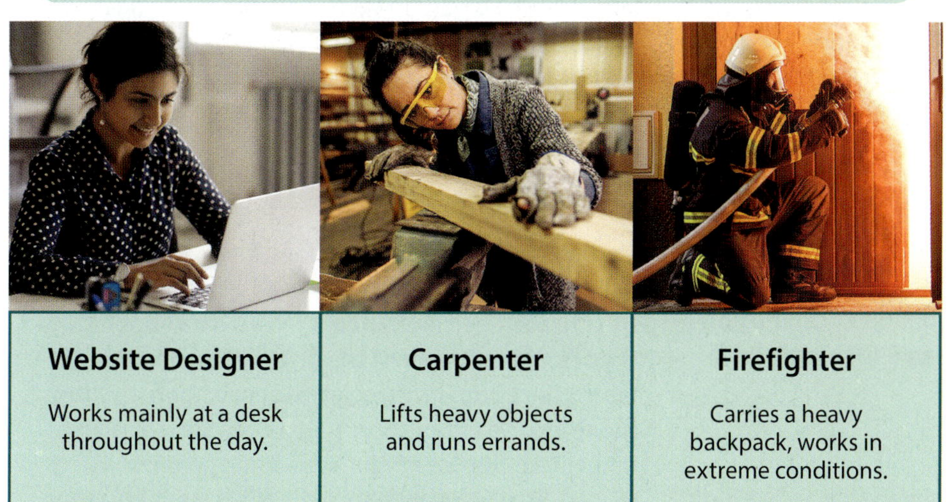

Left to right: fizkes/Shutterstock.com; Dusan Petkovic/Shutterstock.com; urbans/Shutterstock.com

Figure 1.10 Each person requires physical activity to avoid a sedentary, inactive lifestyle that can lead to health conditions. These three females need the same amount of physical activity each day. They differ, however, in how much physical activity they require outside of the workplace. ***Who needs to get physical activity outside the workplace the most? Who needs the least amount of physical activity outside the workplace?***

Family relationships that are unhealthy or abusive increase the risk for health conditions. Teens from these families are more likely to engage in risky behaviors and use drugs and alcohol, experience pregnancy, or contract a sexually transmitted infection (STI). Teens without positive family relationships also have more mental health conditions.

Peers

Positive peer relationships reduce risk for health conditions. Healthy, respectful peer relationships improve self-esteem, contribute to a sense of belonging, and help teens avoid risky behaviors. Positive interactions with friends keep teens physically active and socially engaged.

Negative or abusive peer relationships are risk factors for anxiety and depression. Teens who feel rejected may become socially isolated and less physically active. This can contribute to physical and mental health conditions. Feeling the need for acceptance can make teens more susceptible to peer pressure and risky behaviors such as substance use and sexual activity.

Local and Global Health

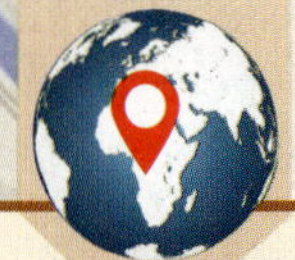

Perceptions and Norms: The Impact on Health

In different cultures, people tend to share certain ideas. This often leads to varying *norms*, or common behaviors and attitudes that are considered "normal." Sometimes people perceive norms to be different than they actually are. For example, a teen may think everyone is in a dating relationship, when in reality, many teens do not feel ready to date. Norms and perceptions of norms in different societies, cultures, and populations impact health.

In Australia, for example, some people from native populations (Australian Aborigines) avoid physical activity due to cultural perceptions. These people tell researchers they fear shame and embarrassment within society. This attitude about physical activity places people at increased risk for developing a variety of physical health conditions.

As another example, India has the world's second largest population and largest medical program for preventing mother-to-child HIV transmission. Many factors, however, keep Indian females from participating. One factor is social and cultural *stigma*, or negative beliefs, associated with people living with HIV. This stigma increases risk for mother-to-child HIV transmission.

In the US, many teens hold the inaccurate perception that sexual activity is the norm among teens. Studies such as the Youth Risk Behavior Surveillance Survey, however, find that reality does not match teens' perceptions. In fact, the majority of teens are not sexually active. Still, inaccurate perceptions can make teens feel pressure to engage in sexual activity.

Practice Your Skills

Analyze Influences

In a small group, brainstorm all the norms you perceive among teens in your community and school. To begin, think about norms related to the following behaviors:

- being physically active
- eating nutritious meals and dieting
- getting help for mental health
- smoking, vaping, and chewing tobacco
- using alcohol and abusing medications and drugs
- being sexually active

List your group's perceptions. Then, assign each person to research one norm using reliable resources. Next to each perceived norm, record data about the actual prevalence of the behavior among US teens. Once you have researched each norm, create a group podcast discussing how perceptions of norms influence behavior in your school and community. Discuss how behavior might change if teens knew the actual data about norms related to these behaviors.

Culture and Community

Your **culture** (the beliefs, values, customs, and arts of a group of people) and community are also part of your social environment. Cultural practices and behaviors affect health and wellness (**Figure 1.11**).

A community's safety and security affects personal health. For example, some communities struggle with violence and crime. In these communities, people may avoid going outside and engage in less physical and social activities. People in these communities also have more chronic stress. They are more likely to experience stress-related health conditions, such as obesity, high blood pressure, high heart rate, anxiety, and depression.

A person's sense of belonging in a community also affects health. Feeling isolated is a risk factor that often affects older adults and people who are new to the community. Immigrants and refugees from other countries may feel isolated because of their new community's language and culture. On the other hand, a sense of belonging and social support improves health.

culture beliefs, values, customs, and arts of a particular group or society

Cultural Practices That Affect Health and Wellness

- Food and taste preferences
- Eating patterns
- Religious or spiritual practices
- Activity preferences
- Medical treatment and customs

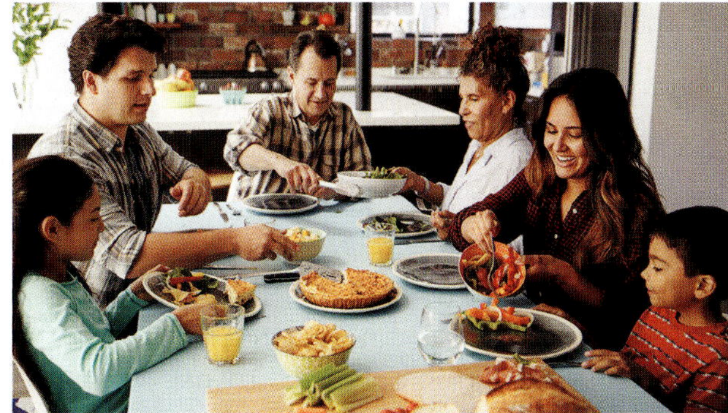

Monkey Business Images/Shutterstock.com

Figure 1.11 The way your family and the wider culture you are part of eats, celebrates, gets physical activity, and treats illnesses affect your overall health and wellness.

Media and Technology

The media and technology in your environment have a significant influence on health. **Media** includes books, TV shows, movies, radio or podcasts, social media, and advertisements in person and online. These communication channels can impact your view of yourself, your family and community, and the world. Media can also encourage you to select certain health products and services over others. These influences, which reflect the society in which you live, can lead to decisions that are healthy or unhealthy (**Figure 1.12**).

media in-person and online communication channels, such as books, TV shows, movies, social media, and advertisements

Questions for Analyzing Media

Question	Reason
Who created this message?	All media messages are created by an author. This author's point of view informs the message.
What techniques does the message use to catch my attention?	Media messages use creative words, images, and sounds to catch the attention of an audience. Media has to get your attention first before you will receive its message.
How might other people understand this message differently from me?	Media has a target audience in mind. You may or may not be the target audience, and people experience media differently.
What behaviors, values, and points of view are included or excluded from the message?	All media has a point of view and communicates certain values. This means media may also exclude certain behaviors and values.
Why is this message being sent?	Most media is produced for a profit. The creator of the message makes money or gains influence from its success.

Source: Center for Media Literacy

Figure 1.12 When you encounter media, you can ask certain questions to identify the message being communicated and why. Analyzing media in this way can help you determine whether representations are realistic or not and manage the influence these messages have on you.

Health in the Media

How Has Technology Affected Health?

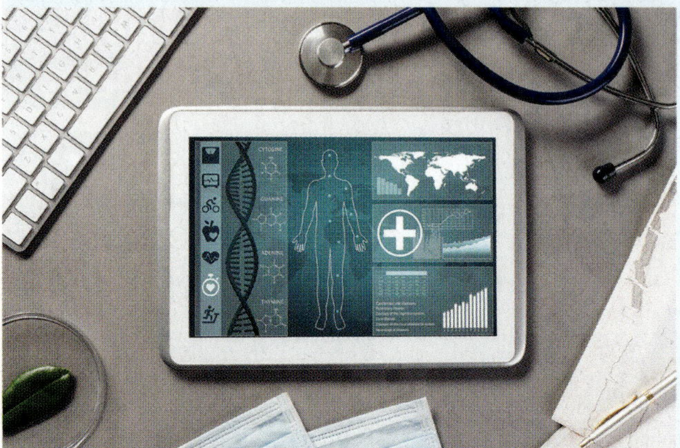
Khakimullin Aleksandr/Shutterstock.com

Over the years, advances in technology have changed life for people around the world. These changes have had both positive and negative effects on the different areas of health.

In healthcare, evolving medical technology has allowed immediate diagnosis, more effective treatments, and new strategies for preventing health conditions. Today, for example, newborns can be screened for many genetic diseases. Artificial intelligence enables the rapid development of safe and effective influenza vaccines, antibiotics, and medications to treat cancer.

New communication technologies enable doctors to collaborate remotely. For example, doctors can share test results and X-ray images with experts anywhere to help diagnose diseases. At the same time, this technology raises concerns about confidentiality. Outside the world of healthcare, communication technologies make it easier to talk with people across distances. Friends can chat at all hours, day and night, and communicate even if they do not live nearby. While these advances make it easier to maintain relationships, they can also lead to more harassment, abuse, stress, and conflict.

The internet also impacts health. Digital devices and the internet have increased access to entertainment, health information, and social support. At the same time, people can also find incorrect health information on the internet and are exposed to more media and advertisements. Social media can spread false information and negative emotions, but also enables more communication. Many public health agencies use social media to inform and educate the public. Excessive use of the internet and technology reduces social and physical activities and has been linked to obesity, trouble sleeping, depression, and anxiety.

Practice Your Skills

Advocate for Health

To understand the impact of technology on your life, have a conversation with someone much older than you. During your conversation, ask questions about how technology has changed since this person was a teen. How did this older person communicate with friends? What did the person do on weekends and during summers off school? How has the person had to adapt to changing technology? After your conversation, create and share a short documentary about how technology makes your life different from the lives older people led as teens. In your documentary, include tips for maximizing the positive effects of technology and minimizing the negative effects.

For example, comparing yourself to a movie star and developing a negative body image can lead to disordered eating and negative health outcomes. On a larger scale, media that glorifies drug use can harm the health of families, communities, and the world.

You have control over what and how much media you consume. Excessive technology use can lead to physical inactivity, overweight, obesity, headaches, and trouble concentrating. It can also lead to declines in social health if you do not spend time building healthy relationships in person.

Continuous exposure to social media can negatively impact mental and emotional health by encouraging you to compare your accomplishments to those of others.

Media and technology also have many positive effects. Media that encourages healthy behaviors can push you to improve health and relationships. Social media and technological devices can help you connect more easily with family members and peers. Technological advances in medicine can also improve health by treating diseases and disorders and screening for health conditions.

Economic Environment

Your *economic environment* includes your family's and community's level of education, income, and resources. Whether you graduate high school, how much money you earn, and what resources are in your neighborhood are all factors in your economic environment. These factors influence a person's understanding of health concepts and access to healthcare and needed resources.

Education and Income

Level of education affects a person's risk for developing health conditions (**Figure 1.13**). In part, this factor is related to knowledge. For example, education improves knowledge about the importance of nutrition and physical activity. The correlation between education and health also relates to income. People with more education tend to earn more money and thus are better able to pay for healthcare, activities, and resources that promote health.

Income itself also influences health. Inability to pay for healthcare can lead to children not having needed vaccinations or screenings. Families with lower incomes often live in low-income communities, which tend to have more violence. This environment and a family's financial difficulties harm mental and emotional health and can cause stress-related health conditions. In low-income communities, people also have less access to nutritious food, fewer affordable healthcare facilities, and fewer opportunities for physical activity.

The education and income of your family members may not be in your control, but you can take steps to pursue your own education. You can also choose to make healthy decisions using the resources you have, take advantage of community assistance programs, and seek out reliable health information.

Percentage of Adults (18 Years of Age and Older) with Certain Heath Conditions

Disease	Education		
	No high school diploma or GED	High school diploma or GED	College degree or higher
Cardiovascular disease	13.7%	12.1%	11.3%
Stroke	4.5%	3.1%	2.4%

Figure 1.13 The risk of developing health conditions like cardiovascular disease or stroke decreases as a person's level of education increases. ***What two factors explain why education decreases risk of health conditions?***

Access to Health Services

Another economic factor is access to health services. Effective health services result from collaboration among a community's healthcare professionals. For example, scientists study how infections spread, and doctors advise patients and administer recommended vaccines.

Skills for Health and Wellness

What Factors Affect Your Health?

Simply by being alive, you possess risk and protective factors that affect your health. You can modify some of these factors; others you cannot. Analyzing the different factors that influence your health can help you make good decisions and practice healthier behaviors. For example, you could eliminate some risk factors or reduce them. You could also increase protective factors. Knowing and understanding these factors will enable you to make changes and decisions that benefit your health.

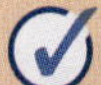

Practice Your Skills

Analyze Influences

Using what you learned in this chapter, create an inventory of the risk and protective factors that influence your health. Start by reviewing the risk and protective factors in the table shown. Indicate all of the factors that apply to you and then add any factors not given in the table.

After completing your inventory of risk and protective factors, look at each factor and determine whether it is modifiable or nonmodifiable. How does each factor influence each dimension of your health? Create a video, essay, song, poem, or artistic representation of the factors in your life.

Risk Factors	Protective Factors
• My family has health conditions I could inherit. • I consume too many or too few calories on a regular basis. • I am not physically active most days. • I spend several hours each day using social media or watching television or videos. • I spend several hours per day playing video games. • I sleep fewer than seven hours per night on a regular basis. • My family cannot afford safe housing, healthcare, or nutritious food. • I smoke cigarettes, vape, or chew tobacco. • I drink alcoholic beverages. • I use medications in ways that are not intended or use illegal drugs. • I often feel stressed, unsafe, or anxious at home or in my community. • I am sexually active. • I perform poorly in school and may not complete high school. • I do not feel safe walking around my community. • I am exposed to bad air quality or noise pollution where I live or work. • I am exposed to hazardous substances where I live or work. • Hazardous or extreme weather are common where I live.	• My family can afford healthcare, and I see the doctor regularly. • I have a healthy body weight. • I am physically active most days. • I use social media, but spend lots of time talking with friends in person too. • My family has access to and can afford nutritious food. • My family has access to and can afford safe housing. • I take precautions to remain safe during recreational or work activities. • My family has clear expectations about not using drugs, tobacco, and alcohol. • I have mostly positive relationships with my family. • I have mostly positive relationships with peers. • I participate in community activities and organizations. • My family and I value education. • I earn good grades and am on track for completing high school. • I feel a sense of belonging in my community and among peers. • My community rarely experiences hazardous or extreme weather. • My environment is relatively free of pollution.

A community's access to health services depends on the location and affordability of healthcare facilities and services. In some regions, people have to travel long distances to get healthcare. For other people, there are many healthcare facilities nearby. In areas that have few healthcare facilities, accessing health services is more difficult. Income, population, and regional policies all affect the availability of healthcare facilities. Low income can make it difficult to afford health services, even if facilities are nearby.

Lesson 1.3 Review

Know and Understand

1. What are the components of a physical environment?
2. How can homelessness affect health?
3. Give one example of a cultural practice that influences health.
4. With a partner, take turns listing the positive and negative impacts of technology on individuals, families, communities, and the world.
5. How does education influence health?

Think Critically

6. Describe the climate and geography in your community. What risk and protective factors do they pose?
7. Why do you think teens with abusive or negative family relationships are more likely to engage in risky behaviors?
8. With a partner, think about your community. How accepting is your community? How safe is it? What evidence do you have for these perceptions, and how do they influence health?

REAL WORLD Health Skills

Communicate with Others Environmental issues impact the risk and protective factors you encounter. These issues can include physical factors, such as air pollution or inactivity at school, as well as social factors, such as respect among your peers or cultural diversity. In a small group, consider your environment and answer the following questions:

- What are some examples of environmental factors you face? How do these factors risk or protect your health? Do these factors also impact others? What factors have the most impact?
- What actions could you take to decrease risk factors in your environment? Would these actions also be useful to others?

Working in your group, agree on one of the actions you identified and commit to carry it out. Pay attention to how this action affects your health. Meet with your group again after a few days and discuss how effective the action you chose was.

Chapter 1

Review and Assessment

Chapter Summary

Health is not just the absence of disease, but a state of complete physical, mental and emotional, and social well-being. This definition is holistic and includes three dimensions of health: physical (related to the body), mental and emotional (thoughts and feelings), and social (relationships). The dimensions of health are not isolated from each other. Each dimension affects the others. Practicing wellness means taking steps to improve health in each dimension.

People often see health as something a person does or does not have. In reality, health is a continuum. At the high end of the continuum is optimal health, and at the low end is illness. The factors in people's lives place them somewhere near the middle of this continuum, and people can take steps to change their place on the continuum.

Many factors affect people's health. Risk factors have the potential to harm health, and protective factors increase health. Some factors are modifiable, and others are nonmodifiable. Individual factors, including genetic and behavioral factors, relate to a person's identity and decisions. Genetic factors are the genes inherited from biological parents. Genes can make a person more likely to develop a disease, though other factors often play a role. Behavioral factors are a person's decisions—about nutrition, physical activity, safety, or sexual activity, for example.

Environmental factors describe the circumstances, relationships, and conditions surrounding a person. In the physical environment, climate, pollution, and conditions at home or school impact health. For example, not having stable housing can increase risk for health conditions. Social environment describes a person's relationships. Supportive family, peer, and community relationships improve health, and unhealthy relationships harm health.

Media and technology are key environmental factors. Media influences people's decisions. Asking questions and choosing media carefully can help people manage this influence. Technology can support communication, but can harm health in excess. The economic environment, including education, income, and access to health services, also influences health. Lack of education or income can lead to worse health outcomes.

Vocabulary Activity

Write each of the terms shown on a separate sheet of paper. For each term, quickly write a word you have learned that relates to the term. In small groups, exchange papers. Have each person in the group explain a term on the list. Work together to properly pronounce the term and take turns until all terms have complete explanations. Ask for assistance, if needed.

behavioral factors	*health*	*physical health*
culture	*homelessness*	*pollution*
deoxyribonucleic acid (DNA)	*illness*	*protective factors*
emotional health	*life expectancy*	*quality of life*
environment	*life span*	*risk factors*
genes	*media*	*social health*
genetic disorders	*mental health*	*well-being*
geography	*optimal health*	*wellness*

Review and Recall

Review the information in this chapter by answering the following questions.

1. What does it mean for wellness to be holistic?
2. Give an example of how one could measure health in each dimension of health.

3. Which of the following is *not* part of positive social health?
   A. honest communication
   B. supportive relationships
   C. threats
   D. interpersonal skills
4. How can people change their place on the health and wellness continuum?
5. Explain the difference between risk and protective factors.
6. Why are genetic risk factors nonmodifiable?
7. Which type of disorder develops from a genetic risk factor, regardless of any other risk factors?
   A. noncommunicable disease
   B. genetic disorder
   C. communicable disease
   D. pathogenic disorder
8. How can decisions about physical activity now impact health over time?
9. What is the leading cause of death among children and teens in the US?
   A. homicide
   B. accidents
   C. diseases
   D. suicide
10. List the components of a person's environment.
11. Explain why continuous computer use is an environmental risk factor.
12. What elements of your social environment can you control? What elements can you not control?
13. How much of what you see or hear each day is media? List all the forms of media you encounter on a given day.
14. What factors can make it difficult for people to access health services?

Standardized Test Prep

Reading and Writing Practice

Read the passage below and then answer the following questions.

Education and income both have a large impact on whether a person gets needed healthcare. Education affects income. Often, having more education means a person will earn more income later in life. Education also helps people make wise decisions when choosing between health products and services.

Income often determines whether healthcare is affordable. Even if they have health insurance, people pay some amount for healthcare. When a person has little income, this amount can become difficult. People with less education can spend as much as 50 percent of their income on housing, leaving little for money for healthcare and other expenses. As a result of not getting needed healthcare, people can develop health conditions or leave health conditions untreated. In fact, studies have found that more than one-half of people in the US have delayed or chosen not to get treatment for a health condition because of cost.

15. According to this passage, how does education affect income?
    A. Education is expensive and decreases income in the long run.
    B. Having more education often leads to more income in the long run.
    C. Education enables good decisions, which save money.
    D. Education has no impact on income.
16. What is the main point of the second paragraph in this passage?
    A. People with less education spend a lot of their income on housing.
    B. Healthcare is a large expense for many families.
    C. Lack of income makes it difficult to get education.
    D. Low income makes it difficult to get needed healthcare.
17. Using the information in this passage, write an essay about the relationship between education, income, and access to healthcare. How do these factors affect each other? How do interactions between these factors influence health?

Chapter 1 Skills Assessment

Critical Thinking Skills

Answer the following questions to assess your knowledge of what you learned in this chapter.

1. What is your level of well-being? What would have to change for you to be more satisfied with life's present conditions?
2. Why does wellness look different among different people?
3. Is it possible for someone to be totally healthy in one dimension of health, but unhealthy in the other dimensions? Explain.
4. With a partner, discuss the following statement: *Achieving health does not mean eliminating all factors that hinder health and wellness.* Why do you think this is? Is it possible for a person to eliminate all factors that decrease health and wellness?
5. How can you tell if a factor is modifiable or nonmodifiable? Can a factor fall somewhere in between? Explain.
6. While factors fall into different categories, they are also closely related. With a partner, discuss how genetic, behavioral, and environmental factors can influence each other. For example, do genes influence behavior? Does behavior influence environment?
7. With a partner, discuss the following question: Is there ever a situation in which a behavioral factor is nonmodifiable?
8. Imagine you have a friend who drives home from parties after drinking alcohol. When you confront your friend, your friend says, "I've done it before and never got into trouble." What could you say to this friend to explain why the behavior is still dangerous?
9. Give four examples of factors in the physical environment that can increase health and encourage wellness.
10. Why do you think a person's sense of belonging in a community affects health and wellness?
11. Think about the media you encounter. How accurately do you think media reflects the society in which you live? What impact does this have on your health?
12. Lack of income, lack of education, and poor health are sometimes described as a cycle. Why do you think this is? What needs to happen for people to break this cycle?
13. Discuss with a partner and use reliable resources to answer the following question: How does access to health services in the US compare to access in other countries?

Health and Wellness Skills

Complete the following activities to practice your skills related to health and wellness.

14. **Analyze Influences.** Write a letter to someone who currently has or has had a positive influence on you. In your letter, explain why you chose this individual and how this person has influenced you. Thank the person for having a positive influence on your life. After writing your letter, make the decision to share or keep it.
15. **Access Information.** In this chapter, you learned that media can have a significant influence on your health. Think about a product you purchased or used recently due to media influence. What was the product, and how did media influence you to use or buy it? Do you feel the influence was positive or negative? Why? Using reliable resources, research the product's risks and proven health benefits. Also research some similar products that might have more health benefits and fewer risks.
16. **Communicate with Others.** Think about the risk factors in your life and choose one factor you want to improve. Think of someone in your life who could help you identify protective factors against your identified risk factor. Then have a conversation with this person, sharing your risk factor and brainstorming ways to improve. During your conversation, practice effective communication skills like maintaining eye contact, being clear and concise about your needs, and giving and receiving feedback.

17. **Make Decisions.** Think about some decisions you have made over the last week. Make a list of decisions that had a positive impact on your health and a list of decisions that were risky or had a negative impact. Cross out each risky decision and replace it with a positive, healthier decision you could have made.
18. **Set Goals.** Think about the diseases that run in your family, diseases that have spread through your school, and diseases your friends have experienced. Then design a plan to delay or prevent these diseases. Identify one action you can take and then outline a specific, measurable, achievable, relevant, and timely goal that will motivate you to engage in a healthier lifestyle.
19. **Practice Health-Enhancing Behaviors.** Think about your own life and choose one unhealthy or risky behavior you would like to change. Write a statement explaining how changing this behavior will help improve your overall health and wellness. Then list several actions you will need to take to change this behavior; several payoffs or positives that will result from your change; and a "significant helper," or factor that will help reinforce this change.
20. **Advocate for Health.** Make a 30-second video or two-minute digital illustration that focuses on a health-related risk. This risk could affect any of the three dimensions of health. The focus of your video or illustration should be to raise awareness about the risk and start a conversation about possible protective factors for prevention or treatment.

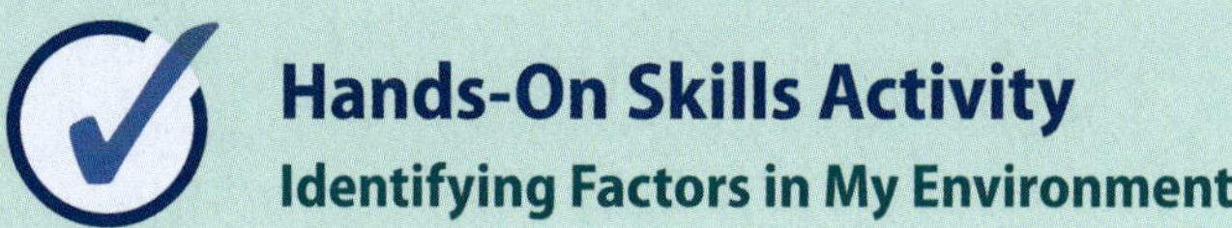

Hands-On Skills Activity

Identifying Factors in My Environment

In this chapter, you read about different types of risk and protective factors. Follow the steps below to identify risk and protective factors that may be present in your own environment.

Steps for This Activity

1. **Analyze Influences.** Your first task is to identify as many potential risk and protective factors as possible in your personal environment—in your home, in your neighborhood, at school, and in your community. Since many of your factors may be the same as those identified by your classmates, focus closely on your own home; your job, if you have one; places your family visits regularly; and any other aspects of your environment that make it unique. Organize your factors in a table like the one shown.

Location	Protective	Risk

2. Take pictures of objects, conditions, and people engaged in activities that represent each factor you identified. Be creative in determining the best possible photo to represent or symbolize a particular factor.
3. **Practice Health-Enhancing Behaviors.** After collecting this information, design a "plan of attack" for how you will keep yourself as healthy as possible while confronting one or two of the most threatening risk factors you found. Keep in mind how you can increase protective factors to make up for risk factors you cannot control.
4. Present your plan, along with the corresponding photos, to your class. Be creative in your presentation. To share information about your environment, you might use a poster, digital presentation, video, or artistic representation, for example. As you listen to other students present, think about the similarities and differences between your factors.

Chapter 2 Health and Wellness Skills

Look for the skills icon throughout this chapter for opportunities to practice your health skills.

Check Your Health and Wellness Skills

In this chapter, you will learn skills for maintaining your lifelong health and wellness and promoting health and wellness in your community and world. To understand the skills you currently use, take the following inventory of your behaviors. Indicate how well you think you use each skill. Use a scale of 1–5, *1* meaning you do not use the skill and *5* meaning you feel completely comfortable using it.

Skill	How Well Do You Use Each Skill?
I evaluate multiple courses of action before making a decision.	
I set goals that have results I can easily measure.	
When I set a goal, I plot a specific and reasonable time line for completing it.	
I leave situations if people pressure me and do not respect my decisions.	
I verify the information I read online with other, reliable sources.	
I check whether information on a website comes from a cited scientific study.	
I compare health products that have the same active ingredients.	
I visit the doctor for an annual checkup or wellness exam.	
I stay home from school and go to the doctor when I need medical care for an illness.	
I keep a list of community resources that are available to provide help and support.	
I participate in community service.	
	Total:

Add up your responses to each statement. The higher your score, the more comfortable you feel practicing health skills related to making decisions, setting goals, evaluating and applying health information, and advocating for health. Which skill do you think is most important for you? Which skill is the most challenging for you? Which skill would you most like to improve? In this chapter, you will learn how to perform these skills better and more often.

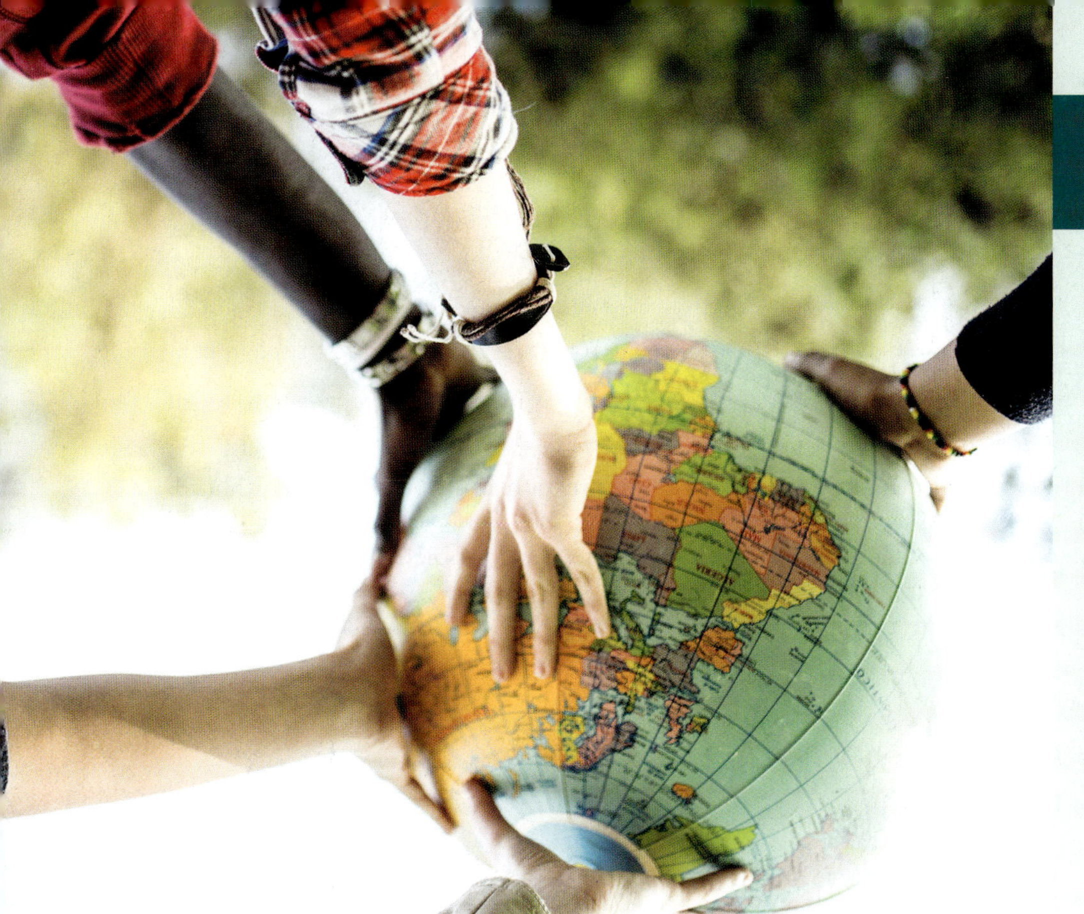

franckreporter/E+/Getty Images

Reading and Notetaking

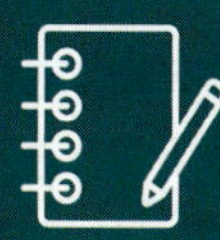

Before reading, skim the headings in this chapter. List the headings to create an outline for taking notes during reading and class discussion. Under each heading, list any key terms. Finally, write two questions you expect to have answered in class. After completing the chapter, ask your teacher any questions you still have about the concepts or terms you learned.

Headings	Notes
Making Healthy Decisions The Decision-Making Process Step 1: Define the Decision or Problem	

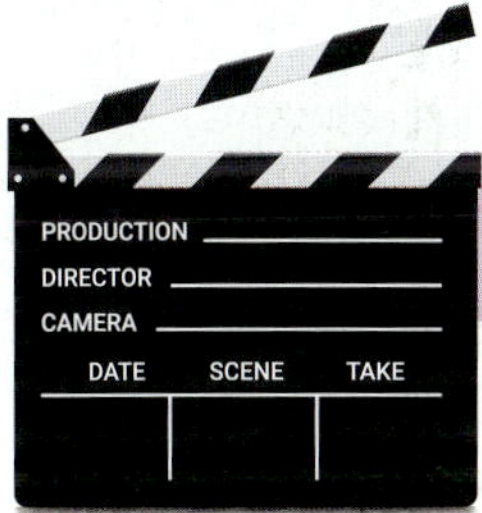

Setting the Scene

Good Information Enables a Good Decision

As the summer comes to a close and a new school year begins, you look forward to seeing your friends in classes again. One of your friends is an athlete. Over the summer, your friend started taking pills to build muscle and lose fat in preparation for a competitive event. Your friend starts messaging you about the pills, saying they will improve your athletic performance and help you lose weight. Your friend offers to give you a few to try if you want.

You do not know much about the pills your friend is taking, but you have seen them advertised online and you know the local drugstore sells them. At home, you research the pills and find websites with conflicting information. Some websites advertise amazing results. Others list frightening side effects. You do not know what to tell your friend, but you know you have to make a decision soon.

Thinking Critically

1. You need credible, true information to make a good decision about the pills your friend is offering you. How can you find reliable information on the internet about these pills?
2. In addition to the internet, what other sources of information or advice can help you make a healthy decision?
3. You know your friend wants you to try these pills. If you decide not to try them and your friend pressures you, what can you do to stick to your decision?

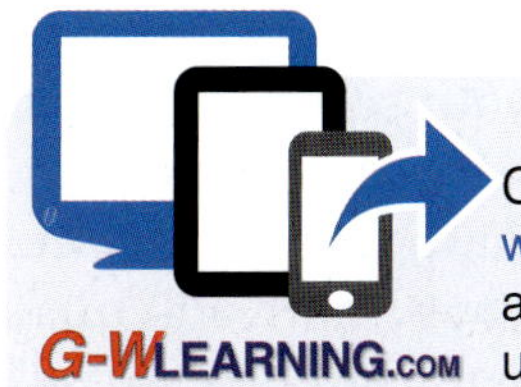

G-WLEARNING.com

Click on the activity icon or visit www.g-wlearning.com/health/4095 to access online vocabulary activities using key terms from the chapter.

Lesson 2.1

Making Decisions and Setting Goals

Essential Question?

What skills do you need to make health-promoting decisions and goals?

Learning Outcomes

After studying this lesson, you will be able to

- explain the importance of taking responsibility for your health and wellness;
- use the decision-making process to solve problems and make healthy choices; and
- develop a plan to achieve short- and long-term SMART goals.

Key Terms 

alternatives
collaborative decision-making
decision-making process
goal
SMART goal
values

Warm-Up Activity

Get Motivated

Analyze Influences In this lesson, you will learn about making decisions and setting goals. Find a quote about setting goals or making decisions that motivates you. Then, write a self-reflection about why you chose that particular quote and what it means to you. Why does this quote appeal to you? What does it tell you about your beliefs and values? Explain how this quote might help you in the future as you make decisions about your health and set short- and long-term goals.

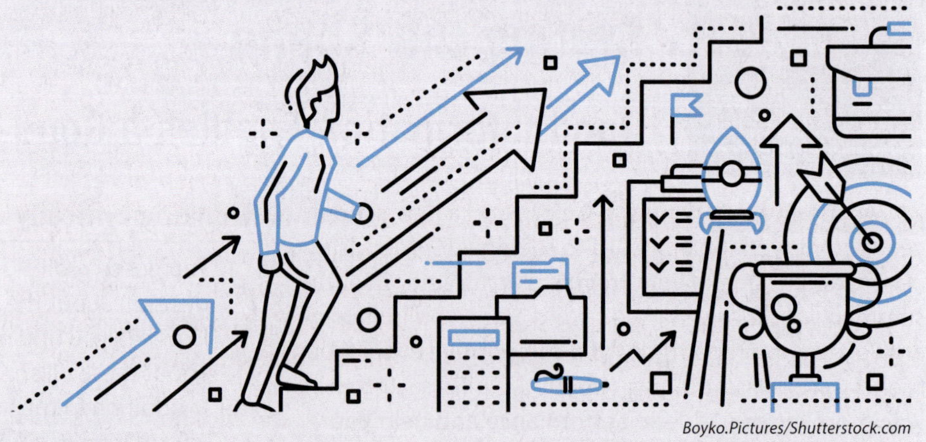

Boyko.Pictures/Shutterstock.com

As a young child, you did not make many choices for yourself—the adults in your life chose for you or gave you alternatives from which you could choose. Now that you are a teen, you make many of your own choices, including choices that affect your health. For example, if your school cafeteria offers pizza and a salad bar, you make the choice between the two. You also choose whether you will be physically active or sit in front of a screen much of the day. These choices and others impact your health and quality of life in either a positive or negative way. Why not learn how to make healthy lifestyle choices now that can help you stay healthy for many years to come?

Making healthy lifestyle choices is not always easy. At times, friends may try to pressure you into engaging in risk-taking behaviors that may actually harm your health.

As you make your own choices, you need to understand how the choices you make can affect your health and wellness. To make healthy choices, you need to demonstrate certain skills. These skills will benefit you today and all through your life.

Making Healthy Decisions

Each day, you make decisions that affect your health and wellness. For instance, should you stay up late playing video games or get a good night's sleep? Should you exercise on a painful knee? Should you eat that second piece of pie? Sometimes, you may need to make decisions to solve problems regarding friendships, dating, substance use, smoking or vaping, and sexual activity.

The Decision-Making Process

How you approach making a decision is important. Do you go with your gut feeling? Do you make the decision that is most convenient or makes you feel good? The best way to make healthy and informed decisions is to use a **decision-making process**. Many different decision-making processes exist. The DECIDE model of decision-making consists of six steps (**Figure 2.1**).

decision-making process steps for making a healthy decision; include defining the decision, exploring alternatives, considering consequences, identifying the best alternative, deciding, and evaluating

Step 1: Define the Decision or Problem

The first step in the decision-making process is to define the problem to be solved or the decision to be made. Depending on the problem or decision, this step can be easy or difficult. You can readily define some problems. For example, maybe you have trouble getting up on time because you stay up too late chatting with friends. You need to make a decision about how to get to bed earlier.

Other times, you may need to think carefully about a situation and examine your own thoughts and feelings to define a problem. For example, maybe you feel unhappy at school, but cannot identify why. The problem could be a relationship conflict or stress at school. If you are having trouble defining the problem, try journaling about your feelings or talking with a trusted adult. Defining the problem accurately is crucial to making a healthy, informed decision.

Step 2: Explore Alternatives and Options

Alternatives are courses of action that are different from the actions you are taking now. Once you have defined the problem, exploring alternatives will help you understand the actions you can take to solve it. In this step, brainstorm all possible alternatives. To learn about different alternatives, you might talk with a friend or trusted adult or research solutions to a problem. Examples of alternatives to a problem are shown in **Figure 2.2**.

alternatives courses of action one can take

As you brainstorm, think of alternatives from multiple perspectives. Do not rule out any ideas, and hold off on making any judgment until after you have identified all alternatives. Listing all possible alternatives can help you envision and remember your options.

Using the Decision-Making Process

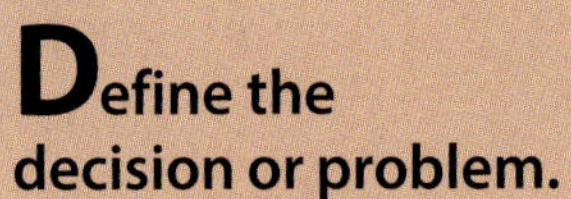

Gabriel meets with his doctor, who advises him to lose weight and then maintain a weight in the healthy BMI range. After his doctor's appointment, Gabriel sits down to make a plan for losing weight. He determines that he needs to lose 20 pounds and wants to lose them in three months.

Explore alternatives and options.

Gabriel talks with his friends and family members about his goal to lose 20 pounds in three months. His friends and family members offer a few ideas, and Gabriel also researches weight-loss strategies online. He keeps a list of possible strategies:

- Exercise 30 minutes three to five times per week for three months.
- Eat two meals per day instead of three for three months.
- Start a fad diet to lose weight quickly for three months.
- Take diet pills for three months.
- Eat lower-calorie meals and exercise 30 minutes three to five days per week for three months.

Consider the consequences.

Gabriel considers the strengths and weaknesses of each alternative. After more research, he learns that skipping meals, taking diet pills, and following fad diets can have serious negative side effects. He learns that experts recommend reducing calories and increasing exercise. He also talks with his brother, who has successfully lost weight in the past. He lists his alternatives in order from most effective to least effective.

Identify the best alternative.

Gabriel chooses to eat lower-calorie meals and exercise 30 minutes three to five days per week for three months.

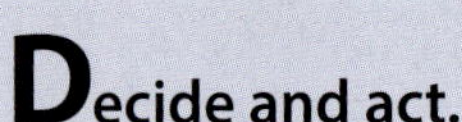

To implement his decision, Gabriel joins an exercise class at a gym nearby. He plans a workout schedule and begins using an app to plan his meals and calorie intake. He plans to weigh himself and track his weight once a week.

Evaluate and revise.

After three months, Gabriel reviews his progress. He has lost 15 pounds. Gabriel has been exercising three days per week and likes how he feels. He decides to continue attending the exercise class. He has noticed he gets hungry between meals and sometimes eats too much for dinner. To revise his plan, Gabriel decides to eat small, healthy snacks between meals.

Figure 2.1 The decision-making process consists of six steps and can be used to help you make your best decisions every day.

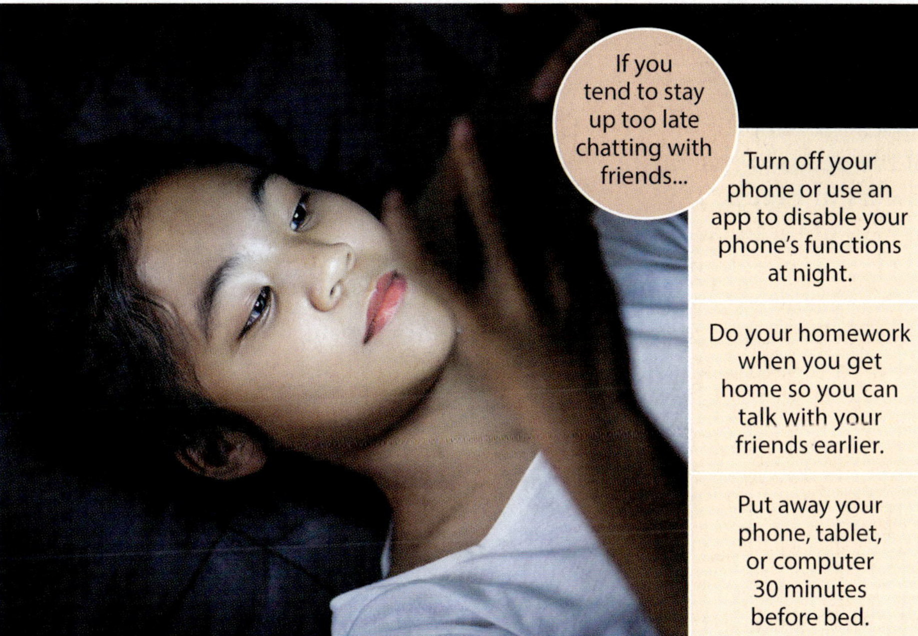

If you tend to stay up too late chatting with friends...
Turn off your phone or use an app to disable your phone's functions at night.
Do your homework when you get home so you can talk with your friends earlier.
Put away your phone, tablet, or computer 30 minutes before bed.
OHishiapply/Shutterstock.com

Figure 2.2 There is almost always more than one alternative decision you can make. Be creative when brainstorming ideas. ***Can you think of other alternative decisions for this scenario?***

Step 3: Consider the Consequences

To select the best alternative from your list of options, consider the consequences of each alternative using relevant data and facts. Imagine choosing each alternative and list any obstacles you might face. Research reliable information about the effectiveness of each alternative and talk with friends and trusted adults about the pros and cons and best- and worst-case scenarios. Also consider how each alternative aligns with your values, goals, and resources and will affect other people. It may be helpful to talk to people who have faced a similar situation. Once you have evaluated each alternative, rank your alternatives from the most effective and favorable to the least.

Step 4: Identify the Best Alternative

After careful evaluation of each alternative, identify the alternative that is right for you and your situation and best solves the problem. Sometimes, you may choose a combination of alternatives that work together to solve the problem. Make sure to select an alternative that aligns with your goals and values and is realistic given your resources.

Step 5: Decide and Act

After you have chosen the best alternative, act on that alternative. In this step, it is important to act on your chosen solution and commit to it for a certain amount of time. Attempting a solution halfway will not give you an accurate idea of how effective the solution is. For example, if you choose to turn off your app notifications before you go to bed to get more sleep, choose a specific time to take this action and have your friends keep you accountable. Ask your friends or a trusted adult to remind you if they notice you responding to messages on your phone after your specified time. Keep a sleep journal to track how much sleep you are getting and how effective your actions are.

Factors to Consider When Evaluating a Decision

- Obstacles you faced in acting on the decision
- What, if any, support you needed to commit to the decision
- Whether the decision solved or just helped with the problem
- Whether you can commit to the decision for a longer time

Figure 2.3 A decision might not be the right fit for your situation if it has too many obstacles, needs too much outside support, does not effectively solve your problem, or if you cannot commit to the decision long term.

Step 6: Evaluate and Revise

Once you have acted on your decision for a certain amount of time, evaluate your decision's effectiveness. An effective alternative is one that solves the problem or resolves the decision you identified in the first step of the decision-making process. When evaluating a decision, consider the factors in **Figure 2.3**.

All of these factors influence whether a decision is right and effective for you. For example, if your friends had to remind you every night to turn off your app notifications and stop messaging them, a different alternative might better help you get enough sleep. Maybe, instead, you want to try turning off your phone and placing it across the room before you go to bed.

If you determine that a decision did not solve your problem, repeat the decision-making process and revise as necessary. Maybe the real problem was not what you thought or you have another alternative. Keep revising until you find the right decision for you.

Collaborative Decision-Making

When you make a decision, try seeking advice from a parent, guardian, trusted adult, or trusted peer. Hearing someone else's perspective might show you a new alternative or change how you think about a problem. In some cases, people use **collaborative decision-making** to make decisions together (**Figure 2.4**). Multiple people might have roles in carrying out the decision and need to know and perform these roles. For example, if you want to change your curfew, talk with your parents or guardians about making the decision. You might make a decision about where to meet over the weekend with several friends. On the other hand, some decisions, like decisions about your personal boundaries, belong only to you.

collaborative decision-making process of working with others to make a decision

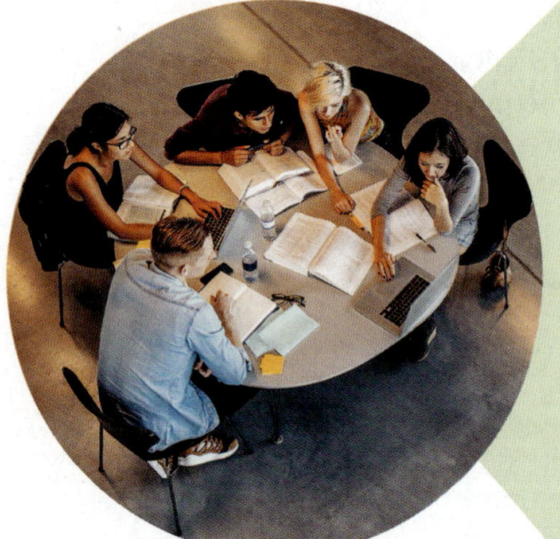

Best Practices for Collaborative Decision-Making

- Decide carefully on who is involved. Include only people who need to weigh in or who can provide relevant ideas.
- Consider choosing someone to keep the group on track.
- Make sure all relevant information and opinions are discussed before selecting an alternative.
- Make sure all members advocate for their own perspectives, but ultimately agree to make the decision that is best for the whole group.
- Determine how the decision will be made. Does everyone need to agree, or will one person decide?
- When you make your decision, schedule a follow-up meeting to evaluate the decision.

Jacob Lund/Shutterstock.com

Figure 2.4 Decision-making becomes more difficult with more voices, more ideas, and more perspectives. Following some basic guidelines can help keep you on track for making an effective decision. ***What should you do if your decision was not right for you?***

Setting and Reaching Goals

A **goal** is a specific endpoint that signifies a condition you hope to reach. Goals motivate you and keep you focused on what you need to accomplish. Setting and working toward goals can help you change situations you do not like or get where you want to be. They can also give you a sense of satisfaction. Do you have goals regarding your physical, mental and emotional, or social wellness? If so, are you working toward them?

goal specific endpoint that signifies a condition one hopes to reach

Goals can be short- or long-term. A *short-term goal* is a goal you want to accomplish in the near future, within days or weeks. A *long-term goal* requires more time—months or years—to achieve. Reaching a long-term goal usually involves achieving a series of short-term goals. When setting goals, consider your **values**, or what you consider important, and your current situation, which includes your resources, independence, and environment. Effective goals are also *SMART*. A **SMART goal** is

values qualities or priorities one considers important

SMART goal endpoint that is specific, measurable, achievable, relevant, and timely

- **Specific**—clearly states what you want to accomplish;
- **Measurable**—has results that can be clearly observed or quantified;
- **Achievable**—can be realistically reached;
- **Relevant**—relates to who you are and what you want; and
- **Timely**—is achievable within a reasonable period of time.

An example of a SMART goal is eating 2½ cups of vegetables every day for three weeks. This goal is more measurable and achievable than the goal of "eating more vegetables." **Figure 2.5** shows more examples of SMART and nonSMART goals. To set a SMART goal, use the following steps:

Step 1: **Assess the situation:** Consider the way your life is right now. What is important to you? What needs improvement? What aspirations and dreams do you want to achieve? Try to think of all the ways you could improve your life or situation.

Step 2: **Identify a specific and realistic goal:** Identify a goal that is important to you and write the specific goal you want to achieve. A goal needs to be measurable so you know when you have reached it. A goal should also be achievable within a specific amount of time.

Step 3: **Define the steps or actions you must take to achieve your goal:** Break big goals into smaller, more achievable steps. These are your short-term goals, which lead to long-term goals. For example, to improve your grade in a class, set short-term goals related to completing your homework, joining a study group, and studying for tests.

Step 4: **Set a reasonable time line:** Look at a calendar and pick a realistic date for completing your goal. If you have a series of short-term goals, set dates for their completion. Enter the dates in your calendar.

Goals
1. Use relaxation techniques to reduce stress.
2. Drink at least 80 ounces of water per day.
3. Join one new club or sport this school year to make new friends.
4. Get into a good college.
5. Make the varsity soccer team next year.
6. Go to sleep before 10 p.m. every night for two weeks.

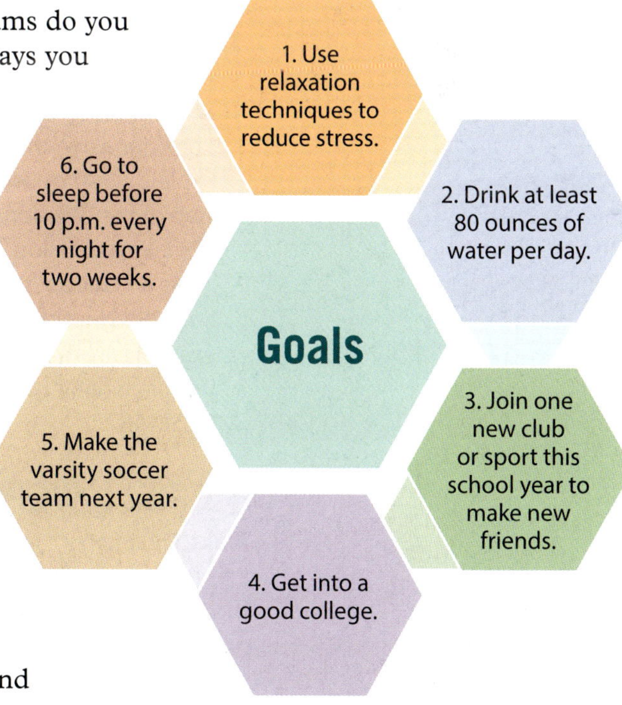

Figure 2.5 All of these goals would help improve your health and wellness, but only some of them are SMART goals. ***Which of the goals shown are SMART goals?***

Step 5: **Act on your goal:** Follow your plan for achieving your goal. If you need help, ask for it. Your relationships and the resources in your community can provide support. Set reminders for yourself to complete each step in your goal.

Step 6: **Monitor your progress and analyze obstacles:** Keep track of your progress. If you are not making progress, determine the obstacles in your way and what you can do to overcome them. For example, if your goal is to pack a healthy lunch every morning and time is an obstacle, you might pack your lunch the night before. If you are unsure what you can do, ask a trusted friend or adult.

Step 7: **Experience the benefits:** Once you have achieved a goal, you can experience its benefits in your life. For example, if you achieve a goal that reduces your procrastination, you might experience less stress and conflict at home. You can also identify a reward for yourself when you reach your goal. Your reward might be a favorite activity or a day out with a friend. Experiencing benefits and giving yourself a reward can help keep you motivated.

Even if you do not achieve a goal you have set, the effort of trying can lead to success in the future. By processing your feelings and revising your goal, you can still learn and experience benefits. Mastering goal-setting skills will help you continually grow and improve yourself, your health, and your overall well-being.

Lesson 2.1 Review

Know and Understand

1. Consider a health issue in your life. Explain how you would use each step of the decision-making process to make a decision.
2. Write an example of a short-term and a long-term goal. Compare examples with a partner and discuss.
3. Explain what it means for a goal to be SMART.

Think Critically

4. Why is it important to take responsibility for your personal health and wellness?
5. Identify one decision you could make in your life today to improve your health.
6. After you have carried out a decision, how do you know if the decision was right and effective for you?

REAL WORLD Health Skills

Make Decisions Imagine these two scenarios: (1) riding to a football game with a friend who texts and drives, and (2) going to a friend's house for a party after the basketball game and discovering your friend's parents are out of town. You do not want to be involved in either of these situations, but you do not want to upset your friend. Using the decision-making process, identify a healthy decision you could make in each scenario and consider the effect on yourself and others. Write a narrative, record a video, or draw a comic strip outlining how the conversation with your friend might go and what you could say or do to exclude yourself from each situation.

Using Health Information

Essential Question?

How can you locate, evaluate, apply, and communicate reliable health information?

Lesson 2.2

Learning Outcomes

After studying this lesson, you will be able to

- explain how to locate reliable sources of health information;
- use criteria to evaluate whether a source of health information is reliable;
- apply reliable health information to make healthy decisions; and
- communicate health information with your family and the community.

Key Terms

advocate
consumer
Food and Drug Administration (FDA)
health fraud
health literacy
health promotion
lifelong learning
pseudoscience
science

Warm-Up Activity

Can You Trust This Website?

Access Information Using online resources, search for information about a health topic of your choice using a variety of different words and phrases. When you use different search terms, do you get different results? Review the list of results. What are some indicators that might suggest if websites listed have a slant, false information, or bias? credible information? Read the information on a few of the websites. Were you correct in your initial assessment? Why or why not?

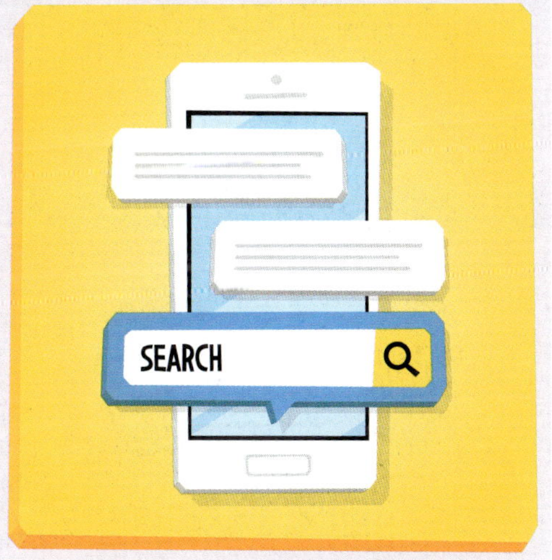

Artyem Dzyuba/Shutterstock.com

What is the best way to control asthma, muscle cramps, or acne? How can you better manage the stress in your life? How can you help a friend with an eating disorder? Do you know how you would find good, reliable answers to these questions? You would not want answers based on rumors or unreliable sources of information.

Health literacy—the ability to locate, evaluate, apply, and communicate information pertaining to your health—is an important skill for promoting health and wellness. How can you make healthy decisions if you do not know how decisions will impact your health? Your health literacy builds on the basic facts and concepts you learn at home and in school. What you learn helps you make informed, healthy decisions. Your health and wellness also depend on your ability to access and use reliable information beyond what you learn at home and in school.

health literacy ability to locate, evaluate, apply, and communicate information pertaining to health

Locating Health Information

Websites, newspapers, magazines, TV, and radio shows often share health-related information. While some of this information is true, some of it is not. By locating *reliable* sources for health information, you can avoid information that is too good to be true, inaccurate, misleading, or not applicable to your situation (**Figure 2.6**).

You can go on the internet to find reliable health information. You will see several websites when you search online for answers to a question about your health, but not all of this information is reliable. In general, you can find *reliable* information through agencies or organizations that provide education, research, or direct healthcare. URL stems that indicate reliable sources include .gov, .edu, and .org.

Websites belonging to businesses that earn profits or organizations promoting a particular cause are often not trustworthy. Since the main goal of businesses is to earn profits, businesses use marketing and advertising strategies to play up the benefits of certain products and play down negative information. Organizations promoting a certain cause may only share information that supports its cause. When searching for information, begin with a reliable, general source.

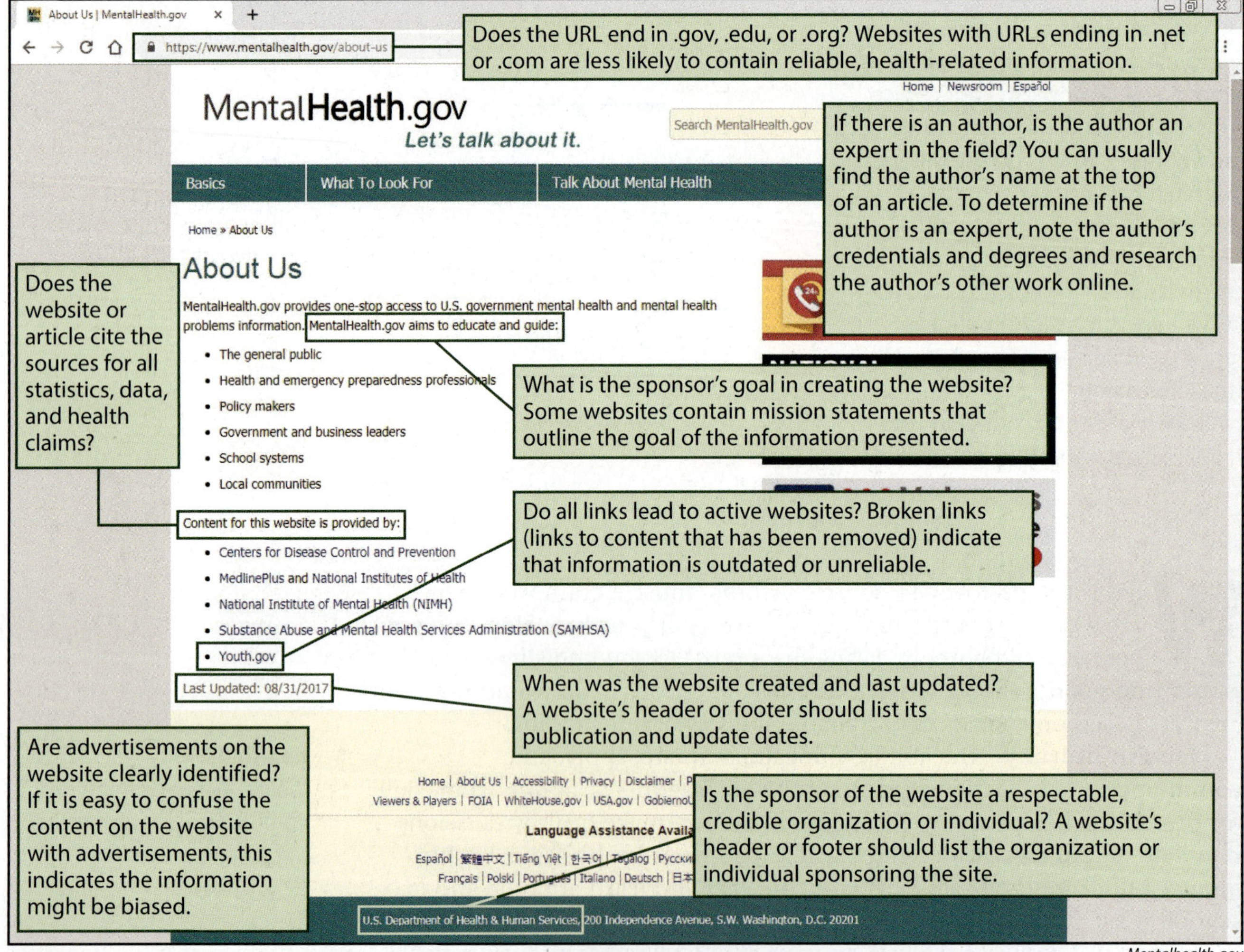

Figure 2.6 The "About Us" page on a health website is often a great place to evaluate the reliability of that source. ***Can some of these tips also help you evaluate printed sources? Explain.***

Research in Action

Debunking Health Claims

You have probably heard claims about the health benefits of certain products, behaviors, and diets. The internet, social media, and advertising spread these claims quickly. Sometimes they even appear on product labels. When you see these health claims, you need to determine: are they true or false? are the products and behaviors advertised genuine or fake? useful or useless? safe or dangerous? Fortunately, reliable health information, based on research done by scientists, can help you verify or debunk health claims.

Health Claim		What Research Says
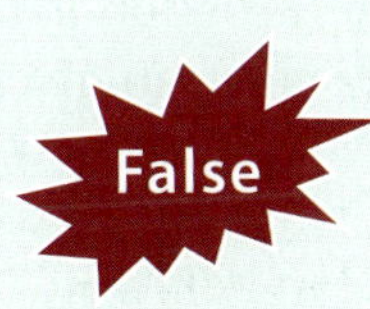 False — Vaping is not harmful.		Vaping devices often contain more nicotine, which is highly addictive, than cigarettes. Nicotine harms the developing brains of teens and children. It impairs learning, memory, and attention and increases the chance teens will smoke. Vaping aerosol contains toxic chemicals that can cause lung damage.
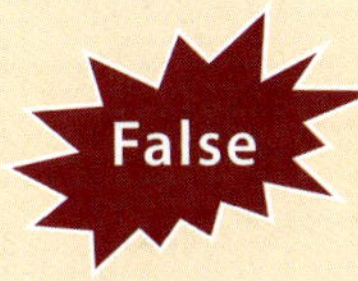 False — Short-term detox diets remove toxins from the body and promote weight loss.	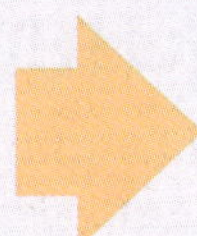	Short-term detox diets are fad diets. There is no evidence they work as promised, and they can lead to dehydration, mineral deficiencies, and malnutrition.
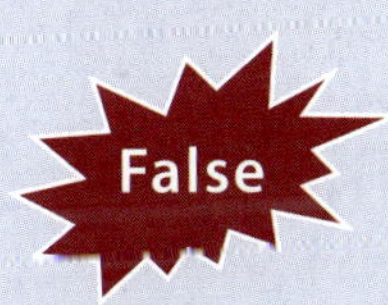 False — Energy drinks improve energy and concentration.		The caffeine in energy drinks may temporarily increase energy, but these effects wear off quickly. Energy drinks contain a large amount of caffeine and other stimulants. These increase heart rate and blood pressure and cause irritability and insomnia. Energy drinks also contain large amounts of sugar and can cause weight gain.
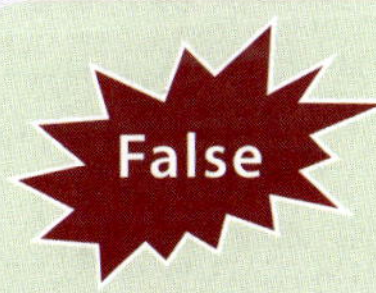 False — Diet soda is a healthy alternative to regular soda.		Diet soda contains less sugar than regular soda, but it is still not a healthy choice. Diet soda has no nutritional value and still increases a person's risk for cardiovascular disease and diabetes.

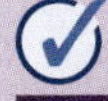

Practice Your Skills

Access Information

Credible sources can help you critically evaluate the health claims you see on product labels, social media, or advertisements. In small groups, consider and evaluate the following health claim: *Eating fat-free or nonfat food helps you lose weight.*

1. In your group, research online, print, and other sources with information about this topic. Compile a list of four credible sources you can consult to evaluate this health claim. The list may include websites, books and articles, trusted adult experts, and other sources.
2. With your group members, discuss why you selected these sources and what makes them credible. Explain whether you should rely on these sources and why.
3. Discuss any possible weaknesses of the sources you chose. Why do you think these are weaknesses? How do they impact the reliability of the information?
4. According to the sources you chose, is the health claim true or false? Explain your reasoning and cite your sources in your explanation.

Newspapers and magazines, whether printed or online, can be good sources for health information. The size or popularity of a newspaper or magazine is not a good indicator of reliability. A better indicator is whether a business that manufactures or sells medications or medical devices produced the newspaper or magazine. Newspapers and magazines produced by businesses that earn profits from the healthcare industry are not reliable. Reliable articles are written by experts and confirmed by other, reliable sources.

When in doubt, ask your school's library media specialist about a reliable media source. Library media specialists specialize in finding and evaluating sources, so you can rely on their advice. Using a library and working with a library media specialist to find health information ensures your sources are reliable.

One of the most reliable ways to get accurate health information is to ask your doctor or another healthcare professional. Your doctor can give you scientifically accurate information about your health and answers to your questions. Talking with your parents or guardians or another trusted adult, and interpreting and evaluating what they tell you, can help you learn more about health.

Evaluating Health Information

"Get six-pack abs in two weeks!"

"You'll catch a cold if you go outside with wet hair."

"The bumps on your skull reveal your character."

"Cell phones cause brain cancer."

"Caffeinated energy drinks will make you perform better on exams."

science body of knowledge based on observation and experimentation; answers questions about the natural world

These are some examples of the thousands of health claims in magazines, on websites, in the media, and in advertisements. Science supports none of these claims. If you act on these claims, you could waste money and time and harm your health.

Health and wellness are science-based disciplines. Your health and wellness depend on reliable information. You need to separate information grounded in science from health claims based on rumor, folk stories, and pseudoscience. Identifying scientifically accurate information will help you maintain your health and make responsible consumer decisions.

Science is a body of knowledge based on observation and experimentation (**Figure 2.7**). Science answers questions about the natural world—including the human body, health, and diseases.

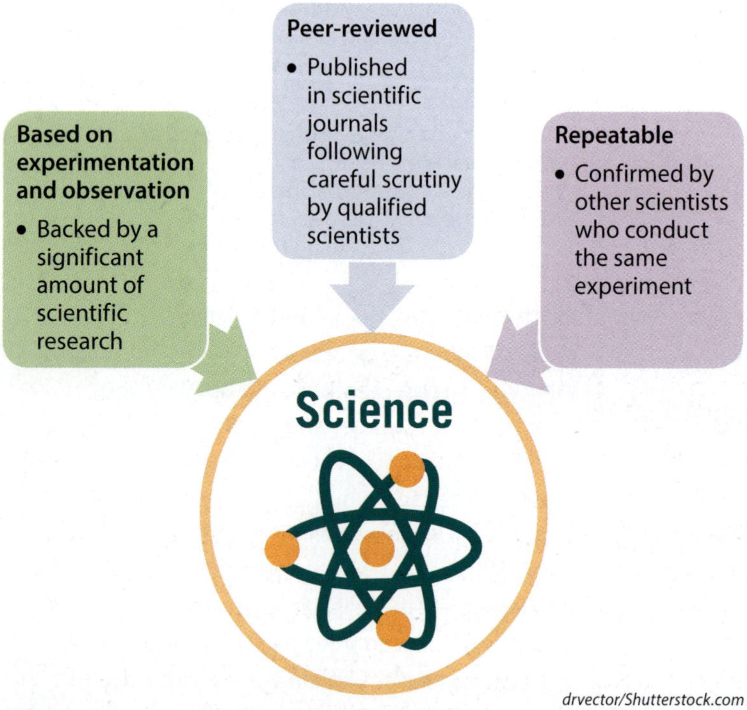

drvector/Shutterstock.com

Figure 2.7 Health-related information that does not meet these criteria is not grounded in science. ***What is the name for theories and health claims that are not science-based?***

In contrast, **pseudoscience** refers to theories and health claims that are described as science-based when they are not. Pseudoscience is not based on repeated experimentation. Other scientists cannot verify it, and scientific journals do not publish it. Pseudoscience is not peer-reviewed and is too good to be true.

pseudoscience theories and health claims that are described as science-based when they are not

When evaluating health information, including health claims about health products, ask yourself the following questions. Answering these questions can help you determine if the information is scientifically accurate:

- Is the source of the information reliable?
- Is the information current?
- Is the information applicable to my life stage and situation?
- Does the source of information have a bias? Is the source making money or promoting a cause by publishing the story or article?
- Does the article refer to research published by medical scientists?
- Does the article give the names of the researchers and the journal that published the original research?
- Can you find other reliable sources with the same information?

Evaluating health information is an ongoing process. Researchers constantly uncover new information about the human body and health, so health information is constantly changing. This should not deter you from keeping up with this fast-growing body of knowledge. View this as an opportunity to engage in **lifelong learning** about how to improve your health (**Figure 2.8**).

Lifelong Learners
• Eagerly accept that knowledge grows
• View learning as an opportunity to improve themselves
• Are confident they can learn and apply knowledge

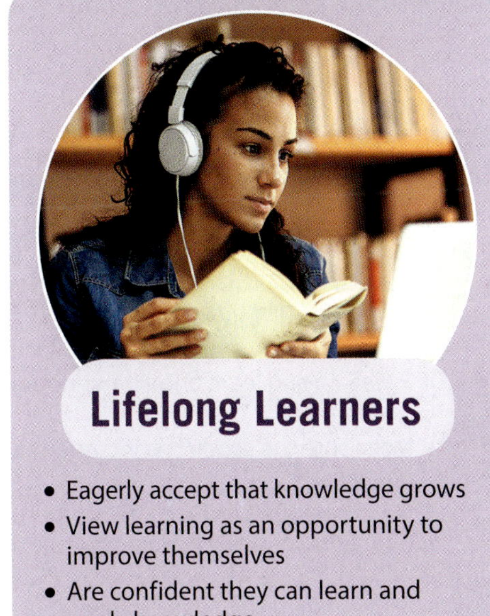

Solis Images/Shutterstock.com

Figure 2.8 Learning does not only occur in a formal environment like a school or workplace. Lifelong learners take information when and where they can throughout their lives.

Applying Health Information

Your health and wellness require your active attention. There is a cause-and-effect relationship between some of your actions and your health. For example, ignoring health information about your diet will result in poor nutrition. Not following safety precautions for using fitness equipment can lead to injury. You can avoid these effects by applying health information.

lifelong learning practice of always seeking to gather new information and learn new skills

In addition to influencing your everyday behaviors, reliable health information can also guide how you choose and evaluate health services and health products, such as medications, supplements, and hygiene and cosmetic products. You can use health information to identify what products and services you need and how effective they are.

Health Products and Services

A **consumer** is someone who purchases goods and services. You are a consumer. As you read this text, you will learn how to become an *informed* consumer. The informed consumer has knowledge and skills to make good decisions about health products and services.

consumer anyone who purchases goods and services

Consumers have rights and responsibilities. *Consumer rights* include the right to be safe from harmful products and deceptive business practices and to have complaints addressed. Regulations and laws protect these rights. For example, *truth-in-advertising laws* require

Food and Drug Administration (FDA) federal organization that regulates and ensures the safety of food, health products, and medications

advertisements and labels to be accurate and not misleading. The US **Food and Drug Administration (FDA)** regulates and ensures the safety of food, health products, and medications. *Consumer responsibilities* are reasonable expectations for consumer actions and decisions. For example, consumers should learn about the products they wish to buy and use products as directed.

When choosing a health product, pay attention to any health claims. The FDA reviews and approves health claims on product labels and in advertisements. If a health claim is not approved, the label should read, "This statement has not been reviewed and approved by the FDA." This tells you the FDA did not review scientific studies of the product's safety and effectiveness. This product may not work and might be harmful, even if used as directed. The best way to choose a health product is to comparison-shop by reviewing different brands and types of products (**Figure 2.9**).

When you are choosing health services, begin by determining your health needs or questions. Do research to learn about alternatives, compare services, and decide which health service best meets your needs. You may consider factors such as cost, convenience, and reviews. For routine healthcare, including regular checkups, vaccinations, medications, treatment, or referrals, visit your doctor. If you need healthcare quickly for a serious illness or injury, go to an urgent care or immediate care clinic or a hospital's emergency room (ER). You will learn more about accessing health services in the next lesson.

Tips for Choosing Health Products

- Be prepared. Know the health issue you want to address.
- Research and learn about your options before shopping.
- Make sure the product is intended for your health issue.
- Make sure the product label states the purpose, directions, and any warnings about the product.
- Read the label to see the product's *active ingredients*, or substances that treat a health issue.
- Compare different products that have the same active ingredients.
- Ask a doctor or pharmacist for advice.

Tyler Olson/Shutterstock.com

Figure 2.9 Evaluating health products carefully can ensure they are safe and will be effective for your needs. ***What organization regulates and ensures the safety of food, health products, and medications?***

Consumer Issues

Sometimes people are dissatisfied or have issues with health products or services. To address these issues, always save receipts to prove your purchases. If you have a complaint, contact the business, store, or healthcare facility in person or online. Politely state the issue and how you would like it resolved. If your issue remains unsolved, ask to speak with a manager. You can also contact organizations that specialize in solving consumer complaints.

health fraud illegal activity related to health products and services; for example, deceptive labeling or advertising

Health fraud is illegal activity related to health products and services. A common example of fraud is a product that claims to treat, diagnose, or cure diseases, when it has not been proven safe or effective. Other kinds of health fraud include fake medical devices and medications, intentionally mislabeled medications, misleading or deceptive advertisements, false medical claims on labels, ineffective treatments, and health services offered by someone without a medical degree and license.

Health in the Media 

Analyzing Health Advertisements

The goal of advertising is to convince people to buy products, including health products. Advertisements use messages and methods to convince people a product is important and necessary. Some advertising strategies try to influence your emotions. The illustration below shows some of these common advertising strategies. Part of applying health information is seeing through these strategies and making an informed decision.

Bandwagon	Appeal to Authority	Scare Tactic	Unproved or Unprovable Claims	Testimonial
XYZ is trending! Don't be the last to try it!	***I prefer using XYZ when I compete.***	***Take XYZ or you could get sick!***	***Using XYZ will improve your study skills and grades!***	***Use XYZ and you could be like me.***
A popular product is not necessarily a good product and might not be right for your needs. Owning a popular product does not make you popular too.	Experts are paid to appear in the advertisement. They might have no experience with the product.	Your decision not to buy a product will not cause bad consequences. Advertisers do not know if you need their product.	Evidence and scientific studies back reliable claims. Vague, unspecified claims cannot be proved.	Companies pay celebrities or other people to be in advertisements. These people may not like or even use the product.
Popularity is not a good reason to buy any product.	**Do not be influenced by the opinion of a person appearing in an advertisement.**	**Do not be scared or intimidated into buying a product.**	**Be suspicious of claims that do not make sense, are not specific, or are not measurable.**	**Know that success does not depend on any product, and be skeptical of people appearing in advertisements.**

 Practice Your Skills

Analyze Influences

With a partner, reflect on the strategies companies use to advertise and sell their products. Choose one advertising strategy discussed and complete the following steps:

1. Tell your partner why you think the strategy you chose encourages people to buy a product. What can people tell themselves to resist the message of this strategy and make good, informed decisions?
2. Reflect on your own experiences with advertising. Have you ever bought a product because of an advertisement? Why did you buy the product, and were you happy with your decision?
3. Suppose you see an advertisement for a new health product. Make a short how-to video describing how you will decide whether you should buy the product, how you will use the advertisements in your decision-making, and how you will gather any other information you need.

advocate to take actions that show support

health promotion process of advocating for the health of families and communities by sharing health information

Communicating Health Information

Once you have reliable health information, you can **advocate** for, or support, the health of your family and community by sharing it with others. This is called **health promotion**. For example, if your mother smokes, consider encouraging her to quit. Research the health risks of smoking and present the information to your mother. If your mother decides to quit smoking, support her effort.

Help your family access health information. For example, if your family members have questions about a health-related topic and do not understand English, help them by researching the topic on the internet and translating the information you find.

You can also advocate for community health. Suppose your state has a high rate of obesity. Begin by learning about existing public health services and write to your elected officials about supporting a healthy eating program.

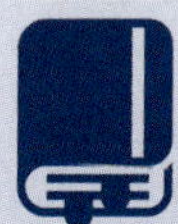

Case Study

Health Resources: What Are Available and How to Access Them

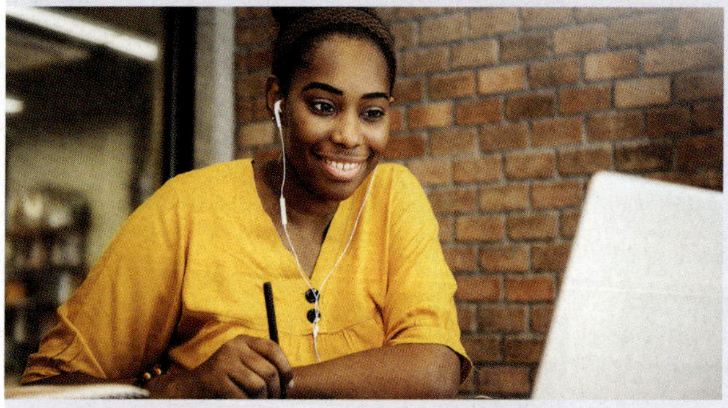

eggeegg/Shutterstock.com

Jasmine knows her poor diet contributes to her difficulty maintaining a healthy weight. She knows the basics: fruits and vegetables have many nutrients, while fast food and sweets have far fewer. Beyond that, she feels a bit lost about what needs to change in her eating habits. Jasmine tries to search for nutrition information online, but worries the information might not be accurate. She finds a lot of information about fad diets and companies selling their products. Instead, Jasmine turns to her school's library media specialist, who helps her find reliable information on the US Department of Agriculture's MyPlate website.

Daniel lives with his grandparents, who are retired. Their only source of income is his grandparents' retirement fund. Money is tight, so Daniel's family is often unable to purchase enough nutritious food for three people. Daniel is not old enough to work, but wants to contribute. One day after school, he visits his state's local Supplemental Nutrition Assistance Program (SNAP) website and finds information about food stamps. Daniel talks to his grandparents about applying. His grandparents decide to sign up for the SNAP program the following day.

Kamal worries about how much fast food his family eats. He knows the portion sizes are often too large and the meals are not that nutritious. Kamal's neighborhood does not have a grocery store. The closest one is about one hour away by car. Kamal's family eats fresh fruits, vegetables, meat, and dairy for a few days after they shop. Once that food runs out, they rely on nonperishable or frozen foods and fast-food restaurants until they go to the grocery store again.

Practice Your Skills

Communicate with Others

In a small group, choose one of the scenarios given and write a role-play in which the teen talks with a trusted adult to get help. In your role-play, the teen should seek to resolve the issue that is hindering health and get support adopting healthy behaviors and using health resources. The teen should state the issue clearly and discuss possible courses of actions with the trusted adult. Use reliable resources to find good advice the trusted adult can give. Perform your role-play for the class and then discuss how effective the conversation was. What, if anything, could have made the conversation more effective?

The Wider Scope of Health Promotion

The government should...

- factor in public health when making policies regarding unhealthy or harmful products, air and water pollution, and safety regulations
- provide people with the opportunity and security to make healthy choices

Schools and communities should...

- teach health literacy to help people understand and make healthy choices
- be a safe environment for people to live and learn

Institutions and organizations should...

- raise awareness of and demand health services and resources
- engage in intentional dialogue with the public to facilitate change

Figure 2.10 Organizations such as local, state, and federal governments; schools; corporations; and community establishments have a responsibility to promote health for the public.

On a local level, start a fitness club at school. Attend community meetings and speak about health issues that concern you. You will learn more about advocating for community health at the end of this chapter. Health promotion can also apply beyond your local community (**Figure 2.10**).

Lesson 2.2 Review

Know and Understand

1. In your own words, define *health literacy*.
2. List four indicators that an online source of health information is reliable. Why do these indicators mean that a source is reliable?
3. How is science different from pseudoscience? Explain how you can tell the difference between them.
4. Go to a drugstore and look at a health product of your choosing. What are the active ingredients in the health product? What other, similar products have the same ingredients?
5. Why is health fraud dangerous for people's health?
6. Give one example of how you can practice health promotion in your community.

Think Critically

7. Using what you learned in this lesson, make a short list of your own criteria for evaluating the reliability of health information. Evaluate a website of your choice using this list.
8. Why is lifelong learning important in health?
9. Why is it dangerous to use health products not approved by the FDA?
10. How does health promotion impact health around the world?

REAL WORLD Health Skills

Access Information Compare two websites with information about a health-promotion strategy or product of your choice. For example, you may want to research dieting, physical activity plans, or energy drinks. Compare one website supported by a reliable organization to a website sponsored by a for-profit company. How do these websites differ? Which website is more reliable? Do you notice any claims of pseudoscience? When you have researched the two websites thoroughly, write a brief summary analyzing the reliability of each website.

Lesson 2.3

Accessing Health Services

Essential Question?

What steps can you take to get needed health services?

Learning Outcomes

After studying this lesson, you will be able to

- summarize how people access health services in the United States;
- explain the rights of minors to seek health services;
- analyze the importance of getting regular checkups and screenings;
- identify when health services are needed to treat a health condition; and
- list the steps in seeking treatment for a health condition.

Key Terms

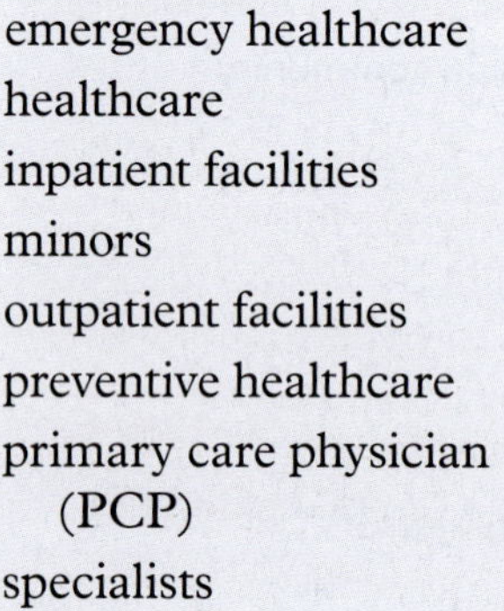

emergency healthcare
healthcare
inpatient facilities
minors
outpatient facilities
preventive healthcare
primary care physician (PCP)
specialists

Warm-Up Activity

Annual Physical Exam

Comprehend Concepts One way to practice prevention and health maintenance is to have an annual physical exam. List some reasons why you should have an annual exam and explain why it would be important to know your family's health history for this type of exam. If you were having an annual exam today, what are three questions related to your present health and well-being that you would want to ask the doctor? List these three questions.

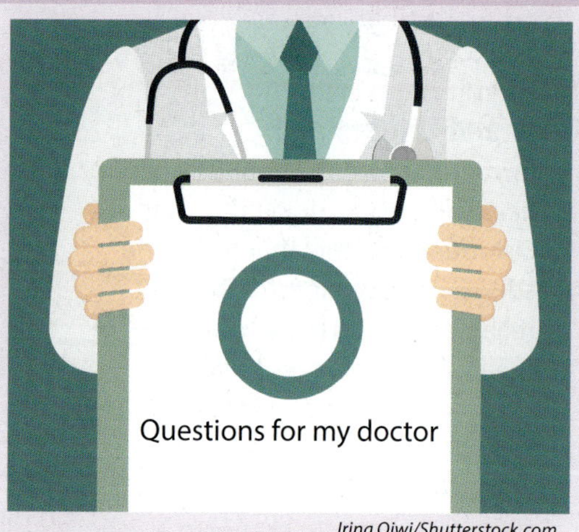

Irina Qiwi/Shutterstock.com

healthcare medical care that seeks to prevent and treat health conditions

An important skill for maintaining your health is getting appropriate **healthcare**. In the healthcare industry, professionals deliver different types of care, including diagnosis, treatment, rehabilitation, prevention, education, and research. At some point in your life, you may need all of these services.

Understanding the Healthcare Industry

The healthcare field employs more people than any other industry in the United States. The field is diverse and includes many types of professions and health services. Some professions provide highly specialized services.

A person's **primary care physician (PCP)**, or doctor, provides *primary care*, including routine checkups, screenings, treatments, prescriptions, and preventive health services. A doctor of medicine (MD) and osteopathic doctor (DO) are two types of PCPs. Physician assistants and nurse practitioners also provide primary care. The *physician assistant* works under the supervision of a PCP and usually provides the same types of health services. A *nurse practitioner* possesses advanced nursing education and can provide many of the same services as a PCP.

PCPs sometimes refer patients to **specialists**, who have extra training and experience with certain types of diseases and disorders (**Figure 2.11**). Within the US government, the Public Health Service of the US Department of Health and Human Services provides leadership, funding, and oversight of the healthcare system.

Healthcare professionals work in diverse settings. In **inpatient facilities**, patients reside in the facility while they receive comprehensive diagnosis, treatment, surgery, therapy, and rehabilitation. Some examples include hospital intensive care units, nursing homes, and addiction recovery programs. **Outpatient facilities** treat patients who do not need to stay in a healthcare facility. Most healthcare in the United States is delivered in outpatient settings. Examples of outpatient settings include

- doctors' offices and private healthcare clinics that provide checkups, physical therapy, day surgery, counseling, addiction treatment, rehabilitation, and eye and dental care;
- hospital emergency rooms;
- urgent care or walk-in clinics;
- health clinics and counseling centers in the school or community; and
- county public health clinics.

primary care physician (PCP) healthcare professional who provides routine checkups, screenings, treatments, prescriptions, and preventive services

specialists healthcare professionals who have additional training in treating certain types of diseases and disorders

inpatient facilities healthcare facilities in which patients reside for the duration of treatment

outpatient facilities healthcare facilities that patients visit for treatment and then leave

Medical Specialists

Specialist	Care
Cardiologist	Heart disease
Dermatologist	Skin conditions
Gastroenterologist	Diseases and disorders of the digestive system
Neurologist	Diseases and disorders of the brain, nerves, and spinal cord
Oncologist	Cancer
Orthopedist	Bone, joint, and muscle conditions
Pediatrician	Medical conditions of children from infancy through adolescence
Psychiatrist	Mental health conditions
Pulmonologist	Breathing conditions and lung diseases
Rheumatologist	Diseases of the joints, such as arthritis
Surgeon	Medical conditions requiring surgery
Urologist	Conditions of the urinary system and male reproductive system

Figure 2.11 This figure lists common types of specialists and the care they provide. ***Which specialist is educated and trained in bone, joint, and muscle conditions?***

The Basics of Insurance

Main Types	Payments
Health maintenance organization (HMO) • Pays for the costs of basic healthcare services and many other specialized services • User must use doctors, hospitals, clinics, and services that are members of the HMO network	**Premium** • A regular fee paid to the insurance company each month • Paid even if you do not receive medical care
Preferred provider organization (PPO) • Pays for the costs of healthcare provided by doctors, healthcare providers, and hospitals • Allows for more flexibility in choosing providers, but is more expensive	**Deductible** • Amount a person pays for healthcare services before the insurance company begins to pay for an agreed-upon portion of healthcare costs
	Co-payment • A fixed amount for medical services • For example, you might need to pay $20 for a visit to the doctor

Figure 2.12 Both HMO and PPO insurance plans involve people making co-payment, deductible, and premium payments.

Healthcare is expensive, and most people cannot afford to pay the full cost of services. Instead, most people buy insurance to help pay for healthcare costs (**Figure 2.12**). Most people get insurance through their employer or purchase insurance from a health insurance marketplace. Other health insurance options, available through the US government, include Medicare and Medicaid. *Medicare* is insurance available for people 65 years of age and older. *Medicaid* pays for healthcare costs of people living in poverty, pregnant people, older adults, and people with disabilities. Because of the *Patient Protection and Affordable Care Act (ACA)*, young people can get coverage through their parents' or guardians' insurance through age 26.

Skills for Health and Wellness

Creating a Health Management Plan

As you get older, you will take more and more responsibility for your health. This might include talking more during doctor appointments, making your own doctor appointments, and changing your behaviors to improve your health today and in the future. To help change your health and behaviors, you can create a *health management plan*, or an outline of actions for improving your health and wellness. This kind of plan includes your health goals related to all areas of health.

Practice Your Skills

Set Goals

A health management plan contains the goals you set for your health and wellness and the actions you take to reach them. To set goals and determine the actions in your health management plan, use the following steps:

1. Assess how you feel in your life right now. How is your physical health? Do you wish you were faster or stronger? How are your mental and social health? How are you managing your stress, and what relationships give you support and love?
2. Make a list of the areas of your health you would like to improve. Then, set four realistic goals about your health. Some examples of these goals might include seeing the doctor once a year, talking to a therapist, choosing not to have sex, running outside to relieve stress, or making two good friends at school.
3. Make each goal SMART:
   - **Specific:** Clearly state what you want to accomplish.
   - **Measurable:** Define the quantifiable result that will mean you achieved the goal.
   - **Achievable:** Break out the actions you will need to take to achieve the goal.
   - **Relevant:** Make sure the goal fits you, your values, and what you want to accomplish.
   - **Timely:** Set a realistic and specific time line for achieving the goal.

Decide how you will monitor your progress and reward yourself for achieving the goal. Once you have all the details about your four goals, go through them with a trusted adult and a trusted friend. Seek feedback from these people and ask them to help hold you accountable to follow your plan. At your next doctor appointment, talk with your doctor about these goals and ask for advice about goals you might set in the future.

Knowing Your Rights

People have certain rights regarding their healthcare. Federal and state laws describe and protect these rights. For example, people who receive healthcare have the right to privacy. According to the *Health Insurance Portability and Accountability Act (HIPAA)*, patients must consent before their private health information can be shared. A doctor would need a patient's consent to share medical information with another doctor.

People also have the right to seek healthcare and to give or withhold consent for treatment. To give consent, a person must be capable of fully understanding the decisions involved. For example, a person with a serious intellectual disability or debilitating physical condition might not be able to give consent. In most states, **minors**, or people under the age of 18, also do not have full rights to consent to healthcare. Instead, parents or guardians usually make these decisions with minors. Even though minors do not have full rights, however, they do have some rights to seek and consent to certain types of healthcare (**Figure 2.13**).

minors people under the age of 18

Minors' rights to access healthcare depend on state laws. If unsure about state laws, teens can ask their doctors for information about consent, decisions, and parent or guardian notification. They can also research this information online.

Minors Can Consent for...			
general medical and surgical care	in 21 states	**medical care and counseling for substance abuse**	in 44 states
outpatient mental health services	in 20 states	**inpatient mental health services**	in 0 states
STI testing and treatment (over 16 years of age)	in all 50 states	**HIV testing and treatment**	in 32 states
reproductive health services	in 25 states	**prenatal care, delivery services, medical care for a baby**	in 27 states

Figure 2.13 In some cases, healthcare providers are authorized or required to notify a parent or guardian about decisions regarding the healthcare of minors.

Getting Regular Checkups and Screenings

preventive healthcare
medical care that seeks to prevent health conditions from developing; includes annual physical or wellness exams, checkups, vaccinations, and screenings

Most people know to visit the doctor if they are sick or have an injury. It is important not to just visit the doctor during these times though. Visiting the doctor regularly can help you stay healthy. This type of healthcare, called **preventive healthcare**, involves getting an annual physical or wellness exam, regular checkups, vaccinations, and screenings for conditions such as hearing or vision loss. Schools and community healthcare facilities offer some preventive healthcare, such as vision and hearing screenings and vaccinations.

To maintain your health, plan to have a physical or wellness exam with a doctor every year. During a physical or wellness exam, a doctor will check your health, screen you for certain diseases and disorders, and give any needed vaccinations. This includes recording basic health information such as height, weight, heart rate, and blood pressure. It also includes examining your body physically to detect signs of any abnormalities.

To find a doctor, talk with your parents or guardians or another trusted adult. Research doctors online, read reviews, and check which doctors are connected with your insurance company. You can also call the doctor's office with any questions.

During the physical or wellness exam, discuss any health-related concerns you may have with your doctor. Together, you might spot a condition and prevent it from becoming worse. If a certain disease is common among your family members, discuss lifestyle changes and behaviors that can reduce your risk. Early detection is an important part of disease treatment, so regular checkups and screenings are important. This health information can be tracked over time, allowing you and your doctor to note any changes.

Be prepared to make the most of your doctor visit. Write a list of questions in case you get nervous or forgetful. If you have symptoms you want to discuss, begin by telling your doctor what is bothering you and for how long. Ask questions about any medications prescribed, when you can expect to feel better, and how you can best protect your health going forward (**Figure 2.14**).

Questions to Ask Your Doctor

- Will you tell my parents or others the information I tell you?
- If I want to, can I talk to you without my parents in the room?
- What is causing my symptoms?
- Is it normal to feel this way?
- What activities should I do or not do while I'm recovering?
- How can I prevent this health issue from happening again?
- How does this medication work?
- Will this test hurt? Can the pain be lessened?
- What side effects should I expect?
- When should I come back to the doctor?

Figure 2.14 When you go to the doctor, remember that your doctor has seen and heard it *all*. Be open with your doctor and ask all of the questions you want to. ***What other questions can you think of to ask your doctor at a physical or wellness exam?***

Local and Global Health

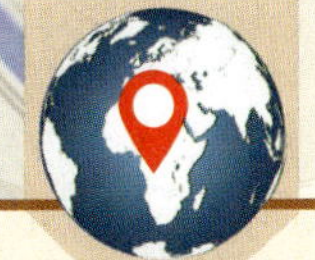

Challenges to Accessing Healthcare

The World Health Organization (WHO), an international health organization, studies the availability and cost of healthcare around the world. Research by the WHO has found that certain countries have a shortage of doctors, hospitals, and healthcare facilities. If these services are not available, people cannot access them. Distance from healthcare facilities, transportation, and laws governing healthcare can also make accessing healthcare difficult.

Even where healthcare is available, it may not be affordable. In most countries, people pay some amount for healthcare even if they have health insurance. In some countries, paying for healthcare drives people into poverty. The WHO recently found the following:

- More than one-half of the world's population does not receive essential health services.
- Each year, 100 million people enter extreme poverty because of healthcare costs.
- More than 800 million people spend at least 10 percent of their household income on healthcare.

Access to healthcare has a major impact on people's overall health outcomes. It affects how healthy people are, how quickly people recover from disease, and how well communities cope.

Practice Your Skills

Advocate for Health

Form a small group with your classmates and discuss the barriers to accessing healthcare in your community. During your discussion, examine the availability of certain services. Also identify challenges related to transportation, finances, and any laws. List all of these barriers and then discuss how your community can help people overcome them. Identify your audience, which should be a population that faces some of these barriers. Then, create a flyer, blog post, or social media post listing these barriers and organizations and programs in your community that can help people access and afford healthcare. Share this information at a health fair or online.

Seeking Treatment for a Health Condition

As you take more responsibility for your health, you need to know how to get help for medical conditions. You should also be able to recognize when you need routine or emergency healthcare.

As you know, early detection and treatment keep many health conditions from getting worse. Regular checkups with your doctor can detect early signs of any health conditions and treat them right away. In addition, you should see your doctor if you have certain symptoms of common diseases. These symptoms include high fever, coughing, extreme fatigue, painful headache, vomiting, diarrhea, unexplained pain, and rashes. You should also see your doctor for any other symptoms that concern you.

Certain symptoms and conditions require **emergency healthcare**. You need emergency healthcare if you experience any of the conditions or symptoms listed in **Figure 2.15**. If you need this kind of care, ask a trusted adult to take you to an urgent care clinic or emergency room. You can also call 911 or your hospital for transport by ambulance.

emergency healthcare
medical care that treats life-threatening health conditions

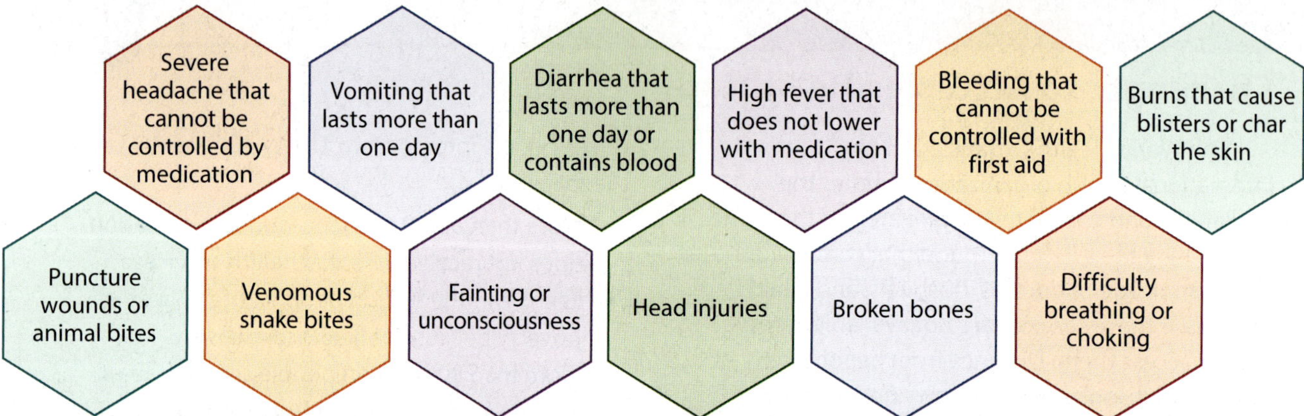

Figure 2.15 If you experience any of the conditions and symptoms listed, seek emergency healthcare in a hospital emergency room or urgent care clinic.

Lesson 2.3 Review

Know and Understand

1. Which healthcare professional provides primary care?
2. Describe the difference between Medicare and Medicaid. How do these programs influence healthcare access?
3. Research your state laws and give one example of a health service to which you can consent.
4. With a partner, take turns explaining the purpose of preventive healthcare.
5. What kind of care is needed to treat animal bites and head injuries?

Think Critically

6. Why do you think minors do not have full legal rights to consent to health services?
7. Give one example of a question you want to ask your doctor.
8. How would you go about getting help if you needed emergency healthcare?

REAL WORLD Health Skills

Make Decisions Think of a time you had a health condition that needed treatment. Did you get the treatment you needed? Why or why not? What factors were part of your decision-making process? Choose one common health condition or issue teens at your school face and write a case study about a teen deciding whether to get healthcare for the condition. Describe the different circumstances and barriers affecting the teen's decision. Then trade case studies with a partner and complete your partner's case study by having the teen go through the steps of the decision-making process.

Advocating for Community and Public Health

Essential Question?

In what ways can you contribute to the health of your community and the world?

Lesson **2.4**

Learning Outcomes

After studying this lesson, you will be able to

- define *community health*;
- analyze the influences affecting community health;
- advocate for community health by identifying community resources, participating in community service, considering organ donation, and understanding environmental justice;
- identify public health goals and organizations; and
- describe health organizations that promote world health.

Key Terms

community health
community resources
community service
environmental justice
food desert
organ donation
public health
world health

Warm-Up Activity

My Community

Analyze Influences Societal factors, as well as environmental factors, affect community and personal health. Draw a map of your community, including areas that are within walking distance or a short drive from where you live. On your map, label different factors you believe affect health in your area, both positively and negatively. Examples could include schools, factories, medical clinics, or pollution. Compare the number of positive factors with the number of negative factors.

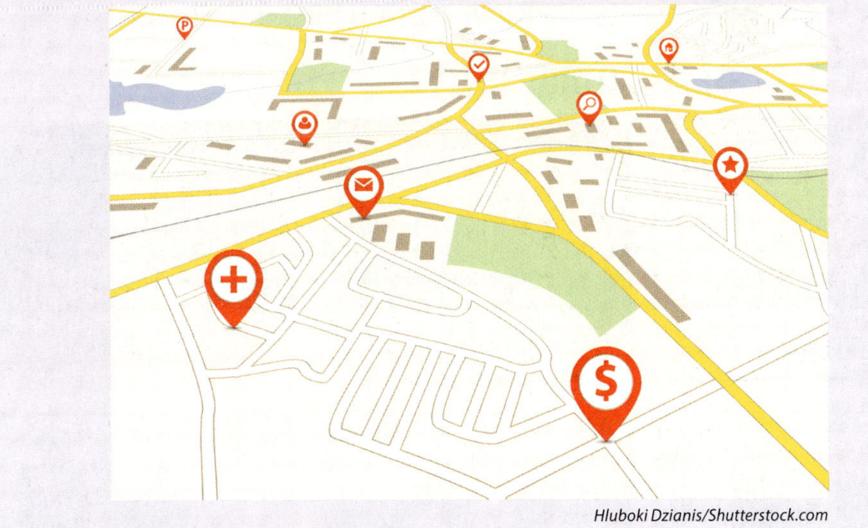

Hluboki Dzianis/Shutterstock.com

Your health and wellness depend on many factors. Some of these factors you can change, and others you cannot. Environment is one example of a factor you can influence, even if you cannot change it. You can have an influence on the characteristics of your community. In this lesson, you will learn how to advocate for community and public health.

community health
overall health of a group of people who live in the same area and interact with one another

What Is Community Health?

Community health describes the overall health of a *community*, which is a group of people who live in the same area and interact with one another (**Figure 2.16**). If a community is healthy, this means there are positive relationships among people and organizations. These organizations include health organizations and local, state, and national governments.

Schools, scientists, healthcare professionals, and community residents work together to promote community health. For example, medical scientists study how diseases spread and how people can prevent them. These scientists advise doctors and governments about how to use vaccines to prevent certain diseases. Government officials use this information to develop laws for the public. Clinics, doctors, and nurses provide vaccines for people in the community.

Factors Affecting Community Health

Several factors can improve or harm the health of a community. Knowing these factors can help you advocate for community health.

Societal Factors

Societal factors are the social aspects of a community. These include access to healthcare, education, housing, safety and security, economic factors, people's sense of belonging, and people's participation in community activities.

The most important societal factor affecting health is education. Completion of high school makes a significant impact on health. High school graduates have a longer life expectancy and better overall health and wellness. They are more likely to get physical activity, stay away from smoking, visit the doctor regularly, know how to access healthcare, and engage in healthy behaviors.

Parts of a Community
Residents
Friends
Neighbors
Relatives
Businesses
Organizations
Schools
Government

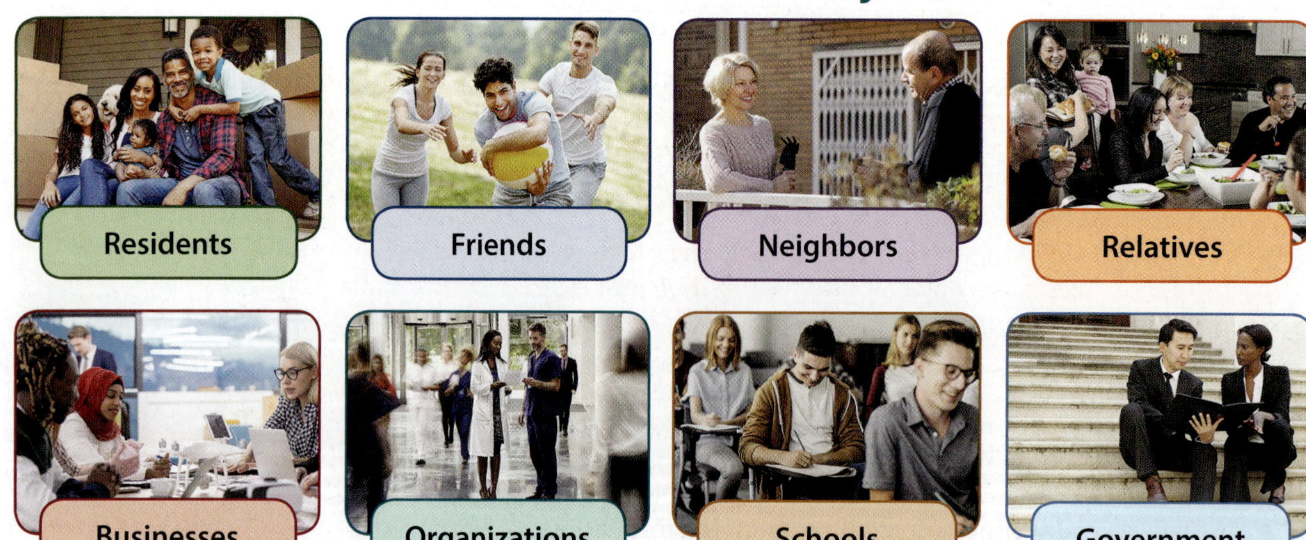

Left to right: Monkey Business Images/Shutterstock.com; Robert Kneschke/Shutterstock.com; Iakov Filimonov/Shutterstock.com; RonTech3000/Shutterstock.com; dotshock/Shutterstock.com; Monkey Business Images/Shutterstock.com; LStockStudio/Shutterstock.com; DW labs Incorporated/Shutterstock.com

Figure 2.16 Some communities are healthier than others, and communities can fall anywhere on the health continuum. ***What types of organizations can affect the health of your community?***

Safety and security have significant effects on a community's health. Concerns about violence prevent people from getting outdoors for regular physical activity. People living in such communities have more anxiety and stress and are more likely to have health conditions such as obesity, high blood pressure, high heart rate, and stress-related disorders.

Economic factors related to jobs and income influence whether people have the resources to maintain their health. People with low income and limited resources have difficulty paying for healthcare in addition to housing, nutritious food, and clothing. This can lead to poor physical and mental health and reduce performance at work and school.

Environmental Factors

Environmental factors come from a community's built and natural environments. The *built environment* includes roads and bridges, buildings and homes, and other structures made by people. The *natural environment* includes naturally occurring animals, plants, water, soils, and other parts of the environment not built by people. The questions in **Figure 2.17** can help you evaluate your current environment. Environmental factors that affect community health include physical layout, food deserts, safe water access, pollution, and population:

- How many public parks are in your community?
- How close are these parks to your residence? Can you get there safely?
- How many fast-food establishments and convenience stores are in your community? How does this number compare to the number of full-service grocery stores?
- Do you have access to clean drinking water?
- Is your community affected by air pollution? (You can research the local Air Quality Index online.)
- Are there safe, public paths for pedestrians, including walkers, runners, and cyclists?
- Is your community a highly populated area?

Evaluating Environmental Factors in Your Community

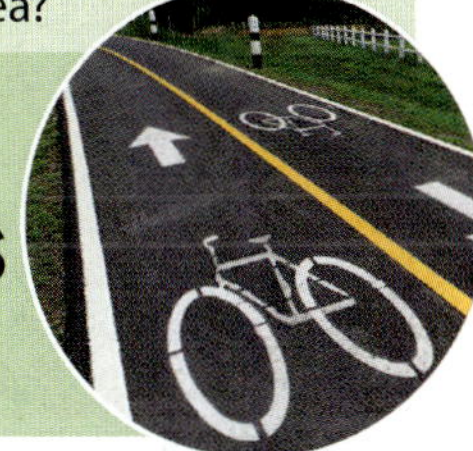

bamgraphy/Shutterstock.com

Figure 2.17 Assessing your access to food, safe public spaces, and clean air and water can help you identify areas you can improve the health of your community.

- **Physical layout:** The physical layout of a community impacts health. For example, in many US cities, buildings and resources are far apart. People may find it difficult or unsafe to walk places and get less physical activity.
- **Food deserts:** A **food desert** is an area without nearby full-service grocery stores. In these areas, people cannot easily get nutritious, fresh vegetables, fruit, and meat. Instead, people living in food deserts may buy their food from convenience stores and fast-food restaurants. These meals are expensive, low in nutritional value, and high in fat, salt, and calories.
- **Access to safe water:** In the US, people depend on their community to provide safe drinking water. A community needs effective sanitation to dispose or treat wastewater. Without sanitation and clean drinking water, people can become sick with waterborne diseases.
- **Pollution:** Pollution is the presence of waste in the environment. Air pollution is one of the most serious environmental factors affecting community and personal health. In large, crowded cities, many automobiles produce harmful air pollution. Air pollution irritates the eyes, throat, and lungs. Breathing air pollution can cause respiratory diseases such as asthma, emphysema, and bronchitis.
- **Population:** Population is an environmental factor that affects nearly all aspects of community health. People living in highly populated areas are exposed to more air and water pollution and are more likely to have unsafe drinking water. They are more likely to experience stress-related disorders, anxiety, and high blood pressure.

food desert area without nearby full-service grocery stores

Promoting the Health of Your Community

Community health depends on the actions of businesses, organizations, and each individual in the community. This means you can promote the health of your community in meaningful ways.

community resources
organizations and programs that help the environment and people within a community

Use Community Resources

Community resources are organizations and programs that help the environment and people within a community. Knowing how to find and use community resources can help you maintain your own health and advocate for the health of others. Examples of community resources include the following:

- **Schools:** Your school may have a nurse and counselor, who can provide immediate medical and mental healthcare. A nurse or counselor can refer you if you need additional or specialized care.
- **Community centers:** Some community centers offer educational workshops about nutrition, physical activity, stress, and other skills for improving and maintaining health.
- **Shelters:** Shelters give people who are homeless safe places to stay. Some shelters specialize in helping adults and children who have been abused and provide counseling, meals, and referrals to health services.
- **Food pantries:** Food pantries store and distribute donated food to people in need. Sometimes a *community garden* grows fresh vegetables and fruits to donate to food pantries and local residents.
- **City and county healthcare facilities:** City and county health clinics may provide free or reduced-cost medical and mental health services.
- **Older adult services:** Some communities offer *adult day care centers*, where older adults can socialize, eat, and rest while their caregivers are away. Other services include *Meals on Wheels*, which delivers nutritious meals to older adults, and *nursing homes*, which care for people who cannot care for themselves.
- **Youth services:** Youth services include care from a school nurse, city and county healthcare clinics, classes on physical and mental health, and physical fitness classes.
- **Crisis hotlines:** Your community might have local offices and services with crisis hotlines you can call for help (**Figure 2.18**).

Crisis Hotlines
Alcohol Abuse & Crisis Intervention Hotline
(800) 234-0246
National Cocaine Hotline
(800) 262-2463
National Runaway Hotline
(800) RUNAWAY or (800) 786-2929
National Youth Crisis Hotline
(800) 442-4673
National Sexual Assault Hotline
(800) 656-HOPE or (800) 656-4673
National Suicide Prevention Lifeline
(800) 273-8255

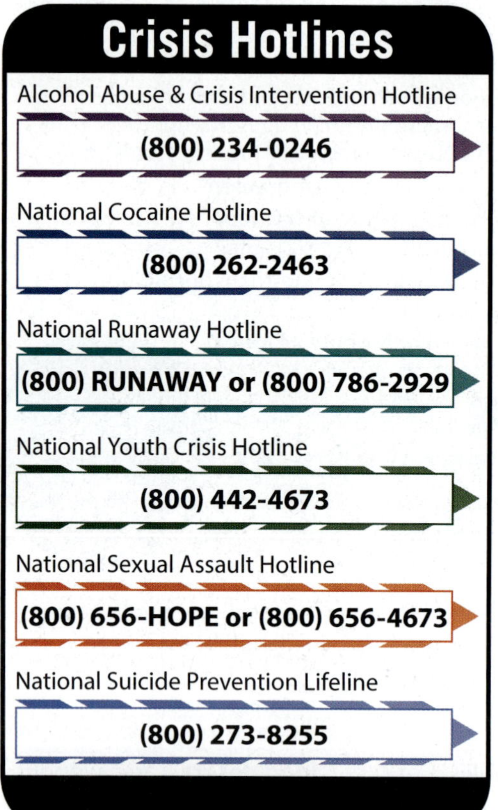

Figure 2.18 National hotlines connect people in crisis to mental health professionals who can help them seek treatment. Your community may have local hotlines as well. ***What additional telephone number connects the caller to emergency responders?***

Participate in Community Service

community service
actions that promote the environment and health of a community

One way to improve your community is to get involved in **community service** by volunteering. Many organizations depend on volunteers. Community service allows you to meet new people and can be rewarding. You can practice valuable skills such as teamwork, leadership, and communication while learning about organizations and your community.

Volunteering shows others you care about your community. By volunteering to help strangers, you demonstrate respect for others and their needs. This promotes a positive and respectful environment, fosters people's sense of belonging, and improves relationships among groups of people.

As you look for volunteer opportunities, consider your interests and skills. You might ask yourself:

- What projects are important to me and my community?
- Do I want to work directly with people or behind the scenes?
- What special skills and time can I offer?
- What do I want to learn when volunteering?

You can volunteer to help people of all ages and backgrounds (**Figure 2.19**). If you do not find a place to volunteer, you can begin your own community service group.

Consider Organ Donation

Organ donation is the act of indicating you allow your organs to be donated and transplanted into another person. Usually, this permission takes effect after a person's death. For example, if you die unexpectedly, organ donation allows a doctor to transplant your organs into someone else.

Organ transplants help people and save lives. Some people have serious illnesses or injuries and require organ transplants to continue living. In the US, more than 100,000 people are on lists waiting for an organ. Unfortunately, the US has a serious shortage of donated organs. Twenty people die each day waiting for an organ transplant.

To sign up for organ donation, you can visit organdonor.gov, ask about signing up at your local department of motor vehicles, or indicate on your driver's license that you would like to be an organ donor. Be sure to let your family members know you have signed up.

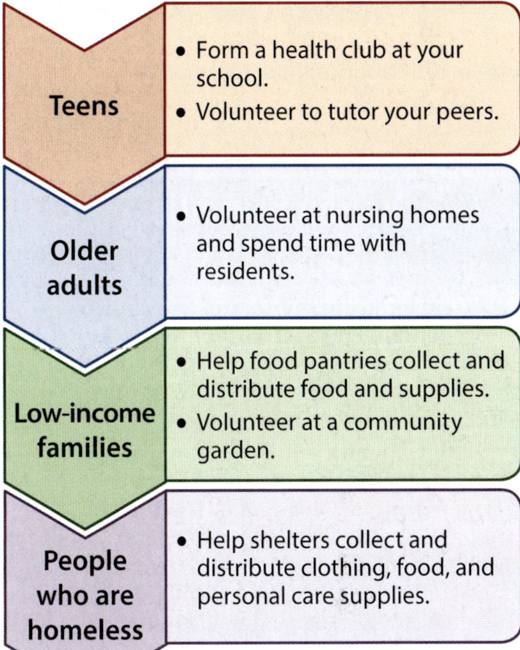

Figure 2.19 You can help these groups of people in your community by volunteering for various programs and donating or distributing resources. ***What is the term for volunteering your time and skills to an organization in your community?***

organ donation act of allowing your organs to be donated and transplanted into another person, typically upon your death

Support Environmental Justice

Environmental justice is an aspect of community and world health concerned with populations exposed to harmful environmental and societal factors through no fault of their own. In many cases, low-income communities cannot protect themselves from environmental hazards caused by others. Environmental justice examines questions such as the following:

- Why are food deserts often located within a city's low-income neighborhoods?
- Do companies build chemical factories next to both low-income and higher-income neighborhoods?
- What can people do about air pollution that originates in one place and affects populations far away?
- Where should people store hazardous waste so it does not harm nearby communities?
- Should a higher-income country send its hazardous electronic waste (e-waste) to a lower-income country for storage or recycling?
- What steps can people take to stop businesses from using forced labor, poor working conditions, or unfair wages?

To learn more about environmental justice programs and how you can help, you can encourage your school to invite speakers from the Environmental Justice Foundation (EJF), become a member of the National Resources Defense Council (NDRC), or report environmental justice issues to the US Environmental Protection Agency (EPA).

environmental justice aspect of community and world health concerned with populations exposed to harmful environmental and societal factors through no fault of their own

public health science-based approach to protecting and improving the health of populations as a whole

Public Health

Public health is a science-based approach to protecting and improving the health of populations as a whole. For example, public health is concerned with the population of a city, state, or country and groups such as teens, children, older adults, pregnant people, and people who are homeless.

National Public Health Goals

- **Attain high-quality, longer lives free of preventable disease, disability, injury, and premature death:** This is the chief goal for public and personal health. The other goals make it possible to achieve this goal.
- **Achieve health equity, eliminate disparities, and improve the health of all groups:** *Health equity* is access to healthcare for all people, regardless of gender, sex, age, race or ethnicity, income, disability, and disease. *Health disparities* are significant differences in the occurrence of disease among groups of people (for example, people who have more or less education). Disparities result from differences in treatment, prevention, and access to healthcare.
- **Create social and physical environments that promote positive health for all:** This goal aims to reduce or eliminate factors that harm community and public health.
- **Promote quality of life, healthy development, and healthy behaviors across all life stages:** This goal aims to improve health at all stages from infancy through older adulthood.

Figure 2.20 These are some examples of national public health goals. These goals influence the work of government health organizations and give guidance to health education programs in schools.

Public Health Goals

The US government provides leadership and develops goals for the country's public health. National public health plans include goals for physical, mental, and social health. Doctors, experts in public health, and leaders of public health organizations help develop these goals. National public health goals have several broad objectives, called *overarching goals*, that promote individual, family, and community health and help prevent disease (**Figure 2.20**).

Health Organizations

Government regulations and organizations also help promote health and prevent disease. Many health organizations employ scientists, doctors, nurses, counselors, medical technicians, and experts in public health. These organizations offer valuable resources for researching, preventing, diagnosing, and treating physical and mental health conditions.

Cities, counties, and states have a *department of health*. Departments of health gather information about health and disease in the community so healthcare professionals can plan public health programs and goals. For example, if a county records increasing cases of a rare disease such as measles, county officials can help local doctors, nurses, and clinics improve vaccination programs. Other local health organizations can also support these efforts.

Large, federal health organizations are responsible for many aspects of US public health. You can consult these organizations' websites for credible, useful information about health (**Figure 2.21**).

The World Community

Your community is part of the larger world community. Advocating for world health is another way to promote your community's health. You can do some good for others and learn about the world's diverse people and cultures.

world health health of human populations around the world

World health is concerned with the health of human populations around the world. World health considers factors such as relations between countries, global climate, war, trade practices, national economies, poverty, and cultural practices.

The chief international health organizations are the *World Health Organization (WHO)*, which promotes health in regions throughout the world, and the *World Bank*, which provides economic support for low-income regions to promote health and safety. Nearly 200 countries are members of each organization. Together, they monitor ongoing health conditions, address health emergencies, and help countries solve underlying factors that lead to health conditions.

Federal Health Organizations	
Centers for Disease Control and Prevention (CDC)*	Is the main US public health agency in charge of the control and prevention of disease, injury, and disability
Department of Health and Human Services (HHS)	Is the largest health organization, run by a member of the US president's cabinet; includes many agencies responsible for ensuring the health and well-being of people in the US
Environmental Protection Agency (EPA)	Creates and enforces rules to protect people from harmful pollution and hazardous substances; protects air and water quality
Food and Drug Administration (FDA)*	Ensures the safety and effectiveness of medications, foods, beverages, and other products
National Institute for Mental Health (NIMH)*	Promotes research and healthcare for mental health
National Institutes of Health (NIH)*	Promotes research in the medical sciences and healthcare
Occupational Safety and Health Administration (OSHA)	Makes and enforces rules to protect workers from workplace hazards
United Network for Organ Sharing (UNOS)	Is a resource for organ recipients and donors; matches people with donor organs; partners with many private and government medical organizations
US Department of Agriculture (USDA)	Regulates food quality and develops nutritional guidelines for people across the life span; protects the health of crop plants and livestock

*A branch of the Department of Health and Human Services

Figure 2.21 Each federal health organization addresses a different health goal with regulations, resources, services, and research. ***What organizations in your city, county, and state gather health information to inform the creation of public health programs?***

Lesson 2.4 Review

Know and Understand

1. What is community health?
2. Write a short slogan that describes how a community's population affects its health.
3. List one overarching public health goal and give examples of how it can be attained.
4. Which federal health organization ensures the safety and effectiveness of medications?
5. What is the purpose of the WHO? How does this organization's work affect your health?

Think Critically

6. Why is there a correlation between economic well-being and health?
7. Which community resources do you use regularly?
8. What steps can you take to become a leader in advocating for community health?

REAL WORLD Health Skills

Practice Health-Enhancing Behaviors In this lesson, you learned about the relationship between community health and personal health. Figure 2.17 lists questions that can help you evaluate your community. Evaluate your community by answering each of these questions. Then, for each question, give your community a letter grade, with A+ being the highest and F being the lowest. After answering and grading each question, give your community an overall grade. List two actions you could take to improve your community's grade or help it maintain a high grade. Explain how these actions would help enhance the health of yourself and others.

Chapter 2 Review and Assessment

Chapter Summary

As you grow older, you will become more responsible for the decisions you make. The best way to make healthy decisions is to use the decision-making process, which consists of six steps: define the decision or problem, explore all alternatives, consider the consequences, identify the best alternative, decide and act, and evaluate the decision. Another key skill is setting goals. Goals should be SMART, or specific, measurable, achievable, relevant, and timely. To set a goal, assess the situation, identify a specific and realistic goal, define the actions you must take to achieve it, set a reasonable time line, act on your goal, monitor your progress, and reward yourself.

You need reliable health information to make healthy decisions. To locate health information, use the internet, talk to a professional, or visit a library. Reliable websites contain .gov, .edu, or .org in the URL and feature expert authors and current information. They are not funded by businesses that earn a profit or organizations that promote a cause. Credible health information is based in science, which is repeatable. This means other sources should confirm what one source says. To apply health information, analyze advertisements critically, read labels on health products, and comparison-shop when choosing health products and services.

Health services in the US are delivered by primary care physicians (PCPs) and specialists, and insurance helps people pay for services. Some states allow minors to consent to specific services. It is important to get an annual physical or wellness exam. You should seek emergency healthcare for certain symptoms, such as a high, uncontrollable fever; difficulty breathing; uncontrollable bleeding or headache; vomiting or diarrhea that lasts more than one day; and fainting or unconsciousness. You also need emergency healthcare for head injuries, broken bones, puncture wounds, animal bites, venomous snake bites, and burns that blister or char the skin.

Community and world health both affect your health. The health of a community is affected by societal and environmental factors, such as income, education, physical layout, population, and pollution. To promote community health, you can use community resources, participate in community service, and support environmental justice. Public health and world health are concerned with larger populations. The US government has several national public health goals. Federal health organizations help research and share health information and regulate health products and services.

Vocabulary Activity

Draw a cartoon for one of the terms shown. The cartoon should express the meaning of the term. After you finish drawing, find a partner and exchange cartoons. Take turns explaining to each other how your cartoons show the meaning of the term you chose.

advocate	*Food and Drug Administration (FDA)*	*organ donation*
alternatives	*food desert*	*outpatient facilities*
collaborative decision-making	*goal*	*preventive healthcare*
community health	*health fraud*	*primary care physician (PCP)*
community resources	*health literacy*	*pseudoscience*
community service	*health promotion*	*public health*
consumer	*healthcare*	*science*
decision-making process	*inpatient facilities*	*SMART goal*
emergency healthcare	*lifelong learning*	*specialists*
environmental justice	*minors*	*values*
		world health

Review and Recall

Review the information in this chapter by answering the following questions.

1. Why is it crucial to define the decision or problem before exploring and deciding on alternatives?
2. Explain why good decision-making requires fully acting on the alternative chosen.
3. Rewrite the following goal to be SMART: *I will manage stress better so I don't feel depressed.*
4. Which URL stem does *not* indicate that a source is probably reliable?
   A. .com
   B. .org
   C. .edu
   D. .gov
5. Why should you be careful about getting information from websites belonging to businesses or organizations promoting a cause?
6. What three qualities separate science from pseudoscience?
7. How do you know if a health claim is approved by the FDA?
8. What is the purpose of health insurance?
9. What happens during a typical annual physical or wellness exam?
10. Where can a person get emergency healthcare?
    A. doctor's office
    B. rehabilitation facility
    C. urgent care clinic
    D. dentist
11. How do concerns about violence impact community health?
    A. increase opportunities for physical activity
    B. reduce anxiety
    C. lower risk of health conditions
    D. increase stress
12. How do food deserts affect nutrition?
13. How does organ donation promote community health?

Standardized Test Prep

Reading and Writing Practice

Read the passage below and then answer the following questions.

The *Patient Protection and Affordable Care Act*, also called the *Affordable Care Act (ACA)*, was signed into law on March 23, 2010, to address rising insurance costs and barriers to obtaining health insurance. The ACA expands access to health insurance in the following ways:

- Insurance companies must provide insurance even if you have preexisting conditions.
- Young adults can be covered through age 26 by their parents' or guardians' health insurance.
- Insurance companies cannot stop insuring customers for no apparent reason.
- Many businesses are now required to provide health insurance for their employees.

14. Which element of the ACA does this passage mostly discuss?
    A. improved healthcare
    B. Patient's Bill of Rights
    C. access to insurance
    D. cost reduction
15. Which of the following does the ACA guarantee?
    A. that healthcare facilities cannot charge high costs
    B. that insurance companies cannot deny people with preexisting conditions
    C. that everyone can afford health insurance
    D. that everyone will receive health insurance through an employer
16. Write a one-paragraph summary of how the ACA improves access to health insurance. What additional protections or laws do you think would benefit people seeking health insurance in the US? Write a second paragraph summarizing your ideas.

Chapter 2 Skills Assessment

Critical Thinking Skills

Answer the following questions to assess your knowledge of what you learned in this chapter.

1. What decisions can you make now that did not belong to you in the past? Did your parent or guardian used to make these decisions? Why are these decisions important for your health?
2. When is it appropriate to engage in collaborative decision-making? When is it not? Explain.
3. Think of a goal in your life you did not achieve. What did this goal teach you, even though you did not achieve it? What were the benefits of trying?
4. With a partner, discuss whether you think websites and the media should be required to only share verified health information. Should websites that share false information be penalized somehow? Explain your perspectives.
5. What factors can make it difficult to comparison-shop for different health products and services? What steps can people take to overcome these factors?
6. With a partner, research a recent example of health fraud. What was involved in the fraud? How did the fraud impact health?
7. Imagine that your older sibling is very depressed and has stopped completing homework because of a mental illness. Your older sibling says treatment is not an option because your family does not have the money for it. How could you engage in health promotion to help your sibling?
8. Why is the privacy of health information important? What could happen if the privacy of health information was not protected?
9. What are the advantages of allowing minors to consent to certain health services? Are there any disadvantages? Explain.
10. Choose one sign that someone needs emergency healthcare and write a case study in which that person recognizes the sign and gets the care needed.
11. Widespread attitudes like racism and sexism can have an impact on community health. Choose one negative attitude in society and explain how it harms your community.
12. Why do you think people in highly populated areas experience more stress, anxiety, and high blood pressure?
13. Give one example of a current environmental justice issue. What factors contribute to this issue? What can people do to help solve the issue and promote world health?

Health and Wellness Skills

Complete the following activities to assess your skills related to health and wellness.

14. **Analyze Influences.** Your decisions affect your overall health and wellness. Often, these decisions are influenced by your day-to-day surroundings, like the availability of parks or grocery stores, bullying, or peer pressure. Think about the specific factors that influence your decisions and behaviors over the course of one day. Create a poster or artistic representation that reflects these surroundings. Identify whether each factor has a positive or negative influence.
15. **Access Information.** Visit the website of the Centers for Disease Control and Prevention (CDC) and explain whether this source is reliable. Give examples of elements that indicate its reliability. Then, on the CDC website, research the leading causes of death among teens (ages 15–24) and adults (ages 45–54). What are the top three causes of death in each age group? What information did you find in your research that might explain these differences?
16. **Communicate with Others.** Imagine you have a health issue and need help. Perhaps a former dating partner persuaded you to take and send nude pictures. After the breakup, this person shared the pictures, which are now going viral. Maybe you have a friend in an abusive situation at home. Your friend feels totally helpless and is thinking about running away or attempting suicide. In these or similar situations, whom in your life or social support network would you go to for help? Explain why and then write a story about how you would go to this person and what you would say.

17. **Make Decisions.** Think about purchases you made over the last week or money you paid for health-related services. Purchases could include food items, vitamins or supplements, hygiene products, or recreational items. Services could include a visit to an emergency clinic, an annual physical exam, or a dental cleaning. List two to four of these purchases or services. For each item, answer the following questions:
    - Was the purchase or service positive or negative for your health?
    - Did advertising play a role in your decision about the purchase or service?
    - Were you satisfied with the outcome of the purchase or service?
    - In the future, would you make a different decision about the purchase or service? Why or why not?
18. **Set Goals.** Think about the opportunities for health promotion in your family, friend group, or community. Then, set a goal for engaging in health promotion. Your goal should be SMART, and you should use the steps of goal setting discussed in this chapter. Compare goals with a partner. Discuss how your strengths, needs, and situation shaped the goals you set. Hold each other accountable for achieving your goals.
19. **Practice Health-Enhancing Behaviors.** In this chapter, you learned that an important skill for health is getting healthcare. With a partner, research doctors, medical offices, and clinics in your area. What resources are available? Are there any facilities or doctors specifically for teens? Choose and compare two doctors, medical offices, or clinics. Are there any differences in the care given? What insurance do they accept? If you needed to choose a doctor, medical office, or clinic, which one would you choose? Why?
20. **Advocate for Health.** Volunteering or getting involved in community service is a way to care for your community. You can meet needs at your school; within your neighborhood, city, or state; or even worldwide. Research volunteer opportunities for teens, identify a need or opportunity that interests you, and then devise a plan. For example, you could plan to start an organization yourself or volunteer with a group. If you decide to start an organization, research the steps you might need to take. If you volunteer with a group, identify the steps for becoming a volunteer.

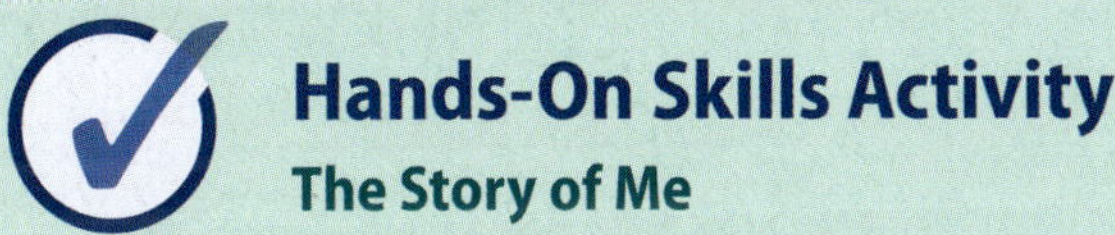

Hands-On Skills Activity

The Story of Me

In this chapter, you have learned about making decisions and setting goals, using and accessing health information, and advocating for community and public health. This activity will give you the opportunity to tell the story of you and reflect on how you can apply these skills to your life.

Steps for This Activity

1. You are going to write a story about yourself. This story can be in a form of your choice—for example, a video, song, or poem. In your story, include details such as where your name came from, your family origin, information about your family members, interests, hobbies, activities, strengths, and weaknesses.
2. After telling this first part of your story, do a personal self-reflection and use the following steps to add a few paragraphs or verses.
3. **Set Goals.** In your self-reflection, identify some areas of your personal health you might want to improve or change. Add one to two SMART goals that will help enhance your health to your story.
4. **Access Information.** Are there school or community resources that can help you fulfill your goals or make changes? Add how available health resources can help you achieve your goals to your story.
5. **Advocate for Health.** Do you have interests or experiences that relate to a school or community group focused on improving health? If so, what is that group? Are you already a part of it, and how could you become a part of it? If not, is there a club or group you could start that would help others with the same interest or experience? Add this to your story.

Chapter 3

Interpersonal Skills

Look for the skills icon throughout this chapter for opportunities to practice your health skills.

Check Your Health and Wellness Skills

In this chapter, you will learn interpersonal skills for communicating, resolving conflicts, and resisting pressure. To understand the skills you currently use, take the following inventory of your behaviors. Indicate how well you think you use each skill. Use a scale of 1–5, *1* meaning you do not use the skill and *5* meaning you feel completely comfortable using it.

Skill	How Well Do You Use Each Skill?
When I'm listening to someone, I make eye contact.	
I repeat back what I think I've heard someone say.	
I clearly express my needs instead of expecting someone else to know them.	
I pay attention to my posture and facial expressions and try to make them match what I'm saying.	
When I disagree with someone online, I follow up in-person instead of settling the conflict publicly.	
I actively resolve conflict instead of avoiding it.	
If I'm too mad to have a conversation, I walk away to cool down.	
During an argument, I really pay attention to what the other person thinks and why.	
I take time to reflect on how I really feel about situations.	
Once I've said I won't do something, I stick with my decision.	
If I see someone being pressured, I step in and tell the person applying the pressure to stop.	
	Total:

Add up your responses to each statement. The higher your score, the more comfortable you feel practicing health skills related to communication, conflict resolution, and peer pressure. Which skill do you think is most important for you? Which skill is the most challenging for you? Which skill would you most like to improve? In this chapter, you will learn how to perform these skills better and more often.

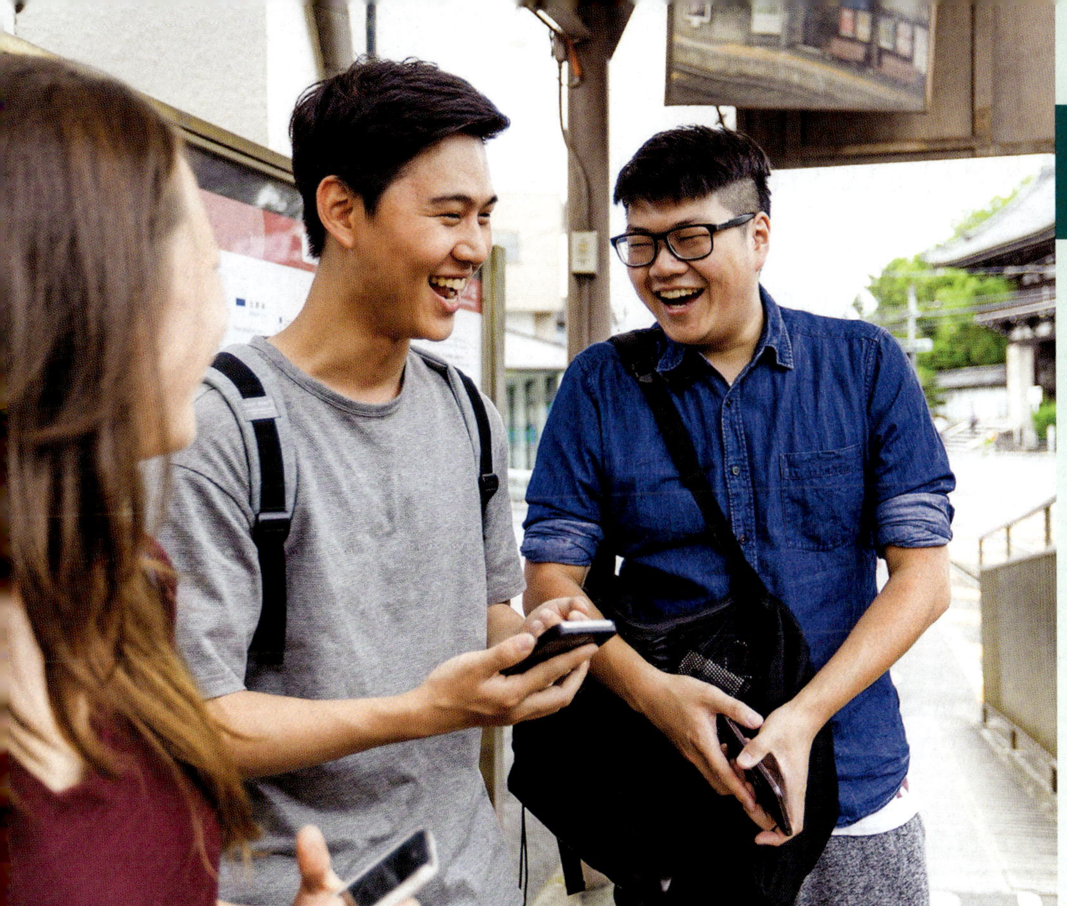
GCShutter/E+/Getty Images

Reading and Notetaking

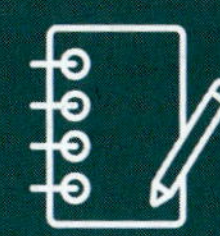

Before reading this chapter, skim the headings and write each heading in a different color or font on a separate piece of paper or electronically. As you silently read the chapter and then listen to your teacher, take notes in the color or font you chose for each heading. After you finish taking notes for each section, draw or copy and paste a small illustration or visual next to the section that will help you remember what you learned.

Lesson 3.1: Communicating Effectively
Types of Communication
Verbal Communication
Nonverbal Communication
Skills for Effective Communication

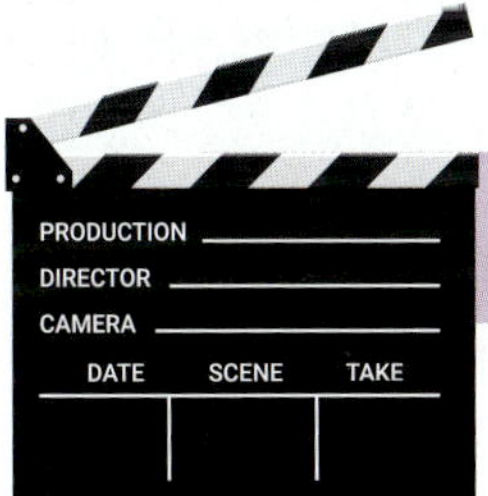

Setting the Scene

Handling Poor Communication

As the fall begins, you are very excited to be starting school. Some of your friends from last year are also going to your school, and you know you want to keep some of your old friendships. You are also very interested in making new friends.

In your first few weeks, you have met some new friends in your math class who always sit together at lunch. They want to spend more time with you, but you are not exactly sure what to do. Whenever they have disagreements, they stop talking to each other and spread embarrassing rumors. When you are talking, some of them do not seem to listen. Sometimes they seem bored even when they say they want to know more. You worry that spending more time with this group will make you adopt some of the same habits. You wonder if it is worth saying how you feel.

Thinking Critically

1. What behaviors would make you hesitant to join this group? Explain.
2. Think about how you could confront this issue. What could you say to tell your new friends how you feel? What boundaries could you set to protect yourself from gossip and rumors?

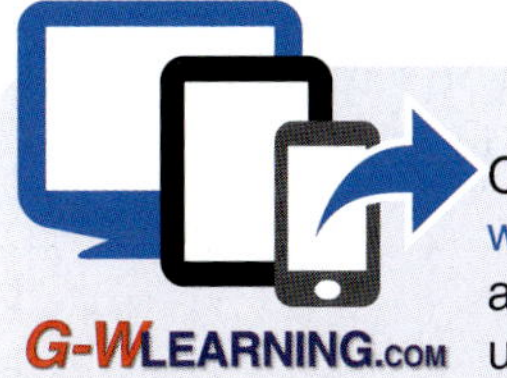

Click on the activity icon or visit www.g-wlearning.com/health/4095 to access online vocabulary activities using key terms from the chapter.

Lesson 3.1

Communicating Effectively

Essential Question?

What skills do you need to communicate effectively with others?

Learning Outcomes

After studying this lesson, you will be able to

- differentiate between verbal and nonverbal communication;
- analyze how active listening improves communication;
- explain the importance of clearly expressing needs and being assertive;
- give examples of effective I-statements;
- explain the importance of matching verbal and nonverbal communication; and
- identify strategies for communicating effectively online.

Key Terms

active listening
aggressive
assertive
communication
communication process
feedback
I-statements
nonverbal communication
passive
passive-aggressive
verbal communication

Warm-Up Activity

Verbal and Nonverbal Communication

Comprehend Concepts Communication between people can be verbal or nonverbal. For example, writing is a form of verbal communication. Facial expressions, posture, and eye contact are forms of nonverbal communication. Based on what you already know, list other examples of verbal and nonverbal communication. Search for images online that illustrate each example you listed. Share the images with your class and describe the type of communication shown in each image.

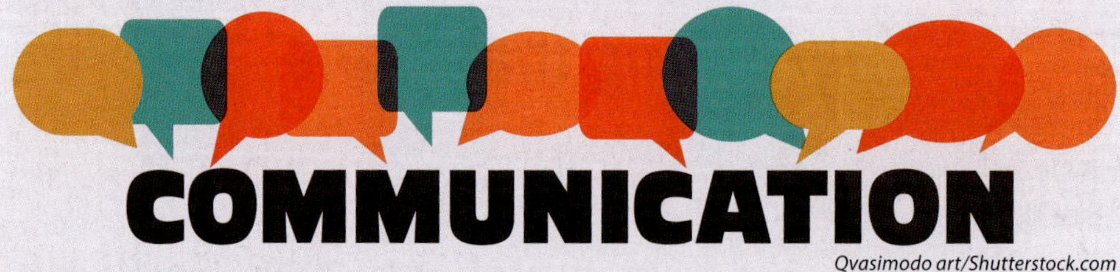

Qvasimodo art/Shutterstock.com

How many times do you talk with your teachers each day? How long do you spend chatting with your friends? Your closest friends are probably some of the people you talk with most often. You probably talk with your teachers to ask or answer questions almost every day. This is because you form and maintain relationships and send and receive information through **communication**, or the exchange of messages between people. Communication not only includes what you say to others. It also includes your tone of voice and the words and images you use and share online.

communication exchange of spoken or unspoken messages between people

Types of Communication

Effective communication is perhaps the most important part of a healthy relationship. It is also an essential health skill for finding and sharing information and defending your decisions and goals. You use communication when you explain a decision to a family member. You also use communication when you share information about resources to promote community health.

The **communication process** involves sending a *message*, which consists of thoughts, ideas, feelings, or information. The *sender* of the message delivers the message to a *receiver*, such as a family member or online friend. Effective communication happens when the receiver understands the message and gives **feedback**, or a constructive response, to communicate that the message was received and understood (**Figure 3.1**). The communication process continues with the further exchange of messages. People send messages using two types of communication: verbal communication and nonverbal communication.

communication process series of actions people use to exchange ideas, thoughts, feelings, and information

feedback constructive response to a message

Verbal Communication

Verbal communication is the use of words to send an oral (spoken) or written message. You use verbal communication all the time in your everyday conversations, through text messages, in-person conversations, phone calls, emails, social media posts, letters, and notes. Telling a family member you will be home at a certain time is a form of verbal communication. So is talking with your friends online.

verbal communication use of words, spoken or written, to send a message

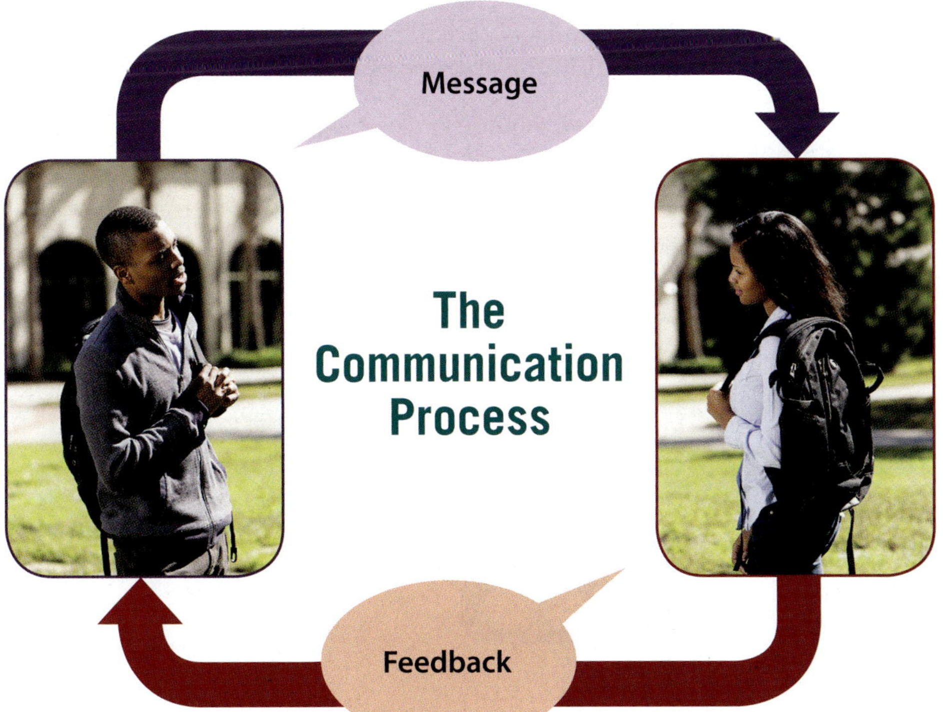

kali9/iStock/Getty Images Plus/Getty Images

Figure 3.1 The communication process involves the exchange of messages and feedback between two or more people. ***What is feedback in the communication process?***

Nonverbal Communication

nonverbal communication
use of body language, tone and volume of voice, and other wordless signals to send a message

Communication involves more than just words. You can also communicate with your face and body. **Nonverbal communication** involves communicating through facial expressions, body language, gestures, tone and volume of voice, and other signals that do not involve words. Your nonverbal communication shows people whether you are paying attention and are interested in a conversation. These signals are an important part of showing respect for the person communicating with you.

Some examples of nonverbal communication include the following:

- eye contact or lack of eye contact
- facial expressions, such as smiling, frowning, or eye rolling
- gestures, such as nodding, shaking the head, or moving the hands
- posture, such as leaning forward, facing away, or slumping in a chair
- tone of voice, which can communicate friendliness, doubt, or sarcasm
- volume of voice, such as loud or soft
- *intonation* (pitch) of voice, such as high-pitched or low-pitched

Nonverbal communication is only possible if you can see or hear the other person. For example, if you are talking with someone at school or video-calling a friend, you can see the other person's facial expressions and hear the person's voice. If you are talking over the phone, you can hear the other person's tone of voice.

Forms of communication where you cannot see or hear the other person (for example, writing letters or emails or sending online messages) can present challenges. The likelihood of miscommunication and conflict increases. Online communication has evolved to incorporate some types of nonverbal communication, such as emoticons, audio messages, pictures, and fonts (for example, capitalizing or italicizing words). These cues help express tone and intent in the absence of body language and voice (**Figure 3.2**).

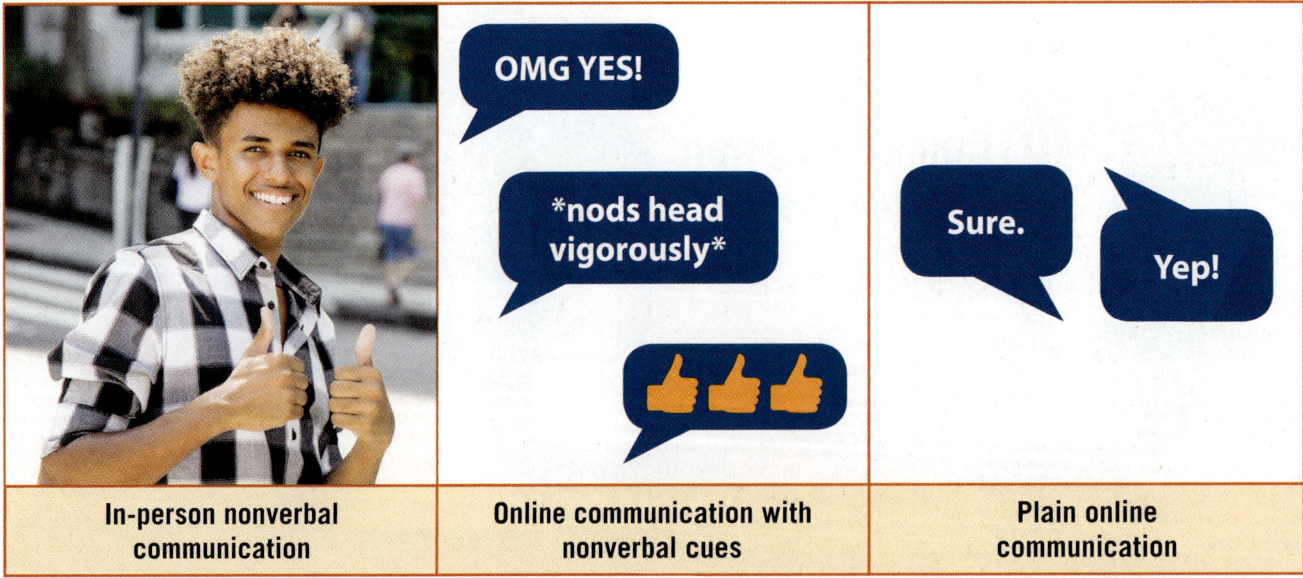

Person: DMEPhotography/iStock/Getty Images; Emoji: Treter/Shutterstock.com

Figure 3.2 Nonverbal elements influence the tone and meaning of a message, whether the communication happens online or in person. ***Are emoticons an example of verbal or nonverbal communication?***

Skills for Effective Communication

In effective communication, people communicate their thoughts, information, values, and feelings. Many communication techniques encourage effective, open communication. You can use these techniques to communicate with care, consideration, and respect for yourself and others.

Use Active Listening

Effective communication requires excellent listening skills. When you listen and focus on what another person is saying, you can better understand the person's point of view and show respect. **Active listening** involves two key steps:

active listening act of concentrating on the person talking and acknowledging what one has heard

1. **Focus your full attention on the person talking:** Make eye contact and face the person talking. Use good posture and do not interrupt. Do not think about your response or something else while the person is speaking.
2. **Acknowledge and repeat what you heard in your own words:** Give feedback by saying, "Oh, wow" or "Yeah, I know." Ask questions about the message and indicate you understand the message. If you paraphrase the message to show your understanding, you allow the speaker to clarify any misunderstandings about the message. Reflect the person's feelings back by relating to and acknowledging the person's emotions (**Figure 3.3**).

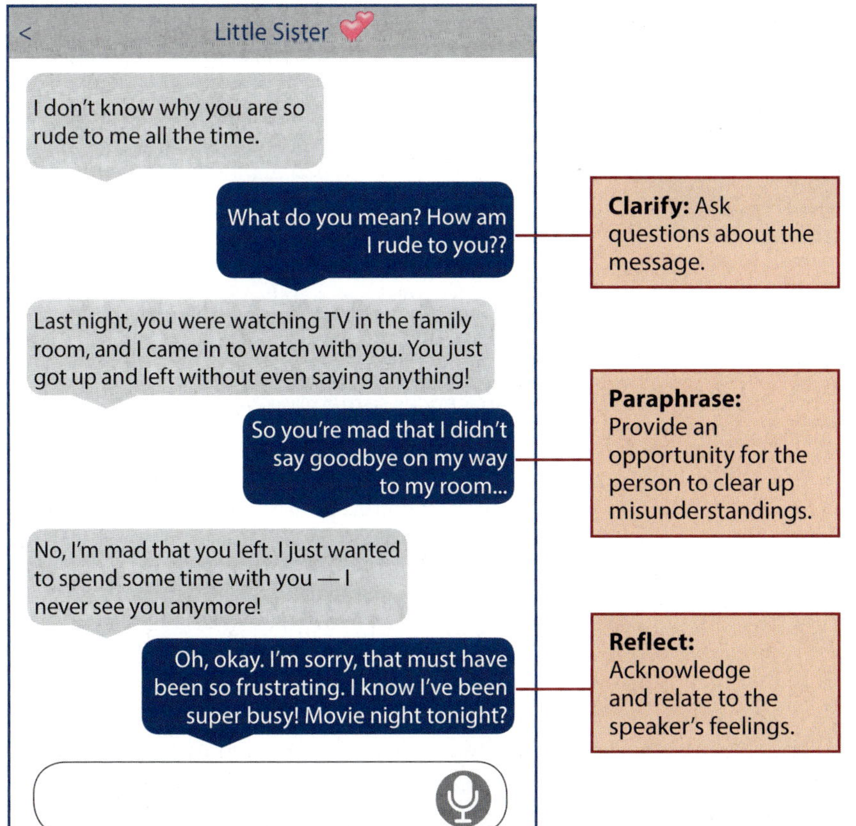

Hearts: Denis Gorelkin/Shutterstock.com; Microphone: Blan-k/Shutterstock.com

Figure 3.3 Let the speaker know you are listening by clarifying or paraphrasing the message and reflecting and acknowledging the speaker's feelings. ***What process involves giving people your attention and letting them know you understand their message?***

Active listening is a great way to avoid misunderstandings. If you carefully listen to what others say, others will be more likely to do the same for you.

Clearly Express Your Needs and Preferences

To communicate effectively, people need to clearly state their wants, needs, opinions, and feelings. Some people assume others should be able to pick up on their subtle hints and know how they are feeling. This is a poor communication strategy. Expecting the other person to be a mind reader is a sign of poor communication. Instead, explain what you want the other person to understand.

Local and Global Health

Culture Affects Communication

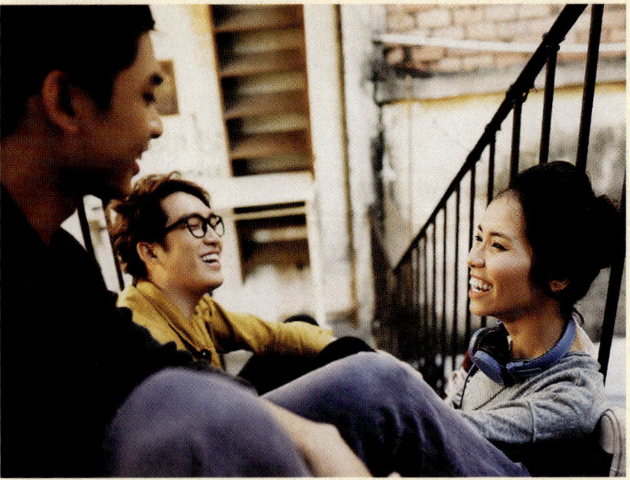

Dragon Images/Shutterstock.com

Many different factors affect communication—from personal preferences to one's background. One factor that influences communication is the culture in which people grow up. Culture shapes a person's verbal and nonverbal communication.

The simplest example of how culture impacts communication is the different languages people speak. Culture also affects how people use and interpret nonverbal communication. For example, in some cultures, making a lot of eye contact with someone when you talk shows respect and attention. In other cultures, direct eye contact is seen as aggressive and insulting. Different cultures also use and interpret facial expressions in different ways. For example, in the United States, smiling is a sign of friendliness. In Japan, smiling at someone you do not know can be seen as inappropriate, especially for females.

Cultures also differ considerably in expectations about touch. In some cultures, people tend to stand close together when they talk and may touch each other. In other cultures, people stand farther apart and rarely touch someone they do not know well. These differences sometimes make communication between people from different cultures challenging. To navigate these challenges, you can recognize and appreciate that cultures vary in communication.

Practice Your Skills

Access Information

In a small group, choose one culture that means something to you. Then, using reliable resources, research the communication strategies people from this culture most commonly use. Make sure to get information about people's verbal communication and body language, including eye contact, facial expressions, and physical touch. What behaviors are considered positive communication in this culture? What behaviors are considered poor communication? What communication barriers might people from this culture face living in your community? In your group, brainstorm effective ways of overcoming these communication barriers while still respecting culture.

Be Assertive

As you communicate with others, you may notice that people use different *communication styles*, or ways of expressing themselves (**Figure 3.4**). Following are four common communication styles:

1. **Passive: Passive** communication does not clearly state needs, wants, and feelings. Someone with a passive communication style may seem to say *yes* to everything, speak very quietly, and let hurt feelings build up. An example of passive communication is agreeing to an activity you do not want to do and thinking that no one cares about your feelings. Another example is not speaking up when someone hurts you.
2. **Aggressive: Aggressive** communication makes demands of another person and insults others. A person with this communication style expresses needs and feelings disrespectfully. Examples of aggressive communication are interrupting or speaking over others, blaming or attacking others, getting frustrated easily, and speaking loudly.
3. **Passive-aggressive: Passive-aggressive** communication uses techniques that do not clearly state needs, wants, and feelings to make demands of or insult others. Examples of passive-aggressive communication are smiling when you are angry, muttering to yourself, spreading rumors, using sarcasm, denying your feelings, and using sabotage.
4. **Assertive: Assertive** communication clearly expresses feelings, needs, and goals in a way that shows respect to the other person. This type of communication values both people and seeks clarity. Examples of assertive communication are calmly and truthfully saying, "It hurts when you say stuff like that," "I really miss you and wish we could hang out more often," or "Sure, let's do it."

passive hiding or not clearly stating needs, wants, and feelings

aggressive making demands of and insulting others

passive-aggressive using techniques that do not clearly state needs, wants, and feelings to make demands of and insult others

assertive clearly stating needs, wants, and feelings

Factors Affecting Communication

Upbringing
Life experiences, values taught during childhood, and cultural traditions affect the way people communicate. People also tend to communicate the same way as the people who raised them.

Self-esteem
People with healthy self-esteem are more willing and able to express their thoughts, opinions, and needs. People with low self-esteem may believe people are not interested in what they have to say or be sidetracked by worries or nervous thoughts.

Environment
A quiet, relaxed environment can promote positive communication. Communication late at night or during a busy part of the day can be more difficult.

Emotional state
Intense emotions make it difficult to accurately express what you mean or understand what others say. With a calmer emotional state, people can avoid upsetting one another further and are more likely to successfully communicate their messages.

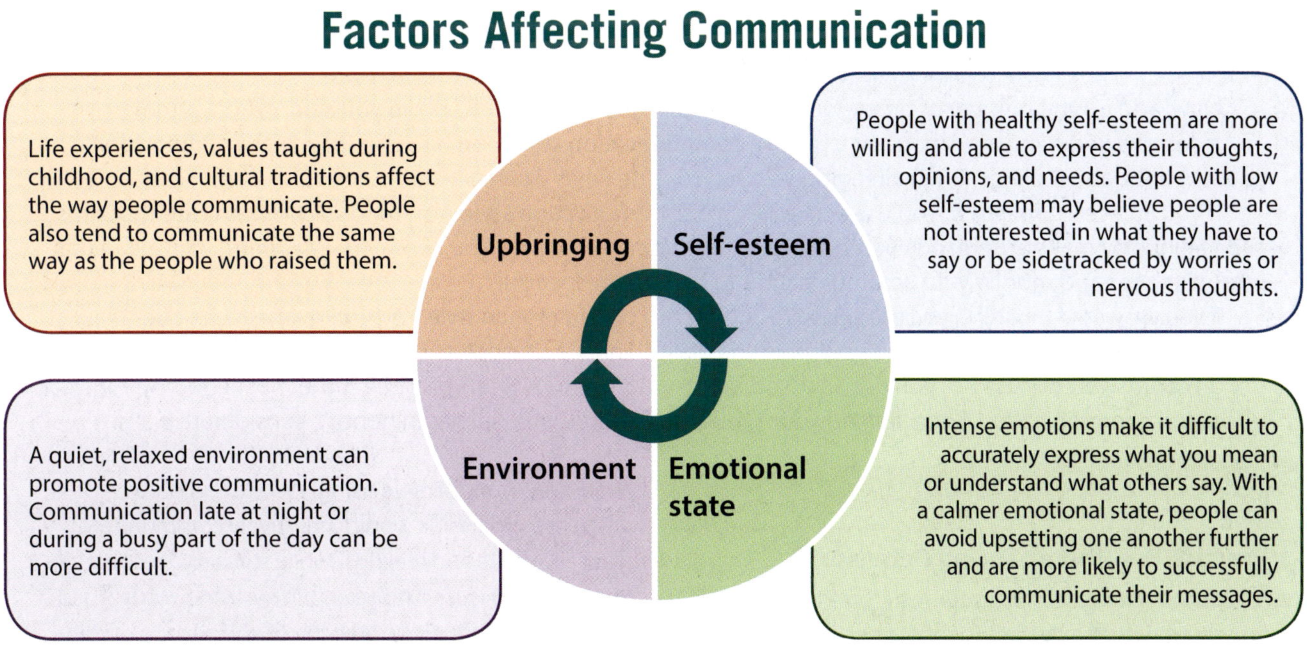

Figure 3.4 Communication styles are influenced by multiple factors in a person's life, including the person's culture, family, past experiences, self-esteem, emotional state, and environment. ***Which communication technique insults others and does not clearly state a person's needs or feelings?***

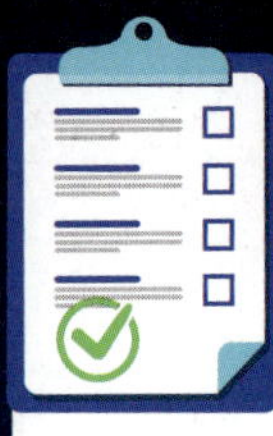

Quiz What Kind of Communicator Are You?

People use different communication styles to express their thoughts, feelings, and desires. The best, clearest style of communication is being assertive. To find out what type of communicator you are, take this quiz. Read the following scenarios. Select the option that best fits how you would react in each situation.

1. You are about to leave home to meet your cousin at the mall. On your way out the door, your parent or guardian asks for your help with some household chores. What do you do?
   A. Message your cousin that you will be late and need to go help with chores.
   B. Say, "What do I look like, your personal servant?" and walk out the door.
   C. Ask, "Why don't you ask your *favorite* child to help?"
   D. Say, "I already had plans to go out. Can I come straight home afterward to help?"
2. In history class, you are working on a group project with three other classmates. You are all debating about which project topic to select. What do you do?
   A. Stay mostly quiet and allow your classmates to make all the decisions.
   B. Take charge and make the final decision without listening to your classmates' opinions.
   C. Persuade your classmates to choose your ideas.
   D. Give your input, listen to your classmates, and work together to come to an agreement.
3. You send a message asking your friend to come hang out at your place. Your friend agrees to come by, but never arrives. What do you do?
   A. Ignore it. Maybe something happened at home, and your friend just forgot to message you.
   B. Send a message saying your friend is awful for ignoring you and is a terrible friend.
   C. Message your friend saying not to worry about it. Ignore your friend the next day at school.
   D. Reach out to your friend to find out what happened.
4. You are meeting your dating partner for dinner at a restaurant your partner chose. The food is *awful*. Your partner asks what you thought about dinner. What do you do?
   A. Say it was okay even though you hated it. You do not want to hurt your partner's feelings.
   B. Say, "It was terrible. How could you make such a horrible choice?"
   C. Say, "It was not the best. We should have gone somewhere else."
   D. Say, "I didn't like the food, but thanks for dinner. We'll try somewhere else next time."
5. Two of your close friends are talking about you behind your back. You catch them talking about you one day after school. How do you react?
   A. Laugh it off with your friends. They were probably just kidding around.
   B. Confront them by yelling insults at them.
   C. Sarcastically say, "Oh, wow, you are really great friends."
   D. Tell your friends you wish they would talk to you because talking behind your back hurts.

Now, add up the number of times you selected each letter. Which letters did you select most often?

If you answered ***mostly A***, you use a passive communication style. You have trouble clearly stating your needs, wants, and feelings. Try challenging yourself to state what you *really* think, even if it seems scary.

If you answered ***mostly B***, you use an aggressive communication style. You tend to communicate thoughts and feelings by making demands of others. Next time someone makes you angry, try imagining yourself in that person's shoes and modify your communication to be more respectful.

If you answered ***mostly C***, you use a passive-aggressive communication style. You use passive techniques that actually make demands of others. Try to say what you really think in a situation and consider the other person's feelings.

If you answered ***mostly D***, you use an assertive communication style. This style is the most effective for clear, respectful communication. Keep sharing your thoughts, feelings, and desires in honest, considerate ways.

Practice Your Skills

Practice Health-Enhancing Behaviors

With a partner, discuss your results from the quiz. Do you agree with the results? Together with your partner, examine each scenario you answered. Brainstorm assertive ways of responding to each scenario that you would feel comfortable using. Write a few phrases or responses you think would assertively communicate your thoughts and feelings, while still being respectful. Afterward, discuss with your partner what you learned from the process. How did both of you have to modify your natural style of communication to be more assertive? What skills helped you in being assertive?

The best style for effective communication is being assertive. Assertive communication allows you to express how you feel and make yourself known. If you do not express your feelings and goals, you are not letting other people truly know you. Assertive communication also helps you express yourself respectfully in a way that is understanding of others. Communicating in a way that disrespects others can be hurtful. Communicating assertively can help you build honest relationships, set healthy boundaries, and defend your decisions and goals.

Use I-Statements

Effective communication uses I-statements to express thoughts, feelings, and desires. **I-statements** explain how the speaker thinks or feels without passing judgment on the receiver. An example of an I-statement is "I feel ignored, which makes me worried. Is something wrong?" This is more constructive than a you-statement, which makes assumptions about and blames the other person (for example, "You don't like me anymore"). Using I-statements can help others understand your point of view without making them feel attacked (**Figure 3.5**).

I-statements words that explain how the speaker feels without judging the receiver

Watch Your Nonverbal Communication

When communicating, be aware of the nonverbal messages you send. What messages do your facial expressions and body language communicate to others? For example, suppose you are having a conversation with your sister.

You-statement
I-statement
You always cancel plans with me at the last minute. Do you even care about me?
I don't like spending time alone. Can I get a heads-up if plans change?
I hate when you leave dirty dishes in the sink.
I feel overwhelmed by the chores I have to do and I would like help.
Why did you have to schedule the party for tonight?
I'm worried it will rain tonight during the party.
First, your rubric for that project was confusing, and then you failed me!
I didn't understand the rubric and I'm upset I got a poor grade.

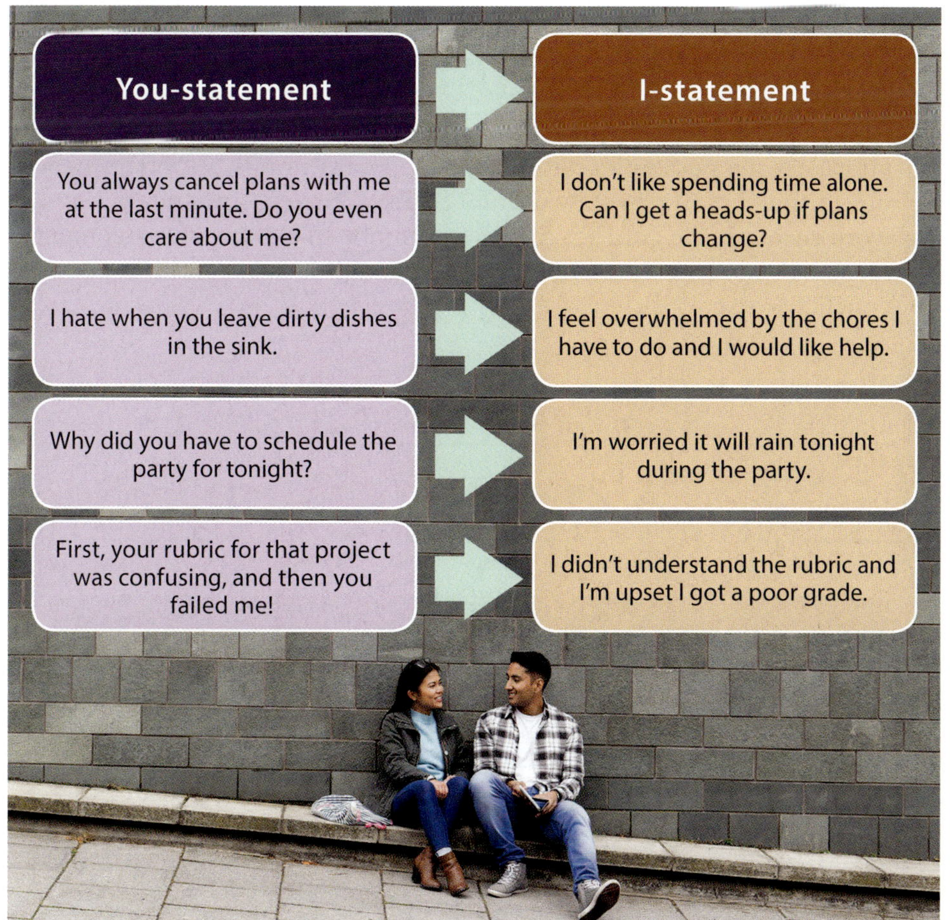

SolStock/iStock/Getty Images

Figure 3.5 I-statements do not blame the other person or escalate emotions. Healthy communication offers your perspective, expresses your emotions, explains your needs, and provides a potential outcome.

As she speaks, you look down at your phone and periodically roll your eyes. These signals do not communicate active listening or respect for your sister. Making eye contact, nodding your head, and leaning forward would communicate you value what she is saying.

Communicate Carefully Online

Most teens regularly communicate online. Online communication occurs on social media and websites and through any digital device, like a phone, computer, laptop, tablet, or gaming system. This type of communication has many advantages, including instant feedback, long-distance communication, and time to think of the best response. Online communication also has some disadvantages.

Miscommunications occur easily online because nonverbal cues, such as gestures and facial expressions, are not always available. Even some features that try to make up for the lack of nonverbal communication do not always succeed. One person may use an emoticon to express one emotion, but another person may associate an entirely different meaning to that same symbol. People can easily misjudge the tone or meaning of online communication (**Figure 3.6**).

Fortunately, there are some strategies you can use to avoid misunderstandings and communicate online safely and effectively. Some of these strategies include the following:

- **Be kind and respectful:** Treat people the way you would like to be treated or the way you would want someone to treat your best friend. If someone is rude or aggressive, you can ignore the message or tell the person to stop. If aggressive behavior continues, block the person or ask an adult or trusted friend for advice about what to do next.
- **Solve conflicts offline:** If you have a disagreement with someone, approach the person face-to-face. If you cannot talk in person, reach out to the person privately online. Share your feelings and try to work through the conflict together. Do not share this disagreement on social media or in a public way. This will just make the conflict worse.

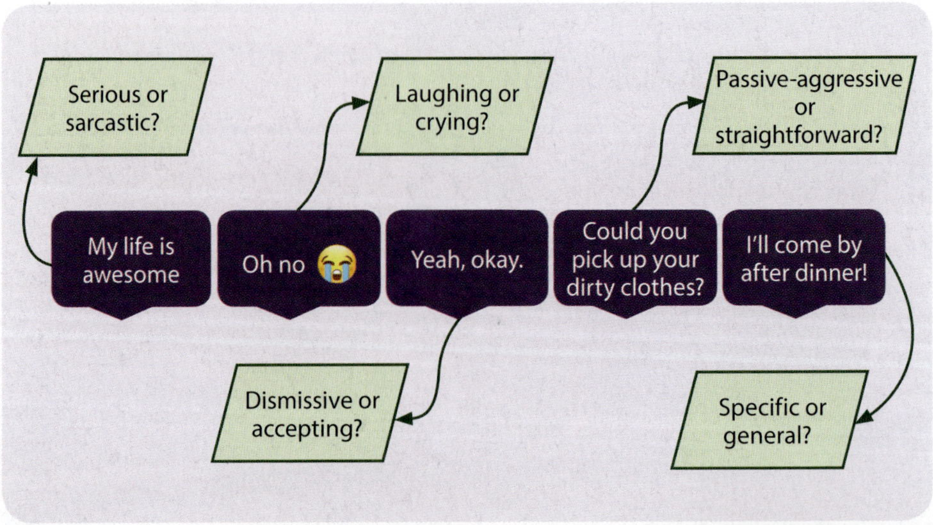

josep.perianes jorba/Shutterstock.com

Figure 3.6 It may be difficult to interpret the tone or meaning people intend in online messages. To avoid miscommunication, clarify if you do not know what someone is saying or how someone means something. ***Why is online communication easy to misinterpret?***

- **Think before you share:** Content you share online—even in private emails or messages—can easily become public and spread. Think carefully before you share anything you would not want other people to see. Even if you are sharing private content only with a friend or dating partner, think about what might happen later on, if you have conflict or if the relationship ends. Assume everyone will be able to see anything you post online, even if you try to remove what you posted.
- **Keep passwords private:** Create a password that you can remember, but that others cannot guess. Do not share this password with anyone, even with friends, and change your password every few months. Sharing a password with a friend can cause issues if that friend pretends to be you, even if it seems like no big deal.

You will learn more strategies for staying safe and communicating online in Lesson 17.3: *Being Safe on the Internet*.

Lesson 3.1 Review

Know and Understand

1. Using Figure 3.1, draw your own diagram to help explain the communication process.
2. Are online messages an example of verbal or nonverbal communication? Explain.
3. Have a conversation with a partner and list all of the types of nonverbal communication your partner uses. What do these cues communicate?
4. What are the steps in active listening?
5. Imagine that, after your friend cancels on you, you message your friend saying, *You like your other friends more than me*. How could you rephrase this feeling into an I-statement?

Think Critically

6. Think of a time you had a misunderstanding with a friend online. What led to the misunderstanding? How did the lack of nonverbal communication affect the misunderstanding?
7. What advantage does assertive communication have over the other three communication styles? Why is this advantage essential for effective communication?
8. Why is it best to communicate about disagreements privately and offline? What qualities of online communication make handling conflict difficult? Explain.

REAL WORLD Health Skills

Practice Health-Enhancing Behaviors One effective strategy for expressing your feelings, thoughts, and desires without the other person feeling attacked is to use I-statements instead of you-statements. For example, you could say, "I feel hurt that everyone knows what I told you," instead of "You told Corby what I said. You violated my trust." To practice this skill, convert the following you-statements into I-statements:

You never ask if you can borrow my clothes, and you know that is my favorite shirt!

You didn't tell me you were going to Charlie's party. You knew I wanted to go.

You always remind me to do my homework. Why can't you just let me try to do it on my own?

Lesson

3.2

Resolving Conflicts

Essential Question?

How can you resolve conflicts in a way that strengthens a relationship?

Learning Outcomes

After studying this lesson, you will be able to

- describe factors that cause conflict;
- analyze the importance of addressing and resolving conflicts;
- explain the steps in effectively resolving a conflict; and
- assess how mediation aids in conflict resolution.

Key Terms

compromise
conflict
conflict-resolution skills
mediation
mediator
misunderstandings
negotiation
peer mediation

Warm-Up Activity

Conflict Comic Strip

Communicate with Others

What is the most recent conflict you had with someone? Illustrate this conflict in a short, six-panel comic strip. Describe what was said and try to show any nonverbal elements of communication such as body language and movement. Then write a paragraph explaining whether this conflict was handled in a healthy or unhealthy way. You will consider your answer again in the *Real World Health Skills* activity at the end of this lesson.

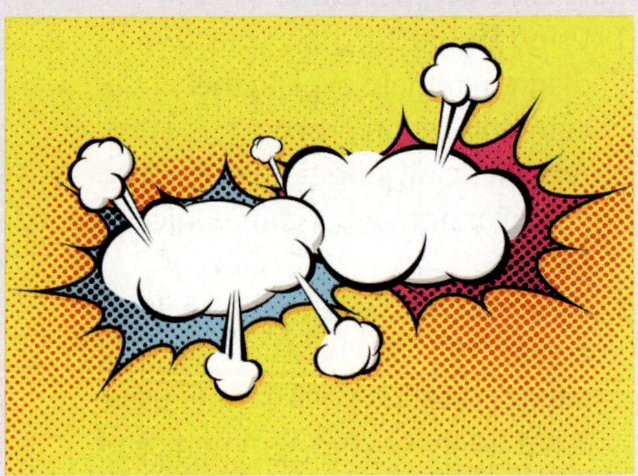

phyZick/Shutterstock.com

conflict disagreement or argument that occurs due to misunderstandings or differing priorities, values, goals, or needs

The disagreements that occur in relationships are known as **conflict**. Conflict is a normal part of everyday life, even for healthy relationships, and is not always negative. Engaging in conflict can have positive outcomes for yourself and your relationships. Understanding conflict—including what causes conflict and how to best resolve conflict—is important.

What Causes Conflict?

Many different factors can lead to *interpersonal conflicts*, which are conflicts between people or groups of people. Conflicts occur when different people have the following:

- **Different priorities:** People may prioritize events, situations, and preferences differently. For example, maybe it is important to you that you see your friend every week, but it is equally important to your friend to attend soccer practice.

- **Different values:** Your *values* are what is important to you. Family, culture, personal views and opinions, and experiences influence your values. For example, maybe your teacher values hard work and is strict with a fellow classmate, but you value your classmate's feelings and disagree with your teacher's approach.
- **Different goals:** People's individual goals can sometimes cause conflict. For example, a goal of your family is to keep you safe, which might clash with your goal to be more independent.
- **Different needs:** People have different needs at different times. For example, maybe you need some time to wind down after school, but your dating partner needs to vent about a fight with a sibling.
- **Misunderstandings:** **Misunderstandings** are failures in communication that lead to conflict. For example, maybe when you complain about your weekend, your friend thinks you are complaining about your time together. If your friend does not clarify your message, this could lead to hurt feelings and conflict.

misunderstandings
failures in communication that lead to conflict

What separates healthy conflict from unhealthy conflict is how conflict is resolved. In disagreements of little importance, it may be best to simply accept differences and agree to respectfully disagree. There is no point arguing with a friend who does not like your favorite TV show, for example (**Figure 3.7**). Other conflicts, such as you and your sibling disagreeing about which movie to see, are easy to settle with no hurt feelings. Many conflicts, however, are more complicated and too serious to ignore.

Conflicts that are not resolved can lead to serious and lasting consequences. Conflicts that go unresolved for a long time often *escalate*, or become major issues. Unresolved conflicts can have negative effects on a person's psychological and emotional well-being. Interpersonal conflict can even impact a person's physical health. Conflict is a type of stress, and people who experience long-term stressors in the form of conflict can develop serious health conditions.

Many people worry that trying to resolve a conflict will destroy a relationship or make the conflict worse. In reality, working through a conflict can actually strengthen a relationship. When people decide to work together to resolve a conflict, they show their commitment to the relationship.

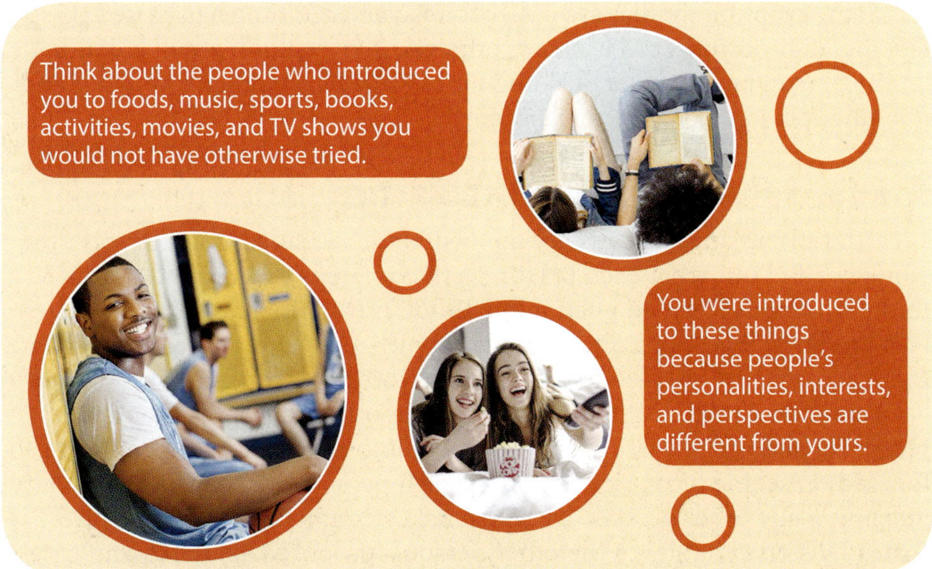

Left to right: SDI Productions/E+/Getty Images; seb_ra/iStock/Getty Images Plus/Getty Images; Lopolo/Shutterstock.com

Figure 3.7 You do not need, or even want, everyone in your life to be identical copies of you. Talking with people who have different interests, experiences, and views of the world can be exciting.

conflict-resolution skills strategies for working through a disagreement or argument in positive, productive ways

negotiation process of working together to resolve conflict and find acceptable solutions; involves identifying the cause, asking for solutions from both parties, agreeing on and carrying out a solution, and evaluating the solution and renegotiating, if necessary

Resolving Conflicts

Your interpersonal interactions may be pleasant most of the time, but conflicts are sure to arise. Learning **conflict-resolution skills**, or strategies for resolving conflict in productive and positive ways, is important because conflict is an inevitable part of life. Settling a conflict requires communication skills, such as assertive communication and active listening. It also requires **negotiation**, a process in which people work together (to think and talk) through a solution to a conflict (**Figure 3.8**).

Step 1
Identify the cause of the conflict.

Step 2
Ask for solutions from both parties.

Step 3
Identify solutions both parties can support.

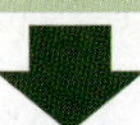

Step 4
Agree on a solution.

Step 5
Carry out the solution.

Step 6
Evaluate the solution and renegotiate, if necessary.

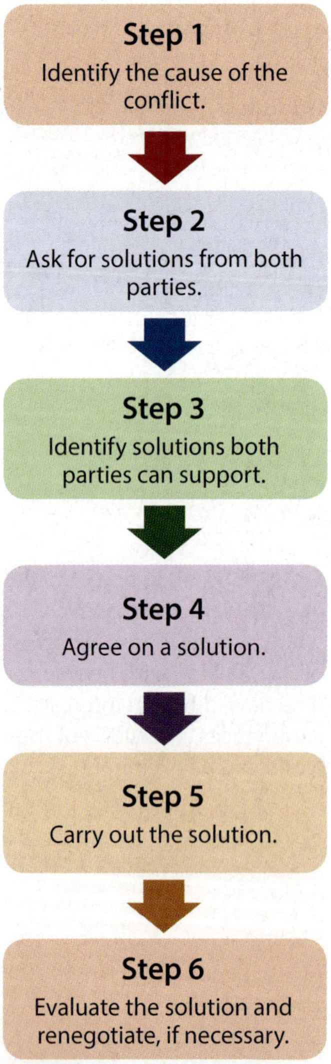

Figure 3.8 Negotiation is an important process for resolving conflicts.

Identify the Cause of the Conflict

The first step in resolving a conflict is identifying what is causing the conflict. This step can start on an individual level, but should eventually involve communication between both people in the conflict. Conflicts continue or grow worse if you do not share your feelings. Instead of trying to pretend you are not upset, plan to talk about the conflict with the other person.

Before setting a time to talk, identify what you think is causing the conflict. Pay attention to your feelings and thoughts to get a clear picture of why the conflict is occurring. Sometimes you may not feel ready to talk directly to the other person in a conflict. In that case, talk to someone else first. Explaining the situation to an adult or friend can help you work out how you feel and what you want. It can also give you a new perspective.

Before starting a discussion with the other person in the conflict, agree with the person on a time and place to discuss the situation. Meet when you both have enough time to focus on the issue. Choose a neutral meeting place away from other people and distractions (**Figure 3.9**).

Remember that when two people are in conflict, they often identify the cause differently. Apply effective verbal and nonverbal communication strategies during this stage. Both people must honestly and clearly state the conflict from their perspectives. Sometimes feelings get heated when people are in the middle of a conflict. Intense feelings, such as disappointment and frustration, can make a conflict worse. To avoid this, learn to manage and control your anger. Use assertive I-statements instead of aggressive you-statements and avoid making accusations or name-calling.

Some types of conflict are easier to resolve after time has passed. If you feel too angry or upset to have a productive conversation about a conflict, let the person know you need some time. Walk away and give yourself and the other person a chance to calm down.

Ask for Solutions from Both Parties

After discussing the cause of the conflict, brainstorm ways to solve the conflict. Find out what each person wants or needs as a desired outcome to the situation. Keep an open mind about everyone's ideas and do not rule out any suggestions. Be creative. People from both parties should state their ideas firmly, but not demand that the other person agree.

People must also listen carefully to what others have to say and recognize and accept the other person's opinions. Sometimes people are so focused on seeing a conflict from their own perspective they have difficulty imagining any other perspective. This makes conflicts harder to resolve. Instead, listen carefully to the other person's proposed solutions and try to understand the person's perspective.

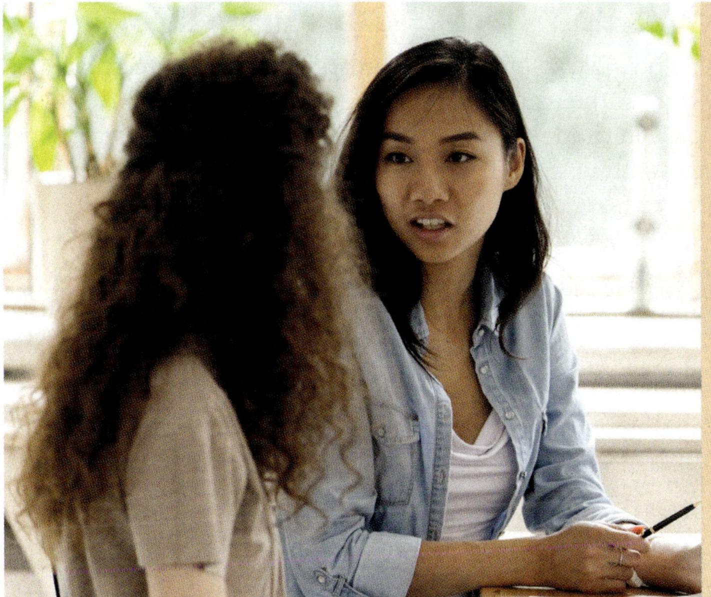

Tips for Identifying the Cause of a Conflict

- State what you think is causing the conflict.
- Speak honestly about your feelings, needs, and goals.
- Have the other person share this information too.
- Do not behave passively or aggressively.
- Listen carefully to what the other person says and try to understand that person's perspective.
- Consider what good points the person is making rather than thinking about your response.
- Pay attention to the person's body language and tone of voice.

fizkes/Shutterstock.com

Figure 3.9 When you meet with the other person in the conflict, use positive conflict-resolution skills, including active listening, to discuss the issue at hand.

Research in Action

The Magic Relationship Ratio

How often do you have conflict with your sibling, best friend, or dating partner? Did you know that some conflict is actually a *good* thing? What matters most is how often people interact positively or negatively when resolving conflict.

Research by Dr. John Gottman at the University of Washington examined how couples resolve conflict and how their interactions impact happiness. In one study, researchers examined videos of married couples trying to solve a conflict in their relationship. They counted how many different positive and negative interactions the couple had during this 15-minute interaction. Positive interactions included behaviors like laughing, teasing, and showing affection. Negative interactions included criticism, anger, and defensiveness. Researchers then contacted these same couples nine years later to see if they were still together.

Researchers found that couples who stayed together had at least five positive interactions for every one negative interaction when they resolved conflict. This led to a so-called "magic ratio" of 5 to 1.

What is the key, take-home point here? Healthy relationships involve conflict, but they also involve lots of positive interactions. Even when people are working through a conflict, people in a healthy relationship show positive behaviors toward each other. Conflict is inevitable in a relationship and is even a sign of a healthy relationship, as long as it is balanced with affection, laughter, and love.

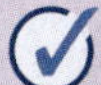

Practice Your Skills

Practice Health-Enhancing Behaviors

Think about the different interactions you have had recently with a friend, dating partner, or family member. What positive interactions have you had? What negative interactions have you had? For one relationship, calculate the ratio of positive to negative interactions in the past two weeks. If your ratio does not include enough positive interactions, think about what you could do differently. What strategies can you use to increase positive interactions with this person? How can you reduce negative interactions? In collaboration with a partner, develop a plan to balance your negative interactions with more positive ones and build a stronger, healthier relationship.

Identify Solutions Both Parties Can Support

After discussing all possible solutions, recommend a solution or combination of solutions. Calmly discuss the issue and possible solutions to reach an agreement both people can support. Both parties should be open to suggestions and focus on finding a solution together, not just on meeting their own needs.

Agree on a Solution

compromise agreement in which two sides come together and each side gives in a little

During this step, both people agree on a solution. Rarely is there a solution that makes everyone happy. Often, both sides agree to give in a little, or **compromise**. Through compromise, each side can reach a solution that is acceptable for all people involved (**Figure 3.10**). Sometimes a compromise is not possible, and the solution involves the two sides simply agreeing to disagree.

Carry Out the Solution

Take action to apply the solution. Ensure that all parties know their designated roles in the solution. Make sure everyone follows through on the agreed-upon solution and consider how each person should overcome any likely obstacles. People are more likely to resolve a conflict with a specific plan outlined.

Examples of Compromises for Common Conflicts

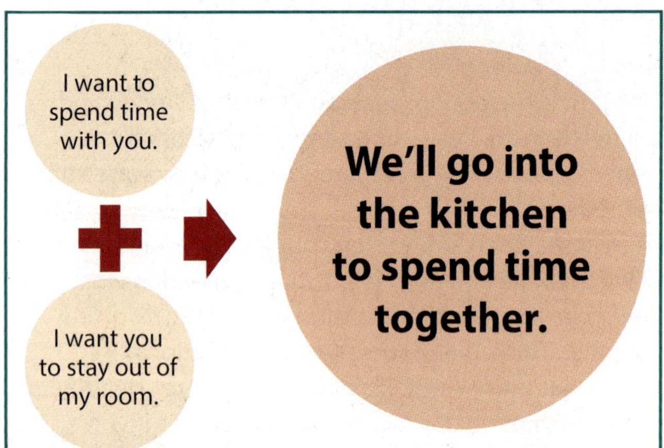

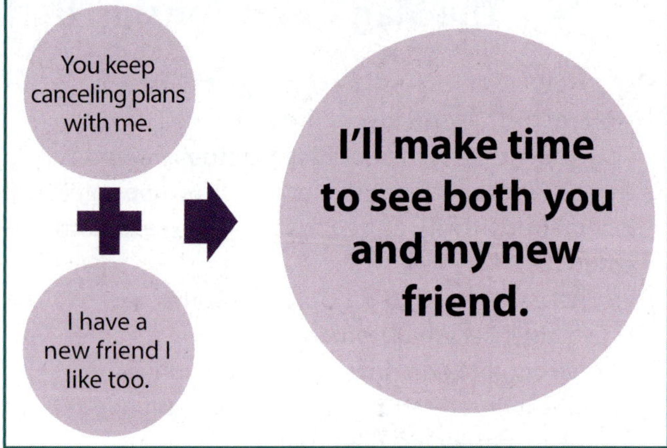

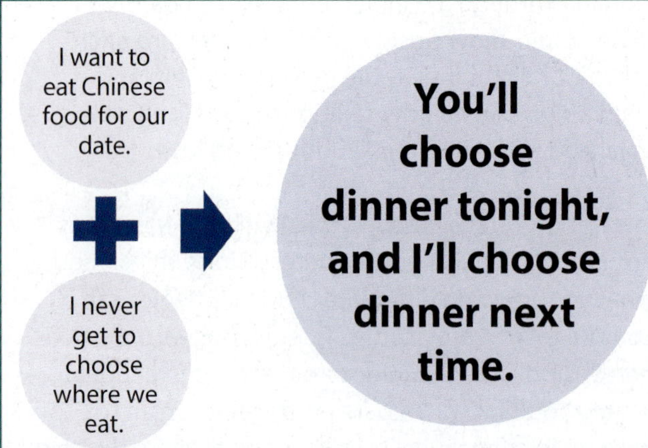

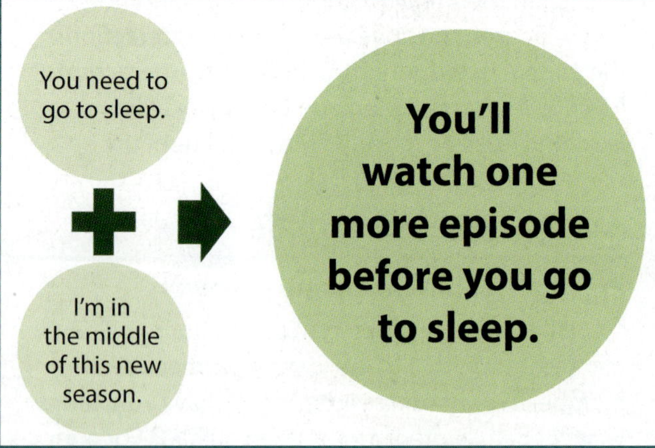

Figure 3.10 Effective compromise is only possible if both people are willing to be flexible. ***Who has to give in a little in a compromise?***

Evaluate the Solution and Renegotiate, If Necessary

Review the outcome of the solution. If for some reason the solution is not working, find out why and renegotiate. Identify which step in the conflict-resolution process failed, go back to that step, and try again.

Using Mediation

In some cases, a conflict is too serious or difficult for the people directly involved to manage by themselves. In this situation, an outside individual with a neutral perspective can help the people or groups find an effective solution.

Skills for Health and Wellness

Solve a Conflict with a Friend

Even in strong, healthy friendships, conflicts occur. When you have conflict with a friend, you have to make a decision about how to respond. Sometimes you may not feel comfortable telling your friend how you are feeling when you are upset. Not saying anything will harm the friendship, however. Working on solving the conflict can help strengthen your friendship.

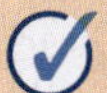

Practice Your Skills

Communicate with Others

Partner with a classmate to role-play managing a conflict with a friend. Choose a conflict one of you recently had. If you cannot think of one, reference Figure 3.10. Then follow these steps to try to work through the conflict in a constructive way:

1. **Set up a time to discuss the conflict** and resolve it. When resolving a conflict, you might want to start by saying something positive about your friendship. For example, express how much you enjoy hanging out with your friend: "I really appreciate our friendship and I enjoy spending time with you."
2. Together with your friend, **identify the cause of the conflict**. State how you feel using an I-statement: "I felt hurt and sad when our plans for Saturday night fell through at the last minute." Acknowledge your own role in the conflict: "I'm sorry I didn't respond when you apologized. I'm sorry I complained about you to some other friends." Ask your friend to also state what your friend thinks is causing the conflict. Listen carefully and acknowledge your friend's feelings and ideas.
4. **Seek solutions** to the conflict from both parties. Suggest a solution: "Next time, I would really appreciate it if you didn't cancel plans, or at least let me know earlier if something wasn't going to work out for you. I will respond to you quickly instead of ignoring you, and make a point of talking to you directly instead of reaching out to complain to other friends." Listen to your friend's ideas as well.
5. Together, **discuss which solutions are best** for both of you. Trade suggestions and try to identify solutions that solve the conflict and address both people's feelings.
6. **Agree on a solution**. Sometimes, this will involve reaching a compromise. If you cannot reach a compromise, agree to disagree.
7. In your role-play, jump forward in time and role-play a situation in which you and your friend carry out the solution. Afterward, **evaluate whether the solution worked** and renegotiate, if necessary.

After role-playing once, switch roles with your partner. Then discuss which statements and communication strategies felt the best to both of you and best resolved the conflict.

mediation strategy for resolving difficult conflicts through a neutral third party

mediator neutral third party who attempts to help people involved in a conflict reach an agreement

peer mediation process in which specially trained students work with other students to resolve conflicts

Mediation is a strategy for resolving difficult conflicts through the involvement of a neutral third party, or **mediator** (**Figure 3.11**). During mediation, both parties in the conflict separately share their perspectives of the conflict with the mediator. The mediator then brings the two parties together to share their views and tries to help them reach an agreement.

Conflict-resolution programs in many high schools provide **peer mediation**, in which specially trained students work with other students to resolve conflicts. Peer mediators learn about conflicts and methods for resolving them. They work under the guidance of faculty advisors. When a conflict arises, the faculty member assigns a mediator to handle the situation. The mediator talks to the people involved in the conflict and helps them work through a solution. If you do not have a peer mediation program at your school, you can talk with a school counselor or teacher about starting one.

Mediators

- make sure everyone is heard
- clarify communication
- illuminate new perspectives
- help find solutions

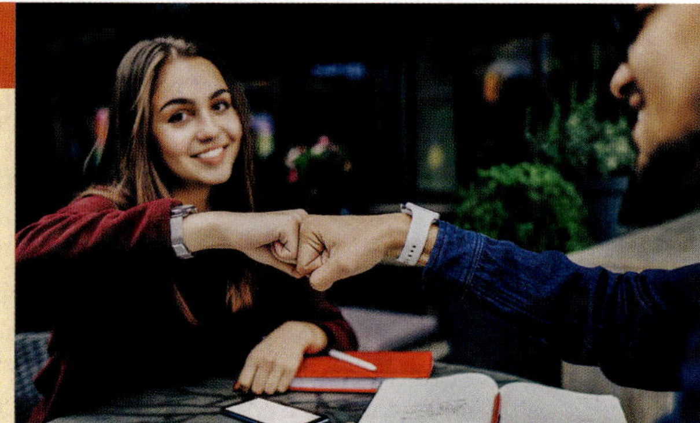

GaudiLab/Shutterstock.com

Figure 3.11 Mediators act as neutral third parties to help people resolve conflict.

Lesson 3.2 Review

Know and Understand

1. Why is it important not to let conflicts go unresolved?
2. With a partner, choose a common conflict and explain how you would resolve it using each step in negotiation.
3. Explain what happens in a compromise.

Think Critically

4. How much conflict do you think is normal in a relationship?
5. Think about a conflict in your life and identify whether it was caused by different priorities, values, goals, needs, misunderstandings, or a combination of these factors.
6. Why do you think the two people in a conflict often identify the cause differently?
7. Why do you think involving a mediator often helps people resolve conflicts?

REAL WORLD Health Skills

Communicate with Others Now that you have learned some strategies for resolving conflict, analyze the comic strip you created for the Warm-Up Activity at the beginning of this lesson. What strategies did you use to resolve that conflict? How healthy were those strategies? What strategies could you have used instead? Choose one or two strategies you think would have resolved the conflict in a better way and then draw a new comic showing how that conflict may have ended differently.

Resisting Pressure

Essential Question?

What skills can you use to resist negative peer pressure?

Lesson 3.3

Learning Outcomes

After studying this lesson, you will be able to

- define *pressure*;
- explain the difference between positive and negative peer pressure;
- identify effective strategies for resisting negative peer pressure; and
- use refusal skills to protect your health and stand up to pressure.

Key Terms

negative peer pressure
peer pressure
positive peer pressure
pressure
refusal skills

Warm-Up Activity

Peer Pressure

Analyze Influences Think about some personal experiences with friends and identify three examples of positive peer pressure and three examples of negative peer pressure. How did you feel when you experienced positive peer pressure? negative peer pressure? In the moment, did you recognize whether the pressure was positive or negative? How did you react? Create an audio journal or video blog entry reflecting on your experiences.

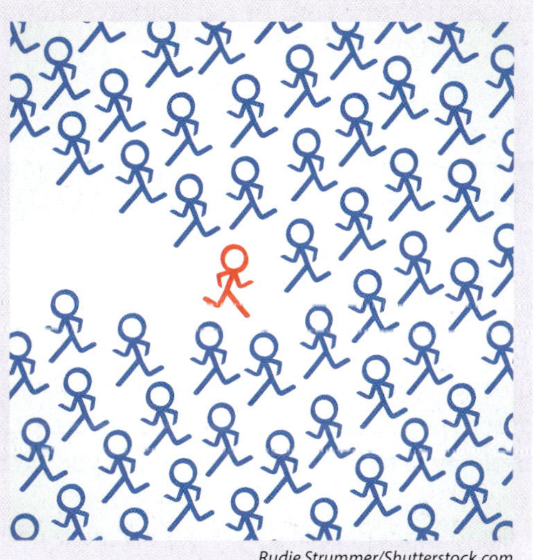

Rudie Strummer/Shutterstock.com

Relationships are a source of support for all people, and the relationships you keep are certain to influence your preferences, activities, and ideas. For example, have you ever noticed that you tend to dress like your closest friends? or that you took up a new activity once a new person entered your life? This is because people naturally try to fit in with their peers and the people in their social groups. This is especially true during the adolescent years, when peer approval is important to teens. The influence your relationships have on your behavior can be positive or negative.

What Is Peer Pressure?

pressure motivation to do an activity or take on certain qualities; can be internal or external

Pressure refers to the motivation to do an activity or take on certain qualities. Pressure can be internal or external. *Internal pressure* is your motivation to complete a task. For example, if you feel pressure to do well in science, this might motivate you to attend a study group or spend more time on homework. *External pressure* refers to outside actions, words, and rewards that influence your behavior. For example, if you hear that most of your classmates are vaping, this might influence you to try vaping despite its harmful effects on health.

peer pressure social pressure among people of the same age or status; can make people feel like they need to do and like the same things to be liked or respected

Pressure exists in all types of relationships. Pressure among *peers*, or people of the same age or status, is called **peer pressure**. Peer pressure is a common element present in friendships, romantic relationships, and casual relationships among acquaintances. Two different types of peer pressure exist—positive and negative.

Positive Peer Pressure

Although people often associate peer pressure with negative activities, peer pressure can have a positive effect on your health. For example, you might feel pressure to participate in community service projects with a

Health in the Media

The Power of Virtual Peer Pressure

Most teens have heard about the effects of peer pressure, but virtual peer pressure can be just as impactful. *Virtual peer pressure* describes the pressure people feel to spend time on social media to fit in with friends—for example, by constantly posting pictures and commenting on or liking other people's pictures and posts. Teens may also feel pressure to post certain types of pictures to feel accepted and valued by friends on social media.

What is so powerful about virtual peer pressure? To test this question, researchers at Temple University in Philadelphia studied teens' brain activity looking at different pictures on social media. Each picture displayed how many likes it supposedly received from other teens in the study. (In reality, researchers assigned the number of likes.) Researchers then measured which photos teens liked and the activity in teens' brains.

Can you predict what researchers found? First, teens were more likely to like a photo if it had been liked by others. Teens were highly influenced by what they believed other teens liked. Second, when teens saw pictures that had many likes, this activated the brain region that processes rewarding experiences—the same region activated by eating chocolate or winning money. In other words, knowing that others like a picture you also like literally feels good in the brain. This shows the power of virtual peer pressure to influence responses on social media.

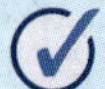

Practice Your Skills

Set Goals

With a partner, discuss why teens are so strongly influenced by what they believe other teens like. Do you think people at other ages would show the same pattern of responses? Why or why not? With your partner, brainstorm strategies teens can use to manage the influence of virtual peer pressure on their thoughts, feelings, and behaviors. Set five SMART goals to put these strategies into action. Act on two of these goals and then evaluate with your partner how successful they were.

school group or athletic team. A friend may encourage you to study harder and improve your grade in a class. In these cases, pressure from peers can help you broaden your perspective, contribute to your community, and succeed. **Positive peer pressure** involves activities that contribute to good health and can benefit you.

positive peer pressure social pressure among people of the same age or status that contributes to good health and can be beneficial

Positive peer pressure is also respectful. It values your opinions, preferences, and individuality. For example, a friend might say, "You're so smart. I think it would be great to study together." The same friend should accept your answer, even if you decline. Peer pressure becomes negative if it makes you feel guilty or harms your self-esteem. Even though encouraging someone to do well in school is positive, if your friend makes you feel bad about yourself or does not accept your answer, this is negative peer pressure.

Negative Peer Pressure

Negative peer pressure refers to peer pressure that encourages unhealthy behaviors or is not respectful (**Figure 3.12**). In some relationships, one person pressures another to do something uncomfortable. A teen may feel pressured to drink alcohol because peers on social media are drinking or skip class because friends encourage it. If the culture at a school is accepting of teasing and bullying, a teen may feel pressured to pick on classmates to fit in.

negative peer pressure social pressure among people of the same age or status that encourages unhealthy behaviors or is not respectful

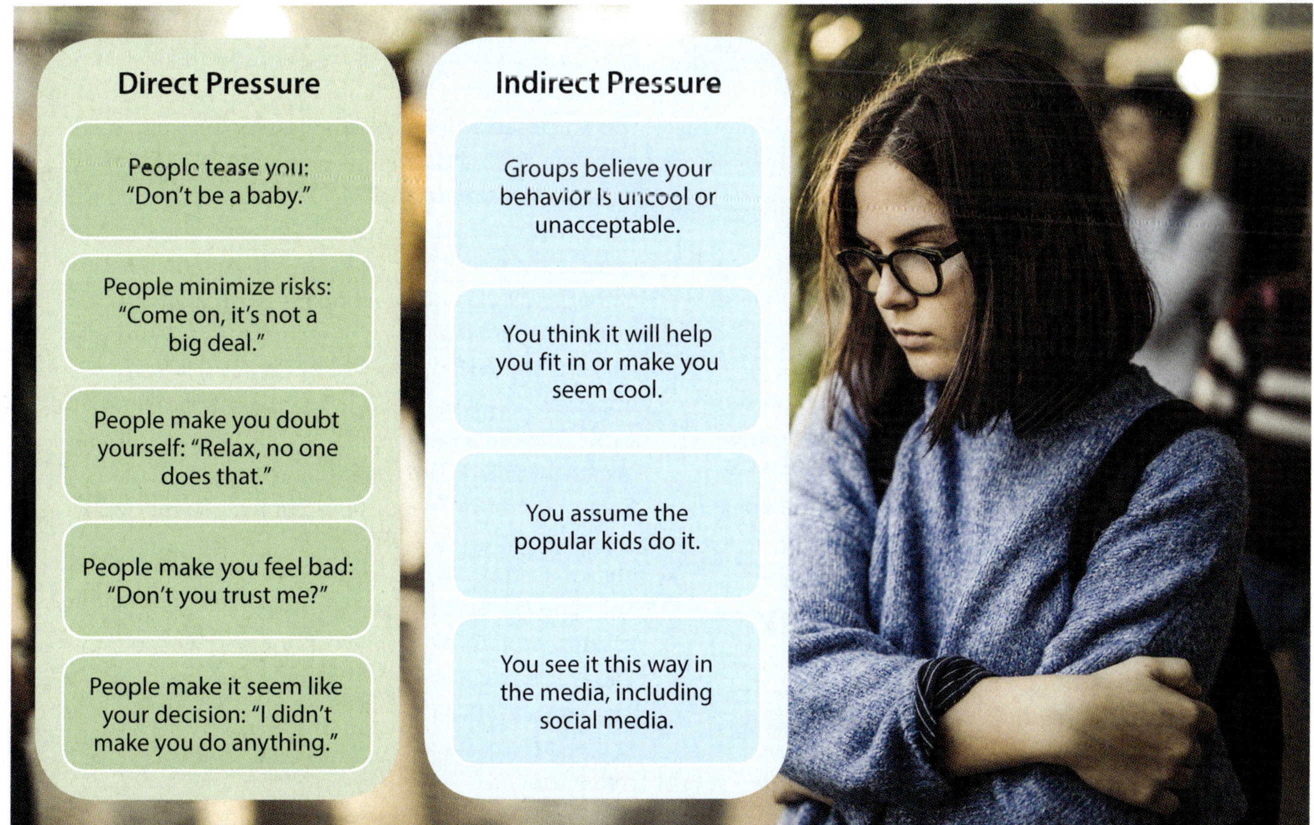

skynesher/E+/Getty Images

Figure 3.12 Trust your instincts. If you feel uncomfortable, even if your friends or classmates seem to be fine, it means something about the situation is wrong for you. ***What type of pressure comes from the words and actions of other people, rather than self-motivation?***

Most people want to be liked and fit in with a group. They may decide to go along with certain behaviors even if they are uncomfortable. They may also give up certain activities they enjoy. They may worry about being ridiculed if they do not join the group activity, go along with culture, or meet expectations in the media. Sometimes teens worry that standing up for their interests or beliefs could cause them to lose a relationship or feel awkward or left out.

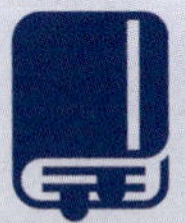

Case Study

Peer Pressure in Action

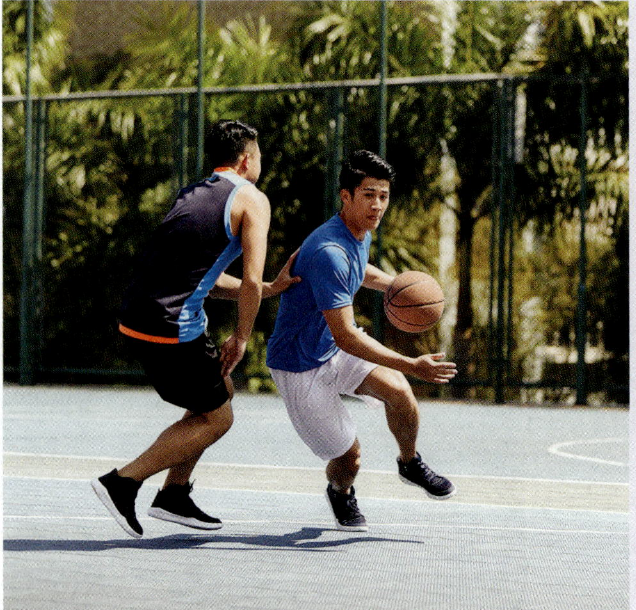

imtmphoto/iStock/Getty Images Plus/Getty Images

Kim is a sophomore and dedicated to her studies. She always does her homework and gets to class on time. Kim's friends do not share these same values, however. Some of her friends wait until the last minute to complete an assignment. Some do not even complete it at all. Lately, Kim's friends have been asking her to skip class with them. Kim thinks it could be kind of fun, but she does not want to get in trouble. Kim's friends reassure her they do this all the time and have never gotten in trouble.

When he was a freshman, Connor used to skip class with his friends all the time. At first, he told them *no*, but he watched how much fun they had on social media. Once he started skipping class, his schoolwork really suffered. He was even suspended from playing basketball until he got his grades up. He wanted to play basketball more than he wanted to skip class, so he told his friends he would not do it anymore. He was surprised when his friend Hassan told him he did not want to skip class either.

As a senior, Hassan really values his friendship with Connor. Hassan appreciates that Connor respects his choices and likes him for who he is, rather than how far he is willing to push boundaries. Hassan thinks that he and Connor drive each other to be better, stronger versions of themselves. Without Connor, Hassan does not know if he would have worked so hard to make the varsity basketball team. He definitely would not have gotten into his dream college if he had not studied with Connor for the SATs and started going back to class.

Practice Your Skills

Make Decisions

Recall a time you experienced a situation similar to Kim or Connor or encountered negative peer pressure. What decisions did you make in the situation? What were the outcomes of your decisions? Were you happy with these outcomes? Thinking back on the situation, use the decision-making process to outline other, healthier decisions you could have made. What could you have done to resist negative peer pressure and stick with your decisions? Create a journal entry of your answers and reflections.

True friends and dating partners respect each other's choices and encourage healthy behaviors. They also appreciate differences between people, including unique interests, opinions, and lifestyles. If you are experiencing negative peer pressure, you have the right to stand up for yourself and to walk away from situations that make you uncomfortable. If a friend or dating partner ends a relationship with you over this choice, that person does not respect you. Standing up to peer pressure is especially important when people are acting in ways that could hurt you or someone else.

Strategies for Handling Peer Pressure

What can you do to stand up to negative peer pressure and build an environment in which peer pressure is positive? How you respond to peer pressure will depend on the kind of pressure, the peers around you, and what skills you are most comfortable using. Strategies you can use to handle peer pressure include the following.

Focus on Yourself

Peer pressure can make you feel like you need to act or think a certain way to fit in. In reality, every person is unique and has different values and goals. To resist negative peer pressure, focus on your own thoughts, feelings, and values and make sure your actions reflect your beliefs and goals. If you feel out of touch with yourself, try journaling or taking time to reflect on how you *really* feel about a situation. Knowing and being confident in yourself and your judgment will give you the strength to walk away from a situation or from people who make you uncomfortable.

Build Respectful Relationships

In healthy, respectful relationships, people recognize each other's boundaries and accept if a person says *no* or is uncomfortable. To resist negative peer pressure, focus on building relationships with people who value you for who you are and do not try to change you. These healthy relationships should be free from negative peer pressure, and sometimes these friends can even help you resist pressure from others.

To reduce negative peer pressure and surround yourself with positive peer pressure, you can also choose friends who have values similar to yours. This will make you less likely to experience pressure to engage in unhealthy behaviors. People who share your values, goals, and beliefs will probably support your decisions.

Use Refusal Skills

Part of resisting negative peer pressure is communicating your decisions, boundaries, and affirmative consent or refusal clearly to other people. Communicating your boundaries can help others know what makes you comfortable or uncomfortable. It can also prepare you to walk away from unhealthy behaviors or dangerous situations.

refusal skills set of skills designed to help someone avoid participating in unhealthy behaviors

Sometimes, you will encounter influences or behaviors that get in the way of your decisions and goals. You might have a friend who wants you to stay up all night messaging back and forth or a dating partner who pressures you to vape. **Refusal skills** help you respond to these influences and behaviors without compromising your own goals, values, and health (**Figure 3.13**). With these skills, you can make independent, informed decisions despite the messages you receive from peers and society.

Examples of Refusal Skills

One day, you visit an older friend, and your friend takes you to a party with alcohol. At the end of the night, your friend is drunk, but intends to drive you home. You know it is not safe for your friend to drive. What do you do?

Skill	Examples
State your refusal	• "No, it isn't safe for you to drive right now. I don't want to ride with you and I don't think you should drive." • "No, that's not safe. Let's get a ride from someone who isn't drunk."
Give reasons	• "Drunk driving can kill people, including you and me." • "You could get arrested and lose your license for driving drunk."
Use your body language	• Stand up straight and look your friend in the eye. • Use a firm, confident voice.
Change the subject	• "Why don't we get some food first instead?" • "Let's go outside and hang out with friends a bit longer."
Tell a story	• "I know someone who almost died because he was hit by a drunk driver." • "Someone in my class lost her license for driving drunk."
Use humor	• "It's dangerous enough to drive around here sober!" • "I don't want you throwing up on the steering wheel."
Make an excuse	• "My parents will never let me visit again." • "Something in your car triggered my allergies."
Repeat your refusal	• Be prepared to repeat your refusal as many times as needed. • Do not waver or let someone convince you to do anything that makes you uncomfortable or is harmful to your health.
Leave the situation	• People may not always respect your refusal. If they continue to pressure you, physically leave the situation and go somewhere safe.

Figure 3.13 These are just a few of the refusal skills you can use. Practicing these skills will help you find the skills you are most comfortable using.

Support Others

Through your actions, you can create a culture of positive peer pressure and support people who are resisting negative peer pressure. The more people who are willing to stand up and say *no* to an unhealthy behavior, the more comfortable others will feel doing the same thing. Sometimes having just one other person say, "I agree, this is a bad idea," is all it takes to change a group's behavior.

If you see another person being pressured to do an activity the person does not want to do, take action. Tell the person who is applying the pressure to stop or offer to do another activity with the person who is being pressured. It may feel hard initially to stand up to negative peer pressure, but you will feel good about yourself for having the courage to do what is right for you.

Ask for Help

Sometimes peer pressure can feel like a lot to handle. Especially if the negative pressure lasts for a long time, you might feel like it is easier to give in. In these cases, do not be afraid to ask for help. Try getting advice from a trusted adult who has some experience handling peer pressure. If negative peer pressure continues over time, talk to someone you trust—a parent or guardian, school nurse, teacher, or school counselor—about the situation. You could also reach out to community resources, such as help lines or organizations, in your area.

Lesson 3.3 Review

Know and Understand

1. Explain the difference between positive and negative peer pressure.
2. How can focusing on yourself help you resist peer pressure?
3. Choose one strategy to refuse unhealthy behaviors and stick to your decision. Practice this strategy with a partner and ask for feedback.
4. Give one example of how you could support others in resisting peer pressure.

Analyze and Apply

5. When you are building a relationship, how do you know if a person values you for who you are or wants to change you?
6. In a small group, discuss what, if any, kinds of peer pressure are appropriate in a healthy relationship.
7. How can refusal skills help you avoid unsafe situations?

REAL WORLD Health Skills

Practice Health-Enhancing Behaviors Review the refusal skills introduced in this lesson. When faced with peer pressure, which refusal skill would you be most comfortable using? Describe how you would put this strategy into action. Which strategy would be the hardest or least comfortable for you? What would have to change for you to feel more comfortable using this strategy? Describe how you might put this strategy into action.

Chapter 3 Review and Assessment

Chapter Summary

Communication is the exchange of messages between people. In the communication process, a sender sends a message. The receiver receives the message and gives feedback to communicate the message was understood. Communication can be verbal or nonverbal. Verbal communication uses words—in person, written, or digital. Nonverbal communication includes all other forms of communication, including facial expressions, body language, and tone and volume of voice.

Effective communication requires positive communication skills. One important skill is active listening, which involves paying attention to the sender's message and giving feedback. A good communicator clearly expresses wants and needs and is assertive, rather than passive, passive-aggressive, or aggressive. Effective communication also uses I-statements, which focus on the speaker's thoughts and feelings without making accusations. Matching nonverbal communication to verbal communication and communicating carefully online, where nonverbal elements may not be present, are also important skills.

Conflict is a normal part of any relationship and results from misunderstandings and different priorities, values, goals, and needs. Conflict-resolution skills include communication skills and negotiation. In negotiation, people identify the cause of the conflict, ask for solutions from both parties, identify solutions they can support, agree on a solution, carry it out, and evaluate the solution. Remaining calm and respectful during this process is important. Mediation, which involves a neutral third party, can be helpful for difficult conflicts.

Peer pressure is the motivation to do certain activities or take on certain qualities to fit in with a group of peers. Positive peer pressure encourages healthy behaviors and is respectful. Negative peer pressure is not respectful and encourages unhealthy behaviors. To resist this type of peer pressure, you can focus on your own qualities and build respectful relationships. You can also use refusal skills—by stating your refusal, using humor, or changing the subject, for example. Supporting others and asking for help can also assist with resisting negative peer pressure.

Vocabulary Activity

Write the definition for each of the terms shown using everyday language and new expressions you have heard during class. Use words that other students will understand and that you will be able to easily remember. Double-check your definitions by using the text glossary.

active listening	*feedback*	*passive*
aggressive	*I-statements*	*passive-aggressive*
assertive	*mediation*	*peer mediation*
communication	*mediator*	*peer pressure*
communication process	*misunderstandings*	*positive peer pressure*
compromise	*negative peer pressure*	*pressure*
conflict	*negotiation*	*refusal skills*
conflict-resolution skills	*nonverbal communication*	*verbal communication*

Review and Recall

Review the information in this chapter by answering the following questions.

1. What is the purpose of giving feedback during communication?
2. Which of the following is an example of nonverbal communication?
   A. spoken words
   B. tone of voice
   C. written letter
   D. social media post
3. Which of the following is *not* part of active listening?
   A. reflecting the person's feelings
   B. making eye contact
   C. paraphrasing the message
   D. thinking about what you will say next
4. What could happen if you share sensitive content, like nude pictures or personal information, online?
5. Explain the difference between healthy and unhealthy conflict.
6. Why should you take some time and walk away from resolving a conflict if you feel very angry and upset?
7. Give an example of a compromise you made recently. What did you "give in" to make the compromise? What did the other person "give in"?
8. What happens in peer mediation?
9. If a friend makes fun of you for not working out after school, is this positive or negative peer pressure? Explain.
10. Which of the following is an effective nonverbal refusal skill?
    A. avoiding eye contact
    B. talking quietly
    C. saying *no*
    D. standing up straight
11. If people do not respect your refusal and keep pressuring you, what should you do?
12. Whom would you talk to if negative peer pressure continued over time to the point of being overwhelming?

Standardized Test Prep

Math Practice

The following results are from a study of US teens' feelings about social media. Review the results and answer the following questions.

81% of teens feel more connected to their friends because of social media.
69% of teens think social media helps them interact with more diverse people.
68% of teens feel friends on social media give them support through hard times.
45% of teens feel overwhelmed by the drama on social media.
43% of teens feel pressure to only post content that makes them look good.
37% of teens feel pressure to get likes and comments.

Source: "Teens' Social Media Habits and Experiences," Pew Research Center

13. Find out the number of students at your school. If these statistics were to hold true for your student population, how many more students feel connected on social media than feel overwhelmed by drama?
14. What percentage of teens did *not* feel social media gave them support through hard times?

Chapter 3 Skills Assessment

Critical Thinking Skills

Answer the following questions to assess your knowledge of what you learned in this chapter.

1. Online communication has evolved to include some elements of nonverbal communication. With a partner, list as many of these elements as you can and assess how effective each element is.
2. Think of situations in which you used or experienced the four different communication styles (passive, aggressive, passive-aggressive, and assertive). How did these styles make the people in these situations feel? What were the outcomes of these situations? How might the outcomes have been different if a different style was used?
3. Ask a trusted friend whether your nonverbal communication usually matches what you are saying. What did your friend say? Do you agree or disagree with your friend's assessment? Explain.
4. With a partner, make a list of guidelines for effective online communication. How do these guidelines differ from guidelines for in-person communication? Why?
5. What are your attitudes toward conflict? Does conflict frighten you? Do you enjoy conflict? What models in your life do you think influenced these attitudes, and how healthy are they?
6. Why do you think ignoring a conflict causes it to escalate?
7. In a conflict, it can be hard to see a situation from the other person's perspective. Why do you think this is? What skills can help people see both sides in a conflict?
8. If you cannot resolve a conflict, even after mediation, what next steps could you take? What resources in your family, school, or community could you use to handle the situation?
9. How does peer pressure compare to pressure in other relationships, such as family relationships?
10. How much do you think teens at your school experience peer pressure? Do most teens experience peer pressure to the same degree? Explain. What types of peer pressure are most common at your school?
11. Which refusal skills do you think are most effective for teens? least effective? Explain.
12. Explain why one person speaking up can change an entire group's behavior.
13. What resources in your school or community are available to help people experiencing negative peer pressure? What elements of peer pressure do these resources target?

Health and Wellness Skills

Complete the following activities to assess your skills related to health and wellness.

14 **Analyze Influences.** Online communication is an extremely popular way of staying in touch with family members and friends and meeting new people. How has online communication influenced you, your family, and teens in general? How has it influenced your communication, conflict-resolution, and refusal skills? Name five positive influences and five negative influences. Give strategies that could turn the negatives into positives.

15. **Access Information.** Sometimes people need outside help to resolve difficult conflicts or emotional situations. Using reliable sources, find out what resources are available in your area. Are there any resources specifically for teens? Research programs that might be available at your school or in your community to help with relationships. Examples might be peer mediation or healthy relationship programs. Make a list of programs and give a short description for each one. Include what services the resource provides and how to access them. Pair and share with a classmate.

16. **Communicate with Others.** Eventually, you will encounter people who disagree with you about certain health topics. When responding to a person you do not agree with, you may find it difficult to effectively communicate your knowledge and opinions while remaining respectful. With a partner, select one controversial health-related topic of your choice. Hold a discussion in which each of you argues different sides of an issue. Practice using strategies for overcoming communication barriers and disagreements.
17. **Make Decisions.** Relationships can affect health in a positive or a negative way. Extreme peer pressure and unsafe situations can cause a lot of harm, and it is important to make decisions and have some exit strategies to get yourself to safety. Make a list of eight to 10 decisions you could use in these situations to protect your own safety and well-being. Some examples might be telling a friend when you are going on a date or having a secret code word with your parent or guardian if you need help. What barriers might get in the way of you using these decisions? How would making these decisions protect your health?
18. **Set Goals.** Part of communicating effectively and building a healthy relationship is having positive interactions in addition to conflict. Think about a relationship you have. Set five SMART goals that involve positive interactions with this person. After you set your goals, reflect on the following question: Once you meet or fulfill your goals, do you think your relationship will change? Will it improve or become more positive? Explain.
19. **Advocate for Health.** Effective communication includes using audio and visual methods to present a message. Work together in small groups to create a public service announcement (PSA) that discusses the value of effective and respectful communication. Target teens with your PSA and include visual messages, such as pictures, graphics, or videos, as well as audio. Adapt your message to your audience and be sure to discuss effective online communication.

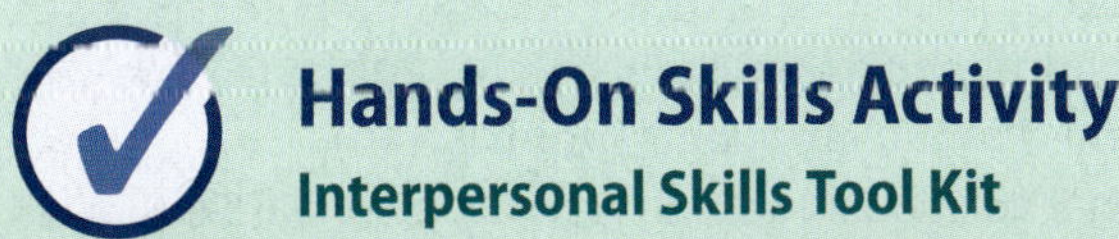

Hands-On Skills Activity

Interpersonal Skills Tool Kit

Sometimes, it can be hard to remember to practice the skills of effective communication and conflict resolution. In the moment, you might feel distracted or angry or have a hard time listening. The more you use effective interpersonal skills, however, the easier it will be. You may want a tool kit to help you when effective communication becomes difficult. This activity will allow you to create that kit with items that symbolize what has been discussed in this chapter. For this activity, you will need a brown paper bag, colored markers or pencils, pictures, and other items that symbolize the skills for effective communication.

Steps for This Activity

1. **Comprehend Concepts.** Review the skills involved in effective communication and conflict resolution. These can include skills for listening, communicating clearly, resolving conflict, and refusing unhealthy behaviors. Then, collect three to five items that remind you of the characteristics of effective communication. These items can be related to any type of communication and can remind you of skills like active listening, I-statements, negotiation, and refusal skills.
2. Decorate the outside of your paper bag with drawings or pictures that reflect the skills you most value and most need to practice. Illustrate how these skills impact health and support healthy relationships.
3. Place your collected items into your bag.
4. **Advocate for Health.** Bring your kit to class. Give a short presentation sharing the meanings behind the items or pictures you included. Use evidence you learned in this chapter to explain why you chose these items and pictures for your Interpersonal Skills Tool Kit.

Unit 2

Being Mentally and Emotionally Healthy

Chapter 4 Promoting Mental and Emotional Health
Chapter 5 Shifting to Positive Thinking
Chapter 6 Managing the Stress in Your Life
Chapter 7 Understanding Mental Illnesses

Big Ideas

- Your mental and emotional health include your internal thoughts and feelings. There is a continuum of mental and emotional health. Any condition that harms mental and emotional health is a *mental health condition*. Assessing your mental and emotional health and getting help are essential skills.
- Part of improving your mental and emotional health is embracing your identity, building self-esteem, and expressing emotions. There are many components of identity, and self-esteem is your feelings about yourself.
- Shifting to positive thinking benefits mental and emotional health. This involves establishing a positive mind-set that focuses on gratitude and sees setbacks as learning opportunities. Mindfulness is one helpful way of doing this.
- Thinking positively also involves developing empathy, which helps you relate to others, and resilience, which helps you recover from stressful situations.
- Stress is a normal part of life and can be positive when it motivates you to achieve your goals. Stress can also be negative if it is constant or poorly managed.
- Learning effective stress-management strategies, such as relaxation techniques and mindfulness-based stress reduction, can help you reduce the negative effects of stress.
- Mental illnesses are long-term mental health conditions that disrupt daily functioning. There are many types of mental illnesses—from anxiety disorders to mood disorders and substance use disorders. Getting treatment for a mental illness may involve taking mental health medications and seeing a mental health professional.
- It is important to seek help for thoughts of suicide in yourself or others. To help prevent suicide, you can promote a positive, respectful environment; recognize warning signs; and act to get help if warning signs are present.

Rawpixel/iStock/Getty Images Plus/Getty Images ▶

Health Management Plan Taking Care of Your Mental and Emotional Health

Your mental and emotional health affect what you feel, think, and do every day. For example, on some days, you might walk outside, spend time with friends, and complete your homework with energy to spare. On other days, you might withdraw from friends and have trouble getting everything done.

Many people talk with friends or turn to the internet to learn about mental and emotional health. This is partly because people sometimes have difficulty talking about this area of health. In this unit, you will learn about characteristics of positive mental and emotional health, skills for maintaining health in this area, and the role of professional treatment.

Open your health management plan. Create a new entry called "My Mental and Emotional Health." Then, work through these steps to make a plan for your mental and emotional health.

1. Answer the following questions based on what you know now. Explain your reasoning for each answer and reflect on the influences that have shaped your thinking:
   - What does it mean to have "positive mental and emotional health"? to be "happy"? Can a person be mentally and emotionally healthy and still have "bad days"?
   - How much control do people have over their mental and emotional health? What factors affect how mentally and emotionally healthy someone is?
   - Is stress a good or a bad thing? Why do some people get more stressed about certain situations than others?
   - What is the difference between having a hard time emotionally or being under stress and having a mental illness?
   - What is the purpose of mental health therapy? Is therapy only for people with a mental illness, or does it also benefit others?
2. Revisit your answers after reading this unit and rewrite them as needed. How has your understanding of mental and emotional health changed?
3. Create three lists. In the first, list questions you can ask yourself to assess mental and emotional health throughout your life. In the second, list skills you personally can use to improve or maintain your mental and emotional health. In the third, list how you would know if you needed professional help and how you would get it.

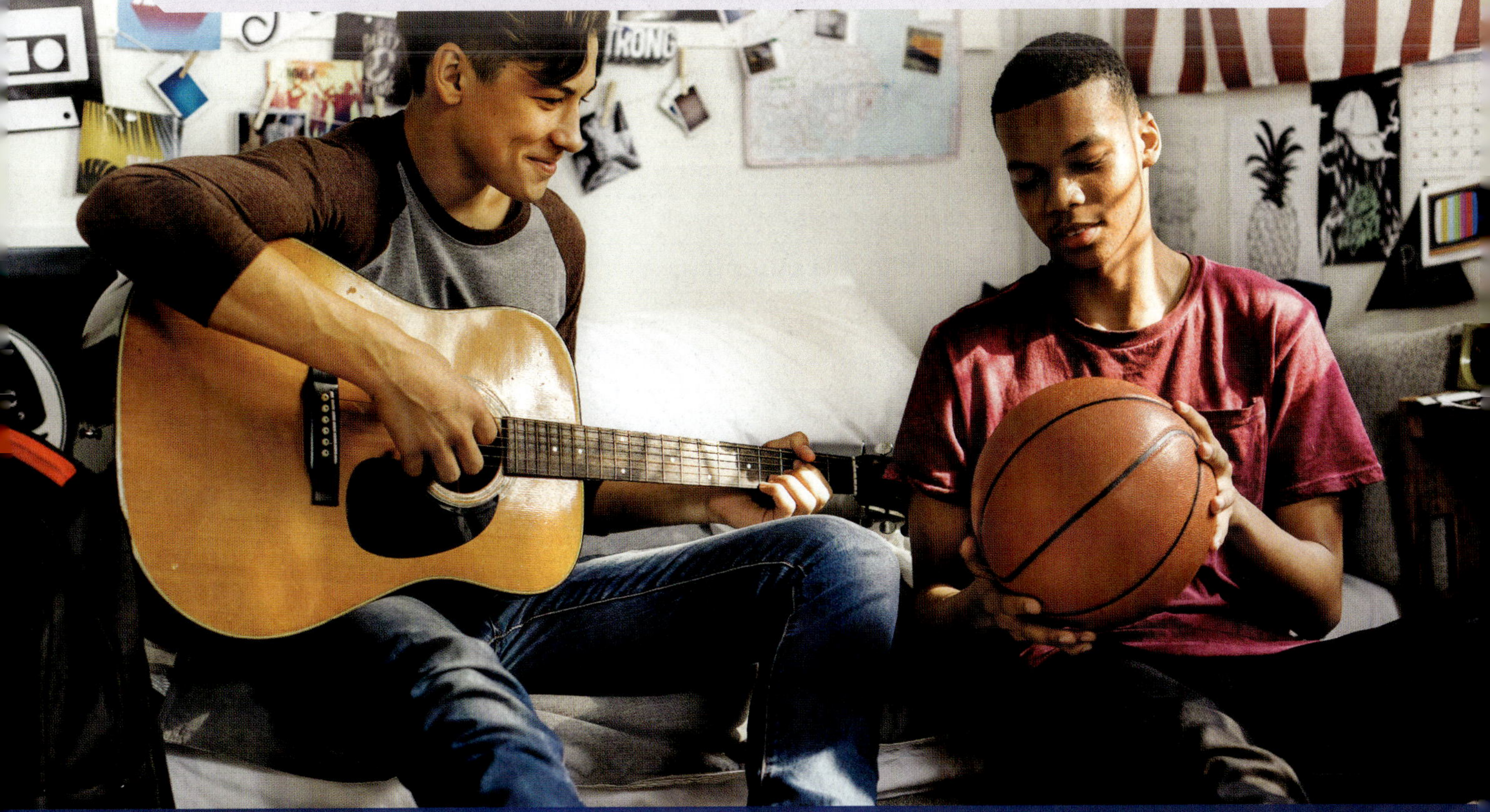

Chapter 4

Promoting Mental and Emotional Health

Look for the skills icon throughout this chapter for opportunities to practice your health skills.

Check Your Health and Wellness Skills

In this chapter, you will learn skills for maintaining positive mental and emotional health. To understand the skills you currently use, take the following inventory of your behaviors. Indicate how well you think you use each skill. Use a scale of 1–5, *1* meaning you do not use the skill and *5* meaning you feel completely comfortable using it.

Skill	How Well Do You Use Each Skill?
I take a break from social media if it's causing me anxiety.	
I know that few situations are "all good" or "all bad." Most fall in between.	
I'm okay with not always being right.	
I know how to get help if I'm depressed or anxious or have thoughts of hurting myself.	
I try new activities and learn from mistakes to discover more about myself.	
I like learning about people's opinions, even if they're different from mine.	
I accept criticism and know it doesn't impact my worth.	
I practice self-care by taking time to do activities I enjoy.	
When I notice an emotion, I try to figure out its cause instead of ignoring it.	
I accept my feelings, even if they aren't how I want to feel.	
When I talk about my feelings, I use I-statements instead of you-statements.	
	Total:

Add up your responses to each statement. The higher your score, the more comfortable you feel practicing health skills related to mental and emotional health. Which skill do you think is most important for you? Which skill is the most challenging for you? Which skill would you most like to improve? In this chapter, you will learn how to perform these skills better and more often.

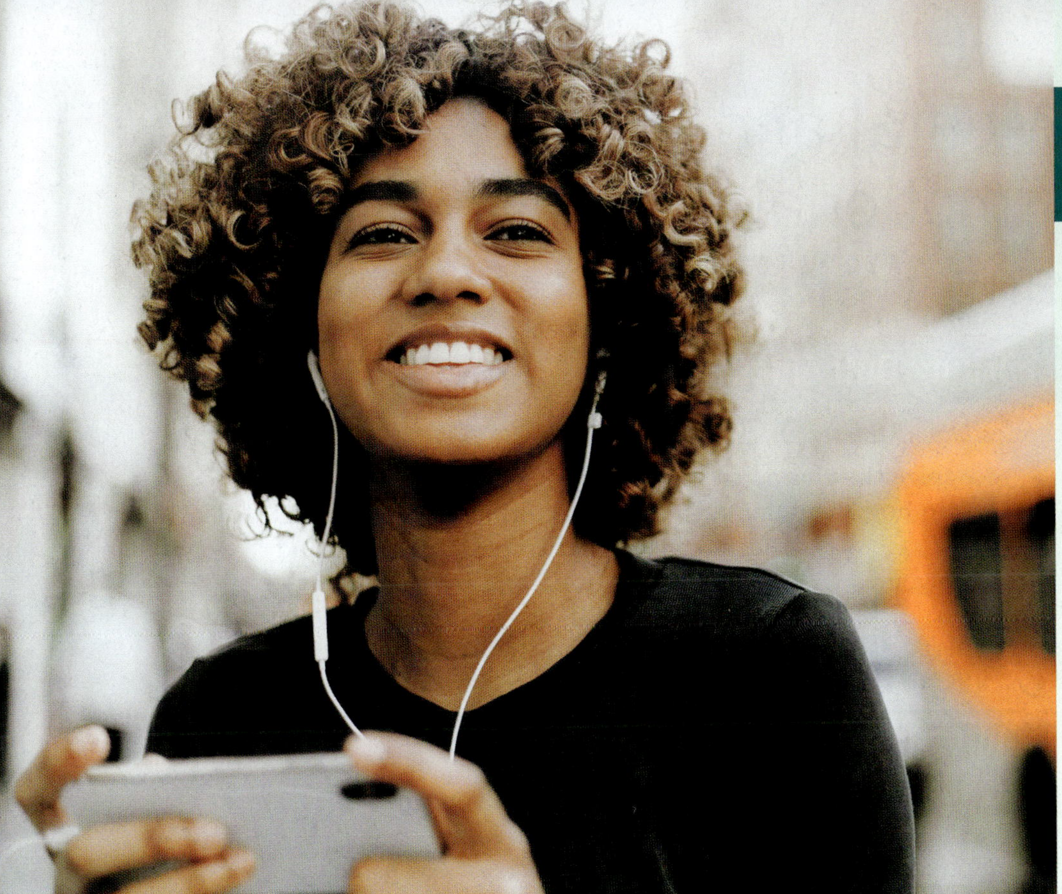

Rawpixel.com/Shutterstock.com

Reading and Notetaking

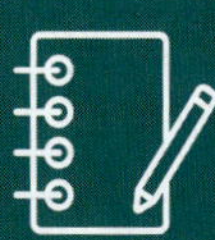

Create a table like the one shown. As your teacher presents this chapter, list the main topics and ways to maintain mental and emotional health. Identify as many details as you need and include information with which you are familiar and unfamiliar. (An example is provided for you.) Then, team up with a classmate to discuss each other's lists. What items do you need to add? If there is anything you do not understand, seek clarification from your teacher.

Main Topics	Ways of Maintaining Mental and Emotional Health
Personal identity	Recognize strengths, seek feedback from others

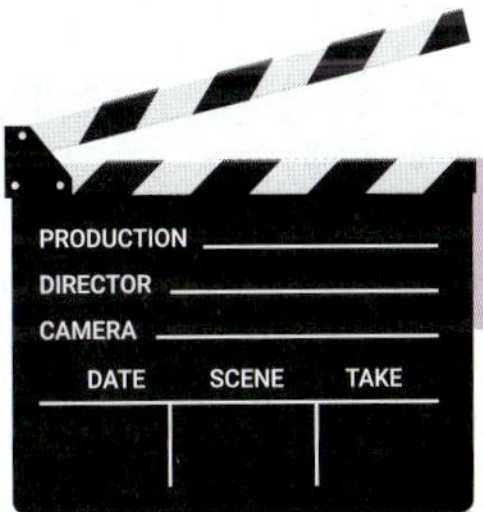

Setting the Scene

Developing Your Own Identity

Lately, you have been trying to figure out your own goals, beliefs, and values. You know that your parents hold certain expectations for you, such as doing well in school. You also feel pressure from friends at school to dress a certain way, listen to particular kinds of music, and participate in specific school clubs. Sometimes it feels hard to figure out who you really are.

This year, your goal is to pay more attention to your own thoughts and feelings. You want to make sure you choose activities that interest *you*, not just those that other people want you to do. You decide to talk to your school counselor and get some advice on learning about your interests and abilities.

Thinking Critically

1. What are some factors that might make it hard for teens to figure out their own identities?
2. What strategies can you use to learn more about your own goals, interests, and abilities?

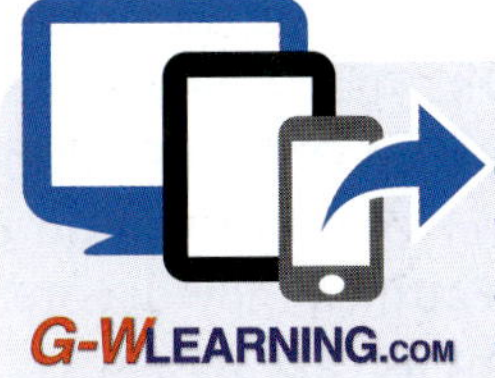

Click on the activity icon or visit www.g-wlearning.com/health/4095 to access online vocabulary activities using key terms from the chapter.

Lesson 4.1

Mental and Emotional Health and Well-Being

Essential Question

What does it mean to be mentally and emotionally healthy?

Learning Outcomes

After studying this lesson, you will be able to

- recognize the characteristics of mental and emotional health;
- explain how mental and emotional health are a continuum;
- identify factors affecting mental and emotional health; and
- assess your own mental and emotional health.

Key Terms

cognitive distortions
genetic predisposition
Maslow's hierarchy of human needs
mental distress
mental health conditions
self-actualization

Warm-Up Activity

Mental and Emotional Health Wheel

Practice Health-Enhancing Behaviors Before reading this lesson, recreate the pie chart shown. Read the statements next to each section of the pie chart and decide what percentage out of 100 percent you accomplish the actions or feel the statements reflect your life. Color in the section of the pie chart with the appropriate color to show the percentage. Which areas were colored in 100 percent? Which areas need work, and why?

A—Blue I have my emotions under control.
B—Red I have people I can trust who trust me back.
C—Green I am not afraid of challenges.
D—Purple I have many activities I enjoy.
E—Orange I treat others with respect and kindness.

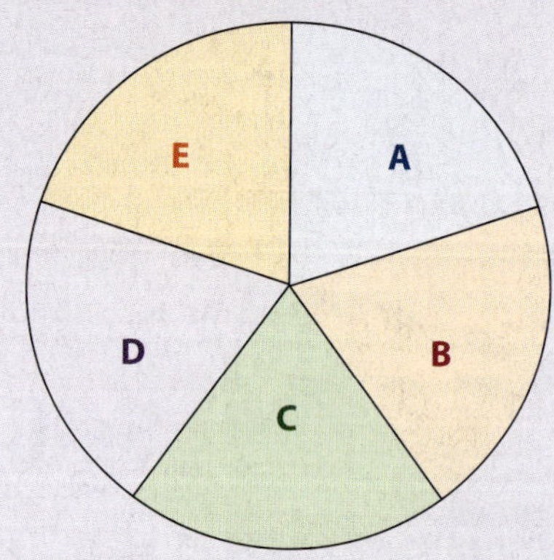

Think about all of the steps you take to stay physically healthy. Do you eat nutritious foods, like fruits and vegetables? Do you get physical activity and try to avoid getting sick and injured? How do you know you are physically healthy? Now, think about your mental and emotional health. How do you know if you are mentally and emotionally healthy? What steps do you take every day to improve your health in these areas? Did you know that taking care of your mental and emotional health is just as important as taking care of your physical health?

Many people do not devote as much time to mental and emotional health as they devote to physical health. Mental and emotional health is not as easy to assess. This may cause people to think their mental and emotional health is not as important. They may feel like this dimension does not matter since it is harder to observe from the outside. In this lesson, you will learn about the importance of mental and emotional health, factors affecting this dimension of health, and ways of assessing your mental and emotional health.

What Are Mental and Emotional Health?

As you learned in Chapter 1, *mental and emotional health* describe the health of your internal life. *Mental health* describes how you observe and interpret information, including events and the world around you. It affects how you make decisions, solve problems, and examine situations. *Emotional health* refers to how you express yourself and your thoughts and feelings. It includes your emotions, mood, feelings about yourself, and way of viewing the world.

People with positive mental and emotional health share several traits and characteristics (**Figure 4.1**). Positive mental and emotional health contribute to *well-being*, or your satisfaction with life.

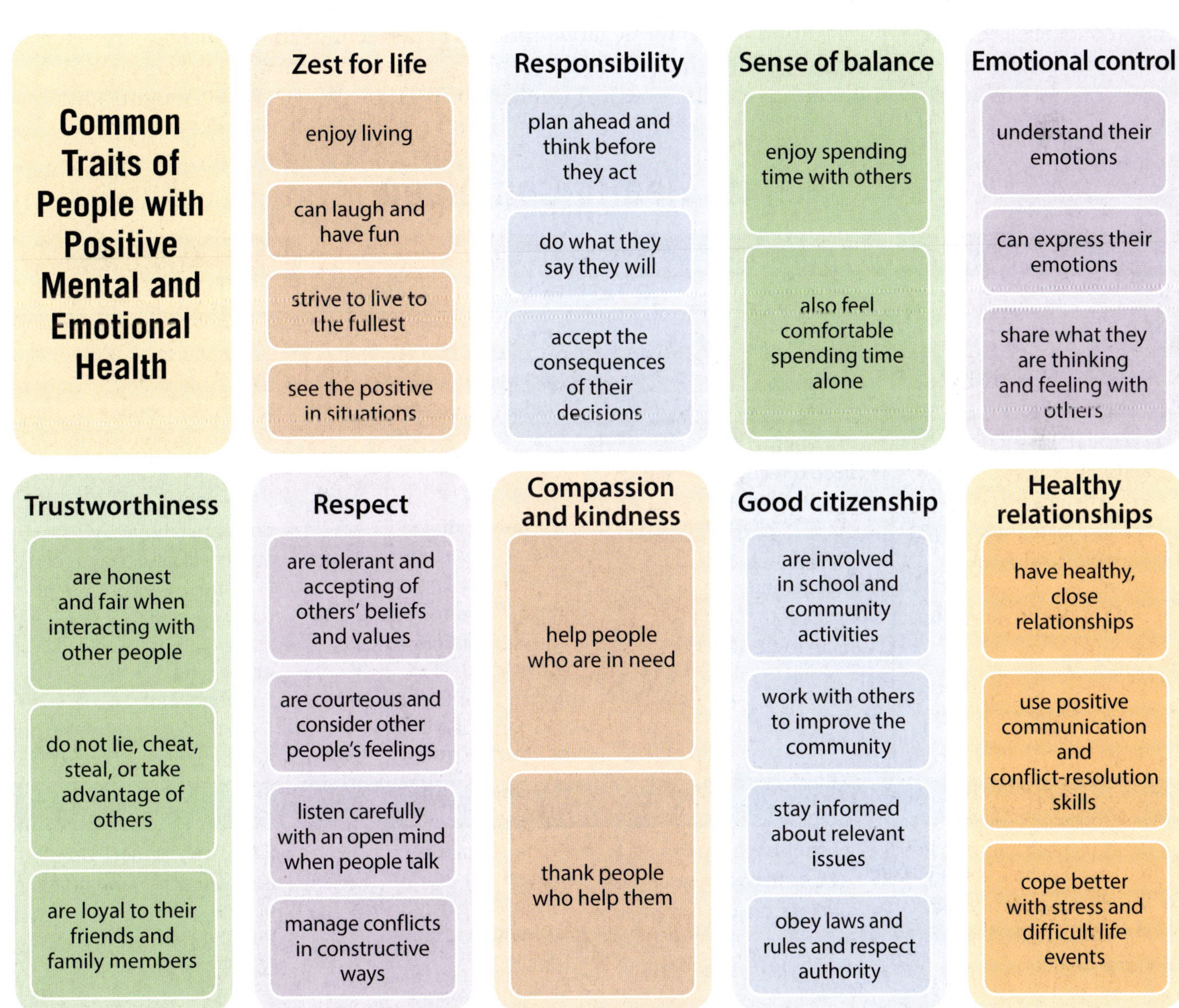

Figure 4.1 Positive mental and emotional health help you think, feel, and behave in ways that support your health and goals. ***What term refers to how you express yourself and your thoughts and feelings?***

Positive mental and emotional health have many benefits. People with positive mental and emotional health are better able to work productively in school and in their careers and are more likely to feel successful and content. They are better able to cope with minor and major stresses. They do not get stuck when difficult situations occur, but can work through them and know when to ask for help. Having positive mental and emotional health also helps people make meaningful contributions to their family, school, and community. In other words, people benefit from feeling good about themselves and also benefit when other people in the community feel positively.

The Mental and Emotional Health Continuum

mental health conditions patterns of thinking and feeling that decrease mental and emotional health; can be everyday worries or serious mental illnesses

Like other areas of health, mental and emotional health exist on a continuum (**Figure 4.2**). Having positive mental and emotional health does not mean feeling good all the time. Similarly, having a mental health condition does not mean a person cannot experience elements of positive mental and emotional health.

All people feel sad sometimes, become tired, experience fluctuations in mood, and have negative thoughts and feelings in response to stressful events. Thoughts and feelings that decrease your mental and emotional health are called **mental health conditions**. When these thoughts and

Mental Health Continuum

Healthy	Reacting	Injured	Ill
• Some mood fluctuations • Typical energy level • Typical sleep habits • Sense of humor • Performance of daily tasks • Social engagement • Confidence in self and others • Little or no substance use	• Sadness • Overwhelmed feeling • Low energy • Sleep difficulties • Procrastination • Forgetfulness • Decreased social engagement • Intrusive thoughts • Regular substance use	• Feelings of pervasive sadness, hopelessness, or worthlessness • Anxiety and anger • Fatigue • Restless sleep • Difficulty concentrating • Difficulty making decisions • Impaired performance • Withdrawal from social activities • Recurring intrusive thoughts • Substance use that is difficult to control	• Panic attacks and excessive anxiety • Aggressive, angry behavior • Numbness • Depression • Constant fatigue • Inability to fall or stay asleep • Inability to concentrate or make decisions • Inability to perform daily tasks • Social isolation • Thoughts of suicide • Addiction to a substance
Actions You Can Take			
• Break problems and goals into manageable chunks • Maintain support system • Maintain healthy lifestyle • Focus on goals	• Recognize personal limits • Use healthy coping strategies • Reduce stressors • Get enough physical activity, rest, and nutritious food	• Examine reasons for distress • Talk with a trusted adult or friend • Seek help • Seek social support	• Seek professional help • Follow recommendations of mental health professional

Figure 4.2 A person's state of mental and emotional health is neither "all good" nor "all bad." Most people fall somewhere in the middle, and people can take actions to improve their health.

feelings temporarily impair your ability to cope with daily life, they are called **mental distress**. Mental distress is a short-term experience. For example, you might feel sad after having a fight with a friend or anxious about an upcoming test. Mental distress may disrupt your life in some way—perhaps you have trouble sleeping or lose your appetite—but is not a diagnosable mental health condition.

mental distress
short-term mental and emotional state in which negative thoughts and feelings impair relationships, daily tasks, and enjoyment of life

Some people have serious mental health conditions that do not go away and involve changes in thinking, emotion, and behavior. These are known as *mental illnesses* or *mental disorders*. Some examples include major depressive disorder, anxiety disorders, bipolar disorder, and post-traumatic stress disorder (PTSD). People with these diagnosable conditions need professional treatment to manage their symptoms. You will learn more about mental illnesses in chapters 6 and 7.

Factors Affecting Mental and Emotional Health

Both internal and external factors help shape your thoughts and feelings. For example, your genetic makeup can influence how happy you feel. The way you think now can shape your thought patterns in the future. At the same time, your relationships may influence how you feel. The stress in your environment can make positive thinking more or less difficult.

Research in Action

Technology and Your Mental and Emotional Health

Did you know that technology use influences your mental and emotional health? Researchers at San Diego State University conducted a large study to examine the link between technology use and mental and emotional health in teens.

In this study, they asked more than one million students in grades 8, 10, and 12 how much time they spent on their phones, tablets, and computers. They also asked how much time these teens spent on in-person social interactions and about students' overall feelings of happiness.

Can you predict the study's findings? First, teens who spent more time on their screens were less happy compared to teens who spent more time on other types of activities, such as playing sports, reading magazines, and interacting face-to-face. Teens who spent less than one hour a day on their screens were the happiest, and every additional hour spent on a screen was linked to increases in unhappiness. This study provides strong evidence that putting away your digital devices and spending time with friends in person is a great way to feel happier and maintain your mental and emotional health.

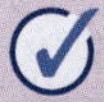

Practice Your Skills

Advocate for Health

Do you find it surprising that spending lots of time using technology is linked to more unhappiness? In small groups, discuss the findings of this study. Why do you think spending more than one hour using a screen each day is associated with fewer feelings of happiness? What factors do you think explain this relationship? In your group, discuss if technology use has any *benefits* for mental and emotional health. How do these benefits compare to the possible negative influences? Based on your discussion, create a short flyer, poem, song, or video highlighting the effects of technology on mental and emotional health. Your target audience should be fellow teens. Share this flyer, poem, song, or video with your class.

Genetics

Do you know some people who always seem to be happy? Research shows that the genes people inherit from their biological parents have a substantial impact on how people feel. As you know, having a genetic risk factor does not always mean a person will develop a condition. It means that person has an increased risk.

For example, genes play a role in your ability to see the good in all situations. Genes also influence a person's risk for mental illnesses. People who have a family member with major depressive disorder or a schizophrenia spectrum disorder, for example, have a greater risk of developing these conditions themselves. This increased likelihood is called a **genetic predisposition**.

genetic predisposition increased likelihood of developing a health condition due to genes inherited from biological parents

Genes also influence how resilient people are in the face of difficult situations. Researchers in one study found that people with one type of genetic makeup can bounce back from stressful life events relatively easily. These people are able to pick themselves up and move on. Other people who experience many stressful events can feel defeated or develop a mental health condition.

Upbringing and Experiences

Life experiences, which include your relationships and the way you were raised, have a substantial impact on mental and emotional health. People who experience stressful life events have a greater risk of developing negative feelings or thought patterns and mental health conditions, including mental illnesses (**Figure 4.3**). Ongoing stressors, such as racism or financial pressure, can also increase this risk.

Fortunately, positive life experiences can work against some of the negative effects of stressful life events. People who grow up with strong support from their family members, trusted adults, or friends cope better with difficult circumstances. This is one reason investing time and energy in developing healthy, close relationships is so important.

Stressful Events
death of a loved one
divorce
significant family conflict
family move
change in a job
natural disaster
abuse or neglect
sexual assault
substance use disorder

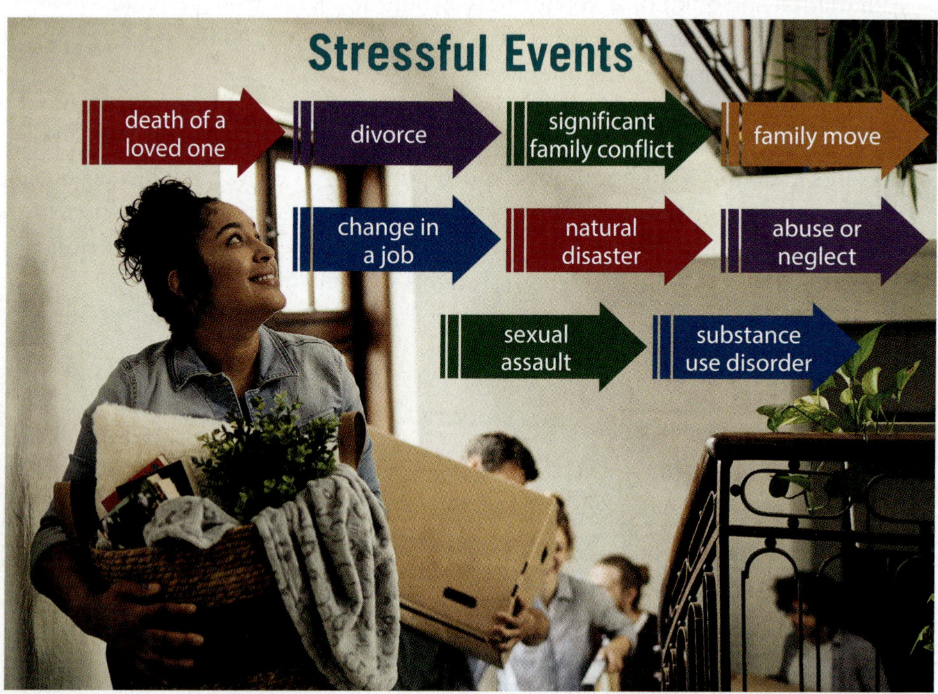

Geber86/E+/Getty Images

Figure 4.3 Common stressful events can negatively impact a person's mental and emotional health.

Environment

Your environment has a large impact on your mental and emotional health and includes your relationships, culture, and community. Part of being mentally and emotionally healthy is working toward **self-actualization**, or the feeling that you are reaching your full potential. According to psychologist Abraham Maslow, meeting other needs helps lead to these feelings.

Maslow's hierarchy of human needs categorizes needs and shows how they progress (**Figure 4.4**). For example, at the most basic level, people meet their physical needs for survival. These needs include having food to eat, water to drink, and shelter from extreme cold and heat. Once basic physical needs are met, people are better able to meet needs listed in the next level.

How well your environment meets needs at each level in Maslow's hierarchy of human needs affects mental and emotional health. For example, not having the resources to meet physical needs can harm a person's feelings of love, acceptance, and esteem. A community with lots of violence can make a person feel afraid. This can reduce a person's feeling of security and make it more difficult to feel love and acceptance. Strong relationships play an essential role in helping people feel good about themselves and live up to their full potential.

self-actualization feeling of reaching one's full potential through creativity, independence, spontaneity, and a grasp of the real world

Maslow's hierarchy of human needs model of understanding human needs, in which basic needs are met before higher-level needs

Social Media and Technology

Media and technology are part of your environment. For example, TV shows and advertisements reflect the beliefs of the culture and community in which you live. Media messages that make you feel good about yourself can improve mental and emotional health. Messages that you need to be richer or more successful, attractive, or accomplished to feel fulfilled harm mental and emotional health.

Social media is an important part of your social environment, including your relationships with friends. This way of communicating can make friendships easier to maintain and offers support, even when you are alone. Close friendships and frequent communication can increase feelings of connection. Social media and the internet can help people get good advice and reach helpful resources.

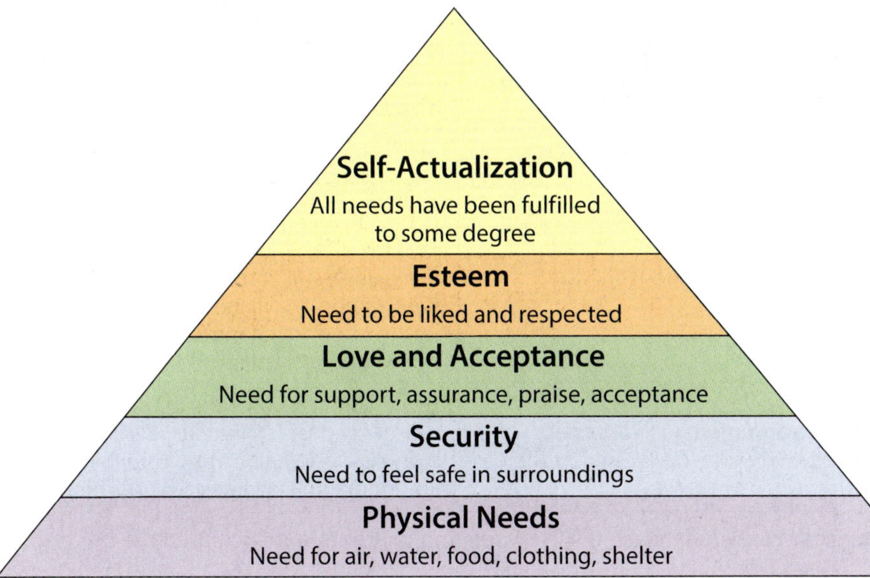

Figure 4.4 Maslow's hierarchy illustrates how people can move from meeting their basic needs for water, food, clothing, and shelter to more complex needs. ***Where would you place yourself on Maslow's hierarchy of needs? Which needs in your life are being met? Which needs are not being met?***

Social media can also negatively impact your mental and emotional health. Research shows that teens who spend more time on social media show more sadness, fatigue, and anxiety and have more negative views of themselves. This is partly because social media creates pressure to present a certain type of image. Teens may feel anxiety trying to respond quickly to online messages, craft perfect posts, and show flattering photographs. Social media can lead to feelings of jealousy and envy. People on social media mostly share the positive aspects of their lives, making it seem like they have exciting—even perfect—lives. This type of comparison leads to worse mental and emotional health.

Patterns of Thinking

People's thoughts about themselves and the world have a significant influence on mental and emotional health. Negative and self-defeating thoughts, for example, generally make people feel worse. An example of a self-defeating thought is thinking you will never be good at science because you performed poorly on a science test. This self-defeating thought about one bad experience creates a negative, unhealthy cycle.

cognitive distortions
unhealthy patterns of thinking that are often not grounded in reality

Over time, unhealthy thought patterns, called **cognitive distortions**, can lead to worse mental and emotional health (**Figure 4.5**).

Cognitive Distortions

Thinking Pattern	Description and Examples	To Challenge This Pattern, Ask Yourself...
Black-and-white thinking	People categorize everything as either *all good* or *all bad*. They do not view situations in more complex ways. They either think *I am perfect* or *I am a failure*.	What is positive about this situation? What is negative about this situation?
Jumping to conclusions	People assume they know what other people are thinking and why they behave as they do. If they encounter people who are unfriendly, they jump to the conclusion that people do not like them. In reality, some people may just be shy.	What evidence do I have for my conclusion? Is there another explanation I am not considering?
Catastrophizing	People believe that every event—even a relatively inconsequential event—has a huge and negative possible consequence. For example, if people do poorly on one exam, they believe they will never get into college.	Will this event necessarily lead to the conclusion I am dreading, and would that be so bad?
Control fallacies (mistaken beliefs)	People believe they are victims of circumstances; they do not see their role in creating situations. If they get a low grade on an English paper because they procrastinated, they blame their teacher for not providing enough time.	What was my role in creating this situation? What could I have done differently to achieve a different outcome? How can I prevent this in the future?
Emotional reasoning	People believe that whatever they feel at the moment is a permanent condition. If they spend a weekend feeling lazy and bored, they believe they are and will always be lazy and bored.	Have I always felt this way in the past? If not, why do I believe I will always feel this way in the future?
Fallacy (mistaken belief) of change	People believe they can pressure or persuade other people to change. In reality, people cannot change anyone except themselves.	Have my efforts to change this person been successful in the past? Can I accept that this person will never change? If the person does not change, do I want to stay in this relationship?
Always being right	People constantly try to prove their attitudes and behaviors are correct. In an argument with another person, they focus more on winning the argument than on issues and feelings.	How would I feel if I were in the other person's shoes? Is this really a right or wrong issue? What is more valuable: being right or maintaining this relationship?

Figure 4.5 Over time, cognitive distortions can cause loneliness, difficulty relating to others, and increased risk of developing a mental health condition.

Cognitive distortions can also create anxiety. People may worry obsessively about upcoming events and imagine bad outcomes. In many cases, these bad outcomes do not actually occur, but repeatedly thinking about negative possibilities creates considerable stress.

Assessing Your Mental and Emotional Health and Well-Being

Everyone has times they feel better and times they feel worse. These fluctuations in mood are a normal part of life. Still, mental health conditions and negative thoughts and feelings can interfere with life and make it difficult to perform daily tasks, maintain relationships, and reach goals. It is important to regularly assess the health of your thoughts and feelings and seek help, if needed.

Seeking help can be as simple as talking to a trusted adult or friend. Mental health conditions can seriously impact a person's health and future, so seeking help is important to prevent negative consequences. Serious mental health conditions and mental illnesses require professional treatment to manage symptoms.

To assess your own mental and emotional health, consider the thoughts and feelings you experience throughout the day. For example, you might keep a journal of your feelings. Identify what events, if any, trigger certain feelings. Are your feelings mostly positive or negative? Are your thoughts encouraging or defeating?

By assessing yourself, you can identify and improve some areas of your mental and emotional health. For example, if you notice that you spend a lot of time criticizing yourself, you can make an effort to pay attention to what is going well. By assessing your mental and emotional health, you can also determine if you need to seek help in this area (**Figure 4.6**).

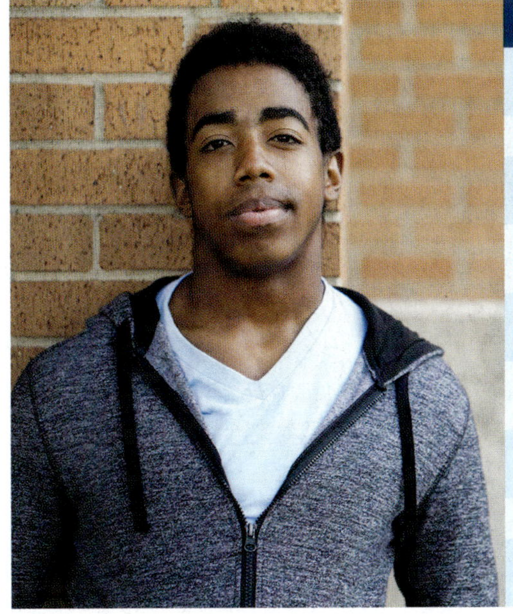

Seeking help would be a good idea if you...

- get really mad about small conflicts or constantly argue with friends and family
- have difficulty sleeping, including getting to sleep or staying asleep
- have difficulty spending time with people and avoid people, in person and online (for example, by withdrawing from social events)
- notice unexplained changes in your weight or appetite (such as overeating or a loss of appetite)
- are unable to relax or have a racing mind or heart, headaches, upset stomach, constant tension, or a persistent feeling of anxiety or dread
- have trouble completing daily tasks because of negative feelings or feelings of numbness
- are using a substance, like tobacco, alcohol, or drugs, to avoid or deal with negative feelings
- think about or have already physically hurt yourself or others
- think a lot of about escaping your current situation or believe others would be better off without you

pixelheadphoto digitalskillet/Shutterstock.com

Figure 4.6 Some common symptoms, such as those listed, indicate a need to seek professional help. ***Why is it important to seek help right away?***

Skills for Health and Wellness

Mental and Emotional Health Checkup

Once a year, you probably get an annual physical and wellness exam to check on your physical health. During the exam, your doctor measures your height and weight, examines your body for symptoms of disease, and answers any questions you have about your health. This yearly checkup helps you track your physical health and make plans to improve it.

Think about this: What similar steps could you take to understand and improve your mental and emotional health? What would be involved in a mental and emotional health checkup? How often do you think people should check on their mental and emotional health?

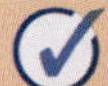

Practice Your Skills

Practice Health-Enhancing Behaviors

Using the questions that follow, perform a mental and emotional health checkup to better understand your own state of mental and emotional health. Consider each question carefully and write or record yourself saying your answer.

- How often do you find yourself worrying about situations? How intense is your worry? Does worrying distract you from tasks you need to be doing?
- How well have you been sleeping? Have you had trouble falling or staying asleep?
- What kinds of statements have you been making about yourself in your own head? Have you been critical of yourself? confident in your abilities?
- Have your friends mentioned any changes in your behavior? If so, what kinds of changes?
- How happy or sad have you been feeling? Do feelings of sadness go away after a while, or do they persist?
- Think about the activities you like doing most. Do you still enjoy them? What, if any, new activities have you tried recently?
- How well have you been maintaining your relationships with your friends? Are your relationships healthy? What conflicts have you experienced? Have you noticed yourself withdrawing or leaning on your friends for support in difficult situations?
- Do you feel in control of your emotions and actions? How do you cope with negative feelings and thoughts? For example, when you feel sad, do you go for a walk? talk with friends? write in a journal?
- Who is part of your support system? When you are having a hard time, whom do you reach out to? Do you feel comfortable communicating your emotions, positive and negative, with the people in your support system?
- Have you noticed any unexplained changes in your weight, appetite, level of energy, or mood? Explain.

Once you have answered all of these questions, read through your answers or listen to your recording. Did any of your answers surprise you? Try to identify the reason for any feelings and behaviors that concern you.

Based on your answers, what areas of your mental and emotional health do you think most need to improve? Talk with your doctor or a trusted adult about the results of your checkup and then brainstorm strategies you can use to improve your mental and emotional health. Make plans to cope in certain ways, such as talking to a close friend, doing an activity you enjoy, getting a good night's sleep, or seeking professional help.

Save the results of your checkup so you can compare results when you perform the checkup again. Regularly checking on your mental and emotional health can help you keep track of your thoughts and feelings, try new strategies, and get help if you ever need it.

If you experience any of these symptoms, or notice them in a friend or family member, talk to a trusted adult about seeking help. Treat thoughts of hurting yourself or others as an emergency. If you experience these symptoms or know someone else who is, call the National Suicide Prevention Lifeline (1-800-273-8255) or 911. You will learn more about suicide and suicide prevention in Chapter 7. Many mental health conditions and mental illnesses are easiest to treat if diagnosed early, so do not wait to get help.

Lesson 4.1 Review

Know and Understand

1. Describe the difference between mental and emotional health.
2. Choose one characteristic of people with positive mental and emotional health and explain how it reflects that someone is mentally and emotionally healthy.
3. What is the benefit of positive mental and emotional health in your life?
4. With a partner, discuss the difference between mental distress, a mental health condition, and a mental illness.
5. How does family influence mental and emotional health? Consider the influence of family genetically and socially.
6. Choose one cognitive distortion and give an example of how it has affected you. What steps can you take to challenge this pattern of thinking?

Think Critically

7. Review the mental health continuum and think about where you would place yourself today. Record a short audio journal or voice memo explaining your reasoning.
8. What are the beliefs surrounding mental and emotional health in your school and community? How does this culture influence you and your peers?
9. Review the list of symptoms that indicate you need to seek professional help for your mental and emotional health in Figure 4.6. What would these symptoms look like in your life? For example, would withdrawing mean you chat with your friends less than once a week? Create a personalized list of symptoms with specific behaviors that would mean *you* need professional help.

REAL WORLD Health Skills

Access Information Mental and emotional health are extremely important, and many people face stress, difficult situations, and feelings that reduce health. Seeking professional help can be extremely beneficial, whether a person is diagnosed with a mental illness or not. Using reliable resources, design a "help sheet" that identifies the names and contact information of mental health resources in your community. Group different types of professional help into categories, such as hotlines, agencies, therapists, and nonprofit organizations. Research each resource to find out the services it offers and how people can access those services.

Lesson 4.2

Embracing Your Identity

Essential Question?

What is identity, and how can you embrace it?

Learning Outcomes

After studying this lesson, you will be able to

- explain the importance of self-discovery;
- describe the different parts of a person's identity; and
- take steps to discover and embrace your unique identity.

Key Terms

biological sex
core values
ethnicity
gender
gender identity
gender roles
gender stereotypes
identity
identity formation
personality

Warm-Up Activity

Who Are You? Collage

Analyze Influences Construct a "Who Are You?" collage. Your collage can be a physical artistic representation or a digital product. In your collage, include pictures, words, and quotes that describe who you are. Once you have added as many items to your collage as you can, answer the following questions in as much detail as possible:

My Past	My Present	My Future
• Which people have had the biggest effect in my life? • What meaningful places have I visited? • What past experiences have had an impact on my life?	• What do I think of myself at this very moment? • What activities do I enjoy? • What makes me happy? • What interests me?	• What do I want to do in my life? • What are my goals and dreams? • What profession would I choose if I had no limitations or barriers in my way?

The teen years are typically a period of self-discovery. As you grow up, you might ask yourself, "Who am I? What do I want to do?" On the quest to learn more about yourself, you might test out different interests, values, and beliefs. You might hang out with different friends, experiment with fashion and music, or join clubs. This process of self-discovery is important. Figuring out your **identity**, or who you are, will help you feel better about yourself and make good decisions. Knowing and being comfortable with yourself is an essential step in improving your mental and emotional health.

identity characteristics and qualities that distinguish who a person is

Components of Identity

Think about how you are similar to and different from your friends. You may be the same age as many of your friends, but have different interests.

Maybe your best friend is in the same activities, but you have different cultural backgrounds and roles in your families. Many different pieces make up a person's identity. The importance a person places on each piece is also part of identity.

Core Values and Beliefs

A person's core values are a key part of identity. **Core values** are the fundamental beliefs and ideals people hold that guide their behaviors and choices (**Figure 4.7**). Often, parents or guardians and other family members teach their children core values. A person's cultural background and experience also influence core values. As people grow older, they examine their own core values through self-exploration and decide which core values are most important to them.

core values part of identity that describes what a person believes and finds important; guide personal behaviors and choices

Your core values impact the goals you set, the decisions you make, and the relationships you maintain. For example, if knowledge is one of your core values, you might decide to pursue education beyond high school and become a professor. If one of your core values is kindness, you might decide to volunteer in your community or prioritize being there for your friends.

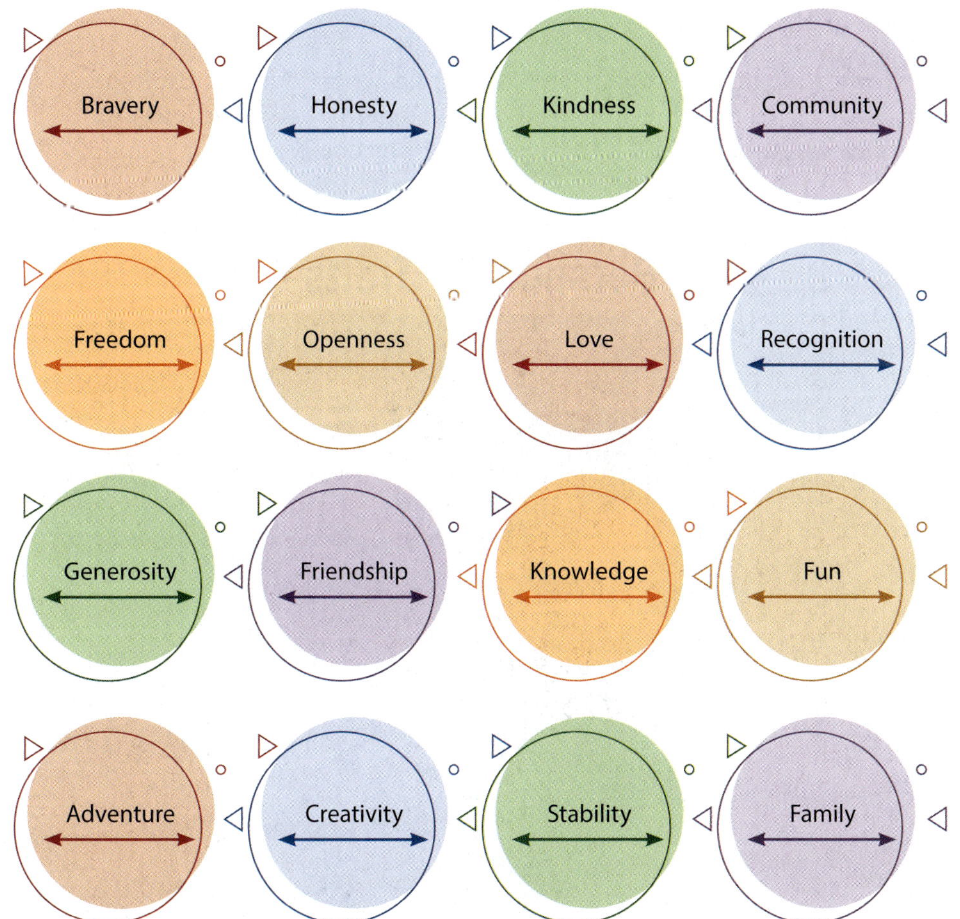

Figure 4.7 All people have a different set of core values, depending on their own life experiences and the influence of their friends, families, and cultures. ***How do family members influence children's core values?***

Personality

personality combination of thoughts, feelings, and behaviors that make a person unique

Another important part of identity is **personality**, or the combination of thoughts, feelings, and behaviors that make you unique (**Figure 4.8**). For example, some people are more *extroverted*, or outgoing and social. Others are more *introverted*, or quiet and reserved. Your personality traits influence how you think about the world, what activities you like, and how you respond to setbacks and disappointments. Personality is generally stable over time. If you were helpful as a child, you will probably be helpful as a teen and adult.

Physical Identity

Your physical identity is made up of your physical characteristics. These characteristics include your biological sex, race, age, height, weight, hair or eye color, and physical abilities. The color of your skin is part of your physical identity. So is your ability or inability to throw a ball, walk, lift weights, and hear a conversation. Your physical identity can influence your behavior. If you are naturally athletic, for example, you may choose to spend time playing sports or being active.

People who have some type of disability may hold a specific type of identity called *disability identity*. Disability identity refers to a person's sense of self and connection to a broader community of people with disabilities. People with a positive disability identity are better able to adapt to challenges and manage stresses.

biological sex label assigned at birth based on physical factors such as hormones, chromosomes, and genitalia

Gender Identity

Your body and biological sex are part of your identity. Biological sex, however, is not the same as a person's gender. **Biological sex** refers to whether you are genetically and physically male or female.

Personality Traits

Talkative
Brave
Friendly
Cooperative
Shy
Polite
Helpful
Sympathetic
Reliable
Curious
Thoughtful
Artistic
Humorous
Analytical
Stubborn
Thoughtful
Organized
Shy
Hardworking
Cautious
Genuine
Practical
Creative
Indecisive
Serious
Intelligent
Loyal
Earnest
Cheerful
Impulsive

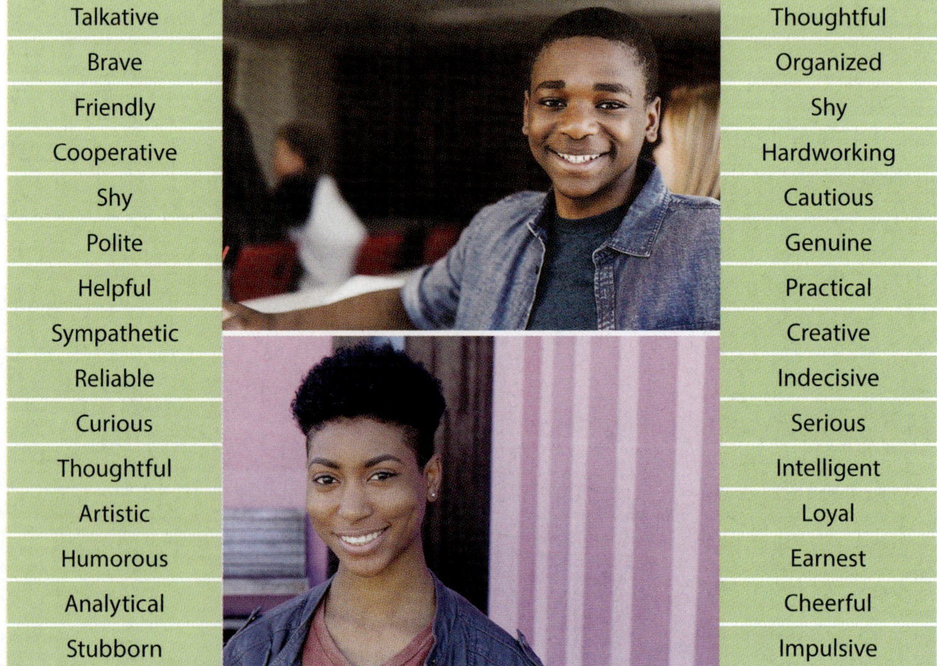

Top to bottom: Stigur Mar Karlsson/Heimsmyndir/E+/Getty Images; ajr_images/iStock/Getty Images Plus/Getty Images

Figure 4.8 Personality traits describe people's thought patterns, emotional responses, behaviors, and interests. Each person has a unique combination of personality traits like these.

A doctor will typically assign a person's biological sex at birth. **Gender** describes the characteristics a society associates with a biological sex. For example, many societies associate certain traits with *femininity* (such as with girls and women) and *masculinity* (such as with boys and men). The societal perception of feminine or masculine traits as the whole of a person's identity is unrealistic. This is because people typically have some masculine and some feminine traits.

gender behavioral, cultural, or psychological traits and roles society associates with a biological sex

gender identity component of identity that describes deeply held thoughts and feelings about one's gender

gender roles societal or cultural expectations about how people of a certain gender should behave, dress, speak, and act

gender stereotypes preconceived ideas, roles, and characteristics people associate with a certain gender

Your **gender identity** is a separate component of identity that includes your deeply held thoughts and feelings about gender. Gender identity influences *gender expression*, or the way you outwardly display your gender. This includes the clothes you wear and your physical appearance and behaviors. People with different gender identities use various words to describe their identification with a gender (**Figure 4.9**).

Gender identity begins developing during childhood and is influenced by a person's culture and environment (including parents, peers, and the media). By three years of age, children usually know their gender. Soon after, young children learn **gender roles**, or the attitudes and behaviors society considers "appropriate" for a certain gender.

Societal assumptions about boys and girls are called **gender stereotypes**. For example, believing that only girls should play with dolls or only boys should play with trucks is gender stereotyping. Another example is thinking that all women are emotional or all men are aggressive. Gender stereotypes influence how people view themselves and others and can lead to unfair treatment of a specific gender.

Gender Identities

Gender Identity	Description
Agender	Having a gender identity that does not align with woman, man, or any other gender; also called *gender neutral*
Androgynous	Exhibiting masculine and feminine traits equally
Bigender	Having a gender identity that includes both man and woman
Cisgender	Having a gender identity that matches one's biological sex assigned at birth
Gender fluid	Having a changing, or *fluid*, gender identity
Gender nonconforming	Having a gender identity that does not follow gender expectations based on a person's biological sex assigned at birth
Gender questioning	Being unsure about one's gender identity or experimenting with different genders
Nonbinary	Having a gender identity that falls outside or between the categories of man and woman; also called *gender queer*
Transgender	Having a gender identity that does not match one's biological sex assigned at birth

Figure 4.9 Each term describes how a person may identify with gender.

Sexual Orientation

A person's sexual orientation is separate from gender identity. *Sexual orientation* describes the enduring pattern of a person's romantic and/or sexual attraction to other people. Sexuality is an important part of a person's identity. You will learn more about sexuality and sexual orientation in Chapter 23: *Understanding Sexuality*.

Social Identity

Your social identity is your connection to other people, including family members, friends, and group members. It also includes the role you play in your community and your relationships with other cultural and socioeconomic groups. For example, your social identity includes your role among friends, religious practices, political beliefs, country of origin, place of residence, and family connections.

Social identity influences how people feel about themselves. Some social identities make people feel good and build confidence.

People who hold social identities that are *stigmatized*, or seen negatively by some people, may feel worse about themselves. Social identity also influences behavior. Your social identity impacts the holidays you celebrate, the foods you prefer, and the community groups or organizations to which you belong.

Cultural and Ethnic Identity

ethnicity one's connection to a particular social group that shares similar cultural or national ties

Your cultural and ethnic identity is your connection to different cultural or ethnic groups. It has probably influenced many parts of your life, including the languages you speak, your traditions and beliefs, and the foods you eat. Your cultural and ethnic identity relates to your **ethnicity**, or your connection to a particular social group that shares similar cultural or national ties. People may define their ethnicity through traditions, language, religious practices, or cultural values. Typically, people go through several stages when discovering their ethnic identity (**Figure 4.10**).

Local and Global Health

Everyone Has a Cultural Identity

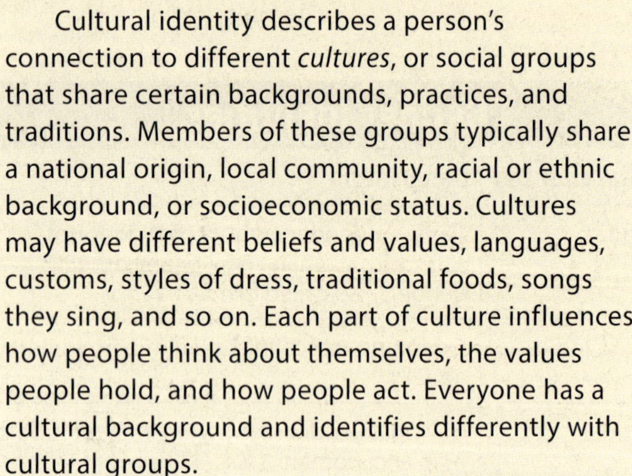

Cultural identity describes a person's connection to different *cultures*, or social groups that share certain backgrounds, practices, and traditions. Members of these groups typically share a national origin, local community, racial or ethnic background, or socioeconomic status. Cultures may have different beliefs and values, languages, customs, styles of dress, traditional foods, songs they sing, and so on. Each part of culture influences how people think about themselves, the values people hold, and how people act. Everyone has a cultural background and identifies differently with cultural groups.

Think about your family's cultural background. What national origins, communities, races, ethnicities, and socioeconomic statuses are represented? Your sense of connection to each of these cultural groups is your cultural identity. For many people, cultural identity describes connections to multiple, different cultures. Parents or guardians may have different cultural backgrounds. In some cases, they may have been born in one country and then emigrated to another.

Sometimes people reject or ignore their cultural identity. They may do this to fit in and feel accepted by another cultural group or because they are uncomfortable with a culture's traditions. Learning to feel comfortable with your cultural identity and proud of your distinct culture and heritage is an important part of embracing identity.

Many teens find it interesting to learn more about the parts of their cultural identity. To learn more about your cultural background, you could talk with family members, read books, watch documentaries and movies, listen to music, or visit another country. Many communities have activities that celebrate different cultures. Community organizations may also provide opportunities to learn more about your culture's traditions and language.

Practice Your Skills

Analyze Influences

With a partner, discuss the different factors that make up your cultural identity. List the different cultures that are part of your cultural background and examine your connection to each one. Then discuss how cultural identity influences your values, traditions, and behaviors, including your health decisions. What strategies could you use to learn more about your cultural identity? What resources are available within your school, family, or community? How can high school students learn to appreciate and respect the cultural identities of other people? How can they recognize and manage the influence of this identity on health?

Stages of Ethnic Identity

1. Unexamined identity
People do not think about the meaning of their ethnic identities.

2. Identity search
People actively search for information about the meaning of their ethnicity, including research about their group's history, language, and cultural activities.

3. Identity achievement
People feel secure in their ethnic identity and see it as an important aspect of who they are.

Figure 4.10 According to Jean Phinney, a developmental psychologist, ethnic identity emerges in these three stages. ***What is ethnicity?***

Discovering Your Identity

Identity formation is the process of discovering and establishing your identity (**Figure 4.11**). This process begins during childhood and continues throughout a person's entire life. Young children typically describe themselves in terms of their height, hair and eye color, and favorite activities. As children become teens, this focus often shifts to social identity. Teens also begin to focus on their unique thoughts and feelings, including personal values, beliefs, interests, personality traits, and attitudes. They may look to *role models*, or people they admire, to influence their identity.

According to psychologist Erik Erikson, figuring out your identity is the primary task of adolescence. Erikson believed that people must develop a sense of who they are before they are ready to join with another person in an intimate relationship. By exploring and testing different interests, values, and beliefs now, you will learn more about who you are. Over time, your identity will likely grow and change further as you mature and develop new interests.

identity formation
process of discovering and establishing one's identity through physical, cognitive, and social changes

Factors Affecting Identity Formation

- Ability to think clearly and reason
- Influence and beliefs of guardians and role models
- Roles within the family
- Relationships with peers and friends
- Cultural background and expectations
- Personal experiences and achievements
- Personality and openness to new experiences
- Environment, including school, home, and community
- Opportunities to grow and explore

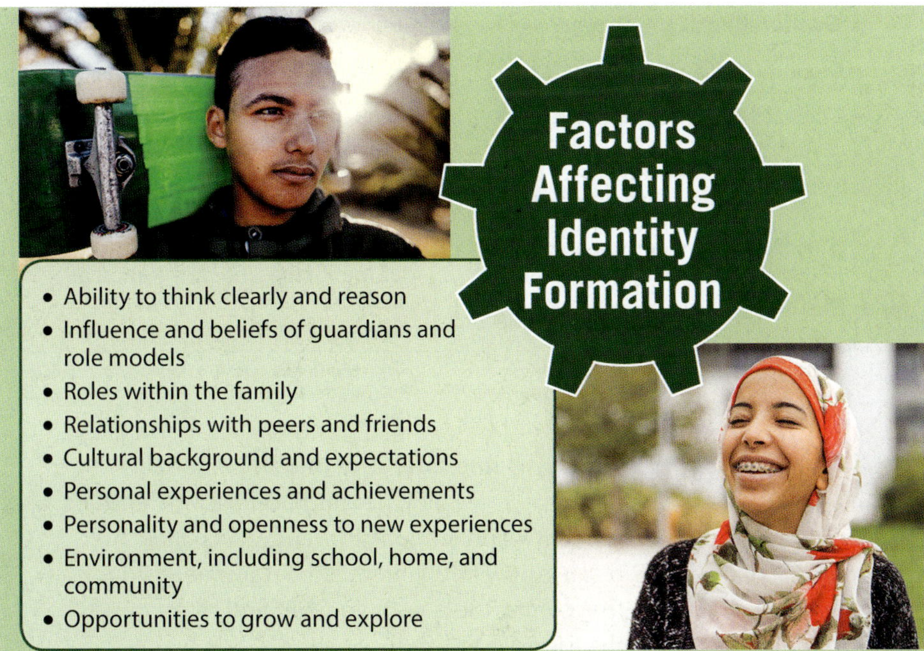

Top to bottom: wundervisuals/E+/Getty Images; LeoPatrizi/E+/Getty Images

Figure 4.11 Identities form as the result of internal and external influences on people.

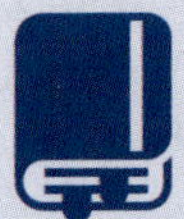

Case Study

Who You Are

There are many components to people's identity, including what they look like, as well as how they act, think, relate to other people, and view the world. The following character profiles describe basic parts of these identities.

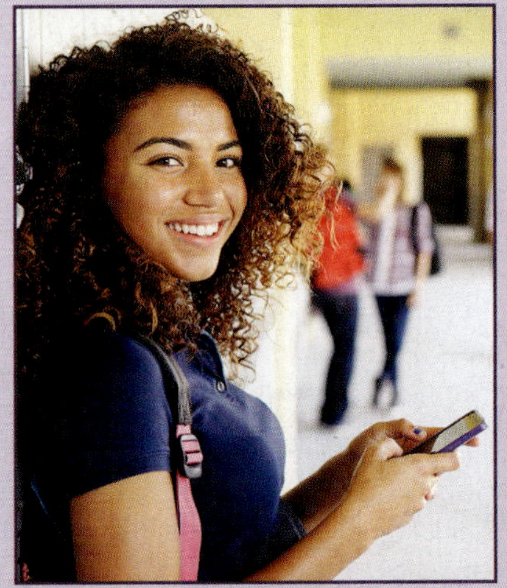

Name: Mikayla

Age: 16

Core Values: Friendship, Fun, Humor, Compassion

Personality: Cheerful, talkative

Physical Identity:
Curly, brown hair
Brown eyes
5′9″
Multiracial (African-American and Caucasian)

Gender Identity: Cisgender

Sexual Orientation: Bisexual

Social Identity: Humorous friend, dependable daughter, blogger, popular among peers

Cultural and Ethnic Identity:
African and German descent, fluent in English and German

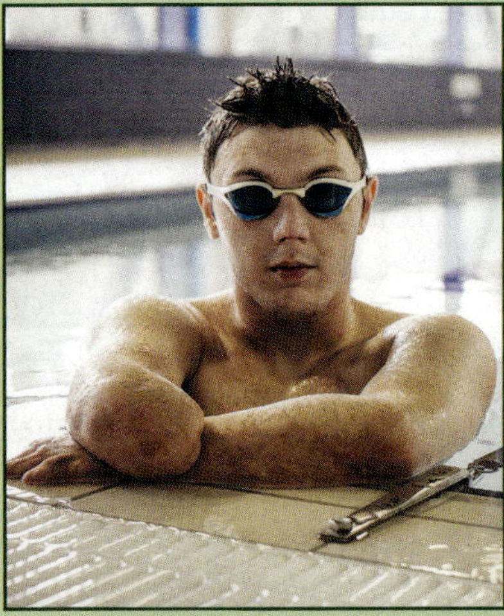

Name: Seth

Age: 17

Core Values: Knowledge, Determination, Optimism

Personality: Loyal, shy, analytical

Physical Identity:
Short, brown hair
Hazel eyes
5′7″
Caucasian

Gender Identity: Cisgender

Sexual Orientation: Heterosexual

Social Identity: Committed varsity swimmer, easygoing brother, environmental advocate, upper-extremity amputee

Cultural and Ethnic Identity:
Polish and Ukrainian descent, fluent in English

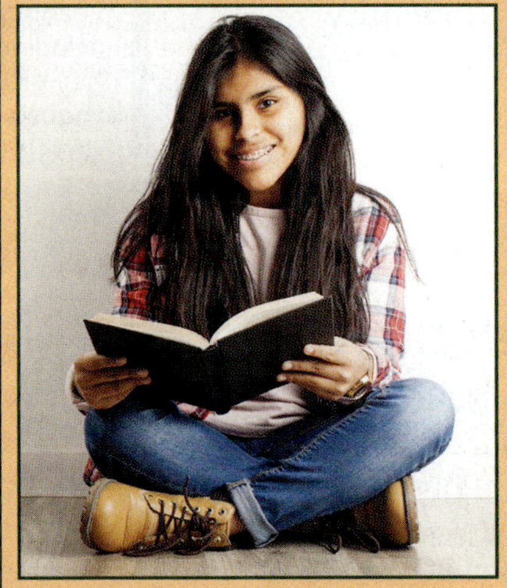

Name: Kai

Age: 14

Core Values: Family, Openness, Knowledge, Generosity

Personality: Sympathetic

Physical Identity:
Long, brown hair
Brown eyes
5′4″
Native American

Gender Identity: Gender fluid

Sexual Orientation: Pansexual

Social Identity: Avid reader, tribe member, painter, nature lover, community volunteer

Cultural and Ethnic Identity:
Member of the Choctaw Nation of Oklahoma, fluent in English and speaks some Choctaw

Left to right: Monkey Business Images/Shutterstock.com; DGLimages/Shutterstock.com; Asier Romero/Shutterstock.com

Practice Your Skills

Comprehend Concepts

Using the profiles shown as examples, create a character profile of your own. Include a photo of yourself, as well as the following components of identity: name, age, core values, personality type, hair type, eye color, height, race, social identities, ethnicity, and language fluency. With a partner, discuss how knowing these details helps you feel comfortable with yourself and make good decisions.

Acknowledge Your Qualities

One way to learn about your identity is to identify the particular qualities and attributes that make you unique. Think about your interests, skills, strengths, and weaknesses, both at school and in your community. To learn about yourself, try paying attention to your reactions throughout the day. You might want to keep a journal or record or film yourself answering the questions in **Figure 4.12** for future reference. Keeping a journal can help you identify the times you feel better or worse. This kind of information can help you understand yourself better. You can also take online or in-person self-assessments to identify components of your identity, including personality traits, interests, and strengths.

Listen to Others (and Yourself)

To learn more about yourself, talk to people who know you well and ask what they see as your strengths. Try asking your parents or guardians, teachers, school counselors, employers, or trusted friends. These people may recognize abilities and strengths you could explore through classes, jobs, or clubs. Advice from people you trust may help you determine where your interests and talents lie. This is one of the benefits of establishing healthy relationships, in which people respect and get to know each other well.

As you gather advice from others, do not stop paying attention to your own feelings and thoughts. Sometimes the advice you get from others may conflict with your own sense of who you are. If this happens, talk to an adult you trust about figuring out what feels right to you.

Questions to Help You Reflect on Your Qualities

1. What activities do you most enjoy?
2. What topics do you like discussing with friends?
3. In what areas do you excel?
4. What tasks do you find difficult?
5. In what situations are you happiest or saddest?
6. What types of activities make you feel most engaged?
7. What types of activities have trouble holding your interest?

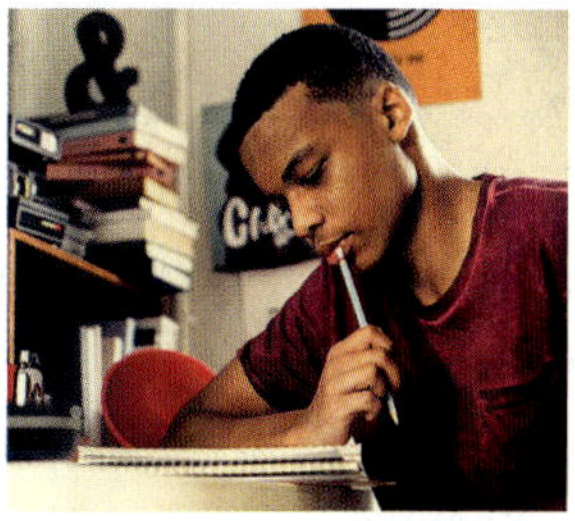

Rawpixel.com/Shutterstock.com

Figure 4.12 Thinking about your answers to these questions can help you understand the qualities that make you who you are.

Try New Activities

A good way to figure out your interests is to have an open mind and try new activities. In trying a new activity, even one you are not sure you will like, you might find a passion you did not know you had. Getting out of your comfort zone and exploring new interests can help you figure out what you do and do not enjoy. Be sure, however, to only try activities that are safe and helpful for your health and well-being.

Learn from Mistakes

When you try new activities, you will inevitably make some mistakes. These mistakes do not mean that you should stop trying new activities or that anything is wrong with you. Avoiding new activities because you are afraid of making mistakes limits your ability to explore new areas of interest. It can also lead to regret later in life. Instead, understand that mistakes are a normal and natural part of life. Research even shows that people who experience mistakes learn valuable lessons and have more resilience. Try to take mistakes in stride and learn from them.

Lesson 4.2 Review

Know and Understand

1. List three factors that influence your core values.
2. Explain what makes up a person's physical identity.
3. What is the difference between biological sex and gender?
4. In your own words, define *ethnicity*.
5. What steps can you take to learn about the different parts of your identity?

Think Critically

6. Think about your own personality. What personality traits do you possess? How stable has your personality remained over time?
7. With a partner, discuss different types of gender expression. How do people with different gender identities express gender differently?
8. What social groups do you belong to? How do these groups influence your social identity?
9. Give an example of a time you learned from a mistake. What did this experience teach you?

REAL WORLD Health Skills

Advocate for Health Using a library or online resources, find a recently published article about cultural or gender stereotypes. After reading the article, write a fully developed paper or record a podcast about your opinion on the topic. Whether you agree or disagree with different parts of the article, state your opinion clearly and support it with detailed reasons. Be sure to cite specific examples and details from the article. Do you think the article correctly identifies norms in the US? perceptions of norms? In your paper or podcast, discuss how teens can resist stereotypes to enhance their own health and the health of others.

Building Your Self-Esteem

Essential Question?
What steps can you take to develop a healthy self-esteem?

Lesson 4.3

Learning Outcomes

After studying this lesson, you will be able to

- describe the difference between self-image and self-esteem;
- explain the importance of self-esteem;
- assess the characteristics of people with healthy and low self-esteem;
- identify factors that influence self-esteem; and
- employ strategies for improving your self-esteem.

Key Terms

affirmations
perfectionism
self-care
self-esteem
self-image

Warm-Up Activity

Understanding Self-Esteem

Comprehend Concepts In this lesson, you will learn about *self-esteem*, or your feelings about yourself. Before reading, think of a fictional character you would say has low self-esteem and a character you would say has healthy self-esteem. Describe these characters in detail and then analyze their self-esteem by answering the following questions:

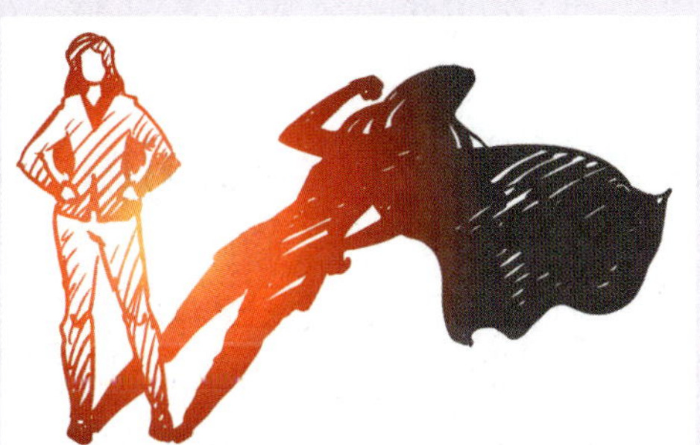

Drawlab19/Shutterstock.com

- How do these characters feel about themselves? What examples demonstrate these feelings?
- What are these characters' flaws? Do the characters know their flaws? How do they feel about their flaws?
- How do the characters' family members and friends affect their self-esteem?
- How would these characters be different if they had different self-esteem?

Many teens feel good about some aspects of themselves and their lives, but feel dissatisfied about other aspects. These sometimes complex feelings are a normal part of adolescence, when many people struggle to figure out what they think of themselves. During this time, your self-image and self-esteem are developing. Self-image and self-esteem have a significant impact on your mental and emotional health.

How do you think others see you? Answering this question can give you a sense of your self-image. Your **self-image** is your mental picture of yourself, including your appearance, skills and abilities, and weaknesses. You are not born with a self-image. Rather, it forms gradually over time, starting in childhood, and is influenced by your experiences and interactions with others. As you experience different events and interact with people, your self-image may change.

self-image mental picture of one's abilities, appearance, and personality based on experiences and interactions with others

self-esteem confidence in one's own worth and abilities

Self-image is closely related to self-esteem. **Self-esteem** describes how you feel about yourself. It also changes with life experiences and new understanding. Building a healthy self-esteem now, during adolescence, will help you transition to adulthood and maintain positive mental and emotional health.

The Importance of Self-Esteem

Your self-esteem has a major impact on many different aspects of your life. It affects how well you do in school, how easily you make friends, and how you manage disappointments and frustrations. Having healthy self-esteem will drive you to care for yourself and take steps to reach your full potential (**Figure 4.13**).

Healthy Self-Esteem

People who have realistic views of themselves have *healthy self-esteem*. If you have healthy self-esteem, you generally feel good about yourself, including your skills and abilities. You know you have worth and feel good about your relationships with other people. You feel loved, appreciated, and accepted by your friends and family members.

Characteristics of People with Healthy and Low Self-Esteem

Healthy Self-Esteem	Low Self-Esteem
• Generally like themselves	• Generally dislike themselves
• Feel secure and worthy of love and respect	• Feel insecure and unworthy of love and respect
• Feel proud of accomplishments and recognize weaknesses	• Criticize their abilities and skills
• Accept correction from others	• Are extremely sensitive to criticism
• Are not worried about acting in certain ways to make other people like them	• Act in certain ways to show others they are worthy of love
• Come to view negative events as learning experiences	• Continue to view negative events as failures
• Ask others for help, if needed	• Are afraid to ask others for help
• Trust their choices and follow their values	• Make decisions to avoid rejection
• Attempt new activities and embrace challenges	• Avoid new activities for fear of failure
• Take responsibility for actions and mistakes	• Blame others for mistakes and problems
• Cope well with frustration and use healthy stress-management strategies	• Avoid painful feelings, sometimes using addictive behaviors
• Are confident in their identity and accepting of others	• Change depending on who is around them and feel threatened by differences
• Live in the present and plan for the future	• Regret the past and worry about the future

Figure 4.13 Whether or not people have healthy self-esteem can affect many aspects of their lives, including how they approach new activities, cope with stress, and feel about their accomplishments. ***What is the term for your mental picture of your appearance, skills, abilities, and weaknesses?***

Some people think that people who brag about themselves or are arrogant have healthy self-esteem. In reality, people with low self-esteem are more likely to show off because they are trying to convince other people of their worth. People with healthy self-esteem feel good about themselves and accept their strengths and weaknesses, so they are not worried about acting in a particular way to make other people like them.

This does not mean that people with healthy self-esteem only experience positive situations and never encounter challenges. They are, however, better able to cope with mistakes and disappointments. People with healthy self-esteem acknowledge their weaknesses and view negative events as learning experiences, not as failures. When they run into obstacles, people with healthy self-esteem can accept reality and make a new plan. They are more comfortable asking other people for help and support when needed.

People who have healthy self-esteem have great decision-making skills. They feel good about themselves, trust their judgment, and follow their values. They are confident they can make the right decision, even in difficult situations. When pressured to follow the crowd, people with healthy self-esteem have the courage to make the choice they believe is right or take responsibility for a poor choice.

Low Self-Esteem

In contrast, people who have *low self-esteem* doubt their worth and may feel negatively about their traits, skills, and abilities. People with low self-esteem may wish they could change their appearance, intelligence, or skills. They may feel left out of social groups and disconnected from other people. They may question whether other people like or respect them, in part, because they do not like or respect themselves.

People with low self-esteem often worry about what other people think of them. Being concerned about others' opinions makes people vulnerable to peer pressure. They can feel unable to resist pressure to engage in unhealthy behaviors. Unfortunately, these behaviors can have long-term health consequences.

Most people suffer periods of low self-esteem from time to time. This is a normal part of life. As teens try to figure out who they are, they can feel uncertain about themselves. This uncertainty can cause teens to feel lost or like they do not measure up to others. Fortunately, teens can learn to work through these issues and accept who they are.

Factors Affecting Self-Esteem

Having healthy self-esteem is harder for some people than it is for others. Many different factors can affect a person's self-esteem. For example, interactions with other people have a major impact on how people see themselves, especially during early childhood. Children with parents or guardians who treat them lovingly and praise them often develop a sense of pride in who they are. On the other hand, children who receive constant criticism and rejection may develop low self-esteem. Social interactions, whether positive or negative, can have a lasting effect on how people feel about themselves.

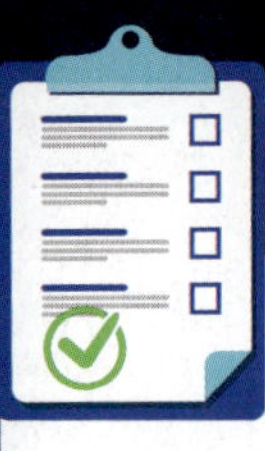

Quiz How Healthy Is Your Self-Esteem?

What level of self-esteem do you think you have? Do you think your self-esteem is healthy? low? To assess your self-esteem, read each of the following statements. Indicate which statements describe your feelings about yourself.

I feel proud of my accomplishments.	☐
I tend to think positively most of the time.	☐
I am not easily embarrassed.	☐
I set goals for the future.	☐
I do not procrastinate often.	☐
I think more about my successes than my mistakes.	☐
I do not often compare myself to others.	☐
I accept criticism and see it as a way to improve in the future.	☐
I rely on myself to make decisions.	☐
I do not let fear or anxiety control my decisions.	☐
I ask others for help when needed.	☐
I know whom to trust and who is part of my support system.	☐
I am always interested in trying new activities.	☐
I embrace change in my life.	☐
I take responsibility for my own actions and mistakes.	☐
I manage stress well and feel in control, even during stressful situations.	☐
I am happy with my appearance.	☐
I usually know how I am feeling.	☐
I would describe myself as optimistic.	☐
Overall, I am satisfied with myself.	☐
Score	

Add up the total number of statements that describe your feelings about yourself. Each statement has a value of 1. Then compare your number to the ranges below.

A score of 0–5 means you have ***very low self-esteem***. Your view of yourself is not positive. You might want to seek professional help to identify why your self-esteem is so low and take steps to improve it.

A score of 6–10 means you have ***low self-esteem***. Low self-esteem may be making it harder for you to maintain healthy relationships and achieve your goals. Try some of the strategies in this lesson for improving your self-esteem and think about seeking help from a trusted adult, friend, or professional.

A score of 11–15 means you have ***somewhat healthy self-esteem***. You know your value and strengths and can put your best foot forward. Keep taking steps to improve your self-esteem and thinking about yourself in positive ways.

A score of 16–20 means you have ***healthy self-esteem***. You have a healthy view of yourself and have the confidence to pursue your goals. Keep acknowledging your strengths and supporting yourself, even when you encounter challenges.

Practice Your Skills

Set Goals

Choose a friend or adult you trust and have a conversation about the results of this quiz. Do you feel like this quiz accurately assessed your self-esteem? Why or why not? What statements did *not* describe your feelings about yourself? Why do you think that is? Together, brainstorm actions you can take to improve your self-esteem. List these actions, and if you had low or very low self-esteem, talk about ways you could get help. Make a long-term plan for building your self-esteem and getting help if you ever need it. Include warning signs you should look out for that mean you have low self-esteem and ways you will address these warning signs. Keep this long-term plan so you can use it now or whenever you need a self-esteem boost.

A person's environment has a significant impact on self-esteem (**Figure 4.14**). A supportive environment can make people feel good about themselves. A negative environment can tear self-esteem down.

Many teens spend a lot of time on social media. Unfortunately, most research demonstrates that social media can impact self-esteem in negative ways. Many people present themselves in very positive ways on social media. This can lead teens to feel that other people have better lives, with more excitement and more friends than they themselves do. That can make people feel worse about themselves.

Personal perceptions also greatly affect how people feel about themselves. Some people constantly criticize and find fault with themselves. This creates a negative mind-set that erodes a person's well-being and lowers self-esteem. For example, some teens may have a very narrow view of intelligence that only focuses on the kind of intelligence assessed by standardized tests and grades. Because of this, they may think they are not smart and may not recognize their intelligence in other areas. This can lead to low self-esteem.

Improving Your Self-Esteem

No matter your level of self-esteem, there are steps you can take to improve your self-esteem and feel better and more confident about yourself. These strategies focus on modifying the factors that affect self-esteem by changing perceptions and bettering your environment.

Know Your Strengths

One of the best ways to have healthy self-esteem is to focus on your strengths and positive qualities rather than what you dislike about yourself. To begin, keep a list of qualities you like about yourself. You might also ask family members and close friends what they see as your positive qualities. Try to think about these strengths, instead of what you do not like about yourself.

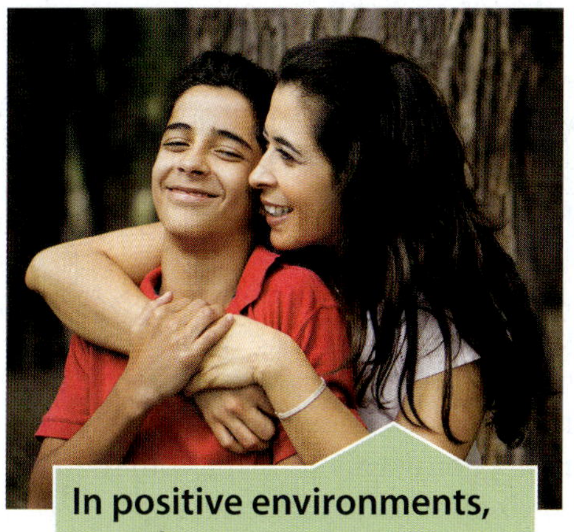

In positive environments, people are

- supported for their successes
- supported when situations do not go their way
- valued for who they are

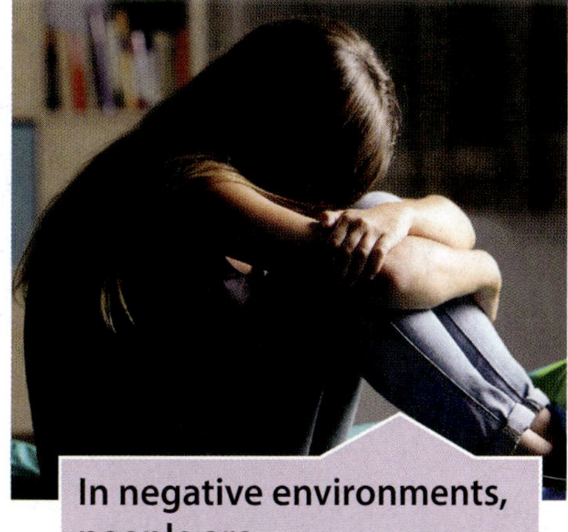

In negative environments, people are

- criticized for any shortcomings
- blamed for failures and disappointments
- held to impossibly high standards

Left to right: Aldo Murillo/E+/Getty Images; Antonio Guillem/Shutterstock.com

Figure 4.14 A person's home, school, community, and culture are all part of environment and can all impact a person's self-esteem.

As you consider your strengths, try not to compare yourself to other people. This can be hard to do, especially since social media makes comparison easier. Keep in mind that happy or successful online posts do not usually represent the whole reality.

Using your strengths and skills can also help you develop healthy self-esteem. For example, you could try volunteering in your community at an animal shelter, soup kitchen, or mentoring organization. Helping others motivates people to focus on other people's needs and not on negative thoughts.

Celebrate Your Successes

Everyone has strengths and weaknesses and succeeds only some of the time. To increase self-esteem, focus on times you have succeeded and recognize and accept areas you could improve. Have you received an *A* on a paper or test? scored a goal? won an award? been hired for a summer job or internship? These are all accomplishments in which you can take pride. You can build healthy self-esteem by celebrating these successes, practicing gratitude, and accepting that all people have weaknesses and experience failure.

You do not have to experience a big success to celebrate yourself and build healthy self-esteem. To celebrate your positive qualities every day, try practicing daily **affirmations**. Each day, write and then repeat what you like about yourself and how you have succeeded. Research shows that writing down these positive statements every day can lessen negative thoughts and feelings.

affirmations statements that acknowledge a person's value and strengths

Avoid Perfectionism

Holding yourself to impossibly high standards is harmful to self-esteem. This habit, called **perfectionism**, is hurtful and unrealistic, since no one can be perfect all of the time. To avoid perfectionism, you can follow these steps:

perfectionism personal standard or attitude that rejects anything less than ideal performance

1. Pay attention to what you are telling yourself. What expectations are you setting for yourself? Write these expectations down and then think about whether they are realistic (**Figure 4.15**). For example, if you find yourself thinking *I have to do perfectly on every math test* or *I always need to have the right words to comfort my friend*, these are unrealistic expectations.
2. Replace each unrealistic expectation with a realistic expectation. For example, you could write *I want to know I've done my best in math* or *I want to help my friend whenever I can.*
3. The next time you notice yourself thinking about an unrealistic expectation, stop yourself. Replace this expectation with a realistic one. Keep doing this to train yourself in setting realistic expectations.
4. Focus on your own strengths and accomplishments and do not judge yourself in comparison to other people. Consider what you feel good about within yourself and recognize your own improvement over time.

What makes expectations for yourself unrealistic?

- Seeking flawlessness and allowing no margin for human error
- Tying achievements to self-worth
- Dismissing past and current achievements as not good enough
- Setting too short of a timeframe for achievement
- Blaming yourself for factors outside of your control

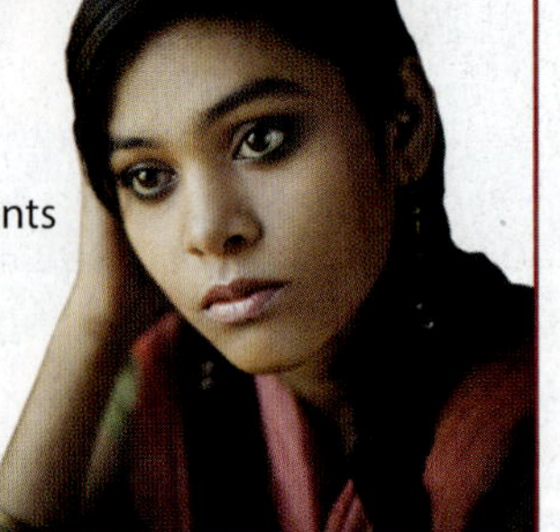

gawrav/E+/Getty Images

Figure 4.15 When people set unrealistic expectations for themselves, they set themselves up for disappointment and failure. ***What dangerous habit involves holding yourself to impossibly high standards?***

Care for Yourself

Another important step in building self-esteem is **self-care**, or taking care of yourself. This can include engaging in physical activity, getting enough sleep, taking time for relaxation, keeping up with personal hygiene, and eating well. People who feel well physically are more likely to feel well mentally. Remember that the different dimensions of health—physical, mental and emotional, and social—are intertwined.

self-care process of actively taking care of one's own well-being and health, especially during periods of stress

If you are not feeling good about yourself one day, practice self-care. Do activities that you know make you feel better, such as watching a funny movie, running outside, or spending time with close friends. Be careful not to do harmful activities, such as binge-eating junk food or drinking alcohol, for a temporary boost. These behaviors may feel good in the moment, but will ultimately leave you feeling worse. Part of taking care of yourself is recognizing when you do not feel well and then taking specific steps to feel better.

Lesson 4.3 Review

Know and Understand

1. What is the difference between self-image and self-esteem?
2. How do people with healthy self-esteem respond to challenges and disappointments?
3. How does a positive environment contribute to healthy self-esteem?
4. Why is it unhelpful to compare your life to the lives others portray on social media?
5. How do daily affirmations improve self-esteem?
6. Why does taking care of yourself physically contribute to healthy self-esteem?

Think Critically

7. Review the characteristics of people with healthy and low self-esteem. With a partner, brainstorm specific behaviors that demonstrate these qualities. Make a list of specific behaviors of people with healthy and low self-esteem.
8. Give one example of how your personal perceptions affect your self-esteem.
9. What unrealistic, perfectionistic expectations do you have of yourself? List two of these expectations and then write realistic expectations you could set instead.
10. What self-care activities could you engage in to help yourself feel better?

REAL WORLD Health Skills

Make Decisions To build self-esteem, you need to make decisions and adopt habits that improve your mental and emotional health. In turn, a healthy self-esteem will make it easier to make decisions. With a partner, list five decisions you could make today to start improving your self-esteem. Use the decision-making process to form each decision and identify barriers that might get in the way of carrying out your decision. Put these decisions into action and record how you feel. Do you notice an improvement in your self-esteem? Explain.

Lesson 4.4

Expressing Your Emotions

Essential Question?

How can you express your emotions in healthy ways?

Learning Outcomes

After studying this lesson, you will be able to

- describe how to understand and uncover your emotions;
- identify defense mechanisms people use to cope with their emotions;
- assess strategies for identifying how you are feeling;
- explain the importance of accepting your emotions;
- discuss healthy ways of expressing your emotions; and
- describe strategies for developing emotional intelligence.

Key Terms

defense mechanisms
emotional intelligence (EI)
emotions
mood swings

Warm-Up Activity

Tally Your Emotions

Analyze Influences Evaluate how you feel throughout the course of three school days. Using a chart like the one shown, indicate how you feel during each period. If a feeling you have is not listed, write it in the box marked *Other*. You may check more than one feeling during a period. After completing a chart for three days, review your three charts. How did your emotions affect your mind and body? Did a particular emotion repeatedly occur at a particular time of day? Why? How did this affect your behavior?

How you feel	Period ___	Period ___	Period ___	Period ___	Period ___	Period ___	Period ___	For one hour after school
Lonely								
Supported								
Sad								
Happy								
Angry								
Content								
Annoyed								
Bored								
Engaged								
Tired								
Energetic								
Other ___								

Adolescence is a time of many powerful emotions. During this time, teens are discovering their identities, forming relationships, and thinking about their futures. Many teens feel happy during some parts of the day, but can quickly shift to feeling angry, sad, or lonely. These **mood swings**, caused in part by chemical changes in the body, are a normal part of adolescence. The increasing pressure many teens face from trying to balance relationships, homework, extracurricular activities, and overall physical health can make emotions and mood swings even more powerful.

mood swings sudden shifts in emotion

In this lesson, you will learn about the types of emotions people experience. You will also learn some strategies for recognizing and managing emotions and using them in a constructive way.

Understanding Emotions

As you know, your mental and emotional health has to do with your internal life (**Figure 4.16**). **Emotions** are the moods or feelings you experience. They reveal to you how you feel about certain situations and events. You can use emotions to understand yourself and make healthy decisions that align with your values.

emotions strong feelings experienced based on one's circumstances, relationships, or moods

Emotions may be comfortable or uncomfortable. Comfortable emotions, such as joy, gratitude, pride, love, and curiosity, make you feel good. Uncomfortable emotions, such as loneliness, anxiety, anger, sadness and grief, jealousy, and guilt, make you feel bad. This does not mean that all uncomfortable emotions are bad for you. Uncomfortable emotions are a natural part of life and can play an important role in motivating change if you manage them well.

Emotions can be complicated and difficult to untangle. Sometimes, the same event or experience can lead to multiple feelings. For example, the end of the school year might make you feel happy because you will not have homework, but sad because you will not see your friends every day. One emotion might mask or hide another emotion. If you try out for a sports team and are not chosen, you might feel angry at the coach for not selecting you. This feeling of anger, however, might be hiding your feelings of sadness because you really wanted to be a part of the team.

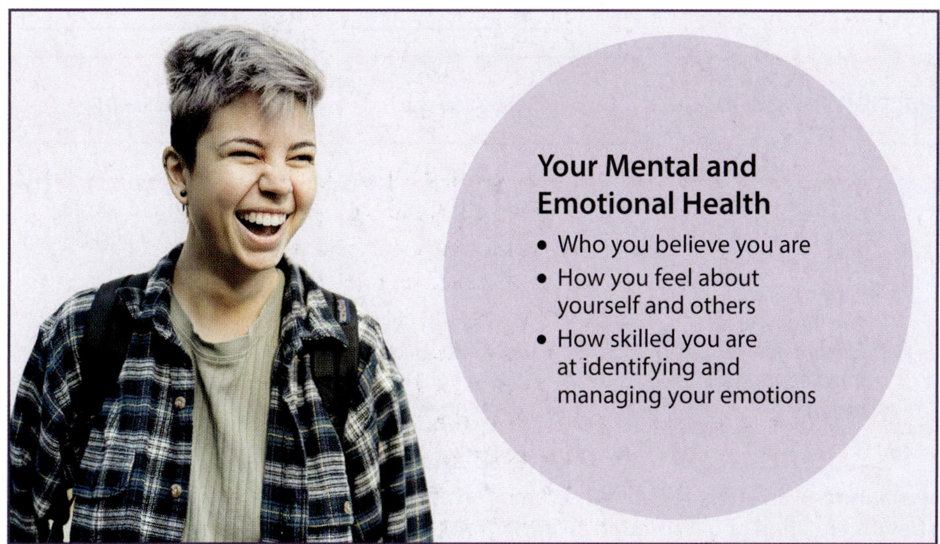

martinedoucet/E+/Getty Images

Figure 4.16
An important part of your mental and emotional health is how well you regularly identify and manage your emotions. ***What are emotions?***

defense mechanisms
mental processes used to avoid conscious conflict, feelings, or thoughts

Some people use **defense mechanisms** to avoid certain feelings and thoughts (**Figure 4.17**). While this strategy might help in the moment when you need to achieve a certain task, overusing defense mechanisms can hurt your mental and emotional health. Many defense mechanisms are unconscious responses. This means you might have to examine your defense mechanisms to identify the emotions beneath them. For example, you might use the defense mechanism of repression to forget about an argument with a friend before a test. While this might help you get through the test, you still need to identify and manage your emotions about the argument. If you keep repressing your feelings, they will build, hurting your mental and emotional health and your relationship with your friend.

Managing Emotions

Identifying and managing your emotions is not easy. As a child, you probably reacted to what you felt without thinking. As you grow up, however, you can learn to control your emotions and express them in healthy ways. Learning how to manage your emotions can have a positive effect on your mind, body, relationships, and overall health.

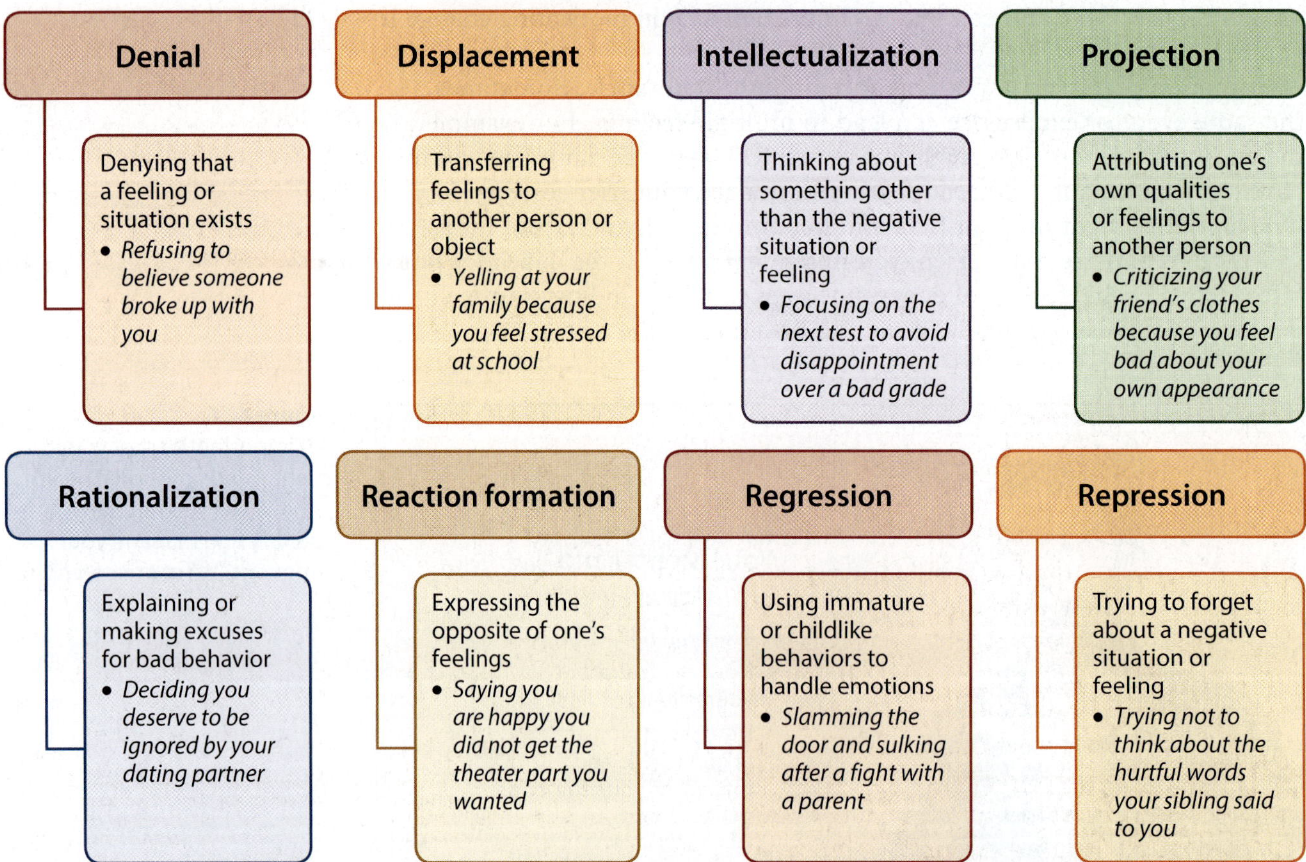

Figure 4.17 People use defense mechanisms in an effort to avoid their emotions. For example, you may need to use a defense mechanism to cope with a stressful situation or get through an important task. Defense mechanisms rarely work in the long run, however, because people eventually need to accept and express their emotions.

Health in the Media

The Rapid Spread of Negative Emotions

How often do people you know share negative emotions on social media? How do you think these emotions then affect other people? In one study, researchers examined how the emotions one person posted on social media impacted the emotions posted by others in that person's network.

Researchers found that relatively few people shared or passed on emotions of sadness or disgust on social media. People did, however, share and pass on joyful emotions, especially with close friends. Anger was the emotion *most likely* to spread through social media. People who posted about angry emotions were much more likely to have that anger shared with others, both within and beyond their social networks.

In another study, researchers at the University of California San Diego demonstrated that negative posts on social media influence other people to also post about negative emotions. In this study, researchers found that people post more about negative emotions on social media when it is raining. Then they examined whether these negative posts impacted posts among a person's friends. This study revealed that people who read negative posts were also more likely to post about negative emotions, even if it was not raining in their area. In sum, negative emotions can spread rapidly on social media and make people feel worse.

Practice Your Skills

Communicate with Others

Why do you think negative emotions spread so easily on social media? What are some factors that may play a role? In a small group, discuss these questions and research explanations. Then, compare your explanations with those of another group. How could you test which factors have the biggest influence? How could you use this information to inform students about the impact of social media on mental health? As a class, arrange an online panel so you can share the information you learned with other students. Take questions about the spread of emotions on social media and answer them using the research you have done.

In the following sections, you will learn about the process of identifying, accepting, and expressing your emotions. You will read about the feelings one teen, Mariana, is experiencing and how she responds to the situation. As you are reading, think about how you would feel if you were in Mariana's shoes. What would you do?

Identify What You Are Feeling

The first step in managing your emotions is identifying the emotions you are feeling. You cannot go through the steps of acknowledging and expressing your emotions if you do not first identify them. As you have learned, understanding your emotions can be difficult. It can be confusing to separate the feelings of sadness from fear or happiness from love. You might need to identify two emotions you are feeling or consider if one emotion might be masking another. If you notice yourself using a defense mechanism, you need to identify the underlying emotion.

Consider Mariana's situation. Mariana started the day in a bad mood. She argued with her sister when her sister said it was Mariana's turn to take the dog for a walk. On the way to school, she yelled at her brother for not keeping up with her. At lunch, Mariana snapped at her best friend, Alia, for no reason. Alia asked Mariana why she was in such a bad mood.

As it turns out, Mariana was reacting negatively to a conversation she had with her mother the night before. Mariana's mother had mentioned she was applying for a new job in another city. If her mother gets the job, Mariana will probably have to move, which she does not want to do. Rather than telling her mother she does not want to move, Mariana took out her frustrations on those around her, which is unhealthy.

Mariana apologized to Alia for snapping at her, and then they talked about Mariana's situation. Mariana identified that she was angry, but as they talked about it, Mariana also identified that she was anxious and afraid. She was anxious about the thought of leaving her friends. She was afraid others would not accept her at a new school. This conversation helped Mariana identify and sort out her feelings.

Several strategies can help you identify the emotions you are feeling. For example, thinking about factors that might be triggering the emotion can help you determine the actual emotion you are experiencing. Keeping a journal can also help you track your emotions and the events that cause them (**Figure 4.18**).

If you are having trouble identifying an emotion, talk with a parent or guardian, trusted adult, or close friend. Sometimes, you might be afraid of realizing you are feeling certain emotions, such as unhappiness. It is important to remember that no emotion is wrong to have. All emotions are a part of life, and it is healthy and important to identify them.

Accept Your Feelings

Once you identify your feelings, the next step is to accept and acknowledge them. Accepting your feelings does not mean that those feelings will go away. It simply means that you allow yourself to experience your emotions. When you accept your emotions, try not to judge or change them.

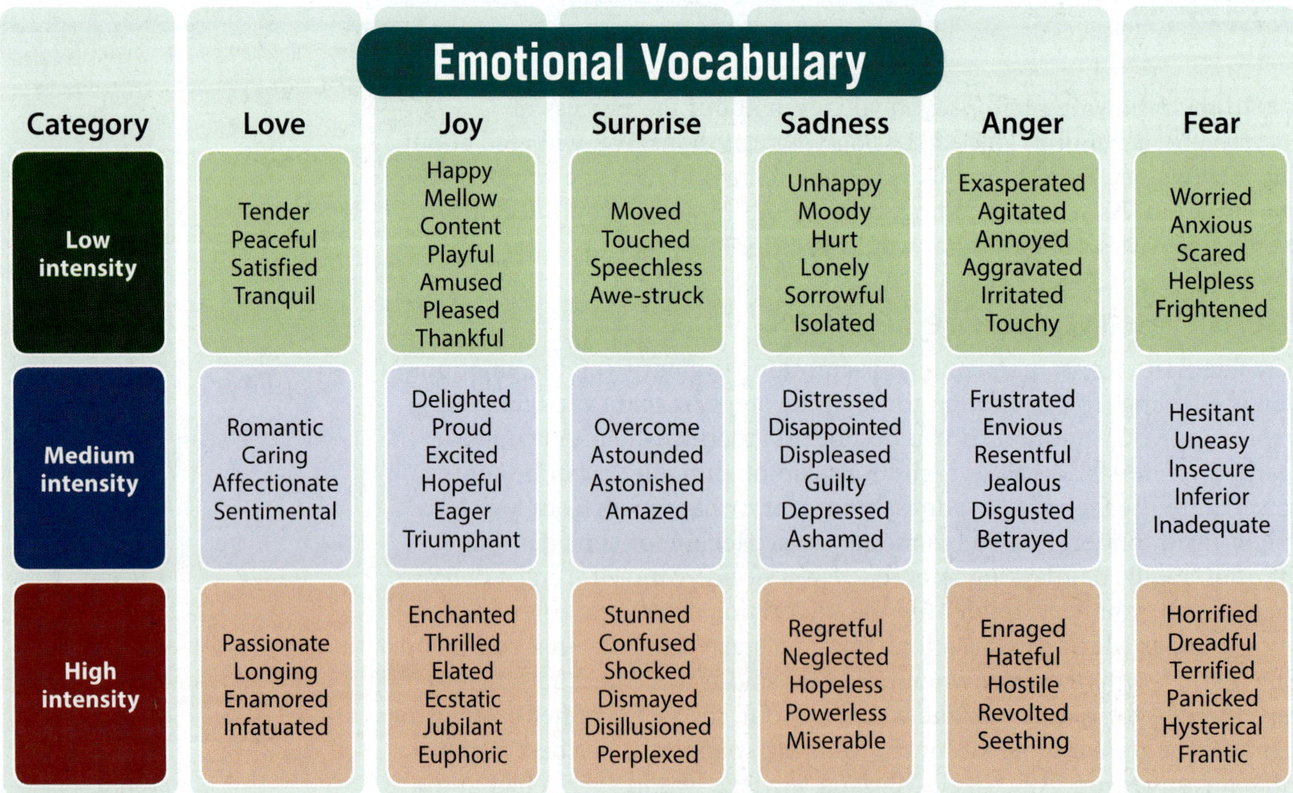

Emotional Vocabulary

Category	Love	Joy	Surprise	Sadness	Anger	Fear
Low intensity	Tender Peaceful Satisfied Tranquil	Happy Mellow Content Playful Amused Pleased Thankful	Moved Touched Speechless Awe-struck	Unhappy Moody Hurt Lonely Sorrowful Isolated	Exasperated Agitated Annoyed Aggravated Irritated Touchy	Worried Anxious Scared Helpless Frightened
Medium intensity	Romantic Caring Affectionate Sentimental	Delighted Proud Excited Hopeful Eager Triumphant	Overcome Astounded Astonished Amazed	Distressed Disappointed Displeased Guilty Depressed Ashamed	Frustrated Envious Resentful Jealous Disgusted Betrayed	Hesitant Uneasy Insecure Inferior Inadequate
High intensity	Passionate Longing Enamored Infatuated	Enchanted Thrilled Elated Ecstatic Jubilant Euphoric	Stunned Confused Shocked Dismayed Disillusioned Perplexed	Regretful Neglected Hopeless Powerless Miserable	Enraged Hateful Hostile Revolted Seething	Horrified Dreadful Terrified Panicked Hysterical Frantic

Figure 4.18 An important part of identifying your emotions is naming them. Writing down your emotions or saying them aloud will help you identify how you feel. ***What other emotional vocabulary do you know?***

They are your emotions, and even if you do not like them, you are not wrong to feel them. Your emotions cannot hurt you as long as you accept them and manage them in healthy ways.

Sometimes people try to cover up or deny their emotions and hope that their feelings will just go away. This denial does not make an emotion go away or lessen. In fact, burying emotions deep inside can increase the intensity of emotions and have a negative effect on your mind and body. When you accept your emotions, you can work through what you are feeling so you can let it go.

Mariana began to accept her emotions when she admitted that her anger was a result of being anxious and afraid about moving. Talking with Alia was a healthy, positive way for Mariana to begin to work through her emotions. Once Mariana acknowledged her feelings and calmed down, she felt that she was ready to express her feelings to her mother.

Express Your Feelings

The third step in managing your emotions is to express your emotions. Expressing your emotions can help you release them and feel better (**Figure 4.19**). If your feelings are overwhelming and difficult to work through, do not hesitate to get professional help.

In a healthy relationship, you do not need to be afraid of expressing your emotions. Your friends or family members will want to hear about how you feel. They may be able to help you by offering support or distracting you.

When you tell others how you feel, stay calm, use I-statements, and keep your emotions under control. If you are negative and lash out at others or try to hurt someone, then you are expressing your emotions in an unhealthy way. You may cause serious harm to the relationship. Instead, be positive and think about the effect your words may have on the other person. Explain how you feel without being hurtful or negative.

Sometimes, you can make a situation worse if you try to confront the person who caused you to feel a certain way while you are still angry. Instead, wait until you cool off before talking about your feelings. By waiting, you can control your emotions and express them in a more positive, healthy way. You are allowing yourself time to work through and get relief from your feelings of anger. This will help you keep your emotions under control.

When Mariana talked with her mother, she had already worked through her anger and was able to remain calm and explain her feelings about the potential move. By talking with her mom, Mariana began to have a more positive outlook about the situation.

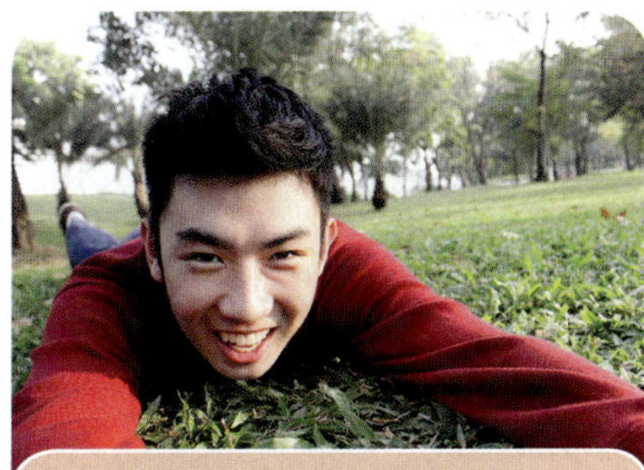

Healthy, positive ways to accept and express emotions

- Sharing with friends, family, or a trusted adult
- Writing in a journal
- Crying
- Taking a walk or run
- Reducing stress
- Doing an activity you enjoy
- Taking a long bath or shower
- Finding a reason to laugh
- Documenting a positive moment

paulaphoto/Shutterstock.com

Figure 4.19 People who allow themselves to express their emotions are better able to release them and move past them.

Emotional Intelligence (EI)

Do you know people who always seem positive, calm, and in control of their emotions in stressful situations? Do you know people who sense that you are feeling down, even before you say anything to them?

emotional intelligence (EI) skill in perceiving, understanding, and managing emotions and feelings

People with this ability have high **emotional intelligence (EI)**. They are skilled at identifying their own emotions and understanding the emotions of others. Having EI is necessary to develop close personal relationships with others (**Figure 4.20**).

People who have high EI have high levels of social awareness and *empathy*, or the ability to put themselves in someone else's shoes. They understand others' wants, needs, and points of view. As a result, they excel at supporting their friends when they are in need. People who have high EI also express their emotions in healthy, positive ways. They openly share their feelings with friends. For example, suppose someone begins a dating

Skills for Developing Emotional Intelligence

Practice identifying, accepting, and expressing your emotions in healthy ways.
Be present in the moment and track what emotions you feel each day.
Accept your emotions and identify them without trying to fix or get rid of them.
Remember there are no wrong emotions. Even uncomfortable emotions serve a purpose.
Use emotions as data to guide your decisions and identify what makes you happy or sad.
Examine your emotional reactions and responses to stress. Modify your behavior, if needed.
Take responsibility for your responses and actions and find ways to improve.
Think about how your actions will impact others and how you would feel in others' shoes.

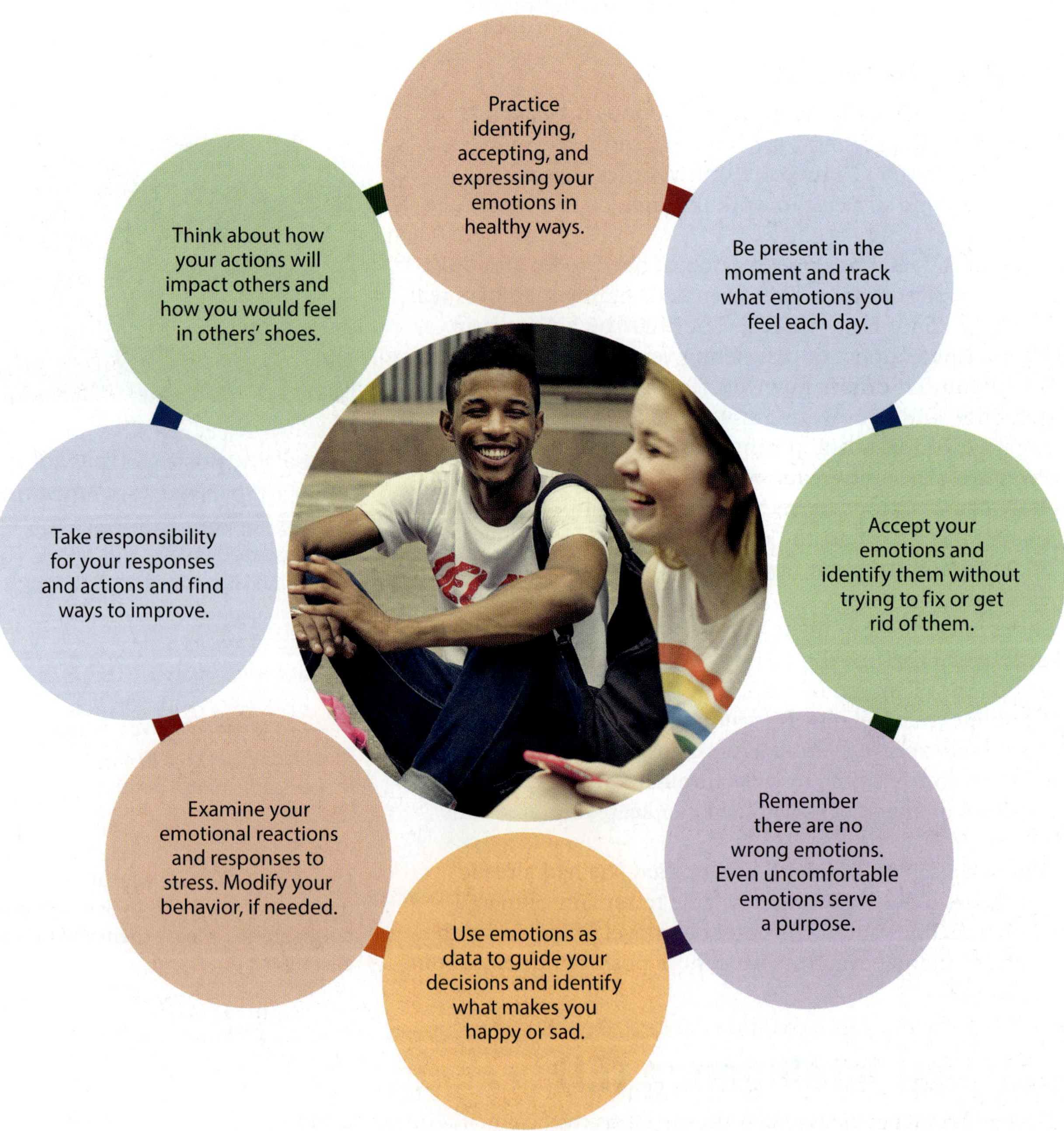

Rawpixel.com/Shutterstock.com

Figure 4.20 Simple actions such as examining your response to stress can help improve EI. ***What aspect of EI means that people can understand others' wants, needs, and points of view?***

relationship that becomes more and more serious. As a result, this person does not spend as much time with old friends. Some of these friends may begin to feel neglected and angry. A person with high EI might speak to the unavailable friend about the situation instead of becoming angry.

People who have high EI also exhibit other characteristics, including the following:

- **Self-awareness:** People with high EI understand their emotions and how those emotions impact people around them. They feel comfortable relying on their intuition and have a good sense of their own strengths and weaknesses.
- **Self-regulation:** People with high EI control their feelings and impulses and act with thought and integrity.
- **Motivation:** People with high EI are willing to work on challenging tasks and are highly productive.
- **Social skills:** People with high EI work well with other people, help build and maintain relationships, and resolve conflicts in constructive ways.

People who have high EI tend to be more successful in school, work, and interpersonal relationships. They also experience greater mental and emotional health.

Lesson 4.4 Review

Know and Understand

1. Explain why uncomfortable emotions are not always bad for you.
2. With a partner, discuss which defense mechanisms you have used in the past. Share your examples with the class.
3. What strategies can you use to identify the emotions you are feeling?
4. Why is it important to accept your feelings and not deny they exist?
5. In a small group, brainstorm healthy ways of expressing emotions. Create a list of techniques and share them with the class.
6. Why is it important to control your emotions when expressing them?

Think Critically

7. Give one example of a time when one emotion masked another for you. How did you uncover the true emotion motivating your behavior?
8. Review the names for emotions in Figure 4.18. Choose three emotions and identify times when you felt each one.
9. How do you know when your emotions have cooled off enough that you can confront someone in a controlled, healthy way?
10. Choose one skill for developing EI and consider practical steps you can take to practice this skill. Give specific examples, such as keeping a log of emotions and identifying their causes. Share these steps in a small group.

REAL WORLD Health Skills

Set Goals Emotions can feel powerful, especially if you are not sure how to manage them. With a partner, assess how well you manage your emotions now. What areas can you improve? Set a SMART goal to manage your emotions better using specific strategies discussed in this lesson. Make sure to set a time line and evaluate whether you achieved your goal at the end of that time. Ask your partner to hold you accountable and assess the impact achieving your goal had on your mental and emotional health.

Chapter 4 Review and Assessment

Chapter Summary

Mental and emotional health describe the health of your internal life. Mental health is how you observe and interpret information. Emotional health refers to how you express yourself and your thoughts and feelings. Mental health exists on a continuum. Mental health conditions reduce mental and emotional health, mental distress disrupts daily function in the short-term, and mental illnesses are diagnosable conditions that require professional treatment. Factors that influence mental and emotional health include your genetics, upbringing and experiences, environment, social media and technology, and patterns of thinking. Assessing your mental and emotional health regularly can help you care for your health in this area and get help, if needed.

A key part of mental and emotional health is embracing your identity, or who you are. There are many components of identity, including your core values, personality, physical identity, gender identity, sexual orientation, social identity, and cultural and ethnic identity. To discover your identity, you can acknowledge your qualities, listen to yourself and others, try new activities, and learn from mistakes.

Self-esteem is your feelings about yourself. Having healthy self-esteem means generally feeling good about and having a realistic view of yourself. People with healthy self-esteem know their worth, view negative events as learning experiences, and make decisions that align with their values. Low self-esteem can lead to negative thoughts and feelings, defensiveness, and concern over others' opinions. To build a healthy self-esteem, you can recognize your strengths, celebrate successes, avoid perfectionism, and practice self-care.

Emotions are often intense during the teen years, and it is important to manage them well. No emotion is wrong to have. Even uncomfortable emotions can help motivate change. Sometimes, people use defense mechanisms to avoid emotions, but using them too much can harm mental and emotional health. To manage emotions, start by identifying them. Accept your feelings without judgment and then express them using effective communication skills like I-statements. Practicing these skills can help you develop emotional intelligence (EI), which will benefit you throughout your life.

Vocabulary Activity

Choose three of the terms shown. Search online for photos, graphics, or videos that show the meanings of these three terms. Create a digital presentation of these photos, graphics, or videos and show them to the class. Explain how they show the meanings of the terms and answer any questions your classmates have. While listening to your classmates' presentations, write down any terms or explanations you do not understand.

affirmations	*gender identity*	*mental health conditions*
biological sex	*gender roles*	*mood swings*
cognitive distortions	*gender stereotypes*	*perfectionism*
core values	*genetic predisposition*	*personality*
defense mechanisms	*identity*	*self-actualization*
emotional intelligence (EI)	*identity formation*	*self-care*
emotions	*Maslow's hierarchy of human needs*	*self-esteem*
ethnicity	*mental distress*	*self-image*
gender		

Review and Recall

Review the information in this chapter by answering the following questions.

1. Create three to five social media posts demonstrating positive mental and emotional health.
2. Write a case study about four people who fall into each category of the mental health continuum. Include details that indicate each person's category and list the actions each person can take to improve mental and emotional health.
3. How does social media influence mental and emotional health?
4. As a class, create a quick reference guide of terms related to gender identity. Brainstorm terms and define them in your own words. Research any terms not discussed in this lesson.
5. How is sexual orientation different from gender identity?
6. What should you do if others' thoughts about you conflict with your sense of who you are?
7. Why are bragging and arrogance *not* a sign of healthy self-esteem?
8. Which of the following is a sign of low self-esteem?
   A. accepting criticism
   B. feeling threatened by differences
   C. asking for help
   D. taking responsibility for mistakes
9. Explain why social media can contribute to low self-esteem.
10. Which of the following is true of uncomfortable emotions?
    A. They are bad for you.
    B. It is best to ignore them.
    C. They are abnormal.
    D. They can help motivate change.
11. Why do people use defense mechanisms?
12. What is involved in accepting your feelings?
    A. making the feeling go away
    B. covering up the feeling
    C. experiencing the feeling
    D. deciding the feeling is wrong
13. When expressing your feelings, you say to your friend, "You have more friends than me, and it isn't fair." Rewrite this you-statement into an I-statement you could use to express your feelings respectfully.

Standardized Test Prep

Math Practice

The following results are from a study of US teens' self-esteem. Review the results and answer the following questions.

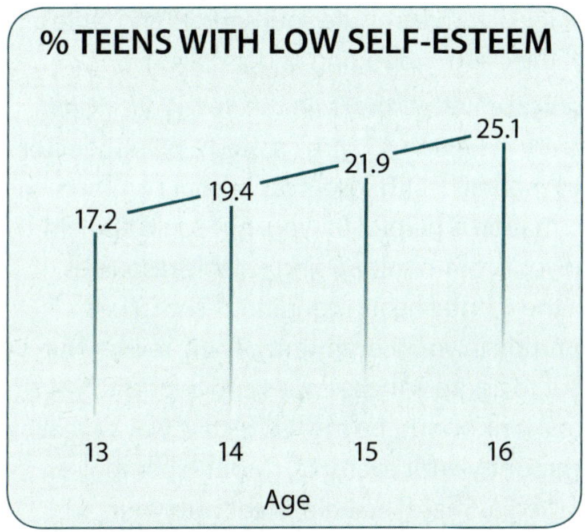

McClure, Auden C et al. "Characteristics associated with low self-esteem among US adolescents." Academic pediatrics vol. 10,4 (2010): 238-44.e2. doi:10.1016/j.acap.2010.03.007

14. Calculate the difference between the percentage of teens with low self-esteem at ages 13 and 16.
15. At age 15, what percentage of teens in the study had normal self-esteem?
    A. 21.9%
    B. 19.4%
    C. 28.1%
    D. 78.1%
16. This study surveyed 883 14-year-olds. According to the results, how many of these teens had low self-esteem? Round to the nearest whole number.

Chapter 4 Skills Assessment

Critical Thinking Skills

Answer the following questions to assess your knowledge of what you learned in this chapter.

1. What messages do you receive from media and society about the importance of mental and emotional health? Are these messages helpful or not? Explain.
2. Think of a time you would have placed yourself in the *reacting*, *injured*, or *ill* categories of the mental health continuum. Write a journal entry about that time in your life and reflect on any actions you took to get help or improve your health.
3. Are there any ongoing stressors in your community that you think increase people's risk for mental health conditions? Explain.
4. Media and technology have many benefits, but can also harm mental and emotional health. With a partner, discuss strategies teens can use to increase the benefits of media and technology and reduce their harm.
5. To learn more about your personality, take a personality test online. After taking the test, reflect on your results. Do you agree or disagree with them? Why?
6. Choose one TV show, movie, book, or online video and explain how it depicts gender. Do you think this depiction is realistic for most people? Why or why not?
7. Why would people need to have a solid sense of who they are before being ready to join with another in an intimate relationship?
8. Is it possible for people to have too high of a self-esteem? Explain.
9. How has your self-esteem changed over time? What factors do you think led to these changes? What strategies could you use to improve your self-esteem in the future?
10. Some people are tempted to label comfortable emotions as "good" and uncomfortable emotions as "bad." Is there such a thing as a "bad" emotion? Explain.
11. Review Figure 4.18 and then create your own emotional vocabulary chart. How would you describe your emotions in each area at each intensity level? Compare your chart with a partner's chart.
12. What feelings are hard for teens to accept? Work with a partner to create a list of these feelings. Then discuss why it is important for teens to accept these feelings.
13. Write a case study about a teen using EI to navigate a difficult situation.

Health and Wellness Skills

Complete the following activities to assess your skills related to health and wellness.

14. **Analyze Influences.** Think about the music you listen to and identify a song that changes your mood somehow. After choosing a song, create an audio journal entry that contains your favorite parts of the song and explains how this song affects your mood. In your entry, answer the following questions:
    - What emotions do you feel listening to the song?
    - What about the song affects your mood? For example, do the lyrics or beat appeal to you? Do you think you interpret the lyrics the way the artist intended? Do you have a connection to the song because of past life experiences?
    - How do you think this song, and the music you listen to, affect your health overall?
15. **Access Information.** Many claims about mental and emotional health spread through media. With a partner, choose a claim about mental and emotional health you recently encountered—through an online video, TV show or film, song, social media post, or trending article, for example. Using reliable resources, evaluate the accuracy of the claim. Cite your sources and write a review of the claim supporting or debunking it.
16. **Communicate with Others.** In the *Real World Health Skills* activity in Lesson 4.1, you created a help sheet for accessing mental health resources in your community. This information is helpful for you, but could also aid others in your community. Using reliable resources, research the mental health conditions and issues most common in your community. Then, revise your help sheet to address these issues and appeal to your audience. Think about the most effective way to reach your community—for example, through pamphlets or social media. Share the help sheet with your community using an effective method.

17. **Make Decisions.** Imagine that one of your friends is acting out because your teacher does not allow students to use phones in class. When the teacher asks your friend to put the phone away, your friend loudly complains, makes a scene, and then sulks for the rest of class. What defense mechanism is your friend using? How could you help your friend handle these feelings without using this defense mechanism? Brainstorm some alternatives your friend could use and write a script in which you talk with your friend about them.
18. **Set Goals.** EI benefits a person's relationships and future success. Developing EI can take time, and people can always improve. To develop more EI, set a SMART goal related to each of the following areas of EI. Act on these goals and evaluate how they impact your emotional health and relationships.
    - *Self-awareness*—become more aware of your emotions and their impact
    - *Self-regulation*—better control your feelings
    - *Motivation*—stay or become motivated
    - *Social skills*—relate better to others
19. **Practice Health-Enhancing Behaviors.** Over the next three days, record at least three successes you had each day. Once you have done this, explain how recording your successes made you feel. What area of health are you improving by celebrating your own success? How could you incorporate this habit into your life on a regular basis?
20. **Advocate for Health.** Imagine you have noticed a lot of tension in your school the last couple weeks. Given what you have learned, you feel it is important for your peers to express their feelings. As a class, create a phone or online hotline your peers can access anonymously. In preparation, research peer hotlines, noting how and why they are created. Recruit other students and then develop a list of questions peer mediators can use while assisting those who access the hotline. Launch your hotline and advertise it at your school.

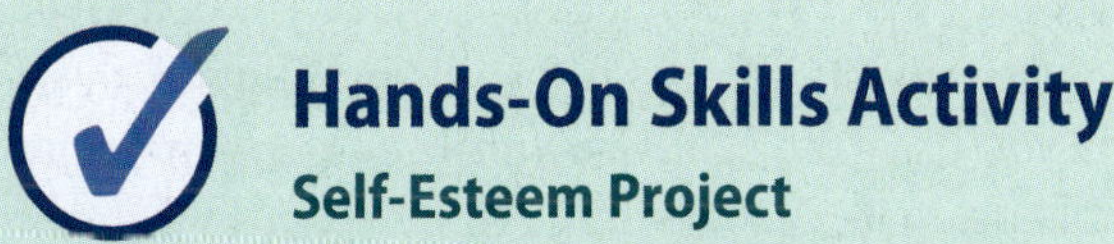

Hands-On Skills Activity

Self-Esteem Project

The term *self-esteem* describes how you feel about yourself. This activity will help you understand what negative remarks can do to a person's self-esteem. For this activity, you will need a container, water balloon, empty 2-liter bottle, water, safety pin, and paper towels.

Steps for This Activity

1. For two days, observe your peers interacting with one another, in person and online. Every time you see or hear a peer make a negative statement toward someone else, even as a joke, record the statement. At the end of the two days, calculate the total number of negative statements you heard or saw.
2. Gather in small groups of about four people. Within your group, add up all the negative statements you recorded. As you discuss these statements, make sure to keep them anonymous.
3. Assign each member of the group a number. Person one will fill the empty 2-liter bottle with water. Person two will fill the water balloon with water from the bottle, tie it, and place it in the container. Person three will be "the reader," and person four will be in charge of the safety pin.
4. After the balloon is full of water, the reader (person three) will begin reading one negative statement at a time. Person four will hold the water balloon over the container. After each statement is read, person four will use the safety pin to carefully poke one hole in the balloon.
5. **Analyze Influences.** After the statements have been read and the holes have been poked in the balloon, consider the following questions:
    - What does the balloon look like now?
    - Imagine that the balloon resembles the person on the receiving end of those negative statements. What has happened to that person's self-esteem?
6. **Communicate with Others.** Go back and examine each negative statement you read. For each statement, discuss the following questions:
    - Was the negative statement necessary? What feelings probably motivated it?
    - How could the person making the statement have expressed those feelings more respectfully?
    - What questions could you ask yourself before making a negative statement to reduce the impact the statement will have on others?

Chapter 5

Shifting to Positive Thinking

Look for the skills icon ✓ throughout this chapter for opportunities to practice your health skills.

Check Your Health and Wellness Skills

In this chapter, you will learn skills for shifting to positive thinking. To understand the skills you currently use, take the following inventory of your behaviors. Indicate how well you think you use each skill. Use a scale of 1–5, *1* meaning you do not use the skill and *5* meaning you feel completely comfortable using it.

Skill	How Well Do You Use Each Skill?
I know how I respond to events has more effect on my happiness than the events themselves.	
I find ways to give to others, such as through volunteering.	
When I'm sad, I try spending time in nature or getting physical activity.	
I try to pay attention to what is happening in the moment.	
I keep a list of things for which I'm grateful.	
When I think something bad about myself, I correct it and think something good.	
I ask questions to learn about other people's opinions.	
I spend the most time with people who make me feel positive.	
I pay close attention to people's body language when they're talking.	
I have confidence I can adapt to change.	
When I make a mistake, I forgive myself and don't beat myself up.	
	Total:

Add up your responses to each statement. The higher your score, the more comfortable you feel practicing health skills related to positive thinking. Which skill do you think is most important for you? Which skill is the most challenging for you? Which skill would you most like to improve? In this chapter, you will learn how to perform these skills better and more often.

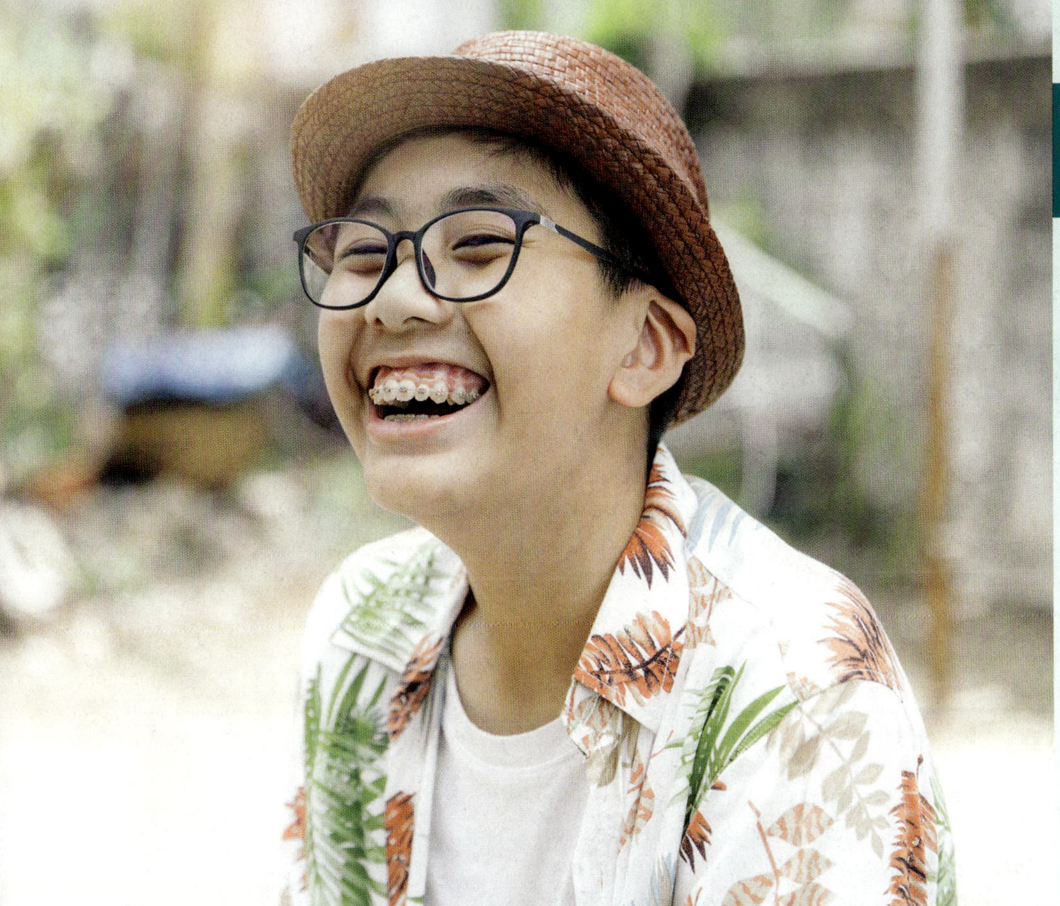

Suriyapong Thongsawang/iStock/GettyImages

Reading and Notetaking

Imagine you are a therapist and your client wants to find a way to be happier. Write a two-paragraph speech recommending steps your client can take to feel happier. Incorporate information you have learned about mental and emotional health and your own experiences. Then record your speech. As you read the chapter, take detailed notes. After reading this chapter, listen to your speech. With a partner, discuss what you would change about your speech based on any new information you have learned. Present your final speech to the class.

My speech → Chapter notes → Revised speech

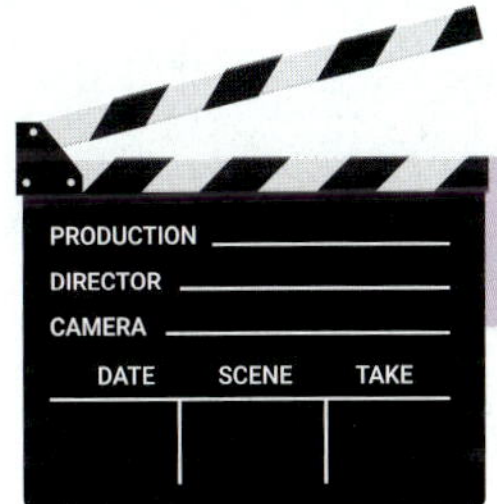

Setting the Scene

Choosing Happiness

Looking back, you have had a difficult past few months. Your parent got a new job, so you moved to a new school and had to leave behind your old friends. Your grandmother, whom you were very close to, passed away last month, and you really miss her. You just do not feel close to anyone in your new school. Sometimes you go all week without really feeling happy.

One day after school, you mention how you have been feeling to your health teacher. Your teacher helps you understand that sometimes difficult life events mean developing new coping strategies. Your teacher also encourages you to think about what activities *do* make you happy. You know you feel happier working out, watching funny video clips, and going for walks with your dog. You feel a bit better after this conversation and decide to start working on finding ways to feel happier.

Thinking Critically

1. What are some factors that can make it hard for high school students to feel happy?
2. What are some strategies you can use to feel happier in your own life?

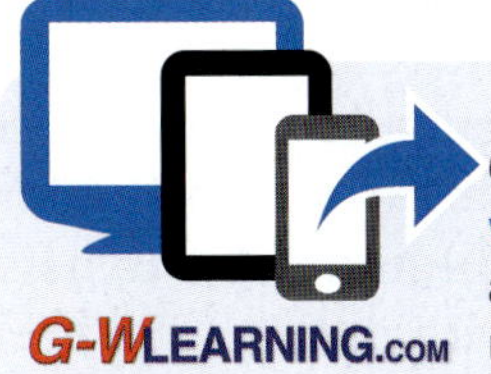

Click on the activity icon or visit www.g-wlearning.com/health/4095 to access online vocabulary activities using key terms from the chapter.

Lesson

5.1

Understanding Happiness

Essential Question?

How does happiness develop?

Learning Outcomes

After studying this lesson, you will be able to

- explain what happiness is and is not;
- identify the factors that influence happiness;
- explain why happiness is a way of thinking and acting; and
- demonstrate skills to increase happiness.

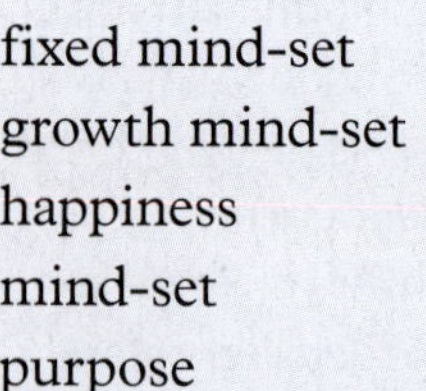

Key Terms

fixed mind-set
growth mind-set
happiness
mind-set
purpose

Warm-Up Activity

What Is Happiness?

Comprehend Concepts What does it mean to be "happy"? Before reading this lesson, create your own definition of *happiness*. Write this definition in the middle of a map like the one shown. Then, think about what makes you happy. In the outer circle of the map, write all the things you can think of that make you happy. Share your map with a partner and discuss how what makes you happy relates to your definition of happiness.

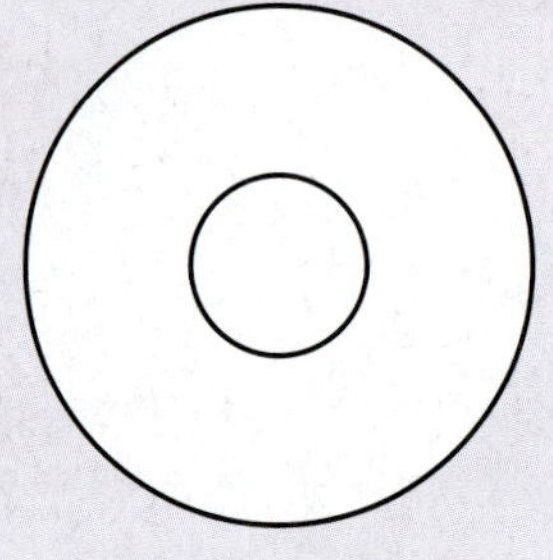

Positive mental and emotional health enables people to cope with stress, make meaningful contributions, and reach their potential. As you know, people with positive mental and emotional health tend to have a sense of balance, emotional control, respect, compassion and kindness, and healthy relationships. People with positive mental and emotional health also tend to experience and pursue happiness. In this lesson, you will learn what happiness is and what factors affect whether a person feels happy. You will also be introduced to strategies for pursuing happiness.

What Does It Mean to Feel Happy?

Most people use the term *happiness* regularly in daily life. You might say you feel happy when you do well on a test, get a summer job you want, or have a fun evening with friends. As these examples illustrate, the term **happiness** refers to experiencing a variety of positive emotions (such as joy, pride, contentment, and gratitude). These emotions are a part of well-being and contribute to positive mental and emotional health (**Figure 5.1**). Experiencing these positive emotions can help people cope with difficult life events and feelings, pursue goals, and connect more strongly with others.

happiness positive emotion linked to well-being and contentment with life

Benefits of Happiness

- Reduced risk of health conditions
- Faster recovery from health conditions
- Longer life
- Better mental and emotional health
- Lower levels of stress and anxiety
- Stronger support system
- Better health habits

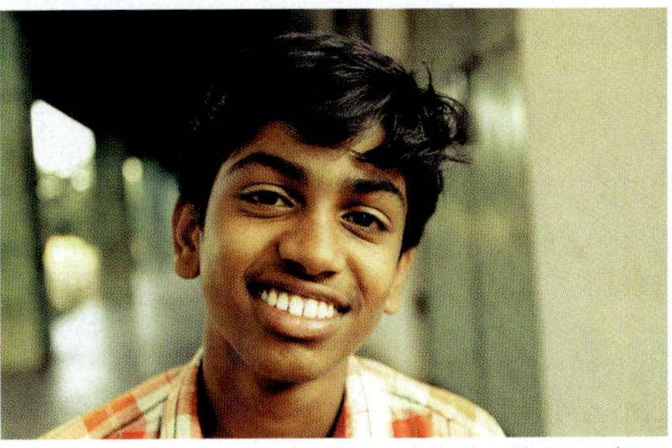

V.S.Anandhakrishna/Shutterstock.com

Figure 5.1 Happiness can benefit a person's physical, mental and emotional, and social health. ***What are some examples of positive emotions related to happiness?***

People anywhere on the mental health continuum can experience the positive emotions associated with happiness. For example, a high school student under considerable stress might feel happy playing soccer or reading a book. A person who experiences extreme anxiety about doing schoolwork, being at home, or seeing a snake may still feel happy spending time with friends.

Some mental health conditions, such as depression, may make it harder to pursue happiness. Even people with these conditions, however, can take some steps to increase happiness. In fact, one study of more than 7,000 people found that 89 percent of those without a mental illness reported they often felt "very happy" over the last four weeks. Sixty-eight percent of those with a mental illness still reported feeling "very happy" during the last four weeks. This study demonstrates that while feeling happy is easier for people who do not have a mental illness, people with a mental illness can regularly feel happy.

Happiness does not mean having only positive emotions all the time. You might feel very happy as you look forward to spending a day at the beach, going to prom, or celebrating your birthday with friends. You might feel sad once these events are over.

Like all people, those who generally feel happy experience times of sadness, frustration, and anxiety. People who tend to feel happier, however, are better able to bounce back from these negative experiences. They can take frustrations and disappointments in stride and move on from them. Instead of giving up, they use coping strategies that help them return to feeling better over time.

Factors That Affect Happiness

Although most people want to be happy, people often make errors in thinking about what will or will not bring happiness. For example, many people think happiness is determined by the events in their lives, such as being asked on a date, having lots of money, or getting an *A* on a project. Although people often feel happy when good things happen, these short-term events have a relatively small impact on lasting happiness. Similarly, when bad things happen, people may think they will never feel happy again. People adjust to negative events, however, and over time, can feel better.

The most important predictors of happiness are not, in fact, what happens to people. People who have many good experiences, such as succeeding at a hobby or making a varsity sports team, may not actually feel happy. Genetics, mind-set, sense of meaning, and relationships have a much stronger influence on people's happiness than the specific events—good or bad—that occur in their lives.

Genetics

Because of genetic makeup, some people find it easier to be happy compared to others. In fact, research shows that about half of a person's happiness is caused by genes (**Figure 5.2**). As a result, some people have a head start finding happiness. The good news is that, no matter their genes, everyone can take steps to increase happiness.

Genetic makeup also contributes to the development of mental illnesses, such as anxiety disorders and major depressive disorder, which can make it harder for people to feel happy. Structural differences in the brain contribute to some mental illnesses. For example, children with anxiety disorders have larger *amygdalas*, the part of the brain that triggers the fear reaction. Chemical imbalances in the brain can also lead to mental illness. Medications that help correct these imbalances can be helpful in treating some mental illnesses. This is why it is important for people with a mental illness to seek professional treatment.

Mind-Set

mind-set person's thought pattern, attitude, and mood

growth mind-set belief that a person's most basic abilities and feelings can be changed through hard work and dedication

fixed mind-set belief that a person's most basic abilities and feelings are permanent and cannot be changed

A person's **mind-set**, or thought pattern, attitude, and mood, influences happiness in real and fundamental ways. When difficult situations happen, some people shake them off or find some good in the situation. For example, if they miss out on getting a part in the high school play they tried out for, they focus instead on how they will have more time to spend with friends. These people approach life with a positive mind-set.

Other people dwell on negative events and cannot seem to let them go and move on. For example, if their partner breaks up with them, they assume they will never find another person to date. These people have a negative mind-set. Not surprisingly, it is harder for people with a negative mind-set to feel happy.

Other types of mind-sets can also influence happiness. Some people have a **growth mind-set**, which means they believe change is possible with time, effort, and practice. Other people have a **fixed mind-set** and believe their current feelings and abilities are basically permanent.

Genes influence traits associated with happiness, including optimism, outgoingness, and resilience.
Genes may also predict factors linked with happiness, such as self-acceptance, a sense of control, and the ability to form healthy relationships.

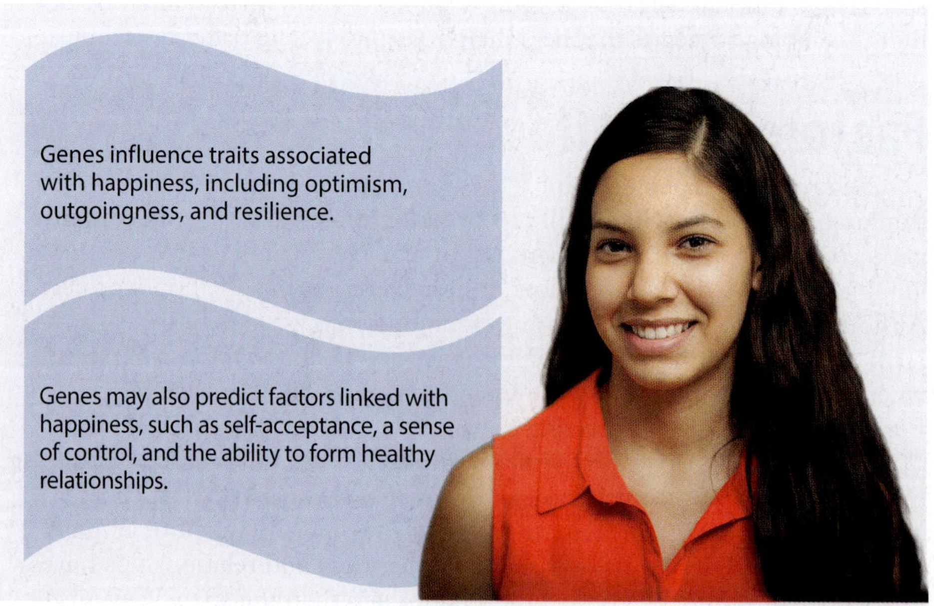

antoniodiaz/Shutterstock.com

Figure 5.2 No single gene predicts happiness, but several different genes play a role.

For example, people who believe their feelings of anxiety and depression cannot be changed, even with professional help, often feel more anxious and depressed. They also have higher levels of worry and sadness and more physical symptoms of anxiety, such as sweaty hands and panic attacks. In contrast, people with a growth mind-set believe that, even if they feel anxious and depressed, there are strategies they can use to feel better.

If adopting a positive mind-set does not come naturally to you, remember that scientific studies show that about 80 percent of people who receive mental health therapy report feeling better. The first step is believing change is possible.

Meaning

One of the most important parts of happiness is feeling a deeper sense of meaning and purpose in life. Researchers describe **purpose** as "a stable and generalized intention to accomplish something that is at the same time meaningful to the self and consequential for the world beyond the self." For example, a person's sense of purpose could be a certain passion or desire to work for a cause. People who feel their lives are good, meaningful, and worthwhile experience the highest levels of happiness (**Figure 5.3**).

purpose stable and generalized intention to accomplish something that is both meaningful to the self and consequential for the world beyond the self

Relationships

All people have different types of relationships in their lives, including relationships with family members, friends, romantic partners, and members of their communities. The single biggest predictor of life satisfaction is the quality of these relationships.

Close relationships have many benefits that contribute to happiness. For example, they provide opportunities for meaningful conversations and allow people to share positive experiences. They also help people cope with the daily stress of life.

Having close relationships also benefits health. People who have high-quality relationships have better physical health, including lower blood pressure, lower body mass index (BMI), and stronger immune systems. They also engage in healthier behaviors, recover faster from surgery, and are less likely to develop a chronic disease.

High school students who focus on finding meaning tend to:

- emphasize internal motivation (doing what they love) over external motivation (doing what they think others want them to do)
- work with other people, instead of competing against them
- find inspiring mentors, such as parents or guardians, teachers, and coaches
- spend time in the community, such as by having a part-time job, doing volunteer work, or becoming involved in local or national causes
- learn from failure, which teaches resilience and persistence
- hold beliefs in causes or ideas bigger than themselves

Figure 5.3 People's senses of meaning or purpose in life relate to their levels of happiness.

Local and Global Health

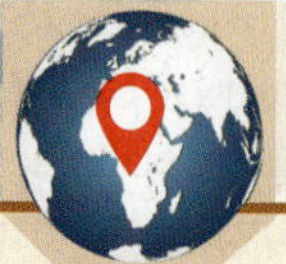

Describing Happiness Around the World

The concept of happiness has different meanings to people in different countries and cultures. In the United States, happiness is commonly associated with positive experiences and personal achievements. Happiness, in this case, is often described in terms of intense emotions, such as excitement and enthusiasm.

In many Asian countries, such as Japan and China, happiness is more commonly associated with feelings of *social harmony*, or getting along with others. People in these countries are more likely to describe happiness in terms of less intense emotions, such as relaxation and calmness.

Cultures also differ in how they think about what happiness really is. In Denmark, the term commonly used to mean happiness is *lykke*. This word describes small moments of well-being in everyday life, such as drinking a nice cup of coffee or eating a slice of bread with cheese. In other countries, such as Germany, France, Poland, and Russia, the terms used for happiness describe much less common experiences.

Still other cultures divide happiness into distinct components. In China, for example, three different words are used to describe happiness: *xingfu* (good life), *you yiyi* (meaning), and *kuaile* (good mood).

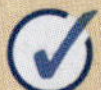

Practice Your Skills

Analyze Influences

What factors do you think explain why people in different countries think about happiness in different ways? Are there other factors that could influence how people think about happiness, such as where they live in a given country, their spiritual beliefs, or their age or level of income? How does a culture's definitions of happiness impact how happy people feel?

Now, think about your own life and values. If you had to define the word *happiness* for yourself, what would your definition be? How does this definition affect how happy you feel? Discuss your definitions in a small group.

Strategies for Increasing Happiness

While some people think that happiness comes from life circumstances, your thought patterns and behaviors have a greater impact on happiness. Sometimes, it can be hard to change your thought patterns and adopt new behaviors. For example, someone with an anxiety disorder or major depressive disorder may have difficulty making decisions that lead to greater happiness and need professional treatment. Someone whose family members encourage a certain thought pattern may have trouble changing this pattern of thinking.

Major steps that can increase happiness include adopting a positive mind-set and developing empathy and resilience. You will learn more about these skills in the next two lessons. Some simpler, smaller steps that can help you feel happier follow.

Set and Work Toward Goals

A great strategy for feeling better about yourself is to set realistic goals and work toward accomplishing them. Think about some goals you would like to achieve, such as keeping your room clean or finding a summer job. Then develop specific strategies for reaching these goals by setting subgoals, such as organizing your closet or preparing a résumé.

Achieving the goals you set for yourself feels good, builds self-confidence, and increases self-esteem. Try to avoid holding yourself to unreasonable standards, however. Each step you take to complete a goal is a positive step. If you miss a goal, reevaluate your progress and adjust your goals as needed.

Maintain Close Relationships

Having close and supportive relationships is an essential part of having a healthy life. There are steps you can take to develop and maintain close relationships with family members and friends. For example, you can join groups in which you can meet people with similar interests or do volunteer work. You can also choose to spend time with people who have a positive outlook on life.

Give to Other People

One of the best ways to find more happiness is to give to other people. In fact, giving to others increases people's happiness, improves their health, and may even extend their lives. Any type of giving counts, from volunteering in your community to donating gently used clothes or performing a random act of kindness (**Figure 5.4**).

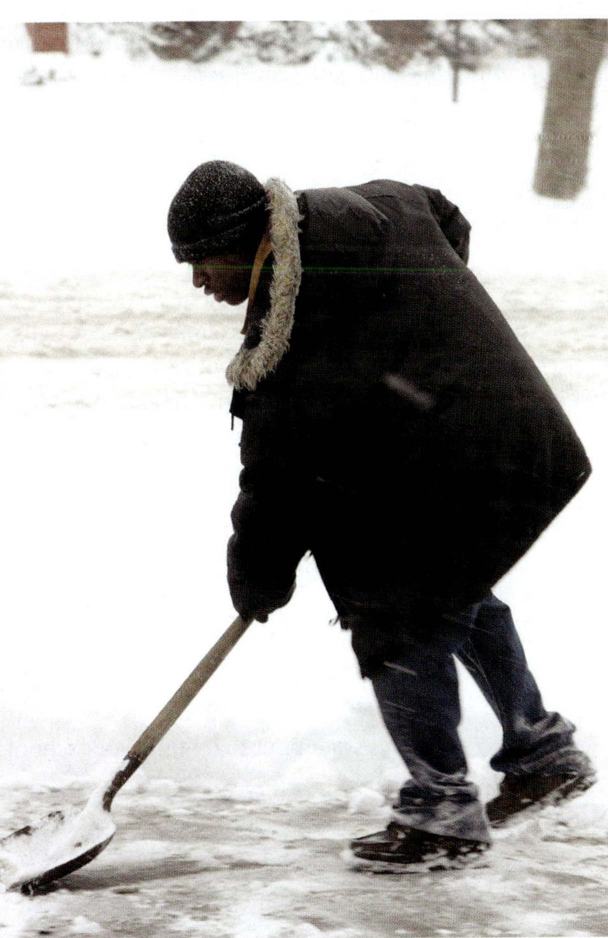

Give help

- Volunteer at a food pantry or other organization
- Pick up litter in community recreational areas
- Donate blood at a blood drive
- Shovel a neighbor's driveway when it snows or mow a neighbor's lawn

Give patience

- Let someone in a hurry ahead of you in line
- Hold a door open for someone
- Let a car merge in front of you
- Actively listen to someone talk without distractions

Give kind words

- Give someone a compliment
- Write a thank-you letter to a teacher or relative
- Write letters to soldiers
- Tell your friends or family members how much they mean to you

Give money or goods

- Donate to a charity or organization that means something to you
- Run or walk a 5K for a good cause
- Donate your clothes, books, movies, toys, or household items
- Buy holiday gifts to give to families in need or children in foster homes

Patricia Marks/Shutterstock.com

Figure 5.4 Giving to other people does not have to be expensive and does not need to take up a lot of time. Simple, free acts of kindness count too.

Adopt Healthy Behaviors

Engaging in a number of simple behaviors can make you feel better and also improve your physical health. For example, getting enough sleep can help you feel happier. People who get the recommended amount of sleep (eight to 10 hours for teens) show lower rates of anxiety, depression, and loneliness.

One behavior that predicts happiness is physical activity. Being physically active can get your mind off difficulties you are facing. It also leads to changes in your body that make you feel better. When you engage in physical activity, the brain releases chemicals called *endorphins*, which improve mood.

Another behavior that can boost mood and improve health is spending time in nature. In fact, simply walking through a garden can lower a person's stress and blood pressure. You can increase your happiness by hiking in the mountains, walking on a beach, or strolling through a park.

Prioritize Experiences

Many people get caught up in the idea that buying items leads to happiness. This is one reason lots of people spend money on the newest smartphone, a particular brand of clothes, or the latest popular electronic gadget. Spending money on belongings, however, only leads to very brief happiness. At first, it is exciting to have this new object, but this excitement wears off quickly.

A better way to use money to increase happiness is to spend money on experiences, such as tickets to a sporting event or concert. When you spend money on an experience, you get to look forward to the event, experience the event, and look back on the experience. This is why spending money on experiences is a better strategy for finding lasting happiness.

Lesson 5.1 Review

Know and Understand

1. How do people who pursue happiness handle negative experiences?
2. Explain the difference between a growth and fixed mind-set. Give an example of each.
3. What does it mean to have purpose in life? Describe your sense of purpose in life.
4. What healthy behaviors can you adopt to help increase happiness?
5. Why do experiences lead to more happiness than belongings?

Think Critically

6. Review the mental health continuum in Figure 4.2. In a small group, discuss the idea that people anywhere on the continuum can experience happiness. Give examples of ways people can pursue happiness, even when they have difficulties with mental and emotional health.
7. With a partner, consider the following statement: *The most important predictors of happiness are not, in fact, what happens to you*. Create a podcast in which you and your partner explain this statement to teens in your school.

REAL WORLD Health Skills

Access Information Refer to the map you created in the *Warm-Up Activity* for this lesson and review the factors you said make you happy. For each factor, use reliable resources to research how the factor is associated with happiness. In a journal entry, reflect on your findings and discuss whether you agree or disagree. Also research strategies you could use to increase the factors associated with happiness.

Establishing a Positive Mind-Set

Essential Question?

What strategies can you use to adopt a positive mind-set?

Lesson 5.2

Learning Outcomes

After studying this lesson, you will be able to

- summarize how mind-set influences happiness;
- explain the difference between optimism and pessimism;
- identify the benefits of an optimistic outlook; and
- demonstrate skills for improving mind-set.

Key Terms

attitude
dignity
diversity
gratitude
mindfulness
optimistic
outlook
pessimistic
rumination
self-respect
self-talk

Warm-Up Activity

Your Mind-Set

Comprehend Concepts Before reading this lesson, answer the following questions:

1. Do you sometimes leave notes for yourself to remind yourself of your self-worth?
2. When you are frustrated, do you stop to assess why you are feeling this way?
3. In hard situations, do you think everything will turn out okay?
4. Do you respect yourself?
5. Are you continually grateful for the good things around you?
6. Do you respect the people around you?
7. When you look at other people's lives, do you feel happy for them?

Aysezgicmeli/Shutterstock.com

Did you answer more questions with *no* or with *yes*? As you read this lesson, think about your answers to these questions. Reflect on how your current actions and attitudes affect your mind-set and think about areas for improvement.

Everyone experiences setbacks and disappointments. This is just a natural part of life. You cannot always protect yourself or the people you love from painful events and negative experiences or emotions. When people feel unhappy after a painful event or experience, they often assume the negative event led them to feel this way. Although it is natural and healthy to feel and cope with negative emotions after a painful experience, people's *mind-set*, or how they think about, feel about, and react to an experience, impacts their ability to recover and feel happy again.

The Impact of Mind-Set

Mind-set affects a person's ability to enjoy life and cope with difficult life circumstances. For example, people with a positive mind-set experience higher levels of happiness and lower levels of anxiety and depression. A negative mind-set can hurt self-esteem and increase anxiety.

People with a positive mind-set not only feel happier, but also experience better physical health. They have fewer physical symptoms, such as coughing, fatigue, and sore throats (**Figure 5.5**). One explanation for the relationship between mind-set and physical health is that people with a positive mind-set may have better coping strategies. They might tackle issues head-on and avoid unhealthy methods of coping with stress, such as eating junk food or drinking alcohol. They might let go of negative events, instead of getting stuck in disappointments. All of these behaviors can lead to better physical health.

People with a positive mind-set often have a stronger social network as well. It is more pleasant to spend time with someone who has a positive mind-set, so people with this approach may develop closer relationships with friends and family members. This type of social support can also help people manage stressful events when they occur.

Positive Versus Negative Mind-Sets

Feeling sad, anxious, and frustrated at times is normal. No one feels happy or hopeful all the time. Having a positive mind-set, however, can help people cope with difficult times and enjoy good experiences. Having a negative mind-set can make these challenges harder and harm health.

Positive Mind-Set

optimistic expecting good outcomes for actions and feeling or showing hope for the future

People who have a positive mind-set are generally **optimistic**. These people view situations positively, even in the face of challenges, and believe they will eventually feel better. They are flexible and adapt, change, and grow as they encounter different life experiences.

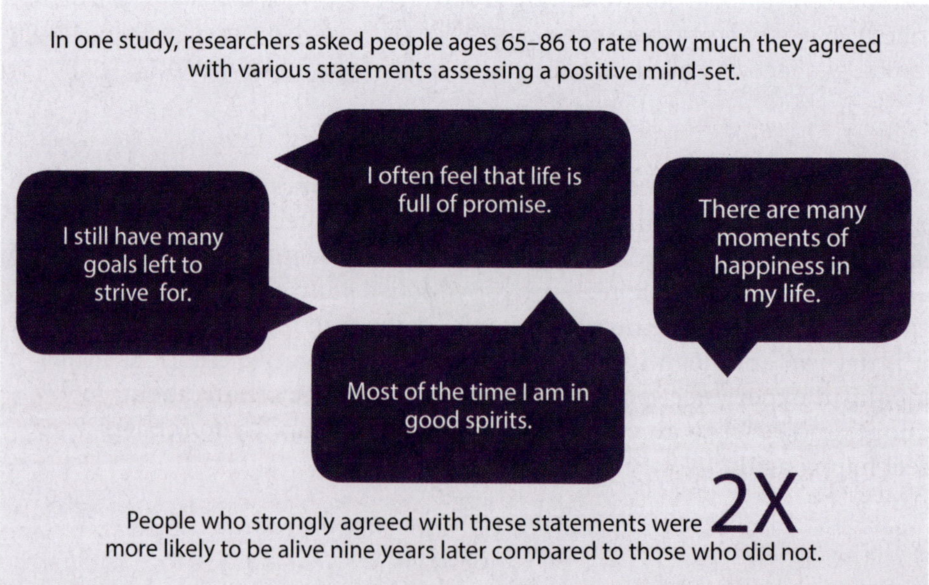

Figure 5.5 Having a positive mind-set is also related to living longer.

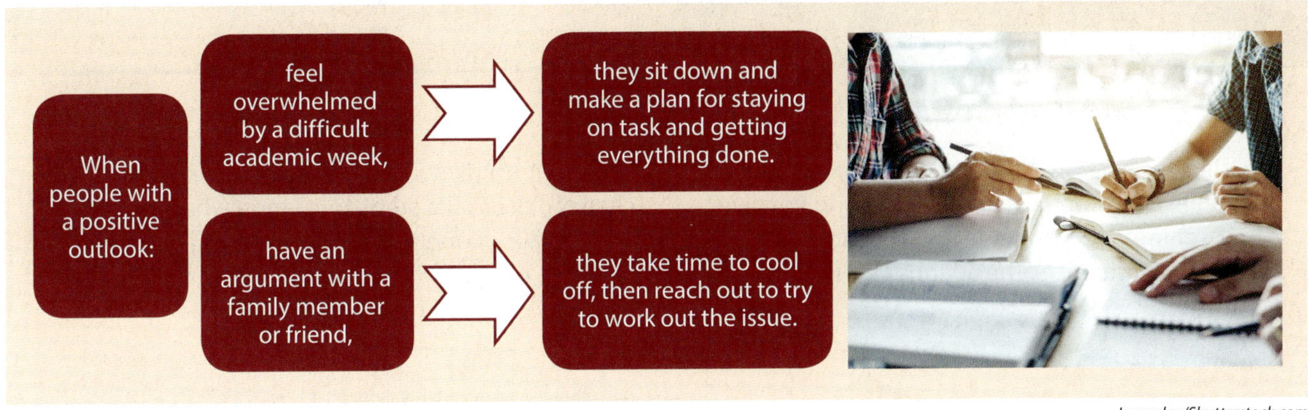

Joyseulay/Shutterstock.com

Figure 5.6 People with a positive outlook tend to have a healthy approach to difficult situations, which helps them manage stress and conflict. ***What type of mind-set involves keeping a positive outlook, even in the face of challenges?***

People who go through life with a positive mind-set have better health in part because they use good coping strategies. For example, these people face and respond to challenges (**Figure 5.6**). This choice to confront challenges head-on helps eliminate, or at least reduce, the challenge. It also reduces the negative physical effects of stress on the body.

People who approach life with a positive mind-set have a remarkable ability to find some good, no matter the situation. This ability to see the glass half full enables them to take negative events in stride and always find some good aspect.

People who have a positive mind-set also focus on what they *can* control, not what they cannot (**Figure 5.7**). This helps people let issues go, especially when they have absolutely no control over a situation. For example, high school students whose parents are getting divorced might recognize there is nothing they can do to fix the difficult situation.

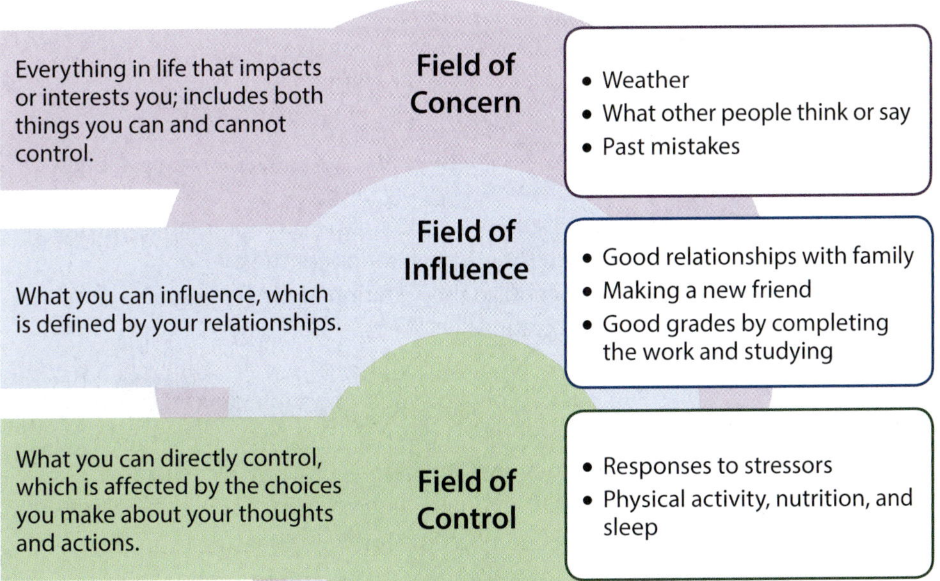

Figure 5.7 Everything within your field of concern interests you and impacts your daily life. Learning what is and is not in your field of control can help you have a positive mind-set. ***What field includes only what you can directly change with your choices about your thoughts and actions?***

Health Across the Life Span

How Does Mind-Set Affect Aging?

Did you know that the mind-set you have about life and aging can affect how long you live? Mind-set impacts your mental and emotional health and influences the actions you take. It can determine whether you give in when facing challenges or take steps to change what you can. The impact of one's mind-set about aging is an example of this.

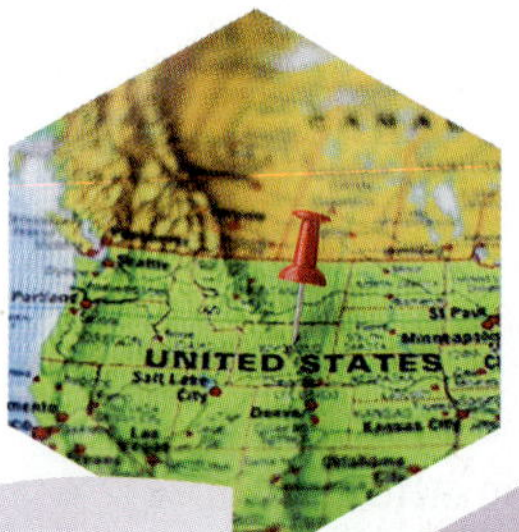

In the US, many people have negative views about aging.

Stereotypes include that older people

- are less attractive
- have a poor memory
- are physically weak

In parts of Italy, Japan, and Greece, retirement is not seen as a natural part of getting older. Older people are expected to stay active and help the community in some way, such as by cooking, gardening, or taking care of children.

In many other cultures around the world, aging is seen in a more positive way.

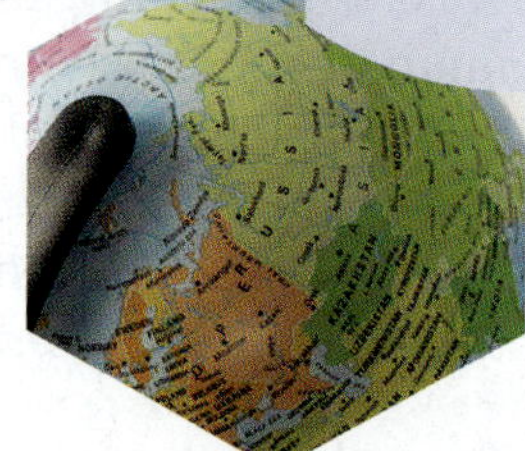

Having positive views about aging can affect how people experience aging as they grow older.

- Researchers at Yale University asked adults ages 50 and older to rate their attitudes about aging.
- Over the next 23 years, they contacted these same people regularly to measure their health.
- **People who had positive attitudes about aging lived, on average, 7.5 years longer than those with negative attitudes.**

Left to right: crazystocker/Shutterstock.com; wael alreweie/Shutterstock.com

Keep these findings in mind the next time you hear someone make a disrespectful comment about an older person or see an advertisement that depicts older adults as weak or sick. Instead of encouraging these ideas, remember to treat older people with respect, show appreciation for their wisdom, and recognize they continue to make valuable contributions.

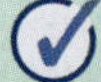

Practice Your Skills

Analyze Influences

Why do you think people in different countries hold different views about aging? How do you think these different views develop? Do they change over time? With a partner, discuss why views about aging impact the health of older people and even how long these people live. What are some strategies that could help people in the US adopt more positive views about aging? Share your ideas with a partner. Then, commit to sharing your ideas for improving views about aging with your friends and family members.

Negative Mind-Set

People with a negative mind-set adopt a very different view and are generally **pessimistic**. These people anticipate negative outcomes and feel fear or dread about the future. When bad events happen, they feel stuck and believe they will never feel better.

pessimistic expecting only bad outcomes for actions and feeling unhopeful for the future

People with a more negative mind-set tend to give up when facing a difficult situation. They may ignore challenges or conflicts and simply hope they will go away. Unfortunately, this "stick your head in the sand" approach means the situation does not get better and could even get worse. When bad events happen, people with negative mind-sets fixate on negative thoughts, even when the situation is beyond their control. Repeatedly focusing on negative thoughts, called **rumination**, can make someone feel even worse and trigger feelings of anxiety or depression.

rumination act of thinking deeply or obsessively about negative feelings or situations

Pursuing a Positive Mind-Set

You may naturally adopt a positive mind-set without much difficulty. Even if this does not come easily to you, however, there are strategies you can use to practice shifting your thoughts in a more positive direction. Over time, using these strategies will help you adopt a more positive mind-set.

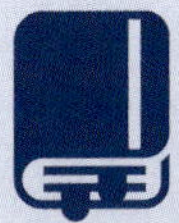

Case Study

Social Media Envy

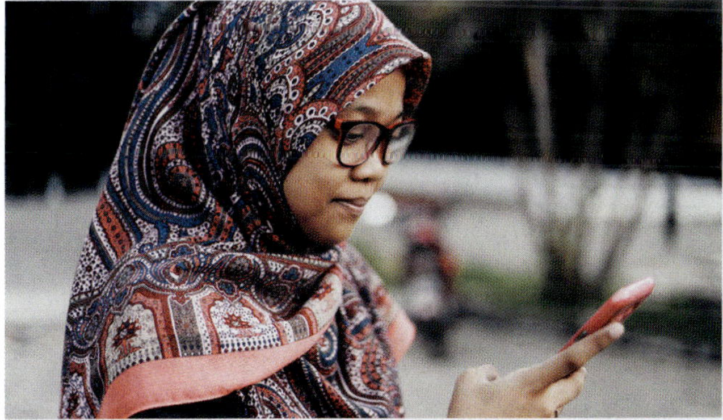

Safwan Abd Rahman/Shutterstock.com

Dimah looks at the pictures people post from their summer vacations and is jealous. Her family did not have the money to go anywhere this year. Instead, they had fun with cheaper outings like going to drive-in movies, barbecuing outdoors, and having family game nights together. Dimah had so much fun this summer, but when she compares her summer to everyone else's pictures, she feels embarrassed. She feels uncomfortable and does not want to talk to her friends about it. She does not want them to feel bad for her.

In his first year at a new school, Matt is struggling to find friends. Sometimes he gets into fights with his parents or feels overwhelmed by school. He wishes he had somebody to talk to about it. The only way he can get people to interact with him is by posting pictures of his family vacation over the summer or his newest pair of shoes. He gets lots of likes, but that does not make going to school every day any easier. Sometimes, Matt thinks he will never make friends.

Practice Your Skills

Set Goals

Create a log and track how much time you spend on social media for one day. Record your feelings and what you tell yourself as you scroll through social media. Do you find yourself comparing your life and experiences with others? What do you say to yourself?

Next, set a few SMART goals for creating a happier social media experience. Determine if your goals should involve spending less time on social media, improving what you tell yourself while using social media, or something else. Include both short-term and long-term goals. Put your SMART goals into action and track your progress for each one you set.

Have a Positive Attitude

When you feel disappointed or your day does not go the way you want, how do you react? Do you immediately become angry or frustrated? Do you withdraw and give up? Do you try to identify some positive aspect of the situation?

attitude pattern of viewing and reacting to events in a certain way

People who adopt a positive **attitude**, or pattern of viewing and reacting to events, can take negative experiences in stride. When they feel disappointment, they can let go of negative emotions instead of replaying the event in their minds. They are also good at maintaining positive expectations about the future. For example, a high school student who gets a *C* on an English paper can feel disappointed, but also have a good attitude. The student can be confident that, with more effort, a better grade on the next paper is possible.

Be Mindful

mindfulness state of concentrated, judgment-free awareness of what is happening in the present moment

Another strategy for feeling more positive is to be aware of your thoughts and feelings. The term **mindfulness** describes a state of concentrated, judgment-free awareness of what is happening in the present moment. People who are mindful show lower rates of stress, depression, and anxiety. Mindfulness can even improve physical health. For example, people who are mindful feel less tired, are less likely to get injured, and have lower levels of pain.

There are many relatively easy ways to practice mindfulness in your own life (**Figure 5.8**). You can become more mindful simply by paying attention to what is happening right now and not letting your mind focus on other thoughts or concerns. For example, while talking with a friend, you can focus intensely on this interaction, instead of thinking about what you will do later or how stressful your day has been.

Strategies for Practicing Mindfulness

Pay Attention
Take time to really experience the world around you, using all of your senses. For example, when you eat a favorite food, make sure to smell it, taste it, and truly enjoy it.

Live in the Moment
Focus on the present and find small moments of pleasure, such as the sound of birds chirping, a beautiful sunset, or the sound of rain on the windows.

Accept Yourself
Appreciate yourself for who you are and treat yourself with compassion, just like you would treat a good friend.

Focus on Breathing
Concentrate on taking deep breaths and feel the air move in and out of your body.

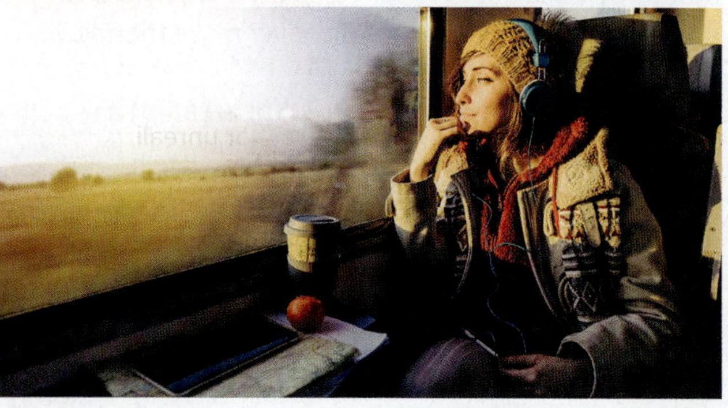

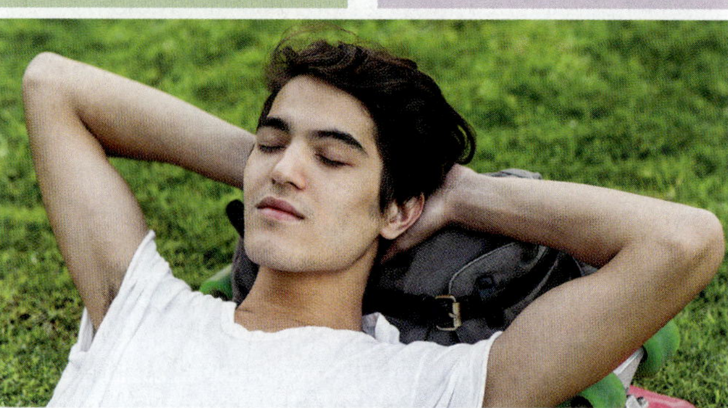

Left to right: martin-dm/E+/GettyImages; PKpix/Shutterstock.com

Figure 5.8 Mindfulness is not used in one individual situation, but is a skill to help people navigate all situations.

Practice Gratitude

It is perhaps human nature to focus often on what is bad in life instead of what is good. Focusing on **gratitude**, or an appreciation for what you have, however, can give you a more positive mind-set. People who focus on gratitude pay attention to what they are thankful for in their lives. They show kindness and compassion to other people, including friends, family members, and even strangers. Practicing gratitude leads to more optimism, as well as increased energy, greater happiness, and better health. People also tend to notice more positive aspects of life the more they focus on being grateful for those aspects.

gratitude appreciation for what one has

Some easy strategies for practicing gratitude in your daily life include the following:

- **Keep a gratitude journal:** Before you go to sleep at night, write several reasons you are thankful in that moment.
- **Write a gratitude letter:** In your letter, thank someone for how that person has made your life better in some way. Then send that person the letter.
- **Carry a gratitude rock:** Find a rock or stone that you like or that already has special meaning for you. Carry it with you in your pocket, purse, or backpack, and whenever you touch it, think about what you are grateful for.
- **Fill a gratitude jar:** Every time you feel grateful, write why on a little piece of paper and put it in the jar. Then, if you are feeling down, go into the jar and remind yourself of what is good in your life.

Remember that you can feel grateful for even small moments throughout the day. You could feel grateful for eating a tasty meal, accomplishing a new weight-lifting goal, or watching a sporting event with friends. Take a minute at the end of the day and just reflect on feeling good about these experiences.

Modify Your Outlook

Another good strategy for adopting a positive mind-set is to shift your **outlook**, or the way you see or think about a situation (**Figure 5.9**). For example, people who adopt a positive outlook try to see challenges as opportunities.

outlook way of thinking or feeling about a situation

On the other hand, adopting an overly negative outlook can make you see situations as far worse than they actually are. This tendency is called *catastrophizing*. People who catastrophize can take a small challenge and make it seem much bigger. For example, a high school student who experiences the end of a dating relationship may believe it means never finding another dating partner or getting married.

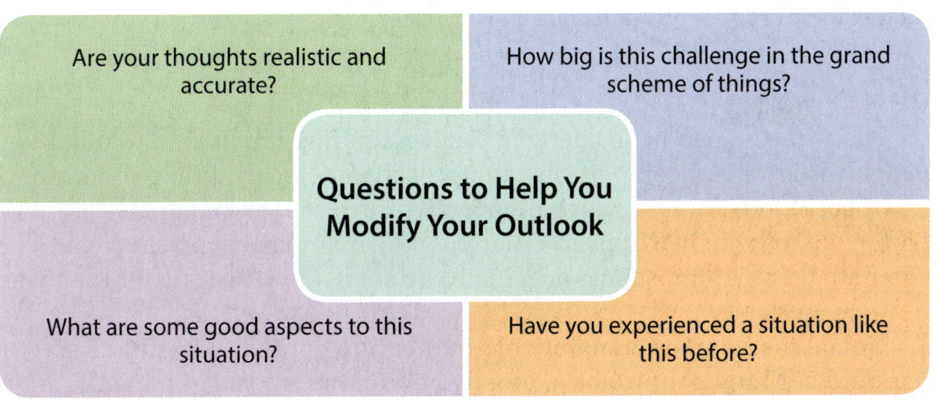

Figure 5.9 Recognizing when your outlook is catastrophized, overly negative, or unrealistic can help you shift to a more positive outlook. ***What tendency means seeing situations as far worse than they actually are?***

If you tend to have a negative outlook, try to become aware of this habit so you can recognize when you do it. Then, replace the negative thoughts with more positive—and realistic—ones. When battling a negative outlook, try to think about a time in which your overly negative expectations were not accurate. This can help you develop a more realistic outlook. For example, maybe you remember a time you did poorly on a test in middle school and thought you would never do better, but actually ended up understanding that material later.

Just like with any habit, it takes time and practice to change your thoughts. Shifting to a more positive outlook, however, is a great way to feel happier.

Watch Your Self-Talk

Everyone has an inner voice that speaks to them regularly throughout the day. For example, you might think to yourself, *I'm so hungry—I should have eaten a bigger breakfast*, or *I should try to speak up in my history class today*. Your thoughts about yourself throughout the day are known as **self-talk**.

self-talk one's thoughts about one's self throughout the day

The type of self-talk you engage in can have a major impact on how you feel. Some types of self-talk are positive and encouraging. For example, you might think about how well your audition for a school play is going to go or how prepared you feel for your science test. These types of positive thoughts feel supportive and enhance your self-confidence.

Other types of self-talk are negative and can undermine confidence and motivation. For example, you might think, *I look terrible in this shirt*, or *I'll never be good at science, no matter how hard I try*. This type of self-defeating self-talk can make you feel worse. It can also lead these negative expectations to become reality. After all, it is hard to do well when you do not have confidence that a positive outcome is even possible.

The first step in replacing negative self-talk with positive self-talk is to pay attention to your thoughts. By paying attention, you can recognize when you start running through pessimistic thoughts and stop the cycle faster.

Once you recognize your negative self-talk, you can replace these negative thoughts with more positive ones. For example, if you beat yourself up over getting any grade lower than an *A*, you might remind yourself that a *B* grade still shows a solid performance. If you feel hopeless as an athlete because you do not start the game, remind yourself of the accomplishment of making the team. This type of positive reframing will take some practice, but gets easier over time.

Respect Yourself

Many teens spend considerable time comparing themselves to other people. This type of comparison can occur in almost any dimension, from how people look, to how much money they have or how smart they are. Unfortunately, comparisons to other people often make people feel bad. After all, there is almost always going to be someone who is better than you in some area.

Social media plays a major role in creating comparisons that hurt happiness. Many people share mostly good news on social media.

Skills for Health and Wellness

Shifting to Positive Self-Talk

If you struggle with negative self-talk, try to practice noticing your self-talk and finding positive alternatives. You can use many different strategies to recognize and stop negative self-talk. For example, you could visualize a stop sign when you notice a negative thought. You could also give the negative voice in your head another name to separate it from yourself. The most powerful strategy you can use against negative self-talk is replacing negative thoughts with positive ones.

I can't talk in front of other people. I'll freeze up or cry if I have to give a speech.

Public speaking is really hard, but maybe it'll get easier with practice.

I'm ugly and awkward. No one will want to date me.

My friends like me for who I am. A dating partner will too.

No one really likes me here, and I'll never fit in.

It's hard making friends, but I've made friends before. I like who I am.

I'm so dumb. Everyone else already understands what we're learning in class.

I *am* smart, even if this subject is not my strong suit.

Other people do homework, have a job, and do extracurriculars. What's wrong with me that I don't?

I can have different priorities from other people. I focus on what I care about.

I look terrible in pictures, especially compared to my friends on social media.

I know my friends' pictures are carefully chosen and edited. Plus, everyone feels insecure sometimes.

Why bother getting good grades when I can't afford college tuition?

If I work hard and achieve my goals, I might get the scholarships I need to go to college.

Practice Your Skills

Practice Health-Enhancing Behaviors

Many teens struggle at times with negative self-talk. Learning strategies to counter negative thoughts is good for all areas of your health. For three days, pay attention to what you tell yourself throughout the day. Use a chart like the one shown to record negative thoughts, such as *My friend doesn't really like me*, *I'll never feel better*, or *It's no use trying when I know I'll fail.*

At the end of each day, review your list of negative thoughts and correct each negative statement with an example of positive self-talk. The next time you tell yourself the negative statement, make a conscious effort to replace it with the positive statement.

Negative Thought	Positive Alternative
I'll never feel better.	*I feel bad right now, but the feeling will pass if I keep going, think positively, and get the help I need.*

After the three days, create a blog post or audio or written journal entry reflecting on whether the exercise helped you. What did you learn, and how will you work to use positive self-talk in the future?

They are likely to share flattering, sometimes altered photographs of themselves; fun times with friends; and impressive accomplishments. A social media account, which presents only the best parts of a person's life, does not accurately portray anyone's life. When you make comparisons based on social media, you compare your life to just one small part of another person's life. This is one reason teens who spend more time on social media often feel more anxious, depressed, and lonely.

self-respect pride and confidence in one's self

dignity recognition that all people have the right to be valued and respected for who they are

diversity people's differences in many areas, such as race, ethnicity, sex, gender identity, sexual orientation, or spiritual beliefs

Instead of constantly focusing on other people, try instead to focus on yourself. People who have **self-respect** feel good about their strengths, abilities, and accomplishments for their own sake (**Figure 5.10**). They value trying their hardest and showing improvement over time. People who respect themselves also show **dignity**, or the recognition that everyone has the right to be valued and respected for who they are. They treat other people with respect and do not put other people down to feel better about themselves.

Respect Others

People who adopt a positive mind-set also respect other people. They recognize that people differ in their backgrounds, experiences, and perspectives. They value this type of **diversity**, which refers to people's differences in many areas, such as race or ethnicity, sex, political ideas, gender identity, sexual orientation, or spiritual beliefs.

Strategies for Increasing Self-Respect

Focus on your strengths, not on your weaknesses.	Do activities you love and that bring you joy.	Avoid comparing yourself to other people, especially on social media.	Be kind to someone else.
Talk to people you trust if you have trouble identifying your strengths.	Examples might include playing basketball or making a video.	Many people tend to share only the impressive, edited versions of their lives, especially online.	Give to others, such as by volunteering in their community or helping a friend.

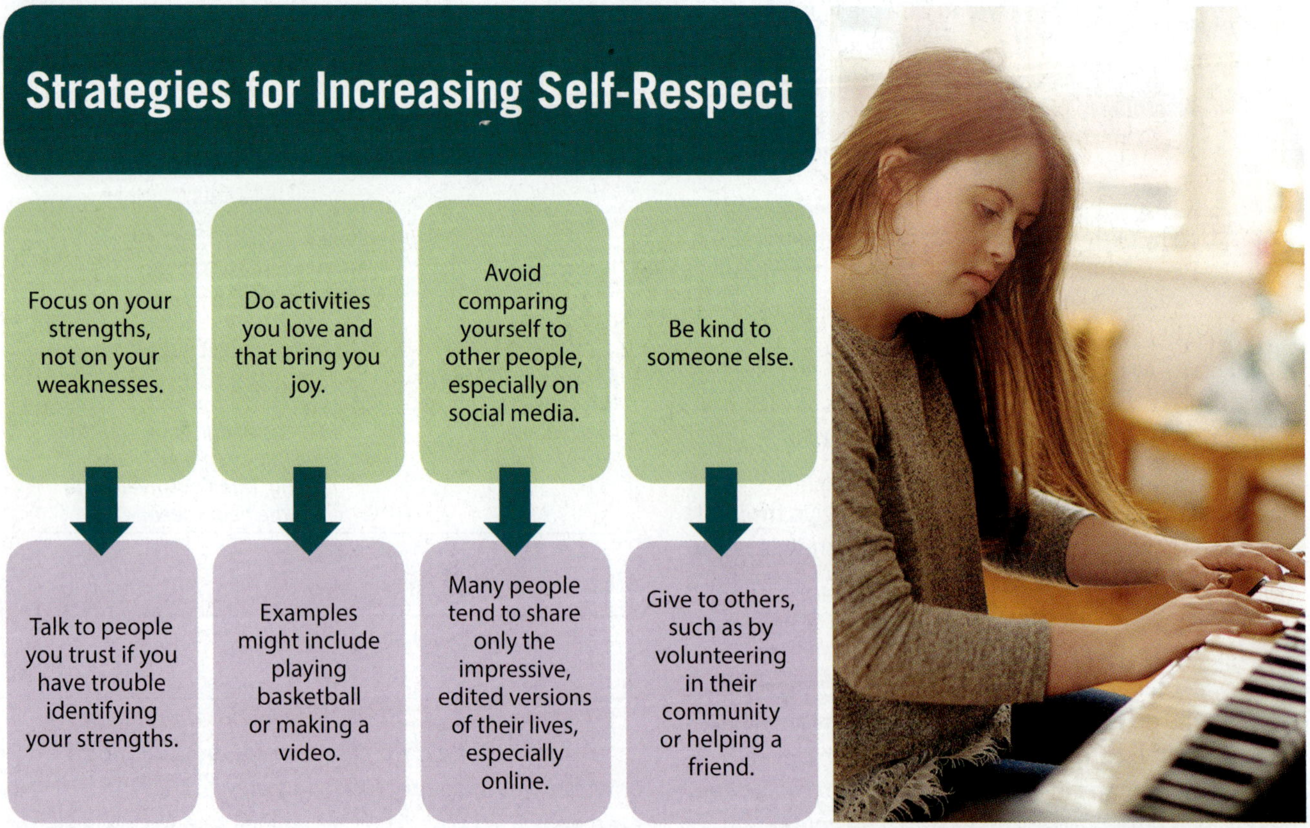

sturti/E+/GettyImages

Figure 5.10 Self-respect helps people understand their value and demand the respect they deserve. ***What idea recognizes that all people have the right to be valued and respected for who they are?***

People who respect themselves and others can get along with people from a variety of backgrounds and benefit from learning different perspectives (**Figure 5.11**).

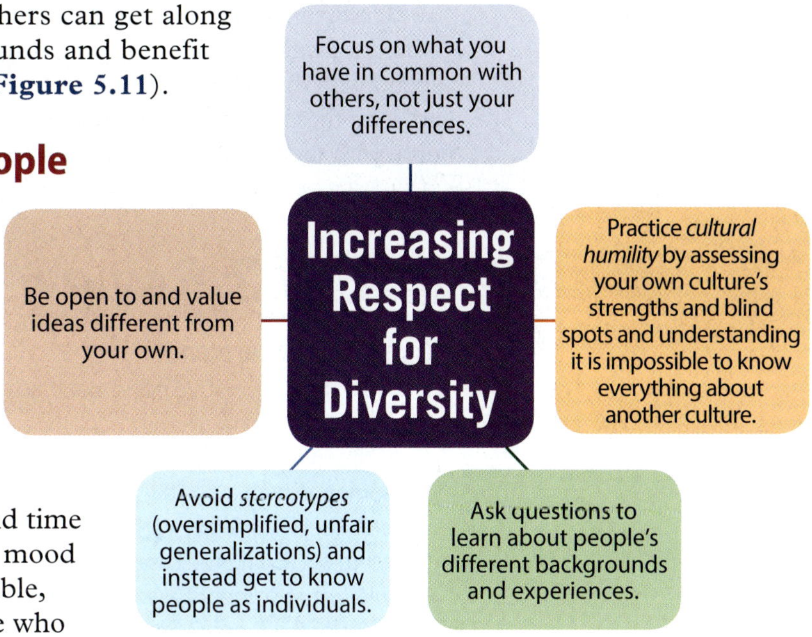

Spend Time with Positive People

Think about the people you spend time with regularly, including friends, family members, and even casual acquaintances. How do you feel when you are with these different people? If you are surrounded by people who generally have a good mood, spending time with them can make you feel better. In fact, happiness is contagious. When you spend time with people who are happy, the positive mood around you lifts you up. Whenever possible, choose to surround yourself with people who make you feel good.

Increasing Respect for Diversity

Focus on what you have in common with others, not just your differences.

Be open to and value ideas different from your own.

Practice *cultural humility* by assessing your own culture's strengths and blind spots and understanding it is impossible to know everything about another culture.

Avoid *stereotypes* (oversimplified, unfair generalizations) and instead get to know people as individuals.

Ask questions to learn about people's different backgrounds and experiences.

Figure 5.11 Respecting the diversity of people helps build a stronger social network and closer relationships.

Health in the Media

Social Media: A Rigged Game of Social Comparison

If you spend a lot of time on social media, you might find it hard not to make comparisons. The constant stream of people looking great and having fun with friends can make you feel your own life does not measure up. This constant comparison helps explain why teens who spend more time using social media and technology have higher rates of depression, eating disorders, and suicide attempts.

In one recent study, researchers from both the University of California, San Diego, and Yale University examined how much time people spent on social media, including "liking" other people's posts and posting their own updates. Researchers then examined whether the frequency of interactions was associated with overall well-being one year later.

Researchers found that people who spent more time on social media each day had lower levels of physical health, mental health, and life satisfaction one year later. A relatively simple strategy for feeling happier is therefore to reduce the amount of time you spend on social media. This choice reduces social comparisons and frees up time you can spend in better ways.

It is important to remember that what people post on social media is not a realistic view of their actual lives. Many teens post only attractive, sometimes edited photos and share mostly good news. This can lead people to feel worse about their own lives. Whenever you are on social media, remember you are seeing what people *choose* to share. Everyone sometimes feels sad, lonely, or less attractive.

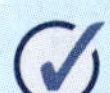

Practice Your Skills

Advocate for Health

With a partner, discuss why social media use can make it hard to feel happy and have a positive mind-set. As you discuss, list the major factors that lead teens and young adults to spend so much time on social media. Then, brainstorm an action you could take to help people in your school and community understand the hazards of making comparisons on social media. What strategies could you use to help people adopt better social media habits? What can you do to support your peers and encourage them to be confident in themselves, reduce time spent on social media, or change what they post? Commit to act on one of these ideas with your partner.

Unfortunately, unhappiness is also contagious. If you have people in your life who are always negative and gloomy, you may want to limit how much time you spend with them. You can also try to assist these people in getting help. When you are with these people, plan to do an activity that lifts your mood after spending time with them. This will help protect you from adopting their negativity.

Lesson 5.2 Review

Know and Understand

1. How does a positive mind-set lead to better health?
2. Write two case studies: one about someone with a positive mind-set and one about someone with a negative mind-set. Exchange case studies with other students in your class and identify the signs of optimism and pessimism in each case study.
3. How does gratitude improve mind-set?
4. Give one example of negative self-talk. Write this example and trade examples with another classmate. Then take turns replacing the negative self-talk with an example of positive self-talk.
5. Why is it unfair to compare your own life to the lives people portray on social media?

Think Critically

6. With a partner, discuss how to focus on what you can control, instead of what you cannot. In your lives, what can you control? What can you not control? Create a diagram to help you focus on decisions and situations inside your control.
7. Why do you think mindfulness helps people have a positive mind-set?
8. Try keeping a gratitude journal for one day. During each class period, write one reason you are grateful. At the end of your journal, reflect on how keeping the journal made you feel.
9. In a small group, discuss what it means to respect diversity. Develop three strategies each of you can use to improve respect for diversity and put these strategies into action.

REAL WORLD Health Skills

Practice Health-Enhancing Behaviors In this lesson, you learned about how changing your mind-set can influence your happiness and mental and emotional health. Imagine you are scrolling through social media, and your friends posted the following pictures with pessimistic captions. For each picture, write a new caption that is more optimistic. Then, discuss with a partner how changing the way you see each event can change your outlook on life. What skills did you use to rewrite these captions?

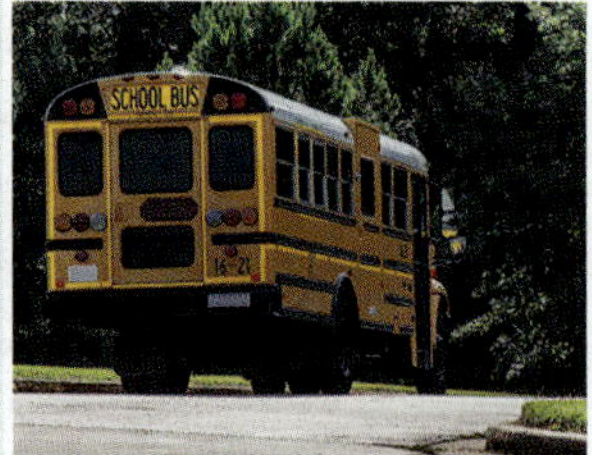

Grandma telling another long story about the old days this morning and missed the bus. #late

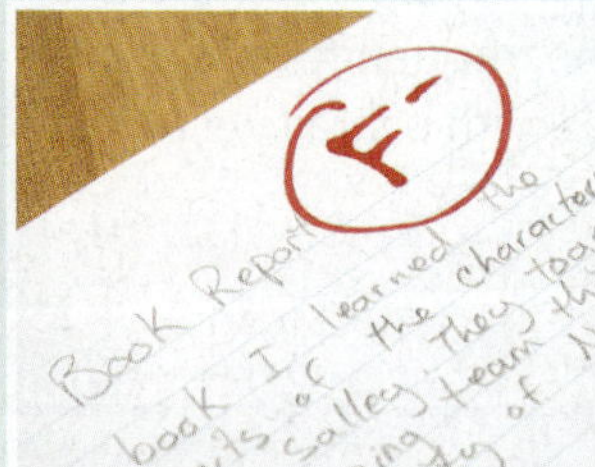

Why do I even study at all? I'll never get it. #procrastination #Iamdumb #theteacheristoohard

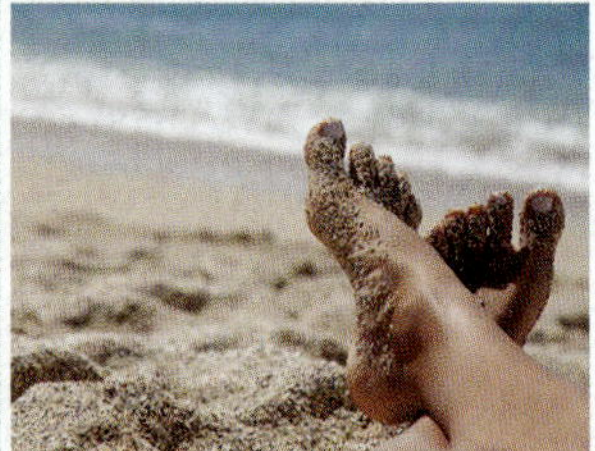

Alone again. Will I ever be good enough? #foreveralone #outofmyleague #didntdeservehim #loweringstandards #wasteoftime

Left to right: Fly Baby Images/Shutterstock.com; Matt Benoit/Shutterstock.com; AbElena/Shutterstock.com

Developing Empathy and Resilience

Essential Question?

What skills do you need to develop empathy and resilience?

Lesson
5.3

Learning Outcomes

After studying this lesson, you will be able to

- identify the benefits of empathy;
- take steps to become more empathetic;
- explain the value of resilience; and
- demonstrate skills to build resilience.

Key Terms

cognitive empathy
emotional empathy
empathy
resilience
self-compassion

Warm-Up Activity

Practicing Empathy

Communicate with Others Imagine your friend sits with you at lunch and is having a hard day. Your friend's dog is really sick and might not make it through the day, and your friend cannot stop crying. You feel stressed, since you and your friend had planned on studying for the test next period during lunch. Write a script in which you respond to your friend, negotiate, and show that you care. Describe what you would say and include what body language you would use to get your message across. How would your response make your friend feel? How would you feel after the conversation?

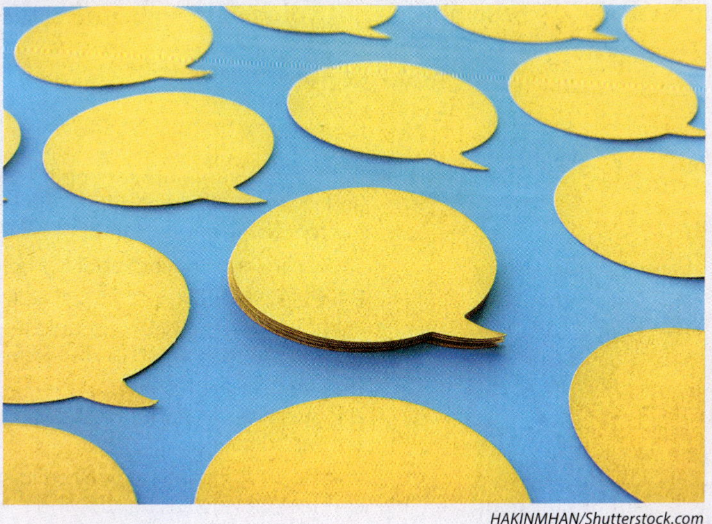

HAKINMHAN/Shutterstock.com

In addition to a positive mind-set, your abilities to relate to others and recover from stressful events also impact happiness. Like mind-set, these are factors you can modify through your actions and the strategies you use. In this lesson, you will learn about the value of empathy and resilience and how you can develop more empathy and resilience in your life.

The Importance of Empathy

empathy ability to understand and share the feelings of another person

The term **empathy** describes the ability to understand and share the feelings of another person. People who have a lot of empathy can easily imagine the world from another person's point of view and can even experience the same emotions a person is feeling. This explains why people who have much empathy may cry watching a fictional character in a movie or TV show. They can clearly imagine being in that person's situation.

cognitive empathy ability to see the world from another person's perspective

emotional empathy ability to experience the emotions another person is feeling

There are two distinct types of empathy. One is **cognitive empathy**, the ability to see the world from another person's perspective. A person with this type of empathy can imagine how it would feel to be bullied, even without experiencing this behavior. The other type is **emotional empathy**, the ability to experience the emotions another person is feeling. This means a person feels truly sad when friends or family members feel sad (**Figure 5.12**).

People who have a lot of empathy often build very close relationships because they can understand how other people are thinking and feeling. This ability may lead them to help other people and show compassion. It may also make other people trust them and feel comfortable confiding in them. People with a lot of empathy are also better able to work through conflict in relationships. This is because they can imagine the conflict from the other person's perspective.

Building Empathy

Some people naturally show more empathy than others. For example, maybe you have always been able to put yourself in someone else's shoes.

People with Empathy

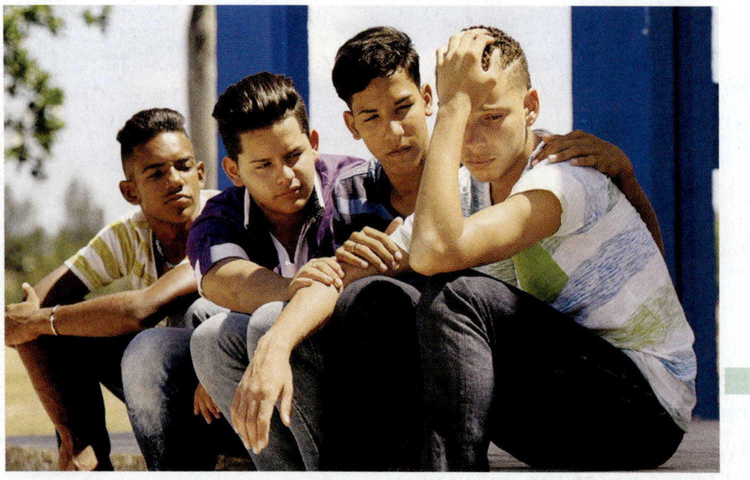

- put themselves in other people's shoes and really see the world from their perspectives
- show care and concern about other people's feelings
- acknowledge how other people feel instead of brushing off or dismissing their concerns
- ask questions to clarify what other people are experiencing
- imitate people's behavior to build a connection (such as by showing the same level of eye contact and degree of sharing)
- stay with other people during challenges instead of rushing ahead to find solutions
- avoid judging and blaming people for their struggles
- give emotional support and reassurance

diego_cervo/iStock/GettyImages

Figure 5.12 People with empathy tend to form stronger relationships because they can better provide support and understand others' feelings and perspectives. ***What type of empathy involves experiencing the emotions another person is feeling?***

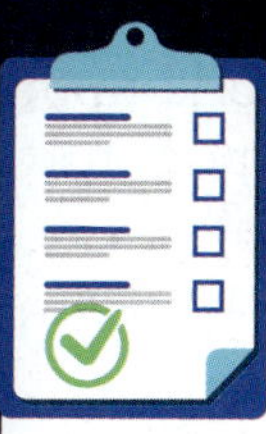

Quiz How Much Empathy Do You Have?

How much empathy do you think you have? To assess your level of empathy, take the following quiz. Consider each statement and indicate whether you strongly disagree, disagree, agree, or strongly agree. Keep track of your answers and tally them at the end to determine your level of empathy.

Statement				
I feel sad when others around me feel sad.	*Strongly disagree*	*Disagree*	*Agree*	*Strongly agree*
I can put myself in another person's place and see the world from that person's point of view.	*Strongly disagree*	*Disagree*	*Agree*	*Strongly agree*
I have a strong urge to help others when they are upset.	*Strongly disagree*	*Disagree*	*Agree*	*Strongly agree*
I provide emotional support and reassurance to others.	*Strongly disagree*	*Disagree*	*Agree*	*Strongly agree*
I feel excited when someone else feels excited.	*Strongly disagree*	*Disagree*	*Agree*	*Strongly agree*
During a disagreement, I listen to each person's side before making a decision.	*Strongly disagree*	*Disagree*	*Agree*	*Strongly agree*
I listen closely when other people are talking.	*Strongly disagree*	*Disagree*	*Agree*	*Strongly agree*
When listening to someone, I pay attention to that person's body language.	*Strongly disagree*	*Disagree*	*Agree*	*Strongly agree*
I do not look at my phone or computer when listening to someone.	*Strongly disagree*	*Disagree*	*Agree*	*Strongly agree*
I ask questions to clarify what others are experiencing.	*Strongly disagree*	*Disagree*	*Agree*	*Strongly agree*
I do not judge or make assumptions about other people.	*Strongly disagree*	*Disagree*	*Agree*	*Strongly agree*
I would describe myself as an open-minded person.	*Strongly disagree*	*Disagree*	*Agree*	*Strongly agree*
I avoid judging or blaming people for my feelings or struggles.	*Strongly disagree*	*Disagree*	*Agree*	*Strongly agree*
I take the time to understand other people's thoughts, feelings, and behaviors.	*Strongly disagree*	*Disagree*	*Agree*	*Strongly agree*

Add up the number of times you chose each response. Which response did you select most often?

If you answered mostly *strongly agree*, you usually demonstrate empathy. You relate fairly easily to the feelings of others and understand their points of view. This makes it easier for you to give emotional support and build close relationships. Keep developing your empathy as you meet and understand new people.

If you answered mostly *agree*, you sometimes show empathy. You may find it easy or difficult to relate to someone, depending on the person. Taking steps to become more empathetic can help you broaden the range of people you understand and build closer relationships.

If you answered mostly *disagree*, you rarely have empathy. You may relate well to some people, but find it impossible to understand others. This might be getting in the way of your relationships and make it harder to value diversity. Try taking some steps to become more empathetic and see your understanding grow.

If you answered mostly *strongly disagree*, you struggle a lot with empathy. Your relationships might suffer from lack of empathy, and you might feel like you cannot understand others. Examine yourself and any biases or beliefs that might prevent you from understanding others. Then take steps to develop your empathy. You might also consider seeking professional help.

Practice Your Skills

Analyze Influences

In a small group, discuss the results of this quiz. Do you agree with the result you got? Why or why not? Then, discuss factors you think may influence your level of empathy. For example, are your family members empathetic? Are your friends generally accepting or judgmental of other people? Who are your role models in the media? Are these people empathetic? As a group, list the top 10 factors you think influence empathy. Share your top 10 with the class and discuss the different factors shared.

On the other hand, maybe you have always struggled to see the world from a different perspective. Empathy can also change depending on a person's life experiences (**Figure 5.13**). Fortunately, no matter your natural tendency or life experience, you can take steps to increase your empathy. Some strategies you can use follow.

Pay Attention

When someone is talking, fully focus on what the person is saying. Empathy requires really paying attention. Do not check your phone or computer or get distracted by other people or activities in the room.

When listening, also pay attention to a person's body language, not just what the person is saying verbally. Observe the emotions in the person's facial expressions. Is the person feeling sad, anxious, or afraid? Sometimes nonverbal messages tell you even more about people's feelings than what they said directly. This is why paying attention is an essential part of empathy.

Listen Well

People with empathy listen well. They are quiet and patient and let the other person finish talking instead of interrupting. They ask questions if they need clarification, but do not judge the challenge or issue the person shares.

Sometimes being a good listener means allowing some periods of silence. People may share because they need to vent. They may not want or need an immediate response or solution. Simply letting people express how they feel can help.

Value Diversity

People with empathy are curious about other people. They have a sincere interest in understanding other people's experiences and perspectives. They understand that people from different backgrounds have different views of the world and enjoy learning about these different perspectives.

Figure 5.13 As you experience hardships, your ability to empathize with people in similar positions grows.

Impact of Life Experiences on Empathy

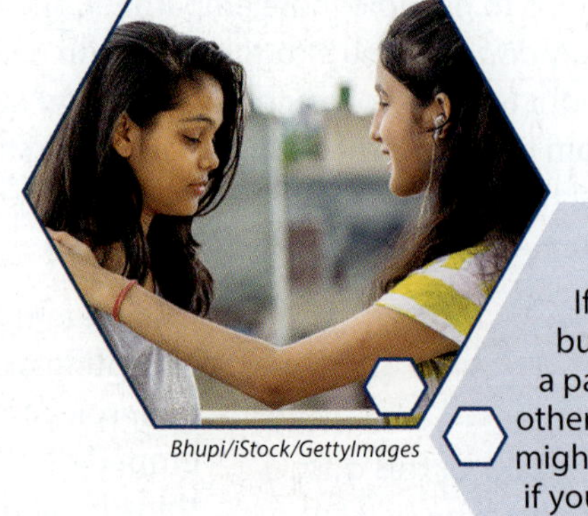

Bhupi/iStock/GettyImages

If you have been bullied or have lost a parent, guardian, or other family member, you might have more empathy if you see someone else having the same experience.

People with empathy also have open minds. They get to know people as individuals and accept them for who they are. They avoid making assumptions about people or relying on stereotypes or *prejudices* (mistaken ideas) based on race, nationality, sex, gender identity, sexual orientation, or other characteristics.

The ability to take the time to understand other people's thoughts, feelings, and behaviors helps empathetic people get along with others from different backgrounds. Empathetic people also focus on what they share with other people, rather than what differences they have.

Read a Book

One simple strategy for increasing empathy is to read a fiction book. Many high school students read mostly for school assignments. Both this reading for school and reading on your own build empathy by helping you practice understanding another person's perspective. When you become absorbed in a novel, you imagine the world through the character's eyes, which increases your ability to take on someone else's perspective in the real world. This skill, in turn, may increase your ability to empathize with others and work through conflict.

The Value of Resilience

No one wants to experience negative or stressful life events, such as a serious injury or illness, violent crime, or the death of a family member. Unfortunately, people cannot always control whether these events occur. **Resilience**, or the ability to recover from stressful events, can help you adapt well even when facing difficult circumstances (**Figure 5.14**). People with resilience show a remarkable ability to "bounce back" from major life stresses, including serious health conditions, financial stress, physical injury, and relationship conflicts.

resilience ability to recover from traumatic and stressful events

Characteristics of People with Resilience
• Ability to make plans and successfully carry them out
• Sense of control over personal actions
• Positive views of themselves and self-confidence in their strengths and abilities
• Skills in communicating with others and solving conflicts
• Strong, healthy relationships
• Ability to manage strong feelings and impulses
• Willingness to ask for help
15

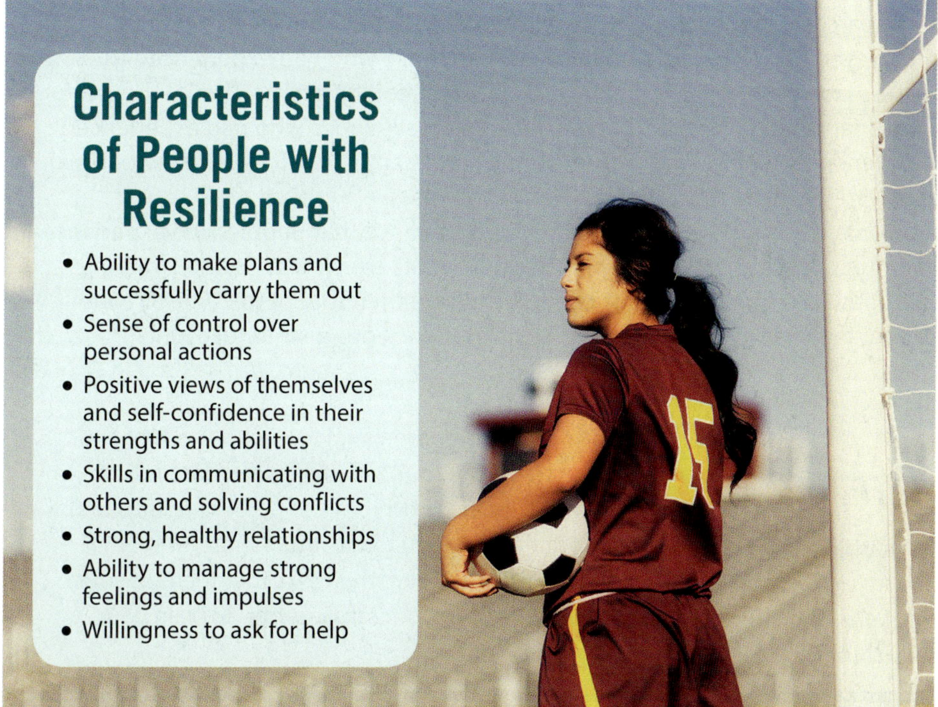

RichVintage/E+/GettyImages

Figure 5.14 People with resilience can recover from stressful events because of certain characteristics. ***Can people build resilience, or is it built-in?***

People can develop the characteristics of resilience with practice. In fact, people who experience difficult life experiences often show high levels of resilience. Experiencing some adversity gives people an opportunity to develop important skills for coping when future challenges arise. This means they can recover better from future difficult events.

Building Resilience

Everyone at some point goes through difficult experiences, including academic disappointments, family conflicts, or health concerns. It is therefore important to build resilience so you can manage such experiences when they do arrive. Some strategies for building your resilience follow.

Maintain Relationships

One of the best strategies for building resilience is to develop and maintain strong, healthy relationships. People who have a strong support network can manage difficult experiences because they know they can rely on close friends and family members for help. For example, if your car breaks down and you cannot get to your after-school job, a close friend or older sibling might be able to give you a ride. This type of support makes difficult situations feel much less stressful.

Research in Action

Resilience's Lasting Power

Did you know that stressful life events do not always make people less happy? In fact, stressful life events can sometimes give people needed coping skills and build resilience. Researchers at the University of Buffalo in New York surveyed nearly 2,000 adults for several years to assess how their well-being changed over time. Participants listed any stressful life events they had experienced prior to the start of the study and then any new ones that occurred. These events included divorce, deaths of loved ones, serious illnesses, and natural disasters. Researchers then measured the link between the number of stressful life experiences and overall psychological well-being.

You might expect that people who had avoided major stresses—who experienced none or only one of these events—would have greater life satisfaction. Those with relatively stress-free lives, however, were no happier than those who had experienced as many as a dozen major life events. Those who were happiest were actually those who had experienced some, but not too many, stressful events (two to six) over the several years.

Researchers believe that people who experience some stressful events develop skills and strategies for coping. They are therefore better able to cope when they experience other stressful events.

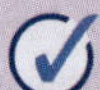

Practice Your Skills

Comprehend Concepts

This study demonstrates that people who have experienced some stressful life events actually feel happier than those who have experienced no or only one such event. List the factors you think may explain this finding. Compare your ideas with those of your classmates. How could you test which factor best explains this relationship? How do the findings of this study affect how you think about stressful events? How would they affect the way other teens in your school think about stressful events? Explain your answer.

High levels of support even help people cope with very serious events, such as major health conditions, natural disasters, or violence in the community. People who have a good social support network show lower levels of anxiety and depression, even after experiencing extremely stressful events.

Embrace Change

Most people find change difficult. High school students may worry about starting a new after-school job, breaking up with a dating partner, or changing schools. Some high school students experience major changes in their families, such as moving to a new home, having a new brother or sister, or having an older sibling leave home.

People with resilience can find positive ways to think about these changes. They see challenges as opportunities and feel optimistic that, over time, they will adapt to change (**Figure 5.15**).

If you have trouble adjusting your thinking to adopt a more positive view, try making a list of any positive effects of change, even if they are very small. Sharing your feelings with a close friend or trusted adult could also help you find some more positive ways to think about hard changes. It is important to remember that change is hard for everyone initially, but over time, you can adjust and feel better.

Practice Self-Compassion

Some people blame the negative events in their lives on themselves, their weaknesses, or their perceived inadequacies. They think long and hard about these bad outcomes and beat themselves up over failures. Not surprisingly, this type of self-criticism makes it hard to be resilient and feel better.

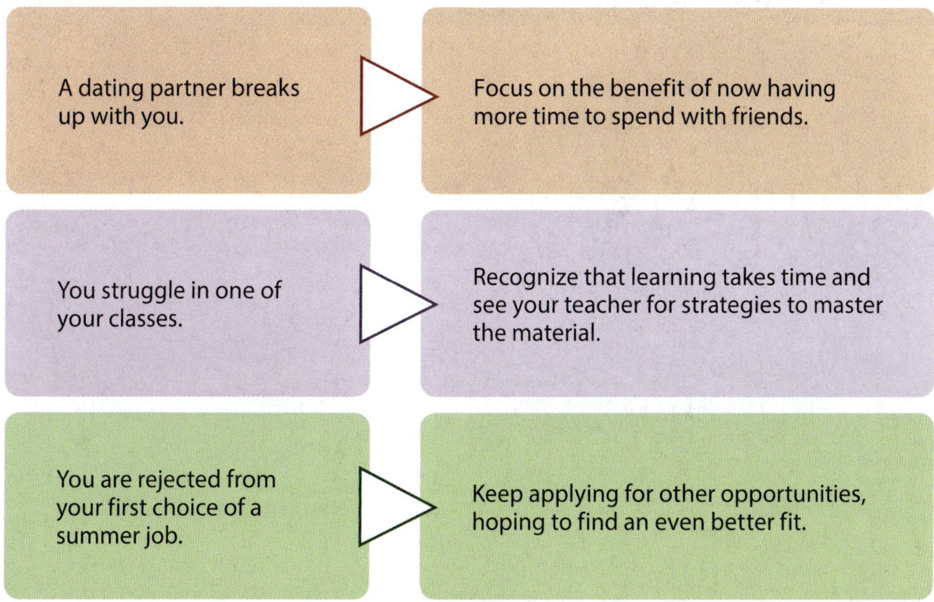

Figure 5.15 People with resilience embrace change as an opportunity for growth or new experiences.

self-compassion attitude of kindness and understanding toward one's self, even when experiencing setbacks and disappointments

A better strategy for developing resilience is to practice self-compassion. **Self-compassion** means treating yourself with kindness and understanding, even when you experience setbacks and disappointments (**Figure 5.16**). People who practice self-compassion recognize that difficulties happen to everyone and forgive themselves when situations or plans do not go well.

People who show self-compassion in the face of negative events feel better. They have lower levels of anxiety and depression and overall feel happier and more optimistic about the future. For example, first-year college students who have more self-compassion during this difficult life transition show greater engagement and motivation with college life. People who treat themselves with kindness when disappointments happen also experience better physical health. An easy way to feel happier and be healthier is to forgive yourself, be kind to yourself, and treat yourself with care and compassion.

Take Responsibility

Another good strategy for building resilience is taking responsibility for your actions and role in the situations in your life. Some people tend to blame negative experiences on others. They may think a test was too tricky, their guardians' rules are not fair, or a coach just does not like them.

Practicing Self-Compassion
Treat yourself the way you would treat a close friend or sibling.
Be mindful of negative self-talk.
Remind yourself that your experiences are normal, human experiences.
Forgive yourself for your mistakes and shortcomings. Remember that nobody is perfect.
Work with a supportive therapist or coach to develop new patterns of thought or behavior.
Comfort your body with healthy foods, sleep, self-massages, or physical activity.

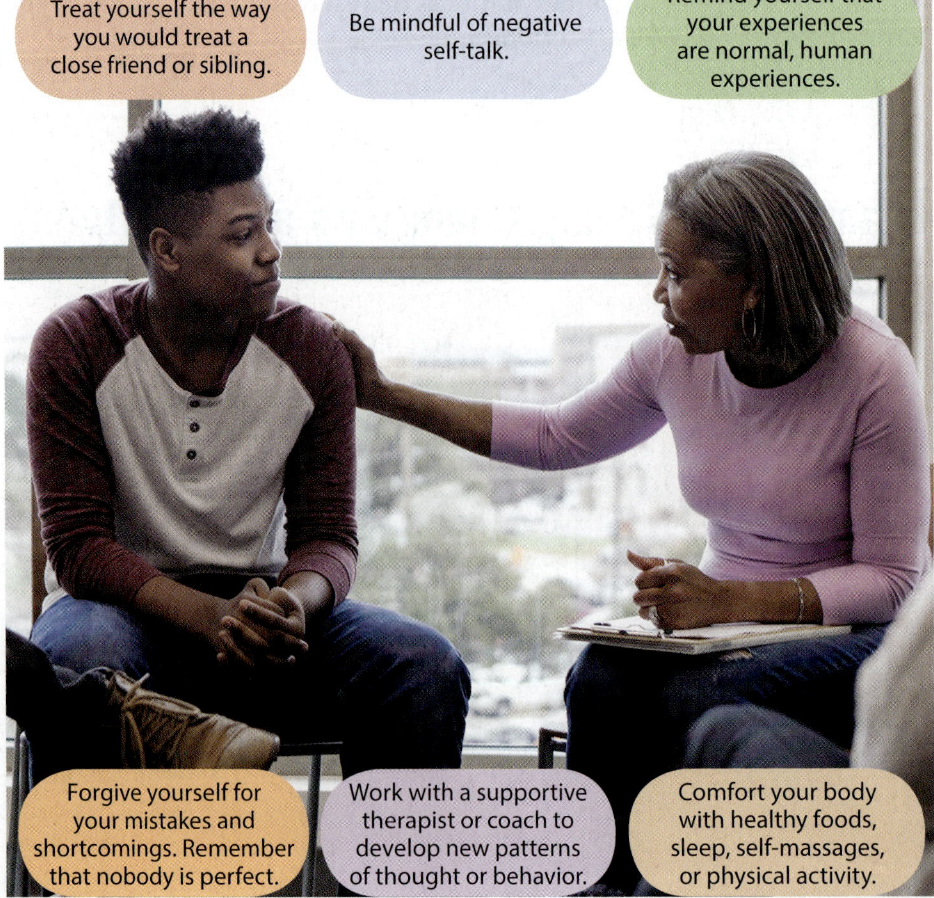

SDI Productions/E+/GettyImages

Figure 5.16 When people practice self-compassion, they learn not to beat themselves up over bad situations, mistakes, or failures. In turn, this increases a person's resilience. ***How does self-compassion impact depression and anxiety?***

Blaming negative outcomes on others, however, does not help people feel better over time. In fact, blaming other people hurts your ability to take control over similar outcomes in the future.

Instead, take responsibility for what you can change in the future. Think about what is in your control and make a plan to work toward a different outcome. For example, if you are disappointed with the amount of playing time your coach gives you or wish you had a larger part in the school musical, think about what you can do differently next time. Talk to people you trust, such as your parents or guardians, teachers, or school counselors, about strategies you could use to work toward these goals.

It is also important to recognize there are some factors you cannot control. For example, you cannot control the specific rules your parents, guardians, or teachers set and expect you to follow. You also cannot control the choices your friends make. Try to recognize what you cannot control, so you can focus your time and energy on what you can.

Lesson 5.3 Review

Know and Understand

1. Explain the difference between cognitive and emotional empathy.
2. How do people who have empathy value diversity?
3. How do relationships increase resilience?
4. What does it mean to have self-compassion?

Think Critically

5. What factors do you think make it hard for teens to pay close attention during conversations? What can teens do to reduce these factors?
6. Since reading a book increases empathy, does watching a movie or TV show or playing a video game also increase empathy? Research this question using reliable resources and write your answer.
7. Why do you think people often fear change? How can people adjust their viewpoint to see change as potentially positive?
8. Think of a setback or challenge you faced recently. In this setback, what could you have done differently to show self-compassion? Could you have done anything differently to take responsibility? Explain.

REAL WORLD Health Skills

Make Decisions As a class, brainstorm 12 events that would require resilience and empathy. Write these events on 12 posters and hang them around the room. Rotate around the room with purple and orange sticky notes. On purple sticky notes, write decisions you could make to respond to an event with empathy. Think about how you could provide support if a friend, family member, or classmate were experiencing the event. On orange sticky notes, write decisions you could make to respond with resilience if you experienced the event. Make sure to respond to at least three posters and explain to the class how one of your decisions would affect health in the short-term and long-term.

Chapter 5 Review and Assessment

Chapter Summary

Happiness refers to a variety of positive emotions. It does not, however, mean feeling positive all the time or only experiencing positive events. Happiness has more to do with how well you cope and how you see the world than it does with what happens to you. Many different factors affect happiness. Genetic makeup can influence how easily someone feels happy and someone's risk for a mental illness. Mind-set, a sense of purpose, and relationships also influence happiness. Some simple ways to increase happiness are to set and work toward goals, have close relationships, and give to others. You can also adopt healthy behaviors like physical activity and spending time in nature and prioritize experiences.

Mind-set is one major factor that influences happiness. A positive mind-set is generally optimistic, while a negative mind-set tends to be pessimistic. People with a positive mind-set cope well, confront issues directly, see the good in situations, and focus on what they can control. People with a negative mind-set tend to think situations will not get better and give up in the face of challenges. To modify your mind-set, you can have a positive attitude. You can practice mindfulness, which involves concentrated, judgment-free awareness. You can focus on gratitude; modify your outlook by seeing a situation differently; and watch your self-talk, or what you say to yourself. Respecting yourself and others and spending time with positive people can also improve mind-set.

Empathy and resilience are important skills. Empathy is the ability to understand and share the feelings of others. Cognitive empathy is the ability to see another perspective, and emotional empathy allows you to feel what others feel. Ways of building empathy include focusing during communication, noticing body language, listening well, valuing diversity, and reading books. Resilience is the ability to bounce back from stressful events. To build resilience, you can maintain relationships, embrace change, and practice self-compassion by forgiving yourself. You can also take responsibility for what you can control.

Vocabulary Activity

Find a video, podcast, or article from a reliable source that discusses one of the key terms from the list. Create a digital presentation to summarize your findings, incorporating other key terms when relevant. Present it to the class and answer any questions your classmates may have. Be sure to cite your media source.

attitude	*gratitude*	*pessimistic*
cognitive empathy	*growth mind-set*	*purpose*
dignity	*happiness*	*resilience*
diversity	*mindfulness*	*rumination*
emotional empathy	*mind-set*	*self-compassion*
empathy	*optimistic*	*self-respect*
fixed mind-set	*outlook*	*self-talk*

Review and Recall

Review the information in this chapter by answering the following questions.

1. Which of the following is part of happiness?
   A. only feeling happy all the time
   B. not experiencing anxiety or sadness
   C. using healthy coping strategies
   D. giving up under pressure
2. How much do events influence happiness? Explain.
3. After a hard week at home, your friend says, "It'll never get better." What mind-set does this show?
4. Why does physical activity help improve mood?
5. Which of the following shows a positive mind-set?
   A. never feeling frustrated
   B. avoiding challenges
   C. focusing on what you cannot control
   D. finding some good in hard situations
6. What is mindfulness?
7. What does it mean to catastrophize?
8. Which of the following is *not* part of self-respect?
   A. putting others down
   B. feeling good about strengths
   C. showing dignity
   D. treating others with respect
9. What does it mean to practice cultural humility?
10. Why do people with empathy often have close relationships?
11. Which of the following helps build empathy?
    A. allowing periods of silence
    B. ignoring body language
    C. believing stereotypes
    D. challenging a person's beliefs
12. What is resilience?
13. How do people with resilience view change?

Standardized Test Prep

Reading and Writing Practice

Read the passage below and then answer the following questions.

In one study, researchers at Stanford University gave people one of two articles to read about empathy. One-half read an article about how a person's level of empathy can change. The other half read an article about how empathy was fixed and could not change.

All of the people in the study were asked to help a group focused on preventing cancer. Some methods of helping were pretty easy, such as passing out information, joining a walkathon, or donating money. Other methods required more empathy, such as listening to patients share their stories.

Can you predict what researchers found? Those who read the article describing how empathy can change were much more likely to help in ways that required more empathy. These findings show that teaching people how empathy can change leads to more helping behavior.

14. In this study, which group helped most in ways that required empathy: the group that read the article about how empathy can change or the group that read the article about how empathy is fixed?
15. How many groups did this study contain?
16. Which statement best summarizes the conclusion of this study?
    A. Reading about empathy makes people have more empathy.
    B. Empathy cannot change.
    C. Reading that empathy can change makes people more likely to help in empathetic ways.
    D. People who think empathy is fixed do not help others.

Chapter 5 Skills Assessment

Critical Thinking Skills

Answer the following questions to assess your knowledge of what you learned in this chapter.

1. Think of a time you felt happy, even though parts of your life were hard. Why did you feel happy, even though life was difficult? What made you happy?
2. Why do you think even some people who have many good things in their life, such as fame, success, or lots of money, are unhappy?
3. What relationships in your life make you the happiest? the least happy?
4. Why do you think giving to others increases happiness?
5. Are teens at your school generally optimistic or pessimistic? Explain.
6. Review the strategies for practicing gratitude in the text and then brainstorm at least three additional strategies for practicing gratitude. Share these strategies with a partner.
7. Think back to the first time you can remember engaging in self-talk. How does that self-talk compare to your self-talk now? Why do you think this is?
8. How much does the culture at your school respect diversity? Explain. What steps could people at your school take to increase respect for diversity?
9. What factors do you think influence how much empathy a person has?
10. How do stereotypes get in the way of empathy? Think of a stereotype you have encountered. How would this stereotype impact your ability to have empathy? What can people do to challenge stereotypes and encourage empathy?
11. Think of a stressful event you have experienced. How did this event impact your resilience? What skills for resilience did it teach you?
12. What does it mean to forgive yourself if you experience setbacks or disappointments? What would forgiveness look like?
13. Think back to the same stressful event you analyzed in question 11. What aspects of the event could you control? What aspects could you not control? What did you do to take responsibility in the situation? If you did not take responsibility, how could you have done so?

Health and Wellness Skills

Complete the following activities to assess your skills related to health and wellness.

14. **Analyze Influences.** For two days, pay attention to what your peers and family members say and do in person and online. Write down statements or behaviors that demonstrate a particular mind-set. Then, write a journal entry or poem or create an artistic representation showing how the influences around you shape your mind-set. Identify strategies you can use to resist negative influences and seek out more positive ones.
15. **Access Information.** Imagine you have the following friends. For each friend, research a book or online resource that provides valid information and helpful advice. Explain why you chose each resource and what information from the resource each friend could apply.
    A. Since her recent breakup, Renee seems withdrawn and does not do her hair and makeup or wear dresses, which she used to love. She has turned down two dates to the homecoming dance because she is "not good enough."
    B. You made the baseball team, while your friend Jacob did not. Jacob also wanted to run track, but only if you did too. Jacob has been unexcited about track and has stopped talking to you. You ask Jacob about coming to a track meet to support him, but Jacob says he wishes he were playing baseball.
    C. Erika is posting a lot on social media, and all of her posts show other people she wishes she looked like.
    D. Lucas is struggling with the loss of his grandfather. He is barely making it to school, is quiet, and dwells on the loss. It has been a few months now.
16. **Communicate with Others.** Create a set of interview questions for a family member who has most likely experienced loss. Your questions should focus on how the person handled the event, how others supported the person, and what the person learned. Then, record yourself interviewing this family member.

At the end of the interview, record yourself summarizing how the person showed resilience and received and showed empathy.

17. **Make Decisions.** This chapter focuses on the decisions people make as they respond to situations that may be out of their control. The sooner people commit to positive thinking behaviors, the more prepared they will be to overcome hardships, stay happy, think positively, and show empathy and resilience. In a journal entry, identify five decisions you can make to commit to positive thinking. For each decision, write a promise to help keep you accountable and make a plan to overcome any barriers in your way.
18. **Set Goals.** Identify three long- or short-term goals you have for your life. Make sure these goals are SMART. For each goal, write two events that could happen in your life and make achieving that goal a greater challenge. Using what you have learned about resilience, explain how you can overcome each event to still accomplish your goal.
19. **Practice Health-Enhancing Behaviors.** Draw two boxes in each of the following colors: red, yellow, and green. In the red boxes, write things you need to *stop* doing to shift to positive thinking. In the yellow boxes, write things you do occasionally, but could do more *consistently*, to think more positively. In the green boxes, write things you are *already* doing that positively impact your thinking and ultimately your life.
20. **Advocate for Health.** As a class, plan an event or social media campaign to promote positive thinking in your school or community. Write a slogan identifying the purpose of the event. Also list the major goals or messages you want to communicate, how you will communicate these messages to your audience, and what tools you will provide. How will you convince your audience that these topics are important? Advertise your event or campaign and then carry it out. Afterward, evaluate how effective it was and what you learned.

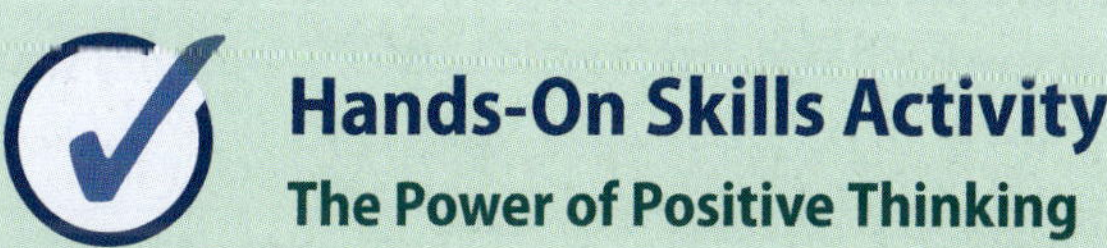

Hands-On Skills Activity

The Power of Positive Thinking

You learned in this chapter that happiness and positivity have a large impact on mental and emotional health. People can experience happiness even if they encounter difficult events, and positive thinking helps people see the good in situations. In this activity, you will learn about how positivity influences mental and emotional health. You will need a cup of paper clips or another small item.

Steps for This Activity

1. Review the following questions and answer each with a numerical value: *1* for never, *2* for every once in a while, *3* for sometimes, *4* for often, and *5* for all of the time.
   A. How often do I feel stressed?
   B. How often do I feel like I cannot accomplish tasks?
   C. How often am I sad or angry?
   D. How often do I feel overwhelmed?
   E. How often do I feel like I am not good enough?
   F. How often am I pessimistic?
   G. How often do I overcome challenges, such as a difficult homework assignment or hard time?
   H. How often do I remind myself that I am capable, even when times are tough?
   I. How often do I show empathy toward others?
   J. How often am I optimistic?
   K. How often do I feel happy?
   L. How often do I stop and acknowledge my feelings so I can handle them?
2. Hold out one hand with your palm facing upward. Then, look at your answers for questions A–F. For each point value you assigned, put that number of paper clips (or another small item) in your palm. If your palm starts to overflow, keep the items in your hand and make a pile under your palm on your desk.
3. Now, look at your answers for questions G–L. For each point value you assigned, remove that number of paper clips (or another small item) from your palm.
4. **Communicate with Others.** If, in this activity, your palm represents your ability to stay positive through life's challenges, what conclusions can you draw? Discuss what you learned with a partner. Using effective communication skills, share ideas about what you can do to stay positive, even when difficult events happen.

Chapter 6 Managing the Stress in Your Life

Look for the skills icon throughout this chapter for opportunities to practice your health skills.

Check Your Health and Wellness Skills

In this chapter, you will learn skills for managing stress. To understand the skills you currently use, take the following inventory of your behaviors. Indicate how well you think you use each skill. Use a scale of 1–5, *1* meaning you do not use the skill and *5* meaning you feel completely comfortable using it.

Skill	How Well Do You Use Each Skill?
I recognize stress can motivate me to achieve my goals.	
When I feel stressed, I make sure to get enough sleep and eat well.	
I stop and take time to think about why when I'm stressed.	
I check my schedule before committing to activities.	
I feel comfortable saying *no* when I don't have time to do something.	
I try to think positively about stressful situations.	
I have activities that help me calm down when I can't control a situation.	
I have people I can talk to when I'm stressed and upset.	
When I feel completely overwhelmed, I stop and take a few deep breaths.	
I help myself relax by concentrating on the present.	
I know how to get help when I can't handle stress on my own.	
	Total:

Add up your responses to each statement. The higher your score, the more comfortable you feel practicing health skills related to managing stress. Which skill do you think is most important for you? Which skill is the most challenging for you? Which skill would you most like to improve? In this chapter, you will learn how to perform these skills better and more often.

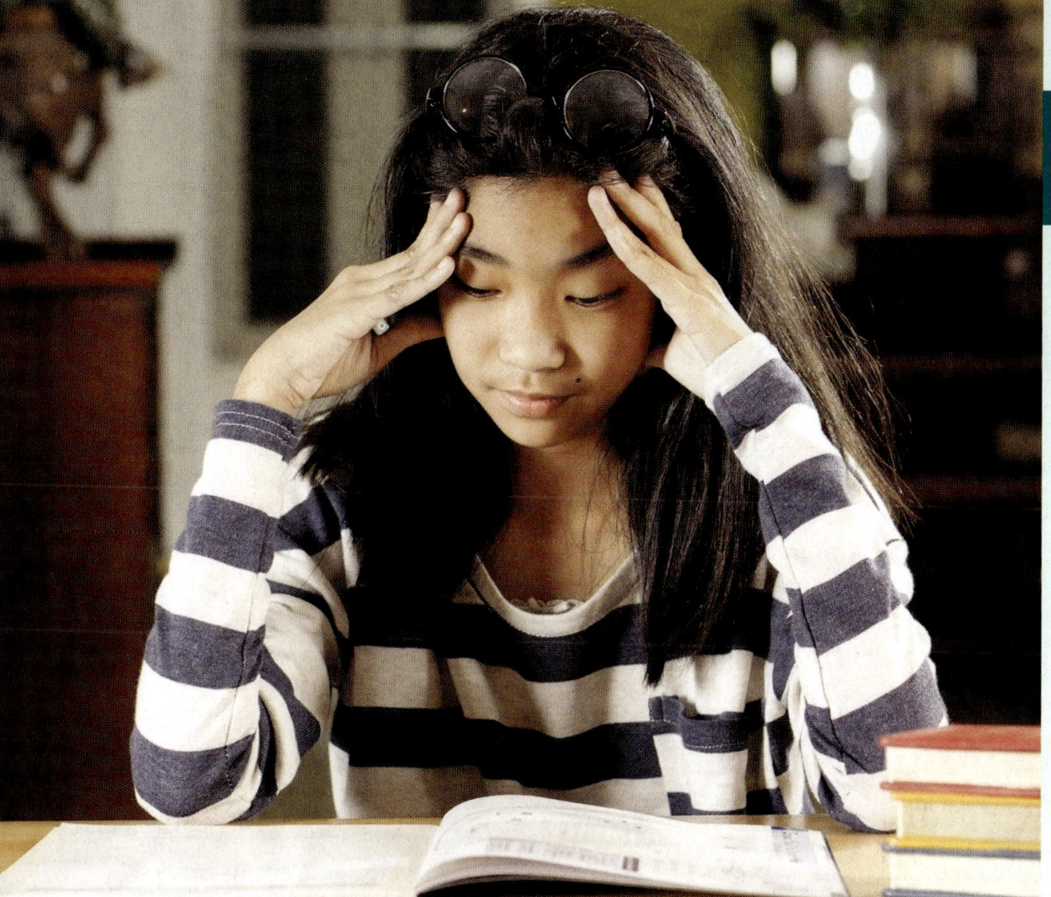
Piti Tan/Shutterstock.com

Reading and Notetaking

Before reading this chapter, scan the chapter and lesson titles. Write a paragraph describing what you already know about these topics. Explain where you got the information you have—from conversations, the media, or research, for example. As you are reading, compare and contrast the information in the chapter with your prior knowledge. Organize your notes around the information you already know. After reading, consider how your prior knowledge of the subject matter helped you understand this topic.

What I Know	Where It Comes From
What I Have Learned	

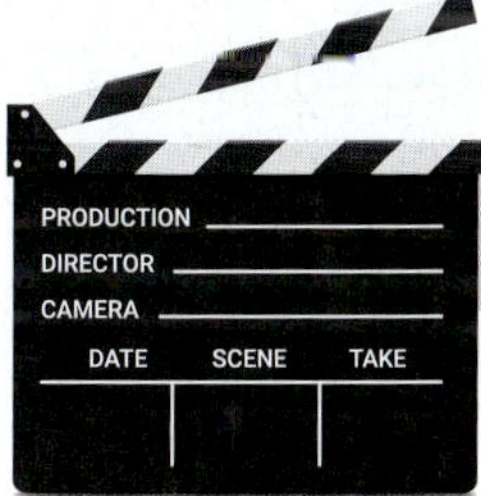

Setting the Scene

Managing Stress in a Healthy Way

This year, you are very busy keeping up with your classes, working a part-time job, and applying to colleges. You sometimes feel overwhelmed by everything you have to do. You often feel like there are just not enough hours in the day. Although you have tried staying up very late to finish homework, you have noticed you are not able to do your best work exhausted. You keep getting sick, which makes it even harder to work effectively.

Your school counselor suggested some strategies you could use to manage the stress you are experiencing. She suggested you try some new time-management strategies, such as creating a schedule, taking on fewer commitments, and reducing the time you spend on social media. She also suggested trying some relaxation exercises, such as deep breathing. You do not know if these approaches will work, but you may as well give them a try.

Thinking Critically

1. When in your life has stress helped you? When has it caused issues in your life?
2. What are some factors that might contribute to the high level of stress many high school students face?
3. What are some strategies you have used in the past to manage stress? How effective were these strategies? What does it look like when you manage your stress well?

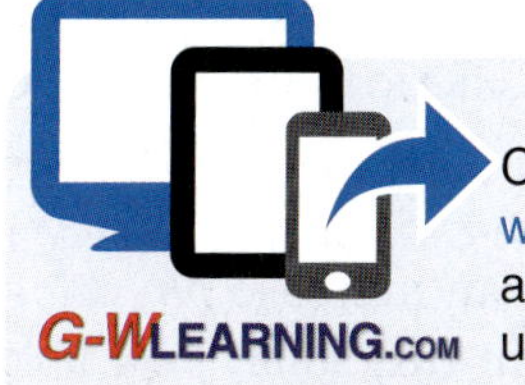

Click on the activity icon or visit www.g-wlearning.com/health/4095 to access online vocabulary activities using key terms from the chapter.

Lesson

6.1

What Is Stress?

Essential Question?

How does the body respond to stressful situations?

Learning Outcomes

After studying this lesson, you will be able to

- define *stress*;
- differentiate between eustress and distress;
- explain the difference between acute, chronic, major, and minor stressors;
- recognize common stressors among teens;
- evaluate how perception influences levels of stress; and
- describe how the body responds to stress.

Key Terms

distress
eustress
fight-or-flight response
relaxation response
stress
stressors
technostress
toxic stress
trauma

Warm-Up Activity

Perception Deception

Analyze Influences On index cards, your teacher will write some events that cause either *eustress* (good stress) or *distress* (bad stress). Some examples might include riding rollercoasters, seeing snakes or spiders, skydiving, public speaking, riding a motorcycle, playing a contact sport, bungee jumping, rock climbing, and singing or playing an instrument in public. Rotate the cards through the class so all of your classmates read each card. When you read a card, write an *E* on the card if you feel the event causes eustress or a *D* if it causes distress. At the end, tally the *E*s and *D*s on each card. As a class, discuss the role of perception in stress.

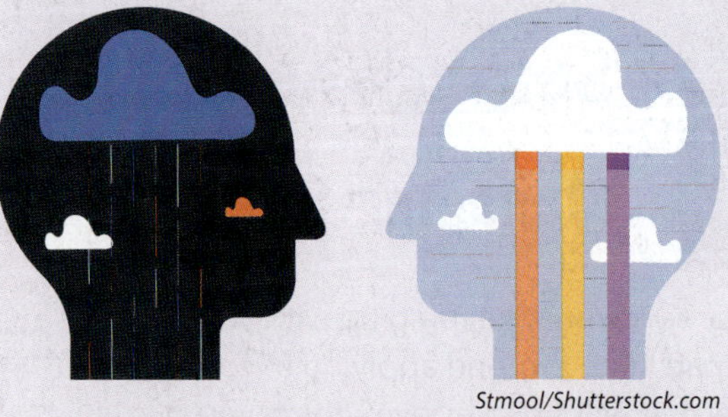

Stmool/Shutterstock.com

stress body's physical and psychological reactions to situations people perceive as threats

Imagine that you are about to give an oral report, confront a friend who let you down, or interview for a job. All of these situations might cause you to feel stress. **Stress** is your body's physical and psychological reactions to situations you perceive as threats. For example, many people find public speaking scary or threatening. Giving an oral report may cause stress, which makes these people feel anxious—a psychological reaction. Physical reactions may include trembling, sweaty palms, and an upset stomach.

Stress is unavoidable. Everyone experiences it at times. Fortunately, stress that is managed properly can be beneficial. Moderate levels of stress can increase *physiological arousal*, or physical and psychological excitement. In this state, people have extra energy to help them perform at their best. Stress can also motivate people to learn and grow. A person may feel stressed giving an oral report due to fear of failure, but use the stress to overcome the challenge.

In this lesson, you will learn about causes of stress. You will also learn about the body's stress response.

Sources of Stress

Have you ever taken a test for a driver's license? gone on a date? been pressured to do an activity you did not want to do? All of these situations contain **stressors**, or factors that lead to stress. Stressors can be positive or negative. Exciting events, like going to your prom, can cause stress by adding to your to-do list and the decisions you need to make. Negative stressors can cause stress that feels unpleasant, like a knot in your stomach.

stressors factors that lead to stress

Stressors can be major or minor events (**Figure 6.1**). Many teens face similar stressors in their lives and have shared experiences of coping with stress. Some of these common sources of stress include the following:

- **Relationships:** Personal relationships can be major sources of stress when disagreements arise. For example, you may feel anxious after an argument with a friend or family member. Feelings of rejection, exclusion, negative peer pressure, sadness after the loss of a relationship, or loneliness can also cause stress. Social media and online communication can intensify some of the stress in teen relationships.
- **School:** Many high school students feel pressure to do well in school. They may worry about their grades, upcoming tests, and homework assignments. Balancing the demands of different teachers, as well as jobs, extracurricular activities, and college applications, can be overwhelming at times.
- **Environment:** People's environments can increase or decrease stress. Some teens live in homes that are crowded and noisy, which can cause stress. Serious financial issues, food insecurity, and homelessness can also cause teens to worry. Some teens feel stress from living in a neighborhood with relatively high levels of crime or going to a school with lots of bullying. Being in an environment where you have little or no control, even for brief periods of time, can also make you feel stressed.

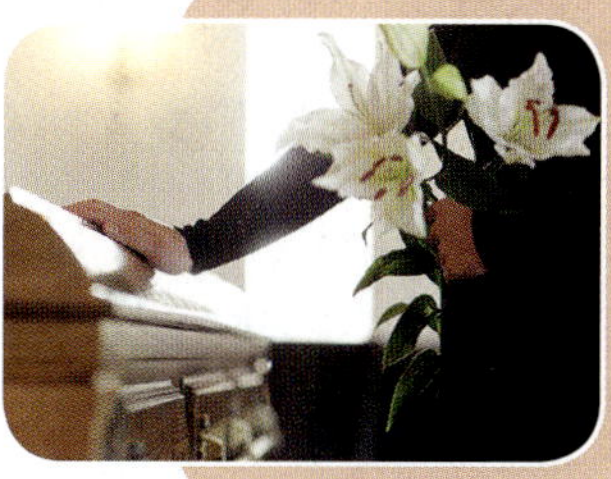

Major, life-event stressors

- Moving to a new school
- Losing a loved one
- Divorce of a parent or guardian
- A new sibling
- An illness or health condition

Minor, daily stressors

- Losing a favorite pair of jeans
- Arriving late for class
- Bad hair day
- Argument with your sibling
- A friend does not text you back

Top to bottom: Syda Productions/Shutterstock.com; Rawpixel.com/Shutterstock.com

Figure 6.1 If minor stressors occur frequently, they can create as much or more overall stress compared to major life events.

technostress type of stress caused by the constant presence of technology

- **Technology:** One type of stress that many teens experience today is **technostress**, or stress caused by the constant presence of technology. Technology can lead to constant incoming messages and pressure to stay active on social media, which contribute to stress.
- **Inner conflict:** The pressure you exert on yourself can cause stress. Have you ever felt stressed about a difficult decision? Making choices, especially choices between two desirable options, can cause stress. So can feeling the need to be perfect or being afraid to make a mistake.

Types of Stress

eustress positive stress that encourages growth and motivation

People of all ages experience many types of stress. Some stress is positive. This type of positive stress, which encourages growth and motivation, is called **eustress**. Experiencing too much stress at once, or being unable to manage stress, however, can lead to harmful health effects.

Health in the Media 

Can Social Media Cause Stress?

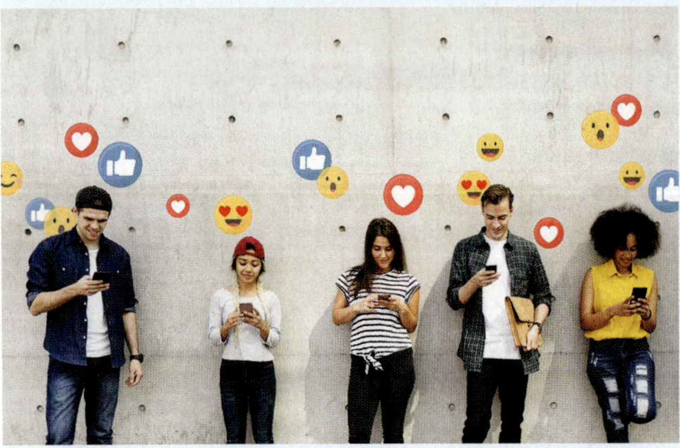

Rawpixel.com/Shutterstock.com

Many teens think social media is a good way to stay connected with friends and family members. Socially connecting through social media can reduce stress by opening communication and increasing social support. Using social media can also create stress, however. One study by the Pew Research Foundation revealed that social media causes stress in several different ways. Teens are likely to feel stress using social media if they

- see people posting about events they were not invited to;
- feel pressure to post positive and attractive content about themselves;
- feel pressure to get comments and likes on their posts; or
- cannot control what other people are posting about them.

These potential stressors may help explain why several studies have found that teens who spend the most time on social media have higher rates of depression compared to those who spend less time. Although social media enables teens to stay connected with friends, this connection does not always provide the same support as face-to-face interactions. Teens who connect more through social media than through in-person interactions may feel socially isolated and lonely.

Practice Your Skills

Advocate for Health

With a partner, brainstorm ways social media can cause and reduce stress for teens. Then, discuss whether you think social media causes the same level of stress for all teens or if some teens are more bothered by it than others. Based on your discussion, list actions you could take to help teens in your community avoid or manage the stress caused by social media. Commit to act on one of these ideas with your partner and share your idea with the class.

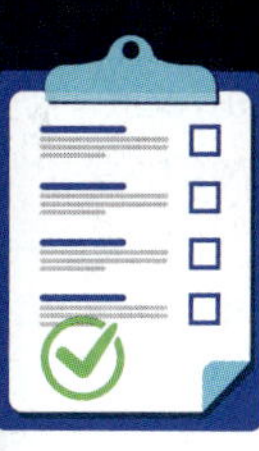

Quiz What Is Your Level of Stress?

Stressors can be positive or negative. Still, no matter the type of stressor, stressors can add up to increase overall stress in a person's life. To understand how stress adds up, review each of the life-event stressors that follow. Indicate all of the stressful events you have experienced within the last 12 months.

Stressful Event	Value
Losing a family member or friend	100
Experiencing divorce or separation of parents or guardians	75
Losing a favorite pet	70
Experiencing conflict with a parent or guardian	64
Having trouble with body changes, such as weight, acne, or height	63
Experiencing conflict with a sibling	63
Experiencing conflict with a teacher or principal	62
Having a family member or friend get very sick or badly injured	60
Getting very sick or badly injured	60
Having an increased workload at school	58
Ending a romantic relationship	53
Preparing for a major project or exam	53
Moving to a new home	51
Quitting or getting laid off from a part-time job	50
Getting a low grade in a class	48
Starting a new school	44
Ending a friendship	40
Balancing academic assignments with extracurricular activities or a part-time job	40
Experiencing a change in financial status of family	39
Experiencing an outstanding personal achievement	37
Starting a part-time job	34
Having new family members move in with you	31
Starting a romantic relationship	27

Add up the point values for all of the stressful events you have experienced in the last 12 months.

A total point value of *150 points or less* means you have a relatively small number of stressful life changes and a low risk of stress causing health-related issues. As you manage stressors, practice healthy stress-management techniques. The more you use healthy strategies, the better you will be able to manage more stressors as they occur.

A total point value of *151–300 points* means you have a moderate number of stressful life changes and have some risk of stress causing health-related issues. Be sure to take care of yourself and reduce stress where you can. Healthy stress-management techniques can help you avoid health-related issues caused by stress.

A total point value of *301 points or more* means you have a relatively high number of stressful life changes and a high risk of stress causing health-related issues. During this stressful time, practice self-care and pay attention to your feelings and what stress-management strategies work for you. Seek professional help if you have trouble managing stress.

Practice Your Skills

Communicate with Others

In a small group, use effective communication skills to debate the point values assigned to each stressor in this activity. Do you agree with the point values assigned? Are there any point values you would change or stressful events you would add? Discuss how group members' perceptions influence how much stress they feel in a given situation. Then, discuss stress-management techniques you have used in the past. Which techniques worked the best? Share healthy strategies that can help group members cope with stress.

distress stress that causes negative feelings and harmful health effects

trauma extreme stress due to deeply disturbing events, such as disasters, sexual assault, or violence

toxic stress stress caused by repeated, long-lasting exposure to severe stressors, such as neglect and abuse, violence, or loss of a loved one

Stress that causes negative feelings and harmful health effects is called **distress** (**Figure 6.2**). Extreme stress due to deeply disturbing events, such as disasters, sexual assault, and violence, is called **trauma**.

Stress can be short-lived or long-lasting. One type of stress, called *acute stress*, is sudden and does not last long. Acute stressors come from the normal pressures of daily life experiences like taking a final exam or having a job interview. People can also experience *chronic stress*, which continues over long periods of time. Chronic stress seems to have no clear end in sight. Examples include feeling unsafe in your neighborhood or worrying about a loved one who has a health condition.

Repeated exposure to severe, chronic stressors can lead to **toxic stress**. Some examples of severe, chronic stressors include exposure to neglect and abuse, family rejection, intimate partner violence, death of a loved one, extreme poverty, substance abuse, a loved one going to jail, or community violence. Toxic stress can lead to negative short- and long-term physical and mental health consequences. If you or someone you know is experiencing toxic stress, it is important to talk to a trusted adult and get professional help.

The Impact of Perception

Your *perceptions*, or beliefs, about the situations in your life can affect how much stress you experience. Even if two people experience the exact same stressor, each person may interpret or think about the stressor in a different way. In fact, the meaning a person assigns to an event is sometimes a better predictor of how stressful it is than the event itself.

For example, suppose Joshua and Colleen both fail a math test. Joshua believes failing the test means the college of his choice will reject him. For Joshua, this event is very stressful, even life-changing. Colleen views failing the test as unfortunate, but plans to study harder and do better next time. The event is therefore less stressful for Colleen.

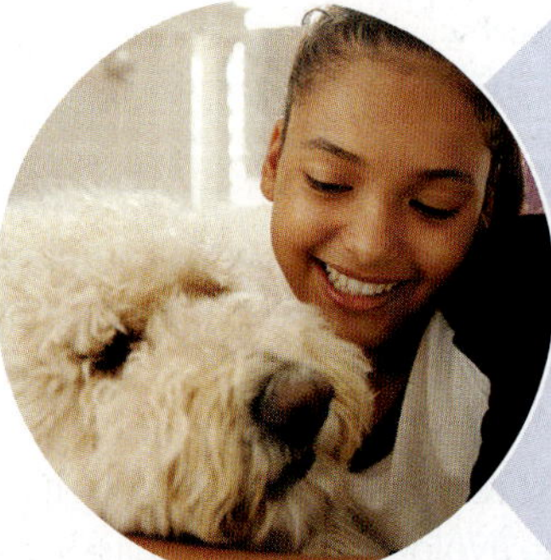

Eustress

- Big events like a school dance, sporting event, or musical performance
- Celebrations such as a surprise party or wedding
- New responsibilities, like a family pet or driver's license
- An energizing workout or physical event like a marathon or obstacle course

Distress

- Major events like losing a loved one or ending a dating relationship
- Annoying daily events like losing your phone charger or getting stuck in traffic
- Conflict with family, friends, or dating partners
- Feelings of rejection or exclusion
- Bullying or aggressive behavior at school

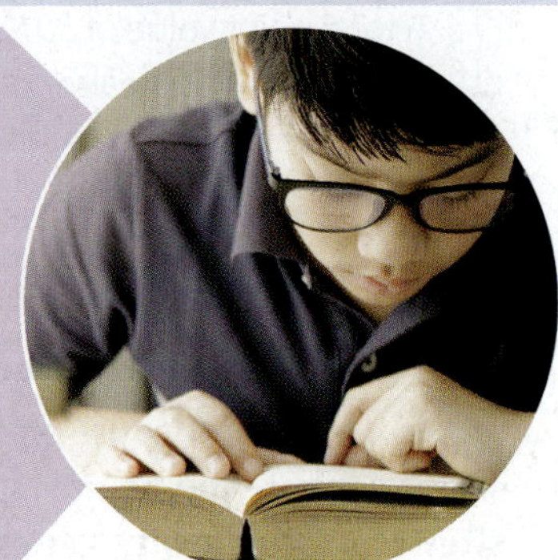

Top to bottom: Monkey Business Images/Shutterstock.com; sirikorn thamniyom/Shutterstock.com

Figure 6.2 Eustress encourages focus, motivation, and growth, while distress can lead to negative feelings and harmful health effects. ***What is the term for extreme stress due to deeply disturbing events?***

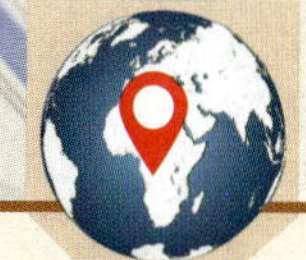

Local and Global Health

Are Some Countries More Stressful Than Others?

According to the 2019 Global Emotions Report by Gallup, people in some countries have higher overall levels of stress compared to people in other countries. In this study, researchers asked people whether they had felt a lot of stress during the previous day. The results show countries with the highest percentage of people who reported a lot of stress.

Researchers also studied which countries had the highest percentage of people experiencing positive emotions. Results show that, out of the top 10 countries that had the highest percentage of people reporting positive experiences, nine are in Latin America. Researchers believe the strong focus on family and social networks in these countries increases positive emotions and buffers the impact of stressors.

Country	Percentage of People Who Reported a Lot of Stress
Greece	59
Philippines	58
Tanzania	57
Albania	55
Iran	55
Sri Lanka	55
United States	55
Uganda	53
Costa Rica	52
Rwanda	52
Turkey	52
Venezuela	52

Practice Your Skills

Analyze Influences

With a partner, review the countries in which the largest percentage of people reported a lot of stress. What patterns do you observe? Do you think the factors predicting stress are the same in different countries? Why or why not? After discussing, compare your thoughts with those of another pair.

How could you test which factors have the most influence? Describe how knowing these factors could help countries reduce stress. In your small group, also discuss the study itself. This study examined stress by asking people whether they felt a lot of stress the prior day. Is this the best way to assess levels of stress? Why or why not? What might be a better way to assess stress in different countries?

People typically perceive stress in two stages. First, people engage in *primary appraisal*. In this stage, people assess their thoughts about a situation and decide what it means. One teen who ends a dating relationship may miss the relationship, but recognize it was not really working well for either person. Another teen might end the relationship and believe it means never having another dating partner again.

Next, people engage in *secondary appraisal* and think about the resources they have to cope with the situation. A teen who just failed a math test might think about talking to the teacher and getting extra help with math. A teen who just ended a dating relationship may think about other sources of emotional support, such as friends or family members. People who have more resources to cope with stressful life experiences are better able to have a positive mind-set about stress.

How the Body Responds to Stress

fight-or-flight response physiological stress reaction in which the body mobilizes its resources to fight off or escape from a perceived threat; also called the *stress response*

Think about a time when you were about to do something very stressful, such as take an important standardized test or give an oral presentation. How did your body react in this situation? Did you start breathing rapidly, feel nauseous, or develop a headache?

This type of reaction to a stressful experience is a natural biological process called the **fight-or-flight response**, or *stress response* (**Figure 6.3**). When a person (or animal) experiences some type of threat, the body's immediate response is to mobilize resources for fighting off or escaping from the threat. During times of stress, the body therefore shifts energy from nonessential processes, such as digestion and reproduction, to those that help the body directly respond to the challenge. This reaction to stress is designed to help people respond to extreme, life-threatening events, such as escaping from a snake or forest fire.

Depending on perception, people can also experience this response to non-life-threatening events, such as taking a test or interviewing for a job. In the fight-or-flight response, a person may not react by literally fighting or escaping. Fighting might take the form of studying hard for a test or confronting a conflict. Flight might take the form of avoiding a task or freezing.

Generally, the body's response to stress progresses through three stages:

1. **Alarm stage:** When faced with a stressful event, your body mobilizes all of its resources to fight off or escape from a perceived threat. To prepare for fighting or escaping, your body undergoes several changes.

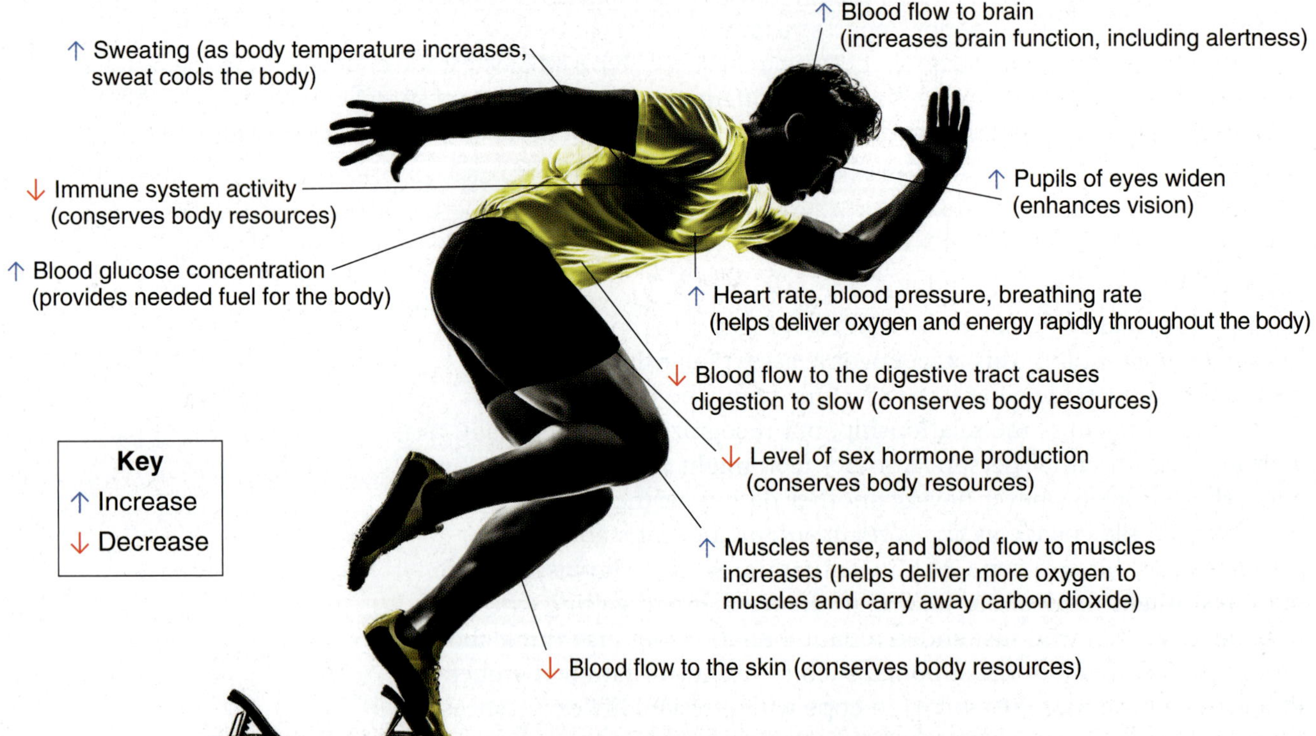

OSTILL is Franck Camhi/Shutterstock.com

Figure 6.3 The body responds to stress by triggering body processes that prepare the body to either fight off or escape from the threat.

Heart rate, blood flow, and breathing increase to supply more blood and oxygen to your muscles, brain, and vital organs. The pupils of your eyes widen to improve your vision. Physiological processes unrelated to fighting off the threat, such as digestion and reproduction, stop or slow down. This allows your body to focus its resources where they are most needed.

2. **Resistance stage:** Your body devotes energy to maintaining its stress response. Heart rate and breathing remain rapid, which helps deliver oxygen and energy quickly to the various parts of your body.
3. **Exhaustion stage:** If the perceived threat persists, the body may continue to maintain its stress response for a long time. Over time, this will use up the body's resources and lead to exhaustion.

After a stressful event is over, the **relaxation response** occurs. This is basically the opposite of the fight-or-flight response. The body gradually returns to its resting state. Hormone levels return to normal, and the cardiovascular system slows down, leading to a lower heart rate and blood pressure. The digestive and reproductive systems start working again. If the stressful event does not end, or if the body maintains the stress response for a long time, however, negative health effects can occur.

relaxation response physiological reaction in which the body returns to its resting state after a stressful event

Lesson 6.1 Review

Know and Understand

1. With a partner, discuss what stressors you think are most common for teens at your school. Compare your list with other pairs in the class.
2. Give one example of eustress and one example of distress.
3. What types of stressors can lead to toxic stress?
4. How does your body prepare to fight or escape in the fight-or-flight response?
5. What happens in the relaxation response?

Think Critically

6. Imagine that a friend of yours is going through a hard time. When you try to help your friend, your friend says, "My dad says I shouldn't be stressed about this." Using the information in this lesson, write a supportive letter to your friend explaining how perception impacts stress.
7. With a partner, discuss the behaviors involved in the fight-or-flight response. What could it look like to "fight" when you are stressed about having too little time? What could it look like to "flee" when you are scared of a situation?
8. What factors might affect whether a person experiences the relaxation response after a stressful event?

REAL WORLD Health Skills

Set Goals Setting goals for how you want to conduct yourself and what you want to accomplish is an important part of a healthy lifestyle. Vision boards are a great way to illustrate what goals you want to achieve. Select three character traits that, if you achieved them, would make you a happier person. Then, create three action steps you would need to take to make each character trait a reality. Lastly, create a SMART goal for gaining each character trait. Remember that SMART goals are specific, measurable, achievable, relevant, and timely. Arrange these traits, action steps, and goals into a vision board and present it to the class.

Lesson
6.2

Health Effects of Stress

Essential Question?
How can stress affect a person's health?

Learning Outcomes

After studying this lesson, you will be able to

- explain how long-term stress affects the body systems;
- describe the cognitive effects of stress;
- discuss how stress affects people's emotions;
- identify mental health conditions associated with stress; and
- summarize how stress influences behavior.

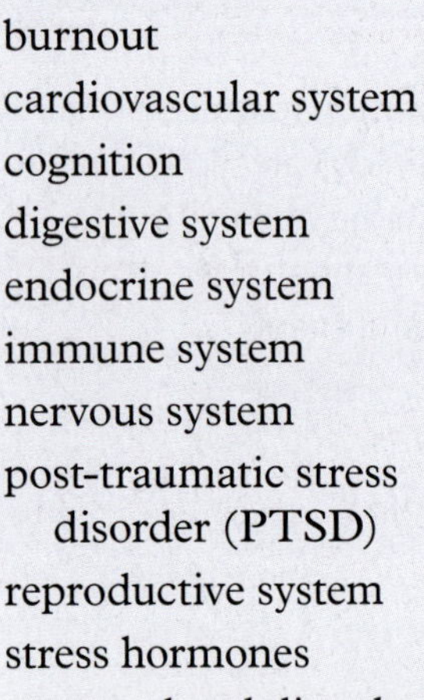

Key Terms

burnout
cardiovascular system
cognition
digestive system
endocrine system
immune system
nervous system
post-traumatic stress disorder (PTSD)
reproductive system
stress hormones
stress-related disorder

Warm-Up Activity

The Stress Effect

Comprehend Concepts Before reading this lesson, discuss with a partner how stress affects your body. Then, using this lesson as a guide, draw an outline of the body and the effects that short-term and long-term stress have on the body. Include effects from all of the major body systems discussed in this lesson, as well as mental and emotional and behavioral effects. Artistically differentiate between short-term effects (the fight-or-flight response) and long-term effects.

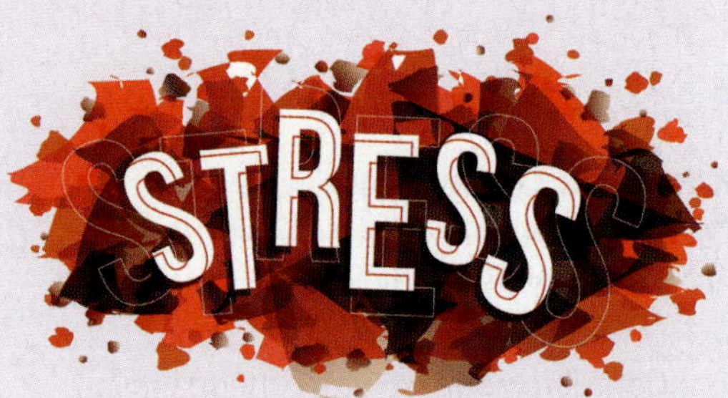

Eightshot_Studio/Shutterstock.com

During times of stress, the body devotes large amounts of energy to reacting to the immediate, perceived threat. This causes physical, cognitive, and emotional changes that help the body fight off the threat. Once the threat resolves, the body relaxes and returns to its original state. If the perceived threat persists, however, the body will maintain its state of physiological arousal and keep devoting energy to fighting off the threat. Over time, this type of chronic stress can cause harmful health effects and make people vulnerable to infections and diseases. In this lesson, you will learn about the health effects of stress in reaction to an immediate threat and long-term.

Physical Effects

In the moment, the body reacts to stress with the fight-or-flight response, which mobilizes body resources to fight off or escape from a perceived threat. This response causes changes in several body systems. If stress resolves, these body systems return to normal functioning.

When stress continues, the body maintains its state of arousal long-term, which can lead to many health conditions. Body systems particularly affected by stress include the nervous, endocrine, cardiovascular, immune, digestive, and reproductive systems (**Figure 6.4**).

Nervous System

The **nervous system** consists of the brain, spinal cord, and nerves that trade information between the brain and the rest of the body. This body system alerts your brain when your body experiences particular sensations, such as touch and pain. The nervous system is also the command center responsible for mobilizing the other body systems to react to a threatening situation.

nervous system body system that consists of the brain, spinal cord, and nerves that trade information throughout the body

In the face of a perceived threat, the nervous system processes the situation and prompts the other body systems to act. These other systems increase breathing and heart rate, decrease digestion and reproduction, and send blood to the muscles. These physiological changes improve your body's ability to respond to threatening situations. If stress persists, however, the nervous system continues to trigger the other body systems, wearing down the body over time.

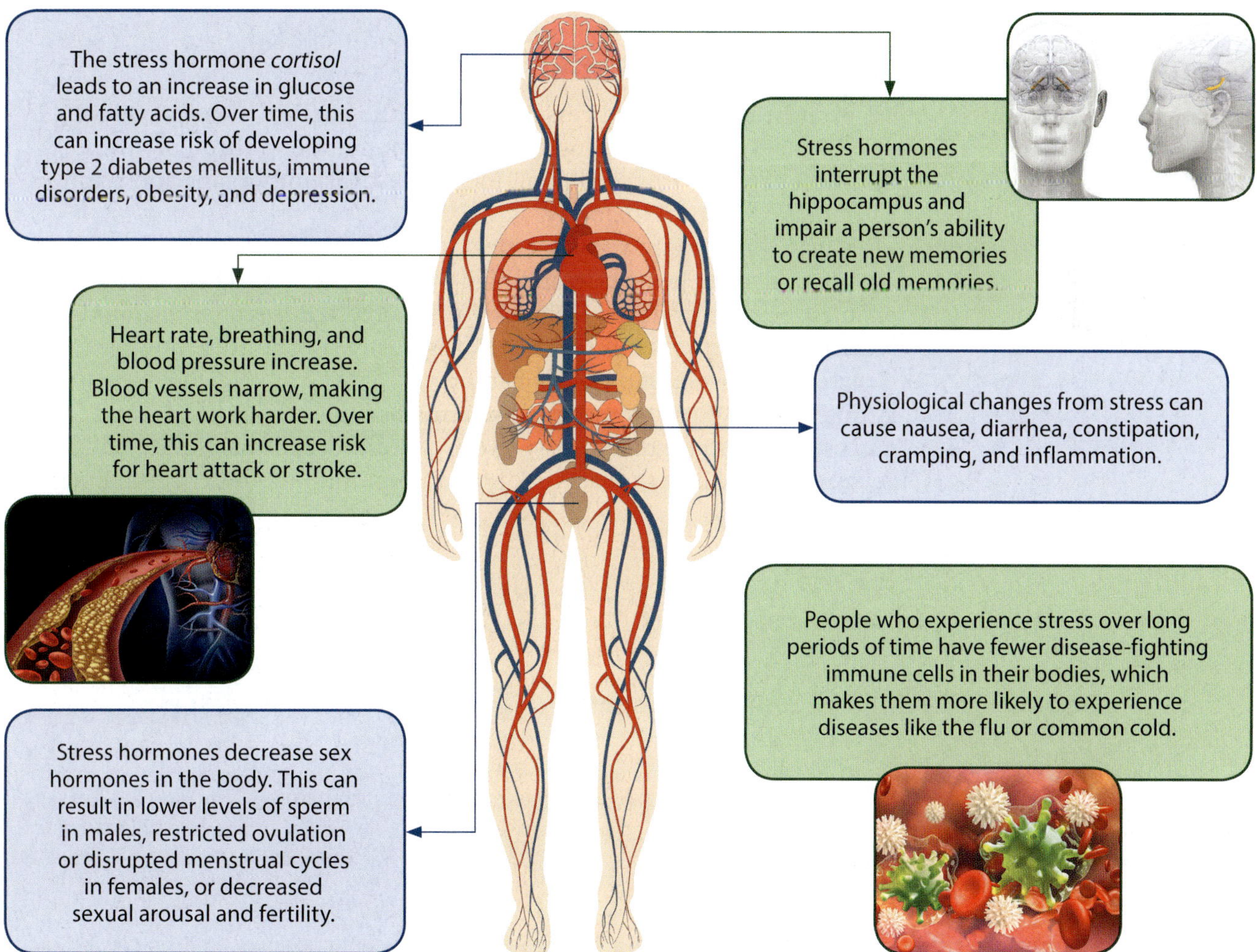

Left: Lightspring/Shutterstock.com; Middle: eveleen/Shutterstock.com; Right, top to bottom: decade3d – anatomy online/Shutterstock.com; Yurchanka Siarhei/Shutterstock.com

Figure 6.4 Stress can cause negative health effects in various body systems. These health effects increase as stress continues over time.

Stress can also cause changes in the brain that lead to forgetfulness, especially if stress is long-term. Hormones released during stress disrupt the functioning of the *hippocampus*, the part of the brain involved in memory. This impairs a person's ability to create new memories or recall old memories.

Endocrine System

endocrine system body system that consists of glands, which secrete hormones to regulate body processes

stress hormones chemicals that coordinate the fight-or-flight response; include epinephrine, norepinephrine, and cortisol

The **endocrine system** is a set of glands that release chemicals called *hormones* into the bloodstream. These hormones travel through the bloodstream and cause changes in particular body tissues or organs.

During times of stress, a part of the brain called the *hypothalamus* stimulates endocrine glands to secrete *epinephrine*, *norepinephrine*, and *cortisol*, which are known as the **stress hormones**. These hormones trigger the changes that help the body respond quickly to a threat.

Higher levels of cortisol in the body lead to increases in glucose and fatty acids, giving the body more energy to respond to stress. Although having extra energy helps manage stress in the short-term, negative health consequences can develop if the body does not return to its resting state. People who experience long-term stress therefore have a greater risk of developing type 2 diabetes mellitus, immune disorders, obesity, and depression.

Cardiovascular System

cardiovascular system body system that transports blood throughout the body; consists of the heart and blood vessels

Your heart and blood vessels make up the **cardiovascular system**. The primary function of this system is to pump blood throughout the body. Blood carries oxygen to all the body's cells and organs and removes carbon dioxide from the body.

The fight-or-flight response causes increased cardiovascular activity, including a faster heart rate and higher blood pressure. This activity enables the body to respond quickly to a perceived threat and should return to normal when the body relaxes. If stress continues, however, elevated cardiovascular activity can have negative consequences (**Figure 6.5**). When blood pressure remains high, fatty deposits and glucose build up on blood vessel walls over time. This narrows blood vessels, and the heart must work harder to pump blood through them.

Impact of Stress on the Cardiovascular System

Initial impact

- Heart rate and blood pressure increase.
- If stress is resolved, the body should relax and return to normal.

Continued impact

- Fatty deposits and glucose build up on blood vessel walls over time, narrowing blood vessels.
- The heart must work harder to pump blood.

Impact over time

- Chronic wear and tear on heart can increase risk for heart attack, stroke, and other cardiovascular diseases.

Figure 6.5 If stress resolves, the body relaxes and activity returns to normal. If stress continues over time, however, a person can experience serious health effects. ***What body parts make up the cardiovascular system?***

This chronic wear and tear can cause considerable damage and increase a person's risk for heart attack, stroke, and other cardiovascular diseases.

Immune System

The **immune system** consists of organs, tissues, and cells that defend against infection. When foreign cells or disease-causing agents enter your body, the cells of your immune system destroy them.

immune system body system consisting of organs, tissues, and cells that defend against infection

During times of stress, your body is focused on escaping from or fighting off a specific threat. As a result, the immune system receives fewer resources as long as the threat continues. This is why people sometimes get sick when they are stressed. People who experience stress over long periods of time have fewer disease-fighting immune cells in their bodies. This makes them more likely to experience diseases like the common cold and flu.

Digestive System

Organs that take in food, pass nutrients from these sources into the bloodstream, and then expel waste out of the body make up the **digestive system**. During times of stress, changes caused by physiological arousal lead the esophagus to spasm. These changes also increase the amount of acid in the stomach, leading to indigestion. This is why stress often leads to nausea, diarrhea, or constipation. Stress can also decrease the flow of blood and oxygen to the stomach, causing cramping and inflammation.

digestive system body system consisting of organs that take in foods, pass nutrients from these sources into the bloodstream, and then expel waste out of the body

For many years, scientists believed that long-term stress led to ulcers. More recent evidence suggests that stress does not cause ulcers, but can make the symptoms of ulcers feel worse. It can also worsen the symptoms of other digestive conditions, including irritable bowel syndrome (IBS) and gastroesophageal reflux disease (GERD).

Reproductive System

The **reproductive system** includes organs that work together to create new human life. During times of stress, levels of particular hormones increase in the body. These hormones decrease levels of *sex hormones*, or hormones related to reproduction, in the body. The result is lower levels of sperm in males, restricted ovulation in females, decreased sexual arousal, and reduced fertility.

reproductive system body system consisting of organs that work together to create new human life; is different between males and females

The effect of stress on the body's hormones can also cause changes in the menstrual cycle in females. This is why females who are experiencing stress may notice disruptions in menstruation, such as a delayed or skipped period.

Mental and Emotional Effects

Stress has significant effects on your mental and emotional health, including how well you think and reason and how you feel. While your body is mobilizing to fight off a perceived threat, your mind is probably thinking about how to resolve the challenge you face and manage your emotions.

Cognitive Effects

cognition ability to think, reason, and remember

Have you ever forgotten about a homework assignment because you were stressed about a test in another class? Have you found it hard to concentrate on school when you are having a conflict with a friend? In addition to affecting your body, stress also affects your **cognition**, or ability to think, reason, and remember.

People facing a stressful event tend to have trouble concentrating or focusing on a task, partly because thoughts about the event distract them (**Figure 6.6**). This can lead to difficulty paying attention and learning. For example, have you ever misread a question on a test and gotten the answer wrong because you were stressed and could not focus? Lack of focus due to stress can sometimes lead to physical injury. For example, a person jogging may be too distracted and trip on something in the road.

Stress increases physiological arousal, which can lead to poor decision-making. When people feel stressed, they are more likely to make impulsive, or quick, decisions. They may forget to consider the advantages and disadvantages of each choice.

People experiencing stress are also more likely to think negative thoughts. Not surprisingly, these thoughts increase stress levels and make it harder to focus on performing tasks.

Emotional Effects

People facing stressful events often experience negative feelings. These feelings can include nervousness, fear, anxiety, helplessness, frustration, irritability, hostility, and anger. Emotional reactions to stressful events vary depending on the person and type of stressor. For example, major losses can lead to disbelief, shock, and numbness. They can also lead to sadness, loneliness, and isolation. Although these emotions can feel overwhelming, they are normal reactions to experiencing stressful events. Managing stress can reduce these emotions and help you feel better.

People who experience chronic stress have a greater risk of developing mental health conditions and illnesses. Researchers have found that the brains of people experiencing chronic stress have lower levels of hormones and chemicals that make people feel good. Lower levels of particular hormones also cause changes in the body, which can contribute to depression. These changes include a lower level of energy, reduced appetite, and difficulty sleeping.

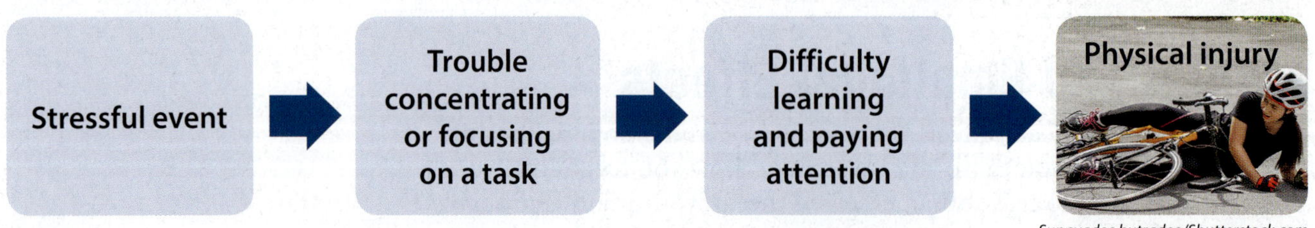

Supavadee butradee/Shutterstock.com

Figure 6.6 A stressful event can lead to trouble concentrating or focusing. This lack of concentration can cause issues learning or paying attention, which in turn can result in physical injuries.

Stress-Related Disorders

In most cases, after people have experienced a traumatic event, they return to a mental and emotional state that is normal for them. In other cases, people have more difficulty returning to their regular lives. These people may develop a **stress-related disorder**, or mental illness that develops in response to a stressful event. People who have experienced multiple traumatic events or have another mental illness are more likely to develop a stress-related disorder.

stress-related disorder
mental illness that develops as a result of stressful events; examples include acute stress disorder and post-traumatic stress disorder (PTSD)

Acute stress disorder is a stress-related disorder that begins immediately after the stressful event occurs and lasts from three days to one month. Symptoms of acute stress disorder include feeling numb, being unaware of surroundings, having repeated thoughts or mental images of the event, and experiencing high levels of anxiety and arousal. These symptoms interfere with a person's ability to go about daily life.

Research in Action

Can Stress Be Passed Through Generations?

Did you know that stressful, traumatic events can affect not just the person experiencing stress, but also that person's children? Researchers at Mount Sinai Medical Center in New York conducted a study to examine the long-term effects of exposure to traumatic events. They collected data from pregnant people who were living in New York City on the morning of September 11, 2001, and experienced the terrorist attacks on the World Trade Center buildings. Researchers measured whether these people developed symptoms of PTSD following the attacks and also collected saliva samples to measure levels of the stress hormone cortisol.

Their findings revealed that those who developed PTSD had lower levels of cortisol than those who did not. Prior research has shown that people with low levels of cortisol have trouble reducing their arousal following a stressful event, since cortisol helps stop the stress response. This inability to bring down intense arousal increases risk of developing PTSD after a traumatic event.

Researchers also examined levels of cortisol in these people's children. Remember, these were children born after the terrorist attacks. Children born to those participants who had developed PTSD also had lower levels of cortisol compared to other children. How are traumatic experiences transmitted by pregnant people to their unborn children? Researchers believe that experiencing traumatic events causes *epigenetic changes*, or changes in how genes are expressed depending on environmental factors. This finding shows how stress can be passed genetically from a pregnant person to an unborn child.

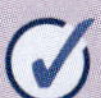

Practice Your Skills

Access Information

With a partner, discuss how traumatic events may lead to changes in levels of stress hormones. Use reliable resources online or talk with a library media specialist to get information to answer the following questions:

- Why do some people react differently to traumatic events compared to others? What factors may lead to these differences?
- What do the findings of this study reveal about the transmission of stress? How is stress transmitted, and what does this mean for future generations?
- What can communities do to help reduce the transmission of stress between generations? What can individuals do?

post-traumatic stress disorder (PTSD) stress-related disorder characterized by flashbacks, feelings of numbness, and difficulty sleeping after an extremely stressful event

burnout state of emotional, physical, and mental exhaustion

Post-traumatic stress disorder (PTSD) may occur after a person experiences an extremely frightening and upsetting event (**Figure 6.7**). These events include natural disasters, war, terrorist events, and violent acts. PTSD is characterized by a strong and lingering reaction to extreme stress. In some cases, these reactions may last for many years.

Burnout

Another mental and emotional effect of stress can be **burnout**, or a state of emotional, physical, and mental exhaustion. Long periods of excessive stress can lead to burnout. When people experience burnout, they feel overwhelmed, emotionally drained, tired, alone, unmotivated, and hopeless. They may experience changes in appetite and sleep habits and lose interest in activities they used to enjoy, such as spending time with friends. Many people with burnout have a sense of failure and self-doubt.

Burnout can lead to significant negative consequences for emotional and physical health. These include difficulty sleeping; negative feelings, including sadness, anger, and irritability; substance abuse; increased risk of developing an illness; and certain health conditions, including cardiovascular disease, high blood pressure, and diabetes.

Behavioral Effects

Think about the last time you felt stressed. How did stress influence your behavior? Many people have difficulty falling or staying asleep, cry easily, do not feel hungry, or lose interest in enjoyable activities when they feel stressed. These changes in behavior can make coping even more difficult. When people who feel stressed do not get enough sleep or proper nutrition, for example, their bodies become even more run-down.

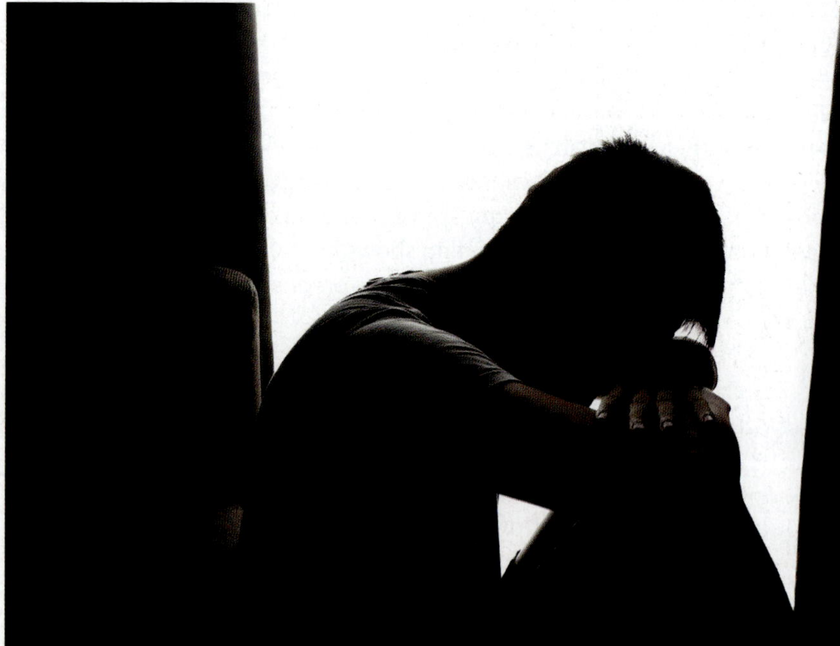

Symptoms of PTSD

- Having nightmares and recurring thoughts about the event
- Feeling detached, numb, and uncaring
- Being unable to remember parts of the upsetting event
- Lacking interest in normal activities
- Avoiding people and situations that are reminders of the event
- Having difficulty concentrating
- Being easily startled
- Feeling irritable and angry
- Experiencing difficulty falling or staying asleep
- Feeling guilty

iphotosmile/Shutterstock.com

Figure 6.7 PTSD symptoms take many forms, and many are easy to overlook as less serious than they are.
What are examples of traumatic events that may lead to PTSD?

People who feel stressed may behave in ways they would not under different circumstances (**Figure 6.8**). High levels of stress, including trauma, make people more likely to engage in health-harming behaviors. Examples include smoking or vaping, using alcohol or drugs, eating unhealthy foods, and not getting physical activity. High levels of stress also make people less likely to engage in healthy behaviors, like taking care of themselves. They tend to get less sleep, for example, which has negative health outcomes.

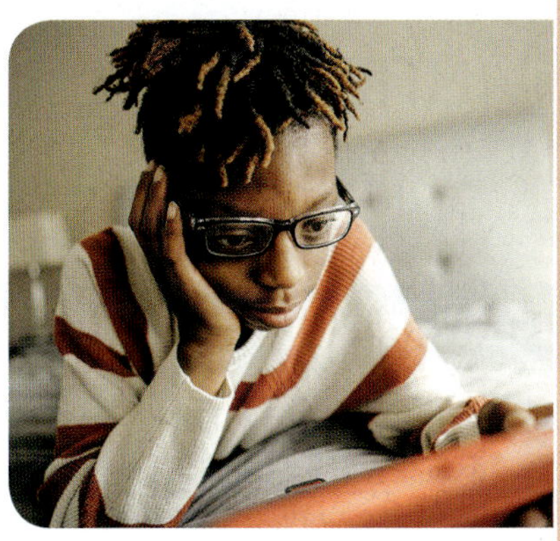

Stress can make people feel

- frustrated and angry, which can lead to conflict
- distracted and overwhelmed, which can cause people to treat others unkindly
- more likely to engage in violence (for example, with major financial stress between romantic partners)

kate_sept2004/E+/Getty Images

Figure 6.8 If you notice someone behaving irregularly, this may be due to stress.

Lesson 6.2 Review

Know and Understand

1. Explain how long-term stress affects the cardiovascular system.
2. Why are people experiencing lots of stress more likely to get sick?
3. Give one example of a time stress made it difficult for you to concentrate or remember something.
4. Write a story in which a person experiences the symptoms of PTSD.

Think Critically

5. With a partner, consider the following question: Are the physical effects of stress always harmful? Why or why not?
6. Why do you think people experience negative feelings when they are stressed?
7. How many teens do you think have experienced burnout? Discuss in a small group and share stories of factors that lead to burnout.
8. How do you behave differently when you experience stress? Share your answer with a friend.

REAL WORLD Health Skills

Communicate with Others Read the "Dear Abby" message shown and then write a short paragraph identifying the potential consequences if Karl does not effectively manage stress. How might Karl's performance in school suffer? Be encouraging in your response and show empathy and good communication skills. Write a response you would want to receive if you were in Karl's position.

Dear Abby,

Hi. The lawn hasn't been mowed in weeks, and my room looks like a war zone. I fell down the steps because my brother left his skateboard on the stairs. My mom is complaining I don't spend enough time with the family, and I have a seven-page paper due on Wednesday. I feel like I'm going to explode.

Sincerely,

Karl

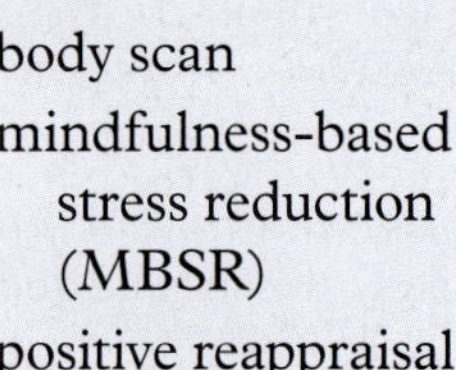

Lesson 6.3 Managing Stress

Essential Question?
What healthy strategies can people use to manage stress?

Learning Outcomes

After studying this lesson, you will be able to

- explain why identifying stressors is the first step in stress management;
- identify ways of reducing stress by managing commitments, time, and thoughts;
- describe the importance of expressing your feelings during a stressful situation;
- identify relaxation techniques;
- use mindfulness-based stress reduction strategies;
- analyze the importance of taking care of yourself; and
- assess when it is necessary to seek professional help.

Key Terms

body scan
mindfulness-based stress reduction (MBSR)
positive reappraisal
progressive muscle relaxation
stress management
time management
visualization

Warm-Up Activity

The Perfect Day

Practice Health-Enhancing Behaviors Imagine you entered a contest and won a "perfect day." As the winner, you choose what you will do and where you will go on your perfect day. Describe your perfect day in detail through the morning, afternoon, and evening. You only have $50 to spend and free public transportation for the day. You must be home by 11 p.m.

After you have outlined your perfect day, share your description with the class. Discuss the importance of free time as it relates to stress management. Also discuss time-management strategies that might lead to more free time and opportunities to have your "perfect day."

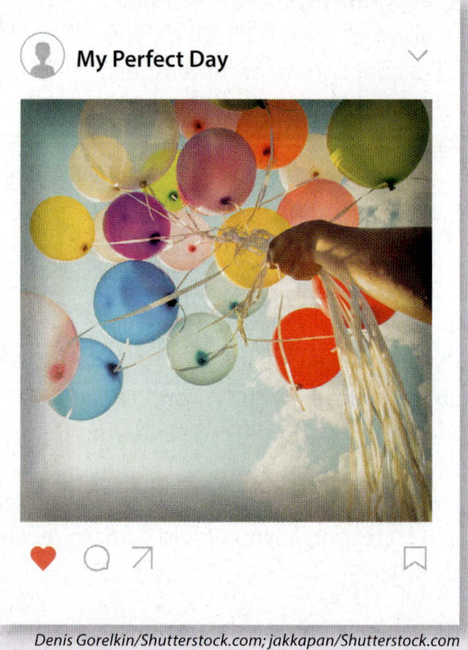

Denis Gorelkin/Shutterstock.com; jakkapan/Shutterstock.com

Think about a stressful situation you faced recently in your life. How did you feel when you were stressed? What did you do to handle these feelings and resolve the situation? Were the strategies you used effective? How did stress affect the different areas of your life?

Stress is a normal part of life. Everyone feels stressed sometimes, and stress can even serve as motivation and help you achieve your goals. Like other emotions, stress can help you learn about yourself and what situations you find threatening. At the same time, stress can negatively affect your health and cause health conditions, negative feelings, and trouble thinking. To avoid these consequences and instead embrace the benefits of stress, you need to learn to manage stress well.

Stress management is the process of using strategies to reduce stress and handle stressful situations in positive ways. Not everyone will find the same stress-management strategies useful. Trying several strategies can help you learn about yourself and identify effective methods of stress management.

stress management
process of using strategies to reduce the impact of the stress response and handle threatening situations in positive ways

Identify Stressors

The first step in managing stress is identifying the stressors, or sources of stress, in your life (**Figure 6.9**). Your stressors could be particular situations you experience, such as taking a test, interviewing for a job, or trying out for the school play or a sports team. Stressors can also be parts of daily life you find challenging. For many high school students, ongoing stressors include managing time, handling interpersonal conflict, and coping with academic pressure. Figuring out what factors cause you stress can help you prepare an effective response.

When identifying stressors, remember that people have different stressors based on their perceptions. Certain events are stressful to everyone. These include major life events, such as the death of a loved one or a serious illness or injury. Other stressors can be experienced in different ways by different people. For some high school students, getting a B+ on a project could be stressful. For others, this might not be stressful at all. How you think about or perceive an event has a major impact on whether you experience stress.

Questions to Help Identify Stressors

- ✔ Are you in conflict with someone in your life?
- ✔ Do you feel you do not have enough money for your needs?
- ✔ Does it seem like there are not enough hours in the day to get everything done?
- ✔ Have you experienced loss recently? of a loved one? of a relationship?
- ✔ Is there an upcoming event you feel pressure about?
- ✔ Are you worried about criticism from others for something you do?
- ✔ Are you or someone you love coping with an illness or health condition?
- ✔ Do you feel unable to express your emotions?
- ✔ Are you under pressure, from yourself or others, to perform well in academics or athletics?
- ✔ Have you recently experienced or are you anticipating a major life change, such as moving or your parent or guardian getting married or divorced?
- ✔ Do you experience discrimination from people based on your race, ethnicity, disability, sex, gender identity, or sexual orientation?
- ✔ Does your neighborhood have safety concerns such as crime?

Figure 6.9 Asking yourself questions can help you identify what stressors are currently affecting you. ***What process uses strategies to handle stressful situations in positive ways?***

Reduce Stress

Once you know what factors cause you stress, you can take steps to reduce the amount of stress in your life. Remember that you cannot eliminate stress altogether or control all sources of stress. Still, there are some steps you can take to reduce your level of stress on a daily basis.

Set Healthy Boundaries

Stress often occurs when people feel like they do not have enough time or energy to fulfill all of their commitments. For example, maybe you agreed to go to a friend's party, but also have a final project due the next day. Maybe you sometimes make commitments you do not have time or energy for because you have a hard time saying *no*, want to have fun, or want to help others. No matter the reason, committing to many events can create stress when your calendar is already full. Learning to set healthy boundaries and limits can help you manage stress.

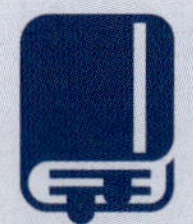

Case Study

Stressful Situations

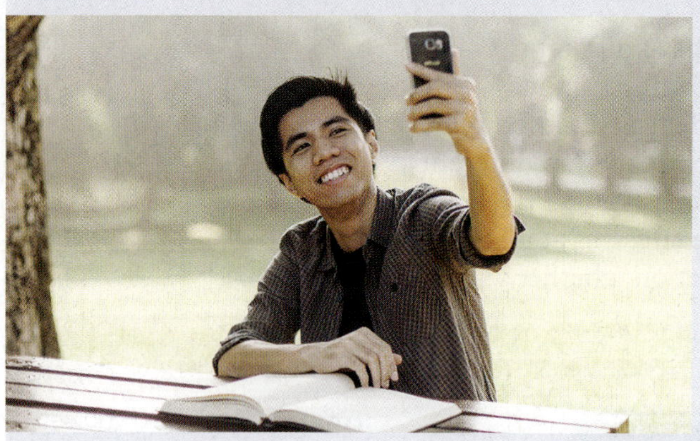

shutterpix/Shutterstock.com

Carlos wants to be a great student, teammate, and big brother, and he does his best to keep up. He makes to-do lists to manage his stress, but seeing everything written out only makes him feel worse. Carlos tries to prepare healthy meals and get enough sleep so he will have the energy he needs, but he worries this wastes time that could be spent doing homework. His mom says, "Cut yourself some slack! Nobody is perfect." Carlos knows she is right, but he still gets an upset stomach when he misses his little sister's events for baseball games. Carlos wonders if talking to a therapist will help him find a better solution.

Elijah's entire life revolves around social media. Elijah plans to work on homework during study hall, but he finds himself talking with friends about who posted what on social media. He also feels pressured to post content for his peers instead of memorizing his lines for the school play. Elijah, finally fed up, vented to his friend about social media. After talking to his friend, Elijah decided it would be best to take a break from social media for a while and focus on school and the upcoming play.

Amelia started high school with high expectations. She felt like she could easily balance school, friends, and her babysitting job. Now, she realizes she was underprepared for how busy she would be. When she has projects due, Amelia procrastinates until the night before. She has started showing up late for her babysitting job and using jokes to deflect attention from her slipping grades. She gets stomachaches in class whenever her teachers announce tests or grades. Amelia hopes that, if she pretends everything is fine, it will all work out.

Practice Your Skills

Make Decisions

Identify the stressors that Carlos, Elijah, and Amelia experience in these scenarios. What are the sources of this stress? What can these students do to manage their stress? With a partner, choose one scenario and use the decision-making process to help Carlos, Elijah, or Amelia make a healthy decision for better managing stress.

To set healthy limits, do not commit to activities too quickly. When someone asks you to do an activity, say you will let the person know later. Then check your calendar and see whether you have time. Sometimes people commit to activities without considering their other commitments. Before you agree to an activity, consider your other responsibilities and be realistic about how much time you have available to commit to something new.

Remember that it is okay to say *no* if you are too busy. If you are unable to do an activity, tell the person as soon as you know and be polite and respectful.

Manage Your Time

Sometimes, feeling like you do not have enough time can result from making too many commitments. Other times, this feeling develops because people struggle to devote the appropriate amount of time to various tasks. Fortunately, you can mostly control how you spend your time. One of the best ways to reduce stress is **time management**, or the practice of managing your time well (**Figure 6.10**). Following are some strategies for time management:

time management practice of devoting the appropriate amount of time to each task, only committing to tasks you have time for, and prioritizing tasks; helps people reach goals and reduce stress

- **Create a time-management plan:** First, make a list of all the tasks you need to do. Then break down big tasks into smaller ones. Create a schedule that describes when you need to accomplish each task and stick to that schedule. If you have more activities than you can possibly do, prioritize them and cancel activities that are less important to make time.
- **Keep a to-do list:** List the tasks you need to work on each day, from studying for a test to mowing the lawn to applying for a summer job. Start each day by reviewing your list and make a plan for tackling each item. If you do not finish the tasks on your list, add them to the next day's list. Keeping a list will ensure you do not forget important tasks you need to accomplish.
- **Make use of a little time:** Sometimes it can be hard to find large blocks of time to work. Take advantage of small blocks of time whenever they arise. For example, you could study for a test while waiting for the bus or in the car. You could read a chapter of your English book at lunch. These small blocks of time can add up if you use them well.

In a case study, researchers examined how college students managed the stress of their schoolwork.

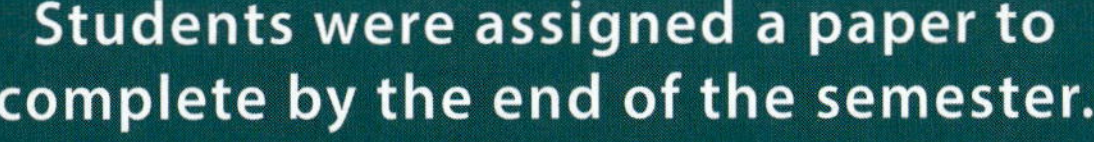

Students were assigned a paper to complete by the end of the semester.

Procrastinating students experienced less stress early in the semester than other students.

They experienced greater stress, however, when postponing the paper caught up with them at the end of the semester.

The procrastinating students had more symptoms of illness and went to the health center for treatment more.

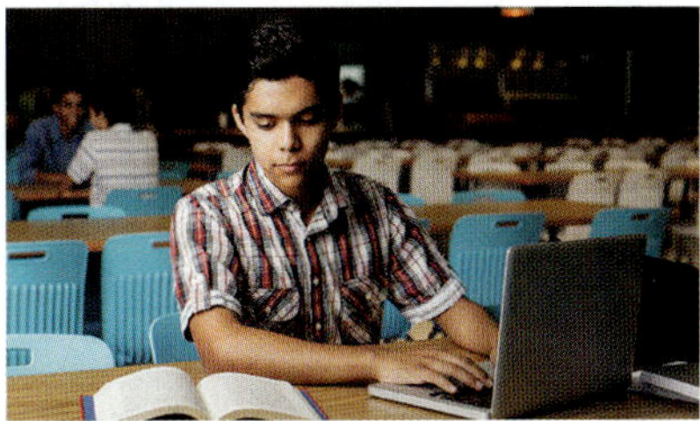

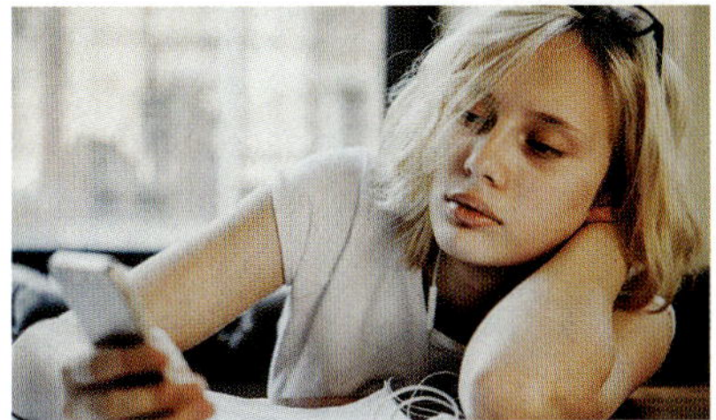

Top to bottom: aldomurillo/E+/Getty Images; Yulia Grigoryeva/Shutterstock.com

Figure 6.10 Managing your time well can help reduce stress. Procrastination does not help reduce stress, but only postpones it.

- **Avoid procrastinating:** Many high school students have a tendency to *procrastinate*, or put tasks off to a later time. Procrastinating just leads to more stress later on, however. Many school assignments are manageable if you work on them for a chunk of time each day. If you put assignments off, however, you might have a huge amount of work to do at the last minute. Make a plan to get your work done over time by creating a schedule. This will reduce stress and also lead to better work and grades.
- **Limit technology use:** Many high school students spend a lot of time browsing social media, playing video games, and watching TV shows or online videos. This can take away from time you could spend getting schoolwork done, seeing friends face-to-face, or doing other activities to reduce stress. Instead, make time for social connections, fun, physical activity, and other enjoyable activities.

Using Positive Self-Talk

"I am lovable."	Remind yourself that people care about you and love you. Think of times family members or friends showed how much they care about you.
"I am capable."	You can always learn new skills and gain new abilities. You just may need to spend more time and effort doing so. Think about a time you mastered something that initially was difficult for you.
"Challenges are opportunities."	Many people experience setbacks and have to learn how to overcome obstacles. Think about disappointments as opportunities to grow and learn. Talk to some adults about times they failed and what they learned from that experience.
"Change is hard."	Remind yourself that change is hard for everyone, so do not beat yourself up for feeling stressed during times of transition. Remind yourself that you have the ability to cope and adapt and that it just takes time to adjust.

Figure 6.11 Positive self-talk reminds you of your positive qualities and your ability to cope with stress and other negative situations.

positive reappraisal act of thinking about the good aspects of stressful events

Maintain a Positive Attitude

Stress is a reaction to situations you *perceive* as threatening. This means your level of stress can change if you alter your perception. Some situations, such as those that threaten your safety or health, are stressful by nature. Other situations, such as those that threaten your view of yourself, plans, or sense of reputation, do not necessarily require a fight-or-flight response.

Often, you can reduce stress by thinking about situations in new, positive ways. For example, being stuck in a traffic jam may make you feel stressed about making your next appointment or wasting time. You could use this time, however, to think through a problem, make a mental list of tasks, or relieve stress by listening to music or a podcast. You cannot control the traffic jam, and others will probably be understanding if you are late because of traffic.

This way of thinking, which looks for the positive aspects of stressful events, is called **positive reappraisal**. As another example, suppose you tried out for a role in a play and were not chosen. Not being chosen means you will have more time to spend with your friends.

Another strategy to help maintain a positive attitude is to engage in positive *self-talk* (**Figure 6.11**). Positive self-talk can go a long way toward helping you keep a positive attitude, even when you are facing stress.

Handle Stressful Situations

When you are in the midst of a stressful situation, you may feel out of control, especially if you cannot immediately change the situation. The effects of stress may get in the way of your thinking, make you feel sick, or stir up negative emotions. Fortunately, you can use certain strategies to manage stress and your reactions to it. These strategies can help you get through the stressful situation and handle its effects in positive ways.

Use Distraction and Humor

Many situations that cause stress are either overwhelming or beyond a person's control. These situations may include family financial difficulties or serious health conditions. Intense focus on these struggles can increase stress. When you cannot control the source of stress, distraction and humor can be good stress-management strategies (**Figure 6.12**).

Finding distractions can be a good way of managing stress. Some distraction strategies include

- going for a walk;
- doing a simple task with your hands, like coloring or woodworking;
- volunteering in the community; and
- reading a good book or listening to music.

You can also distract yourself with laughter and humor. Humor can help you cope with stressors and lighten your mood. If you are feeling stressed, watch a funny video or television show or talk to someone who makes you laugh.

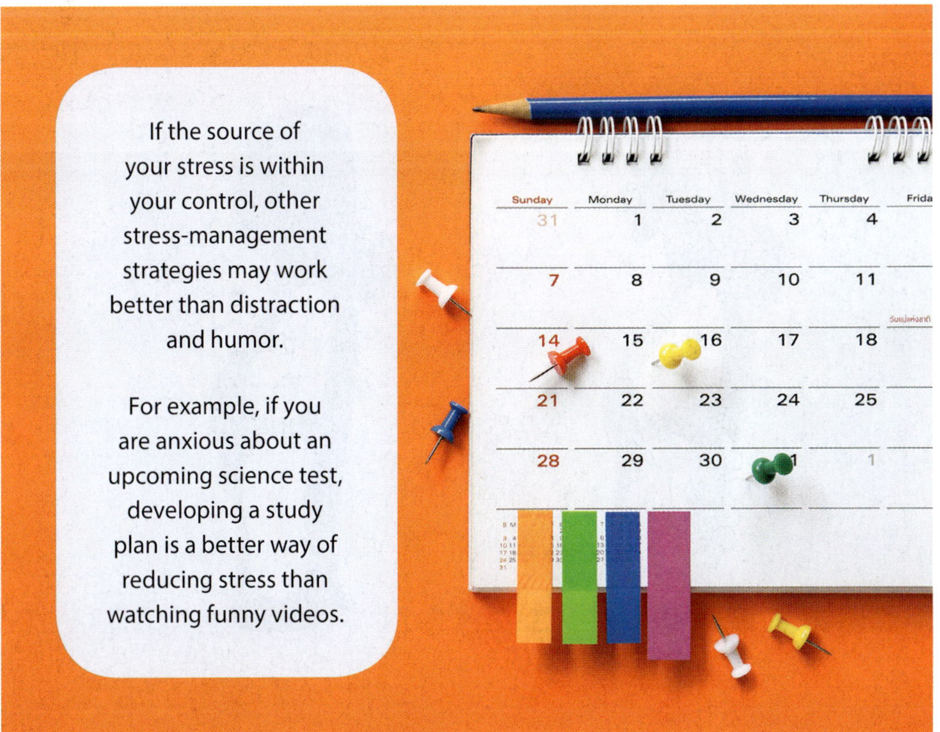

Chutima Chaochaiya/Shutterstock.com

Figure 6.12 Distraction and humor are not stress-management strategies that work for all problems. Be careful not to use stress as an excuse to procrastinate. ***What are two examples of using humor to manage stress?***

Express Your Feelings

Stress causes a lot of feelings, many of which are negative or overwhelming. Holding all of these feelings inside can make the stress worse. Expressing these feelings—verbally or in writing—can make handling a stressful situation easier.

One of the best strategies for managing stress is to talk with people you trust. These people may have helpful insight and suggestions. Even if these people cannot help you resolve the situation, simply talking about your feelings can help you feel better. You can also express your feelings by reflecting on them privately. For example, you might keep a journal about your feelings, track your emotions using a chart or app, or write songs or poems.

Use Relaxation Techniques

Some effective stress-management strategies focus on changing how your body responds to potentially threatening situations. These strategies specifically focus on changing your behavior in response to stress by lowering heart rate, blood pressure, and breathing rate. Instead of becoming tense, you can teach your body to relax using the following techniques:

- **Deep breathing:** Taking slow, deep breaths helps your brain and body calm down and relax (**Figure 6.13**). Deep breathing also lowers your heart rate and decreases blood pressure.

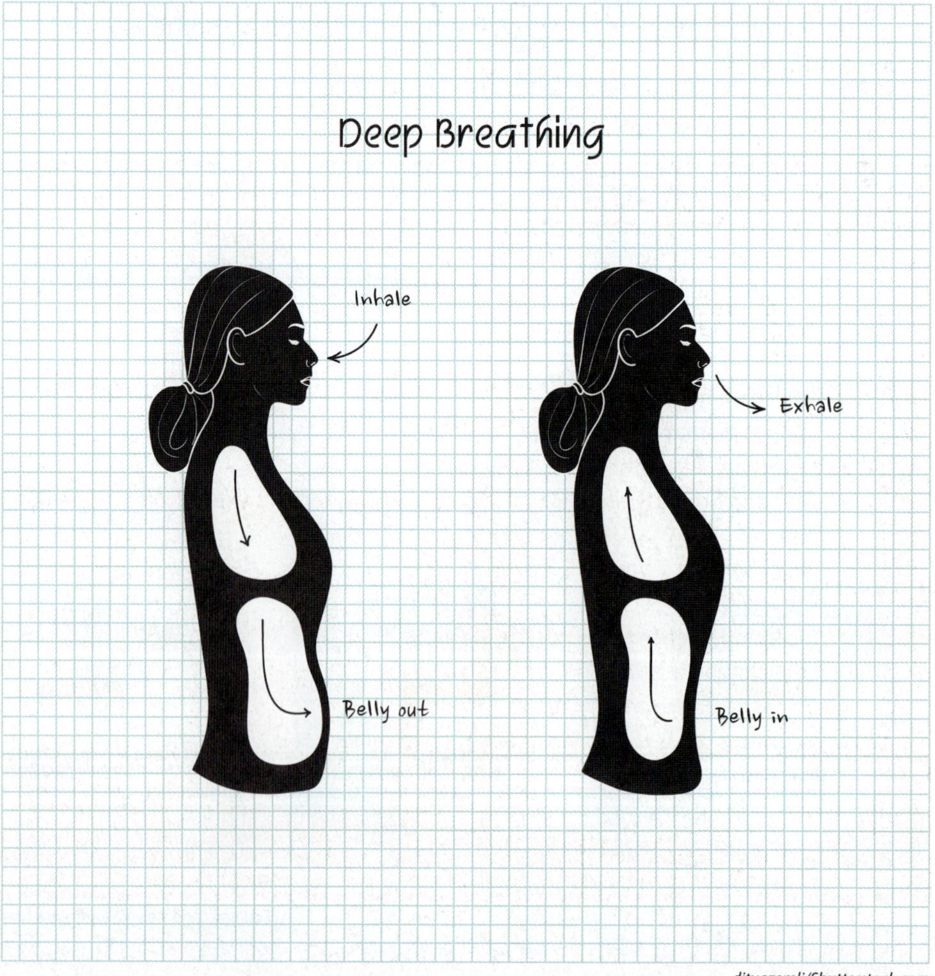

Figure 6.13 Breathing in and out, deep enough that your belly moves with your breathing, can help you relax.

dityazemli/Shutterstock.com

- **Visualization:** Some people have success using **visualization**. This technique involves thinking about or imagining a pleasant environment. For example, if you enjoy the beach, you might imagine the sound of waves crashing and the warmth of the sun on your skin.
- **Progressive muscle relaxation: Progressive muscle relaxation** is a technique in which you tense and then relax each part of your body until your entire body is relaxed (**Figure 6.14**). Deep breathing increases the effectiveness of this technique.
- **Body scan**: **Body scan** is a technique in which you pay close attention and scan your entire body—starting with the head—for any feelings of tension. Then you focus on mentally releasing any physical tension you have in any part of the body that feels tense.
- **Focused attention:** Relaxation techniques that involve focused attention can help reduce negative or stressful thoughts that lead the body to become tense. For example, to practice focused attention, you might clear your mind of all negative and stressful thoughts and concentrate on relaxing your body.
- **Guided movements:** Several relaxation techniques involve using deep breathing while performing a series of postures and movements. For example, certain stretches require balance, flexibility, and intense concentration, which requires both physical and mental discipline. Two examples are *tai chi* and *qigong*. Tai chi and qigong combine rhythmic breathing with movement and require a mental focus that reduces stressful thoughts.

visualization relaxation technique that involves imagining one's self in a pleasant environment

progressive muscle relaxation relaxation technique that involves tensing and then relaxing each part of the body until the whole body feels relaxed

body scan relaxation technique that involves paying careful attention to the body, scanning it for signs of tension, and then releasing that tension

Be Mindful

One of the best strategies for managing stress is to be mindful. As you learned in Chapter 5, *mindfulness* involves fully concentrating on what is happening in the present without judgment. By paying attention to whatever you are doing in the moment, you avoid letting your mind shift to ongoing worries and concerns. For example, being mindful during a conversation with a friend would mean focusing intensely on the conversation instead of thinking about upcoming tasks.

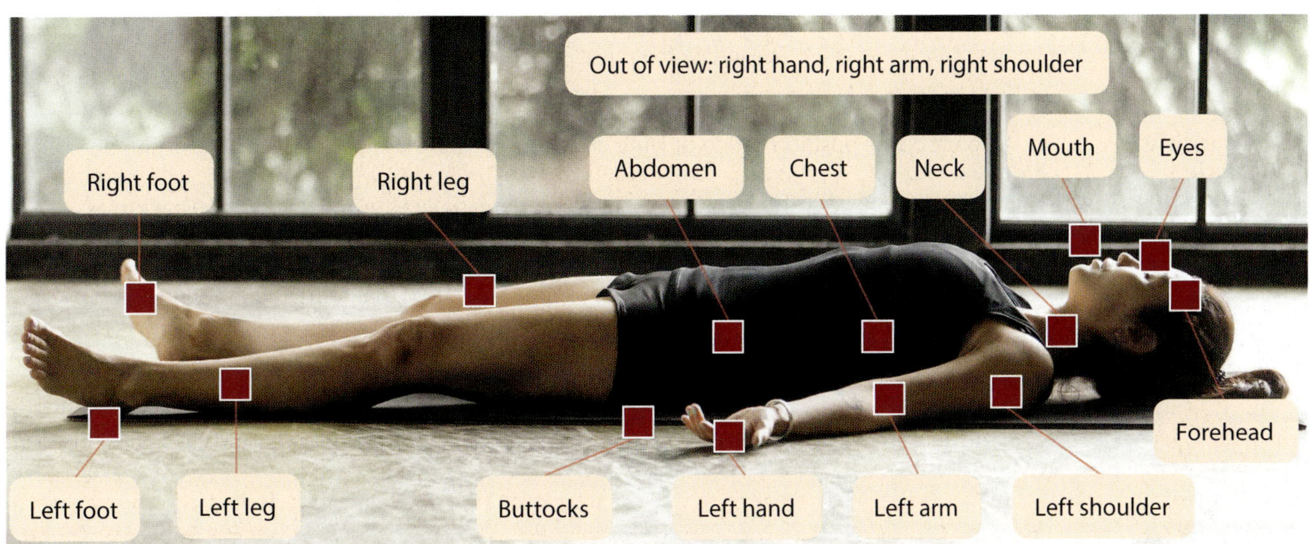

Figure 6.14 Look at the model shown for body parts to tense and relax during progressive muscle relaxation. ***What relaxation technique combined with progressive muscle relaxation increases its effectiveness?***

Skills for Health and Wellness

Trying Relaxation Techniques

Relaxation techniques can help you reduce your body's response to stress. These techniques relieve some of the symptoms of stress and can help you cope better with stressful situations and events. The more you practice these relaxation techniques, the more effective they will be, and different techniques will have varying success with different people. To learn what works for you, try a variety of techniques and notice how they affect your stress level.

Practice Your Skills

Practice Health-Enhancing Behaviors

To try some relaxation techniques, review the steps for the three relaxation techniques that follow. Choose one relaxation technique you want to try and plan to go through the steps. If you want, you can also try all three relaxation techniques.

After practicing at least one relaxation technique, reflect on whether the technique made you feel more relaxed. Share your experience with a partner and create a poster, video, or audio recording of the steps so you can practice this technique whenever you feel stressed.

Technique	Steps
Deep breathing	1. Find a comfortable position sitting or lying down. 2. Place one hand on your stomach. 3. Take a deep breath in through your nose. Count three seconds as you inhale and feel your stomach push out. 4. Breathe out through your nose for three seconds. Feel your stomach move back in and exhale completely. 5. Repeat steps 3 and 4 at least three times. Continue deep breathing as your body and mind relax.
Body scan	1. Find a comfortable position sitting or lying down. Unfold your arms and legs so the body can fully relax. 2. Breathe deeply with your stomach. You should feel your stomach push out and move back in as you breathe. 3. Focus on where your body is in contact with the surface beneath you and keep breathing. 4. Starting at the head, focus on each part of your body. Pay attention to how each body part feels, noticing pain, tightness, relaxation, and tingling sensations. Notice which areas feel tense. Move down your body from the top to the bottom. 5. As you notice areas of tension, move the muscles in those areas to loosen the feeling and relax the body.
Progressive muscle relaxation	1. Find a comfortable position sitting or lying down. Unfold your arms and legs so the body can fully relax. 2. Breathe deeply with your stomach. You should feel your stomach push out and move back in as you breathe. 3. Start with your face. Tense all of the muscles in your face and scalp: make a tight grimace, clench your teeth, squeeze your eyes shut, and move your ears up. Hold that tension and count eight seconds as you inhale. Then exhale and relax all of these muscles completely, feeling the tension fade away. Repeat these steps until your face feels fully relaxed. 4. Repeat this process of fully tensing all of your muscles in a single body part, holding the tension as you count eight seconds, and then releasing all of the tension in that body part. Work your way down the body, moving from your head to your neck and shoulders, abdomen and chest, one arm at a time, buttocks, and one leg at a time.

You can also combine mindfulness with relaxation techniques, such as deep breathing, visualization, guided movements, and focused attention. When these relaxation techniques are combined with mindfulness, they are called **mindfulness-based stress reduction (MBSR)** (**Figure 6.15**).

mindfulness-based stress reduction (MBSR) act of using relaxation techniques, such as deep breathing, visualization, focused attention, and guided movements, while focusing intensely on the present

Take Care of Yourself

During times of stress, many people neglect their physical needs. Not taking care of yourself, however, contributes to more stress. During stressful times, be sure to eat well so you provide your body with the energy and nutrients it needs. Make regular physical activity and adequate sleep a priority. Physical activity reduces heart rate and blood pressure and helps the muscles relax.

Some people who are experiencing stress eat more, use tobacco or alcohol, or abuse medications and drugs to feel better. This approach leads to even more serious difficulties and increases stress. Eating more can lead to weight gain and health conditions. Tobacco products, including vaping devices, contain nicotine, a stimulant that can actually increase anxiety.

Using Mindfulness to Reduce Stress

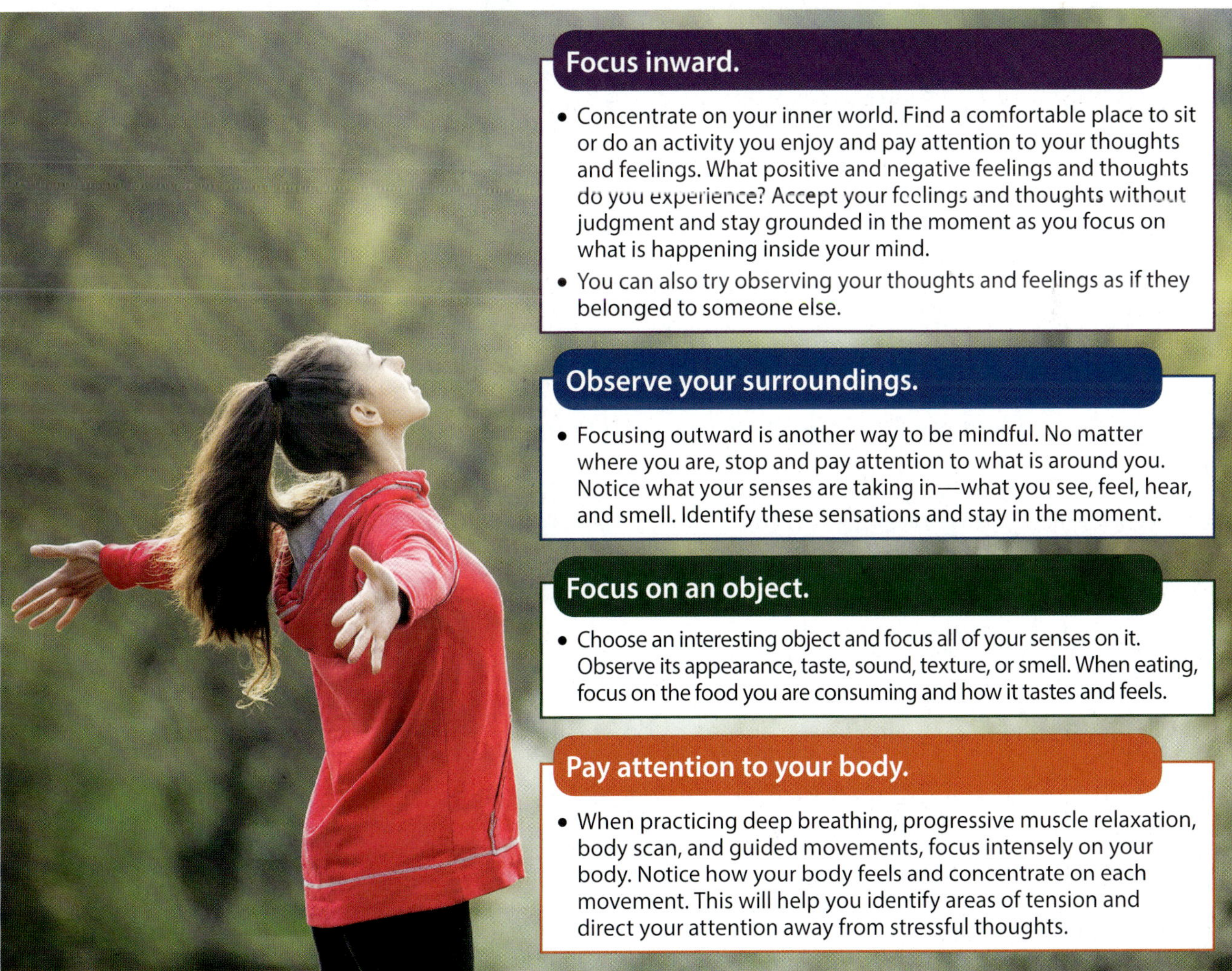

fizkes/Shutterstock.com

Figure 6.15 Mindfulness-based stress reduction strategies are designed to help reduce symptoms of the stress response and develop a feeling of calm.

Health Across the Life Span

The Ups and Downs of Stress

As you go through life, you will find yourself in a variety of stressful situations. How you handle your stress will determine how the situation affects your health. Good stress-management skills reduce the effect of stress, while poor stress-management skills allow stress to continue to impact you in the future. Ride the tracks below by making decisions in response to stressful situations.

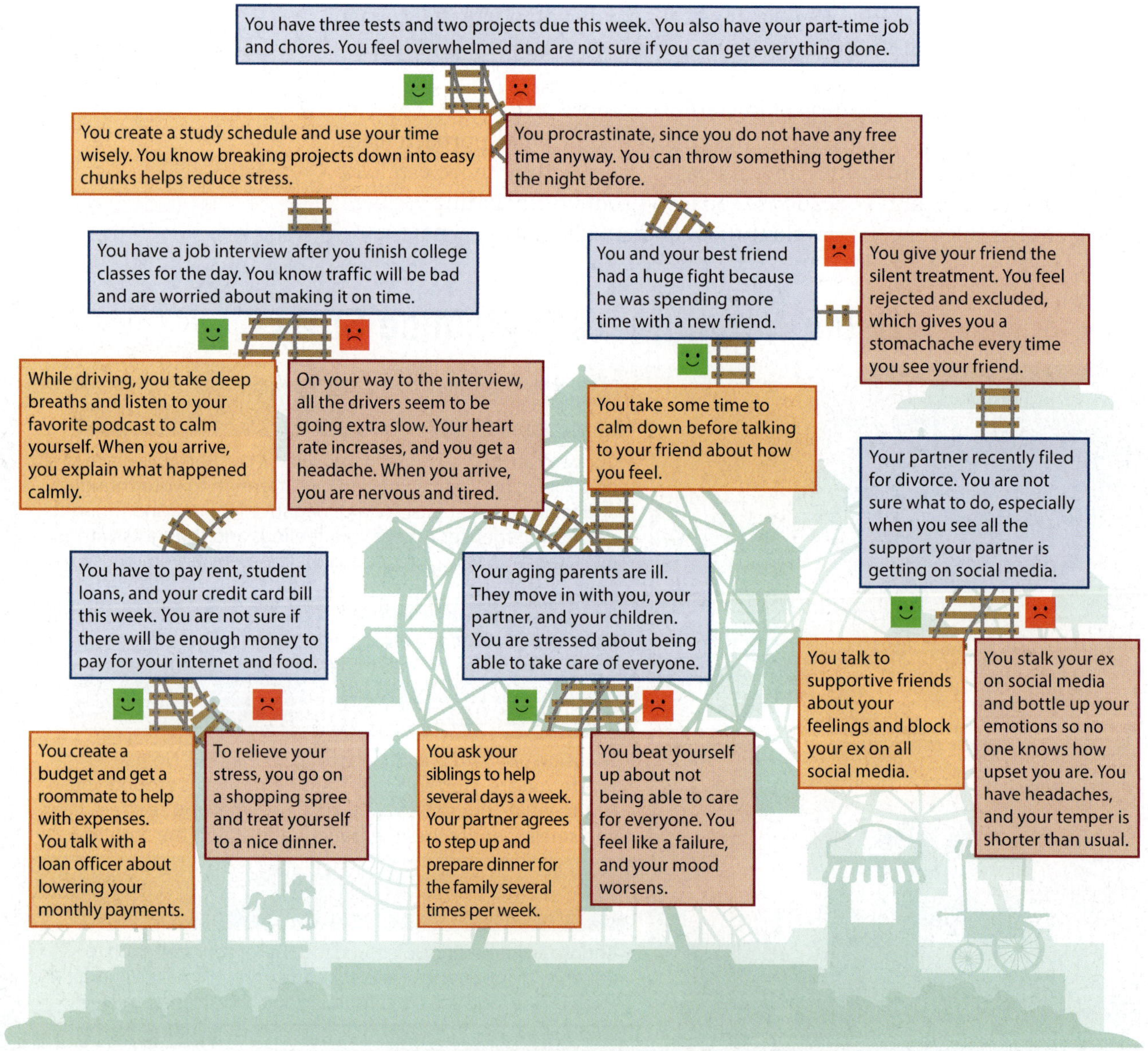

You have three tests and two projects due this week. You also have your part-time job and chores. You feel overwhelmed and are not sure if you can get everything done.

You create a study schedule and use your time wisely. You know breaking projects down into easy chunks helps reduce stress.

You procrastinate, since you do not have any free time anyway. You can throw something together the night before.

You have a job interview after you finish college classes for the day. You know traffic will be bad and are worried about making it on time.

While driving, you take deep breaths and listen to your favorite podcast to calm yourself. When you arrive, you explain what happened calmly.

On your way to the interview, all the drivers seem to be going extra slow. Your heart rate increases, and you get a headache. When you arrive, you are nervous and tired.

You have to pay rent, student loans, and your credit card bill this week. You are not sure if there will be enough money to pay for your internet and food.

You create a budget and get a roommate to help with expenses. You talk with a loan officer about lowering your monthly payments.

To relieve your stress, you go on a shopping spree and treat yourself to a nice dinner.

You and your best friend had a huge fight because he was spending more time with a new friend.

You take some time to calm down before talking to your friend about how you feel.

You give your friend the silent treatment. You feel rejected and excluded, which gives you a stomachache every time you see your friend.

Your aging parents are ill. They move in with you, your partner, and your children. You are stressed about being able to take care of everyone.

You ask your siblings to help several days a week. Your partner agrees to step up and prepare dinner for the family several times per week.

You beat yourself up about not being able to care for everyone. You feel like a failure, and your mood worsens.

Your partner recently filed for divorce. You are not sure what to do, especially when you see all the support your partner is getting on social media.

You talk to supportive friends about your feelings and block your ex on all social media.

You stalk your ex on social media and bottle up your emotions so no one knows how upset you are. You have headaches, and your temper is shorter than usual.

Meter: EgudinKa/Shutterstock.com; Tracks: Shpadaruk Aleksei/Shutterstock.com; Background: Jemastock/Shutterstock.com

Practice Your Skills

Communicate with Others

As you made decisions, did you choose more green paths or red paths? How do you think choosing mostly red paths would affect your health long-term? What effect would choosing green paths have? What would you suggest if you saw a friend making mostly red decisions? Choose one of the scenarios in this activity and imagine you had a friend who was choosing a red path. Create a script in which you talk with your friend and suggest better stress-management strategies. Show effective communication skills in your script.

Seek Professional Help When Needed

Recovery from major stressors, chronic stress, toxic stress, trauma, and burnout can be difficult and take time. People experiencing such stress can become frustrated and discouraged. People who experience stress for more than a couple of weeks should talk to a mental health professional, such as a psychologist, therapist, counselor, or social worker. These professionals are trained to identify mental health conditions and help people cope with the symptoms caused by stress. People can also talk to a doctor, who can identify health conditions associated with stress.

Seeking professional help is especially important if the symptoms of stress last for more than a couple of weeks and interfere with your ability to function in daily life. For example, people experiencing severe stress may have trouble falling asleep at night, concentrating on schoolwork, or enjoying time with friends. They may lose their desire to eat and lose a lot of weight. These are all signs you need to get professional help to manage stress in a healthy way. It is very important to get help for stress-related disorders and burnout so you can feel better. You can talk to an adult you trust for information about mental health professionals in your area.

Lesson 6.3 Review

Know and Understand

1. What are some situations you perceive as stressful that others might not think are stressful?
2. What is the benefit of waiting a while before committing to do an activity?
3. What small blocks of time can you use more effectively to reduce stress?
4. When is distraction a healthy stress-management technique?
5. Which relaxation technique involves imagining yourself in a pleasant environment?
6. What is mindfulness?

Think Critically

7. With a partner, discuss how self-talk affects the stress students at your school experience. How could students change their self-talk to reduce stress?
8. What other relaxation techniques have you heard of, in addition to those discussed in this lesson? Share techniques you have heard in a small group.
9. Why do you think mindfulness helps reduce stress?
10. Write a case study about a teen who needs professional help managing stress. In your case study, include at least three signs the teen needs professional help. Describe how the teen goes about getting help in your community.

REAL WORLD Health Skills

Make Decisions Draw a calendar of the next 30 days, including the month, dates, and any official holidays. Then, for each day, identify one decision you can make to decrease your stress level or manage stress better. Do not repeat any activities. Each day should be different. Display your calendar somewhere in your room and follow through on all the decisions you made. Afterward, evaluate how effective they were and make new decisions, if needed.

Chapter 6

Review and Assessment

Chapter Summary

Stress is the body's physical and psychological reaction to situations perceived as threats. This reaction, called the *fight-or-flight response*, channels energy to your body so you can respond to the threat and overcome the obstacle ahead of you. Often, stress is a good thing (eustress). It can motivate you to take on new challenges and achieve goals. Stress can also negatively influence health (distress) if it is long-lasting or poorly managed. Stress is caused by stressors, which may come from relationships, school, the environment, technology use, and inner conflict. Severe, chronic stressors can lead to toxic stress, which people need professional help to manage.

In the moment, stress prepares the body to respond to a perceived threat. If stress continues over time, it can have many negative health effects. Physically, long-term stress can disrupt memory and cause health conditions such as type 2 diabetes mellitus, immune disorders, ulcers, obesity, depression, and cardiovascular disease. Long-term stress also weakens the immune system. Stress makes it harder to concentrate and reason, which leads to poor decision-making. It can cause negative feelings and mental health conditions and illnesses, including burnout and stress-related disorders such as PTSD. People may behave differently under stress and engage in fewer healthy behaviors, which makes it more difficult for the body to cope.

Managing stress is an essential skill for your health. The first step of managing stress is identifying stressors. Then, you can reduce stress by setting healthy boundaries, managing your time wisely, and viewing stressful situations positively. In stressful situations, you can manage stress by distracting yourself, using humor, and expressing your feelings. You can also use relaxation techniques such as deep breathing and progressive muscle relaxation. Using mindfulness with these techniques is called mindfulness-based stress reduction (MSBR). It is important to seek professional help if you are having trouble managing stress.

Vocabulary Activity

With a partner, review each key term from this chapter and its definition. Then, write a short story, script, or poem about health and wellness in your life using at least 10 of the key terms. Share your short stories, scripts, or poems in class.

body scan	*mindfulness-based stress reduction (MBSR)*	*stress management*
burnout	*nervous system*	*stress*
cardiovascular system	*positive reappraisal*	*stressors*
cognition	*post-traumatic stress disorder (PTSD)*	*stress-related disorder*
digestive system	*progressive muscle relaxation*	*technostress*
distress	*relaxation response*	*time management*
endocrine system	*reproductive system*	*toxic stress*
eustress	*stress hormones*	*trauma*
fight-or-flight response		*visualization*
immune system		

Review and Recall

Review the information in this chapter by answering the following questions.

1. Why is stress sometimes beneficial?
2. What relationship factors can cause stress?
3. What kind of stress comes from the constant presence of technology?
   A. acute stress
   B. toxic stress
   C. technostress
   D. distress
4. Describe the difference between trauma and toxic stress.
5. What body processes slow down during the fight-or-flight response?
6. Why does stress interfere with a person's ability to recall memories?

7. How do high levels of cortisol affect the body short-term and long-term?
8. Why does chronic stress increase a person's risk for mental health conditions and illnesses?
9. Which stress-related disorder develops immediately after a stressful event and lasts a short amount of time?
   A. PTSD
   B. burnout
   C. major depressive disorder
   D. acute stress disorder
10. Which of the following is a common behavioral effect of stress?
    A. not feeling hungry
    B. getting more sleep
    C. having more interest in enjoyable activities
    D. crying less
11. What is the first step in managing stress?
    A. identifying stressors
    B. eliminating stress
    C. reducing stress
    D. using distraction
12. Does procrastination help reduce stress? Explain.
13. Why is it important to express your feelings when you are feeling stressed?
14. Which relaxation technique involves examining your body for any areas of tension?
    A. qigong
    B. visualization
    C. focused attention
    D. body scan

Standardized Test Prep

Math Practice

The following results are from a study of stress among members of generation Z (ages 15–21). This study examined the percentage of generation Z individuals who felt stressed by issues in the US national news. Review the results of this study and then answer the questions that follow.

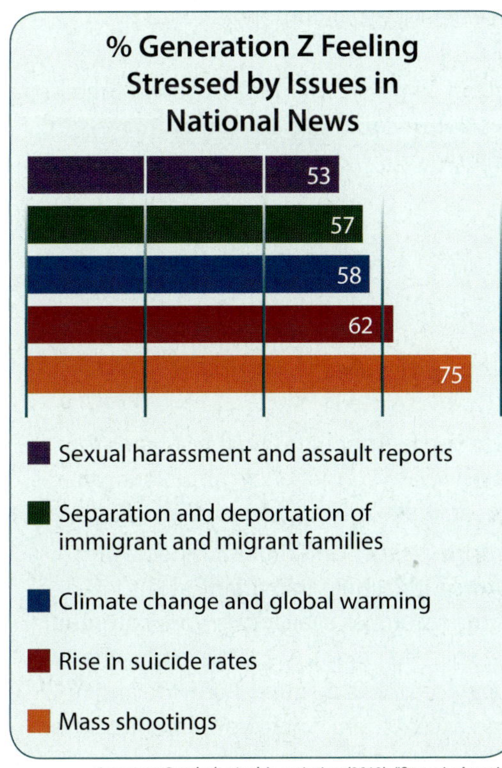

American Psychological Association (2018). "Stress in America: Generation Z." Stress in AmericaTM Survey.

15. Which issue in the national news caused the most stress among generation Z individuals?
    A. sexual assault reports
    B. separation of immigrant families
    C. mass shootings
    D. suicide rates
16. In this study, the percentage of generation Z individuals who said school shootings were a significant source of stress was 3 percent less than the percentage who considered mass shootings a source of stress. What percentage of generation Z individuals considered school shootings a significant source of stress?
17. About seven in 10 millennials have similar feelings about mass and school shootings. What is the percentage difference between millennials and members of generation Z who consider mass shootings a significant source of stress?

Chapter 6 Skills Assessment

Critical Thinking Skills

Answer the following questions to assess your knowledge of what you learned in this chapter.

1. With a partner, discuss when stress can motivate you or help you grow. What determines whether stress is motivating or harmful?
2. What factors in your environment cause stress? In a small group, discuss your environment, including your school environment and community. Identify stressors and discuss their impact on health.
3. Why does the constant presence of technology sometimes cause stress? What do you think teens can do to manage this stress in healthy ways?
4. Give an example of something that causes someone you know stress, but does not cause stress for you. Why is this example a stressor for the person you know? Why do you think it is not for you?
5. Think of the situations that cause you the most stress during a typical week. How helpful is the fight-or-flight response in helping you handle these stressful situations? Explain.
6. Choose one body system and describe a time you experienced the effect of stress on this body system. What did you do to manage these symptoms?
7. What can a person do to make healthy decisions, even under a lot of stress? What steps can a person take to counteract the effect of stress on decision-making?
8. With a partner, write a short story about a teen at your school facing burnout. How does the teen get help for burnout?
9. Why is it hard for people who are under a lot of stress to take care of themselves and engage in healthy behaviors?
10. Ask yourself the questions in Figure 6.9 to identify the stressors in your life. Which stressors cause you the most stress? the least stress? Explain.
11. Review your schedule for the previous month and identify any days or weeks you did not have time to do everything you committed to do. For each time you overcommitted, list a boundary you could have set to protect yourself and reduce stress.
12. On an average day, how much time do you spend browsing social media, playing video games, or watching TV shows or online videos? How does this affect your time management and ability to complete other tasks?
13. Think of a stressful situation you experienced recently. Then, use positive reappraisal to identify positive aspects of the event.
14. Choose one of the relaxation techniques discussed in this lesson and research the exact steps for practicing it. How does this technique help reduce stress? How could you incorporate it into your daily life?
15. Revisit the relaxation technique you researched in question 14. How could you apply mindfulness to this technique?

Health and Wellness Skills

Complete the following activities to assess your skills related to health and wellness.

16. **Analyze Influences.** Tear one piece of paper into 16 squares and arrange the squares in rows of four on your desk. Write the names of four people who mean the most to you on four of the squares. Write your four most important roles, now or in the future, on four more squares. On the next four squares, write your four most treasured material possessions. On the last four squares, write four activities you enjoy. Next, everyone in your class should get up and walk around the room, throwing away one or two squares from other students' desks. Consider which squares are left. How would you feel about losing the squares that were thrown away? Consider how all of your squares affect your ability to manage stress in your life.
17. **Access Information.** Sometimes it is necessary to seek professional help to manage stress levels. Research the resources available in your community to help people manage stress. List exactly what types of services these resources provide and how people can access them. Share your findings with a partner and take notes about the resources your partner found.

18. **Communicate with Others.** Think of a time you had an argument with a friend or family member when you were stressed out and did not use effective communication skills. Create a storyboard illustrating the verbal and nonverbal communication in the argument. How did the outcome of the argument affect your stress? Now, recreate the storyboard showing how you and the other person could have used effective communication skills. Write a few paragraphs analyzing how effective communication strategies could have positively impacted the conversation, your relationship with the other person, and your level of stress. What steps can you take to communicate effectively, even when you are feeling stressed?
19. **Make Decisions.** Chris is a junior in high school and is trying to get accepted into a competitive college next year. Math has always been hard for Chris, and his math grade is at an all-time low. Every weekend is crucial study time to help Chris earn his desired grades. His club is having a big retreat this weekend, and all of his friends are going. Chris has not spent any time with his friends lately because of his stressful academic situation. Using the decision-making process, help Chris make a decision about the trip.
20. **Set Goals.** Lucia has been increasingly disorganized. She has missed a few deadlines and even missed the first day of tryouts for volleyball. She realizes that, if she gets more organized, her stress levels will be more manageable. Create a SMART goal related to time management and organization for Lucia. What steps can she take to put this goal into action and overcome any obstacles?
21. **Practice Health-Enhancing Behaviors.** In a small group, discuss your dream car. How much time and money would you spend taking care of it? Now, consider: How does the amount you would be willing to spend taking care of your car compare to the amount you would spend managing your health and stress levels? Write a short paragraph describing what you could be doing to manage your stress and care for yourself.
22. **Advocate for Health.** Taylor has gone to the school counselor to discuss his increased anxiety. While working with the school counselor, he learns his peers are also coming to the counseling center in record numbers due to stress-related symptoms. Taylor wants to advocate on behalf of all of the students who may have anxiety, but are not coming forward due to fear of judgment. Create a poster advocating the services provided in the counselor's office to the whole student body.

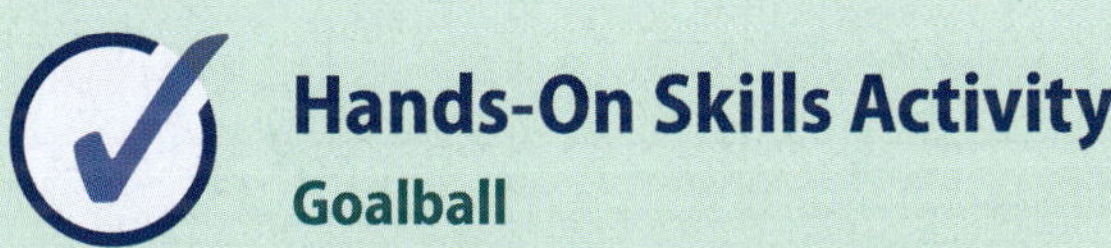

Hands-On Skills Activity

Goalball

Explaining the stressful situations in your life to someone you trust is a good stress-management strategy. Sometimes, a second opinion can help you look at a situation differently or manage stress better. This activity will give you a chance to confide in your classmates and get their feedback on some stressful situations.

Steps for This Activity

1. Write your name on a blank sheet of paper and then describe a task you need to complete by the end of the month. The task could be a set of chores, a homework assignment, or an extracurricular activity. The task should be something that causes you some amount of stress.
2. Crumple up the piece of paper and throw it across the room.
3. **Set Goals.** Walk around the room and retrieve a random piece of paper. Read the task and create a smaller, more manageable goal the person can use to get closer to the large goal. Make sure the goal you write is *SMART* (specific, measurable, achievable, relevant, and timely) and is something the person could accomplish this week.
4. Repeat the second and third steps two to four more times and write a different, smaller goal than the person before you.
5. Return the sheet of paper to the person whose name is written at the top.
6. When you get your paper back, consider the goals your classmates created for you. Then write a short paragraph reflecting on how the smaller goals alter your perception of the larger task, if at all. Why do you think setting small goals is helpful for managing stress?

Chapter 7

Understanding Mental Illnesses

Look for the skills icon throughout this chapter for opportunities to practice your health skills.

Check Your Health and Wellness Skills

In this chapter, you will learn skills for recognizing and getting help for mental health conditions. To understand the skills you currently use, take the following inventory of your behaviors. Indicate how well you think you use each skill. Use a scale of 1–5, *1* meaning you do not use the skill and *5* meaning you feel completely comfortable using it.

Skill	How Well Do You Use Each Skill?
I pay attention to how I'm feeling so I'll know if I need help.	
I know how to access mental health resources.	
I can tell the difference between mental health myths or stereotypes and facts.	
I tell my friends if I'm worried about their mental health and offer to assist them in finding help.	
I know whom I'd talk to if one of my friends talked about hurting someone else.	
I intervene if I see someone being bullied or harassed.	
I know and could recognize the warning signs of suicide.	
If people talk about suicide, I take them seriously.	
I feel comfortable asking my friends about their feelings and expressing concern.	
I know how to get help if I have thoughts of harming myself.	
I listen to and support people who have experienced loss.	
	Total:

Add up your responses to each statement. The higher your score, the more comfortable you feel practicing health skills related to recognizing and getting help for mental health conditions. Which skill do you think is most important for you? Which skill is the most challenging for you? Which skill would you most like to improve? In this chapter, you will learn how to perform these skills better and more often.

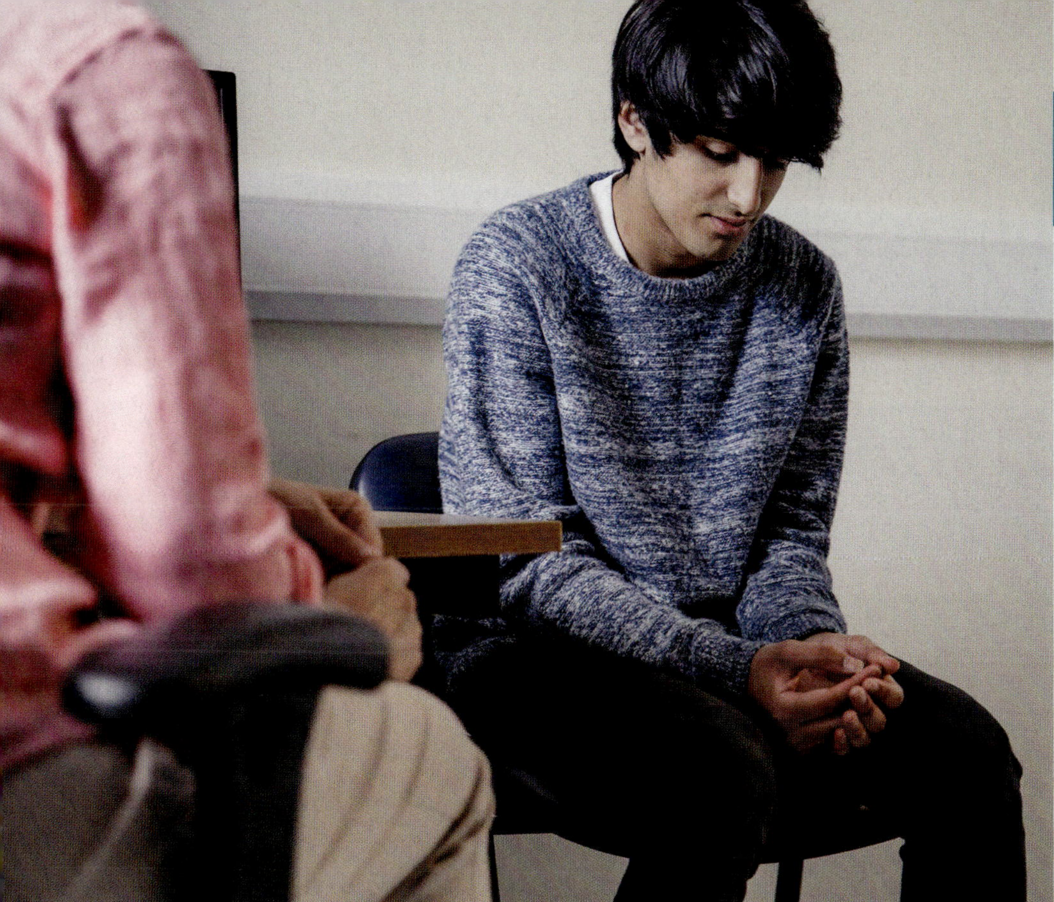

SolStock/E+/Getty Images

Reading and Notetaking

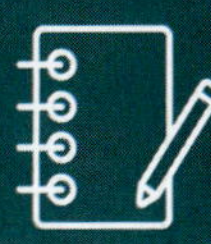

Imagine a friend posted on social media about considering self-harm and suicide. When you commented, your friend said it was just a joke. Before reading this chapter, write a script or short story explaining what you would do in this situation, using language that indicates you take the situation seriously. Trade with a partner and then read the chapter. After reading, mark any errors, such as those related to pronoun agreement, verb tense, subject-verb agreement, or possessives. Also mark any suggestions for handling the situation differently. Trade back with your partner and discuss the changes.

Rashaud Ashur/Shutterstock.com

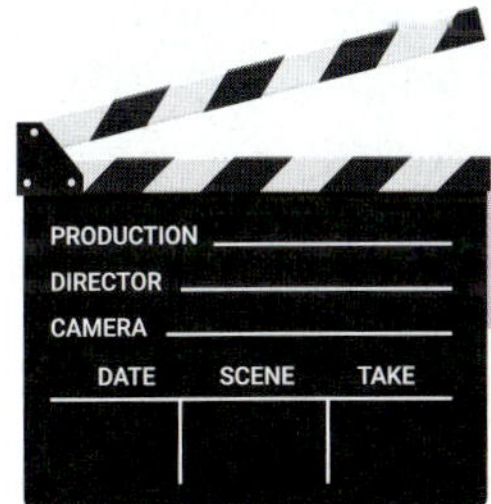

Setting the Scene

Doing the Right Thing for a Friend

Trying to keep up with all of your classes, extracurricular activities, and a part-time job is keeping you busy this year. Still, you are making sure to spend time with your friends. Most weekends, you find at least some time to hang out and catch up. Lately, though, one of your friends has been worrying you.

Before you started your part-time job, your friend used to call you whenever they were sad, and you would sometimes talk or play video games late into the night. Ever since you started your job, you have not had as much time. Now, your friend sometimes does not respond at all when you are trying to make plans. Your friend has also been posting some pretty depressing things on social media. In a recent post, your friend said the world would be better off without them in it. You care about your friend and are getting concerned, but do not know what to do.

Thinking Critically

1. What are some factors that might lead a high school student to act like your friend in this scenario?
2. What should you do? What steps could you take to help your friend?

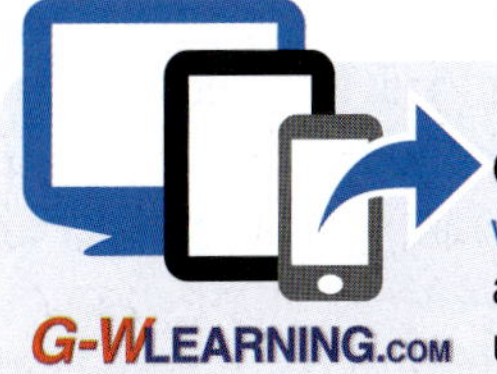

Click on the activity icon or visit www.g-wlearning.com/health/4095 to access online vocabulary activities using key terms from the chapter.

Lesson 7.1

What Are Mental Illnesses?

Essential Question?

What are the symptoms of different types of mental illnesses?

Learning Outcomes

After studying this lesson, you will be able to

- define *mental illness*;
- analyze individual and environmental factors that influence whether a person develops a mental illness;
- explain how anxiety disorders are different from normal anxiety;
- differentiate between attention-deficit hyperactivity disorder (ADHD), executive function disorders (EFDs), and obsessive-compulsive disorder (OCD);
- assess the impact of different types of mood disorders;
- identify types of personality and behavioral disorders;
- list the symptoms of schizophrenia spectrum disorders; and
- explain how substance-related and addictive disorders develop.

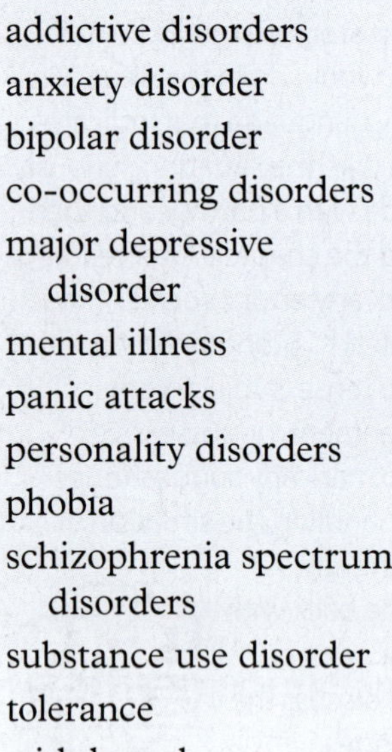

Key Terms

addictive disorders
anxiety disorder
bipolar disorder
co-occurring disorders
major depressive disorder
mental illness
panic attacks
personality disorders
phobia
schizophrenia spectrum disorders
substance use disorder
tolerance
withdrawal

Warm-Up Activity

The Impact of Mental Illness

Analyze Influences Mental illnesses impair people's ability to function in daily life. Before reading this lesson, make a list of what you do every day. This list should include what you need to do as well as what you choose to do for fun. Next to each item on your list, write your answer to this question: *How would being unable to do this affect my physical, mental and emotional, and social health?*

What I do every day	How would being unable to do this affect my physical, mental and emotional, and social health?

Are you surprised to learn that many successful people have mental illnesses? Mental illnesses are surprisingly common. They are also treatable. Many people affected by mental illnesses have active, productive, and fulfilling lives.

Almost everyone experiences feelings of anxiety, sadness, and fear. When these thoughts and feelings decrease mental and emotional health, they are called *mental health conditions*. As you learned in Chapter 4, short-term feelings and thoughts that interfere with a person's ability to perform daily tasks are called *mental distress*. A **mental illness**, also called a *mental disorder*, occurs when mental health conditions do not go away and become so severe that people cannot function in daily life. For example, a phobia of public places could lead a person to avoid going to school or

mental illness health condition in which negative or unhelpful feelings or thoughts become so severe they interfere with daily life

work or visiting family and friends. In this lesson, you will learn about factors that contribute to the development of a mental illness. You will also learn about common types of mental illnesses.

Factors Affecting Mental Illness

Many factors influence whether someone develops a mental illness. As you learned in Chapter 4, genetic makeup plays a large part in a person's mental health. Having a family history of a mental illness increases the risk for that condition, and genes influence levels of chemicals in the brain that control mood and feelings. Fortunately, having a genetic predisposition to a particular mental illness does not mean that a person will develop that condition.

Life experiences and situations play a large role in the development of mental illnesses. For example, people who experience a serious brain injury are at greater risk of developing some mental illnesses, including major depressive disorder, anxiety disorders, and substance use disorders. Sometimes, events that occur even before birth affect the risk of mental illness. Alcohol or drug use, poor nutrition, and trauma or complications during pregnancy increase a baby's risk of developing a mental illness later in life.

Some experts believe that traumatic life events and stressors can trigger the development of mental illnesses in people who are genetically predisposed.

Research in Action

Mental Illnesses: Biology and Psychology

Views about what causes mental illness have changed considerably over the years. The earliest theories attributed mental illness to supernatural forces. More recent theories emphasized the role of early childhood experiences and environmental factors. Today, most scientists believe mental illness is caused by a combination of biological, psychological, and environmental factors.

In one recent study, researchers at the University of California, Los Angeles, examined the brains of 700 people who had known mental illnesses following death. They examined whether these people's brains showed particular patterns of gene activity. The results of this study provide strong evidence that people with particular mental illnesses show some similar patterns of gene activity. Specifically, people with schizophrenia spectrum disorder, bipolar disorder, and major depressive disorder show similar patterns of gene activity. People with other health conditions, such as inflammatory bowel disease, do not show this same pattern. This study provides some evidence that genetics play a large role in mental illness.

Although biological factors such as genetics clearly influence at least some types of mental illnesses, other factors also play a role. These factors include a person's environment, experiences, and patterns of thinking.

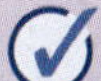

Practice Your Skills

Comprehend Concepts

With a partner, discuss the different factors that could influence the development of a mental illness. Examine how biological, environmental, and psychological factors may all contribute to mental illness. Do these factors have a different impact on different types of mental illness? What questions should future research studies examine to help explain the development of mental illness? How does knowing these different factors help in the prevention or treatment of mental illness?

Social Media and Mental Illness

Certain activities help prevent mental health conditions:
- sleeping
- getting physical activity
- forming and maintaining relationships

Social media use limits time spent doing these activities.

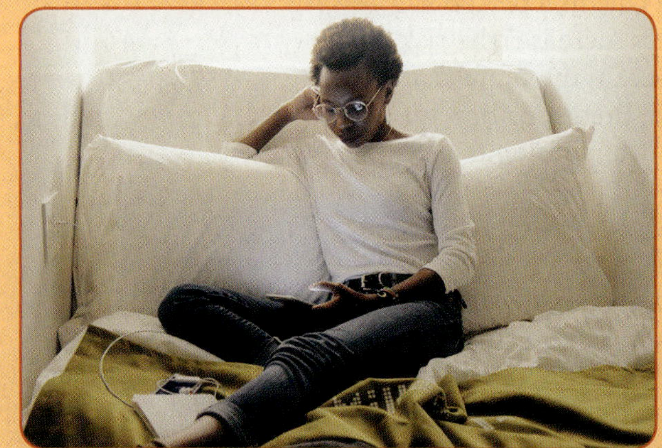

Perhaps as a result, people who spend more time on social media experience more
- anxiety
- depression
- isolation
- loneliness
- disordered eating

Yue_/E+/Getty Images

Figure 7.1 Social media users may experience more symptoms of mental illness because social media encourages them to compare themselves to other people. Since social media presents unrealistic, edited versions of people's lives, users may feel dissatisfied with their own lives.

In fact, social media is one stressor linked with symptoms of mental illness (**Figure 7.1**).

As you know, your own patterns of thinking and views of the world also affect your risk for mental illnesses. Thinking about yourself negatively and not challenging cognitive distortions like black-and-white thinking and catastrophizing can increase your risk for developing a mental illness.

Types of Mental Illnesses

Mental illnesses affect mental and emotional health, including how people process and interpret information, think, feel, and express emotions. All of these factors influence behavior and daily functioning. You already learned about stress-related disorders in Chapter 6. Eating disorders are a type of mental illness you will learn about in Chapter 9.

Anxiety Disorders

Anxiety is a feeling of nervousness and worry about unknown or future situations. Almost everyone experiences anxiety sometimes. You may feel anxious before the first day of school, for example, or after telling a friend or family member about an issue in your life (**Figure 7.2**).

Figure 7.2 When you feel anxious, you may experience different physical responses in your body.

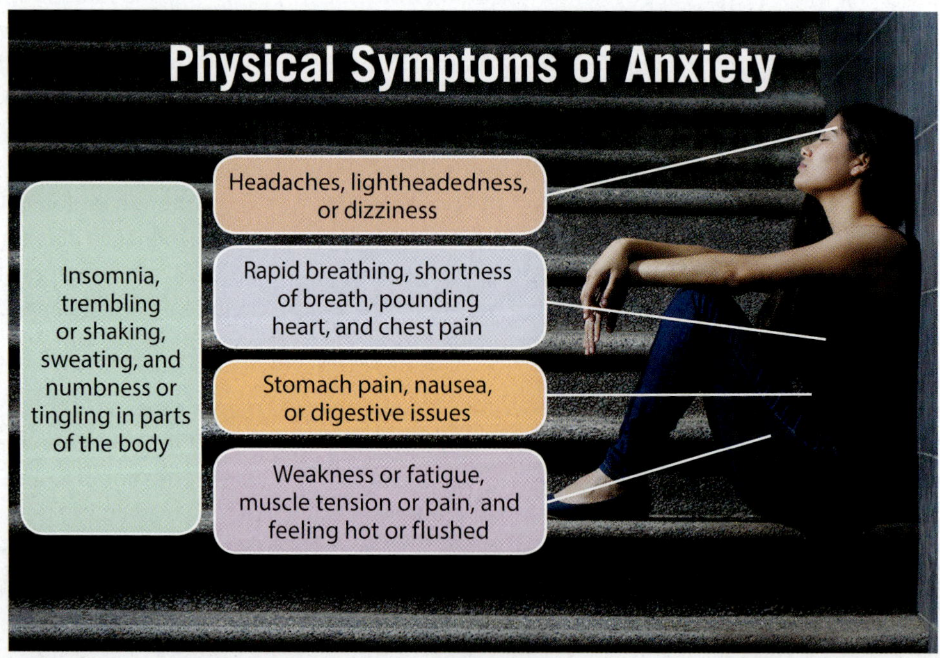

aldomurillo/E+/Getty Images

An **anxiety disorder** is a mental illness characterized by extreme fear or dread that disrupts a person's way of life. In an anxiety disorder, anxiety is unrealistic or exaggerated. A person with an anxiety disorder may worry intensely and consistently about daily life events, experiences, or objects, such as getting through the day or being in a small room. For people with an anxiety disorder, anxiety does not go away on its own and makes it hard to go to school, maintain relationships, and pursue goals.

anxiety disorder mental illness in which feelings of worry and dread interfere with daily life

Anxiety disorders are the most common mental illnesses in the United States. Different types of anxiety disorders include generalized anxiety disorder (GAD), social anxiety disorder, panic disorder, and phobias.

Generalized Anxiety Disorder (GAD)

People with *generalized anxiety disorder (GAD)* feel extreme and constant anxiety about parts of their lives they cannot control. They may feel anxious about school or work, and anxiety persists almost every day for at least six months. People with GAD often experience anxiety in the form of physical symptoms, such as fatigue, muscle tension, and difficulty sleeping. They may also consistently feel on edge, have difficulty concentrating, and feel irritable. Constant, intense anxiety makes it difficult for people with GAD to carry out daily tasks.

Social Anxiety Disorder

People with *social anxiety disorder* feel intensely anxious about social situations in which others might judge them. Situations that may cause anxiety include meeting new people, eating or drinking in public, and performing in front of others. In these situations, a person with social anxiety disorder may worry about being embarrassed or rejected. As a result, people with social anxiety disorder often avoid social situations to the point that it interferes with everyday life.

Some people have a related mental health condition known as *social media anxiety disorder*. People with this disorder feel extremely anxious if they cannot check their social media accounts for a period of time (**Figure 7.3**).

Symptoms of Social Media Anxiety Disorder

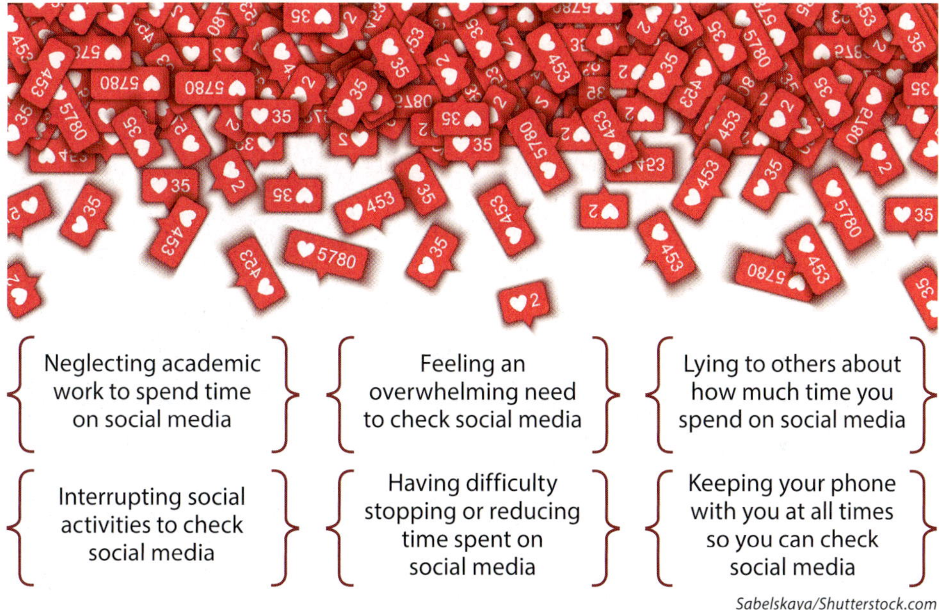

Sabelskaya/Shutterstock.com

Figure 7.3 Social media anxiety disorder may disrupt people's ability to form or maintain healthy relationships and excel academically.

panic attacks episodes of intense fear characterized by fast heartbeat, dizziness, shaking, trouble breathing, and chest pain

Panic Disorder

People with *panic disorder* experience recurring **panic attacks**, or episodes of intense fear. These episodes occur for no rational reason and can be unexpected or develop after exposure to a *trigger* (feared object or situation). They can happen anywhere or anytime without warning. Panic attacks include physical symptoms, such as a fast heartbeat, dizziness, shaking, trouble breathing, and chest pain. During a panic attack, people feel out of control and may have a sense of impending doom.

People who have panic attacks often fear having another attack. They may avoid situations or places they have experienced panic attacks before. Some become so fearful of having another attack they will not leave their own homes.

phobia extreme, unrealistic fear of an object or situation

Phobias

A **phobia** is a strong, unrealistic fear of an object or situation that does not really pose much, if any, danger (**Figure 7.4**). People with phobias take active steps to avoid objects or situations they fear. This can interfere with daily life. For example, a person with a phobia of crowded spaces may avoid public transportation or standing in line at a store. This can prevent the person from getting to appointments or purchasing food. If people with a phobia have to face their fear, they may experience shortness of breath, a fast heartbeat, panic, and a desire to flee.

Attention-Deficit Hyperactivity Disorder (ADHD)

Attention-deficit hyperactivity disorder (ADHD) is a mental illness characterized by difficulty paying attention, *hyperactivity* (overly active behavior), and impulsiveness. People with ADHD consistently experience symptoms such as

- difficulty focusing or sitting still;
- boredom with tasks and activities;
- difficulty organizing and completing a task;
- forgetfulness and losing items;
- difficulty listening to and following instructions;
- nonstop talking or constant motion;
- difficulty waiting; and
- tendency to blurt out inappropriate comments without considering the impact on others.

Different Phobias

Arachnophobia	Acrophobia	Agoraphobia	Astraphobia
• Fear of spiders	• Fear of heights	• Fear of open or crowded spaces	• Fear of thunder or lightning
Claustrophobia	**Cynophobia**	**Ophidiophobia**	**Trypanophobia**
• Fear of small spaces	• Fear of dogs	• Fear of snakes	• Fear of needles

Den Rozhnovsky/Shutterstock.com

Figure 7.4 There are many different kinds of phobias. What they all have in common is that the object or situation does not pose much, if any, danger to the person. ***What is the term for an episode of intense fear?***

Factors such as biological sex influence the symptoms a person with ADHD has. Males with ADHD typically show frequent movement, impulsivity, and physical aggression. Females with ADHD are more likely to show inattentiveness, daydreaming, low self-esteem, and verbal aggression.

For people with ADHD, these symptoms disrupt daily life for at least six months and make it difficult to complete everyday tasks like listening in class, completing homework, or talking with friends. ADHD usually develops during childhood and can continue through adulthood. It can cause difficulty at home, poor performance at school, and strained relationships.

Many of the symptoms of ADHD are also seen in people with *executive function disorders (EFDs)*. People with EFDs show a pattern of chronic difficulty performing daily tasks. This includes struggling to analyze, plan, organize, schedule, and complete tasks in a timely way. People with EFDs have difficulty working toward long-term goals and the steps needed to meet these goals. They have difficulty planning for future events and tend to focus only on the immediate future.

Obsessive-Compulsive Disorder (OCD)

People with *obsessive-compulsive disorder (OCD)* have recurring and uncontrollable thoughts, feelings, and behaviors that make daily functioning difficult. Uncontrollable thoughts are called *obsessions* and often cause anxiety. An example of an obsession is order and symmetry. People with OCD often try to make obsessions go away by engaging in *compulsions*, or repeated actions (**Figure 7.5**). In response to obsessive thoughts about objects being in perfect order, a person with OCD may repeatedly order objects in a specific way.

Obsessions and Compulsions

Obsessions	Compulsions
Order and symmetry	Washing hands or other cleaning rituals
Bad consequences to actions or inactions	Arranging and rearranging items
Contamination and germs	Checking switches or locks
Safety of loved ones	Counting or repeating specific words
	Not throwing anything away

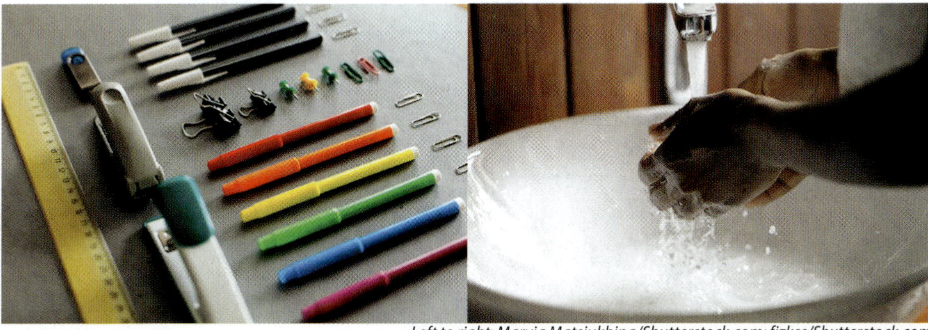

Left to right: Maryia Matsiukhina/Shutterstock.com; fizkes/Shutterstock.com

Figure 7.5 Obsessions are separate from normal, daily events and concerns. Compulsions attempt to eliminate obsessions, but do not succeed.

People with OCD generally cannot control their compulsions and do not get any pleasure or satisfaction from compulsive behaviors. Obsessive thoughts and compulsive behaviors make it difficult for people with OCD to perform tasks and interact with others.

Mood Disorders

A *mood disorder* is a mental illness that causes serious changes in how people feel. Some mood disorders make people feel consistently sad or lose interest in life. Others cause alternating, extreme feelings of intense happiness or sadness. Common mood disorders in the US include major depressive disorder, seasonal affective disorder (SAD), and bipolar disorder.

Major Depressive Disorder

Everyone feels sad sometimes. Feelings like disappointment, boredom, and unhappiness are normal and can help people understand what situations and activities make them happy or upset. These feelings are especially normal during or after stressful situations and difficult life events. For example, grief over the loss of a loved one can cause unpleasant feelings as a person mourns. Often, these feelings of sadness improve and go away over time.

Sometimes, however, negative feelings interfere with a person's life and do not go away, even with time. People who experience ongoing, intense feelings of sadness, worthlessness, and hopelessness have **major depressive disorder**, or *clinical depression*, which is a mental illness (**Figure 7.6**).

major depressive disorder mood disorder characterized by feelings of intense sadness, worthlessness, and hopelessness

Untreated, major depressive disorder can have serious consequences. It disrupts a person's ability to engage in daily life tasks, like maintaining relationships, showering, and going to school. People who have major depressive disorder are more likely to engage in behaviors that are harmful to their health. They also have a greater risk of developing other health conditions. As with other mental illnesses, people who have major depressive disorder need professional treatment with a mental health specialist to manage their condition and feel better.

Seasonal Affective Disorder (SAD)

Seasonal affective disorder (SAD) is a mental illness that causes symptoms similar to those of major depressive disorder. People with SAD

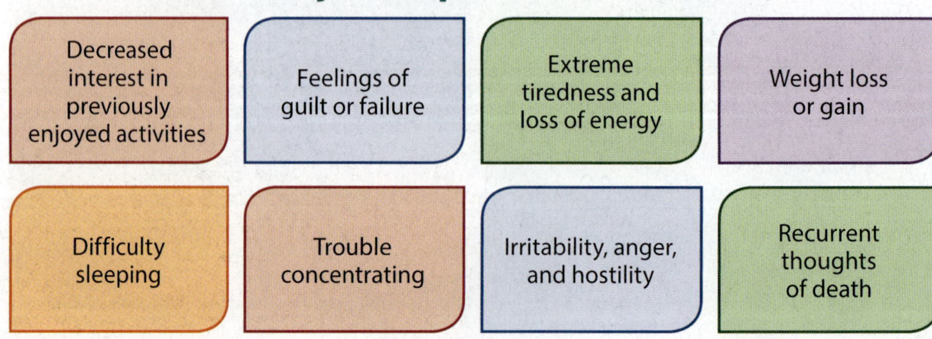

Figure 7.6 People with major depressive disorder experience changes in their patterns of thinking and behavior. ***What is another term for major depressive disorder?***

face depressive symptoms—such as feelings of worthlessness, extreme tiredness, loss of interest, and irritability—in the winter months when there is less natural sunlight. These symptoms are severe enough they make it difficult for a person with SAD to function.

Because depressive symptoms develop during the winter months, they usually go away in the spring and summer. Still, people with SAD often need professional treatment to cope with depressive symptoms. Some people who have SAD may also benefit from light therapy.

Bipolar Disorder

People who have **bipolar disorder** experience intense depressive symptoms that alternate with manic (extremely happy) moods. During periods of depression, people with bipolar disorder experience some of the symptoms of major depressive disorder, including feelings of worthlessness and lack of energy. Symptoms of a manic episode include poor judgment, little need for sleep, hyperactive behavior, and a lack of self-control. This can lead to binge drinking, binge eating, or out-of-control spending. The different episodes of bipolar disorder may last weeks or months. To manage the symptoms of these episodes, people with bipolar disorder need professional treatment.

bipolar disorder mood disorder characterized by extreme highs (mania) and lows (depression)

Personality and Behavioral Disorders

Personality disorders are a category of mental illnesses characterized by consistent patterns of inappropriate behavior. There are many types of personality disorders, and the symptoms of personality disorders interfere with a person's ability to carry out daily life tasks and maintain relationships. **Figure 7.7** outlines some common personality disorders.

personality disorders mental illnesses characterized by consistent patterns of inappropriate behavior

Common Personality Disorders

Antisocial Personality Disorder

- People with this disorder show a disregard for social rules, a tendency for impulsive or aggressive behavior, and indifference to other people's rights and feelings.

Borderline Personality Disorder

- People with this disorder show instability in their self-concept and relationships. They may get very angry at someone for canceling plans because they fear abandonment. They may show extreme shifts in attitudes about people.

Narcissistic Personality Disorder

- People with this disorder have an exaggerated sense of their own importance. They have a deep need for excessive attention and admiration, show a lack of empathy, and experience difficulty in relationships. They appear to have great confidence, but actually have low self-esteem and overreact to criticism.

Obsessive-Compulsive Personality Disorder

- People with this disorder have an unhealthy focus on control, perfection, and order.

Paranoid Personality Disorder

- People with this disorder show extreme *paranoia*, or a deep mistrust and suspicion of others without any reason.

Schizoid Personality Disorder

- People with this disorder avoid social activities and consistently shy away from interactions with others. They often show a limited range of emotional expression.

Figure 7.7 There are many types of personality disorders, but all are characterized by patterns of inappropriate behavior. ***What personality disorder is characterized by an unstable self-concept?***

Most personality disorders are diagnosed in older teens and adults and may be associated with childhood trauma. When children and younger teens show consistent patterns of inappropriate behavior, they are more likely to be diagnosed with a behavioral disorder such as oppositional defiant disorder or conduct disorder.

Oppositional defiant disorder (ODD) is a mental illness usually diagnosed in children. Children with ODD show behaviors that are uncooperative, defiant, and hostile to other people. Symptoms of ODD can include frequent temper tantrums, refusal to obey authority figures, and questioning and arguing. Children with ODD may be easily annoyed by others, speak harshly, and show lots of anger. These behaviors are most common when the child is hungry, tired, or upset.

Conduct disorder is a mental illness that can grow into antisocial personality disorder in adulthood. People with conduct disorder show hostile and sometimes violent behavior toward other people. They disregard other people's feelings and may engage in cruel behavior such as pushing, hitting, or biting others; hurting animals; and picking fights. People with conduct disorder are also more likely to engage in theft, vandalism, or arson.

Schizophrenia Spectrum Disorders

schizophrenia spectrum disorders mental illnesses characterized by irregular thoughts, delusions, and hallucinations

People who have **schizophrenia spectrum disorders** typically experience symptoms such as irregular thoughts, *delusions* (false beliefs or perceptions), and hallucinations. During hallucinations, people with schizophrenia spectrum disorders may hear voices or see objects that are not there. People with schizophrenia spectrum disorders may also experience paranoia and believe that others are threatening or plotting against them. They may show inappropriate emotional reactions, such as laughing when they hear someone has died; appear agitated; talk to themselves; and have difficulty managing personal hygiene tasks.

All of these symptoms help explain why an estimated 20 percent of people who are homeless may have a schizophrenia spectrum disorder. Treatment for schizophrenia spectrum disorders often includes therapy and medications to reduce symptoms.

Substance Use and Addictive Disorders

co-occurring disorders two conditions that affect health at the same time; for example, substance use disorders and other mental illnesses

Substance use and addictive disorders involve people's recurrent use of substances and repetition of behaviors that lead to health issues and an inability to meet responsibilities. Examples of *substances* include nicotine, alcohol, and drugs. *Addictive behaviors* include actions like gambling and internet gaming. Substance use and addictive disorders sometimes occur together with other mental illnesses, such as major depressive disorder and anxiety disorders. This is called **co-occurring disorders**.

Substance Use Disorders

substance use disorder mental illness in which a person continues using a substance despite negative effects on health and life

Substances like nicotine, alcohol, and drugs cause changes in the brain and body that negatively impact a person's health. A **substance use disorder** occurs when a person continues using a substance, regardless of its negative effects on the body and areas of a person's life (**Figure 7.8**). People with substance use disorders often feel

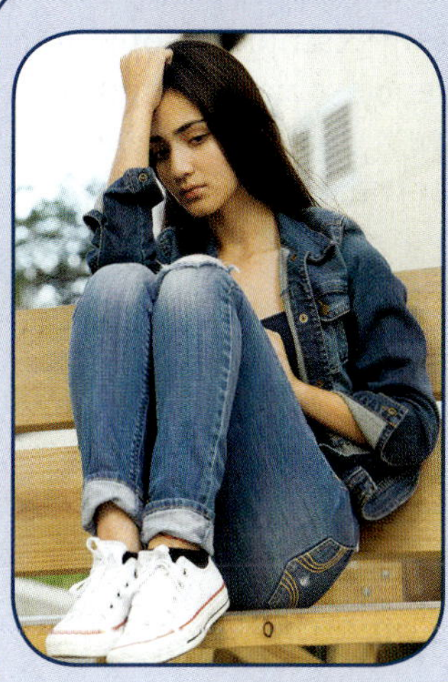

Consequences of Substance Use

- Risky behaviors related to the substance (like using nonsterilized needles)
- Physical health consequences related to the substance
- Injury while intoxicated (motor vehicle accidents and violence)
- Overdose, which becomes more likely with increased tolerance
- Spikes in blood pressure and heart rate, increasing risk of stroke, heart attack, and death
- Loss of hygiene
- Loss of routine, including nutrition, sleep, physical activity, and schoolwork
- Financial instability due to spending money obtaining the substance
- Homelessness, which reduces safety and resources
- Anxiety, depression, loneliness, and suicidal thoughts
- Alterations in the way a person thinks
- Overlooking obligations to or other conflict with family and friends
- Legal consequences of obtaining or using the substance

Juanmonino/iStock/Getty Images Plus/Getty Images

Figure 7.8 If a person continues to use a substance after experiencing consequences like these, it is a sign of a substance use disorder. ***What is it called when a substance use disorder occurs together with another mental illness?***

like they cannot stop using a substance, even if they want to. Several stages of substance use lead to the development of a substance use disorder:

1. **Experimentation:** Initially, people often use a substance "just to try it." Most substances that lead to a substance use disorder cause pleasant feelings, such as happiness and relaxation. These feelings cause a person to want to use more of the substance.
2. **Regular use:** After initially trying a substance, people may continue using the substance and gradually increase the amount they use. For example, over time, people who smoke only a few cigarettes at first may slowly increase how much they smoke in a week. This can lead to a regular pattern of using a substance, as the pleasant feelings associated with the substance reinforce behavior.
3. **Tolerance:** As a person regularly uses a substance, the body develops a tolerance for that substance. **Tolerance** describes an increase in how much of a substance the body needs to experience certain effects. As tolerance develops, people need greater and greater amounts of a substance to achieve the pleasant feelings they once experienced with smaller amounts. As people pursue the pleasant feelings associated with the substance, they consume more and more of it.
4. **Dependence:** If people continue consuming a substance, the body starts to become dependent on the substance's effects. Dependence can be physical and psychological. *Physical dependence* occurs when the body adjusts to a substance and requires it to function normally. For example, because opioids trigger the brain to overproduce chemicals that cause feelings of happiness, the brain begins to produce less of these chemicals on its own. This means the body requires opioids or other substances to reach normal levels of these chemicals. Not using opioids will then lead to **withdrawal**, or negative symptoms associated with no longer using the substance. *Psychological dependence* refers to the cravings and anxiety a person feels when not using or trying to quit the substance. For example, a person who regularly vapes may feel anxious and irritable if a vape pen is not available the next time a craving occurs.

tolerance body's need for an increased amount of a substance to experience the effects once felt with smaller amounts

withdrawal negative symptoms that develop when a person with a physical dependence stops using a substance

5. **Addiction:** Addiction develops when a person continues using a substance despite negative effects on health. For example, people may continue drinking alcohol, even if they experience social isolation. People may keep using drugs, even if they have to turn to dangerous behaviors to afford them. At this point, a person has developed a substance use disorder.

Substance use disorders are serious mental illnesses, and people need professional treatment to overcome them. You will learn more about substance use disorders in Unit 4: *Avoiding Hazardous Substances*.

Addictive Disorders

addictive disorders mental illnesses in which people develop a psychological dependence on certain processes or behaviors

Addictive disorders are mental illnesses in which people become psychologically dependent on a process or behavior. One example is *gambling disorder*, a mental illness in which a person gambles compulsively, despite serious negative effects on health and personal life. Another example is *internet gaming disorder*, in which people participate in online gaming to the exclusion of other activities and experience negative symptoms if they try to stop.

Lesson 7.1 Review

Know and Understand

1. What role do genetics and life experiences and situations play in how mental illnesses develop?
2. How is an anxiety disorder different from everyday anxiety?
3. Describe the difference between ADHD and OCD.
4. Choose one mood disorder and explain how it changes the way people feel.
5. Which personality disorder is characterized by extreme shifts in attitudes about other people?
6. Why is it difficult for people with a substance use disorder to stop using a substance?

Think Critically

7. With a partner, research a story, movie, or TV show about someone with schizophrenia spectrum disorder. How accurate is the portrayal of this mental illness? Explain.
8. How are addictive disorders similar to substance use disorders? How are they different?

REAL WORLD Health Skills

Access Information Use valid and reliable online resources to find an interview with a person who has a mental illness. Listen to or read the interview and examine the characteristics of this person's mental illness and the effect on the person's life. Write a short paragraph about your findings. Make sure to note what characteristics demonstrate that this person has a mental illness.

Getting Help for Mental Illnesses

Essential Question?

What steps can you take to get help or help a friend get help for mental illness?

Lesson 7.2

Learning Outcomes

After studying this lesson, you will be able to

- identify signs that a person needs to seek mental health treatment;
- summarize ways to locate mental health services;
- explain how therapy is used to treat mental illnesses;
- identify types of mental health medications;
- describe why a person might need inpatient mental health treatment;
- assess strategies for overcoming barriers to treatment; and
- analyze strategies for helping someone with a mental illness.

Key Terms

family therapy
mental health medications
stigma
support group
therapist
therapy

Warm-Up Activity

Mental and Physical Health Conditions

Comprehend Concepts With a partner, choose one physical health condition and one mental health condition. Then, list all of the ways the physical and mental health conditions you chose are similar to each other. How are they different? Consider factors such as causes, treatments, and outcomes. Predict why it may be easier or harder for a person to ask for help opening a door due to a physical health condition than to reach out for help with a mental illness.

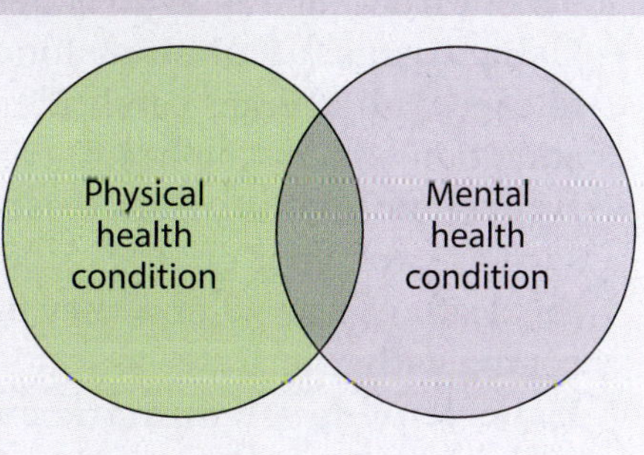

Mental illnesses are health conditions that require professional treatment. The mental nature of these conditions does not make treatment any less important than treatment for a physical health condition. In this lesson, you will learn about ways to seek treatment for a mental illness, treatment options, and strategies for helping a friend or family member with a mental illness.

Deciding to Seek Treatment

Sometimes, people with mental illnesses do not get the help they need. They may assume their negative feelings will go away on their own. Most mental illnesses, however, do not improve without treatment.

Untreated mental illnesses may even get worse and lead to larger difficulties. Knowing when to get help and how to find treatment are essential skills for maintaining your mental and emotional health.

Know When You Need Help

Everyone feels sad, anxious, distracted, angry, or lonely sometimes. These are normal parts of life for everyone, and in most cases, these feelings will fade over time. Sometimes, however, people need help from a therapist or doctor to manage their feelings (**Figure 7.9**). Following are some signs that may indicate you need to seek help from a professional:

- **Feeling sad, angry, or just not like yourself:** These signs could include eating or sleeping more or less than usual, withdrawing from friends and family members, having frequent conflict with family members or teachers, or just feeling "off" in some way.
- **Feeling constantly tense, worried, or on edge:** Signs that it would be a good idea to get help include consistent anxiety that interferes with daily life, a belief that something bad will happen if tasks are not done in a certain way, or sudden panic attacks.
- **Experiencing difficulty paying attention, sitting still, or staying organized:** People who find it difficult to stay focused and organized, constantly lose or misplace items, or become easily distracted may benefit from talking to an expert.
- **Using drugs, alcohol, or food to cope:** Turning to substances to cope with feelings can lead to negative consequences, including addiction and lasting health conditions.
- **Experiencing a serious loss:** People who experience a serious loss, such as parents or guardians getting divorced, a serious illness, or the death of a loved one, may benefit from support from an expert in coping with grief.
- **Experiencing a traumatic event:** People who experience trauma, such as abuse, neglect, or assault, often find it useful to talk to a professional to find healthy ways of coping.
- **Feeling you cannot do activities you used to enjoy:** If you no longer enjoy activities you used to like doing, such as playing sports, hanging out with friends, or watching TV, this is a clear sign you should seek help.

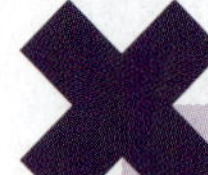

Do Not Need Professional Help	Need Professional Help
• Sometimes feeling sad, anxious, distracted, or lonely • Feelings fading over time	• Being unable to manage feelings individually • Impact on ability to function in daily life • Feelings that do not go away on their own

Figure 7.9 Everyone experiences mental health conditions every once in a while. If these symptoms do not go away, cannot be managed individually, or negatively impact your ability to function, you may want to seek professional help.

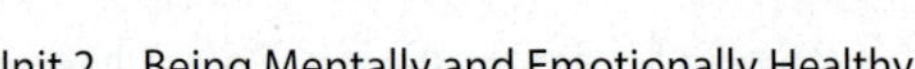

Another sign that someone might need to seek professional help is self-harm. *Self-harm* occurs when people cause injury to themselves in some way on purpose (**Figure 7.10**).

People typically engage in self-harm because they have trouble coping with negative feelings or managing emotions. They may cause injury to themselves because it makes them feel less hopeless, angry, or lonely. Sometimes, self-harming behaviors can become habitual, get out of control, or lead to serious injury. Professional treatment can help people who self-harm cope with feelings and manage their emotions in healthier ways.

Locate Resources

The next step for getting mental health treatment is locating resources. There are many ways teens can get help for mental health conditions and illnesses. Talk to your school counselor, school nurse, or doctor to find a therapist who can help you. Many community agencies and institutions offer some type of mental health counseling. It is often possible to find free or low-cost therapy from local hospitals, colleges or universities, or mental health clinics.

People who provide mental health treatment are required by professional ethics to maintain confidentiality. This means the information you share will not be shared with anyone else, including your family members, school, or even doctor. This confidentiality helps people feel comfortable sharing private information with a mental health professional. Confidentiality can only be broken if people express intent to harm themselves or others or report abuse or neglect that is currently occurring.

In many states, teens have a right to receive mental health treatment without the consent of a parent or guardian. When you call a clinic, hospital, or therapist, ask about whether your state allows teens to receive mental health services on their own.

Even if your state allows mental health treatment without consent from a parent or guardian, it is a good idea to talk to an adult you trust, such as a teacher, nurse, or other relative. This person may be able to support you in other ways, such as helping you find a qualified therapist or driving you to or from appointments.

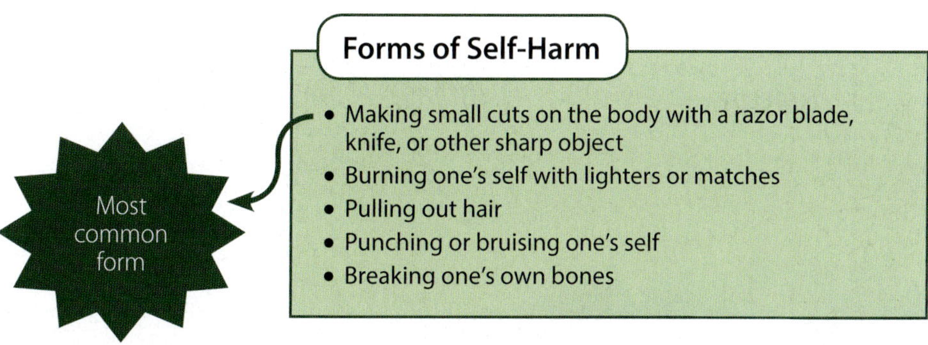

Figure 7.10 Self-harm is a dangerous pattern of behavior that signals the need for professional help.

Treating Mental Illnesses

The purpose of mental health treatment is to help people with mental health conditions and illnesses live healthy, productive, and fulfilling lives. Mental health treatment is not only for people with a diagnosed mental illness. Many people find mental health treatment helpful for managing normal stressors, such as academic pressure, conflict with friends and family members, or challenging life events. To help people handle stress and mental health conditions and illnesses, mental health professionals use several types of treatment. These treatments address mental health's biological and psychological aspects. Methods include therapy, medications, and inpatient treatment.

Therapy

therapy treatment method that changes the way a person thinks, interprets information, behaves, and experiences and expresses emotions

therapist healthcare professional who diagnoses mental illnesses and delivers therapy

family therapy treatment method in which family members meet together with a therapist to build positive, functional relationships and strengthen interactions

support group treatment method in which people who have faced or are facing similar challenges meet together to discuss obstacles and ways of overcoming them

Therapy is a treatment method that focuses on the psychological aspect of mental health. This type of treatment seeks to change the way a person thinks, interprets information, behaves, and experiences and expresses emotions. The type of healthcare professional who diagnoses mental illnesses and delivers this treatment is a **therapist** (**Figure 7.11**). The information people share with therapists is completely confidential in most cases, unless a therapist believes a patient may attempt suicide or hurt someone else. Then the therapist may share that information with a parent, guardian, or other appropriate individual.

Therapists may recommend several different types of therapy, such as the following:

- **Individual therapy:** Individual therapy involves a one-on-one meeting with a therapist to discuss feelings, thoughts, and behaviors. Therapy focuses on strategies for expressing emotions, challenging cognitive distortions, and adopting positive habits.
- **Family therapy:** In **family therapy**, family members meet together with a therapist. The goal is to help families build positive, functional relationships and strengthen interactions. Family therapy can also help members of a family support one member with a mental illness through treatment and recovery.
- **Group therapy:** One form of group therapy is a **support group**, in which a therapist meets with a group of people who share a common experience. Group members discuss strategies for coping and managing difficult situations. Group therapy can also provide the opportunity for people to practice certain skills, such as interpersonal skills or coping with pain, and receive feedback.

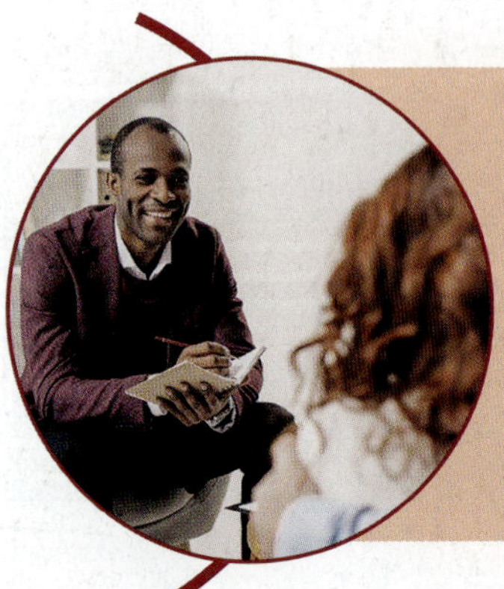

What Does a Therapist Do?

- Helps people understand their feelings and behaviors in an accepting and nonjudgmental environment
- Gives specific suggestions for how people can understand their thought processes, express their emotions, and help themselves feel better
- Helps people learn to cope with difficult thoughts, feelings, and situations in healthy, positive ways

LightFieldStudios/iStock/Getty Images Plus/Getty Images

Figure 7.11 Therapists include professionals such as psychologists, psychiatrists, social workers, and counselors. ***When are therapists allowed to share information provided by a patient?***

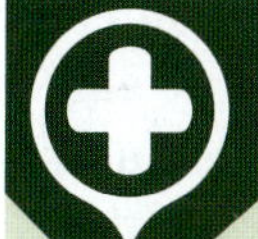

Spotlight on Health and Wellness Careers

Licensed Clinical Psychologist: Linnea Mavrides

When I was a teen, a lot of my friends turned to me to talk about their feelings and challenges. Still, I did not really consider becoming a psychologist until I was in college and worked at a summer camp for children with ADHD. After college, I spent a few years working and then committed to the five years of graduate school it would take to become a clinical psychologist. After graduation, I worked at a Veterans Affairs (VA) hospital, where I provided individual and group therapy for several years while earning my state license. Later, I decided to leave and open a private practice so I could control my schedule and work with different populations.

Today, I spend three days each week providing therapy to clients, mostly individuals and some couples. I also teach and supervise clinical psychology students. My workdays consist of bringing in new clients; providing therapy; writing case notes on clients' progress; and maintaining my schedule and billing statements. I also take time to research treatment issues, develop a deeper understanding of my clients' symptoms, meet with peers to discuss cases, and see my own therapist.

I feel very lucky to have a job that is both intellectually stimulating and emotionally fulfilling. It can be challenging sometimes to hear about upsetting events in people's lives. Fortunately, graduate school prepares you well for managing this through self-awareness, ways of processing, and self-care. In private practice, it is also challenging at times to manage the demands of my business and personal and family life. Still, every day I go to work, I am awed and humbled by people's resilience, desire to do the hard work of therapy, and journeys of self-discovery.

Practice Your Skills

Access Information

Think about your own interests, strengths, and weaknesses. What parts of being a licensed clinical psychologist do you think would interest you? Which elements would be challenging? Using reliable resources like the US Bureau of Labor Statistics' *Occupational Outlook Handbook*, research mental health therapy and related careers. Is the demand for clinical psychologists growing? What are the educational requirements for being a clinical psychologist? Are there related careers that might also interest you? Write a blog post summarizing your thoughts.

In addition, some mental health apps can help supplement more traditional forms of therapy. Many of these are available at either no or low cost. They can also provide some treatment for people who could not otherwise receive it.

Mental Health Medications

As you know, genetic makeup and levels of chemicals in the brain influence a person's risk for developing a mental illness. One treatment method that addresses this aspect of mental health is **mental health medications**. Mental health medications cause changes in the brain to lessen the symptoms of a mental illness and are prescribed by healthcare professionals.

mental health medications substances that cause changes in the brain to reduce the symptoms of a mental illness

Many researchers believe that mental health medications are most effective when used along with some type of therapy. For example, people with major depressive disorder may take medication and also benefit from therapy. Medication can often effectively manage symptoms of a mental illness. Therapy can help people correct unhealthy thought patterns.

Different mental health medications reduce the symptoms of various mental illnesses (**Figure 7.12**). Most medications have some possible side effects. For example, some teens who take certain types of antidepressants can experience *more* thoughts of suicide. Due to side effects, doctors and mental health professionals frequently monitor people who take mental health medications.

Inpatient Treatment

In some cases, people with mental illnesses need care in an *inpatient*, or residential, clinic or hospital. This type of treatment is used only when people are at serious risk of harming themselves or others. People with severe depression or thoughts of suicide may need to be hospitalized for a period of time to make sure they do not attempt suicide. In the hospital, people receive around-the-clock supervision, mental health medications, and therapy.

Figure 7.12 Mental health medications can greatly reduce the symptoms of mental illnesses. They may, however, also cause significant side effects.

Mental Health Medications			
Medication	**Used to Treat**	**How They Work**	**Side Effects**
Antidepressants	Major depressive disorder, anxiety disorders	Make certain brain chemicals, such as serotonin and norepinephrine, more available, which reduces depressive symptoms	Weight gain, nausea, sleepiness, diarrhea, worsening anxiety or depression, agitation, thoughts of suicide
Anti-anxiety medications	Anxiety disorders	Slow down the central nervous system, which makes people feel calmer and more relaxed	Drowsiness, dizziness, nausea, headache, confusion, loss of coordination, frequent urination, thoughts of suicide
Stimulants	ADHD	Increase levels of norepinephrine and dopamine in the brain, which helps improve memory and attention span	Headache, loss of appetite, difficulty sleeping, stomach pain
Antipsychotics	Schizophrenia spectrum disorders, bipolar disorder, severe depression, ADHD, stress-related disorders, OCD, eating disorders	Reduce symptoms of *psychosis*, including hallucinations, delusions, and loss of contact with reality	Dizziness, restlessness, weight gain, nausea, tremors, seizures, dry mouth, constipation, drowsiness
Mood stabilizers	Bipolar disorder, major depressive disorder	Decrease certain activity in the brain to help control extreme high and low moods	Nausea, tremors, fast heartbeat, swelling, loss of coordination, hallucinations, seizures, excessive thirst, frequent urination, slurred speech, blackouts

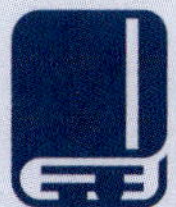

Case Study

Mental Health Medical Record Profiles

The following medical records are for new patients at a mental health clinic. Each teen showed signs that professional treatment might be needed and reached out to get help.

Chart: FISCHER, NATE #7534		New Patient Case
Demographics		Current Encounter
Patient Name	Fischer, Nate	Patient experiences anxiety with speaking or joking in casual social settings. Patient fears rejection by peers. Anxiety extends to interactions on social media, including a compulsive need to check notifications. Symptoms include rapid breathing and increased sweat production during event, as well as interrupted/low-quality sleep. Patient's brother requested information on how to best support the patient.
Sex	Male	
Age	16	
Social History		
Caffeine Intake: Moderate		
Diet: Regular		
Exercise Level: Sedentary		
Stress Level: High		

Chart: SERRANO, JANELLE #7625		New Patient Case
Demographics		Current Encounter
Patient Name	Serrano, Janelle	Patient has difficulty listening to and following directions at home and at school. She finds herself easily bored with tasks, which has led to issues with teachers and parents. Symptoms include impulsive behavior, difficulty waiting, constant motion, and difficulty focusing. Patient tried reducing caffeine intake and getting physical activity to burn off excess energy, but symptoms persisted. Patient went to great lengths to reduce distractions, but realized she needs professional help to control symptoms.
Sex	Female	
Age	15	
Social History		
Caffeine Intake: Low		
Diet: Good		
Exercise Level: Active		
Stress Level: Moderate		

Chart: WYNTER, ALISHA #7452		New Patient Case
Demographics		Current Encounter
Patient Name	Wynter, Alisha	Patient has noticed a decrease in enjoyment of activities. Patient has stopped attending badminton practice and stays in bed most days. Patient feels irritable and has displayed signs of anger in conversations. Patient continues to unconsciously pinch herself during sessions. Symptoms include extreme tiredness, weight loss, and feelings of anger and worthlessness. Patient has recognized that seeking professional help could assist with finding improvement in mood and activity level.
Sex	Female	
Age	18	
Social History		
Caffeine Intake: Low		
Diet: Poor		
Exercise Level: Sedentary		
Stress Level: Moderate		

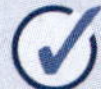

Practice Your Skills

Access Information

Research what mental health resources are available in your area. Where can people with mental health conditions and illnesses get professional help? How many clinics, hospitals, or doctors' offices offer mental health treatment in your community? What online organizations are available to teens? As a class, make a list of these resources with contact or access information. Post the list to your school website. On your own, make a list of the factors that would affect where you would go to get mental health treatment. Make a plan for what you will do if you recognize signs you would benefit from professional help.

Overcome Barriers

Unfortunately, certain barriers can get in the way of people accessing mental health treatment. Examples of these barriers include the social stigma attached to mental illnesses and the cost of mental health treatment.

stigma negative, false, unfair beliefs associated with a circumstance, quality, or person

In the US and around the world, some people attach a social **stigma**—or negative and unfair beliefs—to mental illnesses and those who have them (**Figure 7.13**). Because of stigma, people with mental illnesses may deny they have a condition or feel shame and embarrassment. They may fear losing an opportunity (a job, scholarship, or leadership position, for example) because of their condition.

If you feel stigma about having a mental illness, do not let that stop you from getting the help you need. Many people who hold negative beliefs about those with a mental illness do not understand these conditions. Learning more about mental illness will help you understand your feelings and educate other people.

It is also important to recognize that you are not your mental illness. A mental illness is a treatable condition and does not define who you are.

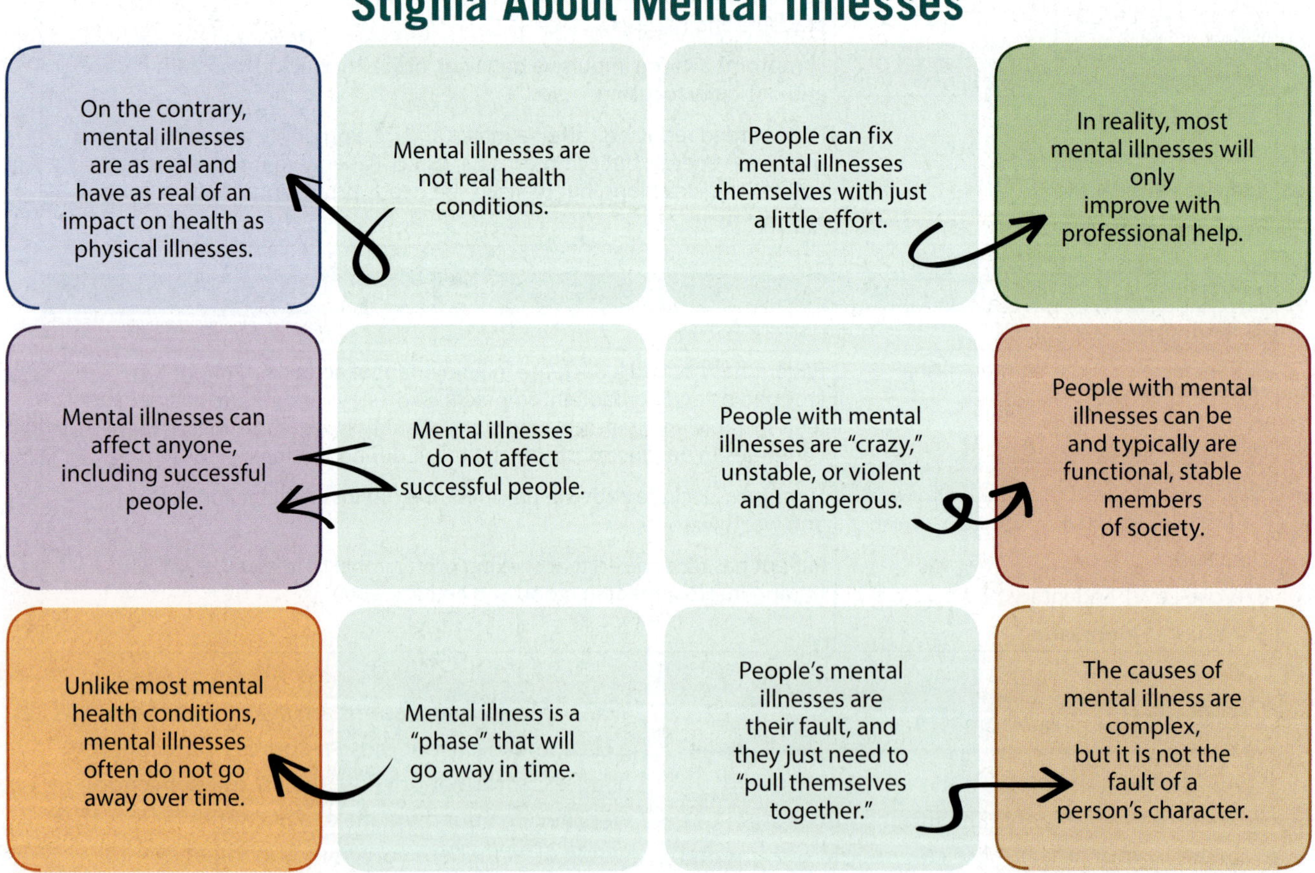

Figure 7.13 Stigma about mental illnesses can discourage people from seeking help, but these harmful beliefs are not true. ***What kind of treatment involves care in a residential clinic or hospital?***

Talking to friends and family members you trust about your mental illness can help give you support. Joining a support group can help you understand that you are not alone and teach you strategies for feeling better.

Another barrier to mental health treatment is cost. People may be reluctant to seek help because they cannot afford mental health treatment. Fortunately, health insurance often covers a portion of the expenses for mental health treatment. Some mental health clinics also provide therapy services at no cost or a reduced rate.

Local and Global Health

Perceptions of Mental Illnesses

One out of every four people in the world will be affected by a mental illness or neurological disorder at some point in their lives. Anxiety disorders, major depressive disorder, and alcohol use disorders are the most common worldwide. Although mental illness occurs in people from all cultures, people from different cultures and even different regions have varying views of mental illness.

People from different cultures describe the causes of mental illness in different ways. Some cultures emphasize the role of biological factors, while others emphasize the role of psychological factors. The prevalence of particular mental illnesses also varies in different cultures. Certain mental illnesses, such as schizophrenia spectrum disorders, are seen in people from all cultural backgrounds. Other mental illnesses, such as eating disorders, are much more common in some cultures than in others.

1 in 4 people
in the world will be affected by a mental illness or neurological disorder

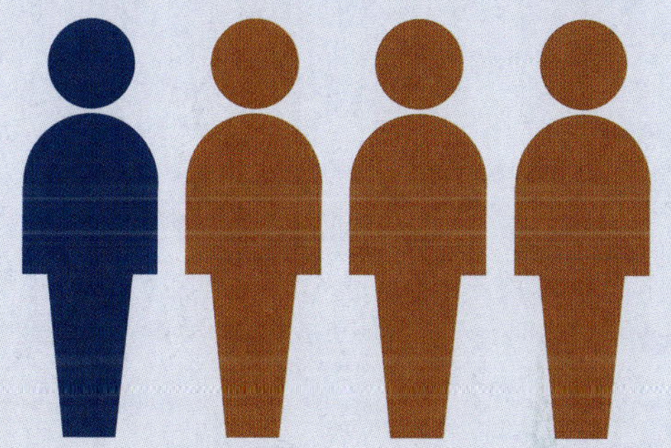

Cultures also differ in how they treat people with mental illnesses. Unfortunately, all cultures have some stigma regarding mental illness. This stigma influences people's willingness to seek treatment. Reducing mental health stigma is therefore an important goal for all cultures.

Practice Your Skills

Advocate for Health

What do you think explains cultural differences in perceptions of mental illnesses? Do you believe these perceptions will change over time? Why do you think people still attach some stigma to mental illness? As you know, stigma can make it harder for people to receive mental health treatment, which is important for managing mental illness.

With a partner, discuss the stigma attached to mental illness in your community. Where do you observe this stigma? How has it impacted you? your classmates? your family members or friends? With your partner, identify some strategies you could use to help reduce stigma in your community. What role could you play in your own school or community to increase acceptance of mental illness and treatment? As a class, share your strategies and choose one to act on together. After acting on this strategy, assess how it impacted the level of stigma in your community.

Helping Someone with a Mental Illness

Many people have a friend or loved one with a mental illness. If you know someone with a mental illness, you may want to know how you can help that person (**Figure 7.14**). To begin, share your concerns with the person in an open and honest way. You can simply say you are worried and would like to help. You could also offer to find a mental health professional who can help and accompany the person to talk to the professional.

Figure 7.14 These strategies can help if you want to support someone with a mental illness, but do not know where to begin.

National Alliance on Mental Illness (NAMI) Strategies for Helping Someone with a Mental Illness
1
Remember that you cannot cure a mental illness any more than you can cure someone's broken leg or high blood pressure. You are not a trained medical professional.
2
Remember that it is not your fault this person has a mental illness.
3
Try to separate your feelings about the mental illness and its symptoms from the feelings you have toward the person.
4
Remember it is often difficult for a person to accept having a mental illness.
5
Recognize that other people may not understand or accept the person's mental illness.
6
Understand that the person's symptoms may change over time.
7
Make sure to take care of your own needs. Do not neglect your health.
8
Talk to a therapist or join a support group for people whose friends or family members have a mental illness. Remember that you are not alone in your experience.

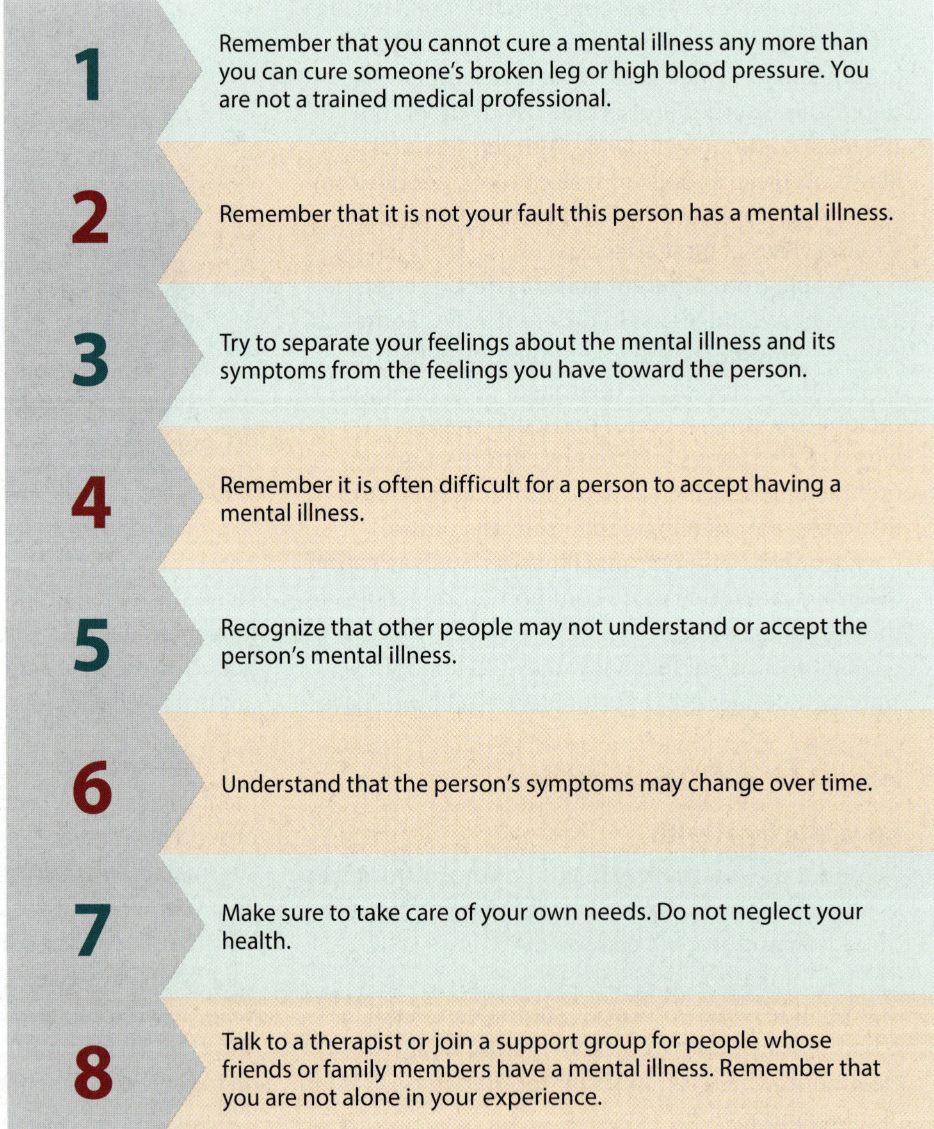

Sometimes a person who is experiencing a mental illness is not interested in seeking help. You must intervene if you suspect someone intends to attempt suicide or hurt someone else. Otherwise, you need to accept it is not your responsibility to make the person seek treatment. It does not help to protect people from the effects of their mental illnesses. This type of protection simply enables people to continue without treatment. For example, if your friend is too depressed to complete her homework, doing her homework for her just helps her hide the seriousness of her condition from people who could help.

Remember that sometimes people just need more time before they are ready to get help. Take immediate action, however, if you suspect someone is contemplating or has taken steps toward suicide. Call 911 or take the person to the hospital right away.

Lesson 7.2 Review

Know and Understand

1. In your state, can teens consent to receive mental health services without a parent or guardian?
2. Describe the difference between individual and family therapy.
3. How do mental health medications help treat mental illnesses?
4. What can you do to help someone who has a mental illness, but does not want to seek help?

Think Critically

5. Review the list of signs that someone might need to seek help with mental health. Then write a case study about a student who shows these signs, but is not seeking help. Trade case studies with a partner and complete your partner's case study by having a friend of the person intervene and assist in getting help.
6. Why do you think some people engage in self-harming behaviors to handle negative feelings? What are some healthier strategies people could use?
7. What are some examples of apps designed to support therapy and promote mental health? Share these apps with the class.
8. Give an example of a time you experienced the stigma attached to mental health. What steps can you take to combat this stigma?
9. With a partner, role-play a situation in which you are trying to encourage your friend to get help for a mental illness. Switch roles so each person gets practice helping a friend.

REAL WORLD Health Skills

Make Decisions Research the resources available in your community to help people with mental health conditions and illnesses. Make a list of these organizations and select one to contact. Find out what services are available and how much they cost. Using this information, write a case study in which someone with a mental illness makes the decision to seek treatment. Show how this person goes through the decision-making process and gets needed treatment from the organization you chose.

Lesson
7.3

Preventing and Coping with Suicide

Essential Question?

What skills do you need to recognize warning signs and help prevent suicide?

Learning Outcomes

After studying this lesson, you will be able to

- explain why suicide is not an effective solution to the challenges in a person's life;
- identify factors that affect whether a person will attempt suicide;
- describe strategies for preventing suicide;
- explain the importance of getting help in response to warning signs of suicide; and
- analyze ways of coping with suicide and supporting survivors.

Key Terms

suicide
suicide clusters
suicide contagion
survivors

Warm-Up Activity

Myths and Facts About Suicide

Communicate with Others Consider what you have heard about suicide— from friends, family members, or the media—and about what you already know. List these ideas in a table and then categorize them as myths or facts. Compare your table with a partner. Did you and your partner list any of the same statements? If so, did you agree which statements were myths and facts? Using effective communication and negotiation skills, discuss any disagreements with your partner. Revisit your statements and discuss again after reading this lesson.

Statement	Myth or Fact?	Why

When you hear the word *suicide*, what do you think of? You have probably heard about suicide in the media—on social media or in TV shows. Maybe a celebrity you admired or someone you know has died by suicide. **Suicide** is the intentional act of ending one's own life. Typically, when people think about attempting suicide, they feel like their lives are never going to change or get better—but they are wrong. Change is inevitable, and treatment can help reduce feelings of hopelessness and despair. Suicide ends life before this change can occur. It also has severe effects on a person's friends, family members, and community.

suicide intentional act of ending one's own life

What Factors Affect Risk for Suicide?

In the US, suicide is the second leading cause of death for people ages 10–34. The most common reason people of any age attempt suicide is severe depression. Severe depression can make people believe life is not worth living, the world will be better off without them, or no one will care if they die.

In some cases, a person who attempts suicide has planned to for some time. In other cases, a person who already feels depressed decides to attempt suicide following some negative life event. This might include the end of a dating relationship, academic failure, or a fight with a friend or family member.

Many individual and environmental factors affect whether a person attempts suicide. *Individual factors* relate to a person's genetic makeup, identity, and thoughts and feelings. *Environmental factors* include social environment (family and peers), community environment, and the media.

Individual Factors

Several individual factors affect a person's risk of suicide. One major risk factor is a previous suicide attempt. A person who has attempted suicide before is more likely to make a future attempt. Other individual factors include mental health and substance use.

Mental health has a profound impact on whether people attempt suicide (**Figure 7.15**). It is important, however, to remember that many people with mental illnesses never attempt suicide. Instead, they seek treatment to eliminate or reduce symptoms and change unhealthy thought patterns to lead fulfilling lives.

Another factor that increases risk for suicide is substance use. People who abuse drugs or alcohol are six times more likely than others to report attempting suicide. Often, substance use is linked to negative feelings, which may cause people to consider ending their lives. People who abuse drugs and alcohol often experience social and financial difficulties, which also increases risk of suicide. Abusing drugs and alcohol can cloud judgment and make people more likely to engage in self-harm or attempt suicide.

Environmental Factors

Environmental factors relate to your family, peers, culture, community, and the media. For example, people who experience long-term stress in their environment, such as abuse or neglect, are more likely to attempt suicide. Exposure to intimate partner violence and substance use is also associated with an increased risk. People whose family members have a mental illness or attempt or die by suicide may be at greater risk for attempting suicide themselves. Crises such as financial hardships, death of a close family member, or divorce, may further strain family relationships and increase risk factors.

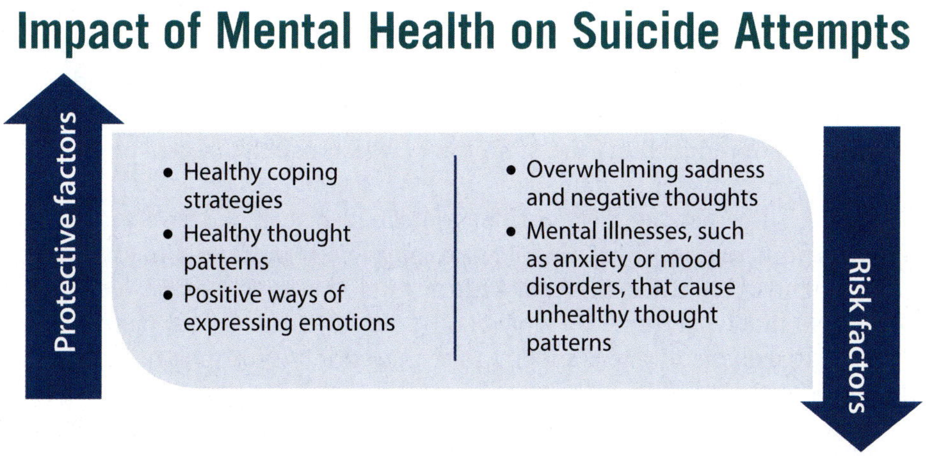

Impact of Mental Health on Suicide Attempts

Protective factors

- Healthy coping strategies
- Healthy thought patterns
- Positive ways of expressing emotions

- Overwhelming sadness and negative thoughts
- Mental illnesses, such as anxiety or mood disorders, that cause unhealthy thought patterns

Risk factors

Figure 7.15 Positive mental health can serve as a protective factor against suicide attempts. Unfortunately, mental health conditions and mental illnesses can become risk factors for suicide. ***What are some other individual risk factors for suicide?***

Severe stress in a person's environment can lead someone with depression to consider suicide. For example, teens who are bullied have a greater risk of thinking about and attempting suicide. Bullying can also lead teens to develop depression. Teens who identify as LGBT+ have a particularly high risk for suicide. Some estimates suggest the rate of suicide attempts for LGBT+ students is two to seven times higher than for other students. This is because LGBT+ students are more likely to experience bullying and may lack support from family members and friends.

The prevalence of suicide in a community also affects suicide risk. Hearing about a suicide—of a friend, family member, classmate, celebrity, or even stranger—can increase someone's risk of a suicide attempt. This increased risk after exposure to suicide is called **suicide contagion** (**Figure 7.16**). Some communities or groups experience a series of suicides or attempted suicides among people in a relatively short period of time. In these **suicide clusters**, one person dies by suicide, and then other people copy this behavior.

suicide contagion copying of suicide attempts after exposure to another person's suicide

suicide clusters series of suicides in a particular community that occur in a relatively short period of time

Another factor in the larger community that affects suicide risk is access to firearms. People who have access to firearms are three times more likely to die by suicide as people who do not. This is partially because access to a firearm increases the risk a person will attempt and die by suicide in response to a stressful life event. Lack of access to a firearm gives people more of a chance to rethink the decision or seek help.

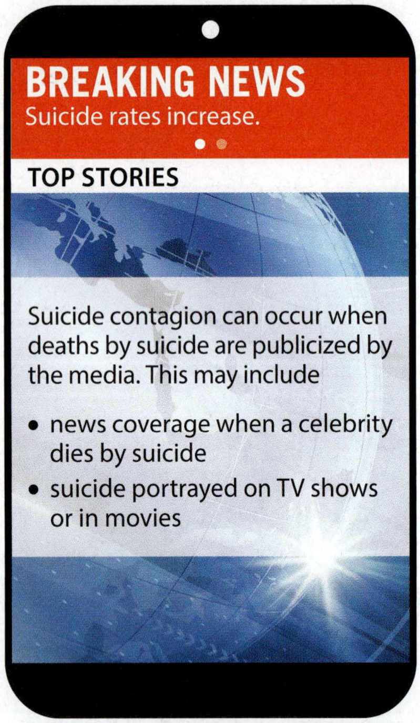

BREAKING NEWS

Suicide rates increase.

TOP STORIES

Suicide contagion can occur when deaths by suicide are publicized by the media. This may include

- news coverage when a celebrity dies by suicide
- suicide portrayed on TV shows or in movies

Phone: Maximon4ik/Shutterstock.com; Background: Bluemoon 1981/Shutterstock.com

Figure 7.16 When a famous person or even a popular character in a fictional show dies by suicide, it can increase the risk of others attempting suicide. ***What is the term for a series of suicides or attempted suicides among a community or group in a short period of time?***

Preventing Suicide

Suicide is a tragedy that affects individuals, families, and communities. It affects those closest to the person who died most dramatically. These people are typically immediate family members and close friends, who grieve intensely. Other people in a community are also impacted by suicide. People in a person's school, workplace, or neighborhood also grieve, even if they did not personally know the individual who died.

All people can take steps to help prevent suicide—on an individual level and in their communities. In this section, you will learn about some of these steps.

Care for Your Mental Health

The most common cause of suicide is untreated depression. Sometimes people consider suicide because of emotions resulting from a mental illness. Anxiety disorders, mood disorders, and other mental illnesses can cause sadness and negative thoughts. To help prevent suicide, get treatment for mental health conditions and illnesses and encourage others to get treatment as well. Treatment seeks to reduce negative symptoms, which usually means people no longer consider suicide.

To protect against suicide, you can also seek and give support in your relationships. People need support from family members, friends, and the community. Simply being able to express feelings and talk with trusted people can be very helpful. Often, people can also encourage someone to seek treatment for mental health conditions or illnesses.

In addition, you can help prevent suicide by using skills to build your self-esteem, shift to a positive mind-set, and manage stress. You have learned about many of these skills already. Practicing them regularly can help you regulate negative feelings and handle stress in healthy ways.

Promote a Positive, Respectful Environment

Because stress in the environment is a risk factor for suicide, improving your environment is another way to reduce risk. A supportive environment is a protective factor against suicide. For example, students who feel connected to the school community, including other students, teachers, and staff, are less likely to experience mental health conditions. They are also more likely to seek help for themselves or their friends.

You can help promote a positive, respectful environment by building supportive, healthy relationships and communicating effectively. You can show empathy and respect to others and stand up to inappropriate behavior. For example, by intervening if you see someone being bullied, you can create an environment in which hurtful behavior is not tolerated. This helps foster a positive school climate, which reduces risk for suicide.

Health in the Media

Media Representations of Suicide

Considerable research demonstrates that suicide depicted in the media may increase the risk of people attempting suicide. After a TV show or movie portrays suicide, rates of suicide attempts increase in the next few weeks after the movie or show is released. For example, in the month following the release of a popular show that focused on a girl who dies by suicide, suicide rates among teens increased. Rates of suicide in older people, who likely did not watch the show, did not increase. Rates of suicide increase similarly after a celebrity or famous figure dies by suicide.

Public representations of suicide do not lead most people to consider harming themselves, but can trigger a suicide attempt in people who are experiencing mental health conditions. For people who have been thinking about suicide, hearing about suicide can make the solution seem okay. People may also see the outpouring of memories and love for the person who died as better than current feelings of grief and isolation.

Many media organizations recognize the unintended negative consequences of reporting on or portraying suicide. These organizations follow careful practices to reduce any potential harm. These practices include not describing the manner of death or showing images of grieving friends and family members. They also include sharing crisis resources and encouraging people who have thoughts of suicide to get help.

Practice Your Skills

Analyze Influences

Why do you think media representations of suicide increase the rate of suicide attempts in people who view them? How are fictional representations of suicide and real-world deaths of celebrities and famous figures similar? different? After reflecting on these questions, compare your answers with those of a partner. How could you test which factors have the biggest influence? What are some of the questions health researchers should be asking to answer these questions? Describe how knowing these factors could help you talk with others and reduce risk for suicide. Is there anything you could do to reduce the negative impact of media representations of suicide on you or your classmates?

You can also contribute to a positive environment by showing tolerance and support for your peers. Students should respect their peers, including those who come from different cultural backgrounds and have different abilities, beliefs, gender identities, and sexual orientations. They should also speak up if they notice others showing disrespect for a student's identity.

Recognize Warning Signs

Most people who attempt suicide show some warning signs about their intentions. They may tell someone about their plans beforehand or hint at their plans in some way (**Figure 7.17**). Some people may say they have no reason to live or may seem obsessed with death. It is very important to take *any* mention of suicide seriously, even if the person seems to be joking.

Warning signs that can indicate a person is considering suicide include the following:

- the person talks about considering or attempting suicide, in person or online
- the person researches or talks about ways of attempting suicide
- the person talks of feeling hopeless or trapped, having no reason to live, or being a burden to others
- changes in eating and sleeping habits
- withdrawal from friends, family, and regular activities and responsibilities
- disregard for personal appearance
- changes in personality, such as irritability, aggression, recklessness, or shame
- the person gives away valued possessions
- the person visits or calls people to say goodbye
- use of alcohol or drugs
- loss of interest in previously enjoyed activities

If you or someone you know is experiencing these symptoms, you need to seek help for yourself or the person you know right away.

Managing Warning Signs Online
It can be hard to tell if online suicidal statements are real. Very real suicidal thoughts may appear like jokes. For this reason, take all suicidal threats seriously.
Taji Rajesh @TajiRaji42 1 hour ago
Today has been the worst day... sometimes I really wish I were dead.
If everyone thinks someone else will ask about the statement, then no one may reach out to help.
Reach out to ask if the person needs help. Encourage this person to talk to an adult, contact a help line, or call 911.

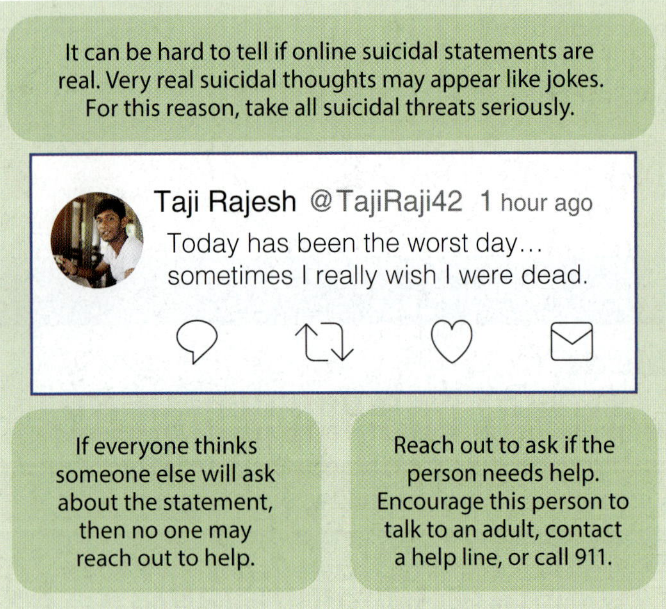

Profile: wong.yu liang/Shutterstock.com; Icons: MAKSIM ANKUDA/Shutterstock.com

Figure 7.17 Most people who attempt suicide talk about suicide beforehand. Even online, jokes or conversations about suicide should be taken seriously.

Get Help

If you ever find yourself considering suicide, there are steps you need to take to get help. First, always take thoughts of suicide very seriously. Talk to an adult you trust immediately. This person can put you in touch with a mental health professional who can help. If you cannot immediately reach a trusted adult, talk to a trusted friend, call 911, or contact a suicide prevention resource, which can assist you in getting help (**Figure 7.18**).

If a person confides in you about considering suicide, or if you think someone is considering suicide, you cannot keep this secret, even if the person asks you not to tell anyone. Keeping this information private could endanger the person's life.

Suicide Prevention Resources

Emergency medical services	Call 911
National Suicide Prevention Lifeline	Call 1-800-273-TALK (8255) or visit suicidepreventionlifeline.org/chat to chat online
Crisis Text Line	Text 741741
The Hope Line	Visit www.thehopeline.com/gethelp to chat online
The Trevor Project (for LGBT+ youth)	Call 1-866-488-7386, text START to 678678, or visit www.thetrevorproject.org/get-help-now to chat online

Figure 7.18 Most suicide prevention resources are available 24 hours every day.

Skills for Health and Wellness

Helping a Friend Who Is Considering Suicide

If someone shares suicidal thoughts or shows other warning signs, it is important to take these actions seriously. Reaching out and talking with this person could save this person's life. Sometimes, talking about suicide can seem awkward or intimidating. Practicing how to start this conversation and find help can make you feel more comfortable helping someone you know.

Practice Your Skills

Communicate with Others

Partner with a classmate to role-play a situation in which someone notices a friend showing warning signs of suicide. Follow these steps for helping a friend in your conversation:

1. **Ask:** Ask directly if your friend has been thinking about suicide. For example, you might say, "You've been talking a lot about wanting to be dead. Have you been thinking about trying to kill yourself?" Sometimes, people fear directly asking this question because they worry it will give the person the idea of attempting suicide. In reality, asking is unlikely to give the person the idea. Most people who are considering suicide are willing to discuss it. They may feel less alone if they know someone cares enough to show concern.
2. **Listen:** Listen to your friend's response. Do not judge what your friend is saying by debating whether suicide is right or wrong or lecturing. Reassure your friend that you are there and that you care and want to help.
3. **Keep your friend safe:** If your friend is considering suicide, do not leave your friend alone. If you are physically with your friend, stay with that friend. If you are talking with your friend online, keep the conversation going. This will give your friend the time and emotional support to rethink the situation and get help.
4. **Tell:** Tell an adult you trust about what the person is saying or sharing online. Even if the person makes you promise not to tell anyone, you still need to get help from a responsible adult. For example, you could say to your friend, "Let's go talk to your dad" or "I'm going to tell the social worker, okay?" If the threat is immediate, you can also help your friend by contacting a suicide prevention resource, taking your friend to an emergency room, or calling 911. Do not leave your friend alone until your friend is getting needed help.

Rotate roles in the role-play so you and your partner get practice asking questions and getting help. Afterward, discuss which statements were most and least effective.

If you learn that someone has made a suicide attempt, or plans to attempt suicide, get help immediately. If you are with the person, do not leave the person alone. If you are talking with the person over the phone or online, keep talking with the person until the person gets help. If you can, take the person to the nearest hospital. Talk to a trusted adult immediately, call 911, or reach a suicide prevention resource.

Supporting Survivors

survivors people who have lost someone to suicide

The term **survivors** describes people who have lost someone to suicide. After a suicide, survivors often feel anger, guilt, and sadness. They may blame themselves because they were unable to prevent the suicide. They may also feel rejected and abandoned by the person who died by suicide. Suicide deaths are often sudden. This means survivors cannot prepare themselves for the loss.

Survivors sometimes feel embarrassed or ashamed by the suicide. Many people are uncomfortable with the topic of suicide. Unfortunately, this means survivors may not get the support they need.

The good news is that there are ways to help survivors. Some survivors may find support groups or therapy helpful. It is important to let survivors grieve. If you know someone who lost a loved one to suicide, learn about the stages of grief (**Figure 7.19**). Knowing what this person is going through can help you be more compassionate.

Survivors may not want to talk about their loss right away. When they are ready to talk, however, just listen. Some people feel better when they talk about difficult topics. Listening is a simple way to help survivors process their loss.

If you have lost someone to suicide, get help for coping with this loss. Even if you were not very close to the individual who died, you may need support managing your feelings. Remember that different people grieve in different ways, and there is no "right way" to cope with loss.

Stages of Grief

Denial

- People may ignore the facts and try to carry on as though nothing has changed.
- Not all people experience denial, but those who do are protecting themselves from emotional pain.

Anger

- Some people become angry with the person who died.
- Although this stage is temporary, it may last a long time, and a person's anger may push family and friends away.

Bargaining

- People often feel out of control and helpless in the face of death.
- Some people may try to bargain to feel they have some control.

Depression

- Deep sadness comes with the reality of the loss.
- This depression is normal and can last a long time and come and go in waves.

Acceptance

- As with other stages, not all people experience this stage.
- When they do, they accept the loss as real and begin to move on knowing life continues.

Figure 7.19 The stages of grief do not happen the same way, in the same order, or for the same amount of time for all people. People may skip certain stages and linger in others. The stages are meant to outline potential emotional responses to loss.

Focus on what you need and get the help that feels right to you. Some other strategies for coping with this loss follow:

- **Accept your feelings:** It is normal to feel a range of emotions after losing someone to suicide. You might feel grief and sadness, but also anger, guilt, shame, anxiety, and confusion. Some people may even feel relief. These are all normal feelings in response to a suicide.
- **Take care of yourself:** It is very important to take care of yourself following a major loss. Get enough sleep and eat nutritious meals. Taking care of your body will give you strength to cope.
- **Rely on friends and family members:** Get support from people who care about you. Talking about your feelings can help you feel better.
- **Join a support group:** Talking with people who have experienced a similar loss can help you process your feelings. This can be especially helpful following a death by suicide, since there is often a stigma about this type of loss, making people feel more isolated.
- **Talk to a professional:** In some cases, people find it helpful to talk with a mental health professional. A therapist can listen to your feelings and help you learn healthy coping strategies.

Lesson 7.3 Review

Know and Understand

1. How do mental health conditions affect a person's risk for suicide?
2. Choose two warning signs of suicide and explain what they might look like in a person at your school. Give details and describe how you could respond to each warning sign.
3. Choose one suicide prevention resource and explain what it is and how to access it.
4. In discussions of suicide, what is meant by the term *survivors*?
5. With a partner, create a video or graph showing the stages of grief and how people act in each stage.

Think Critically

6. Why do you think hearing about a suicide increases a person's risk for suicide?
7. With a partner, discuss the impact suicide has on a person's friends, family, and community. Create an artistic representation showing this impact and share with the class.
8. What are some ways you can promote a positive, respectful environment in your school? Share three strategies in a small group.
9. Why is it important not to leave a person considering suicide alone?

REAL WORLD Health Skills

Set Goals Using reliable resources, research strategies and resources for suicide prevention. These could be personal strategies, strategies for a larger community, or community and national resources. Then, for each strategy, set a SMART goal describing how you could put the strategy into action to enhance your own health and the health of others. Consider your own personal health practices and ways of communicating with others.

Chapter 7 Review and Assessment

Chapter Summary

Mental illnesses are health conditions characterized by negative thoughts and feelings that disrupt daily life and do not go away. Many factors contribute to the development of mental illness. These factors include genetic makeup, life experiences and situations, traumatic life events and stress, and patterns of thinking.

Anxiety disorders involve unrealistic or exaggerated fear or worry and include generalized anxiety disorder (GAD), social anxiety disorder, panic disorder, and phobias. Attention-deficit hyperactivity disorder (ADHD) causes difficulty paying attention, hyperactivity, and impulsiveness. An executive function disorder (EFD) involves chronic difficulty performing daily tasks. In obsessive-compulsive disorder (OCD), people have recurring and uncontrollable thoughts, feelings, and behaviors.

Mood disorders cause changes in how people feel. Major depressive disorder leads to feelings of intense sadness, worthlessness, and hopelessness. Seasonal affective disorder (SAD) occurs when these feelings develop during times of little sunlight, and bipolar disorder includes depressive symptoms that alternate with periods of mania. Personality and behavioral disorders involve consistent patterns of inappropriate behavior, and schizophrenia spectrum disorders lead to irregular thoughts, delusions, and hallucinations. Substance use and addictive disorders develop when a person keeps using a substance or engaging in certain behaviors despite negative consequences.

People need professional treatment for mental illnesses. Recognizing when help is needed, locating resources, and overcoming stigma can help people get needed treatment. This treatment may involve therapy, medications, or inpatient treatment. People can help those with mental illnesses by being supportive and encouraging them to seek help.

Severe depression is the most common cause of suicide. Factors that contribute to suicide include a previous suicide attempt, mental illness, substance use, violence, stress, and suicide prevalence. To prevent suicide, people can invest in positive mental health, promote a respectful environment, and recognize warning signs. They can get help and assist others in getting help for suicidal thoughts. They can also support survivors who lost someone to suicide.

Vocabulary Activity

Consider your prior experiences with and exposure to each of the terms shown. What have you heard about these terms? How have you used them in the past? Then, write the definition of each term in your own words. Double-check your definitions by rereading the text and using the text glossary.

addictive disorders
anxiety disorder
bipolar disorder
co-occurring disorders
family therapy
major depressive disorder
mental health medications
mental illness
panic attacks
personality disorders
phobia
schizophrenia spectrum disorders
stigma
substance use disorder
suicide clusters
suicide contagion
suicide
support group
survivors
therapist
therapy
tolerance
withdrawal

Review and Recall

Review the information in this chapter by answering the following questions.

1. Describe how a mental illness is different from mental distress.
2. Which anxiety disorder is characterized by recurring episodes of intense fear?
   A. GAD
   B. ADHD
   C. panic disorder
   D. social anxiety disorder
3. What are the symptoms of an executive function disorder (EFD)?
4. Which of the following is a symptom of major depressive disorder?
   A. increased energy
   B. irritability and hostility
   C. more interest in enjoyable activities
   D. good concentration
5. Which mental illness can grow into antisocial personality disorder in adulthood?
6. What are the stages of substance use?
7. Which of the following is a sign of needing professional help?
   A. experiencing trauma
   B. feeling occasionally worried
   C. enjoying activities
   D. feeling better after a period of sadness
8. Under what circumstances can mental health professionals break confidentiality?
9. What is the goal of therapy?
10. Why do people who take mental health medications need to be frequently monitored by a doctor or mental health professional?
11. Which type of treatment is most appropriate for someone who intends to attempt suicide?
    A. family therapy
    B. support group
    C. antipsychotics
    D. inpatient treatment
12. What is the most common reason people attempt suicide?
    A. severe depression
    B. attention
    C. traumatic event
    D. revenge
13. Why does substance use increase the risk for suicide?
14. Which of the following is a warning sign of suicide?
    A. collecting valued possessions
    B. more interest in activities
    C. feeling like a burden
    D. improved personal appearance
15. List two suicide prevention resources and how to reach them.

Standstandardized Test Prep

Math Practice

The following results are from a study of substance use and mental illnesses in the US. Review the results of this study and then answer the questions that follow.

In the year 2018,

- 3.5 million adolescents (ages 12–17) had a major depressive episode in the past year
- 358,000 adolescents had a major depressive episode and substance use disorder in the past year
- 1.4 million adolescents who had a major depressive episode in the past year received treatment for depression

Substance Abuse and Mental Health Services Administration. (2019). Key substance use and mental health indicators in the United States: Results from the 2018 National Survey on Drug Use and Health (HHS Publication No. PEP19-5068, NSDUH Series H-54). Rockville, MD: Center for Behavioral Health Statistics and Quality, Substance Abuse and Mental Health Services Administration. Retrieved from https://www.samhsa.gov/data/

16. What percentage of adolescents who had a major depressive episode in the past year received treatment for depression?
17. This study's results show that 14.4 percent of adolescents had a major depressive episode in the past year. What was the total number of adolescents in the study? Round to the nearest whole number.
    A. 24 million
    B. 504,000
    C. 50 million
    D. 243,055
18. What percentage of adolescents had a major depressive episode and substance use disorder? Round to the nearest tenth of a percent.

Chapter 7 Skills Assessment

Critical Thinking Skills

Answer the following questions to assess your knowledge of what you learned in this chapter.

1. How are the factors that contribute to mental illness similar to the factors that lead to physical health conditions? How are these factors different? Explain.
2. Given what you know about stress, how could having constant anxiety impact a person's physical, mental and emotional, and social health?
3. With a partner, discuss the following question: *How do you know the difference between normal feelings of grief, stress, or sadness and major depressive disorder?* After discussing, share your thoughts with another pair.
4. Why do you think substance use and addictive disorders sometimes occur together with other mental illnesses? How could multiple mental illnesses contribute to each other?
5. How are substance use disorders similar to other mental illnesses? How are they different? Not everyone knows that a substance use disorder is a mental illness. Why do you think this is?
6. What do you think are the most significant barriers that prevent teens from seeking professional help for mental health conditions? Why are these barriers significant? What can teens do to overcome them?
7. If you were to seek professional help, what qualities would you look for in a mental health professional? Why would these qualities be important to you? Make a list of these qualities and keep it for future reference.
8. With a partner, discuss the following statement: *Mental health treatment is not only for people with a diagnosed mental illness.* Do you think most teens would agree with this statement? Why or why not? What does this statement mean for your mental and emotional health?
9. In your school, what, if any, stigmas are attached to mental health and mental illness? Why do these stigmas exist? What can you and other students do to reduce them?
10. It is not helpful to protect people from the effects of an untreated mental illness. What is the difference between protecting someone from effects and being a supportive friend? Explain.
11. What thoughts and feelings do you think prevent people considering suicide from seeking treatment? If you had a friend with untreated depression who was considering suicide, how could you help your friend get treatment?
12. With a partner, write a script in which a friend makes a suicidal statement that sounds like a joke. How would you approach your friend? How could you start the conversation and help your friend get help?
13. Imagine that, after your friend shared suicidal thoughts with you, you told your friend's parents. This made your friend angry. How would you navigate this situation? How could you explain to your friend why you did what you did?
14. Search online and read a story about someone who lost a loved one to suicide. How did this person process the grief? How was the grief similar to and different from grief over other types of loss?

Health and Wellness Skills

Complete the following activities to assess your skills related to health and wellness.

15. **Analyze Influences.** Forms of media, such as TV shows, movies, and music, can be extremely influential on how people perceive mental health topics. Think about the shows, movies, and songs you have encountered recently. Choose one that you think helps raise awareness about suicide. Then choose that you think minimizes the seriousness of suicide. Explain why you chose each song, movie, or show and how each could affect someone experiencing a mental illness or considering suicide.
16. **Access Information.** There are many resources for those who have mental health conditions or illnesses or are considering suicide. Research mental health resources available in your community. Note the contact information for these resources, services provided, and how people can get help. Then, as a class, design a digital poster that summarizes the findings of all classmates. Share this poster with the school and save it for future reference.

17. **Communicate with Others.** This chapter identified several strategies for preventing suicide. With a partner, choose one of these strategies to demonstrate. This strategy should involve communicating with someone or reaching out for help. With your partner, record a one- or two-minute advertisement promoting one of these strategies. In your advertisement, demonstrate how the strategy is used and how it can be effective. Share your advertisement with the class.
18. **Make Decisions.** Imagine that you are feeling unusually stressed, and your stress is turning into depression. To feel better, you have started taking some pills a classmate gave you, but the pills do not really help anymore. It is time to make a decision about your next move. What questions should you ask yourself to decide if you need professional help? What decision can you make to get help? Identify three ways you can overcome barriers to getting help.
19. **Set Goals.** Take a moment to think about your life in five years. Write about or illustrate your life and what you want it to look like. How do you look in five years? How do you feel? What are the most important relationships in your life, and what is your career? How do you spend your money and time? Create five SMART goals related to mental and emotional health that will help you build the life you want.
20. **Practice Health-Enhancing Behaviors.** In a written or audio journal entry, identify some of the factors that might contribute to mental health conditions or a mental illness in your life. Then, consider how you might manage each factor to lower your risk for mental illness or improve your mental and emotional health. For each factor, identify three actions you can take this week that will help you control the factor and enhance health.
21. **Advocate for Health.** Imagine that the principal of your school has asked you to lead a program to educate students about the topic of suicide. In a small group, design two different options for a school event you think will give your peers the most important facts about suicide. Your event options should also encourage students to seek help if they need it. Share your event options with the class and agree on several to put into action.

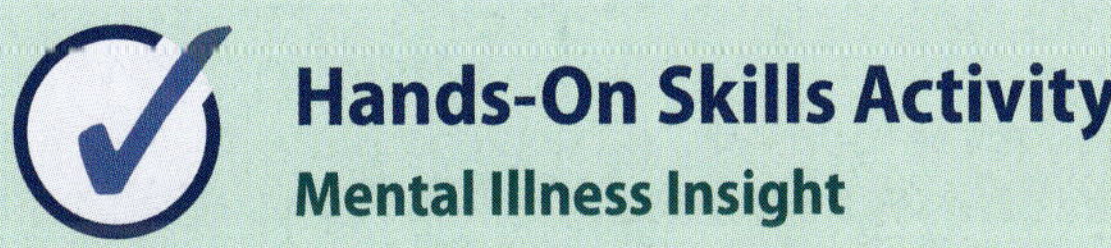

Hands-On Skills Activity

Mental Illness Insight

Mental illness is more common than many people assume. In fact, many extremely successful people have mental illnesses. Some of these people are open about mental illness. Others keep the details of their mental and emotional health to themselves. This activity will help you gain more insight into what people with a mental illness experience.

Steps for This Activity

1. **Access Information.** Using reliable and valid resources, research famous people who have or had mental illnesses. Choose one who is intriguing to you and then research this person's life. During your research, seek to answer the following questions:
   - What are the signs and symptoms of mental illness in this person's life?
   - What, if any, stigma has this person experienced due to mental illness? How has stigma affected this person's life?
   - Does mental illness affect this person physically? If so, how?
   - How does mental illness affect this person's thoughts and emotions?
   - What treatment is this person receiving for mental illness? What treatment options would be available for this person in your community?
   - Has mental illness affected this person's accomplishment? If so, how? Explain.
2. **Advocate for Health.** Make a poster, video, or collage that shares the information you found. Be sure to present this information in a way that will be interesting and engaging for your peers. Your goal in sharing this information should be to reduce the stigma around mental illness and normalize the process of getting help.
3. Present your poster, video, or collage to the class. Be prepared to discuss the ideas you found most interesting in your research.
4. If you can, share your poster, video, or collage with others in your school. For example, you could hang your poster or collage in the school hallway or submit your video to the school administration.

Unit 3

Developing a Healthy Lifestyle

Big Ideas

- The foods you eat and the beverages you drink have a significant impact on health. Your body needs certain nutrients to function and grow. The nutrients and calories you need depend on your age, biological sex, height, weight, and level of physical activity.
- Following a healthy eating pattern requires paying attention to the foods you eat and choosing nutrient-dense foods. You can evaluate the nutritional value of foods by reading Nutrition Facts labels and assessing food claims. Using these skills, you can manage the factors that influence your food choices and prepare nutritious and safe meals.
- Your body image is your thoughts and feelings about how you look. This does not always relate to how you actually look. Many factors influence body image, including environment, the media, race and ethnicity, gender identity, and activities. You can develop a positive body image by viewing media critically and embracing body neutrality, positivity, and compassion.
- A negative body image can sometimes lead to disordered eating, or eating habits that reflect an unhealthy relationship with weight and food. Eating disorders are mental illnesses that cause major disturbances in a person's diet. These disorders have serious health consequences and require professional treatment.
- Physical activity is any activity in which the body uses energy. Getting physical activity has many health benefits, such as a lower risk of disease, a healthier weight, more strength, and better mental and emotional health.
- Setting goals can help people engage in physical activity. Physical activity can be fun and include activities you enjoy. You can fit physical activity even into small amounts of time. Varying FITT factors can help improve fitness, and staying safe will help you improve health and experience physical activity's benefits.

AleksandarNakic/E+/Getty Images ▶

Health Management Plan Building Blocks for a Healthy Lifestyle

The decisions you make every day affect your health. Many of the habits you form now will follow you into adulthood. Over time, these habits have a significant influence on health and can affect your risk for future health conditions.

Many of your habits are probably so normal to you that you hardly think about them. Every day, you eat and get some physical activity. What and how much you eat and how much physical activity you get are major factors, however. In this unit, you will learn how these behaviors can set you up for a healthy life.

Open your health management plan. Create a new entry called "My Lifestyle Behaviors." Then, work through these steps to make a plan for developing a healthy lifestyle.

1. Create a chart like the one shown. Then, in each row, write all the decisions you make and actions you take related to each lifestyle area. For example, how many meals do you eat each day? How do you feel about your body? Be specific and write as many actions as you can.
2. For each lifestyle area, create a time line of your life starting now through adulthood and aging. As you read this unit, take notes on your time line showing how the decisions you are making now will affect you in the future.
3. After reading this unit, review your chart and time lines. Are you happy with your lifestyle behaviors and what they mean for your future? Why or why not? For each lifestyle area, write one long-term SMART goal for either changing your behavior or maintaining healthy behaviors over the course of your life. Divide each long-term SMART goal into smaller, short-term SMART goals you can act on now. Keep these goals and commit to put them into action.

Nutrition
Body Image
Physical Activity

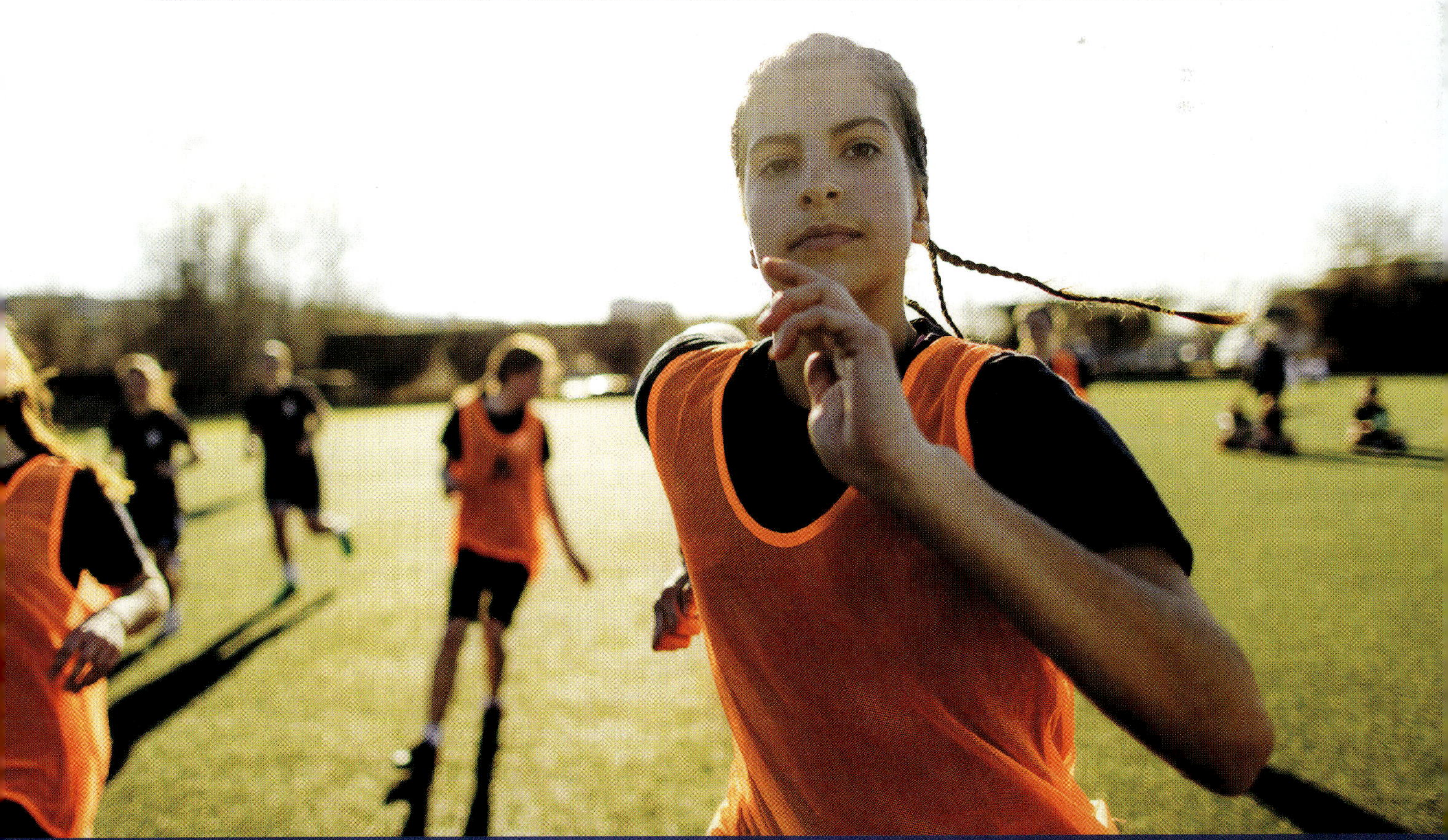

Chapter 8

Following a Healthy Diet

Look for the skills icon throughout this chapter for opportunities to practice your health skills.

Check Your Health and Wellness Skills

In this chapter, you will learn skills for following a healthy diet. To understand the skills you currently use, take the following inventory of your behaviors. Indicate how well you think you use each skill. Use a scale of 1–5, *1* meaning you do not use the skill and *5* meaning you feel completely comfortable using it.

Skill	How Well Do You Use Each Skill?
I drink 11½–15½ cups of fluids each day.	
I use MyPlate to plan how much I should eat from each food group.	
I know how many calories I should be consuming based on my age and level of activity.	
I avoid drinking soda because I know it has empty calories.	
I eat lots of vegetables at lunch and dinner.	
I eat whole-grain bread more often than white bread.	
I eat fresh foods more often than instant or frozen meals.	
I know how to read the information on a Nutrition Facts label.	
I understand why some foods are labeled *organic* or *nonGMO*.	
I wash fruits and vegetables before eating them.	
I avoid fad diets that cut out food groups.	
I keep track of what I eat to help myself maintain a healthy weight.	
	Total:

Add up your responses to each statement. The higher your score, the more comfortable you feel practicing health skills related to following a healthy diet. Which skill do you think is most important for you? Which skill is the most challenging for you? Which skill would you most like to improve? In this chapter, you will learn how to perform these skills better and more often.

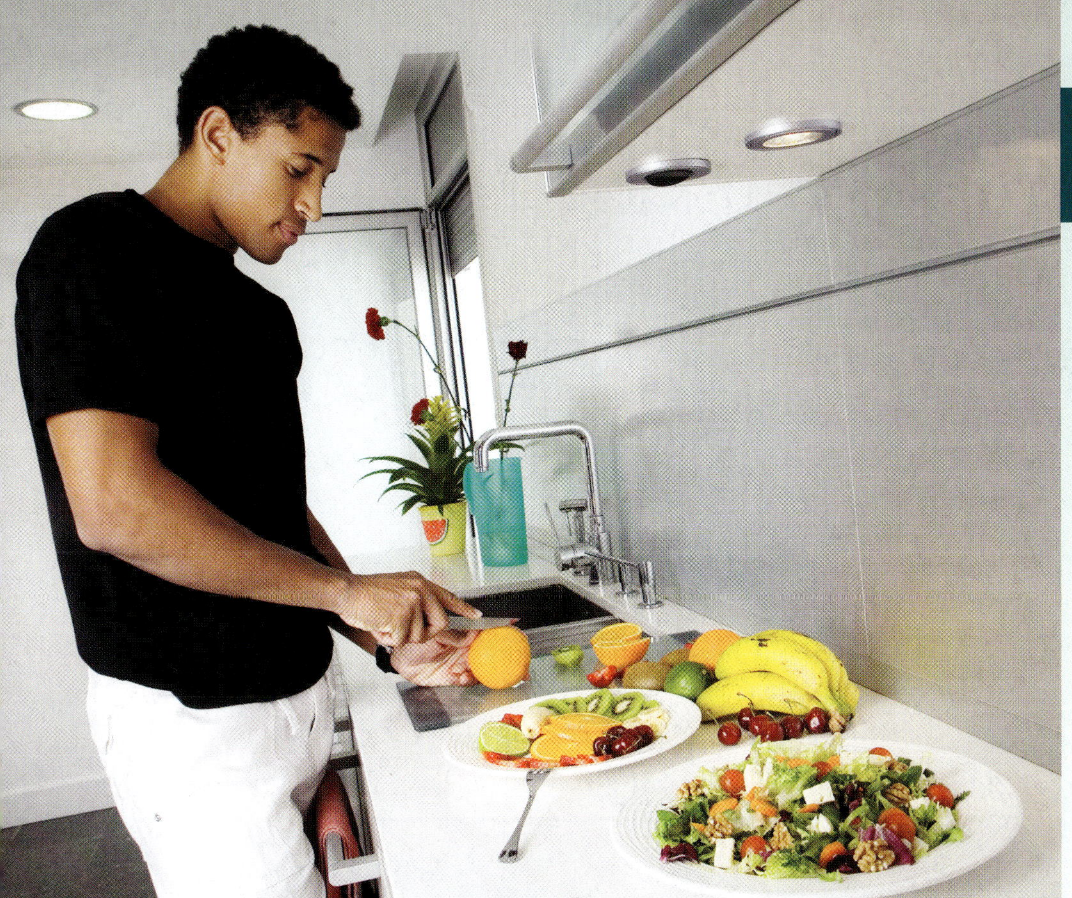

Brosa/E+/Getty Images

Reading and Notetaking

Create a table like the one shown. Include as many rows as you need. Before reading the chapter, list facts you already know about what is included in a healthy diet in the *Give One* column. In the *Get One* column, list facts you learn as you read the chapter. If you have any questions about what you are reading, raise your hand and ask your teacher. After you finish reading the chapter, team up with a classmate and discuss each other's lists. Are there items you would add to your list?

Give One	Get One

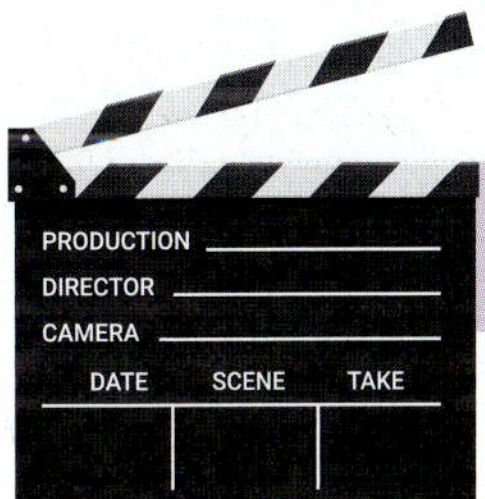

Setting the Scene

Making Nutritious Snack Choices

With your new schedule this year, you eat lunch at school early and are always very hungry at the end of the school day. Some days, you go out with friends after school to get fast food or pizza as a snack. Your older brother suggests bringing along some foods, like chips or a candy bar, to snack on during the day.

Snacking during the day helps, but you worry about eating too many snacks high in saturated fat, sugar, and salt. You have heard these foods are not that good for your health, and eating healthier foods always gives you more energy. You want to make nutritious food choices and keep your body strong, but it is difficult to pack nutritious snacks, and snacks high in fat, sugar, and salt are cheaper.

Thinking Critically

1. What are some factors that might lead high school students to eat foods with little nutritional value?
2. What snacks do you typically eat during the day? How healthy are these snacks? Why?
3. What are some nutritious foods you could snack on when you feel hungry?

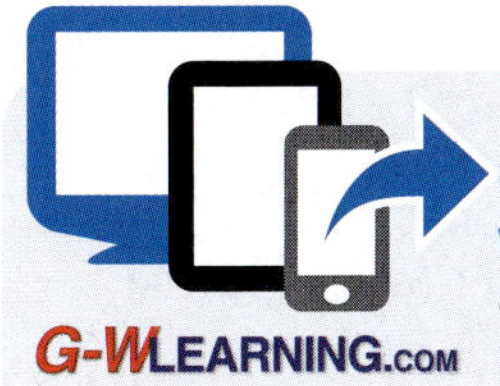

G-WLEARNING.com

Click on the activity icon or visit www.g-wlearning.com/health/4095 to access online vocabulary activities using key terms from the chapter.

Lesson

8.1

What Is Nutrition?

Essential Question?

What nutrients does the body need to function?

Learning Outcomes

After studying this lesson, you will be able to

- define *nutrition*;
- explain how carbohydrates provide energy for the body;
- analyze how to get protein the body needs;
- describe the purpose of fats;
- formulate strategies for consuming vitamins;
- explain why the body needs minerals; and
- assess the importance of water.

Key Terms

carbohydrates
dietary fiber
fats
fat-soluble vitamins
glucose
minerals
nutrients
nutrition
protein
saturated fats
trans fat
unsaturated fats
vitamins
water-soluble vitamins

Warm-Up Activity

The Winning Nutrient

Comprehend Concepts Before reading, fill out a bracket similar to the one shown with key terms from the lesson. To start, skim the chapter to read the definition of each key term. Then, pick a "winner" for each match-up based on which nutrient you think is most important. Write two to three statements expressing why you believe the winner of each match-up is the most important nutrient.

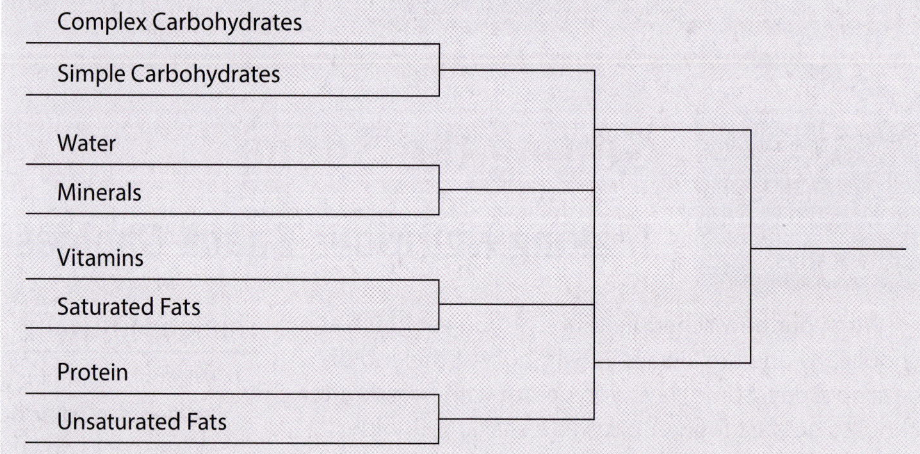

What have you eaten today? Did you eat a nutritious breakfast, such as whole-grain cereal with milk? Did you grab a piece of toast as you raced out the door? Did you skip breakfast completely? Now think about what you ate for lunch. Did you choose a well-balanced meal from the school cafeteria, or did you eat chips you brought from home? Did you skip lunch, planning to grab fast food after school? Although you may not have thought much about the food choices you made today, your diet, or eating pattern, has a major impact on your overall health. Having a healthy eating plan can help you make food choices that benefit your health.

The process of choosing and consuming foods and beverages to fuel your body is **nutrition**. You probably know that foods and beverages are essential to your survival. If you do not eat, you probably start to feel tired and then feel better when you are no longer hungry. This is because foods and beverages contain **nutrients**, chemical substances that give your body what it needs to grow and function.

There are six general types of nutrients. Some provide energy for daily activities. Others enable critical body functions. Nutrition can improve your quality of life and help prevent disease.

nutrition process of choosing and consuming food necessary for health and growth

nutrients chemical substances that provide the nutrition essential for growth, energy, and function

Carbohydrates

Carbohydrates are the body's major source of energy. Fruits, vegetables, grains, and dairy products contain carbohydrates. Carbohydrates are also known as *saccharides* and are either simple or complex. There are three distinct types of carbohydrates: sugar, starch, and dietary fiber.

Sugars include glucose, fructose, lactose, galactose, maltose, and sucrose, which are *simple carbohydrates*. **Glucose** is the body's preferred source of energy that powers your brain and central nervous system. It is the most common sugar found in foods and is usually joined to other sugars. Through the process of digestion, the carbohydrates you eat are broken down to become glucose. Have you ever skipped breakfast and then had trouble concentrating in one of your early classes? Your body running out of glucose causes this (**Figure 8.1**).

Other sugars are found in specific types of food. For example, fructose is sugar that naturally occurs in fruits, and the sugar lactose occurs in dairy products. The table sugar people add to their coffee or use in baking is *sucrose*. This type of sugar is common in processed foods, such as cereal, bread, desserts, and sugar-sweetened beverages. As mentioned earlier, glucose is present in all these foods as well.

carbohydrates nutrients that are the major source of energy for the body; can be found in fruits, vegetables, grains, and dairy products

glucose simple carbohydrate and the preferred source of energy for the brain and central nervous system

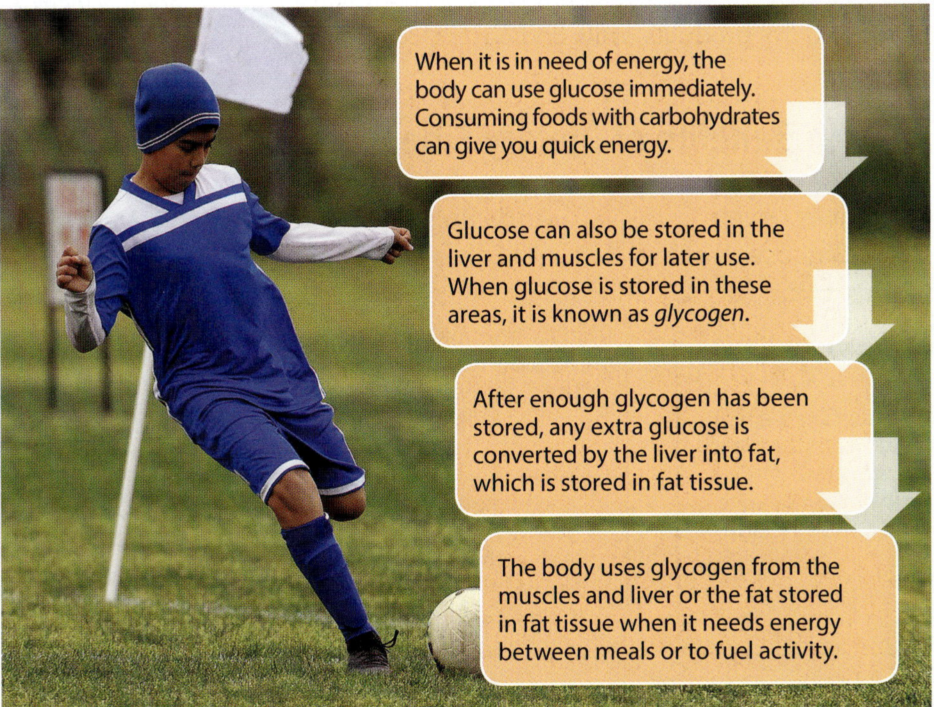

JoeSAPhotos/Shutterstock.com

Figure 8.1 The carbohydrates you eat are broken down to become glucose. ***Which parts of the body are powered by glucose?***

Starches, or chains of glucose linked together, are *complex carbohydrates*. During digestion, your body breaks down starches into smaller glucose units, making the glucose available for energy. Products made from grains, such as bread, cereal, rice, and pasta, are rich sources of starch. Starch is also found in beans and some types of vegetables, including potatoes, peas, and corn.

dietary fiber complex carbohydrate found only in plant-based foods; cannot be completely digested, but has many health benefits

Dietary fiber is a complex carbohydrate that the body cannot completely break down. This type of carbohydrate is found only in plant-based foods, including fruits, most vegetables, whole grains (such as whole-wheat bread or brown rice), and nuts. Although dietary fiber does not provide the body with energy, it has many health benefits (**Figure 8.2**).

Proteins

protein nutrient the body uses to build and maintain cells and tissues and provide energy; may also act as hormones or enzymes

Protein is a nutrient the body uses to build and maintain its cells and tissues, including muscles, bones, skin, hair, fingernails, and other organs. Protein also provides energy. Some proteins act as hormones or *enzymes* (chemicals that cause reactions in the body).

You lose protein when you lose cells—for example, when you brush your hair, shower, trim your fingernails, sweat, and urinate. Since you lose protein every day, you also need to take in protein every day. Though most people in the United States eat more protein than they need, people who do not consume enough protein risk serious consequences. For example, since immune cells are made of protein, individuals who have a protein deficiency are more likely to have weakened immune systems and get infections.

Amino acids make up all types of protein. There are 20 different amino acids, which can join in various combinations. The body produces some amino acids, called *nonessential amino acids*. *Essential amino acids* are not produced by the body in sufficient amounts or at all. You can only get these nine amino acids by eating particular foods.

Protein sources are divided into two types, depending on whether they include all of the essential amino acids. A *complete protein* source contains all nine essential amino acids. Animal-based foods such as meat, poultry, eggs, fish, and dairy products (milk and cheese) are complete protein sources.

Health Benefits of Dietary Fiber

Lowers Cholesterol

Dietary fiber attaches to cholesterol and carries it out of the body during digestion. Cholesterol is a type of fat made by the body and is also present in some foods. Consuming too much cholesterol increases a person's risk of cardiovascular disease, high blood pressure, and stroke.

Balances Level of Glucose

By balancing the level of glucose in the blood, dietary fiber helps control some types of diabetes mellitus.

Adds Bulk to Feces

Dietary fiber maintains the healthy functioning of the digestive system by adding bulk to feces. This prevents issues such as constipation and hemorrhoids (swollen, painful veins in the rectum caused by straining to pass hard feces).

Can Prevent Overeating

Because high-fiber foods take longer to chew, people eating a high-fiber meal tend to eat less. Dietary fiber also slows the movement of food out of your stomach into the intestines. This means you feel full faster.

Figure 8.2 People who do not consume enough fiber may experience several health conditions like hemorrhoids, cardiovascular disease, and diabetes mellitus. ***Can the body digest dietary fiber completely?***

Some plant-based foods, such as soybeans, are also complete protein sources. An *incomplete protein* source lacks one or more essential amino acids. Legumes (dry beans and peas), tofu, nuts and seeds, grains, some vegetables, and some fruits are incomplete protein sources. People must eat a combination of incomplete protein sources to get all nine essential amino acids.

Fats

Fats, a nutrient largely made up of fatty acids, provide a valuable source of energy, particularly for muscles. The fats you consume also play an important role in the absorption and transport of certain vitamins and other nutrients through the bloodstream. Common dietary fats include saturated fats, unsaturated fats, and *trans* fats:

- **Saturated fats** are found primarily in animal-based foods such as meat and dairy products. Saturated fats are typically solid at room temperature.
- **Unsaturated fats** are found in plant-based foods such as vegetable oils, some peanut butters and margarines, olives, salad dressing, nuts, and seeds. Unsaturated fats are liquid at room temperature.
- ***Trans* fats** are created by a process called *hydrogenation*, which makes the fat more saturated and solid. Historically, many processed foods, such as packaged cookies, chips, doughnuts, and crackers, contained this fat. In 2015, the US Food and Drug Administration (FDA) declared that *trans* fats were not *generally recognized as safe (GRAS)*. The FDA gave food companies three years to remove artificial *trans* fats from their food products. Some *trans* fats occur naturally and are found in food from animals, such as cows and goats.

Your body stores the excess calories you consume as *body fat* (**Figure 8.3**). Although fats are important for the body's function, some fats may be better for you than others. Saturated fats are associated with elevated levels of cholesterol in the blood. Eating patterns high in this type of fat may cause long-term health conditions, including cardiovascular disease, stroke, some types of cancer, and type 2 diabetes mellitus.

fats nutrients, largely made up of fatty acids, that provide a valuable source of energy for muscles and help in the absorption and transport of vitamins and nutrients

saturated fats type of fat found primarily in animal-based foods; are typically solid at room temperature

unsaturated fats type of fat found in plant-based foods; are liquid at room temperature

***trans* fat** type of fat historically found in many processed foods; can also occur naturally in animal-based foods

Body Fat
• Supplies energy to the body between meals
• Cushions and protects internal organs
• Insulates your body so you do not get too hot or too cold

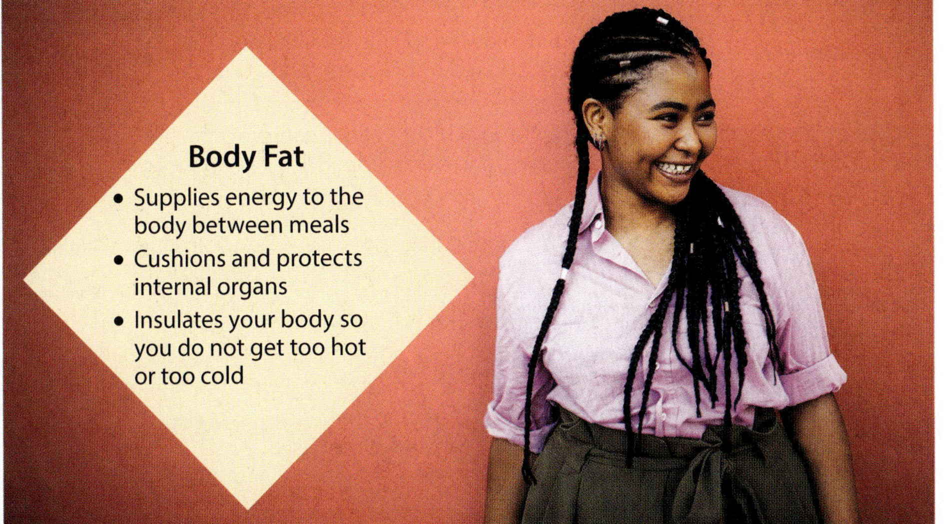

MStudioImages/E+/Getty Images

Figure 8.3 Despite the negative publicity body fat gets, some body fat is important to your body's health.

vitamins organic nutrients that promote growth and development, help regulate body processes, maintain healthy skin, and help the body release energy

Vitamins

Vitamins are organic substances necessary for normal growth and development. They help regulate body processes such as blood clotting, immune system function, and the maintenance of healthy skin. They also help the body release the energy found in proteins, fats, and carbohydrates (**Figure 8.4**).

Your body requires sufficient amounts of 13 different vitamins. Since your body cannot create these vitamins, you need to absorb them from the foods you eat. Unlike carbohydrates, proteins, and fats, your body requires only very small amounts of vitamins to function properly.

Types and Functions of Vitamins		
Fat-Soluble Vitamins		
Vitamin A	Helps fight infection and improve immune function, promotes bone health, supports reproduction, and maintains the health of the retina	Found in some vegetables (carrots, kale, broccoli), dairy products, and meat
Vitamin K	Helps with blood thickening and blood clotting	Found in green leafy vegetables, Brussels sprouts, broccoli, liver, fortified cereal, and cabbage
Vitamin D	Helps the body absorb calcium, which leads to strong teeth and bones; involved in regulation of cell growth, immune function, nervous and muscular function, and reduction of inflammation	Found in fish, egg yolks, fortified dairy products, fortified cereal, and sunlight
Vitamin E	Protects red blood cells from changes caused by oxygen	Found in whole grains, leafy greens, and nuts
Water-Soluble Vitamins		
Vitamin B_1 (Thiamin)	Helps the body change carbohydrates into energy	Found in pork, legumes, enriched or whole-grain products, and cereal
Vitamin B_2 (Riboflavin)	Aids in metabolism	Found in milk, cheese, leafy vegetables, liver, kidney, legumes, tomatoes, mushrooms, and almonds
Vitamin B_3 (Niacin)	Helps maintain healthy skin and nerves and improves circulation	Found in eggs, lean meats, nuts, poultry, legumes, avocado, and potatoes
Vitamin B_5 (Pantothenic acid)	Helps the body use nutrients for energy	Found in beef and chicken liver, potatoes, sunflower seeds, cooked mushrooms, and yogurt
Vitamin B_6 (Pyridoxine)	Aids in the reactions that generate energy from food; is required for proper development of the brain, nerves, and skin	Found in avocado, banana, meat, nuts, poultry, and whole grains
Vitamin B_7 (Biotin)	Assists with metabolism and the production of hormones and cholesterol	Found in milk, nuts, pork, egg yolk, and chocolate
Vitamin B_9 (Folic acid)	Is essential to numerous body functions, including cell division and the growth and production of healthy red blood cells	Found in leafy vegetables, fortified cereal, and bread
Vitamin B_{12} (Cyanocobalamin)	Helps form red blood cells, maintain the central nervous system, and regulate metabolism	Found in meat, eggs, dairy products, poultry, and shellfish
Vitamin C	Promotes healing within the body; is essential for healthy teeth and gums and the production of collagen	Found in citrus fruits and many vegetables (broccoli, cabbage, spinach, and tomatoes)

Figure 8.4 Different vitamins have distinct functions in the body. ***How many vitamins does a human body require?***

There are two types of vitamins: water-soluble vitamins and fat-soluble vitamins. **Water-soluble vitamins** dissolve in water, pass into the bloodstream during digestion, and are used immediately by the body or removed by the kidneys during urination. **Fat-soluble vitamins** dissolve in the body's fats and can be stored in the body for later use.

Obtaining vitamins from your daily eating pattern is preferable to taking vitamin supplements. This is because vitamin supplements do not contain all of the nutrients and other substances your body needs. For example, some substances in food help your body better use vitamins. Vitamin supplements may also provide larger-than-needed doses of vitamins, which can cause unhealthy levels in the body and create waste.

When deciding whether to take a vitamin supplement, consult your doctor. Also be aware that the FDA does not test supplements for safety and effectiveness before manufacturers can sell them.

water-soluble vitamins type of vitamin that dissolves in water; are used immediately by the body or removed during urination

fat-soluble vitamins type of vitamin that dissolves in the body's fats and can be stored for later use

Minerals

Minerals are inorganic elements absorbed by plants from soil and water. Your body needs different minerals to grow and develop normally (**Figure 8.5**). *Major minerals,* or *macrominerals,* are minerals your body needs in quantities greater than 100 milligrams each day. *Trace minerals* are minerals your body needs in very small amounts—less than 100 milligrams daily.

Failing to take in enough of a mineral can lead to negative health consequences. For example, a lack of calcium during childhood and adolescence can lead to *osteoporosis,* a condition in which bones become fragile and break easily. Not consuming enough iron can cause *anemia,*

minerals inorganic nutrients absorbed from plants, water, and animal food sources

Types and Functions of Minerals

Major Minerals		
Calcium	Is necessary for muscle, heart, and digestive system health; builds bone and supports the synthesis and function of blood cells	Found in dairy products, eggs, canned fish with bones (salmon, sardines), green leafy vegetables, nuts, seeds, and tofu
Phosphorus	Is present in bones and cells; assists with energy processing and other functions	Found in red meat, dairy products, fish, poultry, bread, rice, and oats
Magnesium	Contributes to bone health; required for several body processes, such as regulation of blood sugar and immune response	Found in raw nuts, soybeans, spinach, chard, tomatoes, and beans
Sulfur	Promotes metabolism and communication between nerve cells; helps the body resist bacteria and protect against toxic substances	Found in meat, fish, poultry, eggs, milk, and legumes
Sodium	Helps maintain normal blood pressure; regulates the body's fluid balance	Found in table salt (sodium chloride), milk, and bread
Chloride	Assists with maintaining proper amount of body fluids	Found in table salt
Potassium	Assists with heart function, skeletal and muscle contraction, and digestive function	Found in legumes, potato skin, tomatoes, bananas, papayas, lentils, dry beans, whole grains, yams, and soybeans

(Continued)

Figure 8.5 Your body takes in minerals by consuming plants, water, or animal food sources that have absorbed the minerals. ***What health condition can result from a deficit in iron?***

Types and Functions of Minerals		
Trace Minerals		
Iron	Carries oxygen from the lungs to the body's other tissues	Found in red meat, leafy green vegetables, fish (tuna, salmon), eggs, dried fruits, beans, whole grains, and enriched grains
Zinc	Assists with immune function, reproduction, and nervous system functions	Found in beef, pork, lamb, nuts, and whole grains
Iodine	Assists with making thyroid hormones	Found in table salt, some types of fish (cod, sea bass, perch, haddock), and dairy products
Selenium	Protects cells from damage and regulates thyroid hormone action and other processes	Found in vegetables, fish, red meat, grains, eggs, and chicken
Copper	Assists with metabolism and red blood cell formation; helps with the production of energy for cells	Found in shellfish, whole grains, beans, nuts, potatoes, dried fruits, and cocoa
Manganese	Assists with bone formation, metabolism, and wound healing	Found in nuts, legumes, seeds, whole grains, tea, and leafy green vegetables
Fluoride	Prevents dental cavities and stimulates new bone formation	Found in fluoridated water, most seafood, tea, and gelatin
Chromium	Helps maintain normal blood sugar (glucose) levels	Found in beef, liver, eggs, chicken, apples, bananas, spinach, and green peppers
Molybdenum	Helps process proteins and other substances	Found in legumes, grains, leafy vegetables, liver, and nuts

a condition characterized by weakness, fatigue, and headaches. A lack of iodine during pregnancy can result in *cretinism*, a severe disorder characterized by low functioning of the thyroid. A healthy and balanced eating pattern is the best way to provide your body with all the minerals it needs.

Water

Water is necessary for most body functions. In fact, although people can live for several weeks or months without taking in food, they can survive only a few days without water. Water maintains your body temperature, cushions and lubricates joints, and protects the spinal cord and other sensitive tissues. It also gets rid of waste (through urination, perspiration, and bowel movements) and moves oxygen, nutrients, waste, and other materials throughout the body.

Because your body loses water every day through urination, sweat, and even exhalation, you need to consume water to replace what your body loses. Not consuming enough water can lead to *dehydration*, a condition in which the body's tissues lose too much water. Without enough water, the body cannot cool itself, and blood pressure can drop dangerously low as water leaves the blood (**Figure 8.6**).

Fluid needs can change. For instance, people who are pregnant or breastfeeding have increased fluid requirements. Infants also have a greater need for fluids. The body needs more water when a person is outside in hot weather for a long period of time, engaging in vigorous physical activity, running a fever, or experiencing diarrhea or vomiting. Feeling thirsty is a signal that your body needs more water. If possible, drink enough water that you do not get thirsty.

Individuals should drink 11½–15½ cups (2.7 to 3.7 liters) of fluids per day.

Drinking water and other beverages can meet most of your water needs. You can also get some fluids through the foods you eat, like broth soups. Foods such as celery, tomatoes, apples, oranges, and melons also have high water content.

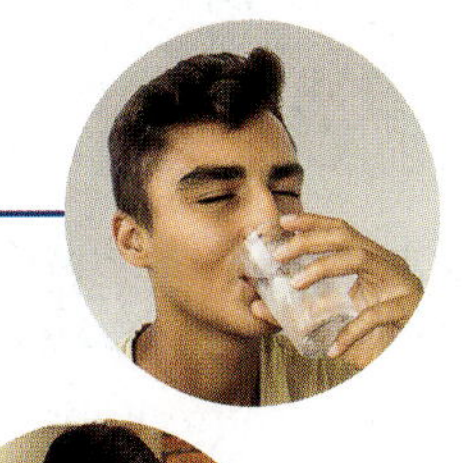

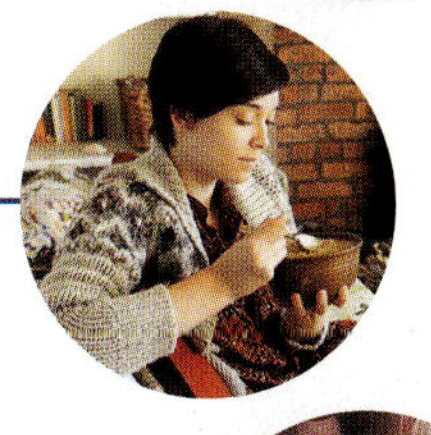

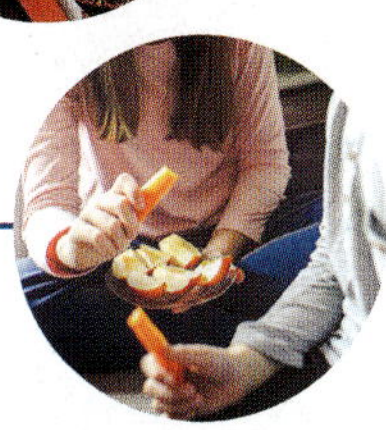

Top to bottom: Ismailciydem/iStock/Getty Images Plus/Getty Images; omgimages/iStock/Getty Images Plus/Getty Images; mixetto/iStock/Getty Images Plus/Getty Images

Figure 8.6 According to the National Academies of Science, Engineering, and Medicine, most people need 11½ to 15½ cups (2.7 to 3.7 liters) of fluids on an average day. They can get fluids through water, other beverages, and foods.

Lesson 8.1 Review

Know and Understand

1. In your own words, define *nutrition*.
2. What is the primary purpose of carbohydrates?
3. Explain the difference between complete and incomplete protein sources.
4. Why is having some body fat important for health?
5. Why is it more dangerous to consume too much of a fat-soluble vitamin than to consume too much of a water-soluble vitamin?

Think Critically

6. Go to a grocery store or examine the food in your home. Which foods are highest in fiber? To find the fiber content of foods that do not have Nutrition Facts labels, use an online nutrient database. Share your observations with the class.
7. With a partner, list as many examples of saturated and unsaturated fats as you can. Which of these fats do you consume on a regular basis?
8. Choose one vitamin or mineral and research how a deficiency in this nutrient could affect health.
9. How much water do you drink on a daily basis? What other beverages and foods with water content do you consume? Are you consuming the recommended amount of fluids each day?

REAL WORLD Health Skills

Make Decisions List the 10 foods you eat most frequently. Next to each food, indicate whether it contains many or few nutrients. For any foods that have few nutrients, suggest two healthier options you could decide to eat instead. Explain why each decision is healthier using information from the lesson, or do your own research to justify your response.

Lesson

8.2

Establishing a Healthy Eating Pattern

Essential Question

What guidelines can help you get the nutrients you need?

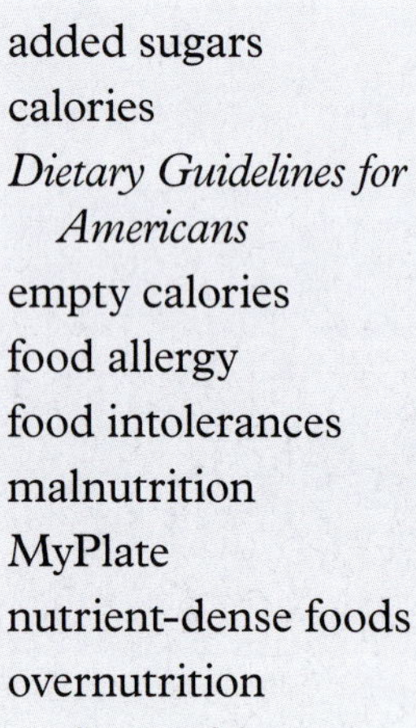

Key Terms

added sugars
calories
Dietary Guidelines for Americans
empty calories
food allergy
food intolerances
malnutrition
MyPlate
nutrient-dense foods
overnutrition
undernutrition

Learning Outcomes

After studying this lesson, you will be able to

- interpret key concepts from the *Dietary Guidelines for Americans*;
- summarize recommendations from the MyPlate food guidance system;
- demonstrate skills for following a healthy eating pattern;
- assess nutrition for people with varying needs; and
- analyze the hazards of poor nutrition.

Warm-Up Activity

Portion Sizes

Practice Health-Enhancing Behaviors Many teens underestimate how much food they eat in a given meal. Analyze the difference between serving sizes and portion sizes, such as those shown in the samples below. Then, identify three strategies to reduce portion sizes to the actual recommended serving sizes. Explain the benefits of eating recommended serving sizes and the dangers of eating too-large portion sizes.

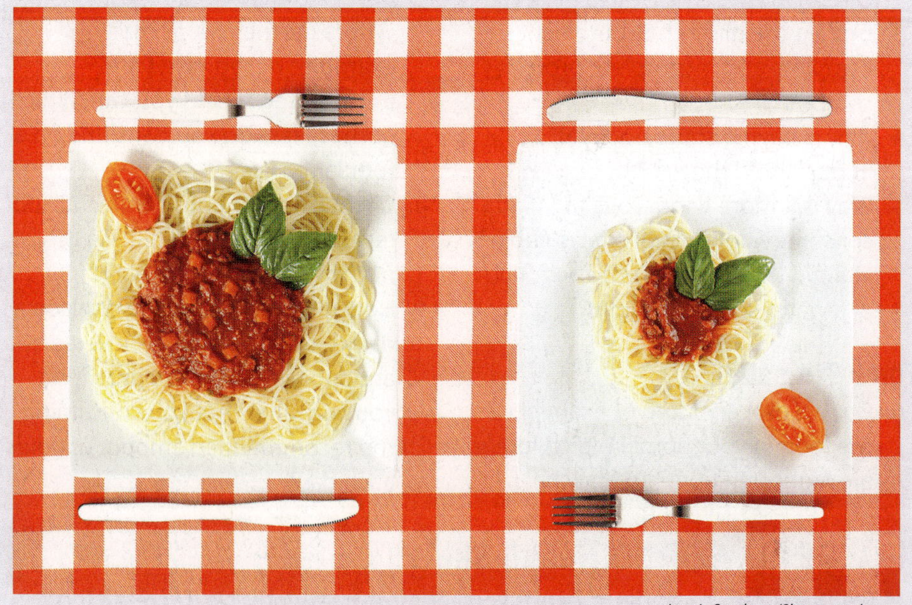

Jose L. Stephens/Shutterstock.com

When you eat nutritious foods today, you lower your risk of developing diseases and health conditions later in life. People who follow a healthy eating plan and maintain a healthy body weight are less likely to develop cardiovascular disease, high blood pressure, type 2 diabetes mellitus, stroke, and cancer. A healthy eating pattern also prevents health conditions such as obesity, cavities, iron deficiency, and osteoporosis.

Overall, the body needs about 45 different nutrients per day. This is why a varied eating pattern full of nutritious foods is important for maintaining good health. A healthy eating pattern includes foods that supply the amounts and types of nutrients your body needs to be healthy. In this lesson, you will learn how to make smart food choices and create a balanced eating pattern. You will also learn about the hazards of poor nutrition.

Guidelines for a Nutritionally Balanced Eating Pattern

Knowing which nutrients your body needs and in what amounts will help you get adequate nutrition. Several sets of guidelines exist to help people make healthy food choices. For example, the US Department of Agriculture (USDA) and the US Department of Health and Human Services (HHS) publish the ***Dietary Guidelines for Americans***, which is revised every five years. The *Dietary Guidelines for Americans* provides recommended dietary allowances (RDAs) for certain nutrients and recommendations for establishing eating patterns to promote health (**Figure 8.7**).

Dietary Guidelines for Americans guidelines published by the USDA and HHS that provide recommendations for establishing eating patterns to promote health

Key Recommendations of the *Dietary Guidelines for Americans*

- Follow a healthy eating pattern across the life span.
- Focus on variety, nutrient density, and amount.
- Limit added sugars, saturated fats, and sodium.
- Shift to healthier food and beverage choices.
- Support healthy eating patterns for all.

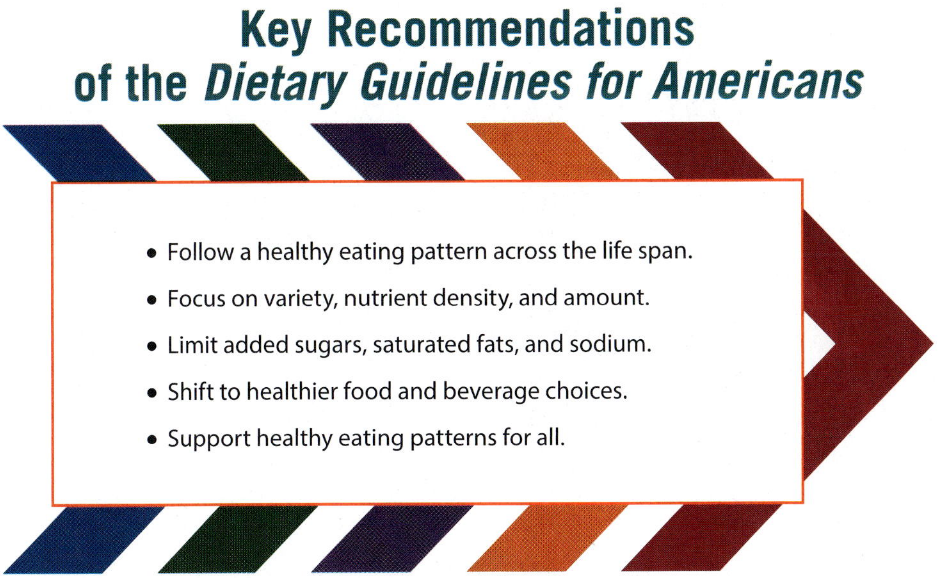

Figure 8.7 The five main recommendations in the *Dietary Guidelines for Americans* help people establish and maintain healthy eating patterns. ***Which government agencies publish the* Dietary Guidelines for Americans?**

MyPlate food guidance system created by the USDA; reminds people about the proportions of the five different food groups they should eat at a meal

In 2011, the USDA created the **MyPlate** food guidance system to help individuals put the *Dietary Guidelines for Americans* into practice (**Figure 8.8**). The MyPlate system includes five food groups:

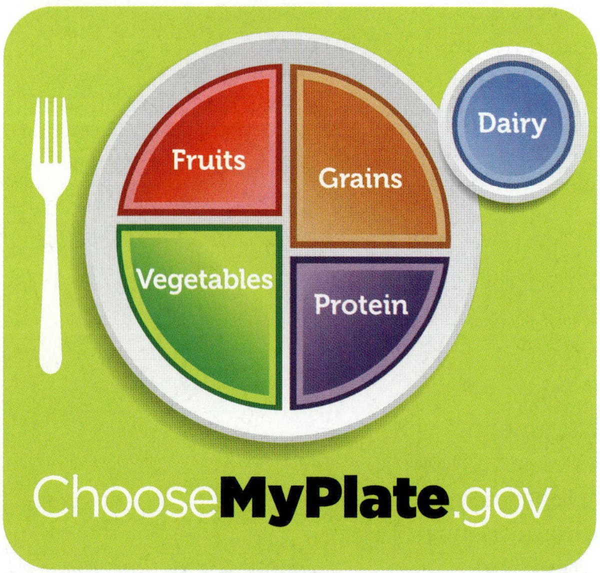

Courtesy of the United States Department of Agriculture

Figure 8.8 The MyPlate graphic is designed to remind people about the proportion of different foods they should eat at a meal.

- **Fruits:** Foods in the fruit group are good sources of potassium, fiber, vitamin C, and folic acid. Fresh, frozen, canned, and dried fruits, as well as 100 percent fruit juices, are in this group.
- **Grains:** This group includes foods made from wheat, rice, oats, cornmeal, barley, or other cereal grains. Whole grains are an important source of fiber and many other nutrients. A food is considered *whole grain* if it contains the entire grain kernel—the bran, germ, and endosperm (**Figure 8.9**). Examples of whole grains include brown rice, oatmeal, whole-wheat bread, and wild rice. *Refined grains*, such as couscous, crackers, and white bread, have been processed to produce a finer texture and improved shelf life, so they no longer contain the whole kernel.

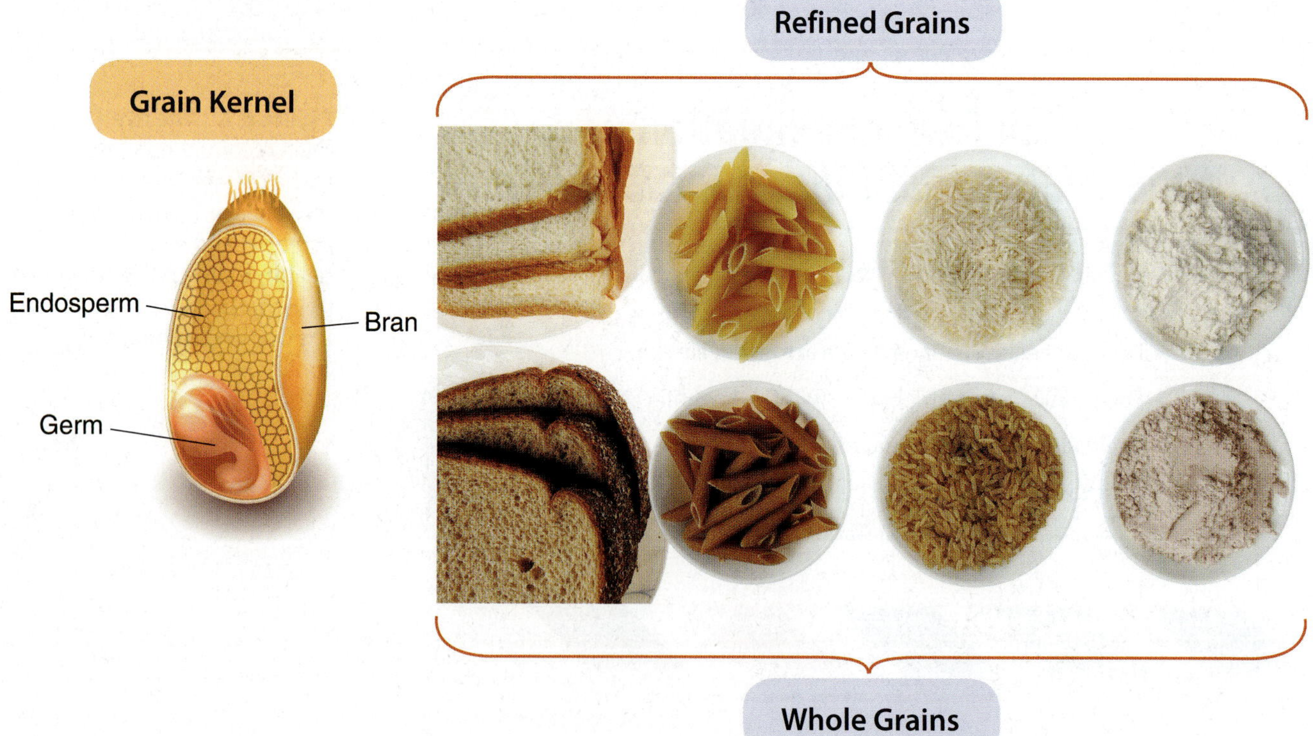

Grain kernel: Tefi/Shutterstock.com; Grains: Ami Parikh/Shutterstock.com

Figure 8.9 The *Dietary Guidelines for Americans* recommends that people make at least one-half of the grains they consume whole grains.

- **Vegetables:** Most vegetables are naturally low in fat and calories and are important sources of many nutrients, including potassium, fiber, folic acid, and vitamins A and C. Vegetables may be fresh, frozen, canned, dried, raw, cooked, whole, cut up, or juiced. They are divided into five subgroups (**Figure 8.10**).
- **Dairy:** The dairy group includes many foods that are high in calcium, including milk and foods made from milk such as cheese and yogurt. This group does not include foods such as cream and butter, which are made from milk, but contain little calcium. Calcium-fortified soy, almond, and rice milk are included in this dairy group as options for those who choose not to consume foods derived from milk. Dairy foods are often good sources of potassium and protein and are frequently fortified with vitamin D.
- **Protein foods:** Protein foods include meat, poultry, seafood, beans, peas, eggs, processed soy products, nuts, and seeds. Foods in this group may also supply niacin, thiamin, riboflavin, vitamin B_6, vitamin E, iron, zinc, and magnesium. Some seafood, such as salmon or tuna, contains fats believed to reduce the risk of cardiovascular disease. Plant-based proteins are often rich in fiber. Try to include at least 8 ounces (227 grams) of cooked seafood in your meal plan each week.

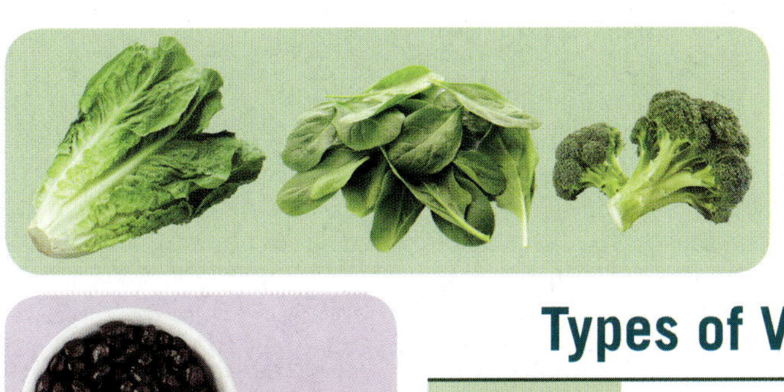
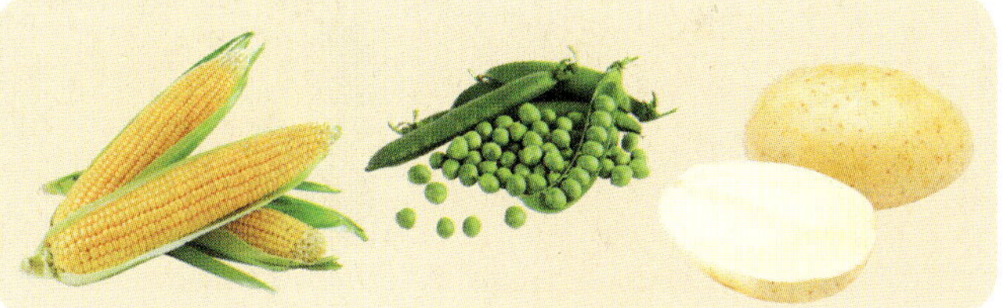
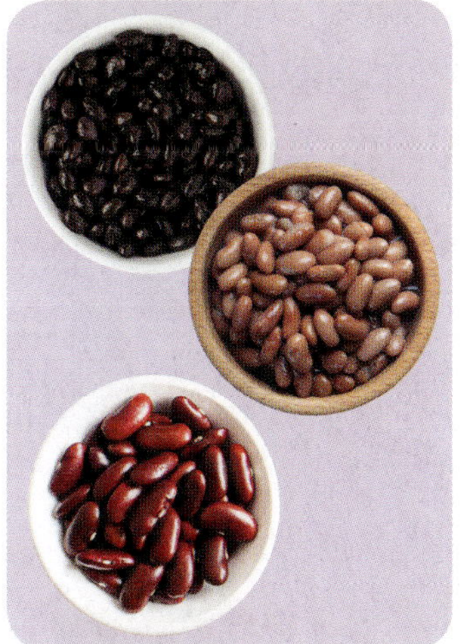

Types of Vegetables

Dark Green	Spinach, broccoli, kale, and dark green and romaine lettuce
Starchy	White potatoes, green peas, and corn
Red and Orange	Carrots, tomatoes, red peppers, and squash
Beans and Peas	Split peas, black beans, pinto beans, and kidney beans
Other	Green peppers, cucumbers, cauliflower, mushrooms, onions, and zucchini

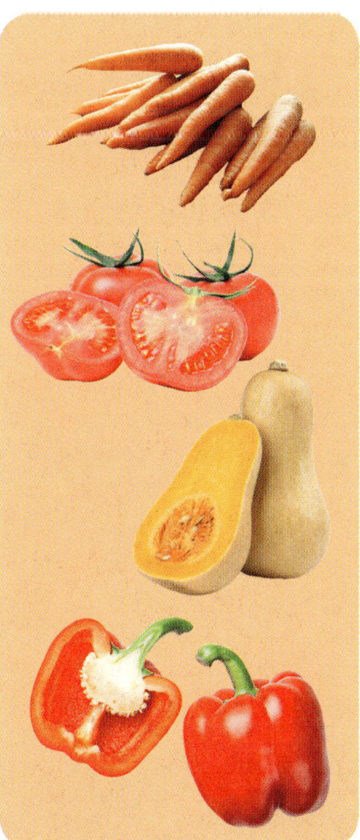
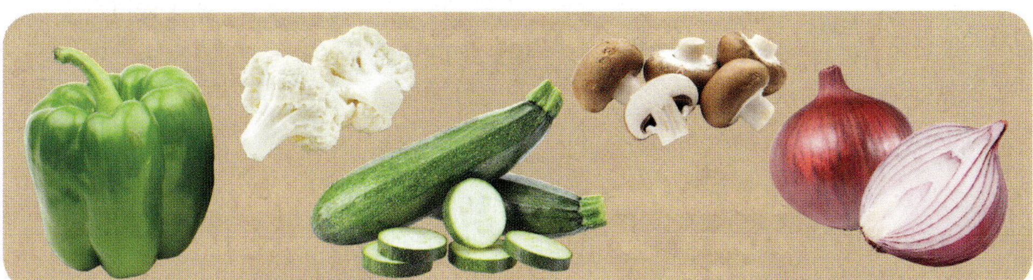

Clockwise from top left: Danny Smythe/Shutterstock.com; Pixel-Shot/Shutterstock.com; Nik Merkulov/Shutterstock.com; Maks Narodenko/Shutterstock.com; morgenstjerne/Shutterstock.com; PhotoStk/Shutterstock.com; 5 second Studio/Shutterstock.com; jiangdi/Shutterstock.com; spixiax/Shutterstock.com; Bozena Fulawka/Shutterstock.com; Kelenart/Shutterstock.com; Gita Kulinitch Studio/Shutterstock.com; SOMMAI/Shutterstock.com; PixaHub/Shutterstock.com; JIANG HONGYAN/Shutterstock.com; Jit-anong Sae-ung/Shutterstock.com; Igor Dutina/Shutterstock.com; Natalia Wimberley/Shutterstock.com

Figure 8.10 People should attempt to consume vegetables from each of these subgroups every week.

- **Oils:** Though they are not considered a food group, oils provide essential nutrients and must be included in your eating plan. Oils are naturally present in many plants and fish. Often, oil is extracted from a food source, such as olives, and sold as liquid oil. Avocados, nuts, and some fish (for example, salmon, mackerel, and trout) are also common sources of oils.

The MyPlate food guidance system provides tools to help you develop a personalized eating plan (**Figure 8.11**). The amount of food you need from each food group is affected by your age, biological sex, height, weight, and level of physical activity. Other factors such as health conditions, pregnancy, and lactation can affect your nutrient needs as well.

Figure 8.11 The MyPlate daily eating plan outlines the amounts a person should consume from each food group and provides information for making nutritious choices. This plan is for someone 14 years of age or older with a 2,000-calorie diet. ***What factors determine the amount of food you need from each food group?***

MyPlate Eating Plan

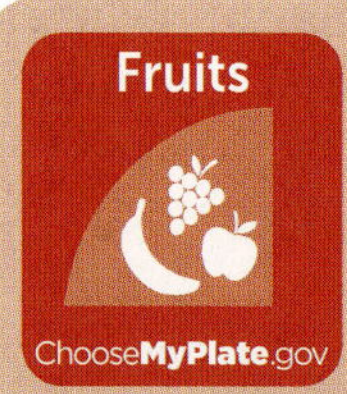

2 cups Fruit

- 1 cup counts as 1 cup raw, frozen, cooked/canned, or fruit juice or ½ cup dried fruit.

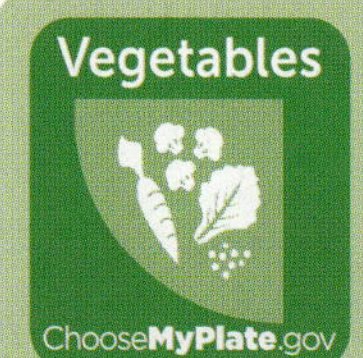

2.5 cups Vegetables

- 1 cup counts as 1 cup raw, frozen, cooked/canned, or vegetable juice or 2 cups leafy salad greens.

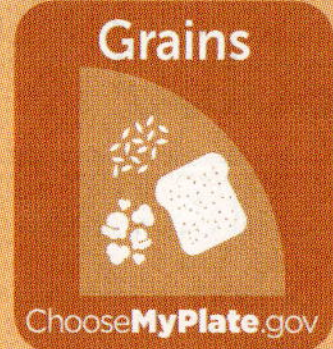

6 ounces Grains

- 1 ounce counts as 1 slice bread, 1 ounce ready-to-eat cereal, or ½ cup cooked rice, pasta, or cereal.

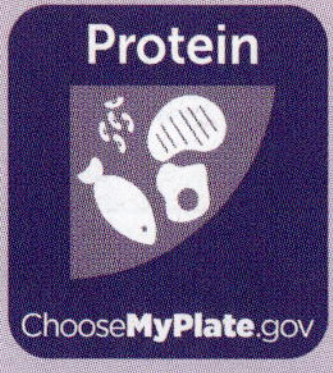

5.5 ounces Protein Foods

- 1 ounce counts as 1 ounce cooked/canned lean meats, poultry, or seafood, 1 egg, 1 Tbsp peanut butter, ¼ cup cooked beans or peas, or ½ ounce nuts or seeds.

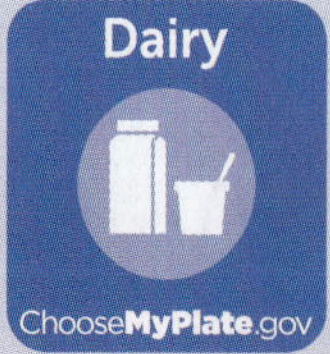

3 cups Dairy

- 1 cup counts as 1 cup milk, yogurt, or fortified soy beverage, 1½ ounces natural cheese, or 2 ounces processed cheese.

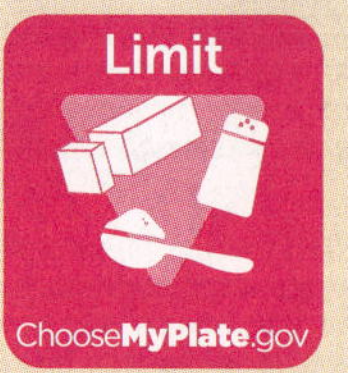

Less sodium, saturated fat, and added sugars

- Limit to 2,200 milligrams of sodium, 22 grams of saturated fat, and 50 grams of added sugars a day.

Courtesy of the United States Department of Agriculture

Skills for Following a Healthy Eating Pattern

A healthy eating pattern provides all the nutrients you need and avoids nutritional excesses that can be harmful to your health. The requirements for a healthy eating pattern change across a person's life span. As a teen, you have different nutritional needs now than you did when you were a child. People who are pregnant or breastfeeding have unique nutritional needs to ensure their health and the health of their babies. Your nutritional needs will also change as you grow older.

Pay Attention to Calorie Balance

Following a healthy eating pattern involves consuming the appropriate number of **calories**, or units of energy in food. Foods that provide larger amounts of energy are higher in calories than foods that provide smaller amounts of energy. The number of calories you need changes over time and is affected by your biological sex, height, weight, and level of physical activity (**Figure 8.12**). Some types of nutrients provide more calories than others. Carbohydrates and protein each provide 4 calories per gram. Fat provides 9 calories per gram, more than any other source.

Recommended Daily Calorie Intake

	Male/Moderately Active	Female/Moderately Active
Age	**Calories**	
10	1,800	1,800
11	2,000	1,800
12	2,200	2,000
13	2,200	2,000
14	2,400	2,000
15	2,600	2,000
16–18	2,800	2,000
19–25	2,800	2,200
26–45	2,600	2,000
46–50	2,400	2,000
51–65	2,400	1,800

Figure 8.12 The recommended calorie intake also changes if you are more or less than moderately active on most days. ***How many calories per gram do carbohydrates, fat, and protein provide?***

calories units of energy in food

Together, the number of calories you consume and the number of calories you burn are called your *calorie balance*. Your calorie balance in a given day depends on the number of calories you

- consume through eating and drinking (this is energy *in* to your body)
- burn through body processes such as breathing, digesting, and growing and your daily physical activities (this is energy *out* of your body)

Your body burns calories to perform the many functions that keep you alive, such as eating, sleeping, and breathing. You also burn calories in the course of daily life—while walking to class, lifting a heavy backpack, and cleaning your room. When your calorie balance is equal (you consume as many calories as you use), you have the energy you need to carry out daily activities and maintain your current weight. You will learn more about calorie balance and weight later in this chapter.

nutrient-dense foods foods that provide vitamins, minerals, and other substances that either contribute to adequate nutrition intake or have positive health effects; contain little or no saturated fats, added sugars, refined starches, and sodium

Choose Nutrient-Dense Foods

A healthy eating pattern includes a variety of nutrient-dense foods in appropriate amounts. **Nutrient-dense foods** are foods that provide vitamins, minerals, and other substances that either contribute to adequate nutrient intake or have positive health effects. Nutrient-dense foods have little or no saturated fats, **added sugars** (sugars that do not occur naturally in foods), refined starches, or sodium (salt).

added sugars sugars that do not occur naturally in foods

empty calories units of energy that supply few or no nutrients to the body

Nutrient-dense foods often have the same calorie content as foods that are not nutrient dense. The difference is that you consume more nutrients for the number of calories in the food. For example, your body gets more nutrients when you eat an apple than when you drink a soda, even though both choices provide 100 calories (**Figure 8.13**). The can of sugary soda contains **empty calories**, or calories that supply few, if any, nutrients to the body. It is best to avoid empty calories, even in foods that have some nutritional value. For example, the most common pizza choices supply needed nutrients, but also contain many empty calories from saturated fats. A more nutrient-dense option might be vegetable pizza with whole-grain crust.

To include more nutrient-dense foods in your eating pattern, use the following guidelines:

- Eat more fruits and vegetables. Try to eat two vegetables (dark green, red, or orange vegetables especially) with your evening meal or have a piece of fruit for dessert. Try making a meal around dried beans or peas (legumes) instead of meat. Substitute pinto or black beans for meat in chili and tacos.
- Choose whole fruits and vegetables more often than fruit and vegetable juices or sauces. Whole fruits and vegetables contain more nutrients. For example, apples with their skins have more fiber than applesauce or apple juice. Whole fruits and vegetables also contain fewer empty calories.
- Eat whole grains more often than refined grains. Whole grains contain dietary fiber and many other nutrients not present in refined grains. The *Dietary Guidelines for Americans* recommends making at least one-half of the grains you consume whole grains. Try substituting whole-grain flour for up to half of the flour in pancake, waffle, and other recipes. You can also choose whole-grain, unsweetened cereal or oatmeal for breakfast.
- Avoid adding empty calories during food preparation. Fried foods, for example, have more empty calories than baked or raw foods because they absorb oil or butter during frying. A grilled chicken leg has 60 calories, whereas a fried chicken leg has 130 calories.

A 100-Calorie Snack
The calories in apples mostly come from naturally occurring sugars.
This snack also supplies fiber, vitamins, and minerals.
Medium Apple
8-Ounce Soda
The calories in soda come from added sugars. This portion has 6 teaspoons of sugar.
This drink has little to no nutritional value.

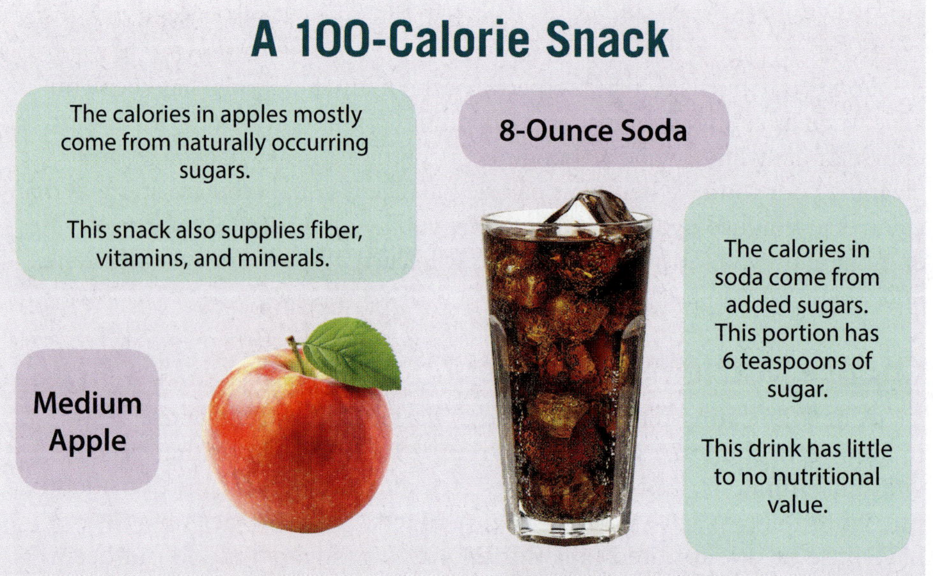

Figure 8.13 When choosing a snack, consider both calories and nutritional value. ***What kind of calories are found in a snack like soda?***

Apple: Dionisvera/Shutterstock.com; Soda: M. Unal Ozmen/Shutterstock.com

Limit Added Sugars, Saturated Fats, and Sodium

Calories from added sugars and saturated fats contribute up to 40 percent of daily calories for children and teens in the US. Approximately one-half of those calories come from six sources: soda, fruit drinks, dairy desserts (such as cheesecake or ice cream), grain desserts (such as cookies or cake), pizza (with meat), and whole milk. According to the *Dietary Guidelines for Americans*, people should limit their intake of added sugars and saturated fats. People should consume less than 10 percent of their calories from added sugars and less than 10 percent of their calories from saturated fats. Consuming more than these recommendations can increase risk for cardiovascular diseases, obesity, and type 2 diabetes mellitus.

People should also limit sodium intake to no more than 2,300 milligrams per day and ideally no more than 1,500 milligrams. To compare, most people in the US, including many teens, consume more than 3,400 milligrams each day. Consuming too much sodium can have health consequences such as high blood pressure and an increased risk of cardiovascular disease and stroke.

Figure 8.14 lists ways you can substitute common foods with foods that are more nutrient dense and contain fewer added sugars, saturated fats, and sodium. To limit your intake of added sugars, saturated fats, and sodium, you can also use the following guidelines:

- When consuming dairy products, choose low-fat or nonfat products. For example, you could drink reduced-fat milk instead of whole milk or use nonfat plain yogurt instead of sour cream.
- Drink water or other unsweetened drinks instead of sugar-sweetened beverages.
- Eat fresh, frozen, and dried fruits if you crave something sweet. Choose fruits canned in water rather than sugary syrup.
- Instead of adding sugar to oatmeal or cereal, use fruit to add sweetness. In some recipes, you can also reduce the amount of sugar or substitute sugar with certain extracts or unsweetened applesauce.
- Limit sauces, mixes, and instant or processed noodles, pastas, cereal, and rice.
- Choose fresh meats, seafood, and poultry rather than processed versions like bacon, hot dogs, or lunch meat.
- Select cuts of meat and poultry that are lean or low-fat more often. Trim away any fat you can see on the cut. For chicken and turkey, remove the skin to reduce fat. When preparing meats, bake, broil, or grill them instead of frying them.

Making Healthier Food Choices

Less Healthy Choice	Healthier Alternative
Whole milk 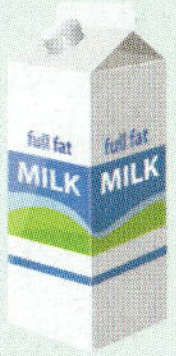	Fat-free (skim) milk 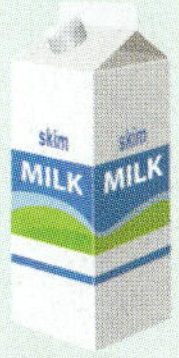
Deep-dish pepperoni pizza 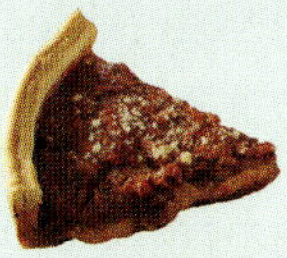	Thin, whole-grain crust veggie pizza 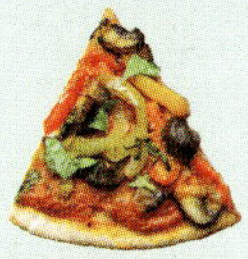
Fried egg rolls or wontons 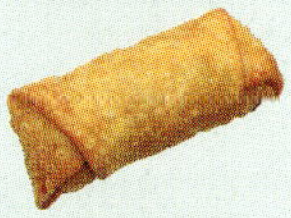	Steamed spring rolls 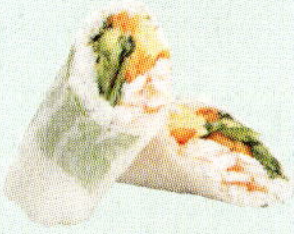
Soups made with cream or coconut milk 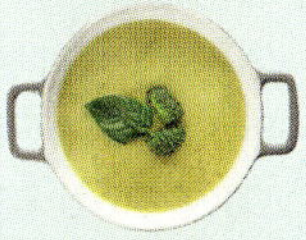	Broth-based soups or soups made with low-fat yogurt 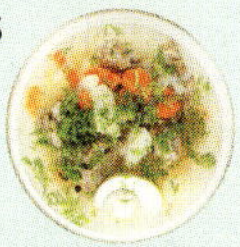
Chorizo (sausage) 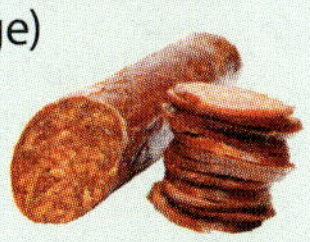	Picadillo (lean ground beef, vegetables, and spices) 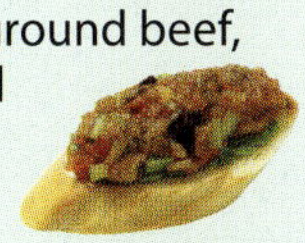
Regular margarine or butter 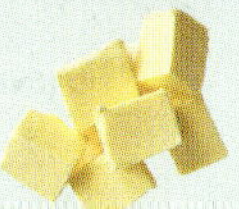	Light spread margarines or olive oil 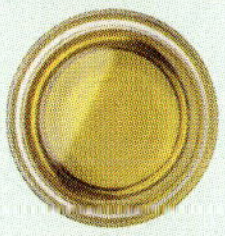
Falafel (fried chickpea cakes) 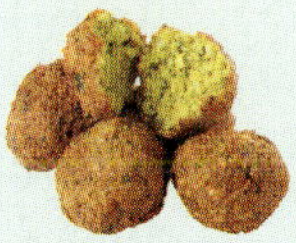	Hummus 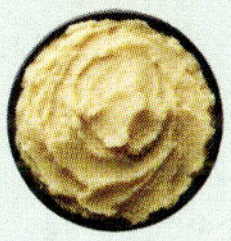

Left column, top to bottom: Netta007/Shutterstock.com; Brent Hofacker/Shutterstock.com; Duplass/Shutterstock.com; Africa Studio/Shutterstock.com; Anatolii Riepin/Shutterstock.com; Rutina/Shutterstock.com; AS Food studio/Shutterstock.com
Right column, top to bottom: Netta007/Shutterstock.com; Olga Nayashkova/Shutterstock.com; margouillat photo/Shutterstock.com; Iakov Filimonov/Shutterstock.com; photokin/Shutterstock.com; Anton Starikov/Shutterstock.com; baibaz/Shutterstock.com

Figure 8.14 Try to include foods with more healthy ingredients or that are prepared in healthier ways. ***What preparation methods are healthier than frying or deep-frying?***

Eat Breakfast Every Day

Eating a nutritious breakfast every day is very important. People need a morning meal to give them energy. Breakfast does more than provide energy for people's bodies, however. It also provides the nutrients people's brains need to learn and grow. Eating breakfast every day is especially important for people who have difficulty getting enough nutrients.

To put together a nutritious breakfast, use whole grains, lean protein foods (like eggs, lean meat, or nuts), low-fat dairy products, and fruits and vegetables. For example, you might make a smoothie, oatmeal with fruit, or a whole-grain tortilla with vegetables and salsa. If consuming cereal, look for cereal that is high in fiber and low in sugar. Making breakfast the night before can make it easier to eat healthy in the morning.

Advocate for Healthy Eating Patterns

Advocating for healthy eating patterns in all settings, including the home, school, work, and community, has major benefits. Knowing the benefits of good nutrition, all people have a responsibility to make nutritious food choices and share health information with others. Even if you cannot make all of your own food choices, for example, you can offer to shop with your family members, help choose healthier foods, and assist with cooking at home.

You can also advocate for healthier food options in your school and community by working with your administration or community organizations to make changes. Some strategies you can use to increase healthy eating in your school include the following:

- Encourage the school administration to increase the number of healthy eating options in the cafeteria. For example, your school could add a salad bar, offer a vegetarian option each day, and provide nutritious snacks (fruit bowls, nuts, or low-sugar trail mix).
- Encourage the school administration to reduce less-nutritious food options, such as deep-fried and highly processed foods (mozzarella sticks, chicken nuggets, or pizza), chips, and ice cream.
- Eliminate school fundraisers that rely on selling less-nutritious foods, such as candy bars, cookie dough, and pizza.
- Encourage the school administration to require that vending machines include only nutritious foods, such as water, nuts, and dried fruit.

The Effect of Individual Needs

Sometimes, specific needs and lifestyles change the way a person makes food choices. For example, certain health conditions and behaviors, such as level of physical activity, can change the balance of nutrients a person needs. Food sensitivities and specific eating plans can also influence how a person makes nutritious food choices.

Food Sensitivities

Food sensitivities impact what foods a person can safely consume. Two types of food sensitivities are food intolerances and food allergies.

Food intolerances occur when a person's body cannot properly digest a particular type of food. Symptoms of intolerance often appear gradually, after someone eats large quantities of a particular type of food or eats the food very frequently. For instance, people who have *gluten intolerance*

food intolerances
conditions in which a person's body cannot properly digest particular types of food; can develop gradually as a person eats large quantities of a certain food frequently

(sometimes as a result of *celiac disease*) have difficulty digesting gluten, which is a protein found in wheat, rye, oats, and barley. People who have *lactose intolerance* may become ill after drinking milk and experience gas, cramps, bloating, heartburn, headaches, and irritability or nervousness. Modifying a food to exclude the ingredient that causes symptoms can help people with food intolerances get adequate nutrition. For example, many gluten-free and lactose-free products are available. People with lactose intolerance can take a dietary supplement called *lactase* that provides the enzyme needed to digest lactose.

A **food allergy** occurs when the body's immune system reacts to a food as if the food is harmful (**Figure 8.15**). The food the body reacts negatively to is called an *allergen*. Symptoms of a food allergy typically occur very suddenly and can be caused even by tiny amounts of the allergen on the skin or in the air. Symptoms of an allergic reaction vary widely. Some common reactions include hives or a rash, swelling in the tongue and throat, difficulty breathing, and abdominal cramps. Currently, no cure exists for food allergies.

food allergy condition in which the body's immune system reacts to a food as if the food is harmful; sudden symptoms can be caused by tiny amounts of the food

The best way to manage allergies is to avoid all contact with food that might trigger a reaction. This is not always as easy as it sounds. Some foods that normally would not contain allergens are manufactured in factories that process other foods containing allergens. For example, an oatmeal cookie that does not contain peanuts may pick up traces of peanut from peanut butter cookies manufactured at the same factory. The manufacturer must indicate on the package whether the oatmeal cookies were manufactured in the same facility as the peanut butter cookies.

Common Food Allergies
Milk
Eggs
Fish
Shellfish
Tree nuts
Peanuts
Wheat
Soybeans

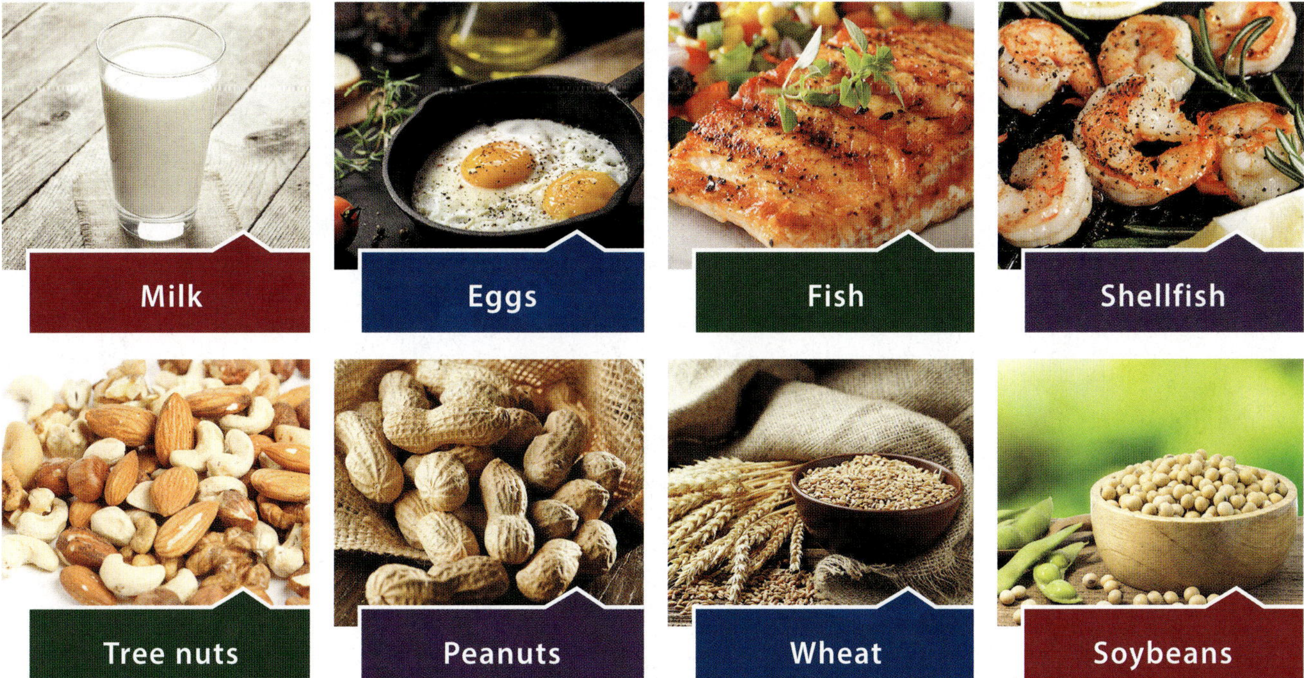

VikramRaghuvanshi/iStock/Getty Images Plus/Getty Images
Left to right, top to bottom: Alter-ego/Shutterstock.com; BorisKotov/Shutterstock.com; AS Food studio/Shutterstock.com; Tema_Kud/Shutterstock.com; Shebeko/Shutterstock.com; HQuality/Shutterstock.com; 5 second Studio/Shutterstock.com; 1989studio/Shutterstock.com

Figure 8.15 These foods account for 90 percent of allergic reactions due to food. ***What is the difference between a food allergy and a food intolerance?***

Vegetarian and Vegan Eating Plans

People who use a vegetarian or vegan eating plan avoid eating all (or most) foods from animal sources, and must rely on plant-based sources to meet their protein needs. With knowledge and planning, a vegetarian or vegan eating plan can easily meet the recommended protein needs for adults and children. People who use a vegetarian or vegan eating plan need to take in multiple types of protein-rich plants to obtain all of the amino acids. Specifically, they need to consume *complementary proteins*, or two or more incomplete protein sources that together provide adequate amounts of all the essential amino acids.

For example, rice contains low amounts of certain essential amino acids. These same essential amino acids, however, are found in greater amounts in dry beans. Similarly, dry beans contain lower amounts of other essential amino acids that are found in larger amounts in rice. Together, rice and beans provide adequate amounts of all the essential amino acids (**Figure 8.16**).

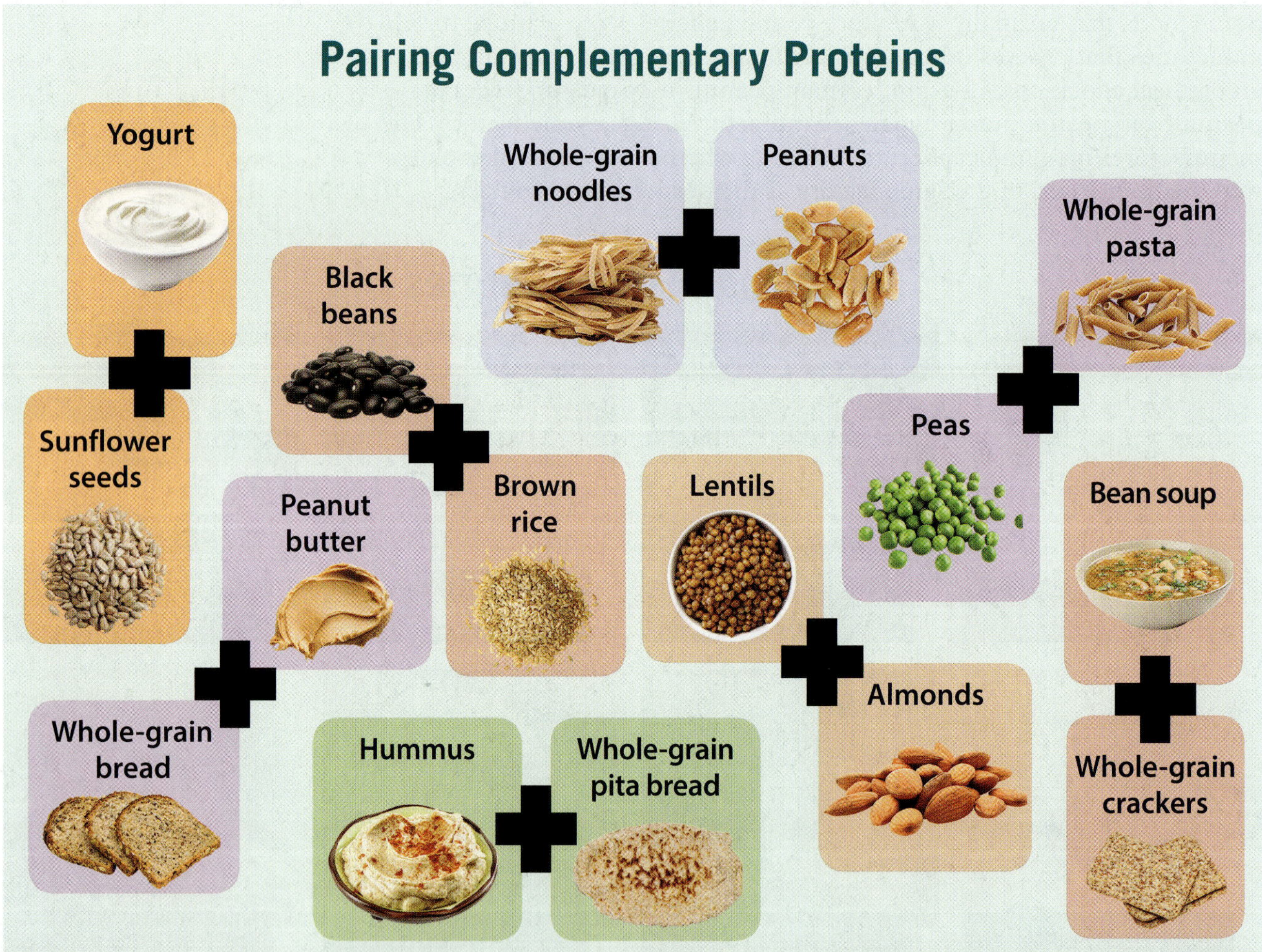

Top row, left to right: baibaz/Shutterstock.com; Galayko Sergey/Shutterstock.com; JIANG HONGYAN/Shutterstock.com; matkub2499/Shutterstock.com; Gita Kulinitch Studio/Shutterstock.com
Middle row, left to right: Anton Starikov/Shutterstock.com; Africa Studio/Shutterstock.com; M. Unal Ozmen/Shutterstock.com; Moving Moment/Shutterstock.com; Chursina Viktoriia/Shutterstock.com; spixiax/Shutterstock.com
Bottom row, left to right: Gita Kulinitch Studio/Shutterstock.com; MaraZe/Shutterstock.com; nito/Shutterstock.com; Africa Studio/Shutterstock.com; Diana Taliun/Shutterstock.com

Figure 8.16 While incomplete proteins do not individually provide all of the essential amino acids, they do when consumed in complementary protein pairs.

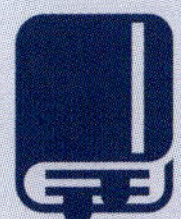

Case Study

Individual Dietary Needs

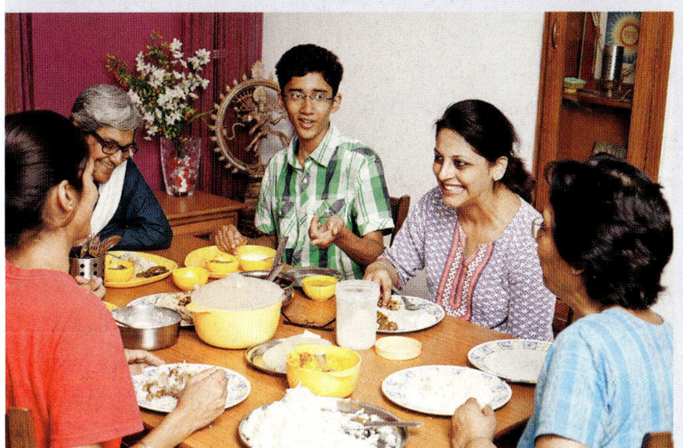

VikramRaghuvanshi/iStock/Getty Images Plus/Getty Images

One morning, Deshawn felt sick after drinking milk with his breakfast, but thought it was nothing. At lunch, he had a turkey and Swiss cheese sandwich, and his symptoms went from bad to worse. He had terrible stomach cramps and was extremely nauseous. He told his mom, who suggested visiting a doctor about it. The doctor informed Deshawn that he is lactose intolerant and will have to eliminate dairy products from his eating plan. Deshawn wonders what he can eat now that he cannot consume dairy.

Imani has a wheat allergy. Sometimes, people tease her about it and tell her to just enjoy some pizza. She does not think they realize that if she ate something with wheat in it, she would break out in hives, and eventually her throat would close up. Imani wishes it were as easy as eating what was in front of her, but she has to be careful to avoid wheat products.

Brody is a vegetarian. When he was 10 years old, he told his parents he did not want to eat meat if it meant harming innocent animals. Brody's parents have supported his decision, and his family has even started participating in "Meatless Mondays" together. At first, Brody's dad worried Brody would not be getting enough iron and protein without eating meat. They have done enough research, however, to know what foods or dietary supplements can provide the nutrients he needs.

Practice Your Skills

Access Information

In small groups, choose one of the dietary needs described in these case studies: Deshawn's lactose intolerance, Imani's wheat allergy, or Brody's vegetarian eating pattern. Use MyPlate to research how much of each food group your teen should eat each day. Assume each teen is moderately active. How can Deshawn, Imani, and Brody get the nutrients they need with their individual dietary needs? Create a meal plan for one day for your student. Include breakfast, lunch, dinner, snacks, and beverages in your plan.

Pregnancy

During pregnancy, people have special nutritional needs. They have to meet these needs for their own health and for the health of the baby they are carrying. People who are pregnant or breastfeeding should avoid seafood that is high in mercury such as shark, swordfish, tilefish, orange roughy, marlin, bigeye tuna, and King mackerel. They should also limit canned white tuna (albacore) to fewer than 6 ounces (170 grams) per week. You will learn more about nutrition recommendations during pregnancy in Chapter 21.

Consequences of Poor Nutrition

A healthy eating pattern is an important part of maintaining your health and reducing your risk for certain diseases. A healthy eating pattern can also help you avoid health risks related to poor nutrition.

Local and Global Health

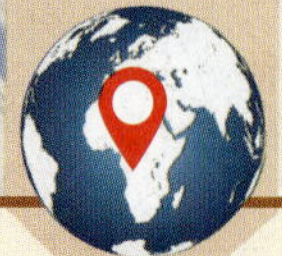

Undernutrition: A Global Problem

Nutrition is essential for normal health and development. Children with well-balanced eating patterns do better in school, have fewer illnesses, and are more likely to become healthy adults. Sadly, an estimated 93 million children under five years of age experience undernutrition worldwide.

Undernutrition is caused by a number of different factors, including

- poverty, which leads to a lack of money to buy food;
- disease, which can cause issues absorbing nutrients;
- food shortages, which agricultural productivity issues can cause; and
- dietary practices, such as an overreliance on a single food source (for example, corn or rice).

Children affected by undernutrition have a lowered resistance to infection. They are more likely to experience underweight and die from common childhood health conditions, such as diarrhea and respiratory infections. More than one-third of child deaths worldwide are caused by not consuming enough nutrients, with approximately 6 million children dying of hunger each year.

Given the serious health conditions caused by undernutrition, several programs are trying to reduce this threat. Some programs provide nutrient supplements to reduce deficiencies in particular vitamins and minerals. Other programs focus on reducing infections, such as intestinal worms, that drain nutrients from the body. Yet another approach is to develop strategies for increasing agricultural productivity, ensuring enough food can be grown to feed people in a given area. This strategy is particularly important, as some research shows climate change may make it harder to grow crops in certain world regions.

Percentage of Child Underweight in Selected Countries

Country	Percentage	Country	Percentage
Bangladesh	32.6	China	2.4
Pakistan	31.6	Morocco	3.1
India	35.7	Peru	3.1
Ethiopia	23.6	Mexico	3.9
Afghanistan	25.0	Bolivia	3.4
Cambodia	23.9	Germany	1.1
Rwanda	9.3	United States	0.5

Practice Your Skills

Analyze Influences

When you look at the rates of underweight in different countries, what do you observe? Research the factors that contribute to undernutrition in these countries. Then, compare your factors with those of a partner. How do you think rates of undernutrition in different countries will change over time? What are some factors that might cause rates of undernutrition to increase in a given country? to decrease? What strategies could governments take to decrease the rate of undernutrition in their countries and worldwide? Which strategies would be most effective, and why?

The following health risks can develop if you do not get the amounts of nutrients your body needs:

- **Malnutrition:** When you do not consume the appropriate amounts of nutrients, **malnutrition** develops. For example, you might eat too much added sugar and too few vitamins. Malnutrition can also occur if your body does not absorb the nutrients you consume properly. Malnutrition can lead to health risks related to nutritional deficiency and excess. Undernutrition and overnutrition are forms of malnutrition.

malnutrition form of poor nutrition in which a person does not get or properly absorb the recommended amounts of essential nutrients

- **Undernutrition:** When people do not take in enough nutrients for health and growth, they experience **undernutrition** (**Figure 8.17**). Undernutrition can lead to issues with growth. For example, children and teens who do not receive enough nutrients may never reach their full height. Undernutrition can also lead to serious health conditions, including brain damage, vision impairments and blindness, and bone deformities. If a person who is pregnant experiences undernutrition, the growing fetus may not receive enough nutrients to develop properly.
- **Overnutrition:** Eating too many foods that contain high amounts of added sugars, saturated fats, sodium, or refined grains or simply too many calories can lead to **overnutrition**. These foods contribute to a variety of health conditions. For instance, evidence suggests limiting sodium intake helps maintain a normal blood pressure, which reduces the risk of cardiovascular and kidney diseases.

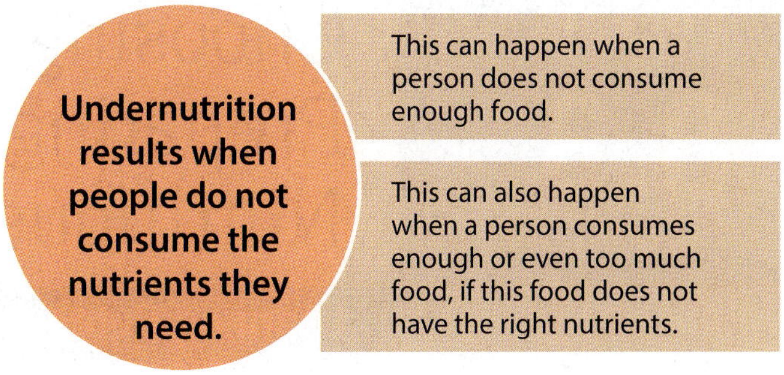

Undernutrition results when people do not consume the nutrients they need.

This can happen when a person does not consume enough food.

This can also happen when a person consumes enough or even too much food, if this food does not have the right nutrients.

Figure 8.17 Undernutrition has to do with the amounts of nutrients a person consumes, not necessarily the amount of overall food.

undernutrition form of malnutrition caused by the body not receiving or absorbing needed nutrients

overnutrition form of malnutrition caused by consuming too many of some nutrients

Lesson 8.2 Review

Know and Understand

1. Explain the difference between whole grains and refined grains. About how much of each type do you consume?
2. Visit the MyPlate website and input the needed information to generate your daily eating plan. How many calories should you consume? How is your plan different from the one in Figure 8.11?
3. What does it mean for a food to be nutrient dense?
4. How can reducing sodium intake improve health?
5. Explain the difference between a food intolerance and food allergy.
6. With a partner, find a recipe that pairs complementary proteins. Share this recipe with the class.

Think Critically

7. Make a plan for eating more vegetables each day. What dishes could you prepare that contain multiple types of vegetables? How easy or hard would it be for you to consume vegetables from each group each week?
8. Think of a food you eat regularly. What modifications could you make to the food to reduce the amount of added sugars, saturated fat, and sodium you consume?
9. With a partner, discuss the following question: Can someone experience undernutrition and overnutrition at the same time? Why or why not?

REAL WORLD Health Skills

Advocate for Health Because you are such a food guru now, write a letter to the food director of your school. This person is responsible for everything served in the cafeteria. In this letter, advocate on behalf of yourself and all your classmates for tools to make nutritious food choices. For example, you could request that each food served have a large food label beside it so students can make more educated decisions in the lunchroom. Do not forget to list the reasons why your new system would be beneficial to student health.

Lesson

8.3

Choosing and Preparing Nutritious Foods

Essential Question

How can you choose nutritious foods and prepare them in healthy ways?

Learning Outcomes

After studying this lesson, you will be able to

- analyze influences on food choices;
- interpret the information on Nutrition Facts and food labels;
- assess claims on food labels;
- follow a recipe to prepare nutritious foods; and
- prepare foods safely to prevent foodborne illness.

Key Terms

Daily Values
food additives
foodborne illnesses
foodborne infection
foodborne intoxication
food preferences
generally recognized as safe (GRAS)
genetically modified organism (GMO)
Nutrition Facts label
organic

Warm-Up Activity

Nutrition Conversion

Comprehend Concepts Choose a packaged food, and before reading this lesson, read the Nutrition Facts label on the food. The information on the Nutrition Facts label is based on a 2,000-calorie diet. Not all people need a 2,000-calorie diet, however. It may be necessary to adjust the values on a Nutrition Facts label. Using the chart shown, convert the values on your Nutrition Facts label to match your energy needs.

	Calorie Needs	
Age	**Male**	**Female**
13	Inactive: 2,000 Moderately active: 2,200 Active: 2,600	Inactive: 1,600 Moderately active: 2,000 Active: 2,200
14–15	Inactive: 2,000–2,200 Moderately active: 2,400–2,600 Active: 2,800–3,000	Inactive: 1,800 Moderately active: 2,000 Active: 2,400
16–18	Inactive: 2,400 Moderately active: 2,800 Active: 3,200	
19	Inactive: 2,600 Moderately active: 2,800 Active: 3,000	Inactive: 2,000 Moderately active: 2,200 Active: 2,400

To follow a healthy eating pattern, you need to make choices and consume foods with nutritional value. Many factors influence the foods you choose. These factors can make it easier or more difficult to choose certain types of food. Nutrition Facts labels and food labels can help you choose foods and know what nutritional value they offer. Preparing your own nutritious food safely can also help you get the nutrition you need.

Analyzing Influences on Food Choices

What are your favorite foods? What tastes do you like? How difficult is it for you to buy and prepare fresh fruits and vegetables? Understanding the factors that influence your food preferences and choices will help you make healthy decisions. Your **food preferences** are your opinions about different types of food. The following internal and external factors influence these preferences:

food preferences
opinions about different types of food; influenced by genetics, age, feelings and thoughts, cultural background, and social environment

- **Genetics:** Research shows that genes may influence people's preferences for different foods. Some people prefer to eat foods high in fats, such as chocolate, doughnuts, and ice cream. Other people prefer to eat salty foods, such as pretzels, French fries, and potato chips.
- **Age:** Food preferences change as people get older. For example, you may have disliked spicy foods as a child, but like them now. Preferences change as people learn about different foods. Changes in the body's taste receptors also influence how sensitive people are to different tastes.
- **Feelings and thoughts:** People experiencing uncomfortable emotions tend to consume more comfort foods. Comfort foods, such as ice cream and candy, make them "feel better." The sugar in these foods triggers the release of chemicals that contribute to pleasure and improved mood. Chocolate also increases production of hormones that generate feelings of happiness. Eating to improve your mood is an example of eating because of a psychological desire rather than a physiological need (**Figure 8.18**).
- **Cultural background:** People in different cultures prefer different foods and tastes. For example, you may not want to eat spiders, snails, or guinea pigs. These foods, however, are delicacies in some cultures. The flavors used in a culture's cooking influence food preferences. Spices such as cardamom are common in Indian dishes, while cumin is a staple in Mexican cooking. Some research indicates taste preferences develop before people are born. Babies born to people who consume particular flavors during pregnancy show stronger preferences for these flavors.

In a study of college students:
62%
of female students
and
29%
of male students
reported eating more when feeling depressed.
People also use food to improve their mood when they feel anxious, angry, or stressed.

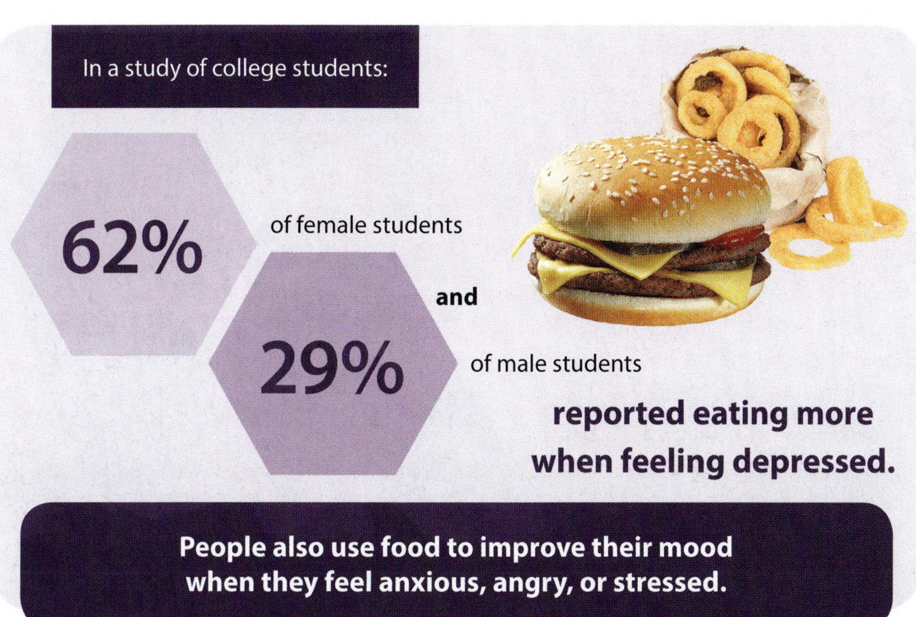

Burger: usaphoto/Shutterstock.com; Onion rings: michelaubryphoto/Shutterstock.com

Figure 8.18 Scientific studies have found that people use food to improve uncomfortable emotions and mood.

Research in Action

How Do Emotions Affect Your Food Choices?

How much do your emotions influence the food you eat? Do you eat certain types of food when you are stressed? sad? happy? Researchers at Cornell University created a study to test how much emotions influence the amounts people eat. They began by creating different moods in different people. To create these moods, they showed people one of two movies:

- a romantic comedy designed to create a happy mood
- a movie in which one of the lead characters dies at a young age, designed to create a sad mood

While watching their assigned movie, people were given a large bucket of hot, buttered, salted popcorn. They were also given water or a diet soda to drink. The researchers then measured how much people ate during each of the two movies.

Can you guess what they found? People who watched the sad movie ate 28 percent more popcorn than the people who watched the happy movie. This study provides evidence suggesting that people eat in part to try to make themselves feel better.

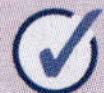

Practice Your Skills

Communicate with Others

With a partner, discuss why you think people ate more popcorn when watching a sad movie than when watching a happy movie. Is this difference a reflection of biological, social, or psychological factors? What do you think researchers would find if they gave people a large tray of celery and carrots instead of a large bucket of popcorn? Would people eat more vegetables during the sad movie than the happy movie? Why or why not? After discussing these questions, think about the foods you and your partner eat when you are happy versus when you are sad. List these foods and then negotiate with your partner to substitute any less-nutritious foods with healthier foods you both would still want to eat.

- **Social environment:** Have you ever craved chocolate chip cookies after seeing a picture of them on social media? The advertisements you see can make you desire certain foods over others. Your peers impact your food choices as well. You may want to eat the same foods as your friends or fit in by ordering a big meal at a restaurant. Controlling this influence can help you make healthier food choices. For example, you could choose not to browse pictures of desserts online (**Figure 8.19**).

Strategies for Eating Healthy in Social Situations

- Eat before the event to prevent yourself from becoming hungry with only less-healthy options to choose.
- Bring a healthy dish with you to share. When eating out with friends, suggest eating healthy snacks or foods.
- When refusing food, be confident and firm, but polite. Try "Oh, thank you, but I'm okay right now." If someone insists, change the subject.
- Pair your refusal of someone's food with a compliment like "This smells incredible, but I couldn't eat another bite."
- Use specific excuses, such as "I'm not hungry," "I can't eat that food," or "That doesn't fit in my diet."

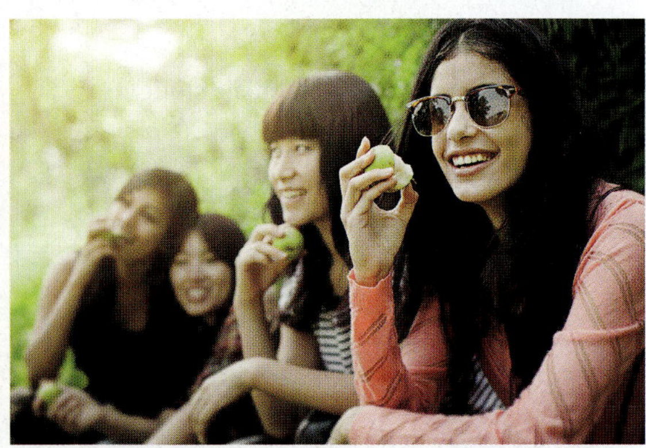

gawrav/E+/Getty Images

Figure 8.19 Social situations, including parties, celebrations, or casually hanging out with friends, often include some kind of food or beverage. Keep these strategies in mind to maintain your healthy eating pattern in these situations. ***What social situations influence your eating patterns?***

In addition to food preferences, the availability of food also affects your food choices. Socioeconomic factors such as income level affect the variety of food available in a community and in the home. If nutritious foods are not easily available to you, or if your community is saturated with fast-food options, you may find it more difficult to make healthy choices. Most communities have programs and services to help people with low incomes obtain nutritious foods. Some examples of these services are food banks and the Supplemental Nutrition Assistance Program (SNAP).

Knowing what influences affect your food choices can help you identify why you want certain foods. You can then determine whether acting on that desire is a healthy choice. For example, if you are feeling stressed and want to eat ice cream, understanding that mood affects your appetite can help you counteract that craving. You can then choose a healthier, more nutritious option.

Health in the Media

Be Wary of Music Star Endorsements

How many foods and beverages advertised in the media do you think are nutritious choices? less-nutritious choices? Researchers at New York University conducted a study to examine the types of foods and beverages promoted by popular music stars. They first gathered data from Billboard Magazine's Hot 100 song charts and the Teen Choice Awards winners to determine the most popular music stars at the time. Next, they examined every advertisement—on TV, in magazines, and on the radio—that included the music stars. They also examined music stars' endorsements on social media and included products promoted at concerts. Researchers found that 65 of the most popular music stars had promoted some type of food or beverage. For each item, researchers then examined nutrition information, such as added sugars.

What types of products do you think the music stars promoted? Researchers found that more than 80 percent of products promoted by these music stars were considered "nutrition poor." Most promotions were for sodas and other sugary drinks, fast foods, and sweets. Only one promotion was for a natural food described as healthy (pistachios). No endorsements were for fruits, vegetables, or whole grains.

Prior research has shown that advertisements for less-nutritious foods make these products seem more desirable and increase people's interest. This study suggests that music stars' promotion of less-nutritious foods and beverages could therefore lead to poor eating habits and increase the risk of obesity.

Practice Your Skills

Advocate for Health

How much influence do you think music stars have on teens? If your favorite music star were to endorse a certain food or beverage, would you want to try it? Think about your favorite music star and then research advertisements in which that music star has appeared. Also research if your favorite music star has endorsed any food or beverage brands at concerts. Examine the nutritional information of the foods or beverages promoted and then write a post reaching out to your favorite music star on social media. Thank your favorite music star for promoting nutritious foods or encourage your favorite music star to consider advocating for nutritious options.

Understanding Nutrition Facts and Food Labels

Nutrition Facts label
FDA-required label on all packaged foods; contains information about serving size, number of servings, number of calories, amounts of different nutrients, and daily values for nutrients

To help consumers make healthy choices about what they eat, the FDA requires any food sold in a package to include a **Nutrition Facts label** (**Figure 8.20**). These labels include the

- serving size (the volume or weight of a single serving of the food);
- number of servings in a package;
- number of calories in each serving;
- amount of different nutrients (including fat, cholesterol, sodium, carbohydrates, fibers, sugars, protein, and some vitamins and minerals) in a serving; and
- percent of daily values for the different nutrients provided in a serving.

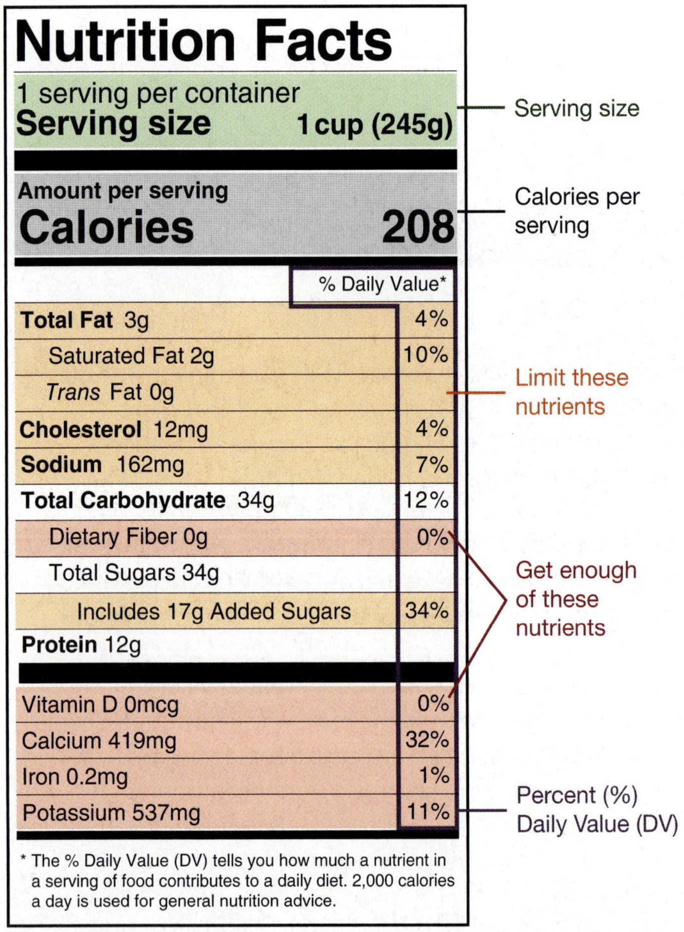

Nutrition Facts	
1 serving per container	
Serving size	**1 cup (245g)**
Amount per serving	
Calories	**208**
	% Daily Value*
Total Fat 3g	4%
Saturated Fat 2g	10%
Trans Fat 0g	
Cholesterol 12mg	4%
Sodium 162mg	7%
Total Carbohydrate 34g	12%
Dietary Fiber 0g	0%
Total Sugars 34g	
Includes 17g Added Sugars	34%
Protein 12g	
Vitamin D 0mcg	0%
Calcium 419mg	32%
Iron 0.2mg	1%
Potassium 537mg	11%

* The % Daily Value (DV) tells you how much a nutrient in a serving of food contributes to a daily diet. 2,000 calories a day is used for general nutrition advice.

Serving size
Calories per serving
Limit these nutrients
Get enough of these nutrients
Percent (%) Daily Value (DV)

Courtesy of the Food and Drug Administration

Figure 8.20 A Nutrition Facts label provides information about serving size, calories, nutrients, and how the food can fit into a person's daily eating plan. ***What does the serving size on a Nutrition Facts label indicate?***

Food packages also must contain labels that list the ingredients and food additives in a food.

Servings and Calories

The number of calories you see at the top of a Nutrition Facts label indicates the number of calories in *one serving* of the food. Because of this, it is important to check the number of servings provided in the *whole container* first.

The number of calories and Percent (%) Daily Values listed on a Nutrition Facts label are based on a single serving size, which is what people customarily consume. This is not a recommendation for what people should consume, and people may consume more than just one serving. For example, if a package contains two servings and you consume the entire package, then you have consumed twice the number of calories and nutrients reported in the Nutrition Facts label.

Can you guess how many servings are in 1 pint of ice cream? Many people would guess one 2-cup serving or two 1-cup servings. Ice cream manufacturers, however, describe a pint of ice cream as three ⅔-cup servings. This means that the calories listed for a single serving of ice cream from a 1-pint container reflect only ⅓ of the container.

Daily Values

Daily Values
recommended daily intake amounts for specific nutrients based on a 2,000-calorie eating plan

Daily Values are the recommended daily intake amounts for specific nutrients. The Daily Values for a 2,000-calorie eating plan are used to calculate the % Daily Values for the nutrients on a Nutrition Facts panel.

These percentages, therefore, could be higher or lower depending on an individual's daily calorie needs.

The % Daily Value signals whether a serving of food contributes a lot or a little of a particular nutrient to your total daily intake. For example, suppose a food item's % Daily Value for calcium is 20. That means one serving of the food supplies 20 percent of the daily requirement for calcium for an individual on a 2,000-calorie eating plan.

You can use % Daily Values to evaluate the overall nutritional quality of a food. Some nutrients on a Nutrition Facts label, such as dietary fiber and calcium, are beneficial. Greater % Daily Values for these beneficial nutrients indicate better nutritional value. For other nutrients, such as saturated fat and sodium, lower % Daily Values are desirable.

A low % Daily Value is 5 percent. Aim for this percentage when eating foods with saturated fat, cholesterol, and sodium. A high % Daily Value is 20 percent or higher. Aim for this percentage when eating foods with dietary fiber, calcium, iron, vitamin D, and potassium.

Ingredients in Foods

Food labels on food packaging list all the ingredients used to make that food. These ingredients appear in the order they contribute weight to a given product. Ingredients listed first make up a greater amount of the final product than ingredients near the end of the list. In other words, the closer an ingredient appears to the top of the list, the more of that ingredient is in the food.

Sometimes ingredients are listed in somewhat confusing ways. This makes it harder to determine exactly what foods are in the product. For example, *corn syrup*, *corn sweetener*, *fructose*, *dextrose*, *high-fructose corn syrup*, *lactose*, *maltose*, *sucrose*, *malt syrup*, *molasses*, *honey*, *glucose*, and *fruit juice concentrate* all describe sugar added to a food. If you see any of these ingredients, you know the food contains added sugars (**Figure 8.21**).

Often, food manufacturers add substances to extend a product's shelf life or improve its flavor. Substances added to food products to cause desired changes are called **food additives**. The government regulates food additives and maintains a list of food additives proven to be safe. Additives on this list are **generally recognized as safe (GRAS)**. Food manufacturers must obtain approval from the FDA to use substances not on the GRAS list. If your goal is to avoid specific food additives, you can find them on the ingredient lists of food labels.

food additives substances added to food products to cause desired changes to flavor, shelf life, or other reasons

generally recognized as safe (GRAS) proven by the FDA to be safe for consumption

One of the best-selling cereals in the United States lists the following five ingredients first on its label:

- whole-grain oats
- sugar
- modified corn starch
- honey
- brown sugar

Four of the top five ingredients in this cereal are a type of sugar. The sixth ingredient is salt.

CLS Digital Arts/Shutterstock.com

Figure 8.21 Checking the ingredient list on food packaging can help you see what foods and food additives are in that package. ***Name a more nutrient-dense cereal.***

Assessing Claims on Food Labels

Sometimes food packages describe a particular food using a specific claim about its health benefits. For example, a label might describe a food as "low-fat" or "organic." To use these terms, the food must meet certain criteria established by the FDA and USDA.

Low-Fat and Heart-Healthy Foods

A "low-fat" food must not contain more than 3 grams (0.1 ounces) of fat in a single serving. For a label to state that a food may reduce the risk of heart disease, the food must contain at least 51 percent whole-grain ingredients and be low in total fat, saturated fat, and cholesterol.

Organic Foods

organic produced without the use of chemical fertilizers, pesticides, or other artificial chemicals

A food described as **organic** must consist of at least 95 percent organically produced ingredients. Organic foods must be grown without the use of any fertilizers or pesticides made from manufactured chemicals, bioengineering, or high-energy radiation. Some people who choose organic foods are trying to avoid consuming pesticides or other substances used in the production of nonorganic foods. Others may choose organic foods because they believe these foods are healthier, although research has not yet confirmed this.

GMO and Non-GMO Foods

genetically modified organism (GMO) living thing with genetic material that has been altered through genetic engineering

Some foods come from **genetically modified organisms (GMOs)**, or living things that have undergone changes to genetic material (DNA). This technology, which uses techniques from genetic engineering, allows the transfer of certain genes from one organism to another. The goal is to create plants and crops with more resistance to disease, more nutritional benefits, and better taste. Foods produced using this technique are often called *GMO foods*. *Non-GMO* foods are those without genetically modified ingredients.

Many countries require the labeling of GMO foods so people know whether the foods they buy have been altered. In 2018, the USDA passed a law that required most genetically modified ingredients to be labeled as bioengineered ingredients. This label can be writing on the package, a symbol, or a digital link. Products that contain very small amounts of genetically modified ingredients, such as high-fructose corn syrup and oils and refined beet sugar, do not have to be labeled.

Preparing Nutritious Foods

One of the best strategies for making nutritious food choices is preparing your own food. Preparing your own food has many benefits. For example, making food at home is usually cheaper than eating at a restaurant or buying premade meals or snacks. Many meals can be made in fewer than 30 minutes, and you can make a large portion of a meal, then eat several small portions or freeze it. You can also make meals or snacks ahead of time so you can take them with you (**Figure 8.22**).

Making food at home is also better for your health. Many foods at restaurants and premade meals and snacks contain large amounts of saturated fat, added sugar, and salt. When you prepare food at home, you know exactly what ingredients you are using. This makes it easier to limit certain substances and manage food allergies or sensitivities.

Make-Ahead Healthy Snacks			
Fruit and low-fat yogurt parfait	Fruit or vegetables with a nut butter	Vegetables and hummus	Smoothie
String cheese and almonds, fruit, or whole-grain crackers	Whole-grain crackers and bean dip	Whole-grain English muffin and all-natural peanut butter	Nuts and dried fruit
Hummus on a whole-grain pita	Edamame	Trail mix (oats, nuts, and dried fruit)	Whole-grain bread with all-natural peanut butter and banana

Left to right, top to bottom: JeniFoto/Shutterstock.com; Robyn Mackenzie/Shutterstock.com; Eywa/Shutterstock.com; Tanya_mtv/Shutterstock.com; JeniFoto/Shutterstock.com; Diana Taliun/Shutterstock.com; Nataly Studio/Shutterstock.com; neung_pongsak/Shutterstock.com; Luella938/Shutterstock.com; CRSPIX/Shutterstock.com; Hong Vo/Shutterstock.com; rodrigobark/Shutterstock.com; dedeejune/Shutterstock.com; P-fotography/Shutterstock.com; gkrphoto/Shutterstock.com

Figure 8.22 Making snacks ahead of time is a great idea when you are in a rush to get to school or do not have much time to eat.

When you make food at home, you can manage portion sizes more easily. Many restaurants offer very large portion sizes, and once you have ordered a meal, you may feel like you have to eat all of it. At home, you can control how much food you serve yourself and save any leftovers for the next day.

Practicing Food Safety

The goal of making healthy food choices is to provide the appropriate amount of nutrients for your body. Another goal is to make sure the foods and beverages you put into your body are safe.

Sometimes, foods can harm your health if they are not handled and prepared safely. **Foodborne illnesses**, or *food poisoning*, refer to illnesses transmitted by foods. Foodborne illnesses are a common, yet preventable, public health issue. Many people experience only a brief period of illness and make a full recovery without medical care. These illnesses can be dangerous, however, for people who are very old, very young, or pregnant. People who already have health conditions or weakened immune systems can become extremely sick and even die from foodborne illnesses.

foodborne illnesses illnesses that are transmitted by food; also called *food poisoning*

foodborne infection foodborne illness that occurs when food is handled or prepared improperly; is caused by bacteria, viruses, or parasites

Types of Foodborne Illness

Some foodborne illnesses are caused by disease-causing microorganisms, called *pathogens*. This type of illness is a **foodborne infection**.

When food is handled improperly, these pathogens rapidly multiply to dangerous levels, causing symptoms such as nausea, vomiting, abdominal cramps, and diarrhea.

foodborne intoxication
foodborne illness caused by toxins, which are produced by organisms present in a food

Toxins in food can also cause a type of foodborne illness called **foodborne intoxication**. In many cases, organisms produce the toxins present in a food. For example, *Escherichia coli (E. coli)* is a bacterium that lives in the digestive tracts of humans and animals.

Skills for Health and Wellness

Following a Recipe

A *recipe* is a set of instructions for preparing a certain food. Once you know how to read and follow a recipe, you will be able to prepare many different types of foods. You will also be able to assess the nutritional value of a recipe and substitute ingredients as needed. Knowing how to follow a recipe and prepare foods will help you eat healthier and get needed nutrients.

Practice Your Skills

Practice Health-Enhancing Behaviors

Think about your favorite meals and snacks and choose one food you want to make. Then, find a recipe for that food. In this activity, you will follow a recipe to prepare the food you chose. To read the recipe and prepare the food, use the following steps:

1. Review the list of ingredients. Most ingredients will include a specific measurement, such as 2 cups or 1 tablespoon, so you know how much you need. If a recipe says to add "to taste" or "a touch," this means you can add as much or little as you like.
2. Assess the nutritional value and number of servings. Some recipes list the nutrients and number of calories in the food you are preparing. Consider the nutritional value of the food and make any substitutions or modifications to make the food healthier. For example, you could use low-fat dairy products, add more vegetables, or choose granola with few added sugars. Also pay attention to the number of servings, which tells you how much food the recipe will make. If you are making food for many people, you might double all the ingredients to make twice as many servings. If you are making food just for yourself, you might want to make fewer servings and halve the amount of all the ingredients.
3. Read the directions before you begin preparing the food. The directions tell you all the steps involved in preparation. Make sure you understand each step. If you do not know what a word in the directions means, look it up in a dictionary or online. You can also ask an adult for help if you do not understand a particular step.
4. Determine the amount of time you will need to prepare the food. All recipes should give an estimate of how long the food will take to prepare.
5. Gather all of the supplies you need. This includes the ingredients listed in the recipe and any cooking equipment, such as a pan, spatula, spoon, or blender. Be sure to wash fruits and vegetables before using them.
6. Prepare the food. Record a video of yourself following the directions in the recipe and adding ingredients in the order indicated. Start by adding a small amount of an ingredient and measure accurately. It is easier to add more of an ingredient than to take out some of an ingredient. During preparation, avoid cross-contamination between uncooked meat and other foods. Wash your hands and any cooking equipment after contact with uncooked meat. If cooking, be sure to cook a food at the appropriate temperature for the amount of time specified.

After following the recipe and recording yourself making the food, share your cooking video with the class and give a short talk about the experience. What were the most challenging parts of following the recipe? What modifications or substitutions did you make to enhance the nutritional value of the food? Did you change the number of servings the recipe made? If so, why? Are you happy with the end result? Why or why not? As a class, discuss some foods you might want to try making next.

Although some strains are harmless, others make a toxin that leads to infection, causing diarrhea, anemia, and kidney failure. The bacterium *Staphylococcus aureus* grows in some foods and produces a toxin that causes intense vomiting.

Toxins in food may result from contamination with chemicals, heavy metals, or other substances. For example, people can become ill if pesticide is added to a food or if naturally poisonous substances are used to prepare a meal.

Preventing Foodborne Illness

Food safety, or safe food handling and preparation, can prevent most foodborne illnesses. Food safety includes strategies for destroying pathogens and toxins in food. It also includes guidelines for not contaminating foods during storage and preparation (**Figure 8.23**).

Preventing Foodborne Illness

- Throw away any food held at room temperature for more than two hours.
- Wash counters, tables, dishes, and eating utensils with hot, soapy water.
- Refrigerate and freeze perishable food and leftovers promptly.
- Keep hot foods hot—above 140 degrees Fahrenheit—since pathogens die at this temperature.
- Keep cold foods cold—below 40 degrees Fahrenheit—since pathogens divide and produce toxins very slowly at this temperature.
- Cook foods to the appropriate temperature.
- Wash your hands with hot, soapy water for at least 20 seconds before cooking and eating and after handling uncooked meat and poultry.
- Avoid nonpasteurized juice, apple cider, and milk.
- Thaw foods in a refrigerator or microwave. Cook meat or poultry immediately after thawing in a microwave.
- Wash fruits and vegetables before preparing them.
- Throw away and do not purchase cans that are leaking or bulging at the top.
- Avoid cross-contamination. Wash cooking equipment, utensils, and surfaces after each use. For example, wash a knife used to cut uncooked meat before using it to cut vegetables. You can also avoid cross-contamination by storing meat and poultry on the lowest refrigerator shelf and using multiple cutting boards—for example, one for meat and one for fruits and vegetables.

Figure 8.23 Keeping foods and food preparation areas clean, handling foods properly, and maintaining the correct temperature for foods can help prevent foodborne illnesses.

Lesson 8.3 Review

Know and Understand

1. Explain why it is important to check serving size on a Nutrition Facts label.
2. In a small group, create an artistic guide teaching other students how to read a Nutrition Facts label. Use real Nutrition Facts labels from foods you see in the grocery store or have at home.
3. Explain what the labels *organic* and *non-GMO* mean.
4. What are the benefits of preparing your own food?

Think Critically

5. What factors influence how healthy you eat on a daily basis?
6. With a partner, research food additives that food manufacturers use to improve food shelf life and taste. Research one food additive more deeply and record a podcast explaining the additive's use, history, and effects.
7. Brainstorm five nutritious snacks you could make ahead to eat at school. Prepare these snacks and try them for one week. Which snacks were your favorite? least favorite?
8. Choose one food safety strategy and create a how-to tutorial video showing students how to use that strategy.

REAL WORLD Health Skills

Practice Health-Enhancing Behaviors Using the MyPlate guidelines, plan, research, and prepare a dinner for your family that features nutritious ingredients you enjoy from all five food groups. Your portion sizes should reflect daily recommended serving sizes. When determining the amount of food to serve, remember dinner is only one of three daily meals.

Lesson

8.4

Managing Your Weight

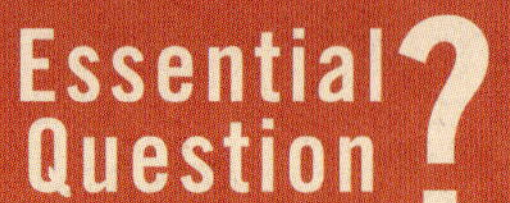

What strategies can you use to maintain a healthy weight?

Key Terms

"all-or-nothing" mind-set
body composition
body-fat distribution
body mass index (BMI)
diuretics
fad diets
food diary
metabolism
obesity
overweight
underweight

Learning Outcomes

After studying this lesson, you will be able to

- summarize the different factors that influence weight;
- explain different strategies for measuring and determining ideal body weight;
- differentiate between healthy and unhealthy strategies of weight management;
- identify healthy strategies for weight loss; and
- describe healthy strategies for weight gain.

Warm-Up Activity

Favorite Foods

Comprehend Concepts Make a list of your favorite foods and explain why each of these foods appeals to you. Read the Nutrition Facts labels or research the nutrition information for these foods. Identify whether each food is helpful for reaching and maintaining a healthy weight. Explain your answers.

Food	Helpful for		
	Losing weight	Maintaining weight	Gaining weight

Many people in the United States have difficulty managing their weight. Among adults 20 years of age and older, seven out of 10 are affected by overweight. From 1980–2008, rates of obesity in the US doubled for adults and tripled for children. Approximately 36 percent of adults and 18 percent of children and teens, from 2 to 19 years of age, are affected by obesity. As you learn more about this topic, you will understand that weight management is a complex and sensitive issue.

Factors Influencing Weight

Evidence increasingly suggests that a number of factors influence a person's weight. Researchers learn more every day about the influence of a person's genetic makeup and social, psychological, cultural, and socioeconomic factors on weight.

Genetics

Researchers have found 32 different genes that may influence weight, including recent evidence that genes may influence obesity. Genetic factors predict a person's height and appear to predict about 40–70 percent of a person's body mass index (BMI), an indicator of body composition (**Figure 8.24**).

Your genetic makeup influences the levels of various hormones in your body. Certain hormones may influence how hungry or full you feel. For example, the hormone *leptin* is an appetite suppressant, meaning high levels of this hormone in your body leave you feeling full. Another hormone, *ghrelin*, makes you feel hungry.

Genes may also influence your **metabolism**, or the rate at which your body uses energy to carry out basic physiological processes such as breathing, digesting, and growing. Some people have a high metabolism. Their bodies use more energy to carry out these processes. As a result, they burn more calories each day. Other people have a lower metabolism, so their bodies do not burn as many calories to perform daily activities.

Influence of Genetic Factors on Weight

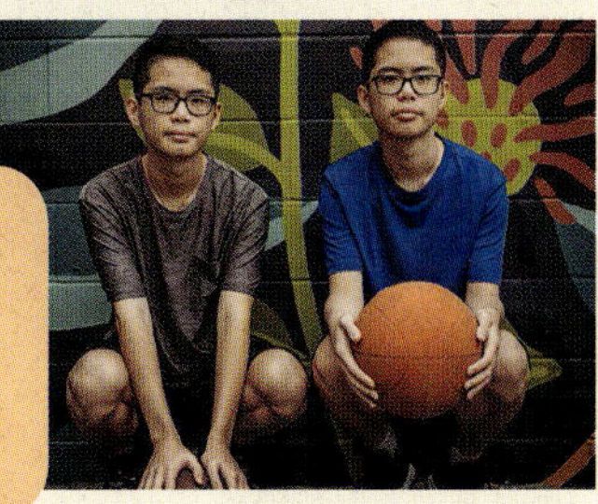

In one study, researchers found that the BMIs of identical twins were very similar whether the twins grew up in the same home or in different homes.

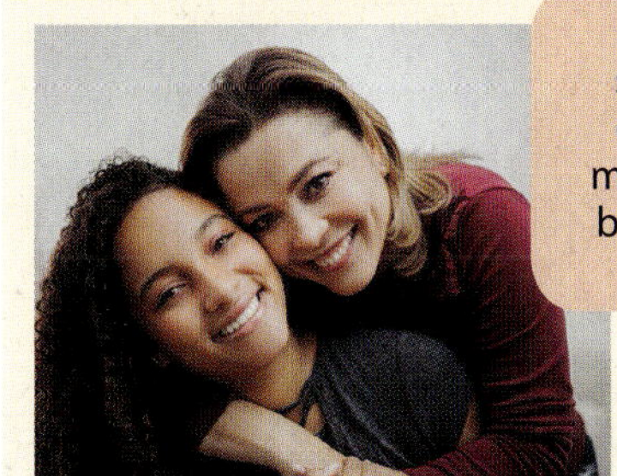

Studies have also shown that the weights of adopted children are much more similar to their biological parents than to their adoptive parents.

Top to bottom: Sisoje/iStock/Getty Images Plus/ Getty Images; oscarhdez/iStock/Getty Images Plus/Getty Images

Figure 8.24 Scientific studies indicate that genetic factors may have a significant impact on a person's weight and body composition.

metabolism rate at which the body uses energy to carry out basic physiological processes

Eating Patterns and Physical Activity

The foods you eat affect your body weight. Specifically, your calorie balance, or the calories you consume compared to the calories you burn, impacts whether you gain, lose, or maintain weight. As you learned earlier in this chapter, *calories* are the units of energy provided in food. When you consume food, you are taking energy *in*. You burn calories through the work of your metabolism and all of your daily physical activities. These calories burned are energy *out*. By comparing energy in and energy out, you can determine how eating and physical activity patterns affect your weight.

- **Maintaining weight:** If your calories consumed equal your calories burned throughout the day, you will maintain your current weight (energy in is equal to energy out).
- **Gaining weight:** If you consume more calories than your body burns, a calorie imbalance occurs. Note that the number of calories you take in and burn does *not* have to balance each day. If you take in more calories than you burn *over time*, however, you will gain weight. The body stores those extra calories, mostly as fat (energy in is greater than energy out).
- **Losing weight:** A calorie imbalance also occurs if, over time, you burn more calories than you take in. If you burn more calories than you consume, you will lose weight (energy in is less than energy out).

Guests attending an ice cream party were given either a large or small bowl. They were also given either a large or small ice cream scoop to serve themselves.
Those with large bowls served themselves
31%
more ice cream than those with small bowls.
Those with large ice cream scoops served themselves
14%
more ice cream than those with small ice cream scoops.

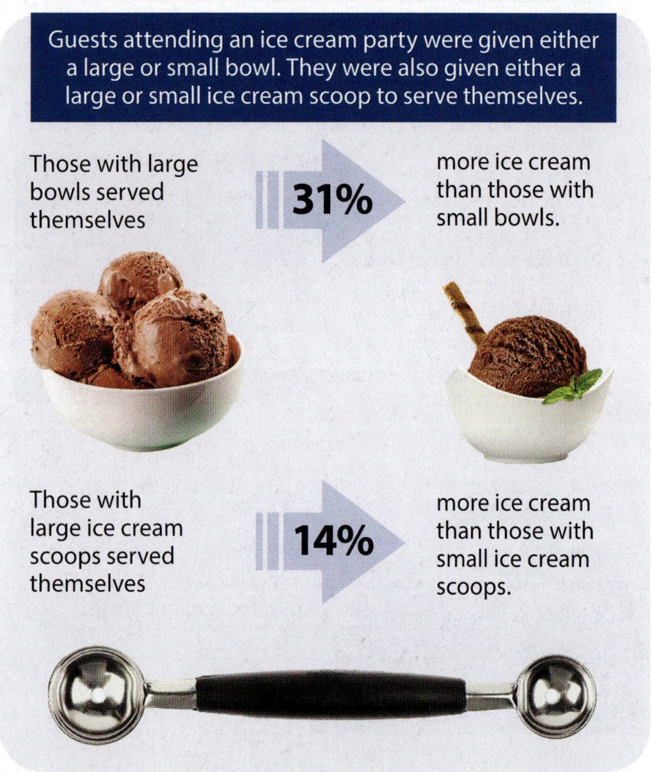

Ice cream, left to right: MaraZe/Shutterstock.com; M. Unal Ozmen/Shutterstock.com; Ice cream scoop: timquo/Shutterstock.com

Figure 8.25 A series of studies demonstrates that even very subtle environmental factors influence the way people eat. This study observed the portion sizes people chose based on environmental cues like dish and serving spoon size.

The influences on your eating patterns, including food preferences, cultural background, social environment, environmental cues, socioeconomic status, and mood, also affect weight (**Figure 8.25**). In fact, research reveals that children who grow up in low-income neighborhoods are 28 percent more likely to be affected by obesity than children who grow up in higher-income environments. This may be because families with a low income have less money to spend on nutritious foods, fewer nutritious foods available in the community, and limited opportunities for physical activity.

What Is a Healthy Weight?

Do you ever wish you weighed more or less? Do you ever compare your weight to the weight of someone else? Sometimes comparisons with other people influence people's beliefs about how much they should weigh. Perhaps you want to weigh what a friend weighs or what your favorite celebrity or athlete weighs. Comparing your weight to the weight of another person, however, is a bad idea. Your ideal weight is the weight at which *your* body is healthy.

Several factors impact the ideal weight for your body. These include your age, height, sex, and body composition. For example, weight is assessed differently for children and teens than for adults because children and teens are still growing. As you grow and become taller, your healthy weight range will increase. Similarly, your biological sex impacts the ratio of fat to muscle and bone in your body. On average, adult males have a body-fat percentage of 15 percent, and adult females have a body-fat percentage of 25 percent. Females have a higher percentage of body fat to support their role in reproduction. This difference, along with other differences in body composition, affects a person's ideal body weight.

Because of these many factors, people use several approaches to identify healthy weight ranges. Some of these approaches are body mass index (BMI), body composition, and body-fat distribution.

Body Mass Index (BMI)

body mass index (BMI) tool used to determine whether a person's weight is healthy for that person's height; BMI = weight (lbs)/height (in)^2 × 703

Body mass index (BMI) is a tool for assessing an individual's weight status. This index is calculated by dividing a person's weight in pounds by height in inches squared. This number is then multiplied by a factor of 703.

BMI = (Weight in pounds/(Height in inches)^2) × 703

To calculate BMI using kilograms and meters, divide weight in kilograms by height in meters squared.

Although BMI is calculated in the same way for children, teens, and adults, the resulting number receives different interpretation for different age groups. Because children and teens are still growing, their BMI values are plotted on growth charts based on age and sex. The BMI percentile for children and teens indicates the relative position of the person's BMI compared with others of the same sex and age.

For children and teens, the Centers for Disease Control and Prevention (CDC) defines **overweight** as having, for a particular height, excess body weight from fat, bone, muscle, water, or a combination of these factors. The CDC defines **obesity** as having excess body fat or excessive overweight. According to the CDC, children and teens who are affected by **underweight** have a body weight that is too low compared with others of the same sex and age (**Figure 8.26**). For adults, these weight categories are based on specific BMI values.

BMI calculation is an easy method for assessing weight status, but it is not perfect. For some individuals, BMI is not accurate due to differences in body composition. Because muscle and bone weigh more than fat, people who are highly fit or muscular may have a high BMI, which incorrectly places them in the overweight category. Likewise, an individual may have a body weight in the acceptable range, but a high percentage of body fat to muscle. BMI would inaccurately place this person in the healthy range.

overweight condition of excess body weight from fat, bone, muscle, water, or a combination of these factors

obesity condition of excess body fat or excessive overweight

underweight condition of a body weight that is too low compared with others of the same sex and age

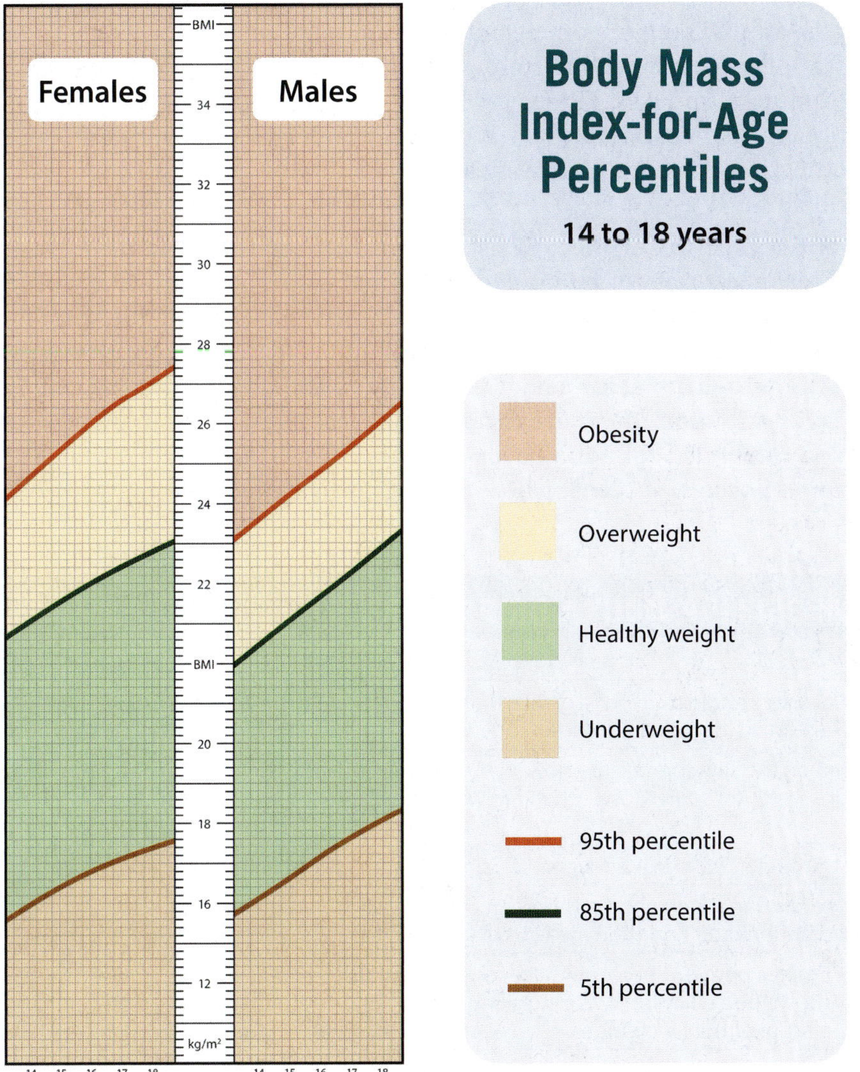

Figure 8.26 The BMI percentiles for teens indicate weight status relative to other teens of the same biological sex and age. ***What is the equation to calculate BMI?***

Body Composition

body composition
ratio of the various components—fat, bone, and muscle—that make up the body; influenced by genetics, eating patterns, and physical activity

Your **body composition** is the ratio of the various components—fat, bone, and muscle—that make up your body. The size and shape of two people who weigh the same, but differ in body composition, can be very different. Genetics, eating patterns, and level of physical activity influence body composition.

To better understand the concept of body composition, try to envision a brick of metal in comparison to a brick of Styrofoam® of the same size. The metal weighs much more than the Styrofoam. In the same way, muscle and bone weigh more than fat. As such, a person with a higher ratio of muscle to fat will weigh more than a person of the same size with a lower ratio of muscle to fat.

Body composition is an important factor in weight. For example, a person may weigh more than others due to being more muscular, not due to being affected by overweight. Athletes often train for long hours, which builds muscle and increases bone density. As a result, athletes often have considerably lower body-fat averages than nonathletes, even though they may weigh as much or more. **Figure 8.27** lists several ways of measuring body composition.

Body-Fat Distribution

body-fat distribution
locations of fat deposits on a person's body

Another factor that influences ideal body weight is **body-fat distribution**, or the location of fat deposits on your body. Some people tend to store extra fat around their abdomen and chest. These people have apple-shaped figures. Other people tend to store extra fat in their lower bodies around their hips, buttocks, and legs. These people have pear-shaped figures. Body-fat distribution can be as important, if not more important, to your health as how much fat you have. Following are two methods for assessing body fat distribution:

- **Waist circumference:** Waist circumference measures waist size. This measurement is simple to obtain and can be an indicator of excess abdominal fat. You can also use this measurement to monitor your progress toward meeting weight-management goals.
- **Waist-to-hip ratio:** The waist-to-hip ratio helps identify a person's fat distribution, or where extra fat is stored. This measurement is recommended for adults over 20 years of age. It is not recommended for children and teens, whose body shapes are evolving.

Measuring Body Composition

Method	Description
Skinfold test	A trained professional uses a *skinfold caliper*, a device that measures the thickness of a fold of fat in specific parts of the body. These measurements are added together to calculate an overall percentage of body fat.
Bioelectrical impedance analysis (BIA)	Electrodes are placed on the skin to measure how the body responds to a small electrical current. Electrical current runs faster through muscle than fat, which helps measure overall body composition.
DEXA scans	An X-ray measures the overall fat in the body, as well as in separate body regions.
Underwater weighing	This method estimates body-fat percentage based on body density. Weight is first measured while a person is submerged underwater and then measured again while the person is on dry land.
Air displacement	This method also estimates body-fat percentage based on density, but uses air instead of water. A person sits in an egg-shaped chamber (wearing skintight clothing or a bathing suit) for several minutes while the pressure of the air changes.

Figure 8.27 Accuracy, availability, time, and cost affect which method of measuring body composition is used. ***What three components are included in body composition?***

For those affected by overweight, distribution of fat on the body is often a better predictor of physical effects than actual weight, BMI, or total body fat. People who have *metabolic syndrome* have extra fat around the waist and high blood pressure, blood sugar, and cholesterol levels. This can lead to a greater risk of developing cardiovascular disease, stroke, and diabetes. Males are more likely than females to store fat in the abdomen, which also increases risk for cardiovascular disease.

How Does Weight Affect Your Health?

Your weight has an impact on your health now and in the future. Underweight, overweight, and obesity can cause a variety of negative health consequences.

When people do not take in enough nutrients and experience underweight, they can develop skin, hair, or teeth conditions. They may also feel tired often and are more likely to get sick, since their bodies are less able to fight off infections. Females who experience underweight may develop *osteoporosis*, a condition in which bones are brittle and more likely to break, and irregular menstrual periods.

Overweight or obesity leads to increased risk of cardiovascular disease. It also increases risk for developing hypertension (high blood pressure), hyperlipidemia (high cholesterol and high triglycerides), and liver and gallbladder disease. It can lead to cancers of the breast, colon, kidney, pancreas, cervix, and prostate. One of the most common health conditions associated with overweight and obesity is *type 2 diabetes mellitus*, a disorder in which the body is unable to manage blood glucose properly. People who are affected by overweight or obesity are more likely to experience respiratory, sleep, and joint conditions and may have trouble getting pregnant.

To avoid the health risks associated with underweight, overweight, and obesity, you need to know how to make healthy food choices and manage your weight in healthy ways (**Figure 8.28**).

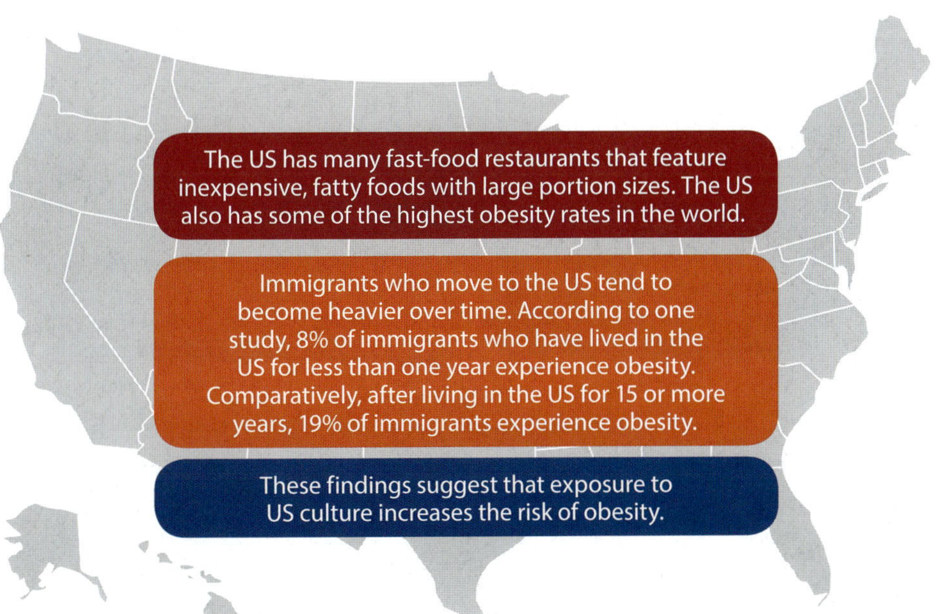

Luchenko Yana/Shutterstock.com

Figure 8.28 A person's culture can impact the availability of certain foods and the temptation to eat them. In the US, for example, quick, high-fat, high-sodium foods and large portions are common, which can result in overweight or obesity.

Health Across the Life Span

Your Food Choices Affect Your Life

Making nutritious food choices is an essential part of sustaining health across your life span. Habits you build now will help you maintain and improve your health in the future. Read each scenario and choose the option you think will provide the most benefit to your health. Follow the path to see the consequences of your decisions and how healthy your decisions are.

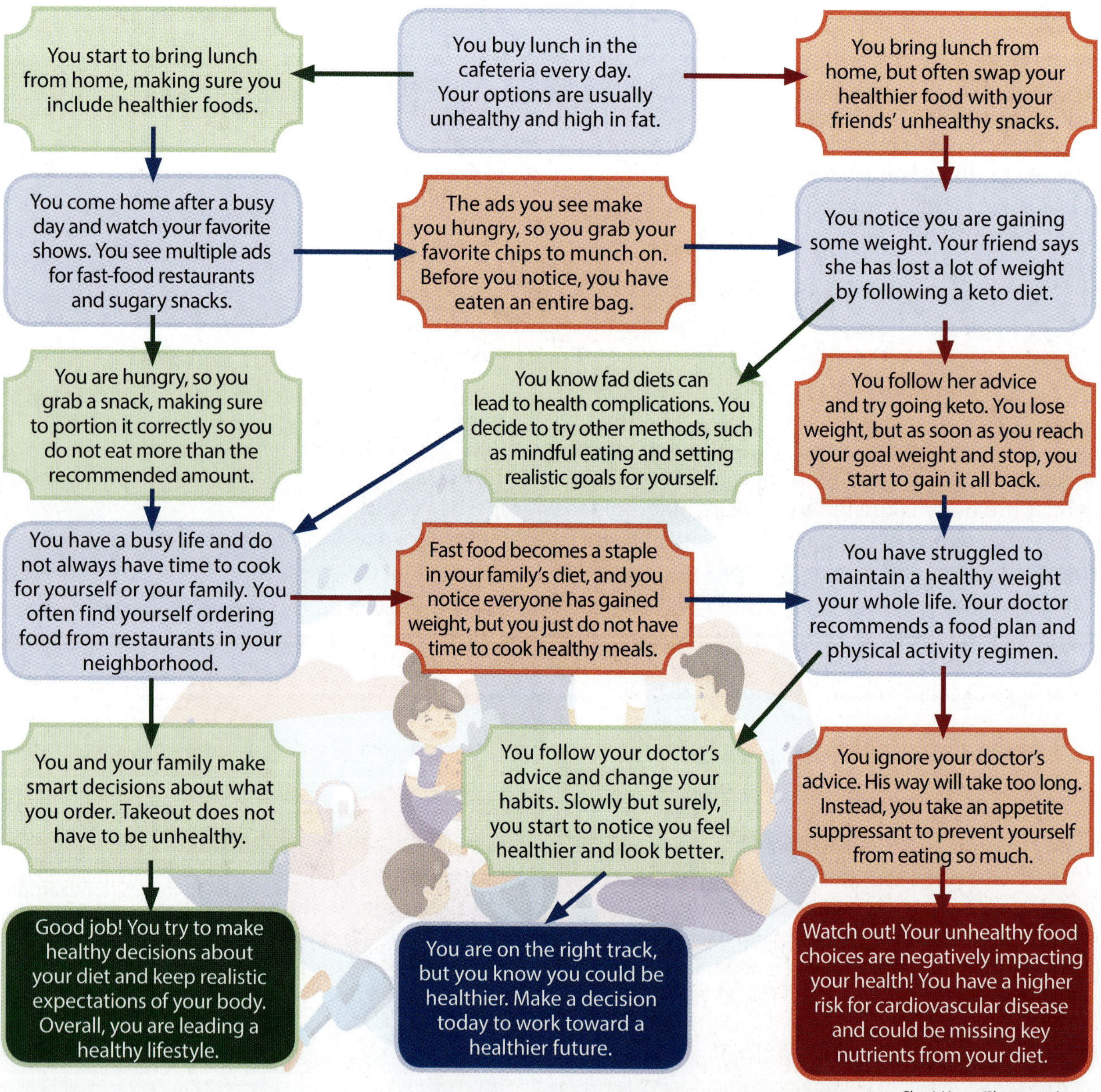

ClassicVector/Shutterstock.com

Practice Your Skills

Analyze Influences

For one week, track what you eat in a food diary. Include what you eat for each meal, as well as snacks. Also track how you feel before, during, and after each meal or snack. Then, analyze how different factors, such as activity level, stress level, or emotions affected what you ate. How can you improve your eating habits? Create a plan to improve one aspect of your eating habits to enhance your health.

Healthy Weight-Management Strategies

Making long-term changes to weight requires a permanent, lifelong change in eating and physical activity habits. To maintain your current weight, you must balance calories you consume with calories used during physical activity. To lose weight, you must consume fewer calories than you burn, and to gain weight, you must consume more calories. All of these activities require a healthy eating and physical activity plan compatible with your daily life. You can use several healthy strategies to lose, gain, or maintain your weight.

Set and Reward Realistic Goals

One effective strategy for managing weight is to set realistic, short-term goals regarding eating and physical activity. For example, you could decide to

- snack on nutritious foods between meals;
- eat an apple instead of chips as a mid-morning pick-me-up; or
- go for a walk with a friend instead of watching videos after school.

This short-term approach helps you experience some success and inspires confidence. Effective weight-loss techniques focus on gradual weight loss of 1–2 pounds (0.5–1 kilogram) a week. Effective weight-gain techniques keep a pace of 0.5–1 pound (0.2–0.5 kilogram) per week. This approach can be especially useful if you reward yourself. For example, after successfully losing 5 pounds or running 3 miles, reward yourself with a new pair of sunglasses or a trip to the movies with a friend.

Avoid Unhealthy Strategies

As many as 45 million adults in the US diet each year. People spend a tremendous amount of money—an estimated $33 billion each year—on weight-loss programs and products. Although these programs and products are highly profitable for the people who sell them, they often promise more than they can deliver.

The amount of weight people lose using any of these programs tends to be small and temporary. As a result, most people who participate in weight-loss programs regain about one-third of any weight lost within one year and return to their initial weight within three to five years.

Some examples of unhealthy weight management are fad diets and the use of appetite suppressants and diuretics. **Fad diets** often restrict certain types of food groups (such as carbohydrates) and may require the purchase of special, and often expensive, premade meals. The goal of these fad diets is to lose a significant amount of weight in a short time. Unfortunately, these types of eating plans can result in muscle loss and nutritional deficits, which is dangerous to your health (**Figure 8.29**). In addition, people often quickly regain any weight lost because the habits that led to the initial weight gain persist.

Some people use appetite suppressants and diuretics as quick-fix strategies that lead to temporary, short-term weight loss. *Appetite suppressants* trick the body into believing that it is not hungry or that the stomach is full. These drugs increase levels of chemicals in the brain that affect mood and appetite. **Diuretics**, or *water pills*, help the body eliminate salt (sodium) and water, mostly through increased urination.

fad diets stylish weight-loss plans that promise significant weight loss in short periods of time, often through cutting out food groups or buying premade meals

diuretics substances that help the body eliminate sodium and water, mostly through increased urination; can cause a drop in weight and dangerous side effects; also called *water pills*

Figure 8.29 Because fad diets often restrict entire nutrients, they increase the risk of health conditions.

Fad Diets		
Fad Diet	**Description**	**Health Effects**
Whole30	Consists of eating meat, seafood, fruits, vegetables, and eggs; avoids eating added sugar, grains, legumes, dairy, processed foods and beverages, baked goods, and junk foods	May lead to nutritional deficits, given limits on dairy, legumes, and whole grains
Keto	Consists of eating high-fat foods, moderate levels of protein, and very few carbohydrates	Is high in saturated fats and may cause nutritional deficits, constipation, and liver and kidney conditions
Atkins	Consists of restricting most carbohydrates and instead eating larger amounts of protein and fat	May lead to side effects, such as headache, dizziness, weakness, fatigue, and constipation; may lead to nutritional deficits and insufficient fiber, which can cause nausea and diarrhea
Paleo and paleo-vegan (pegan)	Consists of eating large amounts of vegetables, fruits, nuts and seeds, as well as lean meats and fish for a paleo diet; limits beans, grains, and dairy	May lead to nutritional deficits, given limits on dairy, legumes, and whole grains
Zone	Consists of eating meals that are 40% carbohydrates, 30% protein, and 30% fat; limits calories; schedules meals at set times throughout the day	May lead to deficits in calcium and other nutrients (fiber, vitamin C, folic acid, and some minerals); can lead to kidney conditions
South Beach	Consists of larger amounts of protein and healthy fat and small amounts of carbohydrates; is a modified low-carbohydrate eating plan	Is generally safe unless carbohydrates are even more severely restricted, which can cause nausea, headaches, and mental fatigue

Loss of water causes a drop in weight. The side effects of these drugs—including blurred vision, dizziness, sleeplessness, and irritability—can be so serious that people need medical treatment or hospitalization.

Eat Mindfully

The term *mindfulness* describes being fully focused on the present moment. You can eat mindfully by paying attention to the foods you consume. Mindful eating helps people make healthier food choices, since people focus on the foods they put into their bodies.

The following are some strategies you can use to practice eating mindfully:

- Appreciate your food. Before starting to eat, take a minute to appreciate the food on your plate. Think about the work that went into bringing this food to the table. Recognize the different colors, smells, and textures of the food.
- Portion out snacks instead of eating straight from the bag or box.
- Take small bites so you can better savor the different flavors and tastes. Try to identify the different ingredients in each bite. Chew each mouthful thoroughly to really taste all the flavors. Put your utensils down between bites. Fully swallow your food before taking another bite.

- Do not skip meals. It is hard to practice mindful eating when you are very hungry. Eat meals when you are hungry. Skipping meals can lead you to overeat just to get something into your stomach.

Monitor Eating

Monitoring when and what you eat is another effective strategy for managing weight. It is easy to forget about some of the calories you consume each day, especially outside a regular meal. For example, you might eat potato chips while you study or have a candy bar as a quick after-school snack. People often overeat at parties because they are not conscious of how much they are eating.

Individuals who keep a **food diary**, or daily record of what they eat, have more success at managing their weight (**Figure 8.30**). After you have determined triggers that cause you to overeat, you can try to eliminate them or substitute another type of food. For example, you could develop new strategies for coping with mood-related factors. If you feel sad or anxious, you could go for a walk, call a friend, or listen to music instead of eating to feel better.

food diary daily record of what a person eats; used to track eating patterns and calorie intake

You can follow through on changes to your eating and drinking behavior by making small but healthy changes. To gain weight, add more

FOOD DIARY

DATE	TIME	ITEMS
T 12/16	8:30a.m.	Nonfat yogurt, blueberries, granola, and glass of orange juice
	11:00a.m.	Baby carrots
	12:30p.m.	Turkey sandwich on whole-grain bread, bell pepper + cheese slices
	3:45p.m	Air popped popcorn
	7:00p.m.	Tacos: corn tortillas, ground turkey, low-fat shredded cheese, lettuce, onions, black beans, tomatoes, corn, avocado
W 12/17	8:30a.m.	Whole-grain toast with peanut butter and banana
	12:30p.m.	Turkey wrap on whole-grain tortilla with lettuce, pickle, onion, and low-fat shredded cheese
	3:45p.m.	Low-fat cheese slices and whole-grain crackers
	6:30p.m.	Salad with strawberries and walnuts

Elena_Nevskaya/Shutterstock.com

Figure 8.30 Recording what you eat each day will help you become aware of what triggers you to overeat, such as coming home from a stressful day at school.

nutrient-dense foods to your eating pattern. To lose or maintain weight, switch from sugary soft drinks to water, take smaller portions of food, and reduce late-night eating. Do not buy foods that will tempt you. Then, when you are hungry, you will grab a nutritious snack instead of a less-nutritious one. Eat healthier foods when you eat out. Order a salad instead of a hamburger or ask for a half-portion of your favorite entree. If you really want to order a dessert, split it with a friend (or two).

Limit Screen Time

People who spend many hours watching shows, playing video games, or scrolling through social media are more likely to be affected by overweight or obesity (**Figure 8.31**). Watching TV and using social media increase exposure to advertisements for less-nutritious foods and beverages. In the US, food and beverage companies spend billions of dollars a year in advertising, often aimed at children and teens. More than one-half of advertisements seen by children and teens relate to food. The majority of these advertisements are for fast foods, snack foods, and sugar-sweetened drinks. Predictably, viewing these advertisements increases children's interest in such products. One study estimated that a ban on fast-food advertising during children's programs could reduce the number of teens affected by overweight by 14 percent.

In one study, researchers found that children and teens who had TVs in their bedrooms, and therefore watched more TV on average, were more than twice as likely to show the highest levels of body fat.

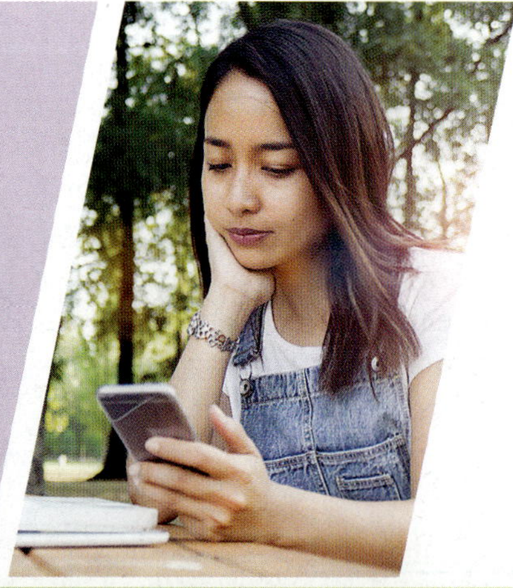

In another study, people who felt more of a compulsive need to check their phones for notifications had a higher BMI and greater percentage of body fat.

This study also indicates a link between digital multitasking and obesity, via factors like food temptations and lack of self-control.

PredragImages/iStock/Getty Images Plus/Getty Images

Figure 8.31 Various scientific studies indicate a link between the use of digital devices and body fat.

Change Your Thoughts

Another way to reach your weight goals is to change negative thoughts about eating and weight. Some people give up on their goals quickly, often because they have negative or unrealistic views about weight management. These people might continually think to themselves, *I will never be able to lose the weight.* These negative views are common among people who have struggled with weight management for some time.

"all-or-nothing" mind-set way of thinking that classifies behaviors as either total successes or total failures

An **"all-or-nothing" mind-set** about eating can also undermine weight-management efforts. This type of thinking occurs when people eat something prohibited by their eating plan and, because they believe they have failed, give up on the plan. For example, you eat chicken nuggets for dinner; think, *Well, I've blown it now*; and proceed to eat brownies for dessert too. Similarly, creating a distinction between "good foods" and "bad foods" and then permanently avoiding all "bad foods" will set you up for failure. Instead, it is best to eat desired foods in moderation as part of a healthy eating plan.

Losing and gaining weight takes time, so you should not expect instant success. Losing or gaining weight gradually through permanent lifestyle changes is more likely to help you achieve a healthy weight long-term.

Also, everyone who is trying to create new eating and physical activity habits experiences slip-ups or lapses. Do not let one lapse lead to a return of your old eating or physical activity habits. If you slip up and eat a food you are trying to avoid, or eat too much, quickly refocus on your plan.

Enlist Support

Changing eating and physical activity behaviors is difficult, so it helps to have support from those around you. Simply having a friend who will go to the gym or go for walks with you can help. Tell friends and family members about your goal and ask them to support or join in your efforts.

Some people participate in formal groups to lose weight. Group approaches are especially effective because they provide social support and healthy competition. Interventions designed to decrease obesity in children and teens are especially effective if family members are involved and supportive. The best results occur when family members change their own habits and provide healthier foods for children.

It is a good idea to consult with a healthcare professional if you are struggling with weight management. These professionals can help you determine the weight-management strategy best for your health.

Lesson 8.4 Review

Know and Understand

1. How do genes influence weight?
2. Explain how calorie balance can lead to weight gain, loss, or maintenance.
3. Why is BMI an imperfect tool for assessing weight status?
4. Why is the waist-to-hip ratio method of measuring body-fat distribution not recommended for teens?
5. What are the health consequences of overweight and obesity?

Think Critically

6. With a partner, discuss the following sentence: *Your ideal weight is the weight at which your body is healthy.* What does this sentence mean? Do you think most teens agree with this sentence? What factors influence whether a particular weight is healthy for someone?
7. Why are fad diets not a healthy method of weight management? Choose one fad diet and research how effectively people are able to maintain the weight change it causes. What risks are associated with the fad diet?
8. For one week, keep a food diary recording everything you eat. At the end of the week, review your food diary. Given what you have learned about nutrition in this chapter, are there any adjustments you could make to have a healthier eating pattern?
9. How does having an "all-or-nothing" mind-set make it difficult to achieve weight-management goals?

REAL WORLD Health Skills

Set Goals Select one factor that can influence a person's weight and then research its impact using reliable resources. In your research, consider how this factor affects you and how a person can use it to maintain or reach a desired weight. Then, using your research, set three SMART goals related to managing this factor. Explain how each goal will help you manage your weight and choose one goal to act on.

Chapter 8 Review and Assessment

Chapter Summary

Nutrition is the process of choosing and consuming foods and beverages to fuel your body. There are six general types of nutrients. Carbohydrates are the body's major source of energy. Protein is used by the body to build and maintain cells and tissues. Fats play an important role in the absorption and transport of nutrients.

Vitamins regulate body processes and help the body release the energy found in proteins, fats, and carbohydrates. Minerals are inorganic elements that help the body grow and develop. Water maintains your body temperature, cushions and lubricates joints, and protects the spinal cord and other sensitive tissues. It also moves oxygen, nutrients, waste, and other materials throughout the body.

The *Dietary Guidelines for Americans* provides recommendations for establishing eating patterns. The MyPlate food guidance system helps individuals develop a personalized eating plan that includes five food groups.

Following a healthy eating pattern involves paying attention to calorie balance and choosing nutrient-dense foods, while limiting intake of added sugars, saturated fats, and sodium. A healthy eating pattern tailored to your individual needs can help avoid health risks, such as malnutrition, undernutrition, and overnutrition.

Food choices are influenced by many factors, including genetics, age, mood, cultural background, and social environment.

Nutrition Facts labels provide information regarding servings and calories, Daily Values, and ingredients in food. Sometimes food packages use terms such as "low-fat" or "organic" to make specific claims about the health benefits of certain foods. Knowing how to prepare foods, assess nutritional value, and substitute ingredients can help you eat healthier and get needed nutrients. Practicing food safety can help prevent foodborne illnesses.

Social, psychological, cultural, and socioeconomic factors, as well as genetics, all affect individuals' healthy body weight. Because of these many factors, several different approaches identify healthy weight ranges, including body mass index (BMI), body composition, and body-fat distribution. To establish a healthy weight, it is important to set realistic, short-term goals, avoid unhealthy weight-management strategies, and eat mindfully.

Vocabulary Activity

Review each of the terms from the list. If there are any terms you do not know how to pronounce, research their pronunciations online. Make flash cards with the phonetic spellings for these terms to help you remember. With a partner, take turns pulling out a flash card from the stack. Look at the word and think about the sounds each letter makes. Then, decode the term by sounding it out from left to right. Check your pronunciation against the phonetic spelling and correct each other if a term is mispronounced. Ask your teacher for clarification, if necessary.

added sugars
"all-or-nothing" mind-set
body composition
body-fat distribution
body mass index (BMI)
calories
carbohydrates
Daily Values
dietary fiber
Dietary Guidelines for Americans
diuretics
empty calories
fad diets
fats
fat-soluble vitamins
food additives
food allergy
food diary
food intolerances
food preferences
foodborne illnesses
foodborne infection
foodborne intoxication
generally recognized as safe (GRAS)
genetically modified organism (GMO)
glucose
malnutrition
metabolism
minerals
MyPlate
nutrient-dense foods
nutrients
nutrition
Nutrition Facts label
obesity
organic
overnutrition
overweight
protein
saturated fats
trans fat
undernutrition
underweight
unsaturated fats
vitamins
water-soluble vitamins

Review and Recall

Review the information in this chapter by answering the following questions.

1. Why is it more beneficial to obtain vitamins through a well-balanced diet, rather than through supplements?
2. Give one example of a negative health consequence of failing to take in enough of a mineral.
3. What is the difference between essential and nonessential amino acids? Which type is more essential to obtain through the foods you eat and why?
4. What are the five main recommendations in the *Dietary Guidelines for Americans*?
5. Which source of essential nutrients is not considered a MyPlate food group, but must be included in your eating plan?
   A. protein foods
   B. oils
   C. grains
   D. dairy
6. What are the five food groups included in the MyPlate system?
7. Which of the following can serve as a plant-based dairy alternative?
   A. goat's milk
   B. water
   C. lactase
   D. calcium-fortified soy milk
8. Which nutrient provides more calories per gram than any other source?
   A. fat
   B. dairy
   C. protein
   D. grains
9. Nutrient-dense foods contain little or none of what substances?
10. All of the following ingredients indicate that a food contains added sugars, *except*
    A. fruit juice concentrate.
    B. high-fructose corn syrup.
    C. ascorbic acid.
    D. maltose.
11. What are the factors that impact ideal weight for individual bodies?
12. What is represented by the % Daily Values listed on a Nutrition Facts label?
13. Which of the following is *not* a method for measuring body composition?
    A. skinfold test
    B. underwater weighing
    C. dividing height by weight
    D. DEXA scans
14. How can TV and social media negatively affect weight-management efforts?

Standardized Test Prep

Math Practice

Review the Nutrition Facts label shown. Then answer the questions that follow.

15. What percentage of the total fat in this food is saturated fat?
16. The Daily Values on this label are based on a 2,000-calorie diet. Calculate the % Daily Value of added sugars for the following diets:
    A. 1,800-calorie diet
    B. 2,200-calorie diet
    C. 2,400-calorie diet
17. If you ate half the food in this container, how many calories would you be consuming?

Nutrition Facts

1 serving per container
Serving size **1 cup (245g)**

Amount per serving	
Calories	**208**
	% Daily Value*
Total Fat 3g	4%
Saturated Fat 2g	10%
Trans Fat 0g	
Cholesterol 12mg	4%
Sodium 162mg	7%
Total Carbohydrate 34g	12%
Dietary Fiber 0g	0%
Total Sugars 34g	
Includes 17g Added Sugars	34%
Protein 12g	
Vitamin D 0mcg	0%
Calcium 419mg	32%
Iron 0.2mg	1%
Potassium 537mg	11%

* The % Daily Value (DV) tells you how much a nutrient in a serving of food contributes to a daily diet. 2,000 calories a day is used for general nutrition advice.

Courtesy of the Food and Drug Administration

Chapter 8 Skills Assessment

Critical Thinking Skills

Answer the following questions to assess your knowledge of what you learned in this chapter.

1. Given what you know about carbohydrates, why do you think it is especially important to include carbohydrates in a healthy breakfast?
2. Can you think of any foods you consume on a regular basis that are high in saturated fats? With a partner, discuss what you can do to reduce your intake of saturated fats.
3. Find a copy of your favorite restaurant's menu. With a partner, take turns imagining you have various dietary needs or preferences, and practice making healthy choices from the menu based on those needs. Were some needs easier or harder to accommodate than others? Which ones?
4. Develop a one-week meal plan. Then compare your plan with a classmate's and discuss the following: How does your meal plan align with the *Dietary Guidelines for Americans* and MyPlate? How did you incorporate variety into the meal plan? Was it difficult to include enough of a certain nutrient in the meal plan?
5. Think about how many whole grains and refined grains are included in your diet. Do you think your diet includes a healthy balance of each? How can you incorporate more whole grains into your diet?
6. With a partner, discuss how your nutritional needs change throughout your lifetime. What nutrients do you think are especially important at your current stage of life?
7. Think of two different snack items with similar calorie content. Which option is the better choice, and why?
8. Do you eat breakfast every day? If so, what do you usually eat? Do you think your breakfast choices tend to be nutritious or not? Why or why not?
9. Imagine you are having a study session with several of your friends after school, and everyone is bringing snacks. Brainstorm some strategies for making sure you maintain appropriate portion sizes and make nutritious choices.
10. At the grocery store, examine low-fat, nonfat, and full-fat versions of various items, such as yogurt or salad dressings. Analyze any corresponding differences on the food labels. Can full-fat versions of an item sometimes be a healthier option than low-fat or nonfat versions? Explain.
11. Calculate your own body mass index (BMI). Do you think your result is an accurate assessment of your body weight status? Why or why not?
12. With a partner, discuss why some people seem to be able to eat whatever they want without gaining weight. Why is it important to follow a healthy diet, regardless of the immediate consequences?
13. With a partner, discuss some negative thoughts a person might have while trying to achieve a healthier weight. Then, discuss some strategies to combat these thoughts.

Health and Wellness Skills

Complete the following activities to assess your skills related to health and wellness.

14. **Analyze Influences.** Each time you watch TV or browse online, the media provides you with persuasive advertising strategies, such as those you learned about in Chapter 2. For this activity, choose one food advertisement you have encountered. Identify what persuasive advertising strategies are being used and analyze how they influence your food choices. Then, create a presentation to share your findings with the rest of the class.
15. **Access Information.** Create a menu that includes all of your favorite foods. Divide your favorite foods into five categories: appetizers (four items), main courses (six items), side dishes (five items), desserts (at least two items), and beverages (at least two items). Once you have listed your favorite foods by category, research the nutrition information for all the items on your menu. Finally, create a visually pleasing menu with your foods listed by category, their nutrition information, your restaurant name, and pictures. Show your menu to the class. At whose "restaurant" would you want to eat?
16. **Communicate with Others.** Learning about nutrition and its effects on the body has made you get serious about your own food choices. At home, your family thrives on fast food and highly processed foods.

You now realize these food choices are not in your best interest. Write a dialogue with your parent or guardian in which you respectfully request to have more say in the food consumed in your home. Do not forget to include all aspects of effective communication in your dialogue.

17. **Make Decisions.** Knowing the different behaviors that lead to an unhealthy weight and body composition enables you to live a healthy life. Using a chart or app, create a daily checklist of decisions you can make to follow a healthy lifestyle. Some examples might include taking a walk after school or packing a nutritious lunch the night before a school day. Try to check off all the decisions on your list each day.
18. **Set Goals.** Healthy eating is a key factor in preventing underweight, overweight, and obesity. Healthy eating also helps you maintain your health so your body can be physically active, fight off infections, and grow. Set one short-term SMART goal for each day of the week to help you adopt healthier eating habits. After each day, record what you accomplished toward your healthy eating goal. Measure the impact of achieving your goal and modify your goals for the next week.
19. **Practice Health-Enhancing Behaviors.** Imagine you have been elected to a Healthy High School Vending Machine committee, and it is your job to determine the foods your high school's vending machines will include. List at least five nutritious criteria foods must meet to be in the machines. Then identify any foods you would remove from the machines based on your criteria and suggest alternatives. Write a paragraph explaining how the new options will enhance student health.
20. **Advocate for Health.** Eating a lot of foods high in added sugars, saturated fats, and sodium can increase your body weight and risk for developing certain diseases. For one week, try to be a true health advocate for your family and friends. Go through the foods in your home and try to substitute nutrient-dense snacks. Encourage your friends to eat nutritious foods and eat mindfully. Record the actions you take to advocate for health. Afterward, evaluate which actions worked and which did not.

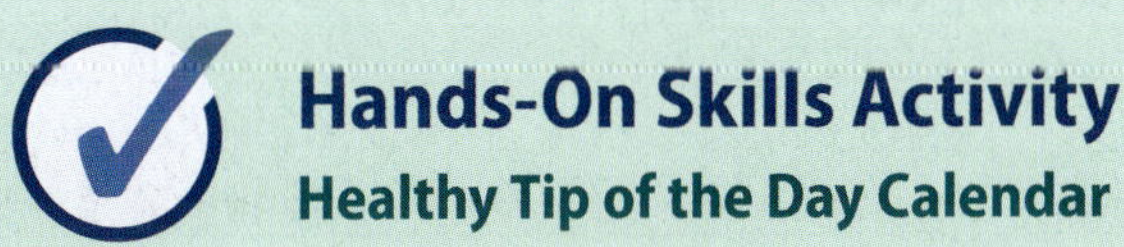

Hands-On Skills Activity

Healthy Tip of the Day Calendar

What you eat every day has an impact on your health. Changing what you eat requires changing your habits. To change your habits, some of which you may have had for a long time, you need to pay attention to what you eat and remember to eat healthy every day.

Steps for This Activity

1. Using a chart or app, create a 30-day calendar. For each day, write a healthy eating tip or slogan, using words you will easily remember. Write a catchy title for your calendar, since you will also be sharing it with other teens. Include at least five pieces of art in your calendar. An example follows this activity.
2. **Access Information.** Before sharing your calendar, verify that all of your tips enhance health. Cite the reliable sources you used to verify your tips on a separate piece of paper.
3. **Advocate for Health.** When you are done with your calendar, put it somewhere you can easily reference it. For example, you might hang it in your locker or save it to your phone. Distribute your calendar to a few of your friends to encourage their healthy eating habits. If they have any questions, give them the list of reliable sources you referenced.

Sunday	Monday	Tuesday	Wednesday	Thursday	Friday	Saturday
21 Wait for 15 minutes to go for seconds; you may find you are already full.	22 Trade in that sugary soda for a glass of milk.	23 Record everything you eat today. You might be surprised how much you are eating.	24 Substitute fruit for a sugary snack.	25 Do not skip meals. Skipping a meal can lower your metabolism by 5 percent, enough to gain 1 pound every month.	26 Sample a new nutritious food today.	27 Sit down with your family and help plan a week of healthy meals.

Left to right: ferie07/Shutterstock.com; Actor/Shutterstock.com; Sudowoodo/Shutterstock.com; Tim UR/Shutterstock.com; MaraZe/Shutterstock.com

Chapter 9

Having a Healthy Body Image

Look for the skills icon throughout this chapter for opportunities to practice your health skills.

Check Your Health and Wellness Skills

In this chapter, you will learn skills for developing a healthy body image. To understand the skills you currently use, take the following inventory of your behaviors. Indicate how well you think you use each skill. Use a scale of 1–5, *1* meaning you do not use the skill and *5* meaning you feel completely comfortable using it.

Skill	How Well Do You Use Each Skill?
I know pictures on social media sometimes use filters that present unrealistic standards.	
I avoid classifying foods as "good" or "bad."	
I could recognize the signs of an eating disorder in a friend.	
I know whom I'd talk to and what I'd say if I needed help for an eating disorder.	
I mostly spend time on media that promotes a positive body image.	
I analyze media images to find out if they're edited.	
I value who I am and what my body can do more than how I look.	
I understand that many different body types are attractive—there is not one ideal.	
When I talk negatively about my body, I correct myself.	
I spend time around people who have a positive body image.	
I encourage others to accept and value their bodies.	
	Total:

Add up your responses to each statement. The higher your score, the more comfortable you feel practicing health skills related to developing a healthy body image. Which skill do you think is most important for you? Which skill is the most challenging for you? Which skill would you most like to improve? In this chapter, you will learn how to perform these skills better and more often.

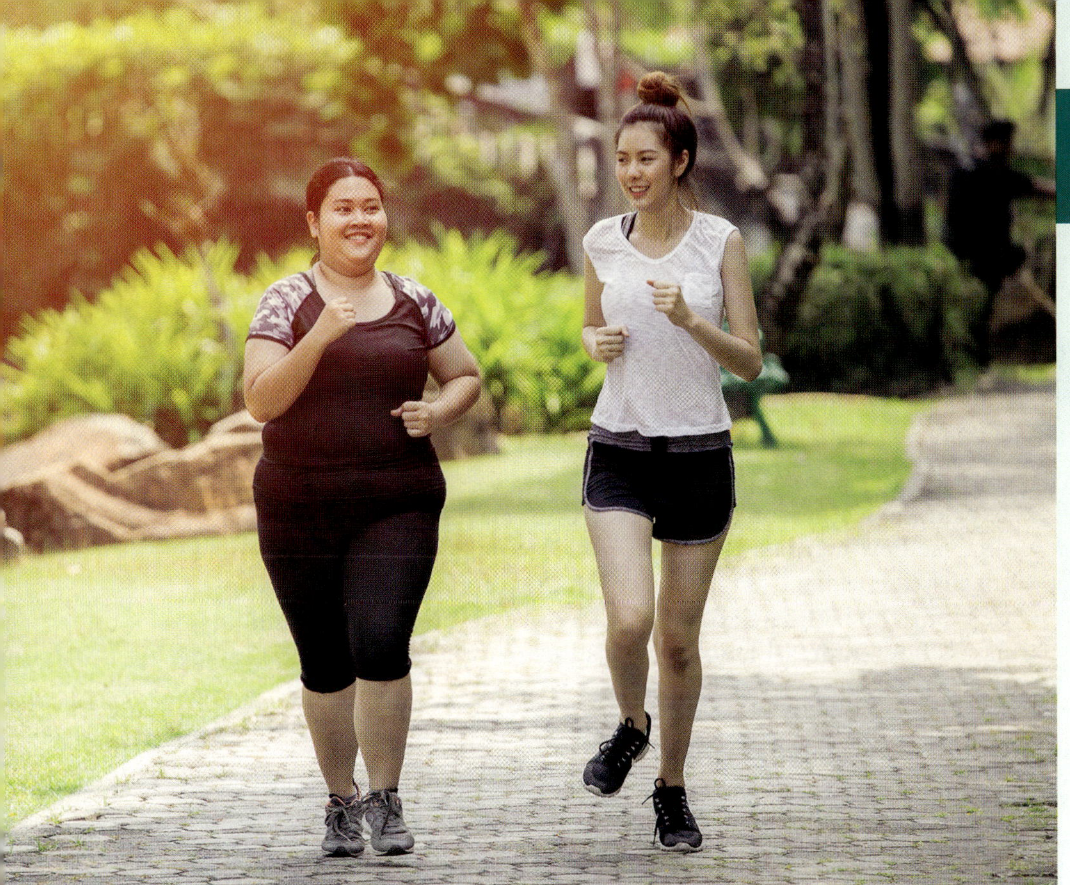

Quality Stock Arts/Shutterstock.com

Reading and Notetaking

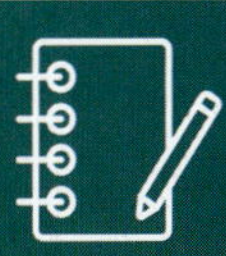

Skim the headings in this chapter and consider what each concept in this chapter might teach you about body image, disordered eating, and eating disorders. Keep a list, placing a star beside any concepts that especially interest you. After reading this chapter, pick three concepts and write a few paragraphs about how these concepts can help you understand yourself. Use proper grammar and spelling in your paragraphs.

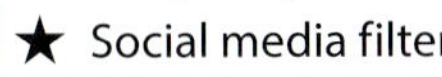

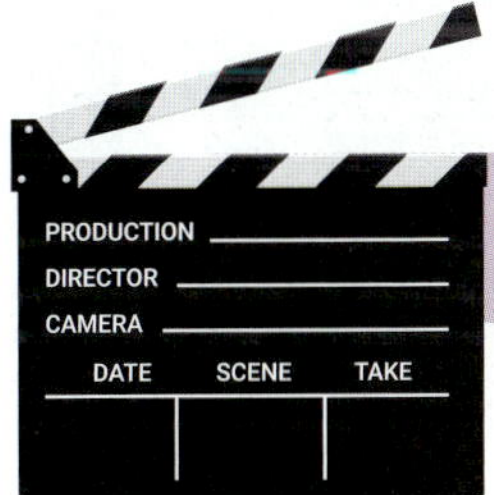

Setting the Scene

Struggling with How You Look

This year, you are excited to make new friends. You have also started thinking about eventually dating. At the same time, you have become pretty self-conscious and anxious about how you look. It seems like the older students at your school always look put together, and you feel like you do not measure up. Sometimes you get acne breakouts on your face. You also wish you were taller. Spending time on social media makes your feelings worse, since everyone's photos look great. Knowing some of these photos use filters does not always help. You still dislike how you look in comparison to everyone else. You do not like feeling so bad about yourself. Your feelings are making it harder to connect with new friends, not to mention potential dating partners. You just are not sure what you can do to feel better.

Thinking Critically

1. What are some factors that might lead teens to feel badly about their bodies?
2. What are some strategies you can use to feel better about your body or help a friend who struggles with these feelings?

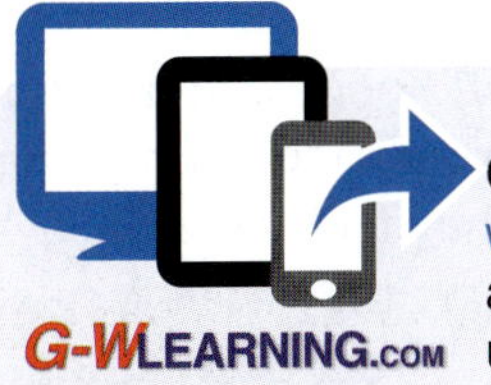

Click on the activity icon or visit www.g-wlearning.com/health/4095 to access online vocabulary activities using key terms from the chapter.

Lesson

9.1

Factors That Influence Body Image

Essential Question?

What influences affect a person's body image?

Learning Outcomes

After studying this lesson, you will be able to

- define *body image*;
- explain how a person's social environment influences body image;
- analyze how media and society affect female and male body image;
- discuss the impact of race and ethnicity on body image; and
- describe the influence of gender identity on body image; and
- assess how some athletic activities influence a person's body image.

Key Terms

airbrushing
body image
muscle dysmorphia
weight stigma

Warm-Up Activity

Social Media Models

Analyze Influences Countless social media advertisements show models selling some type of product. Search for a few different social media accounts that use these kinds of ads. List all of the physical traits that the female models have in common. Then list all of the physical traits that the male models share. What do your findings tell you about the physical ideals presented in the media? How does this influence the way you see yourself?

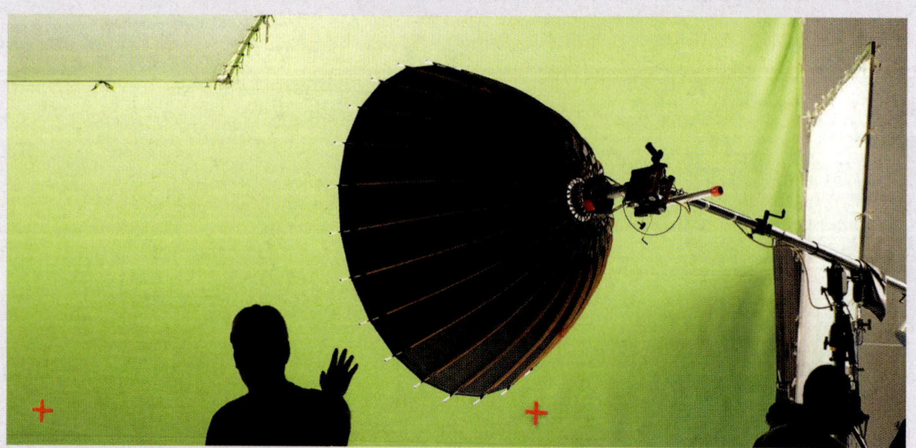

gnepphoto/Shutterstock.com

How do you feel about your body? Do you marvel at its strength and agility? Do you appreciate that the organs in your body accomplish amazing tasks? For example, your heart pumps about 2,000 gallons of blood each day, and your digestive system takes in the nutrients you need from food. Many teens do not think about these aspects when asked how they feel about their bodies. Instead, they worry about a particular body part they wish they could change. These feelings are part of body image.

Your **body image** is your thoughts and feelings about how you look. Your body image is not what your body *actually* looks like, but how you *think* it looks.

body image subjective mental image of one's own body; established based on self-observation and the reactions of others

How your body actually looks and how you feel about it are not necessarily related. All people may like or dislike aspects of their bodies (**Figure 9.1**).

How people feel about their bodies can have a large impact on health. People who have a *positive body image* appreciate and value their bodies. They recognize that a person's physical appearance has no impact on character, value, and worth. People with a *negative body image* dislike their bodies and believe their negative perceptions impact their worth and value.

The effect of body image on mental and emotional health can also influence physical and social health. People who have a positive body image are more likely to take care of their bodies. They are also more likely to feel confident in social situations and build healthy relationships.

In this lesson, you will learn about factors that influence body image, including social environment, media and society, race and ethnicity, and athletic activities.

Many teens feel self-conscious and wish they could change parts of their bodies at some time.
Fortunately, this feeling often goes away with time and age.

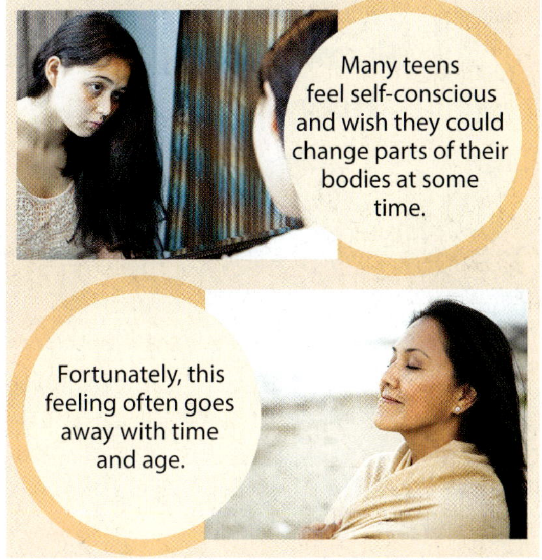

Top to bottom: Phil McDonald/Shutterstock.com; pixelheadphoto digitalskillet/Shutterstock.com

Figure 9.1 People may worry about muscle or breast size, weight, height, skin color, and facial blemishes like acne and pimples. ***Does body image describe what your body actually looks like or how you think it looks?***

Social Environment

Your *social environment*—which includes the relationships in your life and the community around you—influences your body image. For example, family members can affect a person's body image by emphasizing certain physical qualities. These family pressures can lead to a negative body image.

A teen's friends also influence body image. To fit in with a peer group, teens may feel pressured to have a certain appearance (**Figure 9.2**). Teens who hang out with friend groups who have similar physical features can feel pressure to also have those features. Teens may feel extra pressure if they worry potential dating partners will not find them attractive.

Unhealthy Changes to Teens' Bodies

Teen boys, especially those in certain sports, may use steroids or other types of drugs to become more muscular.

These drugs can have very serious side effects, such as increased risk of stroke, heart attack, and kidney or liver damage. In teens, steroids can also cause stunted growth in height and weight.

More than 200,000 teens each year have plastic surgery. Many view this as a way to fit in with their peers.

The most common procedure is *rhinoplasty*, or reshaping of the nose. Risks of this type of surgery include infection, poor wound healing or scarring, numbness or pain in skin, difficulty breathing, and skin discoloration.

Teens of color may use unhealthy products to bleach, or lighten, their skin color.

Toxic chemicals may cause mercury poisoning, dermatitis, or steroid acne. The FDA has stated that over-the-counter skin-bleaching products are not recognized as safe and effective.

Figure 9.2 Teens sometimes make unhealthy choices when attempting to change the different features of their bodies.

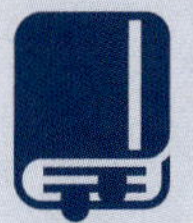

Case Study

How Do I Look?

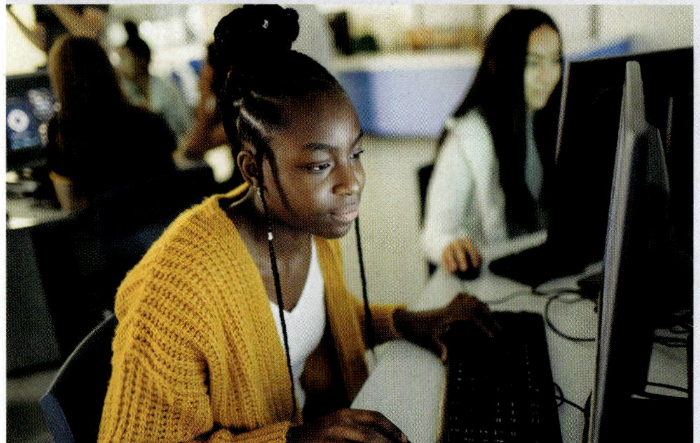

Django/E+/Getty Images

Natalia does not understand how people think she is "lucky" to be skinny. Her friends and other classmates tell her they wish they looked like her all the time. Natalia, however, wishes she could gain weight. Her sister teases her, calling her a "walking bean pole." She struggles to find clothes that give her the fuller, hourglass figure she envies. Natalia has started eating more than she needs to, even after she is full, in hopes that her body will fill out.

Tiffany has come a long way in appreciating her body. When she was younger, she was self-conscious about her height and skin color. No girls at school were as tall or dark-skinned as Tiffany was. She would wear clothes that covered her skin as much as possible and slouch, hoping no one would tease her. All Tiffany ever wanted was to fit in. Since her neighborhood does not have a large African-American population, Tiffany has started following female role models online. Seeing other females who are proud of their height and skin color helps Tiffany embrace her appearance.

Kian is unhappy with how bad his acne has become. What started as a pimple or two has now taken over his face. His close friends do not comment or tease, yet Kian feels like they are always staring. Kian washes his face twice a day, but the acne persists. Kian's friend Aaron recently noticed how upset Kian has been. Kian admitted he has been feeling self-conscious about his acne and is upset that nothing is working. Aaron tells Kian about how his own acne was terrible freshman year, but improved with the help of a dermatologist. Aaron suggests Kian try seeing a professional.

Practice Your Skills

Make Decisions

On your own, make a list of the physical qualities you think are attractive. Next to each quality, note factors you think have influenced your perceptions of attractiveness. Consider the influence of your family members, friends, community, culture, ethnicity, and the media. With a partner, identify 10 decisions you can make to enhance positive influences on your body image and reduce negative influences. Explain how each decision can impact body image and choose five decisions you want to put into action. Act on one decision each day for one week.

Participation in social media can make the pressure from peers worse. Many teens want approval from their friends—as measured in "likes"—and only post pictures in which they look good. Some teens even manipulate images using filters and retouching. These trends make teens feel pressure to be as attractive as possible—to have "perfect" hair, flawless skin, and so on. Social media also makes it hard for teens to avoid comparing themselves to other people. Teens who constantly see idealized pictures of their peers looking great on social media can feel worse about their own appearance.

Media and Society

Every day, people see messages communicating different ideas about attractiveness. Advertisements for products such as cars, deodorant, digital devices, and clothing spread messages that associate certain physical traits with attractiveness, wealth, health, success, and happiness (**Figure 9.3**). Idealized images in the media are different for female and male bodies.

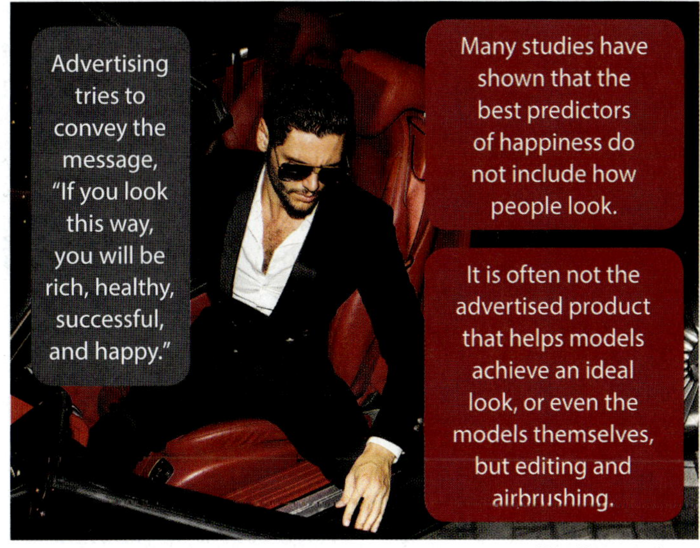

AS Inc/Shutterstock.com

Figure 9.3 Companies use models that represent idealized versions of male and female bodies. These idealized images do not represent most people's bodies.

Female Bodies in the Media

Think quickly: who is the most attractive female TV or film star? Whoever came to mind is almost certainly thin and young. Virtually all images of female bodies in US media—in movies, on TV, in music videos, and on the covers of magazines—show a very thin body type. This preference in the media is relatively new. Movie and magazine depictions of female bodies have become consistently thinner over the years.

Media images of celebrities, actors, and models often set unhealthy standards. For example, the average woman in the US wears a size 12–14, but the average model featured in a magazine wears a size 0–4 (**Figure 9.4**).

In a survey, teen girls said their ideal body size was...
5'7"
100 pounds
but a more accurate range for the average teen girl is...
5'1"– 5'4"
101–126 pounds

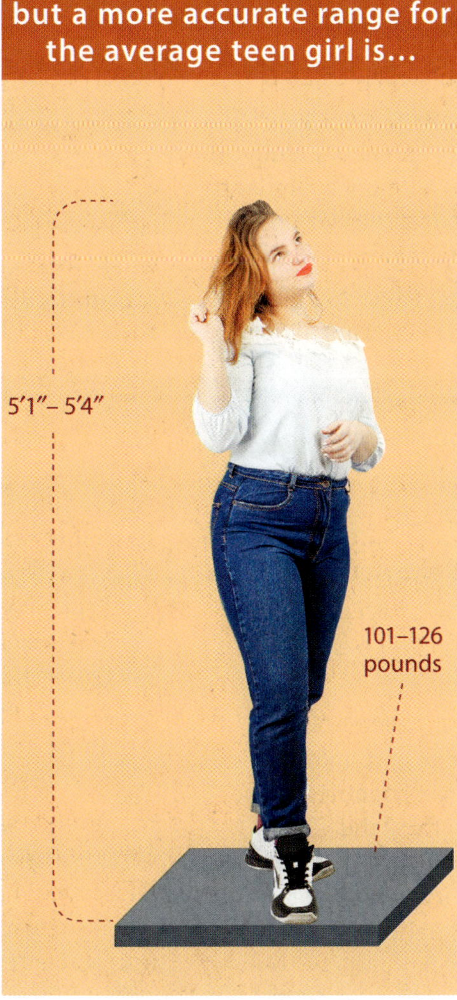

Left to right: Andrei Park/Shutterstock.com; kravik93/Shutterstock.com

Figure 9.4 Because of images in the media, teen girls tend to have a distorted idea of what their bodies should look like. ***What are the health consequences of having this distorted idea of the female body?***

weight stigma flawed belief that having a thinner body or lower weight is always better

airbrushing digitally altering an image to eliminate blemishes, cellulite, bulges, or wrinkles

In one study, women shown female silhouettes of different sizes thought the ideal body size according to *other* women was thinner than their own ideal body size. Women also thought the ideal female body size was thinner than men did. This flawed idea that having a thinner body or lower weight is always better is called **weight stigma** and is a serious risk factor for negative body image and eating disorders.

Media images of female bodies also set unrealistic standards for specific body parts. Female bodies in the media may also have large breasts and butts, long legs, a small waist, clear skin, little body hair, and perfectly styled light hair. In addition, advertisements and media images almost always show females who are young. Many products are advertised to make females appear younger—for example, through cosmetic surgery. These advertisements clearly suggest that attractiveness, at least for females, is linked with appearing young.

Representations of female bodies in the media are not just due to how companies choose models or actresses. Advertising companies and magazines also edit or airbrush images of female bodies. **Airbrushing** involves digitally altering an image to eliminate blemishes, cellulite, bulges, or wrinkles.

Local and Global Health

The Thin Ideal Is Not Universal

In the US, the association between a thin female body and attractiveness is prevalent in the media. This preference for thinness, however, is not seen in all cultures and countries. Researchers in one study asked more than 7,000 people in different countries to rate their own bodies and state what they viewed as the ideal female body. The percentage of participants who preferred a very thin female body was

- 40 percent in the US and in other countries where food is generally plentiful;
- 17 percent in countries where people do not always have enough food; and
- 0 percent in countries where there is often not enough food for all people.

People in countries with limited food supplies, where there is not enough food to satisfy the nutritional needs of all the people, preferred a larger female body compared to people in countries where food is plentiful. Researchers believe that, in societies with limited food supplies, people view females with larger bodies as healthier, more fertile, and possibly wealthier than females with thinner bodies.

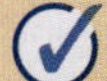

Practice Your Skills

Practice Health-Enhancing Behaviors

With a partner, discuss factors affecting body ideals and create a podcast in which you examine the following questions:

1. This research shows that the preference for a thin female body is stronger in countries where food is plentiful than in countries where food is limited. Why do you think this is true? What factors do you think contribute to these differences? List other factors that could contribute to different preferences in different parts of the world.
2. Do you think the prevalence of a preference for thinness also varies in different parts of the US? What differences do you think there might be? Explain your answer.
3. This study only examined preferences for female bodies. What do you think researchers would find if they conducted similar research about preferences for male bodies in different countries? Explain your answer.

After discussing these questions, work with your partner to identify three strategies you can use to educate your peers and challenge the thin ideal. What healthy behaviors can you adopt to reduce health risks and enhance the health of yourself and others?

This practice is controversial, but still common. Technology has made it easier for people to airbrush and share their own edited images on social media, making it harder to differentiate between real and idealized images.

Because of the standards presented in the media, many girls and women have negative thoughts about their bodies. Society defines girls and women by their physical appearance fairly often. For example, articles and news reports often criticize or compliment women in leadership positions on their outfits, hairstyles, and other physical attributes. In contrast, reports profiling men rarely include such information.

Male Bodies in the Media

Idealized images of male bodies in the media also pressure men to conform to standards that are unrealistic for many people. For example, as images of female bodies in the media have become increasingly thin, images of male bodies have become increasingly tall and muscular. Many images of male bodies in the media show "six-pack" abdominals, muscular chests, and large biceps (**Figure 9.5**). Most male bodies do not look like this, but the bodies of male models, celebrities, and famous athletes portrayed in the media do.

The media portrays males as...
having full facial hair
muscular
tall
lean

but males are still developing throughout adolescence.
25% of males with a normal weight perceive themselves to be underweight, and 90% of teen boys exercise with the goal of bulking up.

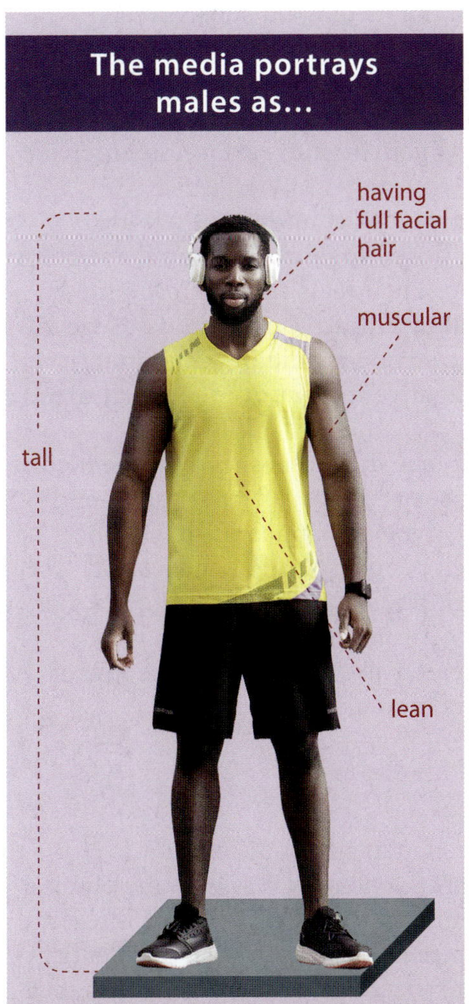

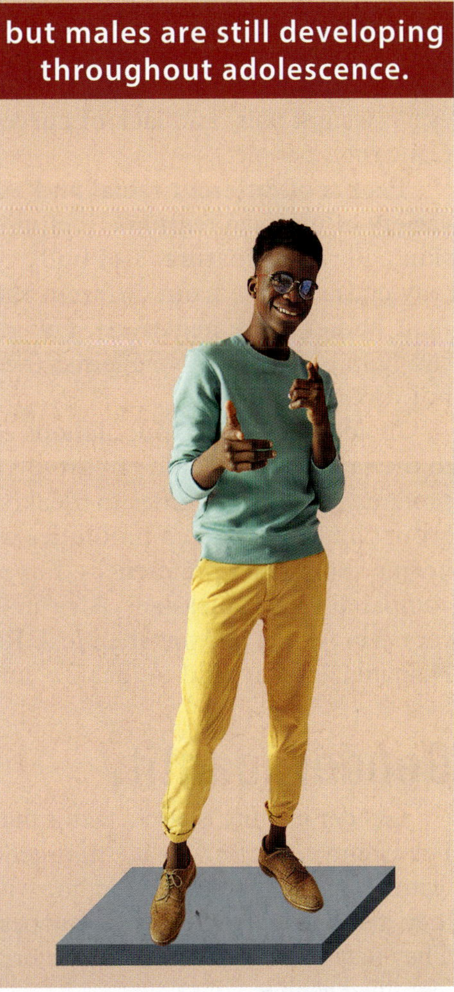

Left to right: Khosro/Shutterstock.com; Olena Yakobchuk/Shutterstock.com

Figure 9.5 The body that the media portrays for males does not represent the reality for most teen boys. ***What is the name of the disorder in which people are extremely concerned with becoming more muscular?***

muscle dysmorphia
disorder characterized by extreme concern with becoming more muscular

As a result of exposure to these ideals, men and boys may feel insecure about their height and figure. Some men may develop **muscle dysmorphia**. This disorder is characterized by extreme concern with becoming more muscular. Boys and men with muscle dysmorphia have a negative body image and are highly focused on making their bodies more muscular.

Recently, media images of males have also begun to portray very thin bodies, which may also be unrealistic. Advertising campaigns often feature males with very thin body types wearing slimming clothes, like skinny jeans. These images can lead men to feel a pressure to be both thin and muscular at the same time.

As with media images of female bodies, media images of male bodies also set standards for other body parts—for example, clear skin and full facial hair. Media images of males may be edited and airbrushed in the same way images of females are. The end result is that idealized, often-manipulated images set a standard that makes many men and boys feel badly about their bodies.

Race and Ethnicity

Idealized images and body types in the media and society reach people from all backgrounds. Unfortunately, US media tends to show mostly Caucasian or light-skinned models. Even when showing models of different races or ethnicities, the media tends to emphasize light eyes, straight hair, and lack of curves, which are more common among Caucasian people.

People of different racial and ethnic backgrounds have a wide variety of physical features, including nose, lip, and eye shape; eye color; skin color; hair texture; and body type. The ideals shown in the media may cause people from different racial or ethnic backgrounds to view their bodies more negatively. Having a strong ethnic or racial identity can help protect people against the negative impact of ideals that are not diverse.

In addition, not all populations embrace the ideals shown in the media to the same extent. Different groups in society have different values and preferences when it comes to ideal body type and appearance. Distinct groups, cultures, and communities teach people specific beliefs and norms about body preferences. For example, some research suggests that, compared with Caucasians, African-Americans are less likely to view a very thin female body as the ideal. Research also suggests that people of Hispanic descent tend to idealize curves more than thinness.

Gender Identity

Gender identity is also a factor that can influence body image. For example, people who are transgender or nonbinary may wish the physical features of their bodies were in line with their gender identity. For this reason, they may choose to change their appearance to better match gender identity. They may also feel pressure to conform to societal ideals associated with their identified gender.

Research in Action

Diversity in the Media and Body Image

How diverse do you think the media you see is? How do you think this diversity impacts people's body image? Researchers at the University of Melbourne examined the images of female bodies seen in 13 different fashion magazines. For each image, they evaluated the model's body size, race, and age. Can you predict their findings? First, most models were quite thin: 74 percent were classified as underweight, 25 percent had a healthy weight, and only 1 percent had a higher weight. Second, 90 percent of the models were Caucasian. Third, only 1 percent of the models showed wrinkles or graying hair. This study suggests that images in magazines overwhelmingly portray females as thin, Caucasian, and young.

Research examining popular movies reveals similar findings. Researchers at the University of Southern California found that more than 70 percent of actors in films were Caucasian. Furthermore, 25 of the top 100 films (as measured by money earned) did not include a single African-American actor in a speaking role. More than one-half of these films did not include a single African-American, Asian, or Hispanic female in a speaking role.

What are the consequences of not commonly portraying diversity in the media? Research shows that media images can influence how people feel about themselves. One study found that, after watching TV, Caucasian males—who often see themselves in the media—experienced increased self-esteem. African-American males and both Caucasian and African-American females felt worse after watching TV. Researchers believe the lack of characters of color and female characters on TV led to this dip in self-esteem. Self-esteem may also have decreased due to negative portrayal of these characters in stereotypical ways.

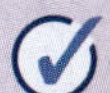

Practice Your Skills

Set Goals

These studies examined media images in magazines and films, but not in other forms of media. What do you think an analysis of images from TV or social media would reveal? Do you think an analysis would show the same patterns or not? Explain your answer.

With a partner, discuss the consequences of the media not accurately representing people of all sexes, gender identities, races, and ethnicities. Make a list of the potential harms of portraying certain types of characters more than others. Then, set five SMART goals you can act on to encourage diversity in the media and help people manage the influence of media diversity on body image. Divide any long-term goals into short-term goals you can act on immediately. Act on your goals and then evaluate how effective they were.

This desire to feel accepted and meet societal ideals is one reason rates of eating disorders among transgender and nonbinary people are much higher than for others. One survey found that transgender students were more than four times as likely to have an eating disorder and twice as likely to have symptoms of disordered eating compared to other students.

Athletic Activities

Another factor that can influence body image is involvement in some athletic activities. Certain athletic activities emphasize particular body types and features, which can negatively impact teens' feelings about their bodies.

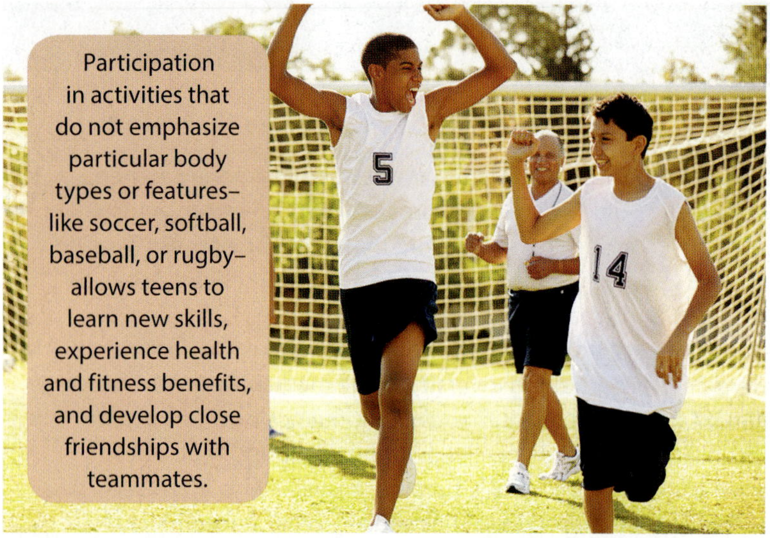

Participation in activities that do not emphasize particular body types or features–like soccer, softball, baseball, or rugby–allows teens to learn new skills, experience health and fitness benefits, and develop close friendships with teammates.

Monkey Business Images/Shutterstock.com

Figure 9.6 Finding an athletic activity that does not emphasize muscle mass, height, or weight can help keep the focus on having fun and being active rather than what your body looks like.

For example, dancers, gymnasts, and ice skaters often face pressure to be thin. Other athletic activities emphasize muscle mass or height. This pressure is common in activities such as football, basketball, swimming, volleyball, lacrosse, and ice hockey.

In contrast, teens who participate in athletic activities that do *not* emphasize particular body types or features may experience less pressure and feel better about their bodies (**Figure 9.6**). People who participate in these activities tend to feel good about what their bodies can do—like hit a home run, score a goal, or make a basket.

Lesson 9.1 Review

Know and Understand

1. What does it mean to have a positive body image?
2. How can social media make body image pressure from peers more intense?
3. Why are images in the media not always realistic? What impact do unrealistic images have on people's body image?
4. How do race and ethnicity influence body image? What impact does gender identity have?
5. What impact can athletic activities have on body image?

Think Critically

6. With a partner, discuss the difference between a person's body image and how a person actually looks. Create a short slogan describing this difference and share with the class.
7. What factors in your social environment have influenced your body image?
8. What factors do you think explain the way media images of female and male bodies have evolved over the years? Why have images of female bodies gotten thinner? Why have images of male bodies gotten more muscular?

REAL WORLD Health Skills

Analyze Influences List your five favorite people and write a sentence or two describing why each person is so special to you. Then read what you have written to determine whether any of the following factors play a role in making these people special to you:

- body size and shape
- clothes
- attractiveness

Write a paragraph describing how important these factors are to you. Write a second paragraph analyzing the difference between the messages the media and your family and friends send to you about physical attractiveness.

Disordered Eating and Eating Disorders

Essential Question?

How do disordered eating behaviors and eating disorders impact health?

Lesson 9.2

Learning Outcomes

After studying this lesson, you will be able to

- explain the difference between disordered eating and an eating disorder;
- give examples of disordered eating;
- identify the short- and long-term health effects of eating disorders;
- recognize warning signs of eating disorders; and
- analyze treatment options for eating disorders.

Key Terms

acid reflux disorder
constipation
disordered eating
eating disorder
lanugo
orthorexia
purging

Warm-Up Activity

The Impact of Eating Disorders

Access Information In a small group, choose one eating disorder to research. Then, locate at least two different *valid and reliable* online resources and research the following topics:

- potential causes of the eating disorder
- physical health consequences
- mental health consequences
- social health consequences
- effects on the family
- effects on personal life
- treatment for the eating disorder

Next, use the outline of a body to illustrate all the effects associated with the eating disorder. Be creative and make your poster and drawing colorful. Be sure to use at least 20 facts from your research. Collect these facts in a worksheet and distribute the worksheet to your classmates.

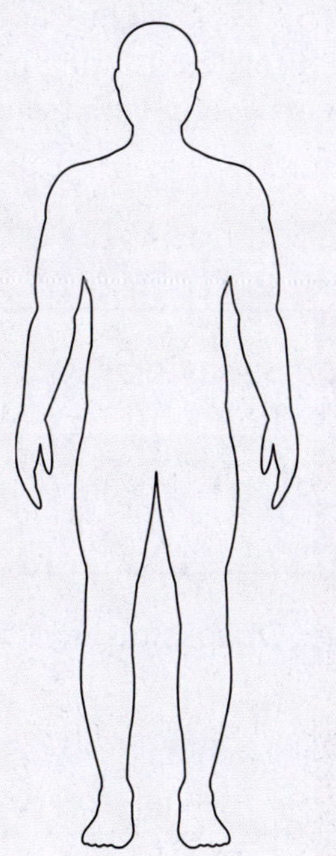

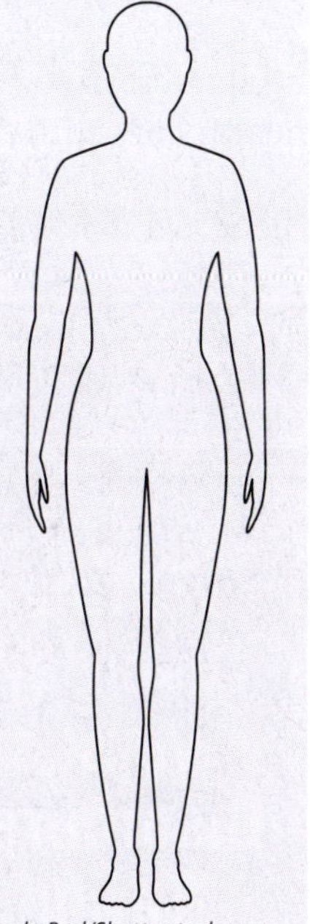

MaskaRad/Shutterstock.com

A healthy diet provides the nutrients your body needs to grow and survive. Not consuming these essential nutrients can significantly affect your health and hurt your body today and in the future. For some people, having a negative body image leads to harmful eating habits.

Although these habits may develop during childhood or later in life, they most commonly begin during the teen years.

Disordered Eating

disordered eating range of irregular eating behaviors; may or may not lead to diagnosis of a specific eating disorder

The term **disordered eating** refers to a range of irregular eating habits that signal an unhealthy relationship with body image and food. These eating habits are similar to the habits of someone with an eating disorder and can sometimes develop into an eating disorder. Some common examples of disordered eating include the following:

- obsessively counting calories
- frequently dieting
- classifying foods as "good" or "bad"
- feeling shame or guilt about eating
- being preoccupied with weight, food, or appearance
- overeating when bored or anxious

Even if the symptoms of disordered eating do not make up an eating disorder diagnosis, they still harm health in many ways. People who engage in disordered eating may develop nutritional deficits from restricting calories or particular foods. They may also lack energy. Most importantly, disordered eating behaviors can develop into an eating disorder if they continue. This is why it is so important for people to recognize symptoms of disordered eating and get professional help at this early stage before an eating disorder develops (**Figure 9.7**).

orthorexia disordered eating pattern characterized by an obsession with healthy eating; leads to negative consequences

One example of a disordered eating pattern is **orthorexia**. Orthorexia is characterized by an obsession with healthy eating that leads to negative health consequences.

Figure 9.7 Disordered eating is different from an eating disorder in several key ways. ***Which obsession characterizes the disordered eating pattern orthorexia?***

Eating Disorders Versus Disordered Eating		
	Behaviors	An eating disorder is associated with multiple types of behaviors and high frequency. Disordered eating occurs less frequently or with fewer associated behaviors.
	Obsession	Obsessive, all-consuming thoughts about food, weight, and exercise indicate an eating disorder. Disordered eating thoughts do not impair focus, sleep, or ability to stay present.
	Functionality	Eating disorders disrupt normal functioning in some way. Disordered eating may not impair social or physical functioning.

Skills for Health and Wellness

Helping a Friend with Disordered Eating

Disordered eating can harm health and lead to an eating disorder. If you recognize signs of disordered eating in yourself or in a friend, therefore, you should take those signs seriously and get help. If you are concerned about a friend who shows signs of disordered eating, there are several strategies you can use to intervene and get that person help. Some of these strategies include the following:

- **Practice what you want to say:** Think about the message you want to share with your friend before you talk. This will help you stay focused and reduce anxiety. You may even want to write out your main points ahead of time.
- **Find a private time and place to talk:** Arrange to talk somewhere you will not be overheard or interrupted by other people. Allow enough time for the conversation so you do not feel rushed.
- **Share your concerns:** Share your feelings openly with your friend. Do not accuse your friend, but instead, communicate your own concern. For example, you might say, "I'm worried about how frequently you're exercising."
- **Focus on the facts:** Talk about the specific behaviors and changes you have noticed. Do not accuse the person of having an eating disorder. Calmly point out why you are concerned. For example, you might say, "I notice you've lost a lot of weight and I'm worried you may be hurting your health."
- **Be prepared for a negative response:** Some people are glad others have noticed their struggles with body image. Others may not appreciate the concern. These people may become angry or brush off your concerns and the danger of their behavior. If this happens, let your friend know you are still concerned and are available to talk.
- **Encourage the person to seek professional help:** Many people with disordered eating behaviors need professional help to get better. You can encourage your friend to seek help and offer to help your friend find treatment options. One resource for getting help is the National Eating Disorders Association (NEDA).
- **Talk to an adult:** It can be really hard to share your concerns about a friend's eating behaviors with someone else, especially if you have promised your friend you will not do so. Still, it is far easier to help someone with disordered eating in the early stages before it becomes more severe and harder to treat. Talk to a trusted adult about what you have noticed. The adult can help you sort out whether the danger is serious and how best to handle it. This approach will give your friend the best chance to seek help and adopt healthier behaviors.

Practice Your Skills

Communicate with Others

With a partner, role-play a situation in which one person shares concerns about another person's potentially unhealthy behaviors. Role-play the situation once and then switch roles so each person practices each part. During each conversation, follow these steps:

1. First, share your concerns. State what you have noticed about the person's behavior and stick with the facts.
2. If the person is angry, defensive, or dismissive of your concerns, express that you still care and are concerned. You might repeat what you have noticed and express how much you care about the person.
3. Try to convince the person to talk to an adult or seek professional help. You could offer to go with the person to talk to an adult or help the person find resources.

After role-playing these situations, discuss which statements were most and least effective in helping the person get help. Think about trusted adults or community resources you could access if you have concerns about a friend's behaviors.

Eating Disorders

eating disorder mental illness characterized by abnormal eating or disturbances in eating habits

An **eating disorder** is a mental illness that causes major disturbances in a person's eating behaviors. People with eating disorders focus so much on these eating behaviors that they have difficulty concentrating on other aspects of their lives. There are several types of eating disorders, which vary considerably in their symptoms. **Figure 9.8** lists the major types of eating disorders.

Risk Factors for Eating Disorders

While experts do not know what specifically causes eating disorders, they believe physical, mental and emotional, and social factors play a role. Physical risk factors include having a close relative with an eating disorder and having a close relative with another mental illness (for example, an anxiety or substance use disorder). Having a history of dieting or restricting calories also increases risk for developing an eating disorder. People who have type 1 diabetes mellitus have an increased risk as well.

Mentally, having an anxiety disorder increases risk for developing an eating disorder. *Perfectionism* (feeling the need to meet unrealistically high expectations), rigidity in following rules, and a negative body image are also risk factors.

A person's social environment affects the risk of an eating disorder. As you know, media images and societal and family expectations can contribute to a negative or positive body image. Unrealistic portrayals of "ideal" bodies, lack of respect for diversity, and *weight stigma* (the idea that having a lower weight is always better) are major risk factors for a negative body image and eating disorders. Bullying, teasing, social isolation, and a history of trauma also increase risk.

Figure 9.8 In each eating disorder, eating behaviors cause significant distress and disrupt daily life.

Types of Eating Disorders

Eating Disorder	Description
Anorexia nervosa	Characterized by severely restricted eating behaviors, intense body dissatisfaction, and low body weight; *atypical anorexia nervosa* is more prevalent than anorexia nervosa and has the same symptoms and health concerns without low body weight
Avoidant-restrictive food intake disorder (ARFID)	Characterized by severely restricted eating behaviors without intense body dissatisfaction
Binge-eating disorder	Characterized by recurrent episodes of *bingeing* (consuming large amounts of food quickly and feeling out of control)
Bulimia nervosa	Characterized by recurrent episodes of bingeing and *purging* (vomiting or using other methods to rid the body of food consumed)
Otherwise specified feeding or eating disorder (OSFED)	Includes eating behaviors that cause great distress, without meeting criteria for other eating disorders; examples are atypical anorexia nervosa, binge-eating disorder and bulimia nervosa of low frequency or duration, purging disorder (purging without binge-eating), and night eating syndrome (frequent episodes of eating at night)

Health Effects of Eating Disorders

Because eating disorders involve disturbances in eating behaviors, they lead to malnutrition and harmful behaviors. In malnutrition, a person does not consume the appropriate amounts of nutrients needed for health and growth. Eating disorders have serious health effects for multiple body systems:

- **Cardiovascular system:** When the body does not receive the energy it needs from food, it breaks down its own tissues for energy. Early in this process, the body breaks down muscle tissues, such as those found in the heart. This can lead to heart damage and heart failure, which can result in death. **Purging** (attempts to rid the body of food) causes electrolyte imbalances, which can disrupt heart rhythm and also lead to heart failure and death.
- **Digestive system:** Restricted eating and purging can cause stomach pain, nausea and vomiting, dramatic changes in blood sugar, dehydration, blocked intestines, inflammation of the pancreas, and infections. Vomiting can also damage the salivary glands and teeth and lead to **acid reflux disorder** (movement of digested food and acid from the stomach into the lower esophagus). Eating disorders can cause **constipation** (infrequent or delayed hard, dry bowel movements) and life-threatening emergencies like stomach rupture.
- **Nervous system:** Lack of adequate nutrition can cause difficulty concentrating, fainting, and dizziness. Eating disorders can also lead to numbness and tingling in the hands and feet. Dehydration and electrolyte imbalance can cause seizures and muscle cramps.
- **Endocrine system:** Without adequate nutrition, levels of certain hormones fall in the body. Low levels of sex hormones can lead to *osteoporosis* (decreased bone density) and *amenorrhea* (lack of menstruation). Metabolism slows down, and body temperature lowers. Bingeing increases a person's risk for developing insulin resistance and type 2 diabetes mellitus.

purging attempts to rid the body of food

acid reflux disorder condition in which a mixture of digested food and acid moves from the stomach to the lower esophagus, resulting in heartburn

constipation infrequent or delayed hard, dry bowel movements

The malnutrition associated with eating disorders can lead to dry skin, thin hair, brittle nails, and **lanugo** (fine hair that grows all over the body). Lack of nutrition also leads to a weaker immune system and *anemia* (an insufficient number of red blood cells), which is characterized by weakness, fatigue, and shortness of breath. Long-term dehydration can cause kidney failure and death (**Figure 9.9**).

lanugo fine hair that grows all over the body as a result of starvation due to anorexia nervosa

Some health effects associated with eating disorders fade once a person gets treatment and returns to healthy eating behaviors.

For example, feeling tired all the time, feeling cold, and having anemia are conditions caused by severe malnutrition and lessen once the person gets adequate nutrition.

Other conditions, however, continue even after treatment.

Adolescence is an extremely important time for bone density growth. Low calcium intake during this stage cannot be made up later, increasing lifetime risk for osteoporosis and bone fractures.

Figure 9.9 Some health effects associated with eating disorders will go away with treatment, but others will not.

Mentally and socially, eating disorders can lead to strained relationships, withdrawal from activities, and worsening mental health conditions. Eating disorders are often associated with low self-esteem and *co-occurring disorders* (mental illnesses that occur together) and increase a person's risk for suicide. You learned about how to get help for people having thoughts of suicide in Chapter 7.

Treating Eating Disorders and Disordered Eating

Eating disorders and disordered eating behaviors rarely go away without proper treatment, so getting help is important. By getting help, people can feel better about themselves and may avoid serious, long-term health consequences. Eating disorders are mental illnesses and should be treated by a multidisciplinary team of professionals. This most often includes a therapist, doctor, dietitian, and sometimes a psychiatrist. Each professional needs to be knowledgeable about eating disorders and their mental and physical effects.

Certain warning signs signal that a person is experiencing disordered eating or an eating disorder and needs professional treatment (**Figure 9.10**). It is important to take these warning signs seriously. The earlier a person gets help for an eating disorder, the more likely the person is to recover and avoid irreversible health effects.

Figure 9.10 Warning signs of eating disorders may be physical, mental and emotional, and behavioral.

Warning Signs of Eating Disorders

Category	Warning Signs
Physical	• Fluctuations in weight • Digestive conditions, such as constipation or acid reflux disorder • Lack of menstruation in females • Dizziness, fainting, and weakness • Feeling cold all the time • Dental issues, such as cavities or tooth sensitivity • Yellow skin, lanugo, and discolored hands and feet • Cuts or calluses on top of finger joints • Impaired immune function and healing
Mental and emotional	• Fixation on appearance, weight, and food • Discomfort eating around others • Lack of interest in previously enjoyed activities • Extreme concern about appearance • Extreme mood swings
Behavioral	• Refusing to eat certain foods • Not eating or eating very small amounts • Frequent dieting • Withdrawal from friends and family • Frequently checking appearance in the mirror

To start the process of getting help, people can talk with a trusted adult, such as a parent or guardian or school counselor. People can also contact the National Eating Disorders Association (NEDA) Helpline to get support and learn about treatment options (**Figure 9.11**).

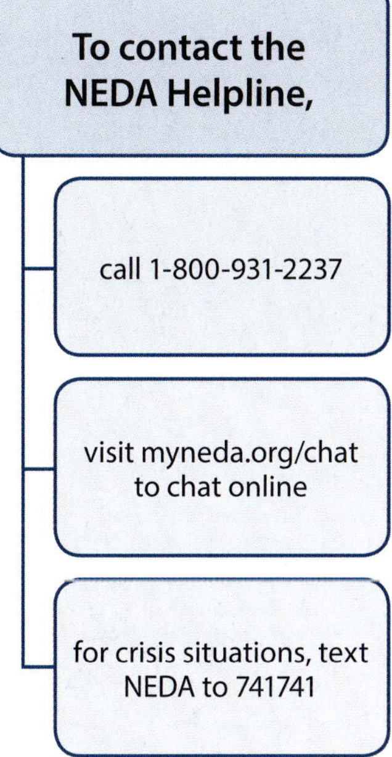

Figure 9.11 The NEDA Helpline provides support and can help people make a plan and find treatment for eating disorders.

Therapy

Talking with a therapist helps many people manage eating disorders and disordered eating behaviors. As you learned in Chapter 7, a *therapist* is a professional trained to diagnose and treat people with mental health conditions. Therapists include psychologists, psychiatrists, social workers, and counselors. There are several types of therapy.

Individual therapy consists of meeting one-on-one with a therapist. Therapists help their patients understand issues that may contribute to their eating disorders using several types of therapy. They employ techniques to

- clarify people's distorted thoughts and behaviors regarding food, weight, and body image;
- help people create healthier eating behaviors;
- expand the types of foods people are comfortable eating;
- change people's faulty beliefs about food, such as *If I gain 1 pound, I'll gain 100* or *Any sweet is instantly converted into fat*;
- help people develop more realistic body ideals; and
- teach people to avoid linking their self-esteem with their weight or appearance.

Many therapists recommend some combination of individual and family therapy for treating eating disorders and disordered eating. *Family therapy* involves parents or guardians, as well as siblings, in treatment. Therapists help parents and guardians separate their child from the disorder and address how this disorder affects the child's development (**Figure 9.12**).

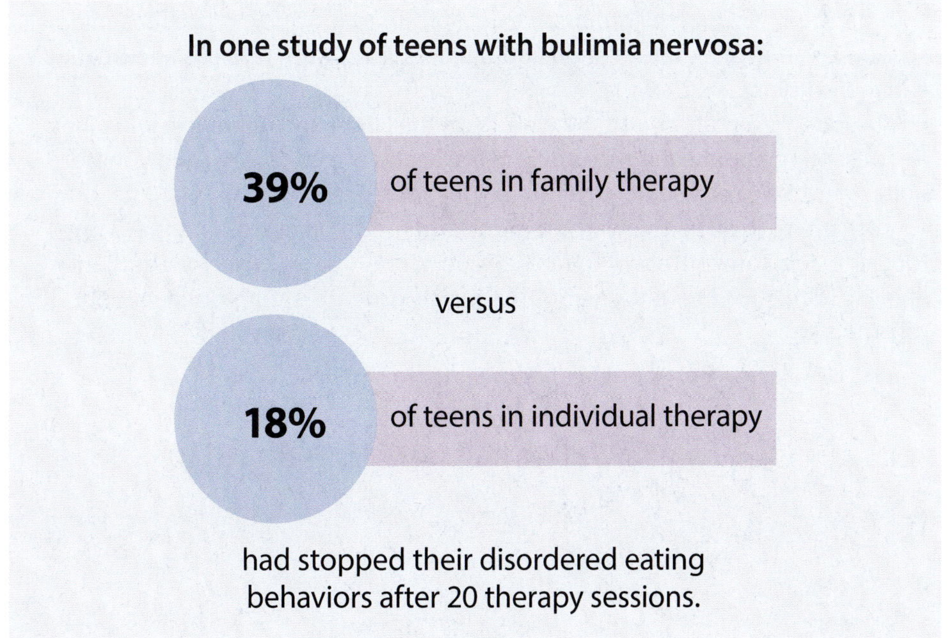

Figure 9.12 Family therapy has been helpful to teens with anorexia nervosa. ***Why is family therapy effective for treating disordered eating and eating disorders?***

Additional Treatment

Depending on the severity of an eating disorder, some people need more advanced treatment. A person's level of care depends on what the person needs to become medically stable and begin the recovery process. These levels of care can include an intensive outpatient program, partial hospitalization program, residential treatment program, or hospitalization. Proper eating disorder treatment can be lifesaving.

Lesson 9.2 Review

Know and Understand

1. Describe the difference between disordered eating and an eating disorder.
2. How is orthorexia different from healthy eating?
3. What kind of eating behavior is characteristic of anorexia nervosa?
4. What are three health consequences of purging?
5. What are the mental and emotional signs of eating disorders?

Think Critically

6. Explain how three examples of disordered eating reflect an unhealthy relationship with body image and food.
7. How are eating disorders similar to other mental illnesses, like anxiety disorders or obsessive-compulsive disorder?
8. Why do you think eating disorders rarely resolve without professional treatment?
9. With a partner, discuss reasons family therapy is often more effective than individual therapy for treating an eating disorder.

REAL WORLD Health Skills

Advocate for Health As a high school student, you can be a great advocate for younger students. In small groups, create a presentation appropriate for a middle school class that gives information about recognizing warning signs and treating eating disorders.

In your presentation, visit the website of the NEDA and reference guidelines for presenting about eating disorders in a safe and effective way. Follow these guidelines to ensure you do no harm to your audience.

Be sure to include the warning signs and methods of treatment. Do not forget to add some interesting facts found in this lesson. Give your audience at least 10 tips for preventing and treating disordered eating or the eating disorder.

Improving Your Body Image

Essential Question?

What skills can people use to develop a positive body image?

Lesson 9.3

Learning Outcomes

After studying this lesson, you will be able to

- analyze media images to identify unrealistic standards and editing;
- demonstrate body neutrality by valuing the whole self;
- advocate for body positivity by celebrating diverse body types;
- modify self-talk to encourage positive messages about the body;
- discuss ways to avoid negative influences; and
- advocate for a positive body image among peers and in the community.

Key Terms

body compassion
body neutrality
body positivity

Warm-Up Activity

"Rules" for Attractiveness

Comprehend Concepts People with a negative body image, and especially people with disordered eating or an eating disorder, often hold extreme standards for attractiveness. Following are several "Attractiveness" Standards people with a negative body image might create and consider important. In groups, develop five Healthy Standards by modifying each statement to reflect healthier behaviors.

"Attractiveness" Standards	Healthy Standards
• You are only attractive if you are thin. • Feeling guilty for what you eat is good. • You have to have clear skin and perfect hair. • You must punish yourself for not going to the gym. • Attractive people have light eyes and straight hair.	

The prevalence of disordered eating is a sign that it is difficult to maintain a positive body image in a culture that promotes idealized standards for female and male bodies. There are, however, strategies you can use to improve your body image and health. These strategies focus on developing a positive, realistic body image, which involves valuing and appreciating your body for how it looks and what it can do. Having a positive body image leads to better mental health and self-esteem. It also motivates people to take care of their bodies in healthy ways.

To improve your body image and see yourself more realistically, you can view media critically, take steps to value your whole self, acknowledge diversity, check your self-talk, and avoid negative influences. You can also participate in campaigns and activities that work to improve body image.

View Media Critically

When you see images of bodies in magazines and advertisements, on TV or social media, or in a movie, ask yourself if the images reflect reality (**Figure 9.13**). Remember that organizations craft advertisements to convince you to buy a product. By making you feel you need to fix or improve some aspect of your appearance, advertisers encourage you to spend money buying their products.

You can protect yourself from the harmful effects of unrealistic media images by thinking critically about the images you see. For example, when reading a magazine, keep in mind that the images in the magazine are carefully posed and constructed. They do not reflect reality. Taking the time to analyze images can also help you on social media. Many teens regularly post edited or filtered images of themselves. These images are also unrealistic. Following are some specific strategies you can use to view media more critically:

- **Limit time spent reading magazines, watching TV, and browsing social media:** The more time you spend viewing advertisements or following social media, the more you will be exposed to unrealistic images. To protect yourself from this exposure, reduce how much time you spend on these activities. Instead of reading a magazine, read a book. Instead of watching TV, spend time with friends.
- **Choose media carefully:** Avoid magazines, TV shows, or social media accounts that make you feel bad about yourself or present unrealistic or idealized images. This might include avoiding certain websites or not following individuals who post edited images on social media. Instead, spend time on media that promotes a positive body image, celebrates diversity, and builds self-confidence.

Figure 9.13 Thinking critically about the images you see can help you remember these images do not reflect reality or improve your body image.

Questions for Reviewing Media Images

Are images digitally edited or airbrushed to present a more idealized image?
Do they make models appear thinner or more muscular?
Do they fix any facial blemishes or smooth out frizzy hair?
Do organizations that produce the images select models who meet an unrealistic body standard?
Do models represent the average person? Do models represent me?

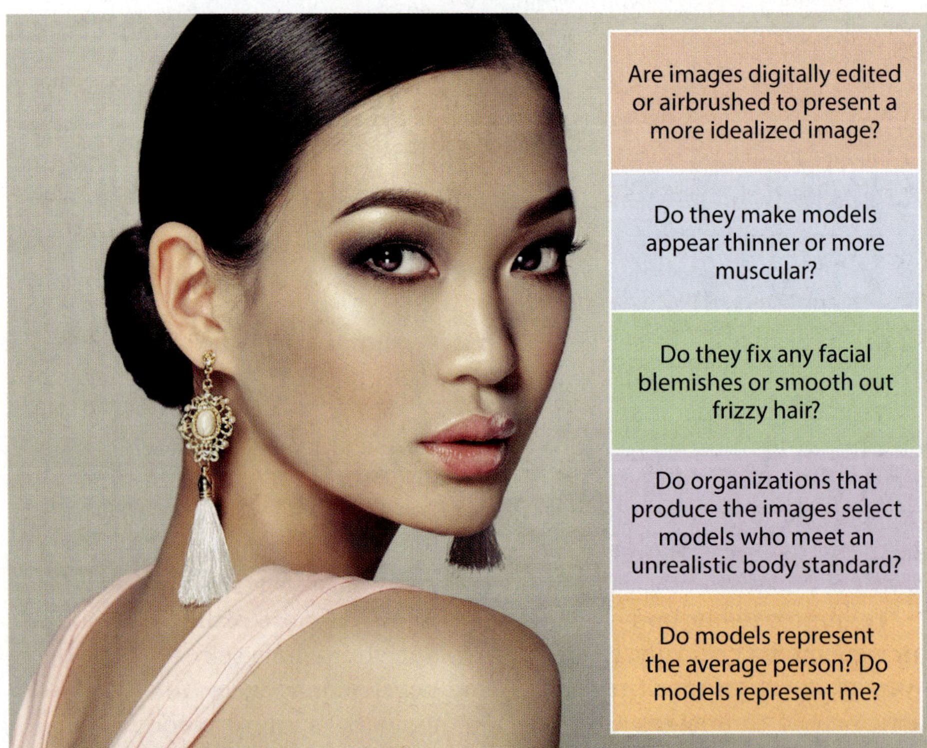

Sofia Zhuravetc/Shutterstock.com

- **Assess whether images have been edited:** Analyze the images you see to determine if they have been altered in some way. Is the background bent or distorted? Editing the person in an image can lead to changes that make the background not look right. Look carefully at the person's face. If you do not see any lines or pores, the image has probably been altered. Is all of the picture sharp and in focus? If so, it is probably two or more pictures spliced together, since no single picture can make the person and background crisp and clear. Another clear sign of alteration is patterning, in which the same part of an image appears several times. This indicates someone has copied part of the picture and inserted it somewhere else.
- **Consider what images you share:** Before sharing photos or videos online, think about whether they promote realistic standards and a positive body image. Will seeing these images make other people feel good or bad? Everyone has a responsibility to consider the effects of what they share on others.

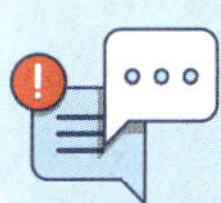

Health in the Media

Editing and Airbrushing Media Images

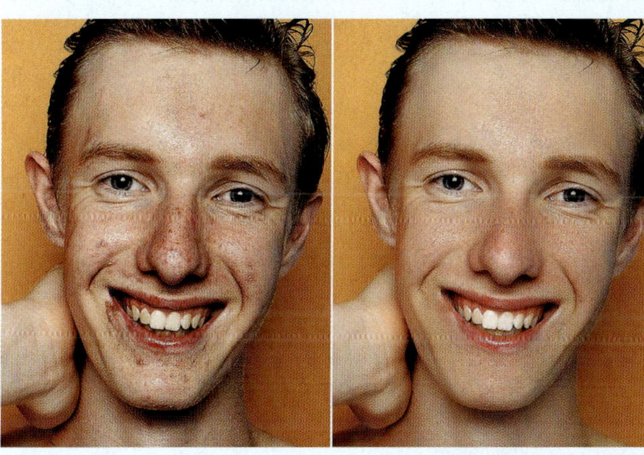

Misha Beliy/Shutterstock.com

In 2011, the British Advertising Standards Authority, which regulates advertising in the United Kingdom, banned the publication of two makeup advertisements. The advertisements violated advertising standards by presenting misleading images of female bodies: one who was a movie star and the other a top model.

Both advertisements promoted the use of skin foundation to cover imperfections and enhance beauty. Images of both women were airbrushed to improve their appearance. This made it difficult for people to determine whether the flawless skin in the advertisement resulted from the products advertised or the altering of the photographs.

While edited and airbrushed images are still common in the media, some companies are responding to criticism and moving away from using altered or retouched images. For example, some fashion magazines no longer alter the body sizes or face shapes of their models. A US drugstore chain now bans photo manipulation in any marketing for its store brand. It will also require other makeup and beauty brands it sells to either stop using photo manipulation or alert customers to the manipulation.

One lingerie company created an entire advertising campaign featuring un-retouched images, which showed models' freckles, beauty marks, and scars. France now requires any advertisers who edit images of models' bodies to add a note that the image has been digitally altered. These are all signs that some advertisers and companies are moving toward presenting more realistic images.

Practice Your Skills

Advocate for Health

With a partner, generate a list of factors you think lead companies to use edited images. Then, for each factor, brainstorm an action you could take to educate members of your community about unrealistic images and their harmful effects. Next, discuss why you think some companies are moving away from the use of digitally altered images. What approaches could you take to encourage advertisers to stop using altered images or require that altered images be specifically labeled? Commit to acting on one of these ideas with your partner.

Value Your Whole Self

Valuing your whole self can help you improve body image. For example, you could make a list of what you like about your body: your hands, hair, or eyes, for example. Try to focus on the features you like instead of dwelling on the parts of your body you do not like. Each day, tell yourself what you like about your body and why. Think about the compliments other people have given you: about your smile, height, or kindness, for example. Recognize that there are lots of good parts about you and focus on these positives (**Figure 9.14**).

Focus on what your body can *do*, not just your appearance. Can you kick a soccer ball, read a book, help others, or laugh at a joke? Reminding yourself of these skills will help you view your body in a more positive light. Recognize even the small activities your body lets you do, such as carrying groceries, comforting a friend, or connecting with your family. This focus on **body neutrality** can help you focus on and admire what bodies can do instead of how bodies look.

body neutrality focus on what the body can do, rather than how it looks

Part of valuing your whole self is also taking care of your body. This includes eating nutritious foods and getting some type of physical or stress-reducing activity every day. You could play a sport, practice mindfulness, go for a run or walk, play wheelchair basketball, or swim. Valuing your whole self also includes getting enough sleep. Go to bed before it gets too late and turn off digital devices even earlier so you can sleep well.

Acknowledge Diversity

Based on the body types and images the media presents, you might assume a specific body type or look is universally considered most attractive. In reality, however, people consider many different body shapes, sizes, and looks attractive.

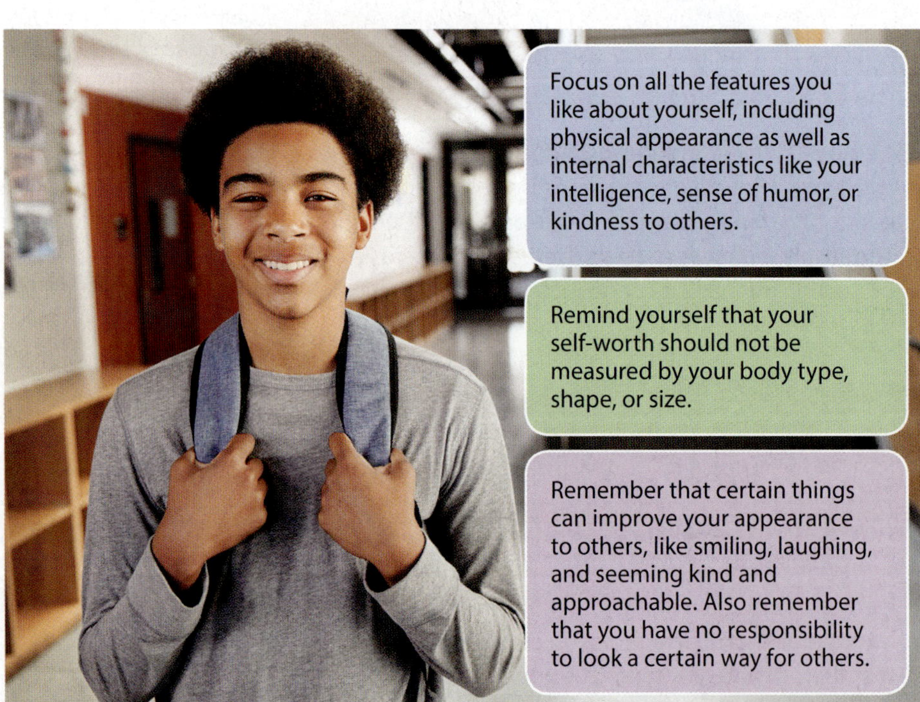

Monkey Business Images/Shutterstock.com

Figure 9.14 One important method for improving your body image is to remember that your body is just one part of your overall identity. ***What focus helps you emphasize what your body can do instead of how it looks?***

Instead of focusing on whether your body matches the media's artificial standards, recognize that people find many different body features attractive. Acknowledging this diversity and appreciating and valuing your body is called **body positivity**. Body positivity also means understanding and accepting that your body will change over time, due to the natural aging process and personal situations.

body positivity
appreciation of body-type diversity; involves valuing the body and understanding it will change

Check Your Self-Talk

Another way to adopt a more positive body image is to change how you talk about your body. This includes changing what you say about your body to other people and changing your *self-talk*, or what you say to yourself. To assess self-talk, consider what you think to yourself when you see your body in the mirror. Are your thoughts positive and encouraging? Do you focus on small flaws and criticize yourself?

If you have a tendency toward negative self-talk, you can improve body image by changing what you tell yourself about your body. This process of developing **body compassion**, or feelings of acceptance, care, and kindness toward your body, takes time and practice. First, you need to become aware of the negative thoughts about your body. Then you can reframe these thoughts into more positive, accepting thoughts (**Figure 9.15**). If you find yourself unable to develop body compassion, a therapist or other professional can help you.

body compassion
feelings of acceptance, care, and kindness toward one's body

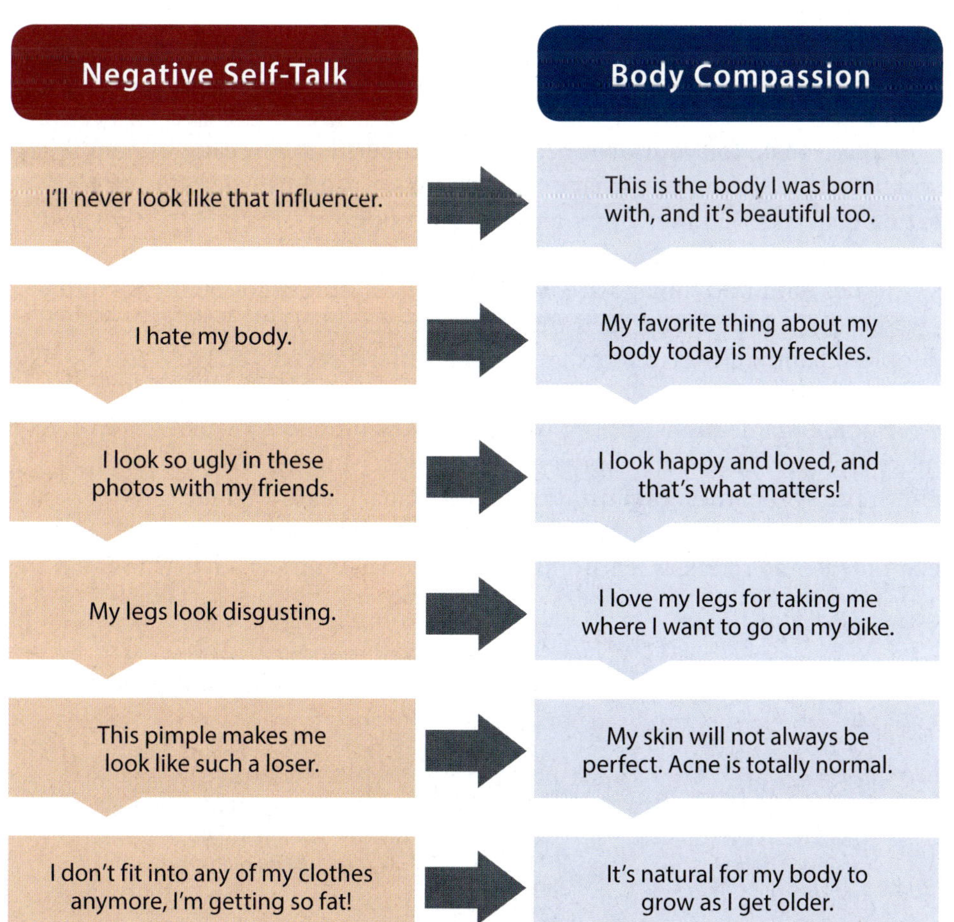

Figure 9.15 Body compassion is a skill that has to be practiced over time. Nobody will get it right every time.

Avoid Negative Influences

To promote a positive body image, avoid idealized images of people in magazines, on TV, and online whenever possible. Remember these images are often manufactured and do not represent most people. If it is difficult to look at these images without making comparisons to yourself, avoid them completely. Making small choices, such as refusing to buy fashion or body-building magazines, can help you feel better about yourself, save money, and send a message of protest.

You can also avoid negative influences in your daily life. Do you have friends who are always dieting or criticizing their appearance? This type of social pressure can make you feel worse about yourself. If you are constantly exposed to conversations about body image, try to shift the discussion to a new topic. In some cases, you may need to walk away or spend less time with friends who focus on appearance.

Some teens have family members who criticize their appearance. In these situations, it can be impossible to just avoid the person or walk away. Instead, you can use the following strategies:

- Remember that the person's intentions may be good, even if the words are hurtful. The person is trying to show care.
- Respond directly and tell the person how the comment made you feel. You could say, "I feel uncomfortable when you mention my weight. Please stop."
- Ignore the comment. Not responding at all to an insensitive comment may help the person recognize it is not a good topic of conversation.
- Get support from someone else. Find a friend or other family member with whom you can share your feelings.

Advocate for Positive Body Image

To advocate for your own health, remember that you can get help if you have a negative body image or warning signs of disordered eating or an eating disorder. Talking with a trusted adult or contacting the NEDA can help you get this assistance.

Issues with body image are widespread, and many governments and organizations have recognized the impact unrealistic images have on people's health. Governments and organizations seek to address this issue in various ways (**Figure 9.16**).

Some organizations are opposing industry practices by using more realistic images and body-positive advertising messages. More and more companies, organizations, and magazines are running advertising campaigns that feature a variety of body types. For example, some retailers feature plus-size models in their advertising.

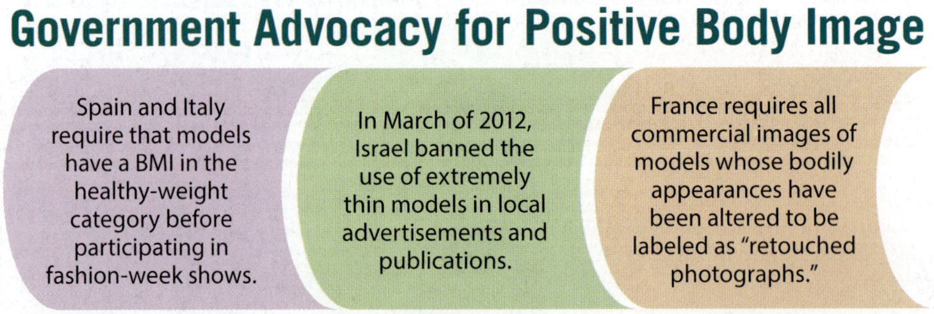

Figure 9.16 The governments of several countries have passed laws to address the impact modeling and advertising have on body image. France, as one of the leading countries in fashion, may inspire other countries to follow suit.

Government Advocacy for Positive Body Image

Spain and Italy require that models have a BMI in the healthy-weight category before participating in fashion-week shows.

In March of 2012, Israel banned the use of extremely thin models in local advertisements and publications.

France requires all commercial images of models whose bodily appearances have been altered to be labeled as "retouched photographs."

Companies are also paying more attention to showing diversity in their models, including racial, ethnic, and age diversity and differences in ability. All of these changes suggest that companies may finally understand the importance of promoting more inclusive and heathier images.

To advocate for a positive body image in your community, you can speak up about idealized images in the media. Let companies, advertisers, and celebrities know how you feel about the images and messages they present. Support those who show diverse body shapes, natural looks, and realistic body sizes. Speak out against those who promote unhealthy body norms. If enough people refuse to buy products advertised using unrealistic images, companies are more likely to change their approach.

You can also promote a positive body image through campaigns that focus on body neutrality and positivity. Many campaigns exist to celebrate realistic and diverse images. Search online for more information about different campaigns and how to get involved. You can even start your own campaign to emphasize healthy, diverse bodies and encourage positive self-talk. Talk to your friends and classmates about starting a positive body image campaign in your own school or community.

Lesson 9.3 Review

Know and Understand

1. What are the signs that a media image has been altered or edited?
2. How does body neutrality promote a positive body image?
3. What thought patterns and behaviors are part of body positivity?
4. Give an example of what it looks like to show body compassion.

Think Critically

5. With a partner, develop a list of criteria for choosing media that promotes a positive body image. Assess five different magazines, TV shows, or social media accounts using these criteria.
6. In a small group, brainstorm what you hear people in your school saying about their bodies. List these statements and determine if they are positive or negative. Convert any negative self-talk into positive self-talk.
7. With a partner, role-play a situation in which your friends are talking about dieting, and their conversation is making you feel worse about yourself. Try different methods of changing the subject or communicating your discomfort. Which methods worked the best?
8. Choose one body-positive campaign that is active right now and research it. Identify the goals of the campaign and how the campaign operates. Share your findings with the class and include ways you and your classmates can participate in the campaign.

REAL WORLD Health Skills

Communicate with Others One of the most powerful contributors to body dissatisfaction and body image issues is exposure to harmful, unrealistic images in the media. Write a letter to one of your favorite brands on social media and express your desire to see models of different shapes and sizes in advertising. Support your argument with at least 10 facts about body image, disordered eating, and eating disorders. Be sure to use effective communication skills, be persuasive, and use correct spelling and grammar. You might trade letters with a partner to proofread each other's work. Once your letter is final, find the appropriate contact information and send your letter.

Chapter 9

Review and Assessment

Chapter Summary

Your body image is your thoughts and feelings about how you look. People who have a positive body image value and appreciate their bodies, while people with a negative body image dislike their bodies and believe their negative perceptions impact their worth and value. Social environment, media and society, race and ethnicity, and athletic activities are all factors that influence body image.

Idealized, often edited images in the media set certain expectations and may cause people from different racial or ethnic backgrounds to view their bodies more negatively. Gender identity is another factor that can influence body image. Certain athletic activities that emphasize particular body types and features can also negatively impact teens' feelings about their bodies.

For some people, having a negative body image leads to unhealthy eating habits. Disordered eating refers to a range of irregular eating habits that signal an unhealthy relationship with appearance and food. An eating disorder is a mental illness that causes major disturbances in a person's daily diet. Eating disorders have serious health effects, many of which result from malnutrition and purging. While some of these effects can fade once a person receives treatment, others last a lifetime. Recognizing warning signs of eating disorders can equip people to get help for themselves or others.

Eating disorders and disordered eating behaviors rarely go away without proper treatment, so getting help is important. Eating disorders are mental illnesses and should be treated by a multidisciplinary team of health professionals. Methods for treating eating disorders and disordered eating include therapy and more advanced treatment programs.

To improve your body image and see yourself more realistically, you can view media critically, take steps to value your whole self, acknowledge diversity, check your self-talk, and avoid negative influences. You can also get help for a negative body image and participate in campaigns and activities that work to help improve body image.

Vocabulary Activity

Working with a partner, choose one key term in this chapter. Watch a video, listen to a podcast, or read an article related to the key term. Make sure the source you access is reliable. In a digital presentation, summarize what you learned and share it with your classmates. Incorporate other key terms when relevant.

acid reflux disorder	*body positivity*	*muscle dysmorphia*
airbrushing	*constipation*	*orthorexia*
body compassion	*disordered eating*	*purging*
body image	*eating disorder*	*weight stigma*
body neutrality	*lanugo*	

Review and Recall

Review the information in this chapter by answering the following questions.

1. What are two common characteristics of females portrayed in the media? of males?
2. Give one example of a sport that does *not* emphasize particular body types or features.
3. Which of the following is *not* an example of disordered eating?
   A. overeating when bored or anxious
   B. feeling good about appearance
   C. classifying foods as "good" or "bad"
   D. frequently dieting

4. What is orthorexia?
5. Which of the following is a good strategy for helping someone who shows signs of disordered eating?
   A. using peer pressure to encourage the person to eat more
   B. confronting the person in a public space
   C. talking to an adult
   D. encouraging the person to recover independently
6. Which eating disorder is characterized by severely restricted eating?
   A. orthorexia
   B. anorexia nervosa
   C. binge-eating disorder
   D. bulimia nervosa
7. What is purging?
8. How do eating disorders affect the heart?
9. Which of the following is *not* a warning sign of an eating disorder?
   A. lanugo
   B. yellowish skin tone
   C. feeling warm all the time
   D. extreme mood swings
10. Name two different types of therapy used to treat eating disorders.
11. What is one way you can protect yourself from the harmful effects of unrealistic media images?
12. What is the difference between body positivity and body neutrality?
13. Which of the following is a feeling of acceptance, care, and kindness toward one's body?
    A. body compassion
    B. body positivity
    C. body neutrality
    D. body image

Standardized Test Prep

Reading and Writing Practice

Read the passage below and then answer the following questions.

Over the years, media organizations have made some progress in showing greater diversity. Movies and TV shows feature more people from different racial and ethnic backgrounds, and characters with different gender identities and sexual orientations are more common. Still, the diversity represented in the media does not reflect the diversity of the US population.

According to the Hollywood Diversity Report 2018, only 1.4 out of 10 lead actors in film are people of color. As of 2016, people of color accounted for 38.7 percent of the US population, but only featured as lead actors in 13.9 percent of theatrical films. Males were also more represented than females, accounting for 68.8 percent of leads in films. Out of all film roles, 78.1 percent of roles were played by Caucasian actors. This is disproportionate, since Caucasians made up only 61.3 percent of the US population.

14. Which statement best describes the main point of this passage?
    A. Diversity in the media is improving.
    B. Media organizations need to make diversity a priority.
    C. Lack of media diversity negatively impacts body image.
    D. Diversity in the media does not match diversity in the US population.
15. In 2016, how did the percentage of lead actors who were people of color compare to the percentage of people of color in the US population?
16. Write a short paragraph discussing how the statistics in this passage compare to your own observations about diversity in the media. Do you think diversity has improved? worsened? Explain.

Chapter 9 Skills Assessment

Critical Thinking Skills

Answer the following questions to assess your knowledge of what you learned in this chapter.

1. Has your body image changed throughout your lifetime? What are some factors that may have caused those changes?
2. Do you think it is possible for someone many people consider attractive to have a negative body image? Why or why not?
3. Look through your social media feed and analyze the diversity of the models in the advertisements. Are certain sexes, races, and ethnicities represented more than others? What physical characteristics are presented as ideal?
4. Create an advertisement that supports a positive body image. What are some characteristics of the models you chose, and how do they promote positive body image?
5. With a partner, discuss some common misconceptions about eating disorders. Then brainstorm ideas for how you can combat those misconceptions in your school and community.
6. What are some factors that might cause someone to be hesitant about asking for help with an eating disorder? What are some resources that may be helpful to someone struggling to ask for help?
7. Select an advertisement to study. Are the images in this advertisement edited or airbrushed? Do the models represent the average person? How do the images affect your body image?
8. Think about the images you share on social media. Do you often use filters to make yourself appear more attractive? Do you select group photos that make you look good, but are unflattering to the others pictured? How do the images you post make other people feel? How do you feel when others post unflattering images of you online?
9. Think about the compliments you have received. Which make you feel better about yourself: compliments on your appearance or compliments on other qualities? How would you feel if you only received compliments on one aspect of yourself?
10. Identify some negative thoughts you have experienced while browsing social media. What are some statements you can use to reframe your negative thoughts and help develop body compassion for yourself and others?
11. Think of a product or company that uses unrealistic or unhealthy images in its advertising, then write a letter recommending specific ways the advertiser might help promote a healthier body image.

Health and Wellness Skills

Complete the following activities to assess your skills related to health and wellness.

12. **Analyze Influences.** Listen to the song "Video" by India.Arie and answer the following questions:
    A. What message is the artist trying to convey to people in this song?
    B. What is your view or opinion about this media message? How does this message influence your health and the health of others?
    C. Pick out your favorite line (a complete thought or sentence) from the song. Write it down and explain why you chose that line.
13. **Access Information.** Review the questions in Figure 2.6 for evaluating websites for validity and reliability. Turn this figure into a checklist and then find a credible website containing strategies for improving one's body image. Evaluate the website using your checklist and then share the website and some of the information it contains with your classmates.

14. **Communicate with Others.** Write a paragraph or record a summary discussing the factors that influence an individual's concept of what is attractive or unattractive. Be persuasive and thorough and use effective communication skills and correct spelling and grammar. Post your paragraph or summary to the classroom website or blog and exchange feedback with a classmate. Then update the paragraph or summary using your classmate's feedback.
15. **Make Decisions.** Lately, Lydia has been very upset about how she looks. She has trouble paying attention in class, and her grades have been dropping. She skips social activities because she feels self-conscious and has experienced more depression, anxiety, and insomnia. Lydia realizes she needs to get help, but would feel embarrassed to be seen in the counselor's office. Work through a formal decision-making process to help Lydia get the help she needs.
16. **Set Goals.** Jerome joined the lacrosse team this year and is quickly earning more and more playing time. He has noticed he is much smaller than the "power players" and feels bad. Jerome talked with the school counselor, who suggested he write and complete a SMART goal to improve his self-image. Write a SMART goal that would help someone like Jerome, or any other student, increase self-image and body image.
17. **Practice Health-Enhancing Behaviors.** With a partner, make a "top 10" list of behaviors or attitudes that help enhance the body image and overall health of teens (for example, *Value what I do more than how I look*). Explain why each behavior or attitude is beneficial (for example, *This helps a person develop body satisfaction*). Present your list and explanations in a poster, video, or podcast.
18. **Advocate for Health.** Use your advocacy skills to produce a school poster that promotes healthy eating and body satisfaction instead of dieting. This poster will be part of an antidieting campaign aimed at teens. Another goal of the campaign will be to boost teens' self-esteem by helping them view their bodies more positively. The poster should be visually engaging and include a catchy slogan, as well as five facts about why dieting is unhealthy.

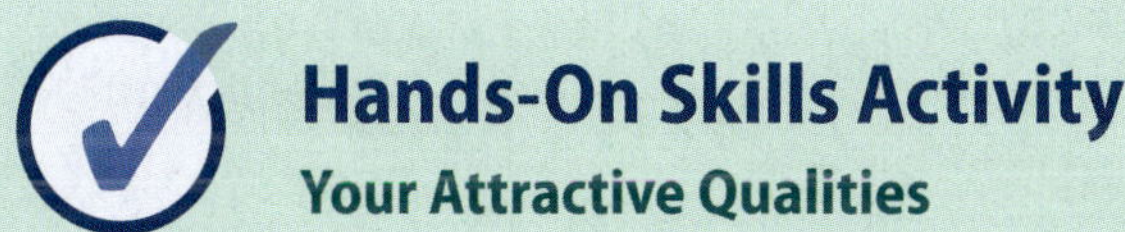

Hands-On Skills Activity

Your Attractive Qualities

You learned in this chapter that body image describes how you *feel* about your appearance. It does not describe how you actually look. If you have a negative body image, you can alter your thinking to view yourself more positively. In this activity, you will take steps to consider your attractive qualities and improve your self-image and body image.

Steps for This Activity

1. On a separate sheet of paper, write seven statements to describe the qualities that make you attractive. This list should include your strengths, talents, physical traits you like, abilities, and other characteristics that make you proud. Next to each statement, try to illustrate the quality with a small drawing or picture.
2. On the back of the sheet of paper, write a few paragraphs to answer the following questions:
   - Did you find it difficult to come up with seven statements about the qualities that make you attractive? If so, why do you think it was difficult? What factors do you think affected how easy or difficult this task was?
   - Think of a time in your life you exhibited or used each quality you listed. Briefly describe these experiences.
3. **Practice Health-Enhancing Behaviors.** Focusing on qualities you like is just one way of improving self-image. With a partner, write a motivational talk analyzing how negative body image can decrease a person's health. In your talk, share 10 action steps people can take to positively improve their body image. Give tips for taking these action steps and explain how they are helpful. Record your motivational talk and share it with the class.

Chapter 10

Engaging in Physical Activity

Look for the skills icon throughout this chapter for opportunities to practice your health skills.

Check Your Health and Wellness Skills

In this chapter, you will learn skills related to getting physical activity. To understand the skills you currently use, take the following inventory of your behaviors. Indicate how well you think you use each skill. Use a scale of 1–5, *1* meaning you do not use the skill and *5* meaning you feel completely comfortable using it.

Skill	How Well Do You Use Each Skill?
I get at least 60 minutes of physical activity each day.	
I choose physical activities I really enjoy.	
I use small windows of time, like when I'm waiting for a ride, to get physical activity.	
I get physical activity with people who hold me accountable.	
I vary the types and intensities of my physical activities.	
I make sure to use proper form during muscle-strengthening activities.	
I set and follow clear SMART goals for physical activity.	
When I begin a new type of physical activity, I start slow.	
I warm up before engaging in physical activity.	
In extreme temperatures, I work out with someone else.	
I know how to treat a sprain.	
	Total:

Add up your responses to each statement. The higher your score, the more comfortable you feel practicing health skills related to getting physical activity. Which skill do you think is most important for you? Which skill is the most challenging for you? Which skill would you most like to improve? In this chapter, you will learn how to perform these skills better and more often.

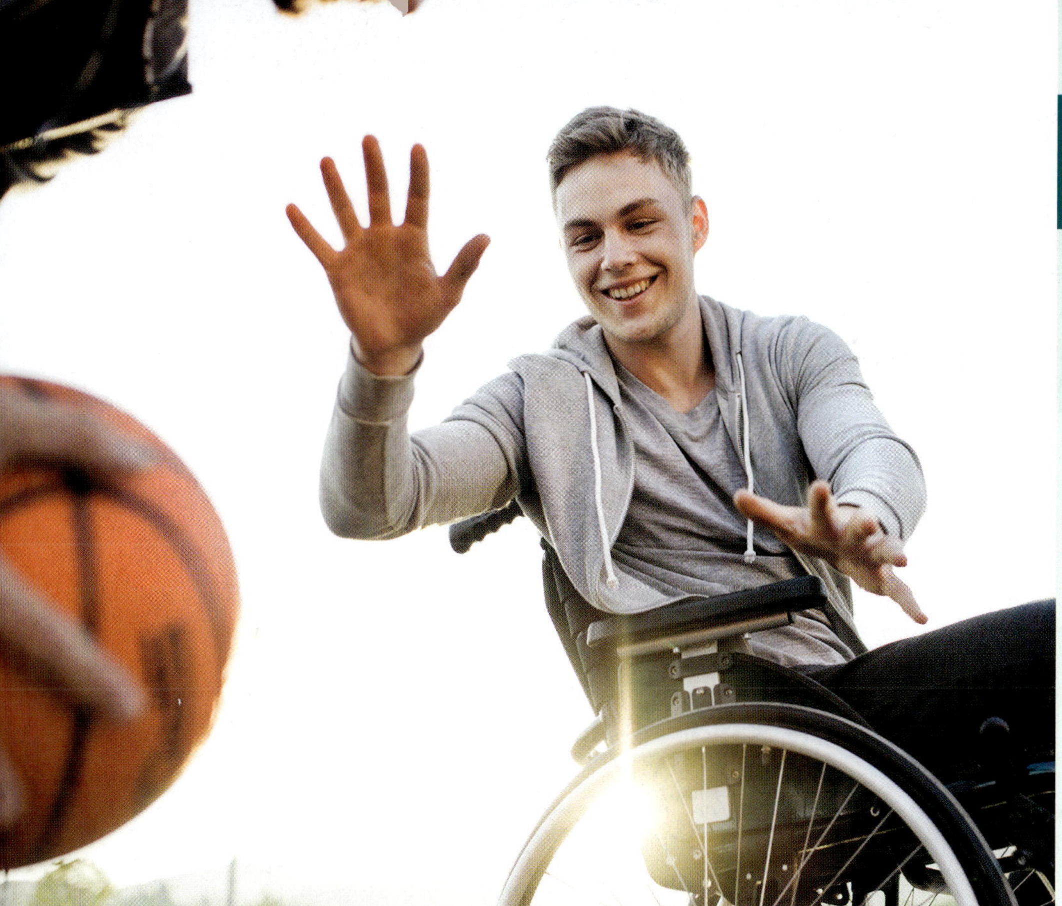

GrapeImages/E+/Getty Images

Reading and Notetaking

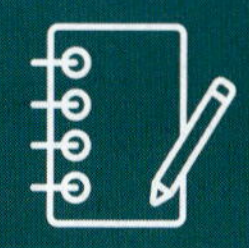

Before you read this chapter, write out all of the chapter's key terms and what you think each term means. Explain your definition for each term by citing your prior experiences, knowledge, and influences. As you read the chapter, compare your definitions to the definitions in the text. Change and highlight any of your definitions that are incorrect. Make flash cards for the terms you highlighted and review them.

Key Terms	My Definitions	Text Definitions

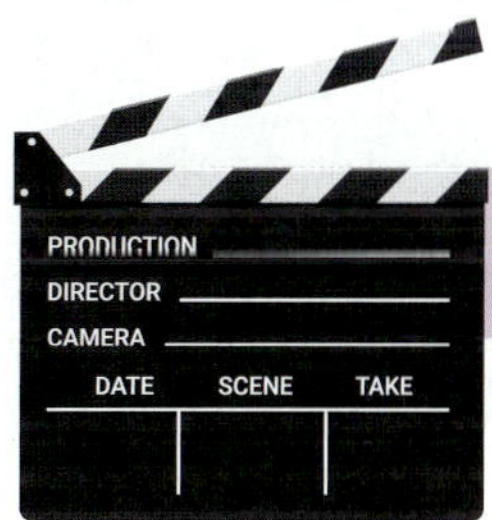

Setting the Scene

Many Ways to Be Active

For a long time, you have been physically active, partly because you know it will maintain your health and partly to reduce stress. Last summer, however, you started having scary symptoms while running outside. You would start coughing and wheezing and even have trouble breathing. Your doctor diagnosed you with asthma.

At first, this diagnosis made you very upset. You thought having asthma meant you could not do the activities you used to do. Talking with your school nurse helped you feel better. Your school nurse said you could still get lots of physical activity, as long as you did so safely. In very hot or cold weather, you need to get physical activity inside. You should also get physical activity inside if levels of pollen are high. When getting physical activity, you need to avoid overexerting yourself and carry your inhaler. You are relieved you can keep getting physical activity, even with this condition.

Thinking Critically

1. What are some factors that require people to modify the types of physical activity they do?
2. What are some strategies teens can use to stay healthy, even if they have some limits on the types of physical activity they can do?

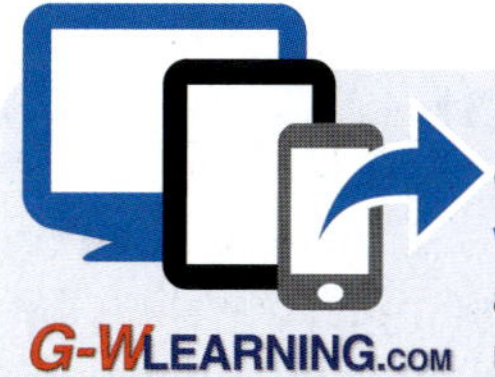

Click on the activity icon or visit www.g-wlearning.com/health/4095 to access online vocabulary activities using key terms from the chapter.

Lesson

10.1

Understanding Physical Activity and Fitness

Essential Question?

What does it mean to be active and fit?

Learning Outcomes

After studying this lesson, you will be able to

- contrast physical activity and exercise;
- analyze the benefits of physical activity on physical health;
- explain how physical activity benefits mental, emotional, and social health;
- define *physical fitness*; and
- differentiate between health-related and skill-related fitness.

Key Terms

aerobic
agility
anaerobic
cardiorespiratory fitness
endorphins
endurance
exercise
flexibility
health-related fitness
physical activity
physical fitness
skill-related fitness

Warm-Up Activity

Agree or Disagree

Access Information Before reading this lesson, record whether you agree or disagree with each statement in the chart shown. Using valid and reliable websites, search for evidence that either proves or disproves each statement. Write down the website and a concise answer. After reading the lesson, consider the statements again based on any new information you read. Then, record again whether you agree or disagree, and check to see whether your opinion changed based on new evidence.

Statements
1. Physical activity mostly benefits physical health.
2. Walking to school and between classes is physical activity.
3. Physical fitness is based on how you look.
4. Cardiorespiratory fitness refers to the strength of your heart and lungs.
5. You cannot be too flexible.
6. Coordination refers to the gracefulness of your movements.

In the past month, have you gone for a walk, run, hike, or bike ride? Have you participated in a team or individual sport? Have you danced with friends at a party or lifted weights? Have you vacuumed, swept the floor, or raked leaves? How did you feel after these activities? Did you have more energy? Were your muscles sore? In this lesson, you will learn about the benefits of being physically active. You will also learn about the different types of physical fitness.

What Are the Benefits of Physical Activity?

physical activity any action in which the body uses energy

Physical activity is any action in which the body uses energy. For example, traveling between classes uses energy. So do swimming with friends, biking to school, carrying groceries, dancing, playing sports, and lifting weights. Many people think exercise is the same as physical activity, but exercise is actually just one type of physical activity. The term **exercise** describes physical activity that is planned and structured and has the purpose of increasing physical fitness. Examples of exercise include doing sit-ups in PE class, practicing for a sports team, or running to prepare for a half-marathon.

exercise physical activity that is structured, planned, and has the purpose of increasing physical fitness

Engaging in physical activity is one of the most important actions you can take to promote your health (**Figure 10.1**). You do not have to participate in structured exercise to experience the benefits of physical activity. Simply being physically active can protect your health today and in the future.

Benefits of Physical Activity

Improved

- Mental health (mood, ability to cope with stress)
- Academic performance and behavior (concentration, focus)
- Strength of muscles and bones
- Sleep quality
- Immune system
- Social interactions and support

Decreased risk of

- Cancers (colon, lung, uterus, and breast)
- Type 2 diabetes mellitus
- Overweight and obesity
- Cardiovascular diseases (heart attack, stroke)
- Depression and anxiety

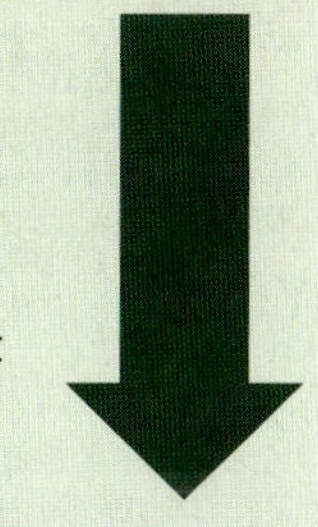

Figure 10.1 Physical activity affects all areas of health—physical, mental and emotional, and social. ***What is the term for a structured and planned physical activity?***

Lower Risk of Disease

Getting physical activity regularly lowers your risk of certain diseases, including cardiovascular diseases (for example, heart disease and stroke), cancer, and type 2 diabetes mellitus. In the US and worldwide, cardiovascular diseases are the first leading cause of death, and cancer is the second leading cause of death. Diabetes mellitus is also a leading cause of death.

Even moderate amounts of physical activity can majorly benefit your cardiovascular system. These benefits include a stronger heart, lower blood pressure, and lower blood cholesterol levels, all of which reduce the risk of cardiovascular disease (**Figure 10.2**). People who get at least 150 minutes (2 hours and 30 minutes) of moderate-intensity physical activity each week are less likely to develop cardiovascular diseases. In this way, engaging in physical activity can add years to your life.

Physical activity reduces your risk for some types of cancer. Physically active people have a lower risk of colon cancer and may have a lower risk of lung cancer. Physically active females may have a lower risk for breast cancer and endometrial cancer (cancer of the uterus). Researchers do not know exactly how physical activity reduces the risk for particular types of cancer. Physical activity does, however, influence the body's production of hormones, rate of metabolism, and immune system. The effects of physical activity on these functions may explain how physical activity reduces cancer risk.

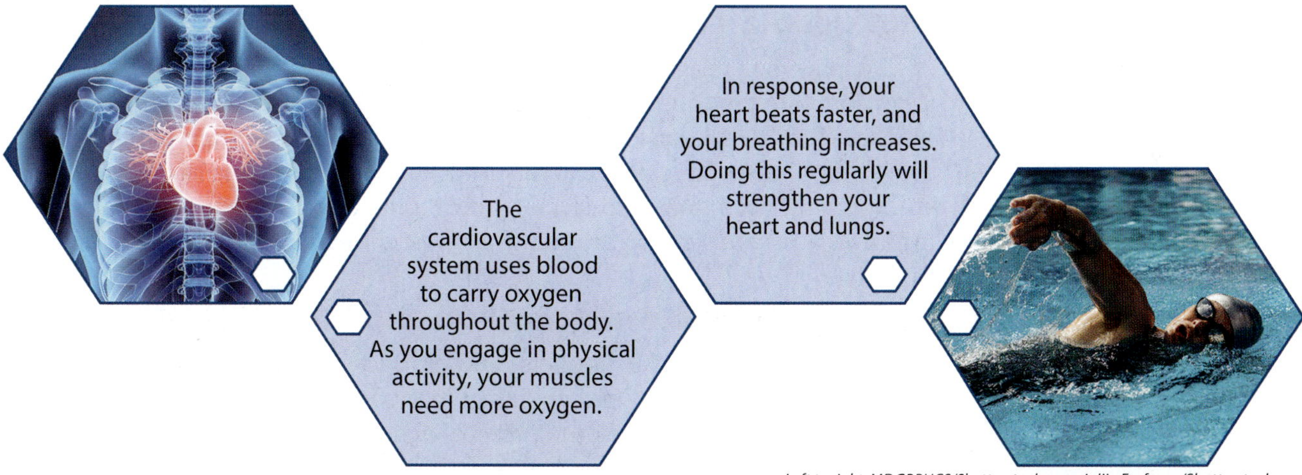

Left to right: MDGRPHCS/Shutterstock.com; Julija Erofeeva/Shutterstock.com

Figure 10.2 Physical activity reduces the risk of developing cardiovascular diseases by strengthening the heart and lungs.

Physical activity reduces a person's risk of developing type 2 diabetes mellitus by lowering blood sugar, blood pressure, and cholesterol. Lower blood sugar decreases the chance that a person will experience insulin resistance, which causes type 2 diabetes mellitus.

Better Weight Management

Physical activity helps people reach and maintain a healthy weight. Getting physical activity means your body burns enough calories to maintain or reach a healthy weight.

Physical activity also helps weight management by changing a person's body composition. People who participate in strength training, including push-ups, sit-ups, or weight lifting, can increase their muscle mass. Muscles are active tissues that consume calories for energy. In contrast, fat stored in the body uses very little energy. This means a person whose body contains more muscle and less fat burns calories at a faster rate. This faster rate can help people reach or maintain a healthy weight. Since muscle weighs more than fat, increased muscle mass can also lead to healthy weight gain.

Physical activity, combined with a healthy eating pattern, can help with underweight, overweight, and obesity. As you know, underweight can lead to frequent infections, osteoporosis, and conditions of the skin, hair, and teeth. Overweight and obesity increase a person's risk for many health conditions, including respiratory conditions, joint pain, trouble sleeping, cardiovascular diseases, type 2 diabetes mellitus, and cancer.

Mental and Emotional Benefits of Physical Activity

- Improved self-confidence and self-esteem
- Distraction from challenges in life
- Increased blood flow to the brain, which contributes to improved mood

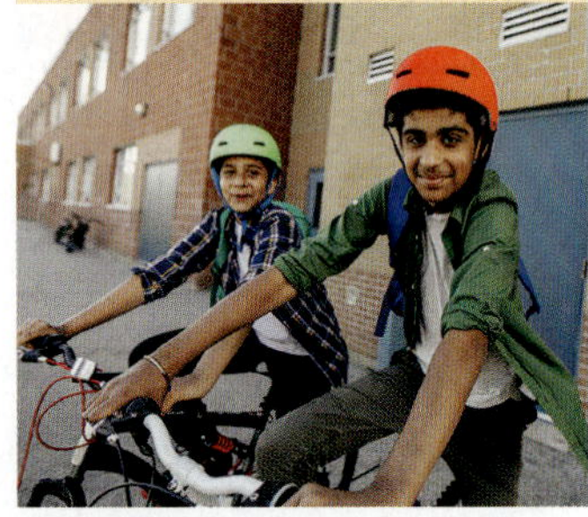

kate_sept2004/iStock/Getty Images Plus/Getty Images

Figure 10.3 Physical activity can improve mental and emotional health in various ways. ***What chemicals are released during physical activity that make you feel good?***

Stronger Bones and Muscles

Engaging in physical activity strengthens your bones and muscles. Physical activity increases the amount of fluid in your joints, which helps strengthen the cartilage covering the ends of your bones. Physical activity also increases the strength of your bones and ligaments, which makes you less likely to become injured or develop *osteoporosis* (health condition in which bones become fragile and brittle). In addition, physical activity improves the strength of your muscles and increases blood flow to and from your muscles.

All of these benefits work together to slow the natural loss of bone density due to aging and increase muscle mass and strength. This can reduce the likelihood of a fall, reduce joint pain, and increase the ability to perform different tasks.

High-Quality Sleep

People who engage in physical activity experience a higher quality of sleep compared to those who do not. Physically active people fall asleep more quickly, enjoy deeper and more restful sleep, wake up less often at night, and stay asleep longer. In fact, research shows strength training is as effective at improving sleep quality as sleep medications. Getting high-quality sleep improves a person's concentration, energy, and mental and emotional health.

Improved Mental, Emotional, and Social Health

Physical activity has benefits for mental and emotional health, including lower levels of depression and anxiety. Have you ever been in a bad mood, but felt better after getting some physical activity? This happens because engaging in physical activity can cause the brain to release chemicals called **endorphins**, which make you feel good (**Figure 10.3**).

endorphins brain chemicals that improve mood; released during physical activity

Physical activity is also an opportunity for people to spend time with others. For example, some teens are part of a sports team or do physical activities, such as hiking, running, or dancing, with friends. All of these activities increase social interactions and help a person build social support.

Better Academic Performance

Physical activity helps improve thinking, learning, and judgment. Not surprisingly, improvements in these areas can lead to better performance in school. Students who participate in physical activity demonstrate improved

- academic achievement, including higher grades;
- academic behavior, such as spending more time focused on a task; and
- concentration and focus in class.

Research in Action

Physical Activity and Mental and Emotional Health

Did you know that engaging in physical activity can have benefits for your mental and emotional health? Researchers at the University of Oxford in the United Kingdom conducted a study to examine the link between physical activity and mental and emotional health. This study used data from 1.2 million adults in the US from all 50 states.

In this study, researchers examined the data to determine whether people who got physical activity regularly during the month experienced better mental and emotional health than people who did not. They also studied if certain types of physical activity were more beneficial than others.

The findings of this study revealed that, compared to people who did not get physical activity, people who were physically active had 1.5 fewer days of poor mental and emotional health during the month. More dramatically, physically active people with major depressive disorder reported having 3.75 fewer days of poor mental and emotional health.

The time spent on physical activity made a difference in these findings. People who were physically active for 30–60 minutes three to five times a week had better mental and emotional health than people who got less or more physical activity. Researchers believe this is because people who get extreme amounts of physical activity may have obsessive tendencies, which interfere with mental and emotional health. All types of physical activity improved mental and emotional health, but people who participated in team sports experienced the greatest benefits.

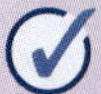

Practice Your Skills

Make Decisions

Working with a partner, make a list of the factors that may explain the link between physical activity and mental and emotional health. What factors could explain the particular benefits of team sports? Are there other physical activities you think could also have more benefits to mental and emotional health?

Use the decision-making process to outline decisions you could make about physical activity that would benefit your mental and emotional health. As you use the decision-making process, be sure to identify plenty of alternatives. Assess how well these alternatives benefit your mental and emotional health. Keep using the decision-making process until you find physical activities that fit in your schedule and help improve your mood.

What Is Physical Fitness?

If your family had to move, and someone asked you to help move a box, could you do it? If your friends wanted to explore the mall for a few hours or go swimming, could you keep up? Can you carry your backpack, travel between classes, participate in any extracurricular activities, and come home with energy to spare? Your answers to these questions describe your level of physical fitness.

physical fitness body's ability to perform daily activities and meet unexpected demands with energy to spare

Physical fitness refers to the body's ability to respond to the physical demands placed on it. People who are physically fit have enough energy to perform daily life activities and also meet unexpected physical demands, like being active with friends. People who are physically fit can meet the day's physical challenges with energy to spare.

There are two types of physical fitness: health-related fitness and skill-related fitness. As people engage in different physical activities, they develop some parts of their fitness more than others.

health-related fitness body's ability to perform daily activities with ease and energy

aerobic using oxygen to break down energy for use in the muscles

anaerobic powering the body without the use of oxygen

cardiorespiratory fitness ability of the cardiovascular and respiratory systems to deliver oxygen and nutrients to muscles and cells

Health-Related Fitness

Health-related fitness is the type of physical fitness you need to perform daily activities with ease and energy. **Aerobic** activities, like dancing or bicycling, use oxygen to break down energy for use in the muscles. In **anaerobic** activities, such as lifting heavy objects or sprinting, stored energy powers the body without the use of oxygen (**Figure 10.4**).

Experts talk about different components of health-related fitness, but major components include cardiorespiratory fitness, endurance, muscle strength, and flexibility. Another component is body composition, which you learned about in Chapter 8.

Cardiorespiratory Fitness

Cardiorespiratory fitness refers to how well the cardiovascular system (heart and blood vessels) and respiratory system (lungs) work together to deliver oxygen and nutrients to muscles and cells. Benefits of cardiorespiratory fitness include a strong heart, improved blood flow, and quick transport of oxygen and nutrients to muscles and cells. These benefits help the body engage in more physical activity for longer.

Many different types of activities (for example, running, swimming, wheelchair propelling, gardening, dancing, and shoveling snow) promote cardiorespiratory fitness. Cardiorespiratory fitness improves as a person becomes physically active for longer periods at greater intensities.

Figure 10.4 Anaerobic activities occur in short, intense bursts, while aerobic activities continue over a longer time. ***Which type of activity uses oxygen to break down energy for use in the muscles?***

Anaerobic Activity Versus Aerobic Activity
Sprinting relies on stored energy to power the body.
Long-distance running uses oxygen to break down energy.

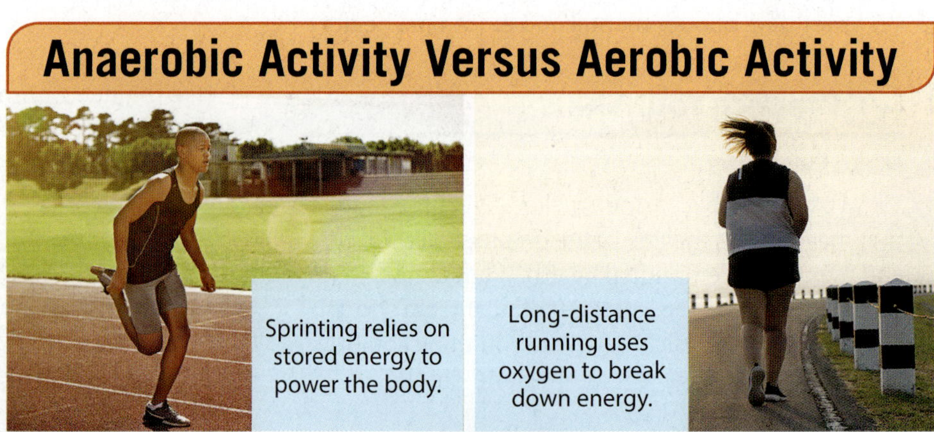

Left to right: kupicoo/E+/Getty Images; x-reflexnaja/iStock/Getty Images Plus/Getty Images

Health Across the Life Span

Steps to a Healthier Life

Physical activity is important for all aspects of your health. Whether you run, bike, dance, swim, or do some other form of activity, you are taking steps to be healthy. Staying active throughout your life can be difficult, as new responsibilities and obstacles arise. Making the healthiest choices you can will allow you to stay moving and improve your health. Follow the paths below by making choices for each situation to see the consequences of your choices and how healthy your future could be.

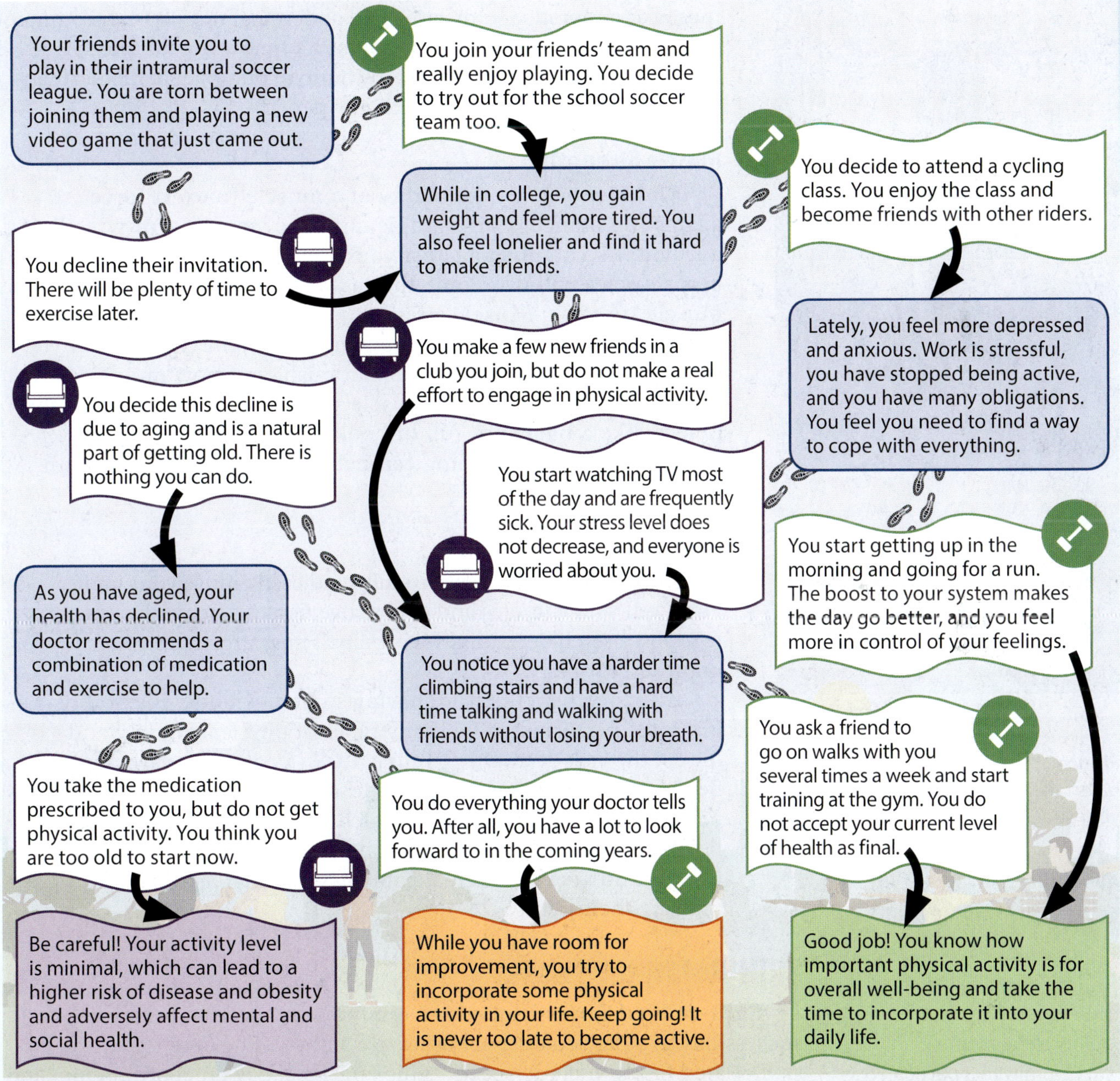

Your friends invite you to play in their intramural soccer league. You are torn between joining them and playing a new video game that just came out.

You join your friends' team and really enjoy playing. You decide to try out for the school soccer team too.

You decline their invitation. There will be plenty of time to exercise later.

While in college, you gain weight and feel more tired. You also feel lonelier and find it hard to make friends.

You decide to attend a cycling class. You enjoy the class and become friends with other riders.

You make a few new friends in a club you join, but do not make a real effort to engage in physical activity.

Lately, you feel more depressed and anxious. Work is stressful, you have stopped being active, and you have many obligations. You feel you need to find a way to cope with everything.

You decide this decline is due to aging and is a natural part of getting old. There is nothing you can do.

You start watching TV most of the day and are frequently sick. Your stress level does not decrease, and everyone is worried about you.

You start getting up in the morning and going for a run. The boost to your system makes the day go better, and you feel more in control of your feelings.

As you have aged, your health has declined. Your doctor recommends a combination of medication and exercise to help.

You notice you have a harder time climbing stairs and have a hard time talking and walking with friends without losing your breath.

You ask a friend to go on walks with you several times a week and start training at the gym. You do not accept your current level of health as final.

You take the medication prescribed to you, but do not get physical activity. You think you are too old to start now.

You do everything your doctor tells you. After all, you have a lot to look forward to in the coming years.

Be careful! Your activity level is minimal, which can lead to a higher risk of disease and obesity and adversely affect mental and social health.

While you have room for improvement, you try to incorporate some physical activity in your life. Keep going! It is never too late to become active.

Good job! You know how important physical activity is for overall well-being and take the time to incorporate it into your daily life.

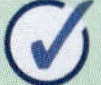
Practice Your Skills

Practice Health-Enhancing Behaviors

As you go through your day, take time to notice where you could incorporate physical activity. Could you park in a farther spot and walk to the store? Do you have the chance to go for a walk or bike ride after school? Then, incorporate one or more of your ideas into your day. Also consider how you can incorporate physical activity into your life as you age. Share your ideas with a partner.

Footsteps: phil Holmes/Shutterstock.com; Background: elenabsl/Shutterstock.com; Icons: Alexander Ryabintsev/Shutterstock.com; phipatbig/Shutterstock.com

Endurance

endurance ability to continue performing a physical activity over time

Another component of health-related fitness is **endurance**, or the ability to continue performing a physical activity over time. *Aerobic endurance* is a person's ability to engage in aerobic activity over a period of time. It depends on the rates at which the heart can continue to pump blood and the body can break down nutrients to produce energy. *Muscular endurance* is the length of time a particular group of muscles can continue to exert force.

Some physical activities require high levels of aerobic and muscular endurance. For example, on a hiking trip, people need muscular endurance so their leg and abdominal muscles can continue working over long distances for hours at a time. They also need aerobic endurance for the heart to continue pumping at higher-than-normal intensity for an extended time period.

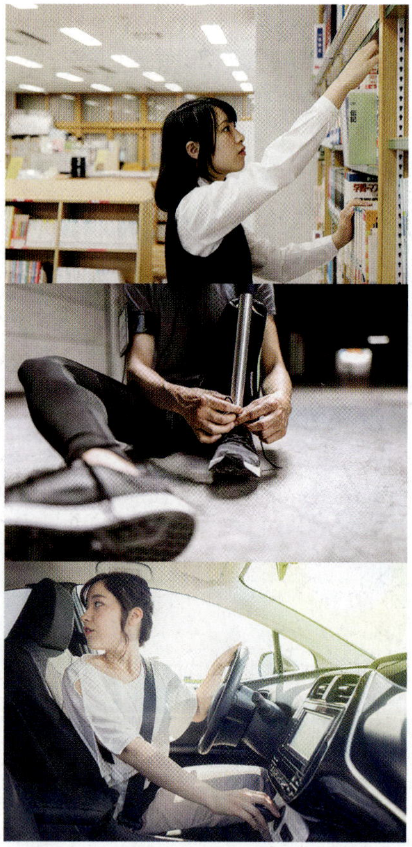

Left to right: urbancow/E+/Getty Images; Pekic/E+/Getty Images; metamorworks/iStock/Getty Images Plus/Getty Images

Figure 10.5 Flexibility means you have full range of motion in joints like your shoulders, hips, and neck.

Muscle Strength

Muscle strength is the ability of a muscle to exert force against resistance. For example, imagine you are arm-wrestling a friend. As you push against your friend's arm muscles, your arm muscles will overcome the resistance if you have more muscle strength. Muscle strength is measured in many ways. For example, you could measure how much weight (resistance) you can lift, how much weight you can push, and how much weight you can pull. With a lot of muscle strength, you can lift heavy objects like a backpack full of books and do high-resistance activities. Strength training can help improve muscle strength and build muscle mass.

Flexibility

flexibility ability to fully and easily move the joints

Flexibility is the ability to fully and easily move your joints. How well your muscles and connective tissues, such as ligaments and tendons, stretch determines flexibility. Thus, stretching your muscles improves flexibility.

Everyone benefits from having some flexibility. Flexibility improves performance in many types of physical activity and lowers the risk of injury (**Figure 10.5**). People who are not very flexible often have tight or stiff muscles. They may have difficulty performing daily life activities, such as tying their shoes. More flexibility is usually good, but you can be too flexible. Some people who are extremely flexible have an increased risk of injuring their joints.

Skill-Related Fitness

skill-related fitness ability to perform successfully in a particular sport or leisure activity

Skill-related fitness is the kind of fitness you need to perform successfully in a particular sport or leisure activity. The components of skill-related fitness include speed, agility, balance, power, coordination, and reaction time.

- **Speed:** If you have participated in or watched sports, you know what speed is. Being fast is an important aspect of many sports. Runners and swimmers must be fast, especially if racing short distances. Sprinting requires more speed than long-distance running or swimming.

- **Agility:** **Agility** is the ability to rapidly change the body's momentum and direction. This skill involves accelerating in a direction or rapidly changing direction. Agility also includes navigating obstacles and going under, over, or around them. A running back on a football team, for example, must maneuver around and away from other players to avoid getting tackled.
- **Balance:** *Balance* is the ability to hold a particular position on a stable or unstable surface. For example, balance determines whether you can do a handstand or ride a bicycle. Balance varies from person to person, and for most people, this skill declines with age.
- **Power:** *Power* is a combination of strength and speed. Power is an important skill in sports such as football and baseball. An outstanding volleyball striker is usually one of the more powerful players on the team.
- **Coordination:** *Coordination* is the ability to perform movements easily and gracefully. Soccer players, hockey players, and other athletes who must have agility and balance also have high levels of coordination. Some people are naturally more coordinated than others. Many athletes who perform complex movements also do so smoothly as a result of practice.
- **Reaction time:** *Reaction time* refers to the quickness of a response. How fast do you react to someone else's movement? If you are faster than most at responding, you might have the qualities to be an outstanding tennis player, batter in baseball, or soccer goalie.

agility ability to rapidly change the body's momentum and direction

Lesson 10.1 Review

Know and Understand

1. How is physical activity different from exercise?
2. What effect does physical activity have on body composition?
3. Explain the difference between aerobic and muscular endurance.
4. Give one example of a physical activity that requires flexibility.
5. Choose one sport or leisure activity and explain which skill-related components of fitness it requires.

Think Critically

6. Think about your family history. What diseases are common among your relatives? Use reliable resources to assess how getting physical activity influences risk for these diseases.
7. With a partner, share examples of how physical activity improves mental, emotional, and social health. Explain why physical activity has this effect in each example.
8. What factors affect what physical fitness looks like for different people? For example, what signs would indicate a person with a physical disability was physically fit? Discuss with a partner.

REAL WORLD Health Skills

Comprehend Concepts Physical activity has many benefits that go even beyond physical health. Identify at least 10 benefits of physical activity, as discussed in this lesson. Indicate whether each benefit affects your physical health, mental and emotional health, or social health. Then, for each dimension of health, identify a challenge you are facing that physical activity might help you solve.

Lesson

10.2 Getting Enough Physical Activity

Essential Question?

What skills can you use to get enough physical activity?

Learning Outcomes

After studying this lesson, you will be able to

- differentiate between active and sedentary behaviors;
- identify recommendations from the *Physical Activity Guidelines for Americans*;
- analyze ways to integrate physical activity into daily life;
- demonstrate ways of varying FITT factors to increase fitness;
- assess strategies for increasing muscle strength and endurance; and
- identify resources for getting physical activity.

Key Terms

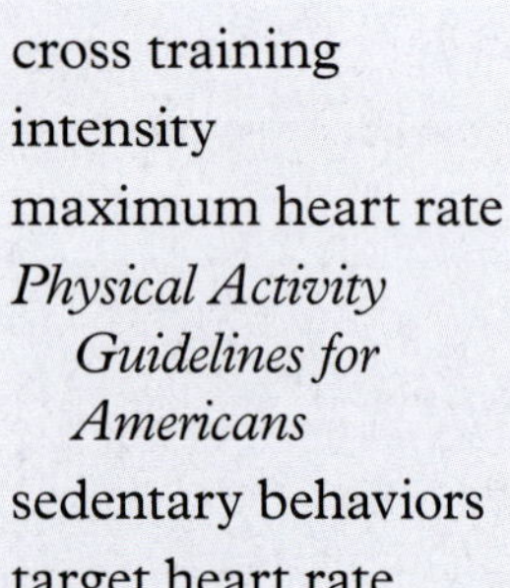

cross training
intensity
maximum heart rate
Physical Activity Guidelines for Americans
sedentary behaviors
target heart rate

Warm-Up Activity

Your Level of Physical Activity

Practice Health-Enhancing Behaviors Before reading this lesson, list all of the physical activity and structured exercise you have participated in over the last seven days. Label each item as a sport, chore, physical education class activity, or physical activity that is part of your daily routine. Write a reflection explaining whether you feel you get enough physical activity. What specific changes could you make to include more physical activity and exercise in your daily life?

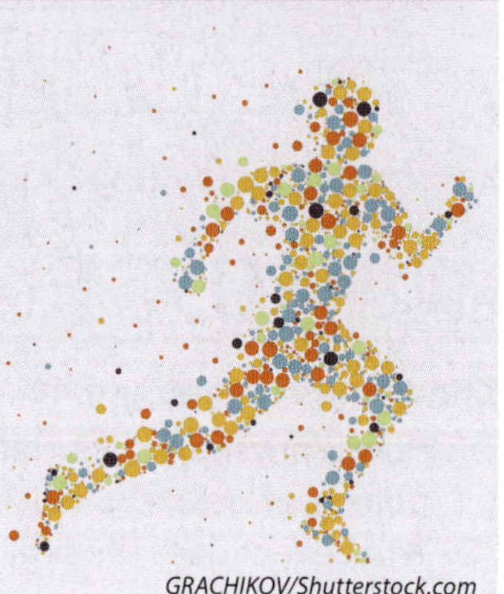

GRACHIKOV/Shutterstock.com

What types of physical activity do you do on a regular basis? Do you jog, play tennis, mow the lawn, swim, or skate? Do you lift weights or do push-ups or sit-ups? Do you stretch or do Pilates? These are all examples of physical activity. Physical activity has many benefits that help people live longer, healthier lives. Different activities improve different components of physical fitness. In this lesson, you will learn ways of incorporating physical activity into your daily life and using physical activity to improve your health.

How Much Physical Activity Should You Get?

sedentary behaviors activities that consist of sitting or lying down and using very little energy

Although the health benefits of physical activity are clear, most people do not get enough physical activity. Many people spend much of their day engaging in **sedentary behaviors**, or activities that consist of sitting or lying down and using very little energy. Examples of sedentary behaviors include driving, watching TV shows or movies, surfing or chatting online, playing video games, working at a classroom desk, and reading.

The US Department of Health and Human Services (HHS) publishes the ***Physical Activity Guidelines for Americans*** to guide people in getting enough physical activity (**Figure 10.6**). These guidelines recommend that children and teens ages 6–17

- get at least one hour of moderate-to-vigorous physical activity every day;
- spend the majority of that time doing moderate- or vigorous-intensity aerobic activities;
- include muscle-strengthening activities at least three days a week; and
- include bone-strengthening activities at least three days a week.

Physical Activity Guidelines for Americans recommendations published by the US Department of Health and Human Services about how much physical activity children, teens, and adults should get

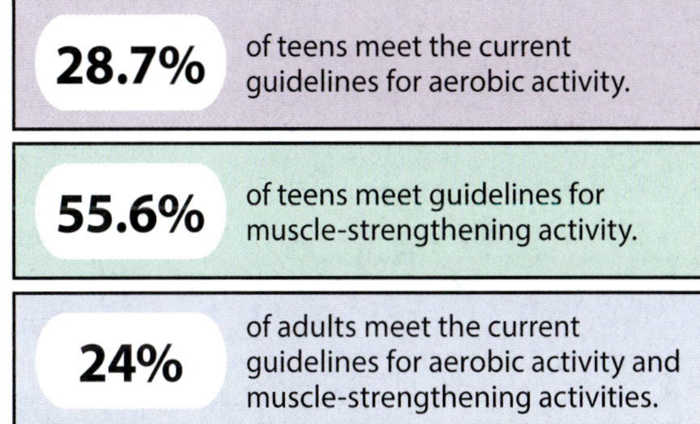

Figure 10.6 Few Americans currently meet the recommendations for aerobic activity and muscle-strengthening activities. ***What publication contains the recommendations for physical activity?***

Examples of aerobic activities include riding a bike, hiking or swimming, doing work at home or in a yard, running or racing, playing sports, doing martial arts, and dancing. As you know, *aerobic activities* improve cardiorespiratory fitness. *Muscle-strengthening activities* improve muscle strength and endurance. Examples of these activities include lifting weights and climbing. *Bone-strengthening activities* promote bone growth. Examples include running and playing sports that involve jumping.

Strategies for Engaging in Physical Activity

There are many ways to incorporate physical activity into your daily life. Setting SMART goals—goals that are specific, measurable, achievable, relevant, and timely—can help you get started. You will need to make time for physical activity and plan activities that are most beneficial for your health. If your goal is to increase fitness, you will need to vary your physical activities and follow the principles in **Figure 10.7**.

Training Principles for Increasing Fitness

Principle	Description
Overload principle	You must put demands on your body to improve it. You will not be able to run a longer distance unless you try to run a longer distance. You will not be able to lift more weight unless you try lifting heavier weights. You need to "overload" your body to strengthen it.
Specificity principle	Certain activities will lead to improvements in certain components of fitness. Stretching your legs improves the flexibility of your leg muscles, but not your arm muscles. If you lift a weight, the muscles used to lift the weight will be strengthened, but that particular activity will have no effect on your other muscles. You need to choose activities that focus on the components of fitness you want to improve.
Progression principle	You must vary the frequency, intensity, time, or type of your physical activities over time to improve fitness. If you want to maintain your current level of fitness, you can develop a consistent plan and stick to it. If you want to improve fitness beyond its current level, you will need to increase frequency, intensity, or time periodically.

Figure 10.7 These training principles will guide you as you monitor and adjust your goals to increase fitness.

Choose Physical Activities You Enjoy

It is much easier to get enough physical activity if you identify types of physical activity you enjoy. Remember that physical activity is any action in which the body uses energy. Physical activity does not have to be structured, like an exercise class or sport. The time you spend traveling between classes, bicycling with friends, swimming, and playing tennis all count toward your physical activity.

Some people enjoy team sports, such as basketball, soccer, or field hockey. Other people prefer to be active alone and might find skateboarding, jogging, or climbing stairs more enjoyable. Consider whether you like to be active outside or inside and whether you like to be active alone or with other people.

Sometimes a person's environment can affect the physical activities a person chooses to do. For example, some teens live in communities where being active outside could be unsafe due to traffic, crime, pollution, or weather. Income level can also affect a person's physical activity choices. Fortunately, there are many physical activities you can do outside or inside with inexpensive or no equipment. Some examples include doing sit-ups, push-ups, squats, or jumping jacks; climbing stairs; running in place; and stretching your muscles.

Local and Global Health

Physical Activity Around the World

Physical activity is an important part of health around the world. The percentage of people who get enough physical activity varies considerably in different countries.

In one study, researchers at the World Health Organization (WHO) asked people in 168 different countries about their activity levels at home, at work, and during free time. They measured the percentage of people in each country who engaged in *regular physical activity* (defined as at least 150 minutes of moderate-intensity or 75 minutes of vigorous-intensity physical activity per week).

In some countries, most people reported getting regular physical activity. The countries with the highest rates of physical activity were in Africa and Southeast Asia. In Mongolia and Benin, 91 percent of people engaged in regular physical activity, as did 93 percent of people in Mozambique. In other countries, relatively few people engaged in regular physical activity. The five countries in which the fewest people engaged in regular physical activity were Malta, Swaziland, Saudi Arabia, Argentina, and Serbia. In the least physically active country, Malta, only about 28 percent of people engaged in regular physical activity.

This study also found other trends in how rates of physical activity differed worldwide. For example, people in higher-income countries were generally less active than people in low-income countries. Males also tended to be more active than females.

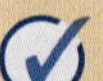

Practice Your Skills

Analyze Influences

What factors do you think might explain why most people in some countries engage in enough physical activity, but most people in other countries do not? What role might environmental factors, such as climate or life in a big city versus small town, have on people's ability to get physical activity? Why do you think people in higher-income countries are less active? Why do you think males tend to be more active than females? After discussing these questions with a partner, think about your community. Make a list of the factors that influence people's rates of physical activity. How can students at your school manage these factors to get enough physical activity?

Physical disabilities, mental illnesses, injuries, and diseases can also impact a person's physical activity. Talking with a doctor can help people make sure particular activities are safe for them. For example, people who use wheelchairs can lift weights and stretch from a seated position or participate in team sports such as wheelchair basketball. People with mental illnesses can be active at home if being in public feels overwhelming or take small steps, such as taking the stairs instead of an elevator. People coping with injuries or diseases can perform activities focused on particular body parts. For example, someone recovering from a shoulder injury could concentrate on leg strength and flexibility.

Integrate Physical Activity into Your Daily Life

To incorporate physical activities that match with your daily life, find ways of being physically active that do not require too much time or money. For example, it is easier and cheaper to jog around your neighborhood than to join an expensive health club or gym.

Most people feel they are too busy to find time for physical activity. They feel they have too many other tasks to accomplish each day. Remember that even a little physical activity goes a long way (**Figure 10.8**). When you make physical activity part of your routine, you will find time for it more easily. The first and most important step is to set aside time each week—even 10 minutes at a time—to engage in some type of physical activity. You can even be physically active while doing other activities. For example, you could do sit-ups or push-ups while watching videos or stretch while doing homework. The more you make a habit of physical activity, the more easily it will become part of your daily life.

Even small doses of physical activity can improve a person's life expectancy and decrease the risk of certain health conditions.
01:00
Do jumping jacks after each TV episode
Walk from class to class
Stretch before breakfast
Take the stairs up to your apartment
05:00
10:00
Clean your room
Shoot hoops with your sibling after school
Play fetch with your dog
Ride your bike to your friend's house
15:00

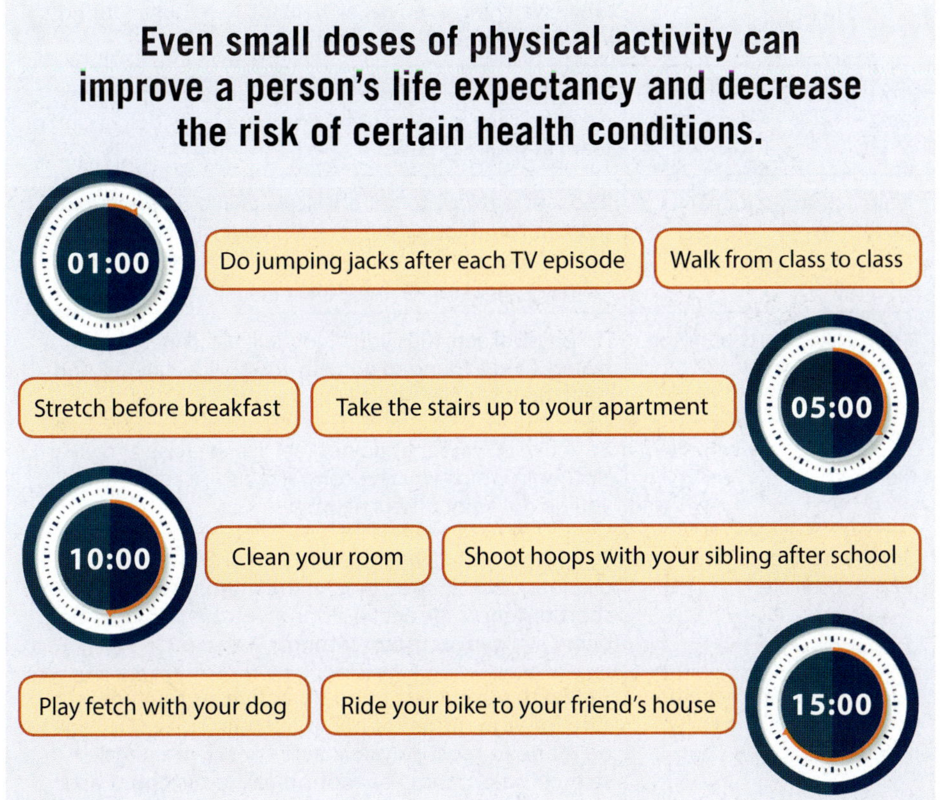

Panimoni/Shutterstock.com

Figure 10.8 Incorporating small activities can quickly add up to 60 minutes a day.

Having the support of friends and family members can help you be more physically active. For example, you could find someone to engage in physical activity with you. Most people find it more difficult to make excuses and cancel plans if they know someone is expecting them to be there. You could also develop new friendships by joining a group of people interested in a particular physical activity. You might meet new people at an aerobics class, pick-up baseball game at a local playground, or hiking club.

As you set goals to be more physically active, consider any obstacles that might get in your way and make plans to overcome them. **Figure 10.9** lists some examples of obstacles and strategies for getting past them.

Vary Frequency, Intensity, Time, and Type

Engaging in many different types of physical activity at different intensities can help you focus on multiple areas of fitness. The FITT principle is one formula for varying physical activity to improve fitness. The acronym *FITT* stands for frequency, intensity, time, and type. Manipulating and varying these factors will help you gradually, safely, and effectively improve your fitness.

Figure 10.9 Remember that physical activity has many health benefits that are worth pursuing.

Overcoming Obstacles to Physical Activity

Obstacle	Strategies to Overcome Obstacle
"I don't have time."	Find easy ways to integrate physical activity into your routine. Take the stairs instead of the elevator, stretch while watching a movie, or walk for 10 minutes during your lunch period or after school.
"My neighborhood isn't safe."	Be active inside, such as climbing stairs, doing chores, jumping rope, or even doing jumping jacks. Join a club or team at your high school.
"I can't afford to join a sport or gym."	Choose free ways to get physical activity. Join a club or team at your high school, stretch your muscles, walk or jog, or explore a local park. Research body weight exercises you can do at home.
"I don't like sports or going to the gym."	Do physical activities you enjoy, such as dancing or hiking. Find a friend to go with you so you can talk and catch up while being active.
"I hate how I look when I exercise."	Be active in ways that do not feel like exercise and wear clothes in which you feel comfortable. Be active alone if you do not want others nearby.
"My mental illness makes it hard to exercise."	Talk with a mental health professional and make small changes, such as stretching in the morning and walking short distances. Be active alone if you are nervous about being in a gym or group setting.
"I can't do certain activities with my disability/injury/disease."	Talk with your doctor and do activities that are safe for you. Adjustments or accommodations can be made to most physical activities. Even gentle stretching or range-of-motion exercises count as physical activity.

Frequency

Frequency describes how often you engage in physical activity—every day or once a week, for example. As you know, the *Physical Activity Guidelines for Americans* recommends spending the majority of time on aerobic activities and engaging in muscle-strengthening and bone-strengthening activities three days a week. When planning physical activity, vary the frequency of how often you do certain activities like running, lifting weights, or doing yard work.

Intensity

Intensity is the amount of energy your body uses per minute during an activity. You can judge the intensity of physical activity based on how it affects your heart rate and breathing. During a moderate-intensity activity, your heart rate and breathing are faster than normal, but you can still carry on a conversation. During a vigorous-intensity activity, your heart rate and breathing are considerably faster than normal, and you cannot carry on a conversation.

intensity amount of energy the body uses per minute during an activity

You can also determine the intensity of aerobic activities by measuring heart rate. **Target heart rate** is the rate of heartbeats that is safe and effective for a given intensity. Your target heart rate is a percentage of your **maximum heart rate**, or your heart's rate when it works its hardest. No single, standard maximum heart rate exists. Maximum heart rate depends on a person's age. You can calculate your maximum heart rate by subtracting your age from the number 220. If you are 16 years of age, your maximum heart rate is

target heart rate number of heartbeats per minute that is safe and effective for a given intensity

maximum heart rate number of heartbeats per minute when the heart is working its hardest

$$220 - \text{age in years} = \text{maximum heart rate in beats per minute (bpm)}$$

$$220 - 16 = 204 \text{ bpm}$$

For moderate-intensity activity, a person's target heart rate should be 50–70 percent of maximum heart rate. For vigorous-intensity activity, a person's target heart rate should be 70–85 percent of maximum heart rate. **Figure 10.10** shows how to calculate target heart rate using maximum heart rate.

To measure heart rate, you can measure your pulse or use a heart rate monitor. Your *pulse* is the feeling of blood being pumped from your heart

Calculating Target Heart Rate		
Maximum Heart Rate (16 Years Old)	**Moderate-Intensity Physical Activity**	**Vigorous-Intensity Physical Activity**
220 – 16 (age in years) = 204 bpm **Maximum heart rate: 204 bpm**	× 50% (0.50) = 102 bpm	× 70% (0.70) = 142.8 bpm
	× 70% (0.70) = 142.8 bpm	× 85% (0.85) = 173.4 bpm
	Moderate-intensity target heart rate: 102–142.8 bpm	**Vigorous-intensity target heart rate: 142.8–173.4 bpm**

Figure 10.10 You can calculate your target heart rate using your age and intensity of physical activity. ***Your target heart rate is a percentage of what measurement?***

Taking a Pulse

1. Find your pulse on the artery of the wrist in line with your thumb.
2. Place the tips of your index and middle fingers over the artery and press lightly.
3. Start counting on a beat. Count the first beat as 0 (not 1).
4. Count the number of heartbeats for a full 60 seconds. You can also count for six seconds and multiply by 10.

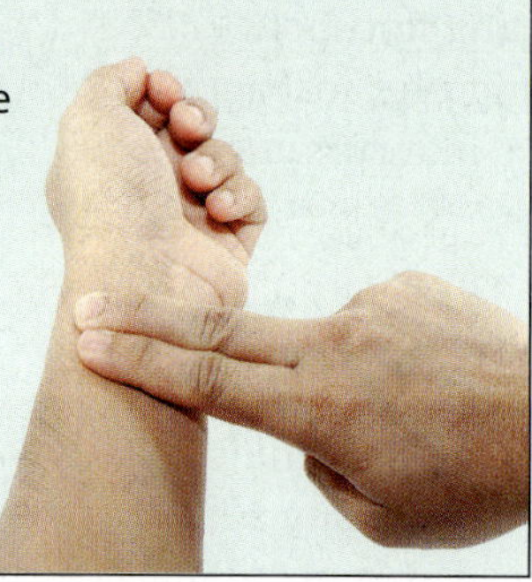

I'm friday/Shutterstock.com

Figure 10.11 You can feel pulse at the neck, wrist, or chest, although the wrist is often the easiest place to find a pulse. ***What is your pulse?***

to the rest of your body. To measure your pulse, follow the steps in **Figure 10.11**.

Heart rate monitors can also measure pulse by shining a light into the blood vessels in your wrist and measuring changes in blood volume each time your heart beats. Less light reflected back into the sensor on your wrist means more blood volume and a faster pulse.

Time

Time refers to the time you spend engaging in physical activity. Maybe you spend 10 minutes biking to the library or 60 minutes working out at the gym. Varying the time you spend being active can help you start with small goals and work toward more and more physical activity. For example, if you cannot find time to jog for 30 minutes, jog around the block once for 10 minutes.

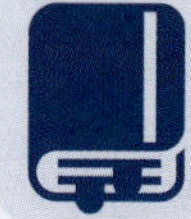

Case Study

Getting More Physical Activity

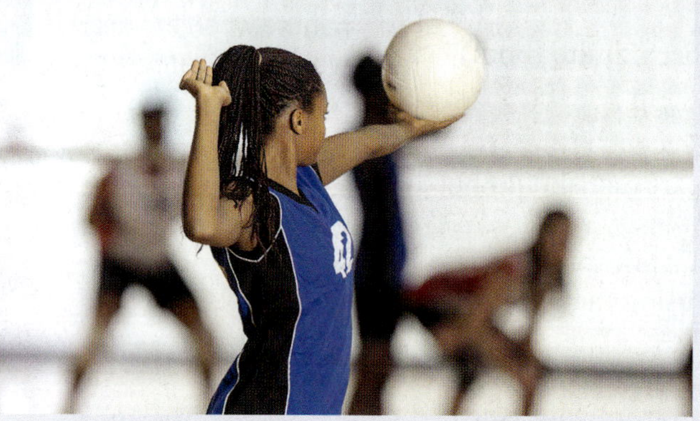

FatCamera/E+/Getty Images

Elise's senior year is very busy. She studies several hours each night, has chorus rehearsals in the afternoons, and has a part-time job at the movie theater. Elise's doctor told her she needs to get more physical activity, but she cannot find the time. Sometimes, she will try a new fitness plan, but will forget about it within a few days. Elise knows she is out of shape because she feels short of breath hurrying to class. She worries her lack of fitness could negatively affect her singing and other activities she enjoys.

Charlie enjoys working out and regularly goes to the gym to lift weights. Recently, he has started getting bored with his gym routine. He wants to maintain his level of fitness, but he does not want to just go to the gym and lift weights. Charlie is not sure how to shake up his workouts, though.

Peyton is on her high school's volleyball team and loves every minute of it. She wishes she could play competitively during the off-season, however. Her coach recommended joining a traveling volleyball team. Peyton talked to her parents about the opportunity. After looking into the expenses, Peyton and her parents decided they were unable to afford the traveling team. Peyton wishes there were another way for her to stay in shape during her off-season.

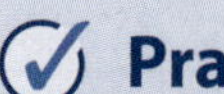

Practice Your Skills

Communicate with Others

In small groups, create a physical activity plan for one of the teens described. List at least three different ways the teen can incorporate physical activity into daily life. Then, write a scenario in which a teen faces a situation that gets in the way of following this physical activity plan. Some examples might include a friend who wants to play video games instead or family members needing the teen to return home at a certain time. Write additional paragraphs in which the teen navigates these situations using effective negotiation and communication skills to meet physical activity goals.

Type

Varying *types* of activities can keep physical activity interesting, increase fitness in several areas, and reduce the chance of injury. If you like several types of aerobic activity, try doing a different activity each time you are active. If you want to lift weights, focus on different muscle groups and methods of strength training. One way to vary your activities is to engage in **cross training**. In cross training, you participate in one activity to help improve another. For example, a tennis player might lift weights to improve upper-body strength and serving ability. A basketball player might take a dance class to improve agility.

cross training act of participating in various types of physical activity to help improve skill in another type

Keep in mind that the types of activities you do might change over time depending on your interests, physical ability, diseases and health conditions, environment, and stage of development.

Engage in Muscle-Strengthening Activities

Muscle-strengthening activities improve muscle strength and endurance. These activities include the use of *resistance*, or a force against which the muscle acts. This resistance can take the form of body weight, resistance bands or tubes, free weights, or weight machines (**Figure 10.12**).

Body weight
Can serve as resistance in various activities
Resistance bands or tubes
Provide tension, increasing with thickness of band

Free weights
Provide maximum resistance; can include barbells, dumbells, and kettlebells
Weight machines
Guide your motion to ensure the target muscle is being exercised

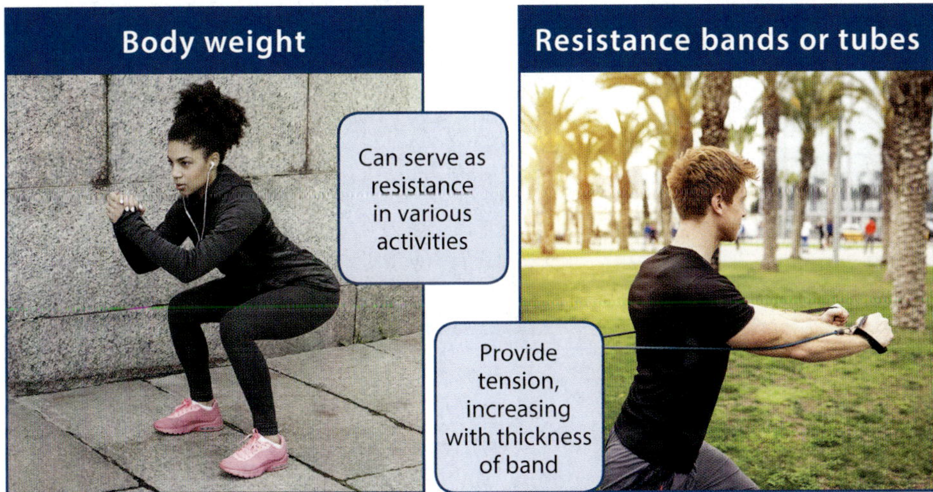

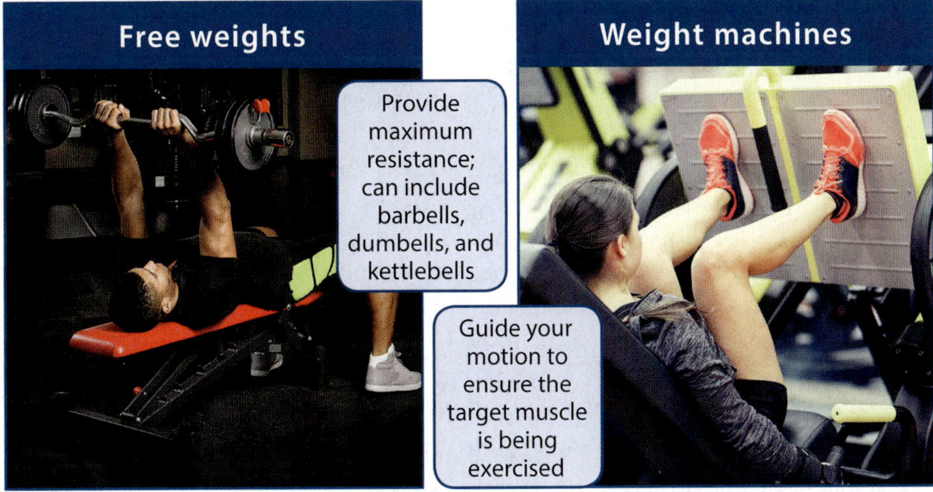

Clockwise from top left: Artem Varnitsin/Shutterstock.com; InnerVisionPRO/Shutterstock.com; Syda Productions/Shutterstock.com; Serghei Starus/Shutterstock.com

Figure 10.12 Various forms of resistance can help improve muscle strength and endurance.

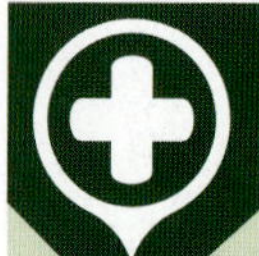

Spotlight on Health and Wellness Careers

Physical Therapist: Courtney Hansen

My path to becoming a physical therapist did not start in high school or even at the beginning of college. Still, I have never regretted it. I was actually an accounting major when I started college—until I got a *C* in my accounting class. I wanted to graduate in four years, so I decided to change my major. My boyfriend at the time was thinking about becoming a physical therapist (PT) and mentioned the profession to me. My mom had a stroke when I was 10 years old, so I was very familiar with physical therapy, and I liked nutrition and my job teaching exercise classes. I changed my major, got my undergraduate degree in Exercise Physiology and Nutrition, and completed my master's degree in Physical Therapy.

My job requires strength, endurance, energy, and positivity. As a PT, I see 10–12 patients for 40 minutes each day. I work in a rural setting and see a variety of patients, including people recovering from wounds, brain injuries, horse accidents, motor vehicle accidents, orthopedic injuries, and surgery. In physical therapy, my goal is to get patients back to their level of function before injury or disease. This is achieved through a variety of manual therapy techniques, therapeutic modalities, aquatic therapy, and a multidisciplinary approach.

I also educate patients and recommend exercises to perform at home. As the Director of Clinical Education for five facilities, I mentor graduates and am responsible for making sure all employees focus on becoming outstanding PTs with continuing education.

I love being a PT and helping people. It is so rewarding to see someone come in using a wheelchair and walk out, return to a sport, or get back to an active lifestyle after a brain injury or chronic pain. The only downfall might be having to stay late or work at home to complete documentation. Being a PT has been a fantastic career for almost 21 years now.

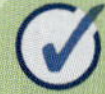

Practice Your Skills

Access Information

Think about your own interests, strengths, and weaknesses. What parts of being a PT do you think would interest you? Which elements would be challenging? Using reliable resources like the US Bureau of Labor Statistics' *Occupational Outlook Handbook*, research physical therapy and related careers. Is the demand for PTs growing? What are the educational requirements for being a PT? Are there related careers that might also interest you? Write a blog post summarizing your thoughts.

Children and teens should engage in muscle-strengthening activities three days a week. During these activities, try to target all of the major muscle groups, including the chest (or *pectorals*), back, arms and shoulders, abdominals, and legs and buttocks. Different activities target different muscle groups.

Do not perform any type of muscle-strengthening activity unless you know the proper form. In addition to correct posture and position, proper form includes finding a consistent tempo and paying attention to your breathing. Improper form can lead to injuries and mean you are not exercising the muscles you intend to. To prevent injuries, lift heavy weights with a partner. Your partner can be your *spotter* and help you avoid dropping a weight on yourself if it becomes too difficult to manage.

To get started with a muscle-strengthening activity, use the following steps:

1. Start with a 5- to 10-minute warm-up, including low- or moderate-intensity aerobic activity, to get blood flowing to your muscles. You will learn more about warm-ups and cooldowns in the next lesson.
2. If using free weights or a weight machine, select a weight (resistance) level that tires your muscles after 12–15 repetitions. This weight will be different for different activities.

3. Do two or three *sets* (groups of repetitions followed by rest) of an activity. For example, you could do three sets of squats, with each set consisting of 10 repetitions. Stop immediately if you feel sharp pain or experience swollen joints. These are signs you have done too much. Some muscle soreness is normal, but intense pain indicates a problem.
4. Rest the muscle group you targeted with a particular activity for at least one full day to give the muscles time to recover. Muscle-strengthening activities work in part by causing tiny tears in muscle tissue, which allows muscles to grow stronger as the tears are repaired.

As you become stronger, the number of sets and repetitions you can do without feeling tired will increase. In response, you may want to increase resistance. To build strength, you may choose to do fewer sets with increased weight. To increase muscular endurance, you may choose to do more sets.

Stretch Your Muscles

Paying attention to flexibility can help you avoid injury during physical activity. The best way to increase flexibility is to regularly (and safely) stretch your muscles. Fitness guidelines suggest that everyone engage in some type of stretching activity at least two or three days each week. To stretch your muscles, use the following steps:

1. Before stretching, engage in 5–10 minutes of low- or moderate-intensity aerobic activity, such as jumping jacks, skipping rope, or light jogging, to increase heart rate and blood flow to the muscles.
2. After your muscles are warmed up, stretch your muscles so you can feel tightness, but not pain (**Figure 10.13**).
3. Hold each stretch for 10–30 seconds, but do not bounce (since bouncing can lead to overstretching or small tears in the muscle).
4. While holding each stretch, breathe naturally to provide oxygen to your muscles.
5. Repeat each stretch two to four times. Repetition will help you work the muscle and increase flexibility.

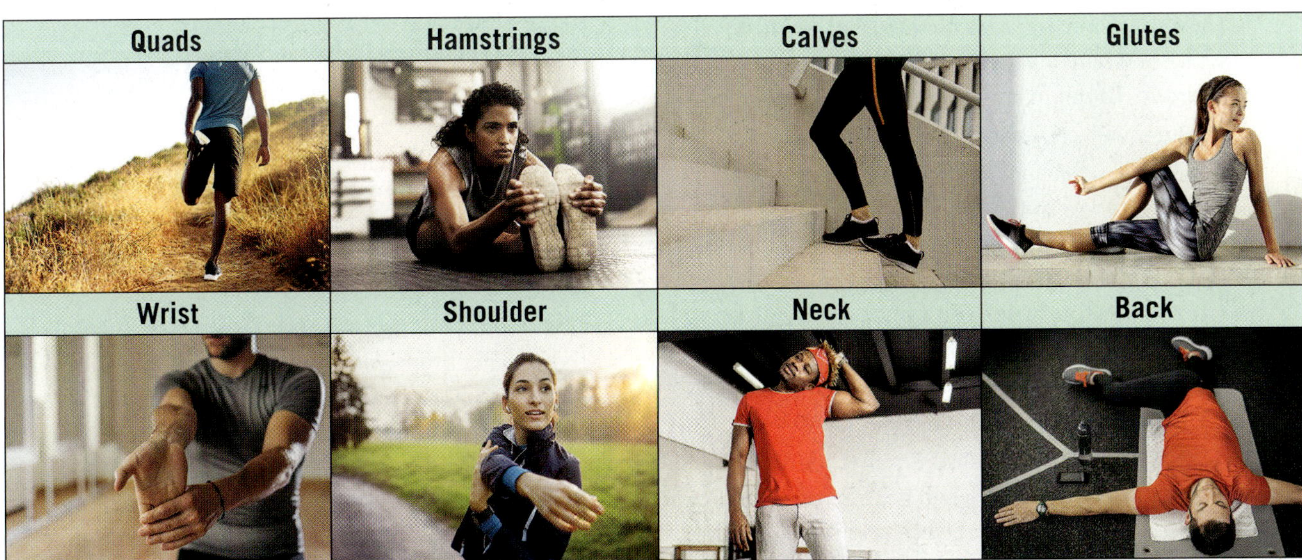

Left to right, top row: PeopleImages/E+/Getty Images; Hiraman/E+/Getty Images; victorsaboya/Shutterstock.com; Maridav/iStock/Getty Images Plus/Getty Images
Left to right, bottom row: emiliozv/iStock/Getty Images Plus/Getty Images; Ridofranz/iStock/Getty Images Plus/Getty Images; Zinkevych/iStock/Getty Images Plus/Getty Images; emiliozv/iStock/Getty Images Plus/Getty Images

Figure 10.13 Different stretches can be used to loosen and warm up different muscles. ***What should you not feel while stretching your muscles?***

Take Advantage of School and Community Programs

School and community programs can help you get the physical activity you need. Most children and teens attend schools that offer *physical education (PE) classes*. Participating in physical activity at school is a great way to increase fitness. Both the National Association for Sport and Physical Education (NASPE) and the American Heart Association (AHA) recommend that high school students participate in 225 minutes of PE per week. Participating in PE classes and advocating for PE at school are great ways to make fitness a priority.

Skills for Health and Wellness

Making a Physical Activity and Fitness Plan

Now that you know strategies for getting more physical activity, you can create a personal physical activity plan for increasing fitness. Most people, even those who are physically fit, can improve some aspects of fitness. This is why physical activity plans are personal. You can work on the parts of *your* fitness most in need of improvement. The components of fitness on which you focus might be very different from those your friends need to prioritize.

Practice Your Skills

Set Goals

In this activity, you will go through the steps of assessing your current physical activity and fitness level and making a plan to be more active and improve your fitness. You can go through these steps on your own or involve a partner in brainstorming.

1. The first step in designing a plan is determining your current level of physical activity and fitness. These baseline measurements will give you a sense of where you are now and what you can improve. To begin, measure the following areas:
   - how much physical activity you get in a given day and week (include all physical activity, structured or not)
   - the time it takes you to walk one mile and your pulse after walking one mile
   - how many push-ups you can do at one time
   - how far you can reach forward, toward your toes, while sitting with your legs straight in front of you
   - your waist circumference, weight, and BMI
2. Next, based on your measurements, identify the areas of physical activity and fitness you would like to improve. Would you like to get at least one hour of physical activity each day? reach a BMI in the healthy range? do 20 push-ups at one time? For each area you would like to improve, set a SMART goal. Be sure your SMART goal is specific, measurable, achievable, relevant, and timely. In your goal, break out the specific activities you will do each day of the week. Consider your resources, time, and any obstacles that might get in your way. These goals will make up your physical activity and fitness plan. Together, all of the goals in your plan should meet or go beyond the *Physical Activity Guidelines for Americans*.
3. Put your goals into action. Work toward your goals and handle any obstacles you encounter. Use your resources to support your goals. Does your school have a gym you can use? Do you have access to a swimming pool? What people in your life can help support your goals? If you have trouble finding time to be active, look for ways to use your time efficiently. For example, you could do lunges or push-ups while watching your favorite show.
4. Document your progress toward your goal. Note the specific times you get physical activity, the activities you do, and any measurements you take. These details will help you assess your progress and modify your goals, if needed.
5. At the end of the specified time for your goal, evaluate your progress. Review your documentation and assess whether you met your goals. Set new goals or modify your goals to get more physical activity and keep improving your fitness.

Many schools and communities also provide free or low-cost opportunities to engage in physical activity outside of school. For example, you could join an intramural club or interscholastic sports team through your school. Your local community center might provide opportunities for noncompetitive physical activity, such as lessons in different types of sports, dance, and strength training.

Many communities contain facilities you can use for free or at a reduced cost. For example, you could engage in physical activity at the following places:

- parks and green spaces for playing Frisbee, throwing a baseball, or playing soccer
- outdoor sports facilities such as baseball or softball fields and tennis and basketball courts
- indoor sports facilities such as weight rooms, fitness centers, and racquetball courts
- walking and biking trails and skate parks
- public pools

Lesson 10.2 Review

Know and Understand

1. According to the *Physical Activity Guidelines for Americans*, how much physical activity should teens get every day?
2. Explain how to measure the intensity of a physical activity.
3. What is the target heart rate for a 15-year-old engaging in moderate-intensity physical activity?
4. What weight should you select when using free weights or a weight machine?
5. What is the purpose of engaging in aerobic activity before stretching?

Think Critically

6. Choose one training principle and explain how you could apply it in your life to increase fitness.
7. What physical activities do you enjoy? Make a list of all the physical activities you enjoy and share them as a class. Identify which physical activities you could incorporate into your routine and explain why you are choosing them.
8. What obstacles get in the way of you getting enough physical activity? What strategies could you use to overcome these obstacles?
9. What school and community programs provide opportunities for physical activity in your community? Choose three programs and identify the area of fitness they improve. Share your findings with the class.

REAL WORLD Health Skills

Advocate for Health In this lesson, you learned about ways to get more physical activity. You read that even getting physical activity during small windows of time can be beneficial. Create an advocacy contest to get your entire school to "Take Time to Be Active" and use even small amounts of time to get physical activity. In your contest, people should identify the short amounts of time they are not doing anything and try to be active during those times. Create a poster or brochure that explains your contest and what people must do to win. Include people of diverse backgrounds and abilities and be sure to include a prize.

Lesson 10.3

Staying Safe During Physical Activity

Essential Question?

What skills do you need to be safe while engaging in physical activity?

Key Terms

amenorrhea
concussion
cooldown
dehydration
dislocation
female athlete triad
fracture
frostbite
heat cramps
heat exhaustion
heatstroke
hypothermia
sprain
warm-up

Learning Outcomes

After studying this lesson, you will be able to

- describe the importance of following rules and showing sportsmanship;
- identify proper equipment for physical activities;
- analyze the best way to start doing a physical activity;
- demonstrate ways of warming up and cooling down;
- explain how to stay hydrated;
- list precautions for being active in extreme conditions; and
- describe ways to reduce health conditions and injuries that can result from physical activity.

Warm-Up Activity

Staying Safe

Practice Health-Enhancing Behaviors This lesson is about reducing the risk of fitness-related injuries. Before reading the lesson, make five predictions about safety strategies you think might be included in the lesson. For each prediction, explain why you think it is an important guideline for avoiding injuries. Use your previous personal experience, as well as information you may have learned elsewhere.

Guidelines	Importance

While physical activity has many benefits, sometimes it can have certain risks. In this lesson, you will learn to reduce these risks and participate in physical activities safely and effectively. Strategies for staying safe during physical activity include conducting yourself respectfully, using equipment properly, pacing yourself, staying hydrated, using caution in extreme conditions, and treating injuries.

Conduct Yourself Respectfully

Conducting yourself with respect during physical activity involves following rules and being a good sport. Many types of physical activity, especially sports, have certain rules that people follow to stay safe. Knowing and following the rules of your chosen activity can keep you and others free from injury.

Rules vary considerably based on the activity. For example, in football, soccer, lacrosse, or ice hockey, a rule states that all activity on the field must stop when the referee blows the whistle. Traffic laws keep people safe during biking, running, or rollerblading. Rules at fitness facilities may include not bringing food or beverages, wiping off equipment after use, and wearing proper clothing and shoes. Because rules change depending on an activity's location or organization, make sure you know the particular rules you should be following.

Another aspect of respectful conduct is *sportsmanship*, or behaviors that play fair and treat people with respect. Sportsmanship includes shaking hands with members of the opposing team at the end of a game, accepting officials' calls (even if you do not believe they were right), and acknowledging performance by members of both teams.

Sometimes it can be hard to congratulate the other team when your team has lost a close game. Remember that sports is about learning new skills and having fun, not just winning. Treating members of the other team how you would like to be treated shows respect for yourself, your teammates, coaches on both sides, officials, and the game.

Use Proper Equipment

Many physical activities involve wearing proper equipment to prevent injury (**Figure 10.14**). Sometimes, laws even require people doing certain physical activities to wear equipment. In the case of riding a bike, for example, some states require people to wear helmets. In the event of an accident, wearing a helmet can save a person's life.

When choosing equipment, make sure your equipment fits well. Do not use hand-me-downs or used equipment that is overly worn or the wrong size.

Fitness Equipment

Equipment	Uses
Helmets	• Organized sports: Baseball, softball, and football • Recreational activities: Biking, skiing, and rollerblading
Mouth guards	• Lacrosse, ice hockey, football, wrestling, boxing, and kickboxing
Eye protection	• Goggles: Swimmers and divers • Face masks: Ice hockey, baseball and softball catchers, lacrosse, and football • Sunglasses, brimmed hats, or visors: Tennis, golf, beach volleyball, softball, baseball, and biking
Padding for wrists, knees, hips, shoulders, and elbows	• Ice hockey, football, soccer, lacrosse, ice-skating, rollerblading, and snowboarding
Reflective gear	• Biking or running along the side of the road

Figure 10.14 Depending on the hazards of a physical activity, different equipment can help keep people safe.

Also be sure to take care of fitness equipment and facilities. Fitness equipment is expensive, so you should keep equipment in good condition and store it in a safe place.

Pace Yourself

Improving fitness is a gradual process that requires steadily increasing your physical activity. When you begin increasing your fitness in an area or try a new physical activity, start slowly. It can be tempting to exert yourself too much when you are first getting started, but overexerting yourself can be harmful. Overdoing any type of physical activity the first couple of days increases your chance of injury.

Once you feel more comfortable with a physical activity, you can increase the time, frequency, and intensity. For example, you could eventually walk, rollerblade, or bike for 30 minutes instead of 10–20 minutes. You could jog instead of walk or increase the amount of weight you lift. Gradually increase the demands on your body and be patient instead of trying to do too much too soon.

Warm Up and Cool Down

warm-up activity that prepares the body for physical activity; gets blood pumping to the muscles and stretches muscles

No matter what type of physical activity you are doing, warming up and cooling down can help you be safe. A **warm-up** is an activity you do before engaging in your chosen physical activity. Warm-ups, even if they only last 5–10 minutes, get much-needed blood to your muscles, which helps prevent injuries. A warm-up should include two distinct components:

1. a low- to moderate-intensity aerobic activity, such as light jogging, jumping jacks, or brisk walking
2. at least five minutes of muscle stretching, starting at the top of your body and moving to your lower body

Some experts recommend warming up by doing a light version of the physical activity you are about to do. For example, just before a basketball game, you could shoot some baskets and retrieve missed shots. Before a tennis match, you could casually hit some balls back and forth with a partner.

cooldown activity that helps the body wind down after physical activity; helps heart rate return to normal level

You should also cool down after engaging in physical activity. A **cooldown** helps your heart rate return to a normal, lower level. Cooldowns should include gentle stretching, which helps prevent your muscles from feeling stiff and sore the next day. Any light activity can serve as your cooldown. Many people simply slow down to low levels of their current activity for a cooldown.

Stay Hydrated

dehydration condition in which the body does not have enough fluid to perform basic functions

During physical activity, you sweat, which decreases the amount of fluid in your body. Fluid loss causes blood volume to decrease, and as a result, the heart must work harder to pump blood throughout the body. Loss of fluid can lead to muscle cramps, dizziness, and fatigue. It can also lead to **dehydration**, in which the body does not have enough fluid to perform its basic functions.

To avoid these consequences of fluid loss, stay hydrated during physical activity. The best way to stay hydrated is to drink lots of water before, during, and even after engaging in physical activity. Make sure to bring water when you are engaging in physical activity and remember to drink frequently. Other types of fluids can also help you stay hydrated (**Figure 10.15**).

Hydration During Physical Activity	
Type of Fluid	**Factors to Consider**
Water	Restores water lost through sweating; does not provide carbohydrates or electrolytes to replace lost nutrients
Sports drink	Restores water and electrolytes lost through sweating; contains some carbohydrates, minerals, electrolytes, and other vitamins and nutrients; contains many calories and large amounts of sugar; provides slower hydration unless diluted with water
Energy drink	May provide a temporary increase in energy, but does not replenish water; may have side effects such as headaches, abnormally fast heartbeat, nausea, and jitteriness
Chocolate milk	Helps build and repair muscles with carbohydrates, proteins, and whey protein; also contains the protein *casein*, which helps reduce muscle breakdown; can be high in sugar and does not work for people who have lactose sensitivities or allergies

Figure 10.15 Each type of fluid has different advantages and disadvantages to keeping you hydrated. ***What form of fluid loss is common with physical activity?***

Use Caution in Extreme Conditions

Physical activity can occur in many different settings. Some settings are prone to outdoor conditions and have certain risks. Getting physical activity in extreme conditions such as high heat and humidity, very cold temperatures, and high altitudes requires extra precautions.

Heat and Humidity

Being active in high heat and humidity can lead to hot weather emergencies unless you are careful. As much as possible, try to avoid being active outside when it is hot and humid. In high heat, your body sweats more, which can more easily lead to dehydration.

Spending too much time in hot weather can lead to **heat cramps** (painful muscle cramps), heat exhaustion, and heatstroke. **Heat exhaustion** is a health condition characterized by nausea, dizziness, weakness, headache, weak pulse, disorientation, and fainting. **Heatstroke** is an emergency that can lead to shock, coma, and even death. You will learn skills for responding to these conditions in Chapter 16.

To avoid these conditions and stay safe while being active in hot weather, use the following strategies:

- Drink at least 8 ounces of fluid—preferably water—every 20 minutes while you are active.
- Drink more water after physical activity to help your body replenish the fluid it lost.
- Wear light-colored and lightweight clothing.
- Use misting sprays to keep cool.
- Try to be active with someone else and be aware of the signs and symptoms of heat-related conditions, including confusion, dizziness, fainting, headache, nausea, and weakness. If you experience any of these symptoms, immediately tell your coach or someone who is with you.

heat cramps painful muscle spasms caused by overheating of the body

heat exhaustion health condition caused by overheating of the body; characterized by nausea, dizziness, weakness, headache, weak pulse, disorientation, and fainting

heatstroke medical emergency caused by overheating of the body; can lead to shock, coma, and even death

Cold Weather

Exercising in very cold weather can also be dangerous. Continuous exposure to very cold weather can lead to **frostbite**, in which the skin and the body tissues beneath it freeze. If untreated, frostbite can lead

frostbite condition in which the skin and the body tissues beneath it freeze

hypothermia medical emergency in which body temperature is too low; can lead to shock, coma, and death

to the death of tissue, infection, and the loss of limbs. Cold weather can also lead to **hypothermia**, an emergency characterized by very low body temperature. Symptoms include uncontrollable shivering, slurred speech, loss of coordination, abnormal or slow breathing, extreme fatigue, and confusion or memory issues. Skills for treating these conditions are discussed in Chapter 16.

Strategies for staying safe during very cold temperatures include the following:

- Check the temperature—including the wind chill factor—carefully before you go outside.
- Dress warmly with several layers of clothing.
- Make sure to protect your head, hands, feet, and ears, which are especially vulnerable to frostbite.
- Drink plenty of fluids, just like you would when being active in hot weather.
- Know the signs and symptoms of frostbite and hypothermia, including numbness, loss of feeling or a stinging sensation, intense shivering, slurred speech, and loss of coordination.
- Try to be active with someone else and be aware of the signs and symptoms of conditions related to extreme cold. If you experience symptoms, immediately tell your coach or someone who is with you.

Health in the Media

Choosing Fitness Products

Fitness products are equipment, supplements, or other objects companies claim will help people get physical activity and increase fitness. For example, some companies advertise fitness products for helping people burn calories, increase strength, or change body shape in some way. These advertisements may not be entirely truthful. Before you buy a new fitness product, such as special shoes, carefully evaluate the evidence showing the product's effectiveness and safety.

One study by researchers at the University of Oxford examined advertisements for a variety of different fitness products, including sports drinks, supplements, footwear, clothing, and fitness devices. Each advertisement claimed the advertised product would enhance performance in some way. Researchers, however, found no evidence that any advertised product improved strength, endurance, or speed or reduced muscle tiredness. In fact, many products had never been objectively evaluated.

This study shows that, if a new fitness product sounds too good to be true, it probably is. To learn more about a fitness product, find information about the product from an objective source. Search for any studies evaluating the effectiveness of the product. Doing your research before spending money and time will help you increase fitness in more effective ways.

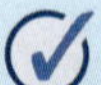

Practice Your Skills

Access Information

Search online or in newspapers and magazines for a fitness product that interests you. This fitness product should claim to improve physical activity or fitness in some way. Look at advertisements for this fitness product and record the information provided in the advertisement. Then check whether scientific evidence supports this information. Using reliable resources, search for studies that prove the information in the advertisement. Has the fitness product ever been objectively evaluated? Have studies confirmed its effectiveness? Does using the fitness product have any risks? After checking the information in the advertisement against the evidence, create a short video in which you review the fitness product and explain whether studies show it is effective.

High Altitudes

Another extreme condition is *high altitudes*, or areas that are high above sea level. Areas of high altitude have lower levels of oxygen in the air, which means you have to breathe faster and more deeply to take in enough oxygen. This can make engaging in physical activity more difficult. High altitude can result in a health condition called *altitude sickness*, or "mountain sickness." Symptoms include dizziness, headache, muscle aches, and nausea.

If you engage in any physical activity at high altitude, take precautions. Ideally, try not to engage in physical activity when you first arrive in an area of high altitude. Give your body a chance to adjust to the change in oxygen level. When you do get physical activity, reduce the time and intensity at first. If you experience altitude sickness, go back down to a lower elevation and seek medical attention, if necessary.

Take Care of Your Back

After colds and the flu, back pain is the third most common reason people see their healthcare providers. Although pain can occur in any part of the back, the most common location for injury is the lower back, which supports most body weight. Many physical activities, especially if they are done improperly, can lead to back injuries. Doing activities like lifting with proper form is important for protecting your back (**Figure 10.16**).

One of the best ways to reduce your risk of back pain is to engage in physical activity regularly. Physical activity reduces the likelihood of back pain by improving your posture, strengthening your back, and improving your flexibility. Doing sit-ups, which strengthen your abdominal muscles, also helps reduce back pain. Strong abdominal muscles strengthen your body's core and give your back more support.

Most back pain goes away on its own over time. If you experience severe back pain that does not improve, or that results from a fall or other injury, talk to a school nurse or doctor.

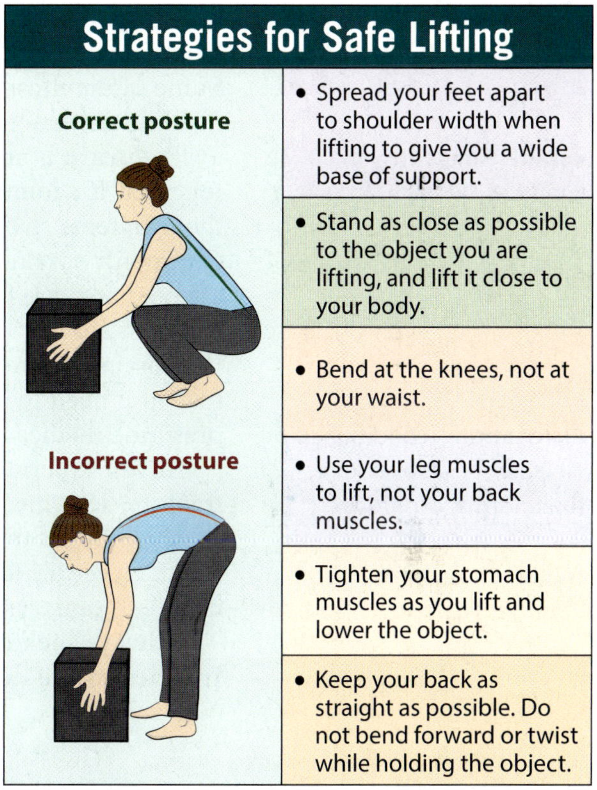

Strategies for Safe Lifting

Correct posture

Incorrect posture

- Spread your feet apart to shoulder width when lifting to give you a wide base of support.
- Stand as close as possible to the object you are lifting, and lift it close to your body.
- Bend at the knees, not at your waist.
- Use your leg muscles to lift, not your back muscles.
- Tighten your stomach muscles as you lift and lower the object.
- Keep your back as straight as possible. Do not bend forward or twist while holding the object.

Lemurik/Shutterstock.com

Figure 10.16 If an object is too heavy or awkward to lift or carry safely by yourself, ask someone for help.

Understand the Female Athlete Triad

Some females who play sports or get intense physical activity are at risk for a set of health conditions called the **female athlete triad**. The female athlete triad is a combination of three conditions:

- *Disordered eating*, which can include avoiding certain foods, eating too few calories, or eliminating consumed calories in an unhealthy way (such as by vomiting or getting excessive physical activity). Disordered eating can develop into eating disorders, such as anorexia nervosa and bulimia nervosa.

female athlete triad
three health conditions related to intense physical activity in females; disordered eating, amenorrhea, and osteoporosis

amenorrhea abnormal absence of menstrual period

- **Amenorrhea** (abnormal absence of menstrual period), which is a sign that the body does not have sufficient fat tissue to function normally. Eating too little or getting too much physical activity can cause amenorrhea.
- *Osteoporosis* (condition of weak bones), which can lead to stress fractures. Getting too little calcium and vitamin D can lead to this condition, which can have a permanent effect on bone strength for the rest of your life.

A female athlete can have one, two, or all three conditions in the triad. If you or someone you know is experiencing any of these conditions, talk to an adult you trust. Each condition can lead to serious, even life-threatening health consequences, so seeking help is very important.

Treat Injuries

Despite precautions, physical activities can sometimes cause injury. Knowing how to treat these injuries is an important part of fitness safety. Some of the most common injuries related to physical activities are sprains, dislocations, fractures, and concussions.

sprain injury to a ligament

A **sprain** is an injury to tissues called *ligaments* that hold joints together. If a joint moves suddenly beyond its normal range of motion, the ligaments stretch and tear. The ankle, knee, and wrist are the most commonly sprained parts of the body. Swelling and pain around the affected area are familiar signs of a sprain.

First aid for a sprain follows the R.I.C.E. treatment (**Figure 10.17**). If a sprain does not improve after two to three days, see a doctor. You may also need to see a doctor if swelling or pain worsens. The doctor may prescribe medication to help reduce the pain and swelling.

dislocation condition in which bones move out of their normal positions

fracture break in a bone

If you experience a more serious injury, such as a dislocation or fracture, seek medical treatment right away. A **dislocation** is a condition in which bones move out of their normal positions. A **fracture** is a broken bone. Never try to force a bone back into place. This can seriously damage muscles, joints, and nerves.

Always seek medical treatment right away for head injuries. Injuries to the head can result in *traumatic brain injuries (TBIs)*.

Figure 10.17 When following the R.I.C.E. treatment, do all four items at the same time. ***A sprain is an injury to which tissues?***

The R.I.C.E. Treatment

Rest	Limit movement of the limb to allow recovery and healing.
Immobilize	Wrap the injury with an elastic bandage to prevent or reduce swelling.
Cold	Cover the injury with a cold compress for 15 minutes several times a day for two to three days.
Elevate	Raise the injury above the heart to control swelling.

A **concussion** is a type of brain injury that results from a blow or jolt to the head or upper body (**Figure 10.18**). Contact sports injuries, such as those from football, soccer, wrestling, or hockey, can result in concussions. Concussions lead to disorientation, confusion, nausea, weakness, memory loss, or unconsciousness. Concussions are usually temporary, but they can lead to serious permanent complications.

concussion brain injury that results from a blow or jolt to the head or upper body

If you do experience an injury that requires medical treatment, see a doctor. Before engaging in physical activity, you might also want to see a doctor if you have an ongoing health condition, such as arthritis, diabetes mellitus, or high blood pressure. Be sure to follow your doctor's instructions. These instructions could include taking medications, performing recommended exercises and stretches, or receiving physical therapy. Be sure to follow the doctor's recommendations regarding amount of time to refrain from certain physical activities. Returning to the activity that led to your injury too soon increases your risk of re-injury.

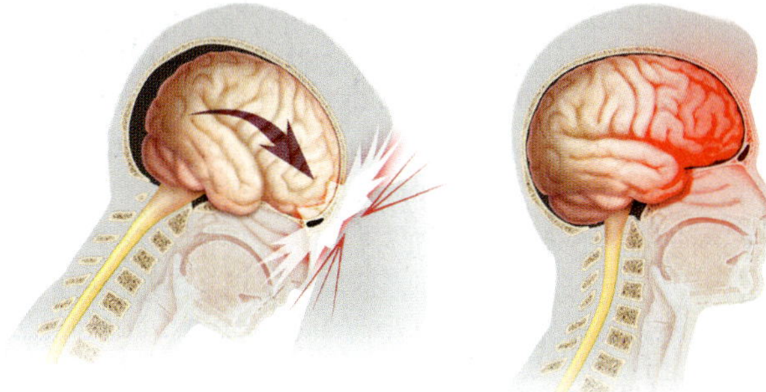

Figure 10.18 The force of impact from a severe blow or jolt to the head causes the brain to slide back and forth in the skull. ***What type of injury is a concussion?***

Lesson 10.3 Review

Know and Understand

1. Give one example of sportsmanship.
2. Why is it important to start slowly when beginning a new physical activity?
3. Why is it important to consume fluids before, during, and after physical activity?
4. What extreme conditions are common in your community? Create a public service announcement (PSA) with tips to help teens stay safe getting physical activity in your community.
5. What are the steps of treating a sprain?

Think Critically

6. What is an example of a physical activity that requires certain equipment? List the equipment required and describe its purpose.
7. Choose one physical activity and identify a warm-up and cooldown you could do before and after the activity. Explain why you chose each warm-up and cooldown.
8. Proper form can vary depending on the type of physical activity. Choose one physical activity you have done and research proper form for doing it. Share this information with the class and explain how the proper form ensures safety.
9. With a partner, research a story about someone who has experienced the female athlete triad. What were the signs and symptoms of the conditions the person experienced? What steps did the person take to resolve the conditions? Turn your findings into a fact sheet with steps female athletes can take to avoid these conditions.

REAL WORLD Health Skills

Set Goals Staying hydrated is important whether you are engaging in physical activity or not. As you learned in Chapter 8, you should drink 11½–15½ cups of fluids each day. Set a SMART goal for how much water you will consume each day and include strategies that will make this possible. Make a chart and record how much water you drink daily.

Chapter 10

Review and Assessment

Chapter Summary

Physical activity is any action in which the body uses energy. Exercise is planned, structured physical activity, which has the purpose of increasing physical fitness. Getting regular physical activity has many physical health benefits, including lower risk of certain diseases, healthy weight, strong bones and muscles, and better sleep. Physical activity also has benefits for mental, emotional, and social health.

Physical fitness refers to the body's ability to respond to the physical demands placed on it. Health-related fitness is the type of physical fitness you need to perform daily activities with ease and energy, while skill-related fitness is the kind of fitness you need to perform successfully in a particular sport or leisure activity.

Most people do not get enough physical activity, but rather spend much of their day engaging in sedentary behaviors. The *Physical Activity Guidelines for Americans* helps guide people in getting enough physical activity.

You can incorporate physical activities into your daily life by finding activities that do not require too much time or money and by setting aside time each week to engage in physical activity. Having the support of friends and family members can also help you be more physically active.

The acronym *FITT* stands for frequency, intensity, time, and type and provides a formula for varying physical activity to improve fitness. Manipulating and varying these factors will help you gradually, safely, and effectively improve your fitness. Practicing muscle-strengthening activities improves muscle strength and endurance, and paying attention to flexibility can help you avoid injury during physical activity.

Strategies for staying safe during physical activity include conducting yourself respectfully, using equipment properly, pacing yourself, staying hydrated, using caution in extreme conditions, and treating injuries.

Improving fitness is a gradual process that requires steadily increasing your physical activity over time. Always start slowly when you try a new physical activity. Doing a warm-up before engaging in your chosen physical activity gets blood flowing to your muscles, and a cooldown helps your heart rate return to a normal, lower level after physical activity.

Despite precautions, physical activities can sometimes cause injury. Knowing how to treat these injuries is an important part of fitness safety. Some of the most common injuries related to physical activities are sprains, dislocations, fractures, and concussions.

Vocabulary Activity

With a partner, make flash cards of the chapter terms. On the front of the card, write the term. On the back, write the phonetic spelling as written in a dictionary. Practice reading aloud the terms, clarifying each other's pronunciations where needed.

aerobic	*endurance*	*intensity*
agility	*exercise*	*maximum heart rate*
amenorrhea	*female athlete triad*	Physical Activity Guidelines for Americans
anaerobic	*flexibility*	*physical activity*
cardiorespiratory fitness	*fracture*	*physical fitness*
concussion	*frostbite*	*sedentary behaviors*
cooldown	*health-related fitness*	*skill-related fitness*
cross training	*heat cramps*	*sprain*
dehydration	*heat exhaustion*	*target heart rate*
dislocation	*heatstroke*	*warm-up*
endorphins	*hypothermia*	

Review and Recall

Review the information in this chapter by answering the following questions.

1. How does physical activity benefit your bones and muscles?
2. All of the following are components of health-related fitness, *except*
   A. muscle strength.
   B. cardiorespiratory fitness.
   C. flexibility.
   D. coordination.
3. What is the difference between aerobic activities and anaerobic activities?
4. How is power different from muscle strength?
5. Which FITT factor refers to the amount of energy your body uses per minute during an activity?
   A. intensity
   B. frequency
   C. time
   D. type
6. What is maximum heart rate, and how is it calculated?
7. Why is it important to know the proper form before performing any type of muscle-strengthening activity?
8. What are the two components of a warm-up?
9. When engaging in physical activity, when is the best time to drink water?
   A. before engaging in physical activity
   B. during physical activity
   C. after engaging in physical activity
   D. All of the above.
10. List three conditions that can result from being active in high heat and humidity.
11. When being active in hot weather, how much fluid should you drink and how often?
12. Which body parts are especially important to protect when active outside in very cold temperatures?
13. What can people do to prevent back pain?
14. Which condition is *not* a member of the female athlete triad?
    A. back pain
    B. disordered eating
    C. amenorrhea
    D. osteoporosis

Standardized Test Prep

Math Practice

Review the table shown and then answer the questions that follow.

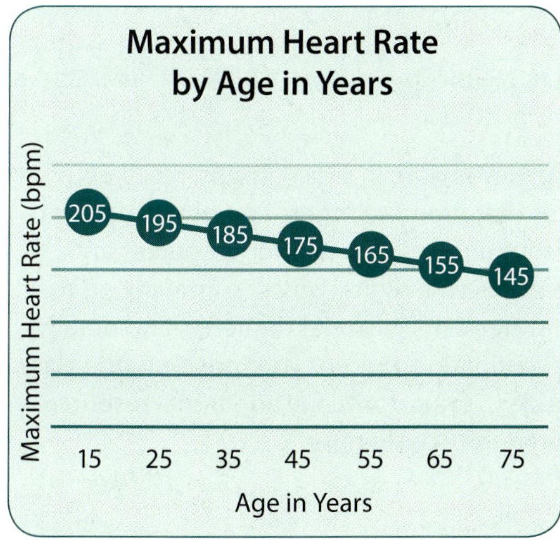

15. In general, maximum heart rate over the years
    A. increases.
    B. stays the same.
    C. decreases and then increases.
    D. decreases.
16. Calculate the maximum heart rate for a person who is 10 years old and a person who is 85 years old.
17. What is the target heart rate of a 15-year-old engaging in vigorous-intensity physical activity? Round to the nearest whole number.

Chapter 10 Skills Assessment

Critical Thinking Skills

Answer the following questions to assess your knowledge of what you learned in this chapter.

1. Think of one common physical, emotional, and social health challenge and discuss ways that physical activity and exercise might help solve each one.
2. Do you think it is possible for someone who gets physical activity quite often to still not be physically fit? Explain your answer.
3. Choose one component of skill-related fitness and research five exercises someone could do to improve that component. Do you think that improving one component of skill-related fitness can help improve another? Why or why not?
4. With a partner, discuss the possible effects of focusing on one component of fitness over the others. List five ways you could avoid doing so in your physical fitness plan.
5. How much is too much physical activity? What are some ways your body might tell you that it is time to stop or slow down physical activity? How can you tell if you are just getting tired or if it is time to stop an activity?
6. How much time each day do you spend engaging in sedentary behaviors? Do you think this is a healthy or unhealthy amount? What is one way you could incorporate physical activity into a part of your day when you would typically be engaging in sedentary behaviors?
7. Do you think physical education should be required in schools? If so, how many times per week should the class meet? Support your answer.
8. Make a list of obstacles to physical activity you have faced. With a partner, discuss how you might overcome those obstacles.
9. Choose a sport and then list five activities that could be used in cross training for that sport. What fitness components do these activities strengthen, and how are they used in the sport you selected?
10. How can technology help you achieve your fitness goals? Have you ever used an app or wearable technology to help you with your fitness routine? Describe your experiences.
11. Research a common sports injury. What is the course of treatment for this injury? How can this injury be prevented?
12. Research one piece of exercise equipment commonly found in a gym. What are some ways the equipment could be used improperly, and what are the possible results? Do you think there should be minimum age limits for certain exercise equipment? Explain your answer.

Health and Wellness Skills

Complete the following activities to assess your skills related to health and wellness.

13. **Analyze Influences.** Everyone has a different level of physical fitness. Place a picture of yourself on the middle of a page and draw a mind map showing all of the different influences that make you more or less likely to be physically fit. If there are influences that decrease your level of fitness, how can you manage them? What steps can you take to increase fitness, given your influences?
14. **Access Information.** In small groups, research resources that promote fitness and physical activity in your community. Choose three resources and create a physical or digital poster summarizing their mission statements, histories, benefits, and details about participation. Present your poster to the class, and as a class, brainstorm one additional resource your community could offer.

15. **Communicate with Others.** Choose one of the skill-related components of fitness and research five activities someone could do to improve this component. Create a presentation containing this information. For each activity, include an explanation of how it is done, an illustration of the activity, at least three steps for performing the activity safely and correctly, and an explanation of how the activity improves your chosen component of fitness. Make sure your explanations are clear and appropriate for your audience of fellow teens. Share your presentation with the class.
16. **Make Decisions.** Ky wants to join the track team, but feels he is too out of shape to be running with his peers. He feels he could meet new friends and get in shape, but his fear is really holding him back. Using the decision-making process, help Ky come up with a healthy decision for handling this situation.
17. **Set Goals.** Reference the influences and strategies you identified in question 13. Choose several steps for improvement you identified and then write a SMART goal that will allow you to increase your fitness levels.
18. **Practice Health-Enhancing Behaviors.** Physical activity and nutrition are key factors in maintaining a healthy weight. For each day of the week, list one or two activities you can do to get active. This could include going to sports practice, walking your dog, jogging with friends, walking to class, or playing Frisbee. After each day, make a note of whether you engaged in physical activity at all. What can you do to become more physically active in your daily life?
19. **Advocate for Health.** Imagine you have been asked to create a fully developed fitness app for an app developer. This is an app teens and adults will use to stay on track with their fitness programs. When presenting your app to the class, include its name, an explanation of how it works, a drawing of the icon used for the app, the app's cost, and an analysis of how the app would be effective in helping people track their fitness progress.

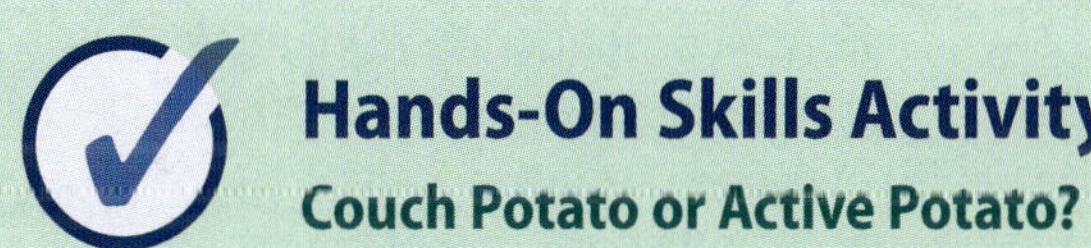

Hands-On Skills Activity

Couch Potato or Active Potato?

In this chapter, you learned about the benefits of physical activity for all three dimensions of health. You also learned about how the physical activity habits you develop now are likely to follow you into your future. In this activity, you will examine these health effects, as well as the influences and strategies that lead someone to be a "couch potato" (sedentary) or "active potato" (physically active).

Steps for This Activity

1. Form a small group to complete this project. In your group, collect all the notes you have from this chapter to guide you during this activity.
2. In your group, create a visual illustration or animation of one "couch potato" and one "active potato." These illustrations should be on the same poster, page, or screen so you can show the relationship between them.
3. Around each person, illustrate and label at least 10 physical, mental and emotional, and social effects of the person's level of activity. Be creative in your illustration, and if you can, show how the different effects are related.
4. **Analyze Influences.** Around each person, illustrate and label at least five influences that might lead someone to be a "couch potato" or "active potato." Identify whether factors are modifiable or nonmodifiable.
5. **Practice Health-Enhancing Behaviors.** To complete your illustration or animation, brainstorm and show five realistic strategies a "couch potato" could use to slowly turn into an "active potato." Share your illustration or animation with the class.

Unit 4 Avoiding Hazardous Substances

Big Ideas

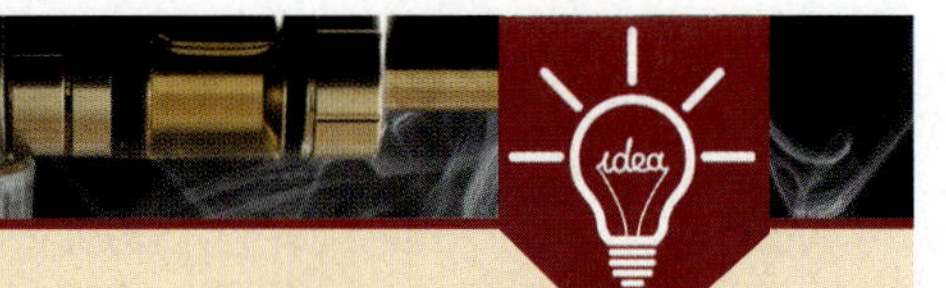

- Nicotine is an addictive substance that comes from the tobacco plant. Tobacco products (for example, cigarettes, vaping devices, and smokeless tobacco) contain nicotine in a natural or synthetic form. Nicotine harms multiple body systems and has consequences for mental, emotional, and social health.
- In addition to the effects of nicotine, tobacco use has other physical health consequences. Cigarette smoke and aerosol from vaping contain chemicals that can lead to respiratory conditions and cancer. Secondhand and thirdhand smoke and aerosol can harm the health of others.
- To avoid using tobacco, you can find alternate ways of managing stress, build healthy relationships, and use refusal skills. Nicotine addiction requires treatment.
- Alcohol is a depressant that reduces inhibition and coordination. Drinking alcohol can damage the brain and other body systems and lead to an alcohol use disorder and chronic health conditions.
- Alcohol use increases risk for dangerous behaviors and serious accidents and injuries. Drinking alcohol can also worsen mental health conditions, harm relationships, and lead to legal consequences.
- Many factors influence whether a person decides to drink alcohol. To refuse alcohol, people can promote mental health, resist pressure, and use refusal skills. People with an alcohol use disorder need professional treatment.
- Medications are used to treat diseases or relieve symptoms. They can be beneficial if taken correctly according to a doctor's instructions.
- Medication abuse occurs when someone intentionally misuses a medication. Medication abuse is dangerous and can lead to substance use disorders, physical health conditions, and consequences in other areas of health. Opioids are one example of a commonly abused medication.
- Using drugs can quickly lead to substance use disorders, death by overdose, and serious consequences for each area of health. Commonly abused drugs include marijuana, cocaine, methamphetamines, bath salts, hallucinogens, heroin, club drugs, and inhalants.
- Several influences affect a person's risk for abusing drugs and medications. Medication and drug abuse often lead to addiction, which requires professional treatment. Ways of preventing medication and drug abuse include caring for mental health, planning ahead, and using refusal skills.

bodu9/iStock/Getty Images Plus/Getty Images ▶

Health Management Plan Where Do You See Yourself?

Whether you are starting high school or preparing for graduation, you have probably thought about your future plans. These plans could include getting into your top choice of college, landing your dream job, or traveling to a different state or country. No matter the plan, your health can impact whether you reach your goals.

For example, imagine you want to hike the Appalachian Trail. To prepare, you begin walking more and improving your endurance to tackle the uneven terrain of the trail. Now, imagine trying to accomplish this goal if you develop an addiction to a hazardous substance like nicotine, alcohol, or drugs. Maybe your lungs are damaged, and you have shortness of breath from inhaling harmful chemicals. Completing the trail now seems impossible.

Open your health management plan. Create a new entry called "My Future Plans." Using the following steps, consider how hazardous substances can impact your health, goals, and future.

1. Create a list of at least 10 plans or goals you want to accomplish in your lifetime. These can be plans for activities in a few months or 20 years from now. An example is "I would like to travel across Europe for a month."
2. Now, imagine what would happen if you started using a substance—by smoking or vaping, drinking alcohol, abusing medications, or using drugs. As you read the information in this unit, take notes about how each of your plans could be affected.
3. Record your thoughts about how using a substance and developing an addiction could decrease your chances of reaching your future goals.
4. After reading this unit, create a list of decisions you can make and SMART goals you can set to advocate for your health. What skills or steps can you take to ensure you live a substance-free life and reach your future goals?

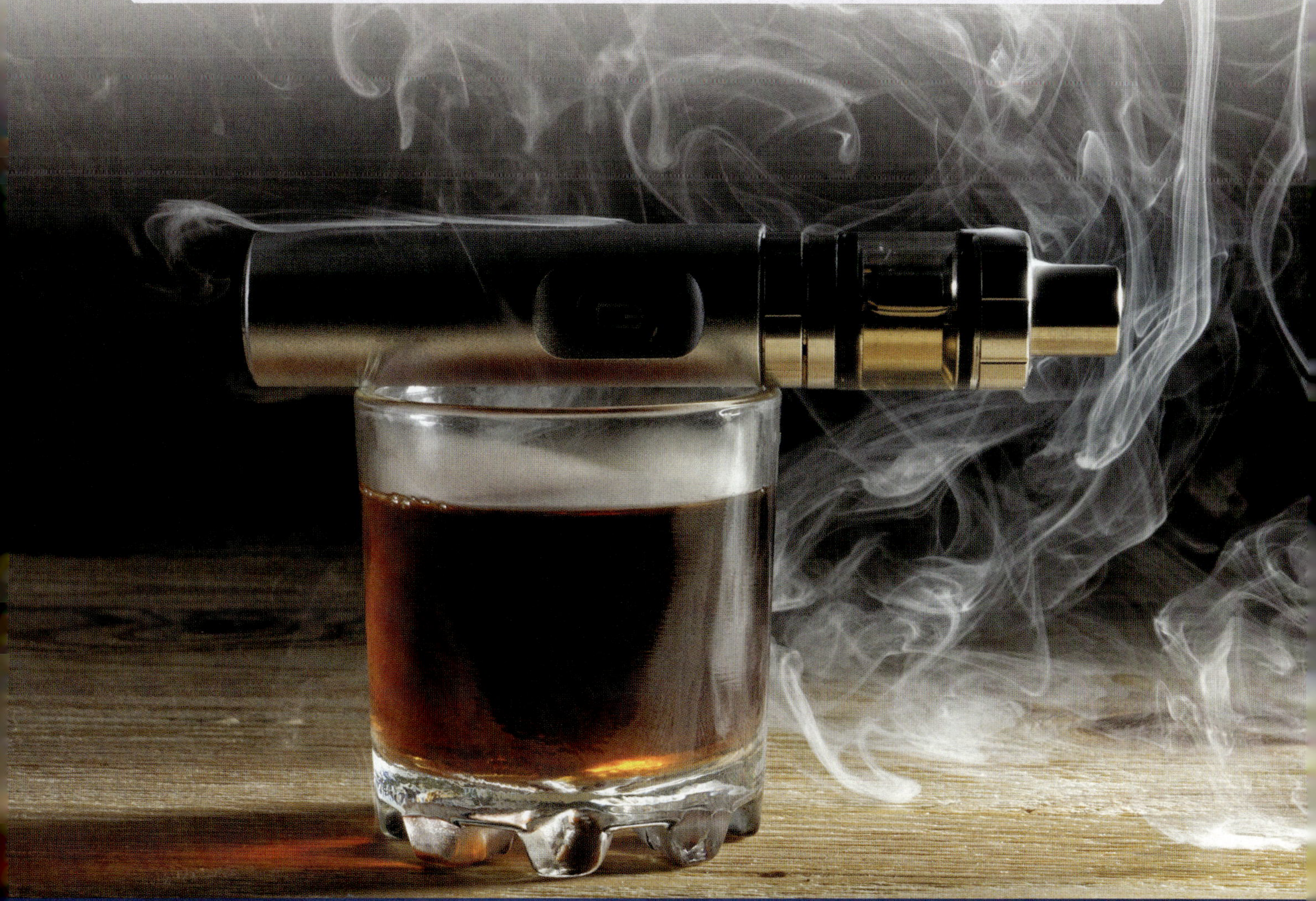

Chapter 11

Vaping and Tobacco

Lesson 11.1 Health Effects of Vaping and Tobacco

Lesson 11.2 Preventing and Treating Tobacco Use

Look for the skills icon throughout this chapter for opportunities to practice your health skills.

Check Your Health and Wellness Skills

In this chapter, you will learn skills for protecting your health from the harms of nicotine and tobacco. To understand the skills you currently use, take the following inventory of your behaviors. Indicate how well you think you use each skill. Use a scale of 1–5, *1* meaning you do not use the skill and *5* meaning you feel completely comfortable using it.

Skill	How Well Do You Use Each Skill?
I try to limit my time around people who are smoking cigarettes.	
When I spend time with someone who is smoking, I shower soon after.	
I feel comfortable saying *no* when my friends tell me I should try vaping.	
I manage stress well—by getting physical activity or listening to music, for example.	
I surround myself with people who respect my decisions and do not make fun of me.	
I know tobacco companies sponsor people to encourage vaping on social media.	
I recognize that depictions of people smoking in movies do not show tobacco's long-term health effects.	
I encourage my friends and family members who use tobacco to quit.	
I do not accept car rides from people who smoke or vape.	
If people do not respect my decision not to use tobacco, I leave the situation.	
	Total:

Add up your responses to each statement. The higher your score, the more comfortable you feel avoiding the harms of nicotine and tobacco. Which skill do you think is most important for you? Which skill is the most challenging for you? Which skill would you most like to improve? In this chapter, you will learn how to perform these skills better and more often.

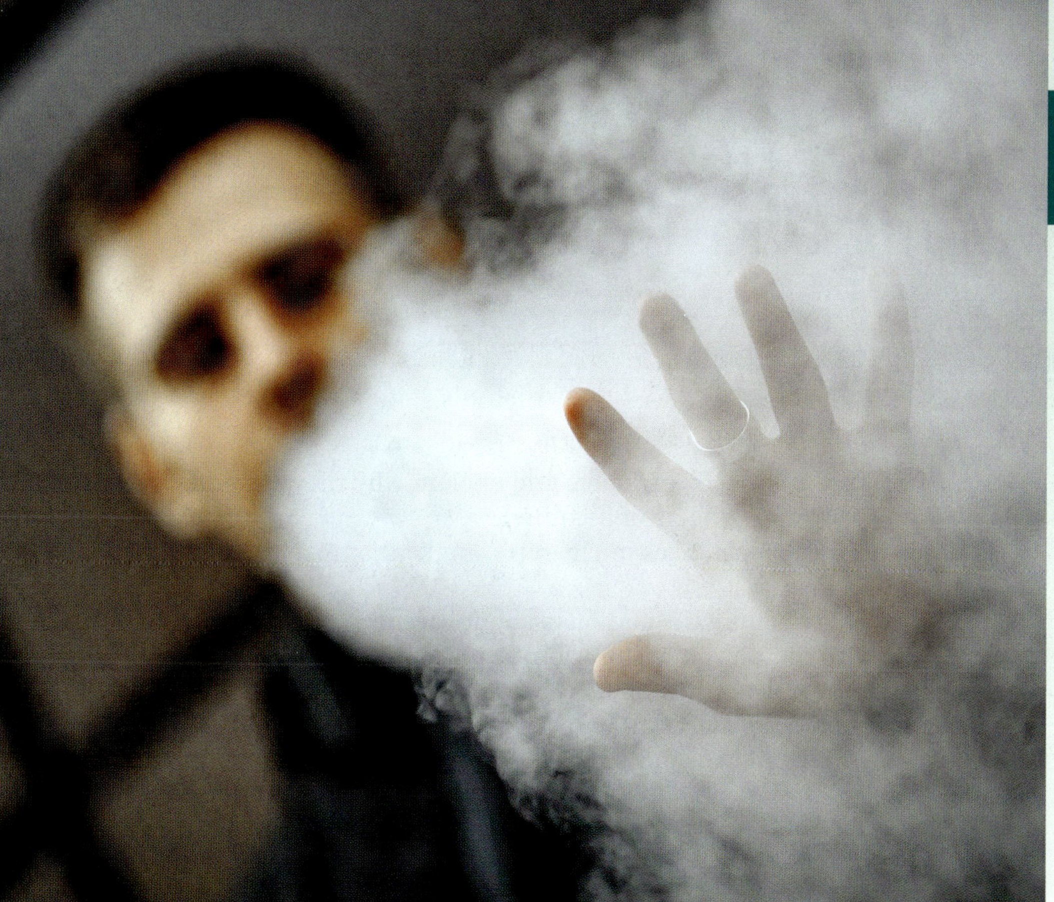

Aleksandr Yu/Shutterstock.com

Reading and Notetaking

As you listen to your teacher present the information in the chapter, record any comments or questions you may have about the content on a separate sheet of paper or electronically. Then, review your comments and questions with a partner. Try to answer each other's questions using information your teacher shared and content in the chapter. If you have any questions you cannot answer, discuss them with the rest of the class. Use reliable resources to pursue and verify the answers to your questions.

My Comments	My Questions

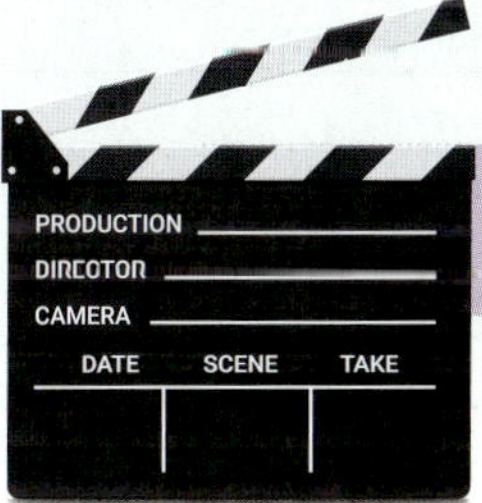

Setting the Scene

Vaping Is Just a Bad Idea

As a high school freshman, you are excited to meet new people and expand your social circle. You have enjoyed hanging out after school with some older students and getting invited to parties with them on the weekends. Some of these older students vape and keep asking you to try it. They say that vaping is not as bad for you as smoking regular cigarettes, but you really do not want to develop an addiction. You remember your uncle smoked cigarettes for years and had a very hard time stopping. Also, some of the older students who vape are always coughing. A few are now even smoking regular cigarettes in addition to vaping.

One Saturday night, you walk into a party where two of your new friends are vaping. One of them passes you a vape to try.

Thinking Critically

1. What would you do in this situation? Use the decision-making process you learned in Lesson 2.1 to think through the decision you face and the consequences of each alternative. What is the healthiest decision you can make in this situation?
2. If you choose not to vape, what are some strategies you can use to stick with your decision? How can you explain your decision to people who might pressure you?
3. Think about what you can do to advocate for the health of those who choose to vape and pressure others. If you were in this situation, what would you say to your new friends to have a conversation about the consequences of vaping?

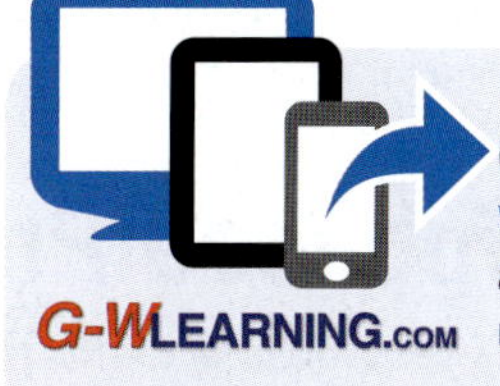

Click on the activity icon or visit www.g-wlearning.com/health/4095 to access online vocabulary activities using key terms from the chapter.

Lesson

11.1 Health Effects of Vaping and Tobacco

Essential Question?

How would deciding to use tobacco products today affect your lifelong health?

Key Terms

aerosol
asthma
carbon monoxide
carcinogens
chronic bronchitis
chronic obstructive pulmonary disease (COPD)
e-liquid
emphysema
leukoplakia
nicotine
popcorn lung
secondhand aerosol
secondhand smoke
smokeless tobacco
tar
thirdhand smoke
tobacco
vaping devices

Learning Outcomes

After studying this lesson, you will be able to

- identify different tobacco products and explain why they are addictive;
- assess the hazardous effects of nicotine;
- describe harmful substances in cigarette smoke that result in serious illnesses and diseases;
- distinguish between myths and facts about vaping;
- analyze the dangerous effects of vaping on the body's systems;
- summarize the risks of smokeless tobacco;
- identify mental, social, and legal consequences of using tobacco products; and
- analyze the impact of secondhand and thirdhand smoke and aerosol.

Warm-Up Activity

Tobacco Use and Death

Comprehend Concepts The table that follows shows the top 10 leading causes of death for adults in the United States, according to the Centers for Disease Control and Prevention (CDC). Before reading this lesson, review the table and consider how each leading cause of death might relate to smoking, vaping, and using smokeless tobacco. As you read, take notes about how tobacco and nicotine relate to each cause of death. If everyone made the decision not to use tobacco products, would the leading causes of death change? Why or why not?

Leading Causes of Death	
1	Cardiovascular disease
2	Cancer
3	Accidents (unintentional injuries)
4	Chronic lower respiratory diseases
5	Stroke
6	Alzheimer's disease
7	Diabetes
8	Influenza and pneumonia
9	Kidney disease
10	Suicide

Smoking is the leading cause of preventable death in the United States. Still, every day in the US, about 2,000 people younger than 18 smoke their first cigarette. Some people who smoke cigarettes start by vaping, which increases their risk for smoking by seven times. Using any tobacco product can lead to nicotine addiction and a lifetime of health issues. Friends and family members of people who smoke or vape can also develop health conditions from inhaling secondhand or thirdhand smoke and aerosol. In this lesson, you will learn about the health effects of tobacco products.

Tobacco Products

According to the Food and Drug Administration (FDA), a *tobacco product* is any product made or derived from tobacco and intended for human consumption.

This definition includes products made from tobacco or from *synthetic* (manmade) substances derived from tobacco. **Tobacco** is a plant with leaves that contain the chemical **nicotine**, a toxic substance that gives tobacco products their addictive quality. Historically, cigarettes were the most commonly used tobacco product among teens. Today, vaping is the most common form.

Cigarettes are an example of a combustible tobacco product. Combustible tobacco products are *smoked*, or burned and then inhaled. Other combustible tobacco products include rolled tobacco, cigars, cigarillos, pipes, blunts, hookah and water pipes, and bidis and kreteks (clove cigarettes). Smokeless tobacco products are noncombustible and include chewing tobacco, dipping tobacco, snuff, gutka or gutkha, and dissolvables.

Unlike other tobacco products, **vaping devices** heat tobacco or synthetic nicotine without burning it. Examples of these devices include e-cigarettes, vaporizers (also called *vapes* or *vape pens*), hookah pens, e-cigars, and e-pipes. Often called *electronic nicotine delivery systems (ENDS)*, these tobacco products are noncombustible and contain either tobacco or an **e-liquid** made of nicotine (or another drug) and other chemicals. Some people believe that vaping devices are safer, healthier, or less addictive than regular cigarettes. The reality is that all tobacco products can lead to addiction and serious health consequences (**Figure 11.1**).

tobacco plant with leaves that contain the chemical nicotine

nicotine toxic substance that gives tobacco products their addictive quality

vaping devices tobacco products that heat tobacco or synthetic nicotine without burning it, producing an aerosol

e-liquid substance made of nicotine (or another drug) and other chemicals; is heated during vaping

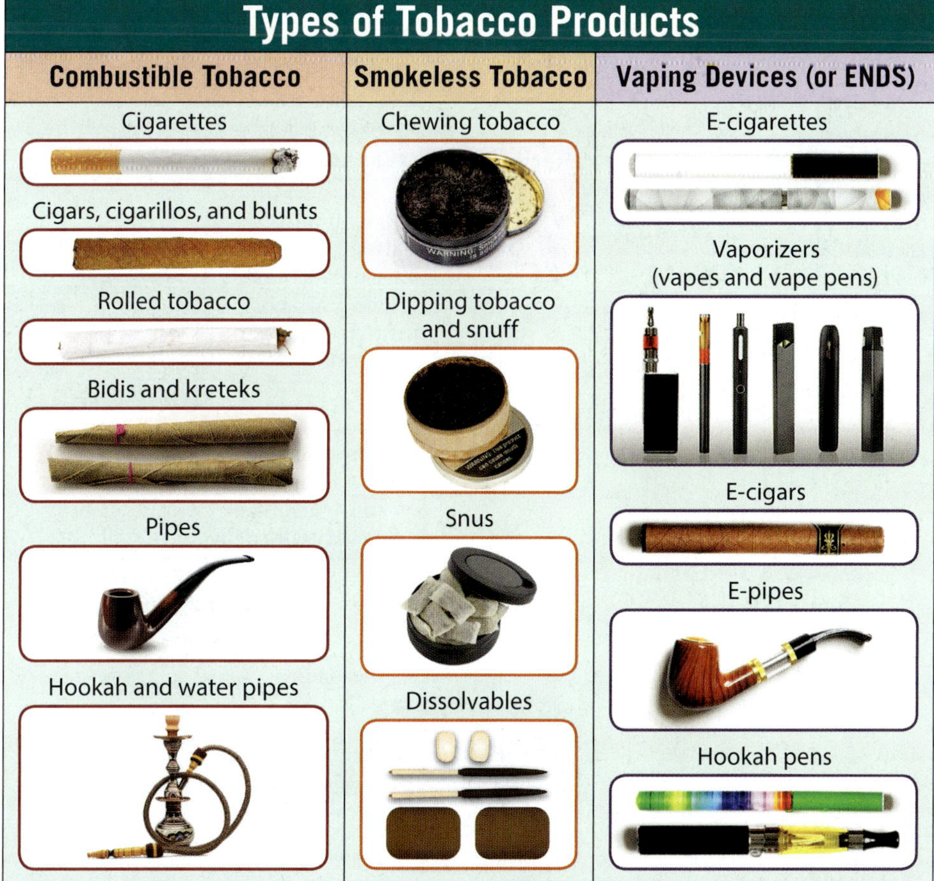

Combustible Tobacco, top to bottom: Voronina Svetlana/Shutterstock.com; domnitsky/Shutterstock.com; Andris Tkacenko/Shutterstock.com; Claudine Van Massenhove/Shutterstock.com; dimpank/Shutterstock.com; Gerisima/Shutterstock.com
Smokeless Tobacco, top to bottom: J.A. Dunbar/Shutterstock.com; Rob Hainer/Shutterstock.com; gopixgo/Shutterstock.com; Goodheart-Willcox Publisher
Vaping Devices: United States Food and Drug Administration

Figure 11.1 Tobacco products may be combustible, smokeless, or electronic, but all can have serious health consequences. ***Do all of these tobacco products contain nicotine?***

The Impact of Nicotine

One thing almost all tobacco products have in common is that they contain nicotine. Most combustible tobacco products contain nicotine from the leaves of the tobacco plant. E-liquids with nicotine contain a synthetic form. In fact, e-liquids in vapes sometimes contain *more* nicotine than cigarettes.

Nicotine is a highly addictive substance, which means it is difficult to stop using. In fact, in 2010, the US Surgeon General identified that nicotine was as addictive as cocaine and heroin. As a result, a person who uses nicotine is at serious risk for becoming addicted and developing a *substance use disorder*. As you learned in Chapter 7, the stages of substance use are experimentation, regular use, tolerance, dependence, and addiction. Once someone has an addiction to nicotine, that person will experience unpleasant withdrawal symptoms without the substance.

On top of being addictive, nicotine is toxic and extremely harmful to a person's health (**Figure 11.2**).

Cardiovascular System

The *cardiovascular system* includes the heart and blood transportation system in your body. When people use any tobacco product, nicotine enters their bloodstream. Nicotine's presence triggers the release of the hormone *adrenaline*.

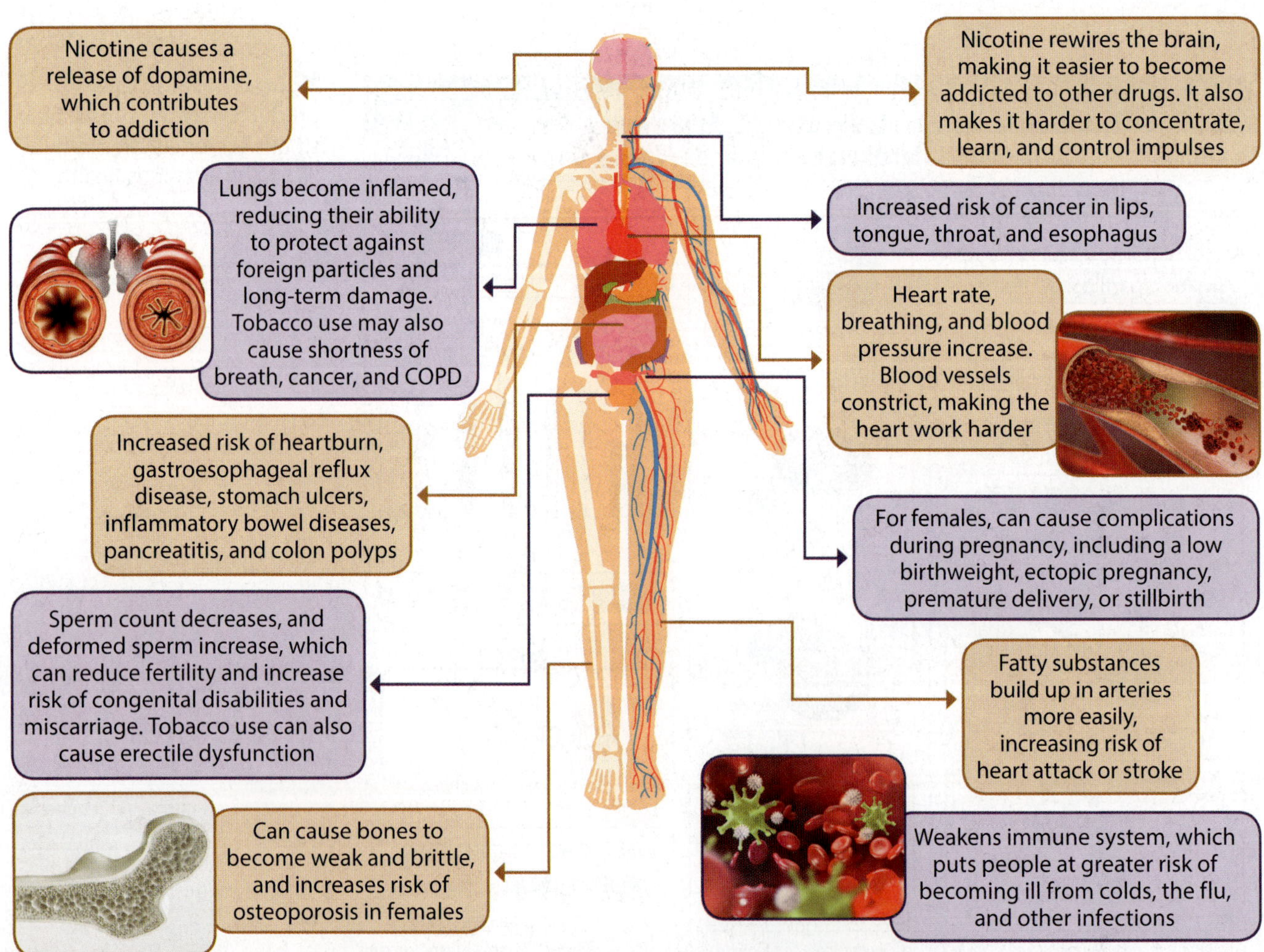

Left, top to bottom: Lightspring/Shutterstock.com; Crevis/Shutterstock.com; Middle: Lilanakani/Shutterstock.com; Right, top to bottom: Christoph Burgstedt/Shutterstock.com; Yurchanka Siarhei/Shutterstock.com

Figure 11.2 Nicotine is highly toxic to a person's body systems, and its harmful effects are not always reversible.

Adrenaline causes an increase in heart rate, breathing, and blood pressure. This makes the heart work harder to pump blood faster around the body.

Nicotine also causes the blood vessels to constrict. This means the heart works harder to pump blood through increasingly narrow vessels. Over time, this can lead to high blood pressure and cardiovascular disease. It also makes it more difficult for oxygen and nutrients to reach the skin, nails, hair, and mouth. As a result, people who use nicotine develop more wrinkles in their skin, brittle nails, thin hair, bad breath, and diseases of the mouth.

Gradually, nicotine leads to changes in the walls of blood vessels, causing fatty substances such as cholesterol to build up more easily in the arteries. This disrupts the flow of blood through the body as fatty deposits restrict blood transportation. Over time, this buildup can cause cardiovascular disease, which is the leading cause of death in the US.

Respiratory System

The *respiratory system's* primary function is to enable breathing. Nicotine causes inflammation of the lungs and also reduces the lungs' ability to protect against foreign particles, which can lead to long-term damage. As a result, people who use nicotine may experience shortness of breath. Nicotine use also increases risk for developing chronic obstructive pulmonary disease (COPD) and cancer, which are also leading causes of death in the US.

Nervous System

The *nervous system* consists of the brain, spinal cord, and nerves. Nicotine usually acts as a stimulant, increasing heart rate, blood pressure, and breathing. In large doses, it can also act as a sedative, reducing anger and anxiety.

Nicotine causes the release of a chemical called *dopamine* in the brain. Dopamine leads to a pleasurable sensation, just like when people use heroin or cocaine. People continue to use nicotine because they want this good feeling. Over time, the body develops a tolerance to nicotine, and people need higher levels of nicotine to enjoy the same effects. Using nicotine disrupts the brain's natural production of dopamine. As a result, people become dependent on nicotine to experience dopamine's positive sensations. This is why addiction happens so easily.

Teens are especially sensitive to the effects of nicotine because their brains are still developing. Using nicotine rewires the brain and makes it easier to develop an addiction to other drugs. Nicotine also makes it harder to concentrate, learn, and control impulses.

Digestive System

Nicotine has harmful effects on the digestive system. The body is not able to process food as easily. Common conditions such as heartburn, gastroesophageal reflux disease, and ulcers may develop due to nicotine use. Nicotine use also increases the risk of Crohn's disease (a form of inflammatory bowel disease), as well as pancreatitis and colon polyps.

Immune System

Using nicotine also leads to a weakened immune system. Your *immune system* includes organs, tissues, and cells that defend against disease-causing bacteria, parasites, and viruses. People who use nicotine have a greater risk of becoming ill from diseases like the common cold, flu, pneumonia, and meningitis.

Reproductive System

Nicotine affects the male and female reproductive systems. Males who use nicotine have a lower sperm count and more deformed sperm. This can reduce fertility and increase risks for congenital disabilities and miscarriage. Nicotine use can also damage blood vessels in the penis, leading to erectile dysfunction. In females, nicotine use can damage egg cells, reducing fertility. Pregnant people who use nicotine are more likely to experience complications, including a low-birthweight baby, ectopic pregnancy (a pregnancy that develops outside the uterus), premature delivery, or stillbirth.

Health Effects of Cigarettes

Did you know that, on average, long-term users of cigarettes die 13–15 years earlier than people who do not use cigarettes? According to the US Surgeon General, people who smoke have a higher risk for developing type 2 diabetes mellitus, colorectal and liver cancers, vision loss, tuberculosis, and arthritis. Smoking cigarettes also leads to stained teeth and hair and clothes that smell like smoke. In addition to nicotine, cigarette smoke contains toxic, cancer-causing chemicals and can lead to respiratory conditions.

Toxic Chemicals

carbon monoxide
poisonous gas that interferes with the ability of red blood cells to carry oxygen throughout the body

Cigarettes and cigarette smoke contain thousands of chemicals and toxic substances that harm the body (**Figure 11.3**). Nicotine is just one of these harmful substances. Cigarette smoke contains high levels of **carbon monoxide**, a poisonous gas. When inhaled, carbon monoxide interferes with the ability of red blood cells to carry oxygen.

Chemicals Found in Cigarette Smoke

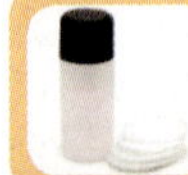
Acetone
- Found in nail polish remover

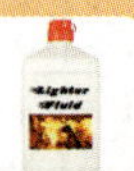

Butane
- Used in lighter fluid

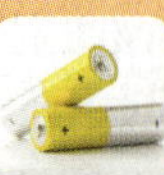
Lead
- Used in batteries

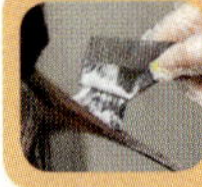
Acetic acid
- An ingredient in hair dye

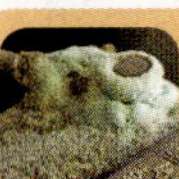
Cadmium
- Active component in battery acid

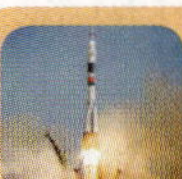
Methanol
- A main component in rocket fuel

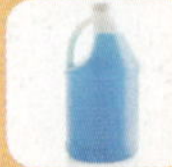
Ammonia
- A common household cleaner

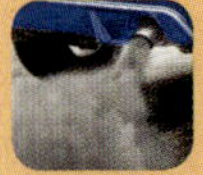
Carbon monoxide
- Released in car exhaust fumes

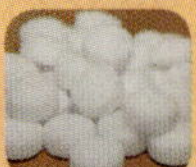
Naphthalene
- An ingredient in mothballs

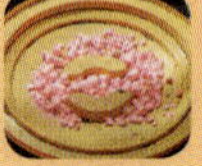
Arsenic
- Used in rat poison

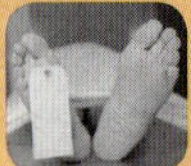
Formaldehyde
- Embalming fluid

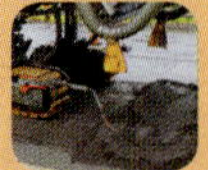
Tar
- Material for paving roads

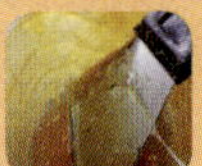
Benzene
- Found in rubber cement

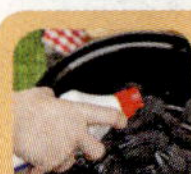
Hexamine
- Found in barbecue lighter fluid

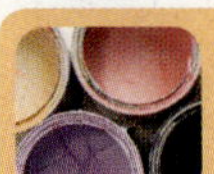
Toluene
- Used to manufacture paint

A–Z: Nadiia Ishchenko/Shutterstock.com; schankz/Shutterstock.com; gowithstock/Shutterstock.com; JR AK/Shutterstock.com; shinja jang/Shutterstock.com; Joe Belanger/Shutterstock.com; Charles Knowles/Shutterstock.com; Toa55/Shutterstock.com; John Gomez/Shutterstock.com; Arina P Habich/Shutterstock.com; Kenishirotie/Shutterstock.com; STEFANY LUNA DE LINZY/Shutterstock.com; Vera Larina/Shutterstock.com; ungvar/Shutterstock.com; Kyle Lee/Shutterstock.com

Figure 11.3 These are among the thousands of toxic chemicals and substances found in cigarettes and cigarette smoke. ***Would you otherwise ingest any of these chemicals?***

This reduces the amount of oxygen in the blood and the amount of oxygen that reaches the heart. As a result, after beginning to smoke, someone who once ran one lap around the track without becoming out of breath may be breathless after running half as far.

Cigarette smoke also contains more than 70 **carcinogens**, or cancer-causing substances. These increase a person's risk for developing cancers of the mouth, throat, esophagus, lung, and bladder. Cancerous cells grow rapidly and form a mass of cells, called a *tumor*. These tumors can spread to other parts of the body.

carcinogens cancer-causing substances

Due to the toxic chemicals in cigarette smoke, people who smoke have a higher risk for developing osteoporosis, ulcers, fertility issues, and gum disease. Cigarette use can interfere with eating by changing the shape of taste buds. When food does not taste as good, some people who smoke long-term lose their appetite and interest in eating.

Respiratory Conditions

Smoking damages the respiratory system and makes breathing more difficult. Burning tobacco produces a residue known as **tar**, which consists of small, thick, sticky particles. Over time, as smoke repeatedly passes through the bronchial tubes, tar builds up in the lungs. Tar disrupts the ability of fine, hair-like projections called *cilia* to effectively clear the lungs of foreign particles.

tar residue consisting of small, thick, sticky particles; builds up in the lungs as a result of smoking

Smoking-related damage to the lungs contributes to chronic (long-lasting) respiratory diseases and can trigger asthma attacks. **Chronic obstructive pulmonary disease (COPD)** is a group of conditions that make breathing more difficult (**Figure 11.4**). Most people who develop COPD have a combination of chronic bronchitis, emphysema, and asthma.

chronic obstructive pulmonary disease (COPD) group of conditions that make breathing more difficult; includes chronic bronchitis, emphysema, and asthma

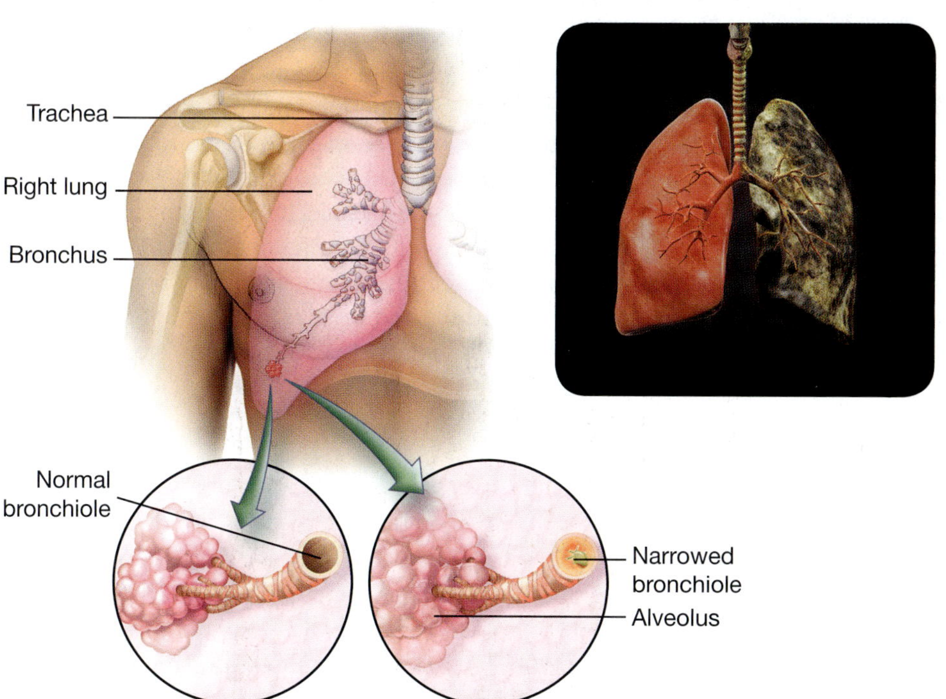

Left: © Body Scientific International; Right: iStock.com/Nerthuz

Figure 11.4 Chronic obstructive pulmonary disease (COPD) clogs the bronchioles and damages the lungs, making it more difficult to breathe. On the left is a normal, healthy lung. On the right is a smoker's lung, which shows the cumulative effects of COPD. ***What three lung diseases are grouped in COPD?***

chronic bronchitis condition in which the bronchial tubes become swollen and irritated, narrowing the pathway to the lungs

emphysema condition that causes the lungs to lose elasticity; permanently enlarges airways and destroys the alveoli in lung tissue

asthma chronic condition in which airways constrict and fill with mucus; blocks airflow to and from the lungs

Chronic bronchitis is an ongoing condition in which the bronchial tubes become swollen and irritated, narrowing the pathway to the lungs. This makes it increasingly difficult for the lungs to take in enough oxygen. People with bronchitis experience coughing spells and have difficulty catching their breath.

Emphysema is a disease that causes the lungs to lose elasticity, permanently enlarging the airways. Emphysema destroys the *alveoli*, or sacs of air, that make up lung tissue. The destruction of alveoli makes breathing difficult. As a result, a person has to breathe faster to get enough oxygen into the lungs and bloodstream.

Asthma is a chronic disease caused by blockages of airflow to and from the lungs. Inhaling cigarette smoke irritates the lining of the airways, which can cause an asthma attack. Because cigarette smoke damages the cilia, the lungs cannot eliminate unwanted particles. These particles stay in the airways and continue to trigger asthma attacks.

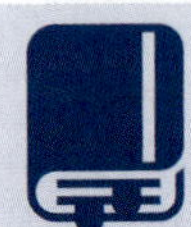

Case Study

"Just" a Vape

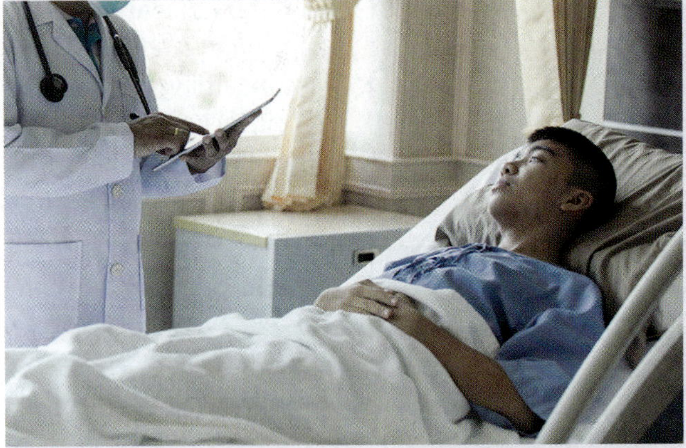

Silarock/Shutterstock.com

While Dwayne is in the hospital with pneumonia, his doctor tells him that a likely factor for his illness is his daily vaping habit. She warns him of the harmful effects on his respiratory system. Dwayne is stunned—he did not realize vaping was harmful to his health. He grew up knowing that cigarettes were dangerous; he has seen pictures of damaged smokers' lungs in his health classes. Vaping seemed safe, especially since he was using nicotine-free vape.

Ximena has loved playing basketball since she was a kid. Lately, however, she has coughing fits during practice and gets out of breath more quickly. Ximena does not vape, but she sits with her friends while they do. She knows that is probably what is causing her coughing fits. Ximena does not want to spend less time with her friends, but she worries about not making the varsity team next year if she does not get away from the aerosol.

Audrey is around people who use tobacco all the time. Her mom smokes cigarettes, and her older brother vapes. One day, a boy at school offers Audrey a vape. Audrey thinks to herself that one time cannot hurt. Audrey remembers her mother's stained yellow teeth and fingers and her brother's worsening asthma and smelly clothes. Audrey shakes her head, gives the vape back, and says, "No, thanks. I've seen what smoking has done to my family and I don't want to start."

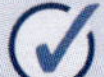

Practice Your Skills

Make Decisions

Consider the stories of Dwayne, Ximena, and Audrey. Are they making healthy decisions? What, if anything, can they do to be healthier? Rewrite each person's story to include a healthier decision and include any necessary knowledge or refusal skills each person would need to make these decisions. Share your new stories with a partner and discuss how a few small decisions can affect your health. Then, write a story about your own personal experience with tobacco. If you could go back in time in your story, what decisions would you make?

Health Effects of Vaping

Some people see vaping, or the use of vaping devices, as a harmless alternative to smoking cigarettes. While vaping is less harmful than cigarette smoking, it is *not* harmless (**Figure 11.5**). Many people believe that vaping produces a water vapor that people inhale. In reality, vaping produces an **aerosol**, or a suspension of fine particles or droplets in the air—like dust, smoke, deodorant spray, or bug spray.

aerosol suspension of fine particles or droplets in the air

Vaping introduces nicotine (or another drug) into a person's body and poses significant health risks. E-liquids with nicotine contain large amounts of nicotine. Even some e-liquids that claim to be nicotine-free contain nicotine. As you have learned, nicotine is a dangerous, addictive substance that harms the body's systems.

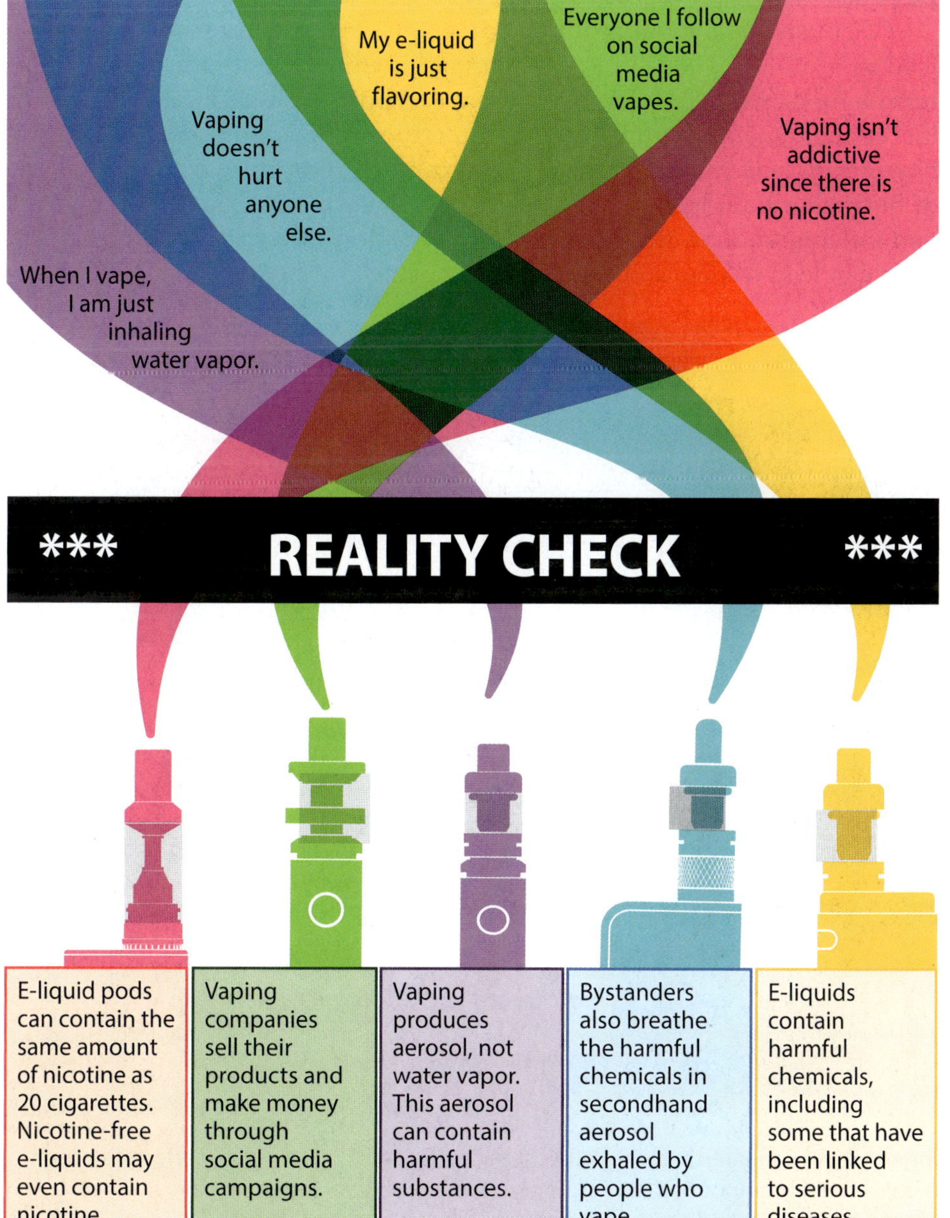

smartboy10/DigitalVision Vectors/Getty Images

Figure 11.5 The statements at the top show common misconceptions about vaping. Read each accompanying explanation to see why these ideas are incorrect. ***Did you previously believe that vaping was harmless?***

In addition to the dangers posed by nicotine, vaping also harms health in other ways. Vape battery explosions can cause serious injury and even death. Some people use vaping devices to consume other drugs like marijuana, which you will learn about in Chapter 13. Vaping any e-liquid can have serious health risks.

Most of the time, when people vape, they are consuming an e-liquid made of many chemicals. The vaping device heats the e-liquid into an aerosol that people inhale (**Figure 11.6**). When someone vapes, these chemicals enter the body and affect its organs and systems.

Scientists are still studying the long-term effects of inhaling the chemicals contained in aerosol. This research is difficult because companies that manufacture e-liquids are not required to list all the ingredients in the e-liquid. This means people who vape do not know what exactly they are inhaling into their lungs. Some people may claim that the chemical flavorings in e-liquids are *generally recognized as safe (GRAS)*. This means the FDA has approved that they are safe for ingestion. It does *not* mean the FDA has stated they are safe to inhale.

popcorn lung condition that damages the lungs' smallest airways; leads to coughing and shortness of breath

Scientists do know that inhaling the chemicals in aerosol can lead to respiratory conditions, including inflammation and long-term lung damage. As more people vape, reports of lung diseases are increasing. One rare lung disease related to vaping is **popcorn lung** or *bronchiolitis obliterans*. Diacetyl, a flavoring found in more than 75 percent of flavored e-liquids, causes this disease. Popcorn lung causes scarring and inflammation in the *bronchioles*, the smallest airways in the lungs. This can lead to persistent coughing, shortness of breath, and difficulty breathing.

Volatile organic compounds
Heavy metals, such as nickel, tin, and lead
Flavorings, including the chemical diacetyl
Nicotine
Carcinogens
Ultrafine particles

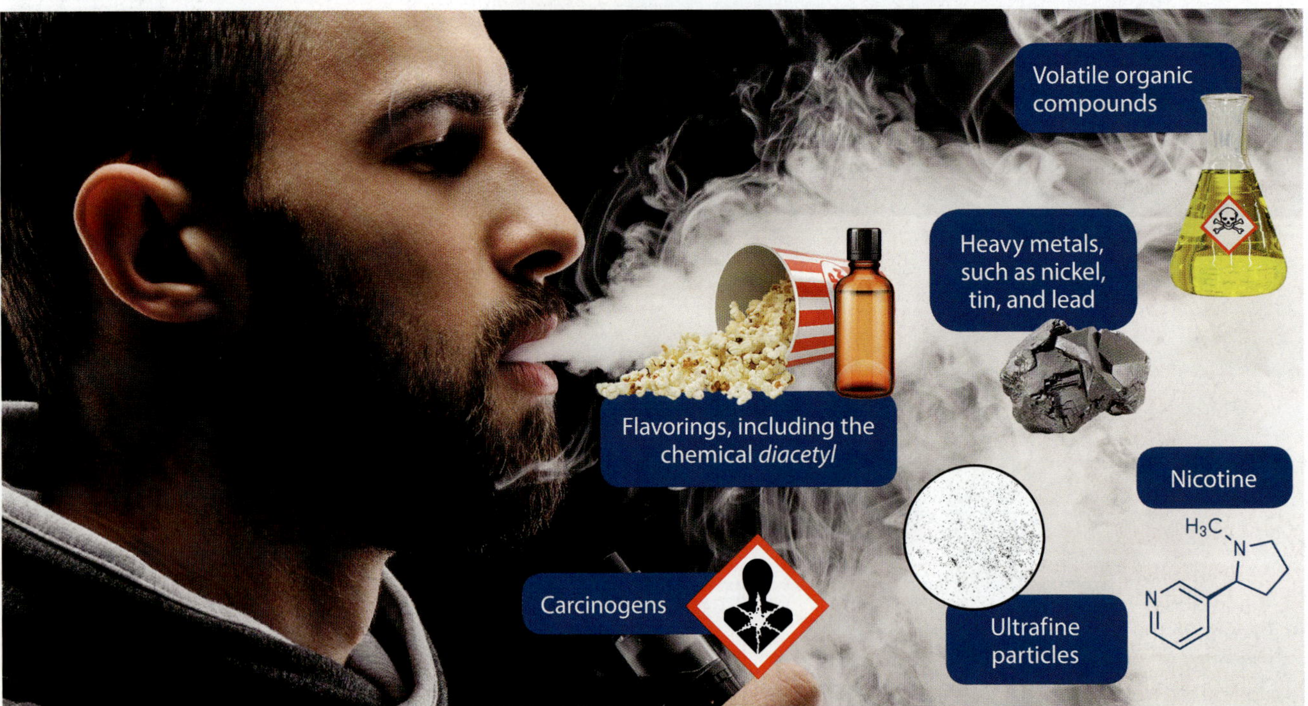

Person: Prostock-studio/Shutterstock.com; Top row, left to right: urfin/Shutterstock.com; Sensvector/Shutterstock.com; BrankoG/Shutterstock.com; mewaji/Shutterstock.com; Bottom row, left to right: ASAG Studio/Shutterstock.com; mexrix/Shutterstock.com; molekuul_be/Shutterstock.com

Figure 11.6 Aerosol created by vaping devices contains many harmful chemicals that are connected to serious health consequences. Chemicals include volatile organic compounds (VOCs), or pollutants that evaporate in the air; ultrafine particles that can be inhaled deep into people's lungs; and cancer-causing substances.

Health Effects of Smokeless Tobacco

Forms of **smokeless tobacco** include chewing tobacco, snuff, *snus* (a form of snuff), and dissolvable tobacco. Chewing tobacco involves placing wads, or *plugs*, of tobacco leaves between the cheeks and gums. Snuff is a finely cut or powdered tobacco that people inhale or place between the cheek and gums. Dissolvable tobacco comes in the form of flavored mouth drops or strips.

smokeless tobacco tobacco product that is chewed or snuffed rather than smoked

All forms of smokeless tobacco contain nicotine and carcinogens. The harmful effects of these substances are the same as if they were smoked. The presence of nicotine makes smokeless tobacco just as addictive as cigarettes. In fact, because people place smokeless tobacco directly into the mouth, people who use these products actually absorb even more nicotine than people who smoke (**Figure 11.7**).

Because using smokeless tobacco does not involve inhaling smoke, people who use these products are less likely to develop lung diseases than people who smoke. People who use smokeless tobacco do, however, increase their risk of developing other serious diseases. When using smokeless tobacco, people absorb nicotine through their mouth tissues. Nicotine stains the teeth and can lead to gum recession. Using smokeless tobacco can also lead to **leukoplakia**, a condition characterized by thickened, white, leathery spots inside the mouth. This condition can develop into oral cancer. Smokeless tobacco use leads to an increased risk of cardiovascular disease, respiratory irritation, gum disease, and tooth decay.

leukoplakia condition characterized by thickened, white, leathery spots inside the mouth; can develop into oral cancer

Mental, Social, and Legal Consequences

Using tobacco impacts not just a person's body, but also a person's mind and social relationships. As you know, the different dimensions of health are interconnected. Consequences in one area of health also affect other areas of health. The effects of tobacco use are long lasting and can shape your future in serious ways.

Smokeless Tobacco Bans in Baseball

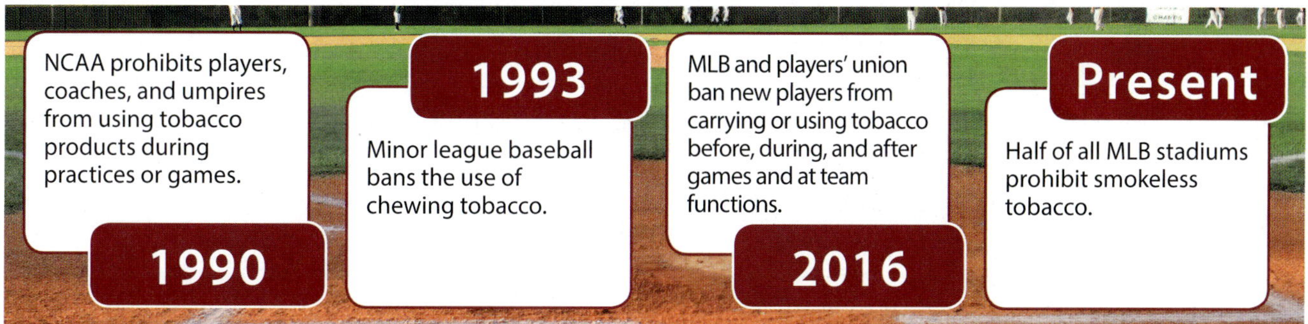

World in Hand/Shutterstock.com

Figure 11.7 Though chewing and dipping tobacco have long been associated with baseball, this trend has been on the decline for a few decades. Recognizing the dangers to players' health, various organizations and many players support the ban of smokeless tobacco. ***Do users of smokeless tobacco absorb more or less nicotine than people who smoke? How?***

Research in Action

Tobacco Use and Risky Behaviors

Did you know that engaging in some risky behaviors makes you more likely to try others as well? Risky behaviors are actions that can have negative health consequences. They include behaviors like smoking cigarettes, vaping, being physically violent, texting and driving, and engaging in high-risk sexual activity that can result in sexually transmitted infections (STIs) and unplanned pregnancies.

Many teens tell themselves that risky behaviors are not harmful if they are less risky compared to other behaviors. For example, some teens justify their decision to vape by saying that vaping is safer than smoking cigarettes. What teens do not realize is that vaping makes them much more likely to smoke cigarettes in the future. A 2017 study by researchers at the Centers for Disease Control and Prevention found that students in grades 7–12 who had ever tried vaping were *more than twice as likely* to start smoking.

Students who use tobacco products also have a greater risk of engaging in other risky behaviors. Researchers in one study compared the rates of risky behaviors among high school students who had or had never used tobacco products. Students who used tobacco products were more likely to engage in risky behaviors, including getting in a physical fight, texting and driving, and having more sexual partners. They were also more likely to use other health-harming substances, such as alcohol, marijuana, and illegal drugs.

Practice Your Skills

Practice Health-Enhancing Behaviors

Research shows that teens who vape or smoke have riskier health-related behaviors than those who do not. With a partner, discuss what factors you think explain this association. Why does making one risky choice lead to other risky choices? What barriers prevent some teens from making better health choices? With your partner, brainstorm ways teens can end a habit of making risky choices. What resources and support could teens use? What information can arm them to resist negative influences and make healthier choices? Create an infographic that illustrates the influences leading to a pattern of risky behavior and steps teens can take to interrupt the pattern.

Mental Consequences

Most teens believe they can smoke, vape, or chew tobacco occasionally or even regularly for a few years and then easily quit. The reality, however, is that addiction happens very quickly and makes it very difficult to stop using tobacco products (**Figure 11.8**).

Mental Consequences of Addiction

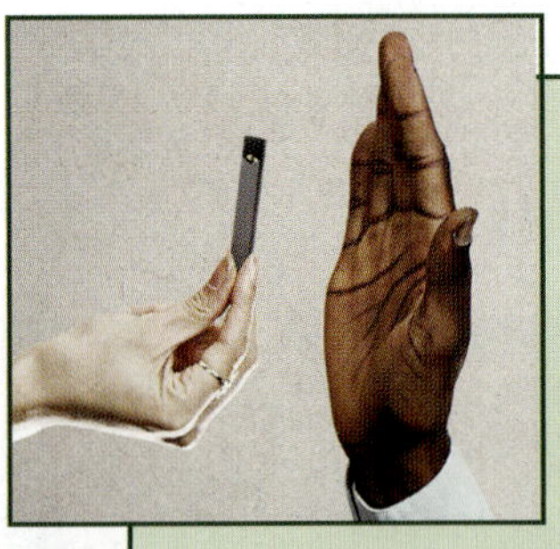

If they cannot smoke or vape, or if they are trying to quit, people may experience intense cravings, sadness, anxiety, or irritability.

pathdoc/Shutterstock.com; United States Food and Drug Administration

Figure 11.8 Even if people want to, the consequences to their mental health make it very hard to quit vaping, smoking, or chewing tobacco.

Using nicotine can rewire your brain so you are more likely to develop addictions to other drugs. Nicotine can also make it harder to concentrate, learn, and control impulses. People who use nicotine are more likely to engage in other risky behaviors, such as sexual activity and illegal drug use. Nicotine can also make mental health conditions and mental illnesses worse if people use nicotine to relieve symptoms instead of seeking treatment.

Social Consequences

Tobacco use can seriously harm a person's social relationships. An addiction to nicotine hurts not just the person with the addiction, but also everyone around that person. When people feel dependent on a substance such as nicotine, getting more of that substance can seem more important than anything else. As a result, teens may lie to their parents, guardians, or friends or steal money to buy cigarettes, smokeless tobacco, vaping devices, or e-liquid. Lying and theft can cause long-term trust issues in a relationship and the community. In addition, teens who use tobacco model this behavior for others, which can lead others to develop addictions too.

Because tobacco use harms people's health, people may withdraw from teens who use tobacco products. People who use tobacco products may have to leave a social situation to smoke or vape and feel left out.

Legal Consequences

Teens who use tobacco can experience serious legal consequences. In the US, all states prohibit people under the age of 21 from buying tobacco products. Some cities, such as Beverly Hills in California, have banned the sale of tobacco products altogether. Teens who try to buy tobacco products or ask someone else to buy them may have to pay fines or perform community services. Some states suspend driving privileges for teens who illegally buy or possess tobacco products.

Many schools have policies that prohibit use of cigarettes, smokeless tobacco, and vaping devices. Students who bring tobacco products to school or use them at school-sponsored events may face disciplinary actions and even suspension. Teens can also face legal consequences for using tobacco products in public places, including restaurants and workplaces.

Secondhand Smoke and Aerosol

People who use tobacco products are not the only ones at risk for negative health outcomes because of nicotine. Smoking and vaping both release substances into the air other people breathe. In the case of cigarette smoking, this substance is called **secondhand smoke**. People who regularly inhale secondhand smoke because they live or socialize with people who smoke have a greater risk of developing lung cancer or heart disease. Secondhand smoke is especially dangerous for fetuses, infants, and children (**Figure 11.9**).

secondhand smoke smoke that people inhale involuntarily when someone nearby is smoking

Secondhand Smoke During Pregnancy and Childhood

Fetuses exposed to secondhand smoke during pregnancy
- receive nicotine and carbon monoxide through the placenta, which reduces the amount of oxygen passed to the fetus
- experience increased risk of death, premature birth, or low birthweight

Babies and children exposed to secondhand smoke during pregnancy
- have an increased risk of sudden infant death syndrome (SIDS)
- commonly experience behavior-related issues, including attention deficit disorders, hyperactivity, and aggression

Children exposed to secondhand smoke during childhood
- experience more respiratory conditions such as pneumonia, bronchitis, and asthma attacks
- have higher rates of sore throats and ear infections
- are more likely to develop smoking habits of their own

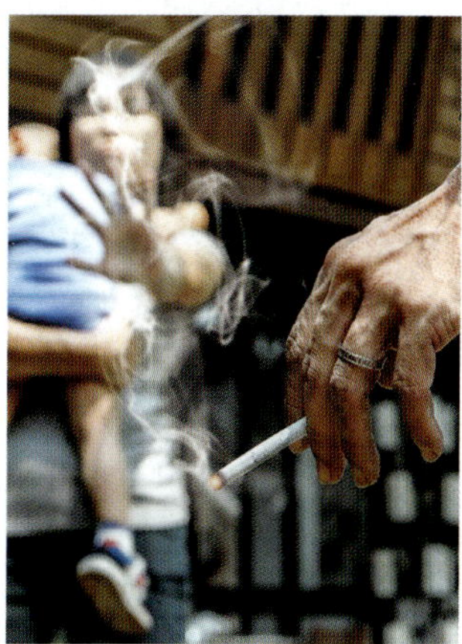

Anucha Naisuntorn/Shutterstock.com

Figure 11.9 Fetuses, infants, and children are especially vulnerable to secondhand smoke, throughout pregnancy and while they grow. Smoking also increases a pregnant person's risk of miscarriage. ***Is secondhand aerosol dangerous for fetuses, infants, and children too?***

Health Across the Life Span

Choose Your Future: Vaping and Tobacco

Right now, you may have a hard time seeing how small decisions impact your health. It is important to remember, however, that choices you make regarding your health have far-reaching impacts on your future. Starting with the box at the top of the flowchart, walk through hypothetical decisions you could make during your life. Certain lifestyles are associated with a higher risk for negative health consequences, while other lifestyles have a lower risk for those same consequences. Choices made at each step have impacts that ripple out toward your future.

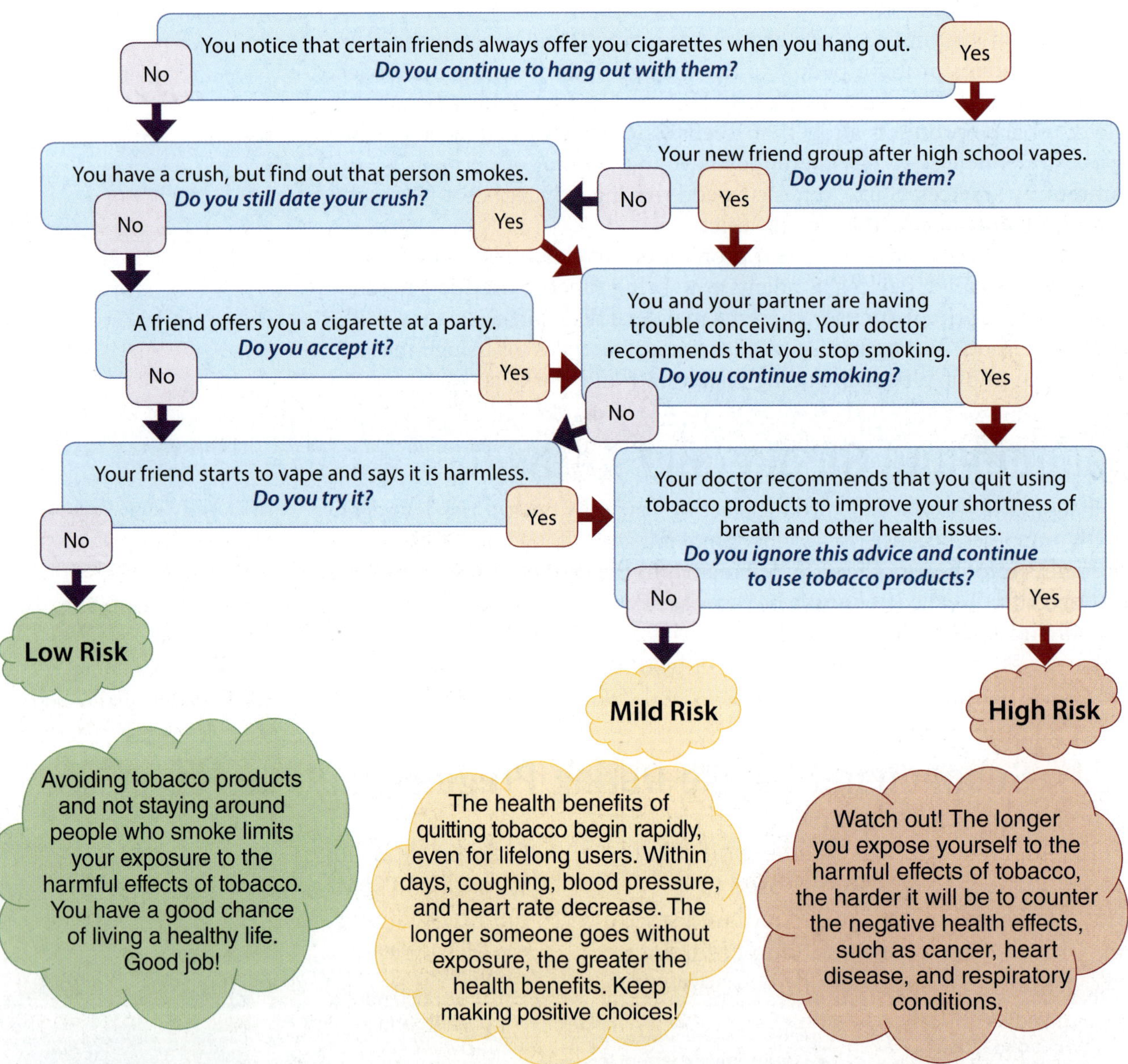

Practice Your Skills

Make Decisions

Answer the questions in the flowchart and determine your level of risk in the activity. Look at each decision and analyze why you chose the path that you did. What influenced your decision to make one choice over another?

For each scenario in the flowchart, write a short scene in which you decide to make the healthier decision. Use refusal skills and the facts you learned in this lesson to back up your decisions.

Vaping produces **secondhand aerosol**, which people nearby inhale. According to the US Surgeon General, secondhand aerosol from vaping can contain harmful chemicals such as nicotine, diacetyl, and heavy metals.

secondhand aerosol suspension of fine particles that people inhale involuntarily when someone nearby is vaping

Concerns about the dangerous effects of secondhand smoke have led a number of states to pass laws banning smoking in many public areas. These laws protect the health of customers and staff. Some states have enacted similar laws to protect people from secondhand aerosol.

If you share the air with people who are smoking or vaping, taking certain steps can reduce your risk of exposure to secondhand smoke and aerosol:

- Avoid spending time in places that allow smoking and vaping.
- Do not accept car rides from people who smoke or vape while driving.
- Ask that people smoke or vape only outdoors or in a particular room sealed off from the rest of a home or building.
- Increase air circulation in buildings where people smoke or vape by opening the windows to let in fresh air.
- Perhaps most importantly, encourage a friend or family member who smokes or vapes to stop and support the person's efforts toward quitting.

Thirdhand Smoke and Aerosol

Thirdhand smoke refers to the particles and gases left over after a cigarette is extinguished. Similarly, the particles and gases left over from a vaping device are called *thirdhand aerosol*. The particles in thirdhand smoke and aerosol land and remain on virtually any surface in the area where someone has smoked or vaped (**Figure 11.10**). Exposure to thirdhand smoke and aerosol can lead to serious diseases such as asthma and cancer. These chemicals can even become more dangerous over time.

thirdhand smoke particles and gases left over after someone smokes a cigarette; remains on surfaces nearby

Thirdhand Smoke and Aerosol

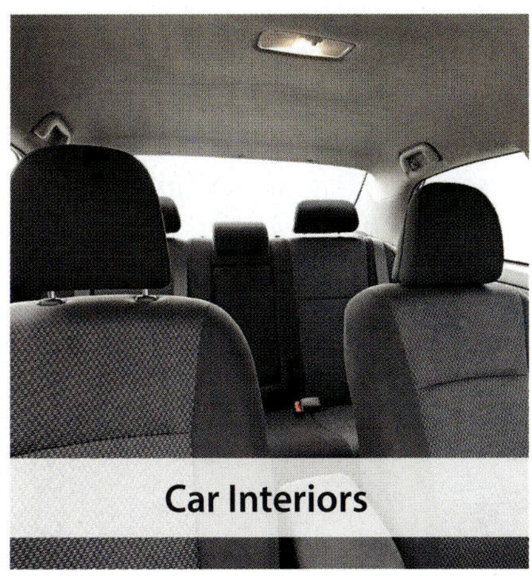

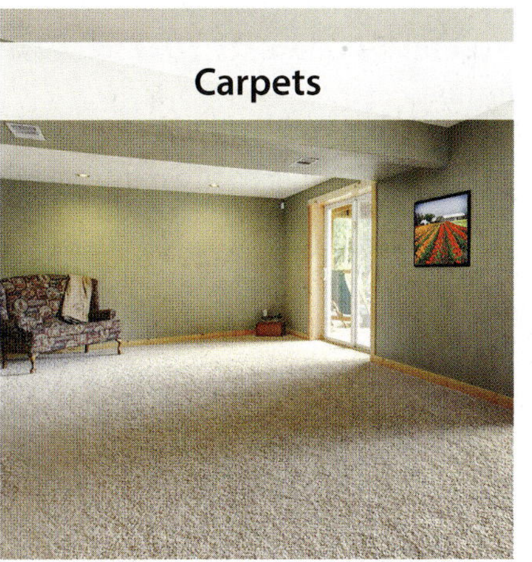

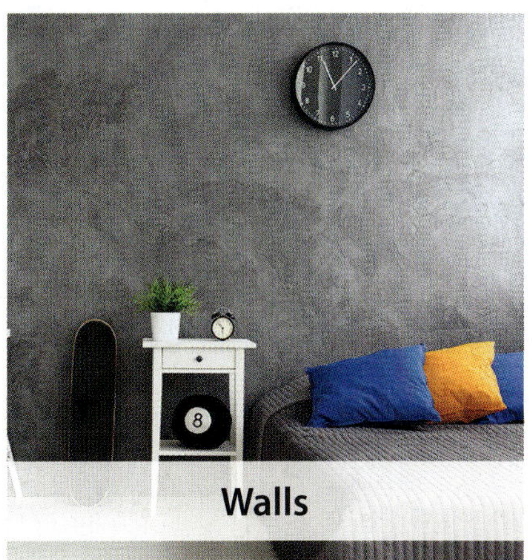

Left to right: Peter Gudella/Shutterstock.com; Artazum/Shutterstock.com; Photographee.eu/Shutterstock.com

Figure 11.10 The particles and gases left over from cigarettes and vaping devices remain on nearby surfaces and are difficult to clean away.

Eliminating thirdhand smoke and aerosol is extremely challenging. Common cleaning methods such as vacuuming, wiping down surfaces, and airing out rooms do not eliminate the residue. Particles remain behind, even after the smell fades. This means that people often are not aware of their exposure to thirdhand smoke and aerosol.

The best way to avoid thirdhand smoke and aerosol is not to allow someone to smoke or vape around you, including in your home or car. You can also protect yourself by showering after exposure to thirdhand smoke or aerosol and opening the windows in your car or home if someone is smoking or vaping. In addition, tell other people about the dangers of thirdhand smoke and aerosol. Many people who smoke or vape do not realize they are harming those around them.

Lesson 11.1 Review

Know and Understand

1. Explain the difference between combustible and noncombustible tobacco products.
2. How does nicotine use impact cardiovascular health, immediately and in the future?
3. Describe how nicotine use leads to addiction.
4. What respiratory conditions does smoking cigarettes cause? Choose one condition and describe it in your own words.
5. Which chemical in vaping aerosol can cause popcorn lung?
6. What kind of cancer is associated with using smokeless tobacco?
7. Describe the difference between secondhand and thirdhand smoke and aerosol.

Think Critically

8. Why do many teens think vaping is harmless?
9. Explain how using tobacco products negatively impacts mental health and social relationships.
10. How could the legal issues associated with using tobacco products affect your future?
11. How does tobacco use impact a person's community?

REAL WORLD Health Skills

Advocate for Health Talk to your parent or guardian about any relatives who have been affected by diseases associated with using tobacco. Use effective communication skills to start this conversation and ask questions to clarify information.

Then, using the information you learn, write a letter to your fellow students about the impact tobacco use can have on a person's life. Use vocabulary your peers will understand and tell the story of one of your family members to influence your peers to make positive health choices.

Preventing and Treating Tobacco Use

Essential Question?

What can you do to protect yourself from nicotine addiction?

Lesson 11.2

Learning Outcomes

After studying this lesson, you will be able to

- analyze the influences that affect whether or not a person uses tobacco;
- analyze the government's role in preventing tobacco use and encouraging quitting;
- practice skills for resisting tobacco and preventing tobacco use;
- assess the difficulty of quitting tobacco use; and
- summarize strategies used to quit tobacco use.

Key Terms

laryngectomy
nicotine replacement
public service announcements (PSAs)
response substitution
stimulus control

Warm-Up Activity

Differences in Smoking Rates

Analyze Influences The table that follows shows differences in smoking rates among US adults based on gender, race, education, and income. Working in groups, choose one of the four factors and brainstorm reasons your group thinks these differences exist. Discuss the listed reasons and explain how the factor can Influence a person's likelihood of using tobacco. Present your complete list of reasons and summary of the factor's influence to the class.

Gender	Race/Ethnicity
15.8% adult men 12.2% adult women	24% American Indians/Alaska Natives 15.2% Caucasians 14.9% African Americans 9.9% Hispanics 7.1% Asian Americans
Level of Education	**Income**
36.8% GED certificate 18.7% high school diploma 7.1% undergraduate degree 4.1% graduate degree	21.4% income less than $35,000 15.3% income $35,000–$74,999 11.8% income $75,000–$99,999 7.6% income greater than $100,000

The many negative health consequences of using tobacco products discourage people who prioritize their health from smoking, vaping, and chewing tobacco. Still, some people choose to use tobacco products despite the consequences. Fortunately, there are strategies you can use to prevent tobacco use in your personal life and community. Knowing about treatment options for people with an addiction to nicotine can help you advocate for the health of your family, friends, and community.

Factors Affecting Tobacco Use

People choose to use tobacco products for a number of reasons. The environment and a person's experiences influence these reasons. Risk factors and protective factors for tobacco use include the following.

Individual Factors

Individual factors are the factors related to your identity and behaviors. These factors include genetic makeup, mental health, and stage of development.

Genetic makeup influences how likely a person is to develop an addiction to nicotine. Researchers have identified several genes that impact risk for nicotine addiction. This means that having a family history of nicotine addiction increases a person's risk for developing a substance use disorder using tobacco products.

Some teens smoke, vape, or chew tobacco in an attempt to manage their mental health. Teens may feel stressed at school and turn to smoking or vaping as a way to relax. They may also be trying out a new identity. Teens may associate using tobacco with maturity, sophistication, glamour, rebellion, or toughness. Mental health conditions can increase the risk of nicotine addiction in teens. Rather than turning to tobacco products, people with mental health conditions and mental illnesses need to seek professional treatment.

Another individual factor that influences risk is stage of development. Teens are at increased risk for addiction because their brains are still developing.

Environment

Your environment includes your family, culture, peers, community, and the media (**Figure 11.11**). All of these components affect your risk for using tobacco.

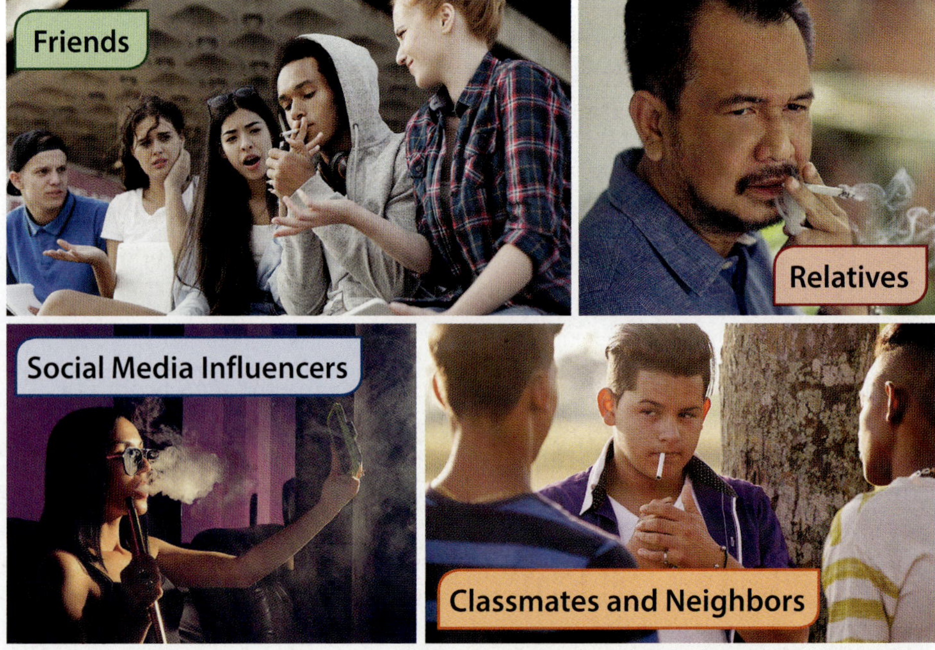

s/Shutterstock.com; Diego Cervo/Shutterstock.com; andrey_l/Shutterstock.com

Figure 11.11 You are much more likely to use tobacco if celebrities you follow or people in your friend groups, culture, school, family, or neighborhood use tobacco or are open to using tobacco. ***What other people in your environment may influence your perspective on tobacco?***

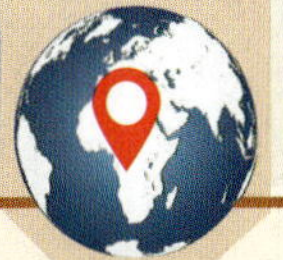

Local and Global Health

Rates of Tobacco Use Around the World

Many factors influence rates of tobacco use around the world. Rates of tobacco use vary by country, sex, race and ethnicity, and age, to name a few.

Rates of smoking vary considerably by country. People who live in higher-income countries are less likely to smoke than those who live in low-income countries. One explanation for this difference is that people with higher incomes tend to have higher levels of education. People with higher levels of education may be more aware of the health hazards of using tobacco.

Rates of smoking also vary by sex. In most countries, males are more likely to smoke than females. Health experts believe these differences may reflect different gender roles. For example, some parts of the world may view females smoking as less acceptable than males smoking. In addition, females may not have access to money or be able to afford cigarettes in some countries.

Rates of smoking are higher in some age groups than in others. Only about 10 percent of adults ages 18–24 smoke, compared to about 16 percent of adults ages 25–64. Smoking is less common (8.2 percent) in adults ages 65 and older.

Vaping rates around the world are growing rapidly. The US, Japan, and the United Kingdom currently have the highest rates. Given the health risks of vaping, some countries have banned the use or sales of vaping devices completely. These countries include Chile, Nicaragua, Egypt, and Singapore.

Practice Your Skills

Analyze Influences

Study the illustration of smoking rates in different regions of the world, according to the World Health Organization (WHO). What do you observe? What are the similarities between different world regions? What are the differences? List the reasons you think may contribute to different rates of smoking in different parts of the world. Then, compare your reasons with those of a partner. How could you test which factors have the biggest influence? What are some questions health researchers could be testing? Describe how knowing these factors could help reduce tobacco use.

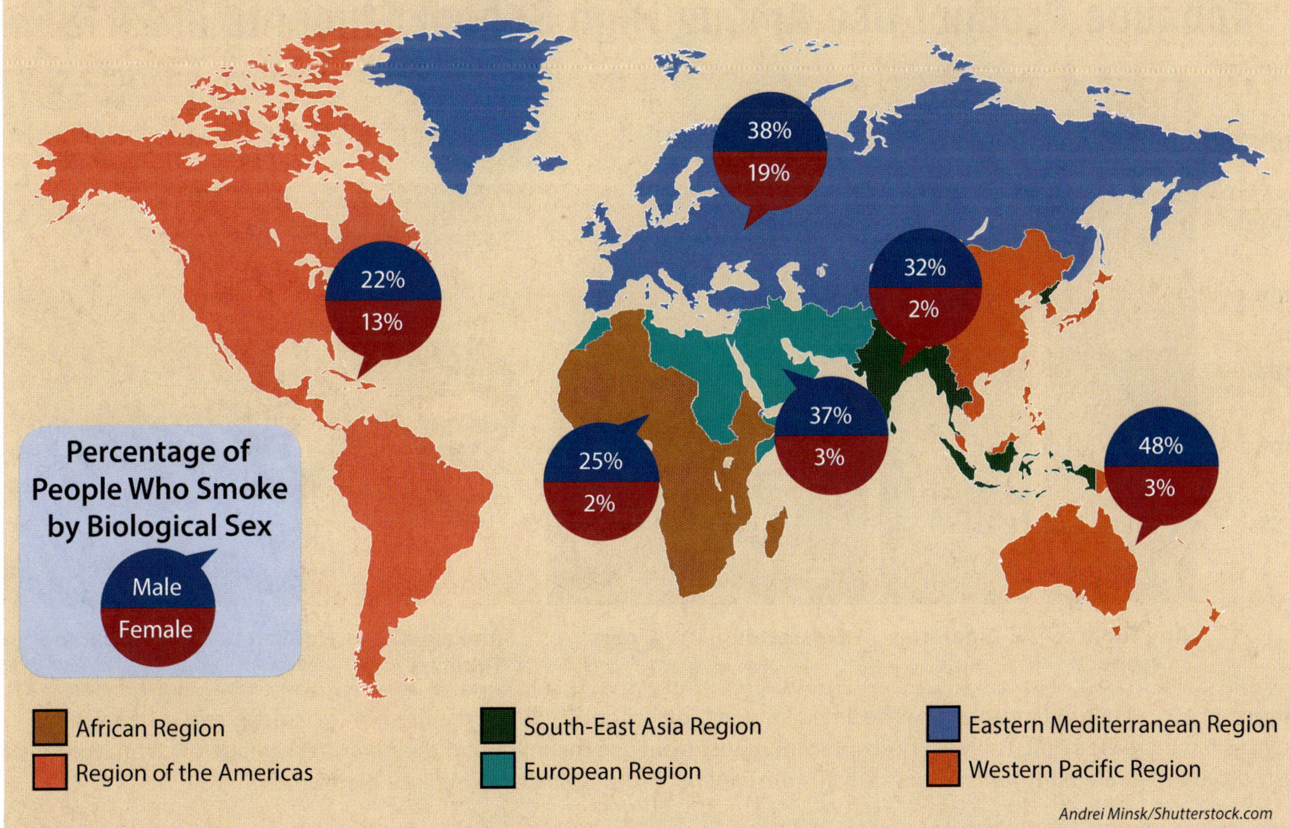

Andrei Minsk/Shutterstock.com

Family members' attitudes and behaviors about tobacco use influence whether teens smoke, vape, or chew tobacco. Teens are much less likely to use tobacco products if their families set clear expectations. Teens whose family members or cultures strongly oppose tobacco use are less likely to use tobacco products.

Teens with friends who smoke, vape, or chew tobacco are also much more likely to use tobacco products themselves. Teens may experience peer pressure to use tobacco. They may worry others will not like or accept them if they choose not to (**Figure 11.12**). Real friends, however, do not want their friends to endanger their health.

Another environmental factor is the community in which people live. Communities with violence, less education, and financial struggles often show higher rates of tobacco use. The availability of tobacco products within a community also affects whether teens and adults will use tobacco.

The media is an important part of people's environment. People often look to celebrities for ideas about fashionable clothing, new hairstyles, and lifestyle choices like tobacco use. Teens also imitate the behaviors of their peers on social media. Social media, however, only tells a small portion of a person's story. It may not capture the serious health consequences of tobacco use immediately and in the future.

Preventing Tobacco Use

Did you know that most adults who smoke picked up the habit when they were teens? Avoiding a lifetime of tobacco use starts now, with the decisions you make today.

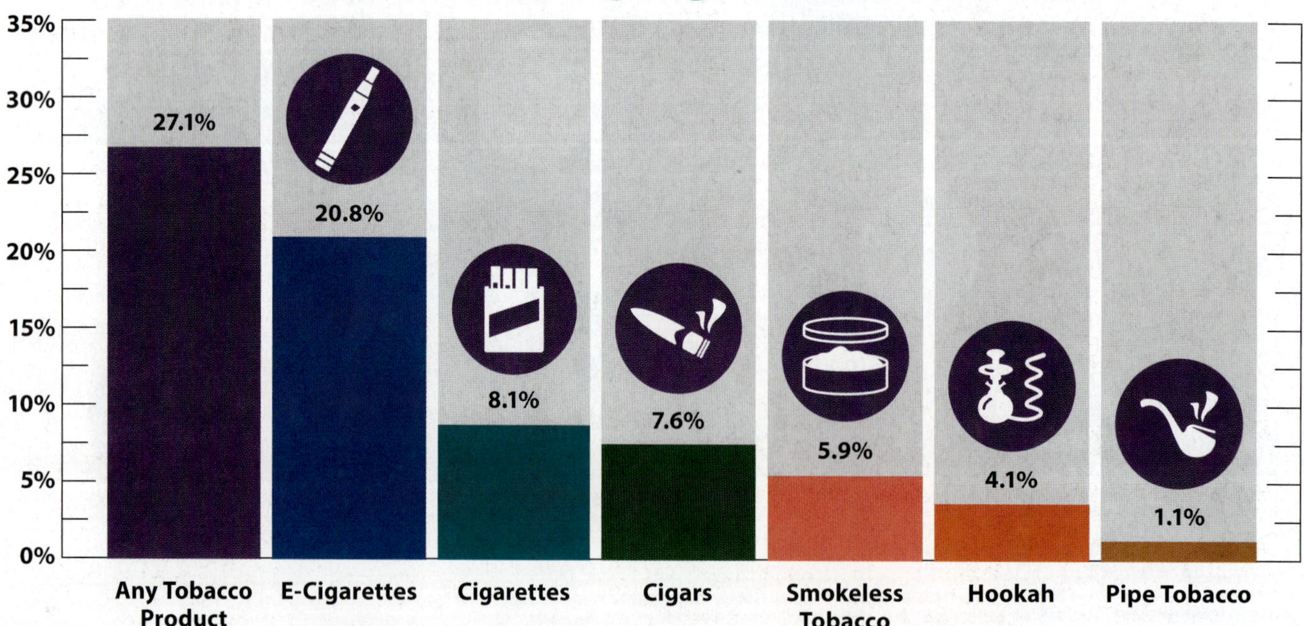

Gentzke AS, Creamer M, Cullen KA, et al. Vital Signs: Tobacco Product Use Among Middle and High School Students — United States, 2011–2018. MMWR Morb Mortal Wkly Rep 2019;68:157–164.

Figure 11.12 While cigarette use has declined among high school students, the use of e-cigarettes and other vaping devices has increased drastically. Sixty-six percent of teens believe the myth that their e-liquid is made of just flavoring. ***Why do you think so many high school students are willing to use vaping devices like e-cigarettes?***

Smoking costs society an estimated $289 billion a year in healthcare costs. Given the serious threat to public health, governments have strategies to regulate the sale, use, cost, and advertisement of tobacco products (**Figure 11.13**). Organizations have created mass media campaigns and **public service announcements (PSAs)** discouraging tobacco use. Successful campaigns emphasize short- and long-term health effects, strategies for refusing tobacco, and the fact that most teens do not use tobacco. Teens who regularly see these advertisements and campaigns are less likely to use tobacco products.

public service announcements (PSAs) media messages that support public health

Ultimately, the decision about whether or not to use tobacco products lies with you. You can use several skills to protect yourself from tobacco use and refuse tobacco products. These include building healthy relationships, learning strategies for managing stress, thinking critically about the media you see, and using refusal skills.

Build Healthy Relationships

Many teens feel pressure to use tobacco products if they have close friends who engage in this behavior. Fitting in during social situations if other people are smoking, vaping, or chewing tobacco and you are not can be difficult. In healthy friendships, however, your friends respect the choices you make and do not pressure you. People choose friends because they enjoy spending time with them, not because they use tobacco products.

If your friends do not respect your decision to avoid tobacco products, focus on developing other friendships. Perhaps you have grown apart from some of your other friends. Try to form friendships with people who respect you and accept your choices.

Learn to Manage Stress

Some people start using tobacco products to relieve stress. Smoking, vaping, or chewing tobacco may help them relax or not worry about a difficult situation. Using tobacco ends up increasing stress, however. An addiction to nicotine causes more issues than it solves and has negative mental and social consequences. Fortunately, there are many ways of managing stress that are more effective and do not have negative health consequences. You learned about some of these strategies in Lesson 5.3. Instead of using tobacco products, try the following methods for managing stress:

- **Listen to music:** Create a playlist of songs that help you relax and feel good. Listen to this playlist when you are feeling anxious or need to reduce stress.
- **Talk to a friend:** Find a friend who is a good listener and reach out to that person when you are feeling stressed. Social support is one of the best ways to manage stress.

Government Regulations on Tobacco Products

Bans on the sale of tobacco products

The sale of tobacco is prohibited to anyone younger than 21 years of age. Government programs also banned the sale of all candy- and fruit-flavored cigarettes and the sale of cigarettes in vending machines in places where minors are allowed.

Bans on smoking and vaping in public places

Some states have laws banning smoking and vaping in public places. These laws reduce exposure to secondhand smoke and aerosol and reduce triggers for people trying to quit nicotine.

Taxes on tobacco products

Federal, state, and municipal governments have set high taxes on the purchase of tobacco products, decreasing their sale, especially among teens.

Warnings on packages and advertisements

All tobacco product packaging and advertisements must contain warnings stating the risks associated with tobacco use.

Bans on advertising

Tobacco companies are banned from producing TV, radio, magazine, and newspaper advertisements for their products.

Figure 11.13 Restricting the ability for teens to buy and use tobacco products is an effective way for the government to prevent nicotine addiction.

- **Get physical activity:** All types of aerobic physical activity—from jogging to playing basketball to dancing—cause your body to release *endorphins*, or chemicals that make you feel better. Physical activity is also good for physical health.
- **Do a simple activity:** Focusing on a simple activity that is not stressful can help relieve stress. Try doing an activity with your hands, such as coloring or woodworking. This will distract you from whatever is stressing you and help you relax.

Think Critically

Advertisements for cigarettes, vaping devices, and smokeless tobacco try to make these products look attractive. Companies that sell tobacco products cannot advertise on TV, radio stations, or billboards. Because an estimated 480,000 people die every year from diseases caused by tobacco in the US, tobacco companies have to use sneaky strategies to persuade people to use their products. Fortunately, critical thinking can help you recognize the tobacco industry's sneaky practices and avoid being tricked.

Most people today know that cigarettes are dangerous. Since this knowledge has spread, tobacco companies have changed the types of products they sell to appeal to young people. Some tobacco products look like mints, toothpicks, electronic devices, breath strips, and flavored candy. These products have names that resemble sugary snacks more than addictive tobacco products. To advertise these products, some tobacco companies mimic popular social media trends to appeal to young people.

To resist these strategies, use critical thinking skills to analyze tobacco products and the messages from tobacco companies (**Figure 11.14**). People who understand the manipulative nature of tobacco advertisements resist them better. Analyzing advertisements can remind you about the serious consequences of tobacco use.

Analyzing Advertisements

1. Identify that the content is an ad. Sometimes, especially on social media, it can be difficult to tell what content is sponsored.
2. Identify the product or service being sold.
3. Identify the target audience for the ad. How old are the actors?
4. Identify the advertising techniques used. What mood or feeling is portrayed? Does the ad use happy or fun, fast music? flashy graphics? modern culture references?

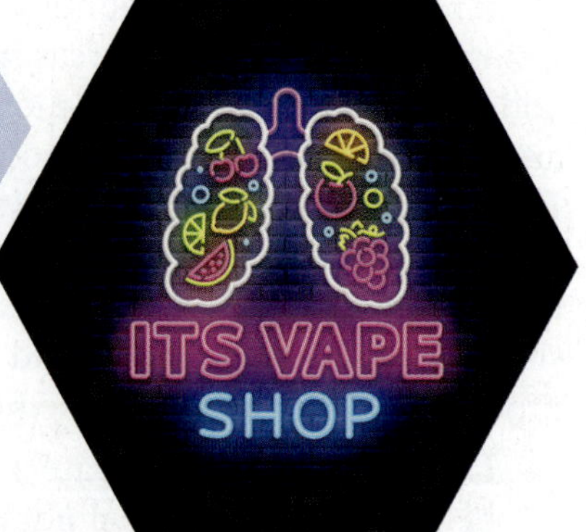

Left to right: Mike Orlov/Shutterstock.com; Soifer/Shutterstock.com

Figure 11.14 Smoking and vaping advertisements are designed to make tobacco products appear cool and harmless. ***What about the advertisements shown makes vaping seem harmless?***

Use Refusal Skills

Refusal skills can help you avoid using tobacco and make decisions that benefit your health now and in the future. If you do not want to use tobacco products or want to quit using tobacco, spend time with people who feel the same. Make sure the people around you know you do not want to use tobacco products or inhale their secondhand smoke and aerosol. Firmly explain the reasons behind your decision. Then stick to your decision and refuse to give in (**Figure 11.15**).

Sometimes teens worry that people will not like them if they choose not to use tobacco. Remember that your true friends will support your decision. If you have a friend who judges or leaves you out because you do not use tobacco, that friendship is not worth keeping. True friends will support your decision and respect you for who you are.

Treating Tobacco Use

A nicotine addiction is hard to break. Even people who experience life-threatening, smoking-related illnesses have difficulty quitting. For example, about 40 percent of people who have had a laryngectomy continue to smoke. A **laryngectomy** is a surgical procedure that removes the larynx, requiring a person to breathe through an opening in the neck.

laryngectomy surgical procedure that removes the larynx, requiring a person to breathe through an opening in the neck

Approaches to Refusing Tobacco

Change the subject.

Have you seen this video? It killed me, I can't stop laughing.

Is anyone else hungry? I could go for some tacos.

Try shifting the focus in some way. This approach can be easiest when you do not know a person well.

Share your reasons.

I don't want my breath to smell like cigarettes.

No thanks, I want to keep my lungs clear for track season.

There are many good reasons not to use tobacco products, and you can be honest about your personal reasons.

Emphasize health risks.

Vaping is still nicotine, and I don't want to get addicted.

My aunt got lung cancer from smoking, so no thanks.

Say you are too worried about the health effects of tobacco products to even try them. Use real examples if you have them.

Exit the situation.

My brother just texted me that he needs a ride, so I gotta go.

I'm meeting a friend to work on a school project.

If you believe the person will keep nagging you, make an excuse and leave.

Figure 11.15 Before you face situations in which someone offers you tobacco, imagine various situations and how you might respond. Play out each situation in your mind and practice different responses.

This procedure is typically performed when a person has cancer of the larynx. Similarly, more than one-half of people who have had a heart attack or surgery resulting from lung cancer continue to smoke. Despite these statistics, it is never too late to stop using tobacco. People who successfully quit smoking experience many health benefits (**Figure 11.16**).

Although quitting tobacco is difficult, nicotine addiction can be treated. Treatment methods include nicotine replacement, medication, and self-management techniques.

Benefits of Quitting Smoking Over Time
1 hour
Heart rate returns to normal, blood pressure begins to drop, and circulation may improve.
12 hours
Body cleanses itself of excess carbon monoxide and increases oxygen levels.
1 day
Risk of heart attack decreases.
2 days
Nerve endings heal, and senses of smell and taste are heightened.
1 month
Lung function improves, coughing and shortness of breath subside, and endurance increases.
9 months
Cilia recover to help push mucus out of the lungs and fight infections.
1 year
Risk for coronary heart diseases has decreased by half and will continue to drop.
10 years
Risk of lung, mouth, throat, and pancreatic cancers have all decreased significantly. Arteries and blood vessels widen again, reducing risk of stroke.
20 years
Risk of developing coronary heart disease, lung disease, and cancer drop to the level of a person who has never smoked.

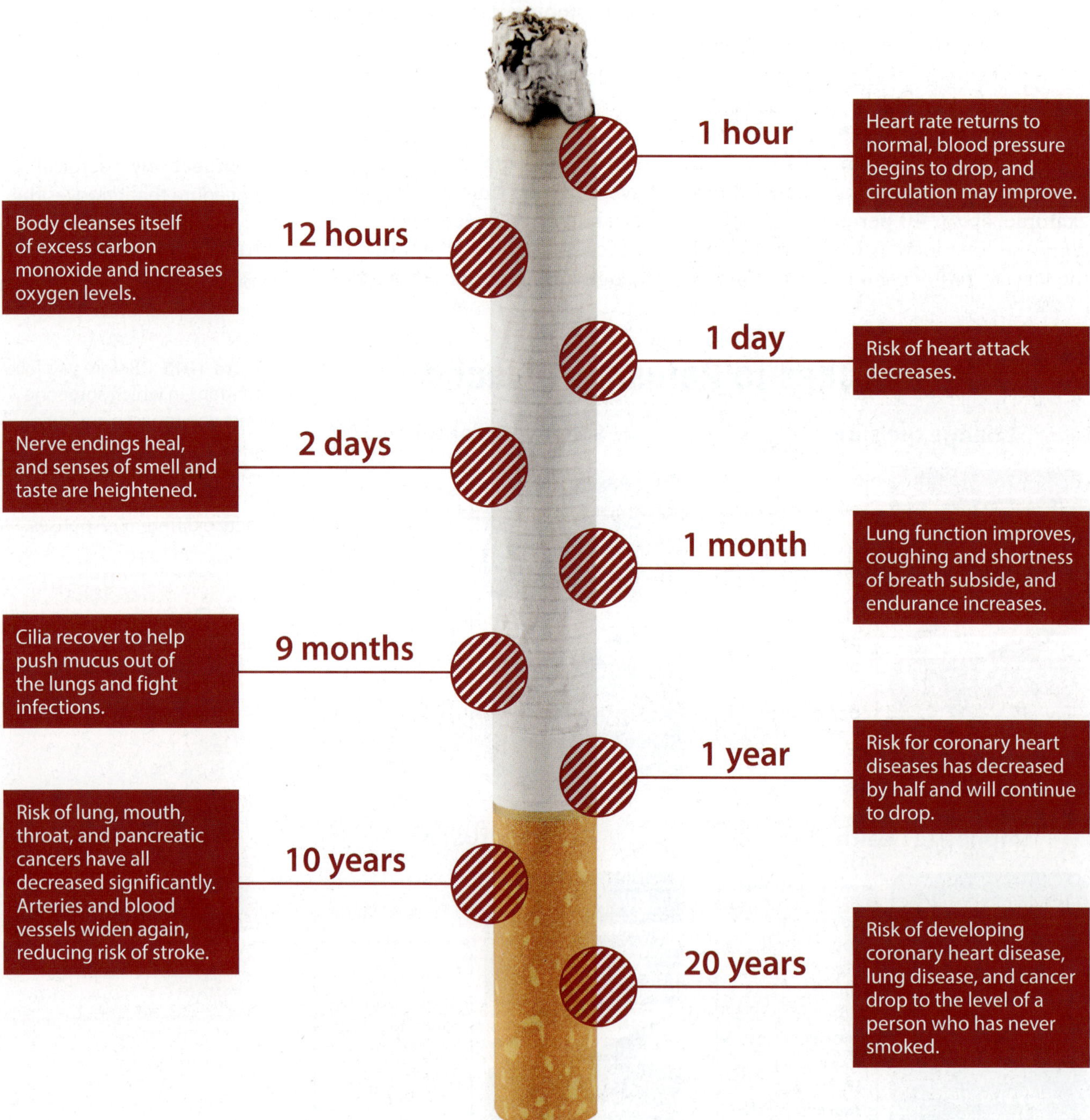

Voronina Svetlana/Shutterstock.com

Figure 11.16 Some benefits develop after just a few hours or days of quitting smoking. Other benefits accumulate within a year or more after quitting. These benefits increase the longer a person goes without using tobacco.

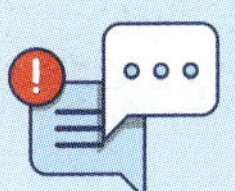

Health in the Media 

Tobacco in the Media: Then and Now

A long time ago, tobacco companies advertised their products on TV and the radio, as well as in magazines and newspapers. After scientific data clearly demonstrated the very serious health consequences of tobacco use, however, bans forced tobacco companies to stop this type of advertising.

Today, tobacco companies still cannot advertise using these methods. Instead, they try to avoid these laws by using social media. On social media, tobacco companies pay *ambassadors* and *influencers* to post content and link followers to tobacco products. Sometimes, posts by influencers do not even mention tobacco, but advertise upcoming parties or events where people promote or give away tobacco products. Teens may see these posts and not even recognize they are attempts at getting people to try tobacco products.

TV shows and movies also expose many teens to smoking, vaping, and chewing tobacco. In fact, 26 percent of movies rated G, PG, or PG-13 show tobacco use. It may seem harmless to simply see smoking or vaping in a movie. Research shows, however, that children and teens who see tobacco use in movies are more likely to start smoking.

Practice Your Skills

Set Goals

Take a few minutes to think about why so many companies now use social media to advertise tobacco products. Then discuss with a partner why these ads lead to increased rates of tobacco use. Do you think these ads should be legal? Why or why not? Do you think most teens recognize that these social media posts are advertisements designed to make money for tobacco companies? What strategies could help teens see through these techniques? With your partner, set five SMART goals to protect yourself from the impact of these advertisements. Share these SMART goals with the class, act on them, and evaluate how helpful they are.

Nicotine Replacement

Some approaches to treating nicotine addiction rely on **nicotine replacement**. In this treatment, people who use tobacco continue to put nicotine into their bodies, which lessens their withdrawal symptoms and cravings, making it easier to quit. In this way, people who use tobacco gradually treat their addiction by using smaller and smaller amounts. Eventually, people find they are no longer dependent on nicotine. Commonly used nicotine replacement strategies are nicotine gum, the nicotine patch, and nicotine lozenges.

nicotine replacement treatment for nicotine addiction that continues to put some nicotine into the body; lessens withdrawal symptoms and cravings, making it easier to quit

Companies sometimes market vaping devices like e-cigarettes as a nicotine-replacement tool for people who want to quit smoking. Unlike nicotine patches and lozenges, vaping devices have not been approved by the US government as a successful and safe form of smoking cessation.

Medications

Sometimes medications prescribed by a doctor help people quit using tobacco. These medications usually simulate *dopamine*, the chemical the brain releases in response to nicotine. People who take these medications cope better with withdrawal from nicotine.

Skills for Health and Wellness

Refusing Tobacco

Even if your friends do not smoke, vape, or chew tobacco, you may find yourself in a situation where others want you to use tobacco products. In a situation like this, the choice you make will impact your health in the moment and for years to come. Smoking, vaping, or chewing tobacco even one time can harm your health and lead you on the path to a serious addiction. Do you know what you would say if one of your classmates offered you tobacco?

Practice Your Skills

Communicate with Others

Partner with two of your classmates to form a group of three. Then, in your group, role-play a situation in which two of your friends want you to smoke, vape, or chew tobacco. During your refusal, follow these steps:

1. Reflect on what you have learned about the harmful effects of tobacco and nicotine.
2. If your friends are using tobacco, express concern. You might say, "I don't want to see you get sick."
3. State your refusal. Sometimes a simple "No, I don't smoke" is enough to end the conversation. If it is not, try giving a reason, telling a story, asking a question, or changing the subject. Make eye contact and speak firmly. You might say:
   - *"My dad has lung cancer because he smoked. There's no way I'm trying that."*
   - *"If my family finds out, I'll get grounded and won't be able to go to the concert."*
4. Stick to your refusal. Think about the consequences of tobacco use. Are the long-term health effects really worth trying a new vape flavor or fitting in? State your refusal as many times as you need to and leave the situation, if needed.

Rotate roles in the role-play and practice using three to five different phrases to state your refusal. Afterward, discuss which statements were most and least effective. Also discuss what it means if you have to leave a situation because your friends keep pressuring you to use tobacco. If your friends do not respect your decision, are they really your friends?

Self-Management Strategies

Self-management strategies involve identifying situations that trigger the desire for tobacco use and developing techniques to resist temptation. Once people who use tobacco understand situations or feelings that lead them to want to use tobacco, they can respond with two techniques—stimulus control and response substitution. **Stimulus control** is trying to avoid tempting situations and managing feelings that lead to nicotine use. With **response substitution**, people respond to difficult feelings and situations using stress management, relaxation, and coping skills instead of tobacco use.

stimulus control
treatment for nicotine addiction that involves avoiding tempting situations and managing feelings that lead to nicotine use

response substitution
treatment for nicotine addiction where people practice responding to difficult feelings and situations using stress management, relaxation, and coping skills instead of tobacco use

If you are trying to quit using tobacco, you can take the following steps to use self-management strategies:

1. Set a "quit date" within the next month and note that date on your calendar. Make a strong commitment to actually stop using tobacco on that date.
2. Tell friends and family members about your quit date and ask them to support your efforts. Ask people who smoke, vape, or chew tobacco not to do so around you.
3. Get rid of tobacco products and their accessories in your environment. Avoid exposure to tobacco advertisements on social media.

4. Develop strategies for coping with nicotine cravings, such as getting physical activity, chewing gum, or keeping busy with other activities.
5. Develop strategies for refusing offers of tobacco products from other people.
6. Remind yourself of the benefits of quitting, including a longer life, more spending money, and increased stamina.
7. Reward yourself for quitting. Buy something with the money you saved by not using tobacco (**Figure 11.17**).
8. If you slip up, quickly renew your focus on the goal of quitting. Do not let one lapse lead to a return of the old behavior.

Some people need additional support to break a nicotine addiction. People can find this support through individual or group counseling; a school counselor, doctor, teacher, or trusted adult; telephone or online helplines with free counseling; and online resources.

The average person who smokes goes through **14** cigarettes per day.
There are **20** cigarettes in a pack. One pack costs on average **$6.28**.
Giving up cigarettes would save this person:
$31 each week
$942 each month
$11,304 each year
$113,040 each decade

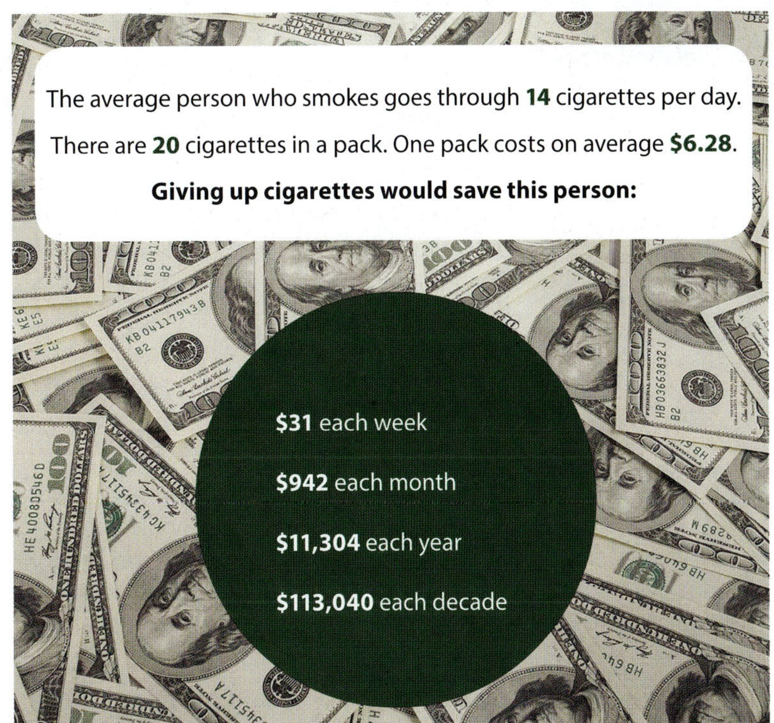

Goskova Tatiana/Shutterstock.com

Figure 11.17 Depending on the price of cigarettes in your area and how often you smoke, smoking can be a costly habit. ***What would you spend $942 on every month instead of cigarettes?***

Lesson 11.2 Review

Know and Understand

1. Analyze the influence of a person's social relationships on tobacco use.
2. List one step your state's government has taken to reduce tobacco use.
3. Identify one effective stress-management strategy that does not involve using tobacco.
4. What three methods are used to treat nicotine addiction?
5. What support is available for people who have trouble quitting nicotine?

Think Critically

6. What role has your family and culture played in influencing whether you use tobacco?
7. Give one example of a refusal you could use to avoid using tobacco.
8. What do you think schools and communities can do to help reduce tobacco use among teens?

REAL WORLD Health Skills

Access Information Visit a local store or search online to determine the average prices of vaping devices. If an individual vapes one pod each day, how much money would the person spend on vaping for one week, one month, one year, and five years? Also include the initial cost of purchasing a vape starter kit. What other activities could you do with the money spent on vaping? Write a social media post about your findings.

Chapter 11 Review and Assessment

Chapter Summary

A tobacco product is any product made or derived from tobacco and intended for human consumption. One thing almost all tobacco products have in common is they contain nicotine, which is a highly addictive substance. Nicotine is also toxic and has severe effects on multiple body systems.

Cigarettes and cigarette smoke contain thousands of chemicals and toxic substances that harm the body. People who smoke have a higher risk for developing osteoporosis, ulcers, fertility issues, and gum disease. Smoking also damages the respiratory system and makes breathing more difficult.

While some people see vaping as a harmless alternative to smoking cigarettes, vaping poses several health risks. Vaping devices heat e-liquid, which is made of many chemicals, into an aerosol that people inhale. Inhaling the chemicals in aerosol can lead to respiratory conditions, including inflammation and long-term lung damage.

The harmful effects of the nicotine and carcinogens found in smokeless tobacco are the same as if they were smoked. When using smokeless tobacco, people absorb nicotine and other chemicals through their mouth tissues. This can lead to leukoplakia, oral cancer, cardiovascular disease, respiratory irritation, gum disease, and tooth decay.

Using tobacco impacts not just a person's body, but also a person's mind and social relationships. In addition, teens who use tobacco can experience serious legal consequences and may face disciplinary actions at school. Smoking and vaping can also impact the health of other people by releasing substances into the air they breathe. Exposure to secondhand and thirdhand smoke and aerosol can increase the risk of developing serious diseases and health conditions.

People's choices to use tobacco products can be influenced by their environment and experiences. You can use several skills to protect yourself from tobacco use and refuse tobacco products. These include building healthy relationships, learning strategies for managing stress, thinking critically about the media you see, and using refusal skills.

A nicotine addiction is hard to break. Treatment methods include nicotine replacement, medication, and self-management techniques. Some people need additional support to quit using nicotine. People can find this support through individual or group counseling; a school counselor, doctor, teacher, or trusted adult; telephone or online helplines with free counseling; and online resources.

Vocabulary Activity

As a class, divide into two groups and assign each group one lesson in this chapter. In your group, review your assigned lesson and the main ideas and key terms introduced. Ask your teacher if you are not sure which ideas are most important. Create a multimedia presentation that uses text, photos and illustrations, and music to summarize the main ideas in the lesson. Use all of the key terms from the lesson in your summary. Present your interactive summary to the class and adapt your vocabulary as needed to respond to questions and clarify information. Then switch roles.

aerosol
asthma
carbon monoxide
carcinogens
chronic bronchitis
chronic obstructive pulmonary disease (COPD)
e-liquid
emphysema
laryngectomy
leukoplakia
nicotine
nicotine replacement
popcorn lung
public service announcements (PSAs)
response substitution
secondhand aerosol
secondhand smoke
smokeless tobacco
stimulus control
tar
thirdhand smoke
tobacco
vaping devices

Review and Recall

Review the information in this chapter by answering the following questions.

1. The addictive, toxic substance present in all tobacco products is called
   A. carcinogen.
   B. carbon monoxide.
   C. adrenaline.
   D. nicotine.
2. What is the most common form of tobacco use among teens today?
3. What is tolerance, and how does it drive a nicotine addiction?
4. Define *adrenaline*. How does nicotine affect adrenaline and the body?
5. How can tobacco use affect appearance?
6. Which chemical does nicotine cause the brain to release, leading to a pleasurable sensation?
7. Why are teens especially sensitive to the effects of nicotine?
8. Describe how tar affects the lungs.
9. Why is it difficult for scientists to study the long-term effects of inhaling the chemicals contained in vaping aerosol?
10. Why is it misleading to say that the chemical flavorings in e-liquids are generally recognized as safe (GRAS)?
11. Why is it difficult to eliminate thirdhand smoke and aerosol?
12. What is one commonly used nicotine replacement strategy?
13. Which of the following is *not* an effective self-management strategy to help stop using nicotine?
    A. setting a "quit date"
    B. punishing yourself if you slip up
    C. asking friends and family to support your efforts
    D. rewarding yourself for quitting

Standardized Test Prep

Reading and Writing Practice

Read the passage below and then answer the following questions.

Many teens do not realize how harmful vaping is to health. According to a survey conducted by Gallup in 2018, 82 percent of people ages 18–29 think smoking is very harmful to health. In contrast, only 22 percent considered vaping very harmful to health.

Contrary to these beliefs, research shows that vaping increases the risk a teen will smoke cigarettes. In fact, high school students who vape are seven times more likely to report smoking six months later. In addition to nicotine, which can lead to addiction, vaping e-liquids contain harmful chemicals. The number of reported lung illnesses related to vaping has been growing. Some of these illnesses have occurred in people vaping nicotine, and others have developed in people vaping marijuana. Typically, symptoms of these lung illnesses include shortness of breath and chest pain.

14. Which of the following is *not* a health risk associated with vaping?
    A. nicotine addiction
    B. increased likelihood of smoking
    C. tar in the lungs
    D. shortness of breath
15. Do lung illnesses related to vaping only occur in those vaping nicotine? Defend your answer.
16. Which statement best describes the main point of this passage?
    A. Vaping is more dangerous than smoking.
    B. Most people do not know vaping is harmful.
    C. Contrary to people's beliefs, vaping can harm health in several ways.
    D. Scientists are still studying the health effects of vaping.

Chapter 11 Skills Assessment

Critical Thinking Skills

Answer the following questions to assess your knowledge of what you learned in this chapter.

1. Why do you think vaping devices might be more appealing to teens than regular cigarettes?
2. Explain how exposure to nicotine during pregnancy can impact the developing fetus.
3. Consider the effects of tobacco use on healthy behaviors such as physical activity, nutrition, and sleep. What negative effects might tobacco use have on healthy behaviors? Explain.
4. Can you think of any places where you might frequently encounter secondhand smoke or aerosol? What are some ways you can protect yourself from it?
5. Discuss the connection between tobacco use and mental illness. Do you think people with mental illnesses are more likely to use tobacco? Do you think people who use tobacco are more likely to develop mental illnesses? Explain your answer.
6. What other behaviors and characteristics do you associate with smoking or vaping? How do you think those associations could affect your decisions?
7. Do people in your community have mostly positive or mostly negative perceptions of tobacco use? How might people's perceptions of tobacco use change in different types of communities?
8. Talk with your family to find out about relatives who have been affected by diseases associated with tobacco use. Make a list of family members, their diseases, and whether or not they used tobacco. Discuss the influence that tobacco use may have had on these family members and their health.
9. How do parents' behaviors and attitudes about tobacco influence their children's future decisions about tobacco use?
10. Do you think there is any value in banning the sale of tobacco products across all media platforms? Why or why not?
11. Create a public service announcement (PSA) about the dangers of vaping. Make sure to include at least two of the following: short- and long-term health effects, refusal strategies, or usage statistics.
12. Research a product or medication commonly used to help people quit tobacco use. How effective do you think this product is? Explain your reasoning.
13. Over time, the health consequences of tobacco use have become better known. How do you think this information might relate to the number of people who use or used to use tobacco in different age groups? Do you think rates will change over time? Explain.

Health and Wellness Skills

Complete the following activities to assess your skills related to health and wellness.

14. **Analyze Influences.** Friends, family, and the media can have a strong influence on whether people use tobacco. Over the last two or three days, what factors have influenced you to use or not use tobacco products, including vaping devices? Identify and list the factors you have observed. Has there been any recent national or state legislation to reduce risk factors and decrease tobacco use? Is there any new legislation you would propose to one of your local, state, or national officials? If so, what would that legislation be and how would it affect tobacco use?
15. **Access Information.** E-liquids in vaping devices contain many harmful chemicals. Using valid and reliable online and print resources, identify five chemicals commonly found in e-liquids and choose one to research. Evaluate the resources you find and use the most credible source. List other products that contain the chemical you chose and explain how this chemical can harm the body.
16. **Communicate with Others.** Peer pressure in schools can create a *social multiplier effect*, which is the concept that the behavior of peers establishes a perceived norm, which influences behavior. Because of this effect, it is difficult for people to defy the perceived norm. In small groups, research this effect and discuss how it is present in your school. Using communication skills, film a video in which you role-play ways to resist peer pressure (including the social multiplier effect) to make healthy decisions about tobacco use.

17. **Make Decisions.** List four myths you believed about tobacco use (including vaping) before reading this chapter. Then, list factual information from the chapter or other valid resources that dispels each myth. Reflect on how this newfound information will help you make healthier decisions regarding tobacco. Create a journal entry discussing your disproved myths and how they will affect your decisions.
18. **Set Goals.** Imagine one of your close friends confides in you about needing help. Your friend is very stressed about school and started vaping after someone said it would help with the stress. Now, your friend needs to vape more often than before to feel the same effect. Create a script in which you help your friend set a SMART goal to find needed help and make healthy decisions about vaping.
19. **Practice Health-Enhancing Behaviors.** Imagine that, during an after-school extracurricular activity, you go to the restroom to take a break. Two other students are in the restroom vaping. One offers you the vaping device and asks if you would like to try. Complete the dialogue that follows, using appropriate terminology and refusal skills to avoid this situation.

    Student 1: "Hey, wanna take a hit? It's cotton candy flavor."

    Your Response: ________________________________

    Student 2: "Don't be lame. It won't hurt you. Just try it."

    Your Response: ________________________________

    Student 1: "Come on. It's safer than smoking. It's not even addictive."

    Your Response: ________________________________

    Student 2: "You don't know what you're missing. Don't tell anyone we're here."

    Your Response: ________________________________

    After completing the dialogue, find a partner and read and share your responses. Exchange feedback and critiques to make each response stronger.
20. **Advocate for Health.** Research some popular PSAs and choose three of your favorites. Consider why these PSAs are effective and then create your own PSA about the health effects of vaping, smoking, or using smokeless tobacco. Consider your target audience for the PSA and present it to the class.

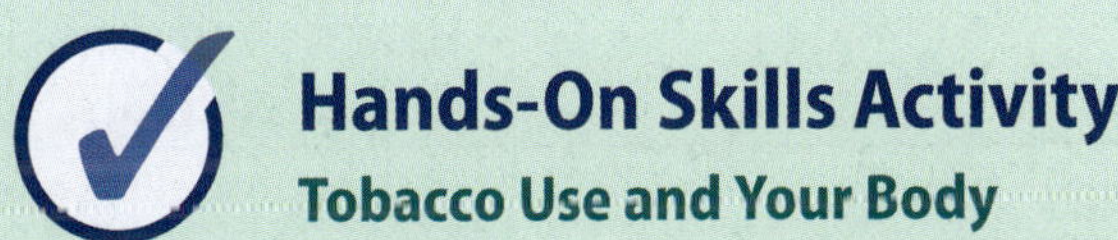

Hands-On Skills Activity

Tobacco Use and Your Body

All tobacco products, including many e-liquids, deliver nicotine into the body. Nicotine is toxic and extremely harmful to a person's health. Body systems affected by nicotine include the cardiovascular, respiratory, nervous, digestive, immune, and reproductive systems. This activity will illustrate how using tobacco products can affect these body systems. For this activity, you will need craft paper, markers, pens or pencils, and reliable resources.

Steps for This Activity

1. Choose several classmates to work with and, as a group, choose one of the six body systems affected by nicotine. Your teacher may also assign a body system to your group.
2. **Access Information.** Using reliable resources, research the parts and pathways of your chosen body system and how nicotine affects this body system. Include whether or not nicotine's effects are reversible once tobacco use stops. Your school's library media specialist can help you find resources, which might include books, journals, magazines, or websites. Remember to use websites with medically accurate information. You can use the guidelines in Chapter 2 to assess the credibility and validity of your resources.
3. Draw an outline of the human body on a long, wide piece of craft paper.
4. Inside the body outline, draw and label the parts and pathways of your group's body system.
5. Outside the body outline, illustrate how nicotine affects this body system. Note whether or not the effects are reversible.
6. **Advocate for Health.** Hang your group's body poster in the hallway of your school to show other students the dangers of using tobacco. Obtain permission, if needed. You may also take a picture of your body poster and share it online. Use your poster to start a discussion with other students and support them in making positive health choices.

Chapter 12

Alcohol

Lesson 12.1 Health Effects of Alcohol

Lesson 12.2 Preventing and Treating Alcohol Abuse

Look for the skills icon throughout this chapter for opportunities to practice your health skills.

Check Your Health and Wellness Skills

In this chapter, you will learn skills for protecting your health from the harms of alcohol. To understand the skills you currently use, take the following inventory of your behaviors. Indicate how well you think you use each skill. Use a scale of 1–5, *1* meaning you do not use the skill and *5* meaning you feel completely comfortable using it.

Skill	How Well Do You Use Each Skill?
I understand how drinking alcohol can lead to addiction and risky behaviors.	
I get help for feelings of anxiety and depression instead of trying to self-medicate.	
When movies and TV shows depict alcohol use, I know they aren't showing the whole picture.	
I try to think positively and cope by journaling or being active when I feel sad.	
I stay away from parties where alcohol is available.	
I build relationships with people who respect my decisions.	
I know how to say *no* if someone offers me alcohol.	
I encourage my friends to make healthy decisions and stay away from alcohol.	
I know whom I'd talk to if a friend of mine had an addiction to alcohol.	
I don't protect people who drink alcohol from the consequences of their decisions.	
	Total:

Add up your responses to each statement. The higher your score, the more comfortable you feel avoiding the harms of alcohol. Which skill do you think is most important for you? Which skill is the most challenging for you? Which skill would you most like to improve? In this chapter, you will learn how to perform these skills better and more often.

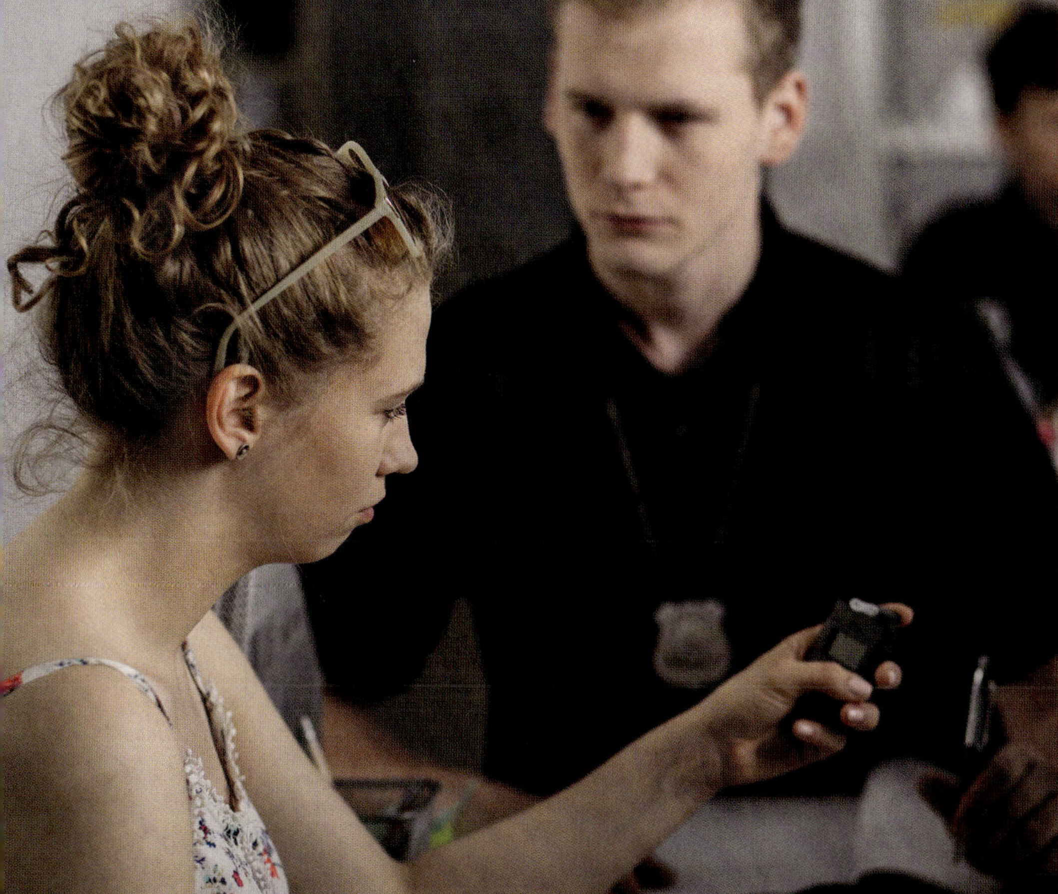

KatarzynaBialasiewicz/iStock/Getty Images Plus/Getty Images

Reading and Notetaking

In what ways do you think drinking alcohol is harmful to your health? Before reading the chapter, write a two-paragraph essay explaining some of the health effects of alcohol use. Consider how alcohol affects physical, mental and emotional, and social health. After you finish reading the chapter, consider what information you might add to your essay. Share your essay and any additions with a partner.

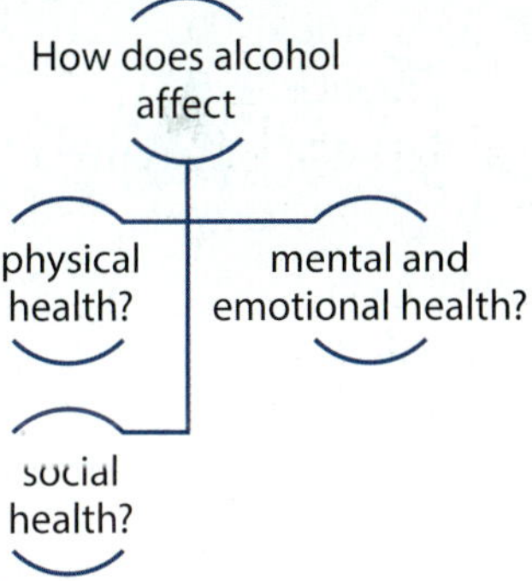

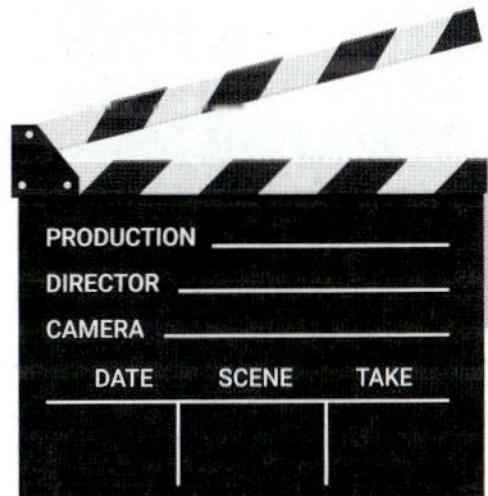

Setting the Scene

Affected by Alcohol

For all of your life, you have looked up to your older sibling. Your sibling includes you in time with friends and has always been willing to talk with you and give advice. Lately, however, your sibling has been acting differently. Your sibling goes out every weekend night with friends, and you have heard your sibling talk about drinking a lot of alcohol. Every weekend morning, your sibling wakes up feeling awful and talks about not drinking anymore. The same night, your sibling goes out anyway and drives home after drinking.

You are worried about your sibling developing an addiction to alcohol. You are also worried your sibling is going to get hurt in an accident or get in trouble with the law. You care about your sibling very much, but also feel like your sibling really needs some help. What should you do?

Thinking Critically

1. In this scenario, what are some strategies you could use to talk with your sibling and get help? What might happen if your sibling does not get help?
2. What are some factors that might lead high school students to drink alcohol?

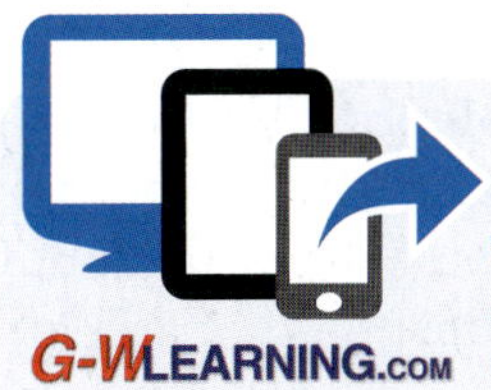

Click on the activity icon or visit www.g-wlearning.com/health/4095 to access online vocabulary activities using key terms from the chapter.

Lesson

12.1

Health Effects of Alcohol

Essential Question?

How does consuming alcohol affect a person's physical, mental and emotional, and social health?

Learning Outcomes

After studying this lesson, you will be able to

- explain the characteristics of alcohol;
- describe the concept of blood alcohol concentration (BAC);
- identify different patterns of alcohol consumption;
- assess how alcohol affects the brain and leads to addiction;
- describe hangover, alcohol poisoning, and chronic health conditions associated with alcohol use; and
- analyze the mental, social, and legal consequences of alcohol use.

Key Terms

alcohol
alcohol poisoning
alcohol use disorder (AUD)
blood alcohol concentration (BAC)
cirrhosis
depressant
driving under the influence (DUI)
fetal alcohol spectrum disorders (FASD)
hangover
inhibition

Warm-Up Activity

Alcohol Underage

Access Information Years ago, the drinking age for alcohol was lower in the United States. In some states, people as young as 18 years old could drink. This age was raised to 21 due to research about how alcohol affects the brain. Using reliable and valid resources, research the reasons the drinking age was raised to 21. Use the guidelines in Chapter 2 to make sure your resources are credible. Then, draw a person and label the person's body with the health consequences of drinking alcohol before age 21. On the outside of the body, list risk factors for consuming alcohol before age 21.

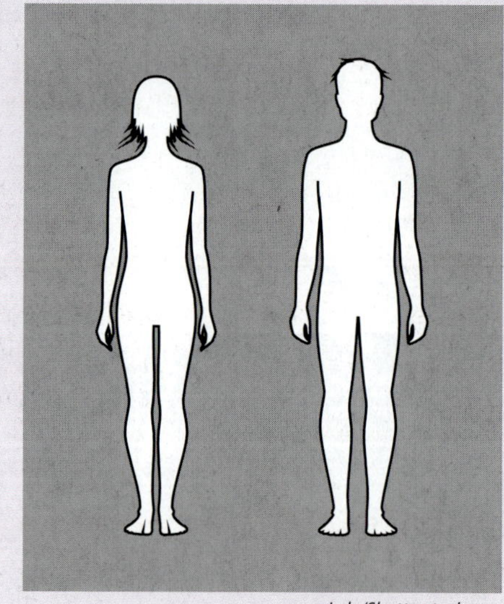

Lole/Shutterstock.com

In the United States, you must be 21 years of age to buy alcohol. Some teens may not understand why this age limit exists. After all, at 18 years of age, you can vote in a presidential election or join the military. Many teens do not know that alcohol is the third leading cause of preventable death in the US. Alcohol use can be extremely dangerous, contributing to the deaths of more than 4,300 Americans under the age of 21 each year. **Alcohol** is an addictive drug that alters brain function and has substantial effects on the body and a person's thinking and behavior. In this lesson, you will learn about the health effects of alcohol—in the moments after consumption and long-term.

alcohol addictive depressant with the active ingredient ethanol; alters brain function

Understanding Alcohol

The active ingredient in alcohol is *ethanol*, which is also known as *pure alcohol*. Ethanol is also used as a component of gasoline in some cars. When experts talk about alcoholic drinks, they are describing any drink that contains at least 0.6 ounces (14.0 grams) of pure alcohol. Different alcoholic drinks have different percentages of pure alcohol (**Figure 12.1**). A drink is determined by the amount of alcohol, not by the amount of liquid, which means that one standard drink can be different sizes.

When someone consumes an alcoholic drink, the alcohol passes from the stomach into the small intestine, where it is quickly absorbed into the bloodstream and distributed throughout the body. This means that drinking alcohol affects every single cell in the body, including cells in the muscles and brain (**Figure 12.2**).

What Counts as One "Standard Drink" of Alcohol?
12 ounces of beer, hard cider, hard lemonade, or hard seltzer
=
5 ounces of wine
=
1.5 ounces of liquor, such as rum, vodka, or whiskey
BEER
5% ABV
12% ABV
40% ABV

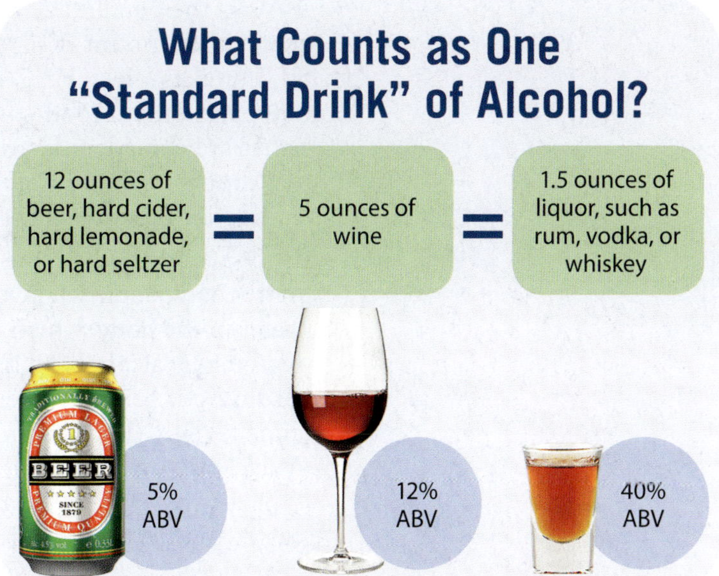

Left to right: Oleksiy Mark/Shutterstock.com; EHStockphoto/Shutterstock.com; OlegSam/Shutterstock.com

Figure 12.1 Alcoholic drinks contain varying amounts of pure alcohol. The amount of alcohol in a drink is labeled as *alcohol by volume (ABV)*. ABV describes the percentage of a drink's volume that is alcohol. The label on an alcoholic drink should list its ABV. ***How many ounces of pure alcohol are in one standard drink?***

Blood Alcohol Concentration (BAC)

Once a person consumes alcohol, alcohol stays in the body until the liver can break it down. Generally, alcohol leaves the body at an average rate of 0.015 grams (100 milliliters) per hour. This is about one standard drink per hour.

When someone drinks a lot of alcohol in a short period of time, the body cannot break down the alcohol fast enough. As a result, alcohol builds up in the bloodstream. The measure of this alcohol in the blood is called **blood alcohol concentration (BAC)**.

blood alcohol concentration (BAC)
percentage of alcohol in a person's blood

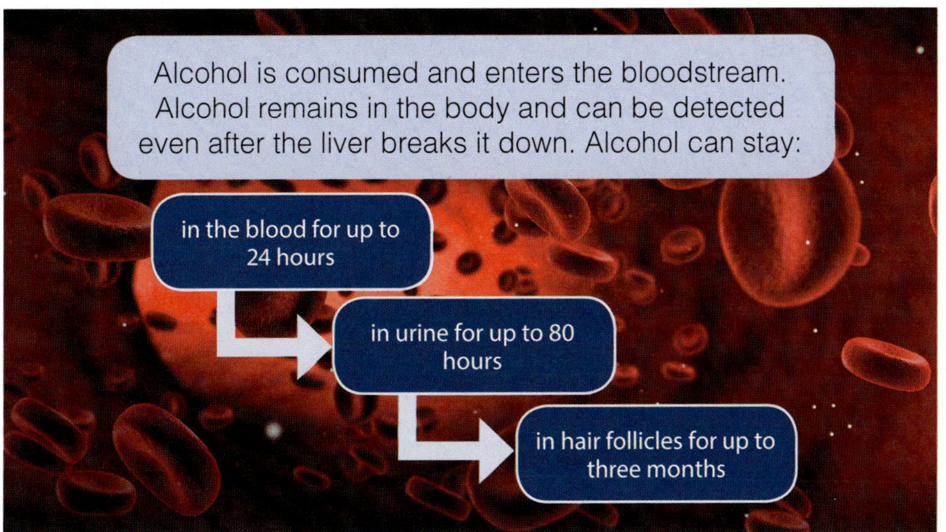

donfiore/Shutterstock.com

Figure 12.2 Since alcohol is absorbed into the bloodstream, it is distributed throughout the body. This means alcohol can continue to be found in various body parts up to three months after consumption.

BAC is the percentage of alcohol in a person's blood. This percentage compares the amount of alcohol in a person's body to the amount of blood. For example, a BAC of 0.08% means there are 8 parts alcohol to 10,000 parts other blood components. People who have a BAC of 0.08% or higher are considered *legally impaired*, also known as *intoxicated* or *drunk*. About two to four alcoholic drinks would result in a BAC of 0.08%, depending on the following factors:

- **Body weight:** The same amount of alcohol affects people who weigh less more than people who weigh more. Someone who weighs more has more water in the body, which dilutes alcohol and lowers BAC. This is one reason why alcohol can have a stronger impact on females than males.
- **Biological sex:** Females often feel the effects of alcohol more quickly and strongly than males and have a higher BAC (**Figure 12.3**). Muscle tissue absorbs alcohol more easily than fat. Because females typically have more fat and less muscle, alcohol is not absorbed as easily and becomes more concentrated. In addition, females have lower levels of a particular enzyme that helps process alcohol. This means that alcohol is processed more slowly in females than in males.

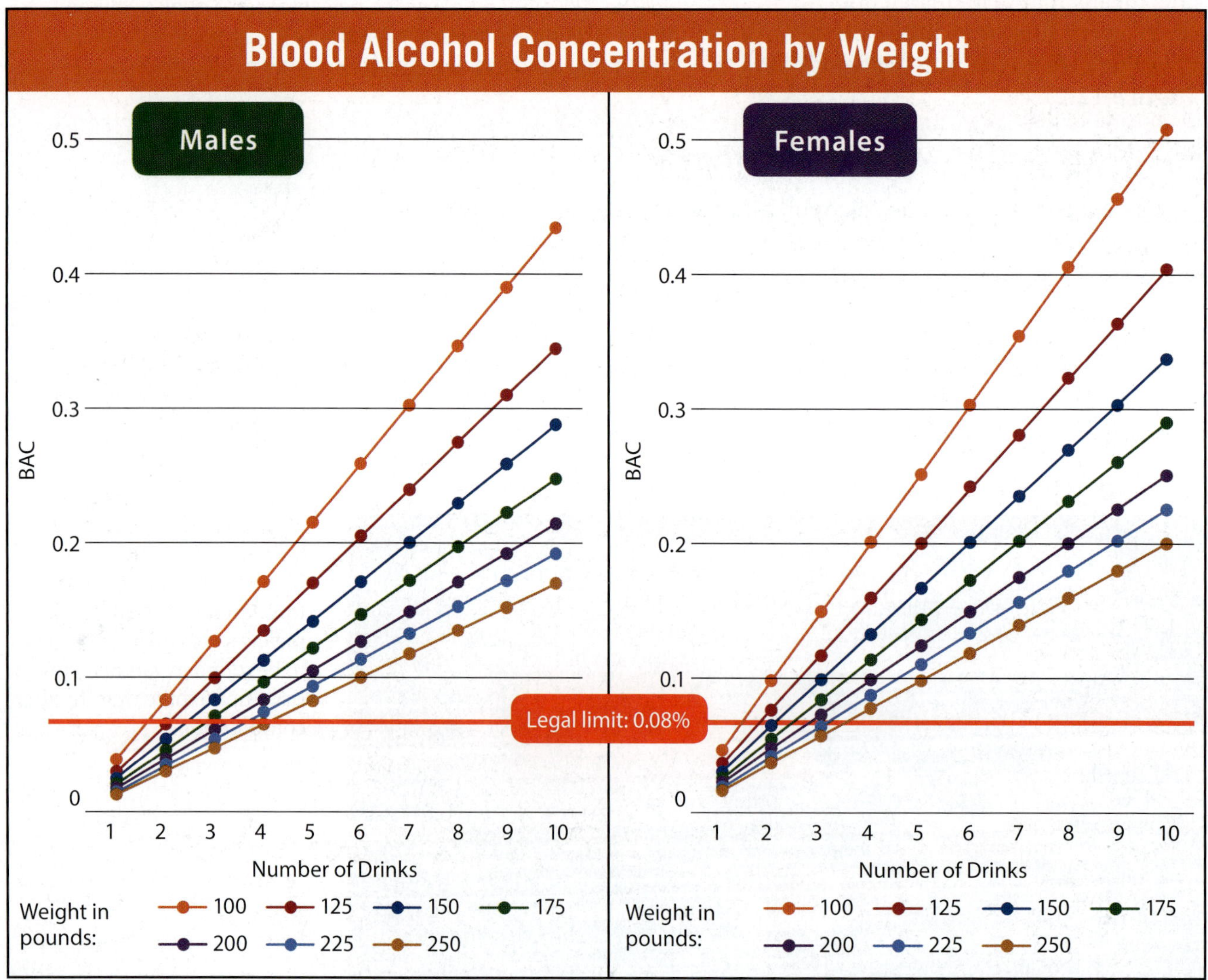

Figure 12.3 Body weight and biological sex often have the biggest impact on how much alcohol will affect an individual's body.

- **Food consumption:** When a person consumes alcohol while eating food, or shortly after eating food, BAC increases more slowly because the digestive system digests alcohol while it digests food. This gives the liver more time to break down alcohol and results in a lower BAC. The type of food consumed can also impact BAC. For example, it takes longer to process foods high in fat, which slows the absorption of alcohol into the bloodstream. In one study, the bodies of people who drank alcohol after eating a full meal took three times as long to absorb the alcohol compared to people who drank alcohol on an empty stomach.
- **Ethnicity:** Ethnicity may also influence a person's BAC. Some research suggests that up to 50 percent of people of Asian heritage have difficulty processing alcohol due to a difference with an enzyme that processes alcohol. This difference can mean the liver processes alcohol more slowly, resulting in a higher BAC.

Patterns of Alcohol Consumption

Drinking alcohol can have serious effects on a person's body, decisions, and future. These effects mean that some people should not drink alcohol under any circumstances. These people include anyone under the age of 21, people who are or may be pregnant, people who are driving or operating equipment, and people who are taking certain medications. People who cannot control their alcohol use or have a family history of alcohol use disorders also should not drink alcohol.

Adults who decide to drink alcohol need to consider the harmful effects. Certain patterns of drinking alcohol can increase or decrease a person's risk of experiencing negative consequences (**Figure 12.4**).

Patterns of Alcohol Consumption

Underage drinking

- Consuming any alcohol under the age of 21; has serious physical, mental, social, and legal consequences

Moderate drinking (also called *social drinking*)

- Consuming no more than one drink on the same occasion for females and no more than two drinks on the same occasion for males; involves *occasionally* consuming alcohol, not consuming alcohol every day

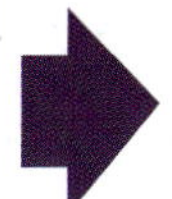

Binge drinking

- Consuming four or more drinks on the same occasion for females and five or more drinks on the same occasion for males in a short amount of time; can cause serious health consequences

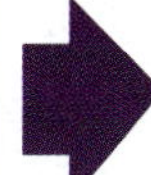

Heavy drinking

- Consuming eight or more drinks in one week for females and 15 or more drinks in one week for males; can easily lead to psychological and physical dependence

Figure 12.4 Moderate drinking can lead to binge drinking or heavy drinking. Underage drinking at any rate has serious consequences to health. ***What groups of people should not drink alcohol under any circumstances?***

Effects of Alcohol on the Brain

depressant substance that slows down the central nervous system, including the brain

Consuming alcohol has immediate and long-term effects on the brain. Alcohol is a type of drug called a **depressant**, which slows down the central nervous system, including the brain. When alcohol reaches the brain, it changes levels of certain *neurotransmitters*, or chemicals that affect body processes and cognition. These changes affect thinking and behavior.

Immediate Effects

As soon as alcohol reaches the brain, it impacts particular parts of the brain in different ways (**Figure 12.5**):

inhibition psychological restraint that keeps people from acting in dangerous ways

- **Cerebral cortex:** The cerebral cortex controls thinking. In the cerebral cortex, alcohol reduces the brain's ability to process information. This makes it difficult for a person to think clearly and accurately observe surroundings. Alcohol also reduces **inhibition**, the psychological restraint that keeps people from taking dangerous risks. Reduced inhibition can lead to poor decision-making and aggression.
- **Cerebellum:** Alcohol disrupts the cerebellum, which controls movement and balance. Consuming alcohol can make it difficult for a person to walk steadily and coordinate other body movements. This leads to longer reaction times, slurred speech, and accidents, including motor vehicle accidents and falls.
- **Hypothalamus and pituitary gland:** The hypothalamus and pituitary gland control the release of hormones in the body. Alcohol's effect on these structures changes hormone levels in ways that may increase sexual arousal. Reduced inhibition and increased sexual arousal can lead to poor sexual decision-making, which can result in pregnancy or a sexually transmitted infection (STI).

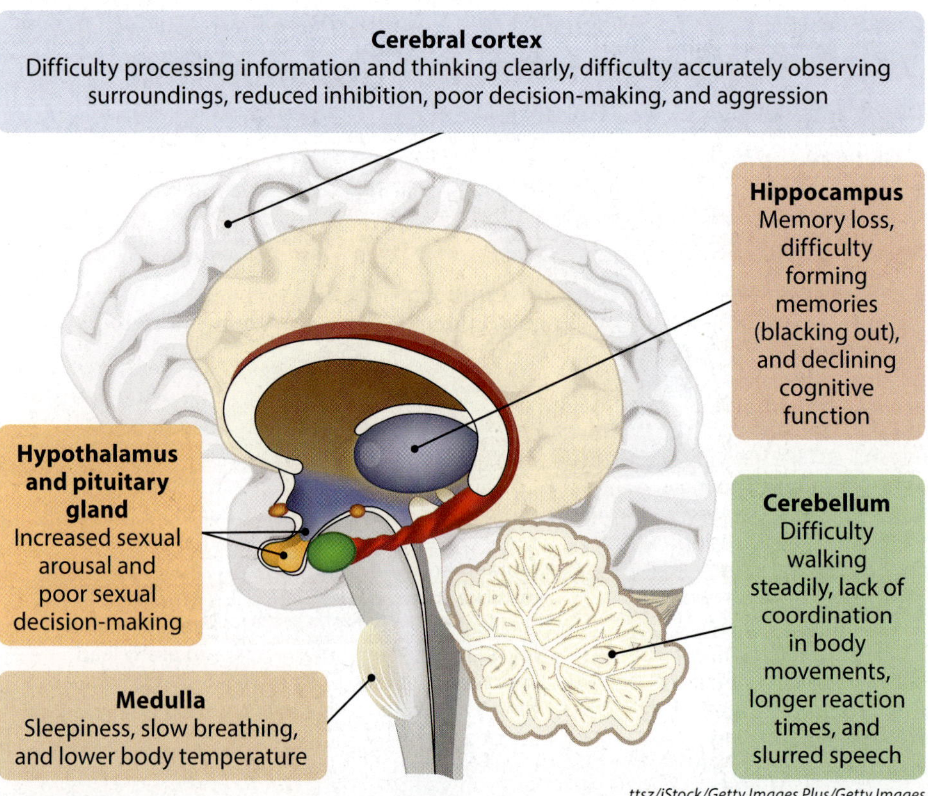

Figure 12.5 Certain structures of the brain control thinking, movement, balance, hormones, breathing, consciousness, learning, and memory. Alcohol disrupts each of these body functions.

- **Medulla:** The medulla controls automatic functions in the body, such as breathing and consciousness. Alcohol disrupts the medulla and causes sleepiness, slow breathing, and lower body temperature. Large amounts of alcohol can cause a person's breathing to slow dramatically and body temperature to drop. This can lead to life-threatening health conditions and even death.
- **Hippocampus:** The hippocampus is a brain structure linked to learning and memory. Alcohol interferes with how the hippocampus forms memories. Consuming a lot of alcohol can lead to memory loss, sometimes called *blacking out*. Long-term alcohol use can increase risk for *dementia*, a neurological condition characterized by memory loss and declining cognitive function.

The more alcohol a person consumes, the more significant effects alcohol will have on the brain. At low levels, alcohol usually leads to relatively minor changes in the brain's functioning. People who have had one drink may feel less inhibited, speak more loudly, and use more body movements. When a person consumes larger amounts of alcohol, especially in a short period of time, there are corresponding large changes in the brain (**Figure 12.6**).

Path to Addiction

Like nicotine, alcohol is an addictive drug. Consuming alcohol can cause changes in the brain that lead to physical and psychological dependence. People who are dependent on alcohol can develop an **alcohol use disorder (AUD)**, which is a type of substance use disorder. As you learned in Chapter 7, *substance use disorders* are mental illnesses in which people keep using a substance despite its negative effects.

alcohol use disorder (AUD) substance use disorder in which a person has an addiction to alcohol and continues to consume it despite negative health effects

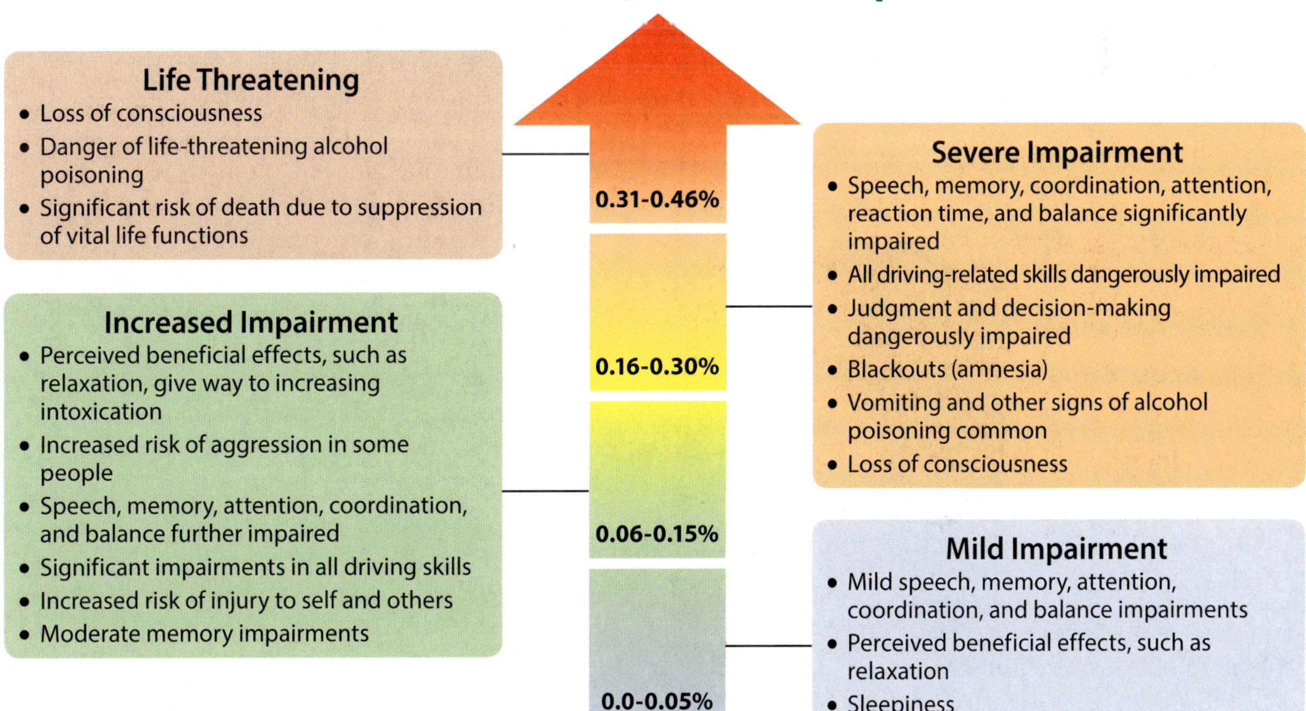

Figure 12.6 Remember that BAC increases faster for females than males and slower for heavier people than for lighter people. ***What neurological condition is associated with the long-term impact of alcohol on the hippocampus?***

Local and Global Health

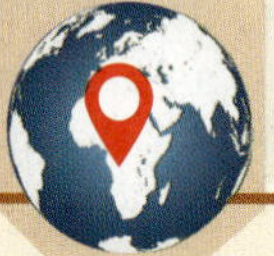

Consequences of Alcohol Use

A recent scientific study examined the health risks of alcohol in 195 countries around the world. Its findings revealed that alcohol use causes nearly three million deaths each year, including 12 percent of deaths in males ages 15–49. Alcohol use was linked with deaths caused by

- cardiovascular diseases, such as stroke;
- cancer, including breast, colorectal, and liver cancer;
- diabetes, pancreatitis, and tuberculosis;
- unintentional injuries, including drowning, poisoning, and motor vehicle accidents; and
- intentional injuries, including self-harm and interpersonal violence.

Many of the countries with the lowest rates of death caused by alcohol were in the Middle East—for example, Iran, Syria, and Saudi Arabia. Many of the countries with the highest rates of death caused by alcohol were in Eastern Europe or Central Asia—including Russia, Ukraine, and Mongolia.

Researchers noted that, in addition to physical health consequences, alcohol use can have negative social consequences. For example, alcohol use can cause harm to family members, friends, coworkers, and strangers. It can also have harmful effects on a country's economy.

Practice Your Skills

Access Information

In a small group, choose one of the consequences associated with alcohol use. This consequence can relate to physical, mental and emotional, or social health. Research this consequence using reliable resources and examine how alcohol use leads to it. Then research how common this consequence is in the US and in two other countries. How common is this consequence in the US compared to the two other countries? What factors do you think might explain this difference? What can people do to reduce their risk for this consequence? Share your findings with the class.

No one who drinks alcohol intends to develop an addiction or substance use disorder. As you learned in chapters 7 and 11, addiction develops gradually, through a series of stages. During the experimentation stage, a person may drink alcohol with friends or drink occasionally. A person may also use alcohol to feel more relaxed or less self-conscious and start drinking more frequently. Someone who regularly uses alcohol may not drink every day, but may drink in a predictable way, such as on weekends, at parties, or when stressed.

As the stages progress, the brain adapts to the presence of alcohol in the body. To counteract how alcohol slows the central nervous system, the brain produces more chemicals that speed up activity. This is an attempt to compensate for the influence of alcohol. Once this happens, the brain has to readjust if the person stops drinking alcohol. This leads to unpleasant withdrawal symptoms. Even drinking small amounts of alcohol during the teen years can lead to long-term alcohol issues (**Figure 12.7**).

People who start drinking alcohol before
15 years of age
are
5x
more likely to develop an alcohol use disorder than those who begin drinking as adults.

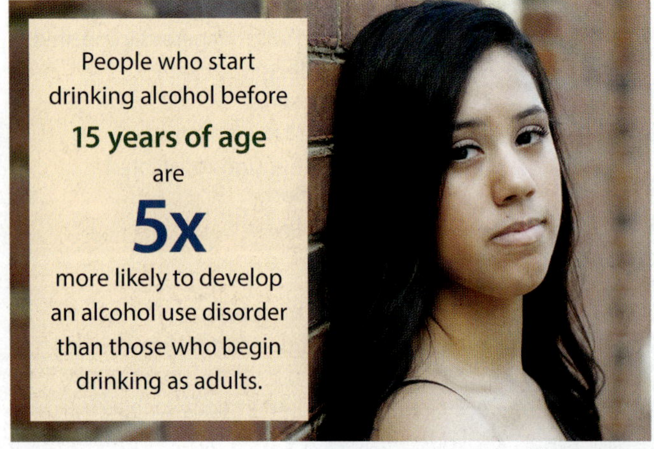

tammykayphoto/Shutterstock.com

Figure 12.7 Experimenting with alcohol early increases the risk of developing an alcohol use disorder later in life.

Long-Term Brain Damage

Excessive alcohol use over time can have negative effects on the brain and cognitive functioning. People who begin drinking early in life experience changes in brain development. One recent study found that young people who binge-drink show permanent changes in their brains, including learning and memory difficulties. People who drink heavily or binge-drink on a regular basis can experience neurological conditions, including dementia, stroke, difficulty remembering, disorientation, and drowsiness.

Binge drinking during adolescence permanently changes how the brain functions. Teens who drink heavily show damage in the *white matter* of the brain, which allows information to travel between different parts of the brain. Damage to the white matter of the brain can lead to long-term issues with thinking, learning, and memory. Alcohol use also damages the *prefrontal cortex*, which controls attention, concentration, decision-making, and self-control.

When these parts of the brain are damaged, people find it harder to control their behavior. This increases risk of engaging in dangerous behaviors, such as drinking excessively or driving after drinking alcohol. This is one reason scientists consistently say there is "no known safe level of binge drinking."

Other Physical Health Effects

Because alcohol is distributed throughout the entire body, it affects every organ and body system. Regular consumption of excessive amounts of alcohol is, therefore, associated with serious and sometimes life threatening consequences.

Hangover

The consequences of alcohol consumption continue even after alcohol has left a person's body. Most people who engage in heavy drinking experience a **hangover**, or negative symptoms caused by excessive alcohol use (**Figure 12.8**).

The negative symptoms of a hangover develop because of the changes alcohol causes in the body. When alcohol reaches the brain, it causes the pituitary gland to stop producing the hormone *vasopressin*. This hormone helps the body reabsorb liquids. Without enough vasopressin, liquids go straight to the bladder and leave the body. This means the body expels about four times as much liquid as it consumed, causing dehydration. This dehydration may result in thirst, headaches, and muscle aches.

The body reacts to dehydration by moving water from other parts of the body, including the brain. When water is removed, the brain gets smaller, which places pressure on the membranes connecting the brain to the skull. The overall result is a headache, dizziness, and sensitivity to light and sound. Loss of liquid also causes the loss of essential substances, including salt, potassium, and magnesium. Low levels of these substances cause feelings of tiredness, lack of coordination, and overall weakness.

In addition to these effects, alcohol irritates the lining of the stomach by increasing stomach acid. This can lead to stomach pain, nausea, and vomiting. Alcohol use disrupts REM sleep, leading to difficulty sleeping. Alcohol use also decreases blood sugar, which leads to weakness, shakiness, difficulty concentrating, anxiety, depression, irritability, and fatigue.

hangover negative symptoms caused by excessive alcohol use; for example, nausea, fatigue, and headaches

Symptoms of a Hangover

- Tiredness
- Dizziness and feeling that the room is spinning
- Sensitivity to light and sound
- Headaches
- Muscle aches
- Nausea and vomiting
- Difficulty sleeping
- Dehydration and thirst
- Shakiness
- Depression, anxiety, and irritability
- Difficulty concentrating

Figure 12.8 As alcohol leaves the body, a person may experience these symptoms.

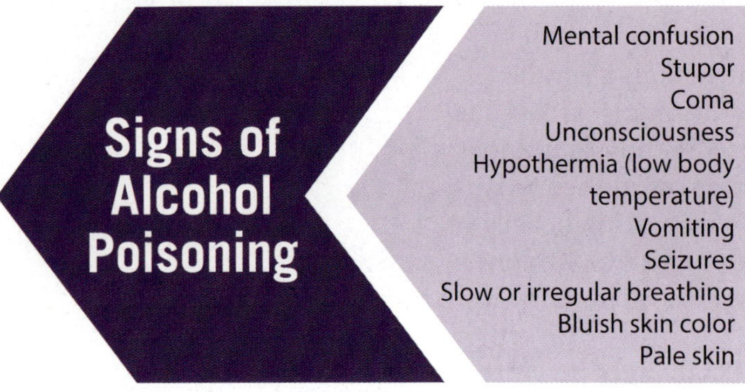

Figure 12.9 Alcohol poisoning can lead to loss of consciousness, low blood pressure and body temperature, and difficulty breathing. ***What should you do if you suspect someone has alcohol poisoning?***

Alcohol Poisoning

Alcohol slows down the nervous system and suppresses various body functions. If a person consumes too much alcohol, these body functions can become suppressed to the point of serious danger. **Alcohol poisoning**, also known as an *alcohol overdose*, is a medical emergency that occurs when a high concentration of alcohol in the blood has life-threatening effects (**Figure 12.9**). Extreme levels of alcohol consumption, usually a BAC of 0.40% or higher, can lead to permanent brain damage and death. If you suspect someone has alcohol poisoning, seek help immediately by calling 911.

alcohol poisoning medical emergency in which a person consumes more alcohol than the body can break down; alcohol suppresses the nervous system and vital body functions to dangerous levels; also called *alcohol overdose*

cirrhosis buildup of scar tissue in the liver

fetal alcohol spectrum disorders (FASD) set of health conditions that affect the baby born to a person who has consumed alcohol during the pregnancy

Chronic Health Conditions

Alcohol use over time and during pregnancy can lead to the development of chronic health conditions. Consuming large amounts of alcohol causes fat to build up in the liver, which blocks blood flow. Eventually, this can cause **cirrhosis**, a buildup of scar tissue in the liver (**Figure 12.10**).

Heavy drinking, including binge drinking, can lead to cardiovascular health conditions, including an irregular heartbeat, high blood pressure, and heart attacks. Digestive health conditions and some types of cancer are associated with alcohol use. Alcohol use is also linked to several types of oral cancer, including cancers of the esophagus, larynx, lips and oral cavity, pharynx, and nasopharynx.

Alcohol use can cause reproductive health conditions. In males, heavy drinking lowers testosterone levels, reduces the amount and quality of sperm, and makes it harder to get an erection. In females, even small amounts of alcohol, such as one to five drinks a week, can reduce fertility.

Alcohol use during pregnancy can cause serious health conditions for the baby. These health conditions are called **fetal alcohol spectrum disorders (FASD)**. Typically, these conditions are present at birth and include

- poor growth (before and after birth);
- decreased muscle tone and poor coordination;
- delayed intellectual, speech, physical, and social development;
- heart conditions; and
- changes in facial development.

For these reasons, people who are pregnant, may become pregnant, or are trying to become pregnant should not consume any alcohol at all.

Figure 12.10 Cirrhosis is a leading cause of death in the US. ***How does alcohol use lead to cirrhosis?***

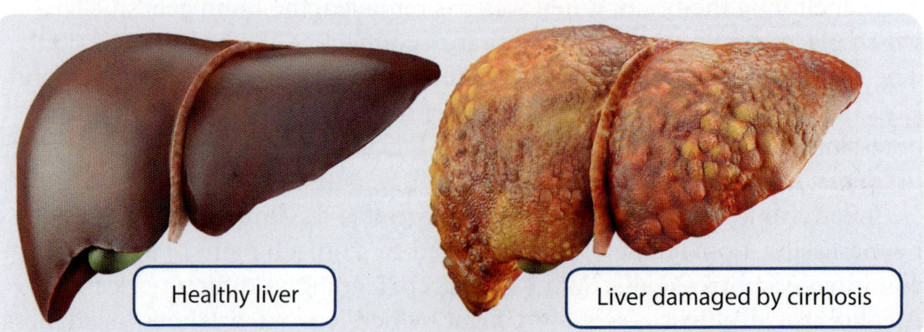

iStock.com/eranicle

Mental, Social, and Legal Consequences

Alcohol use affects not just a person's physical health, but also mental, emotional, and social health. Consuming alcohol can also lead to legal consequences that follow a person throughout life.

35%
of people who have experienced some kind of violent attack report that the person who assaulted them was under the influence of alcohol.

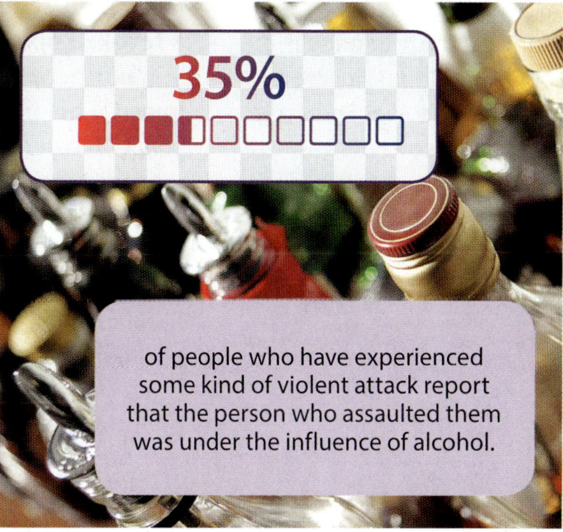

Bottles: Marcio Jose Bastos Silva/Shutterstock.com; Percentage: LVM/Shutterstock.com

Figure 12.11 Alcohol use can result in increased aggression and reduced inhibitions. This increases risk of engaging in acts of violence. ***Which part of the brain can cause aggression and reduced inhibitions when impaired by alcohol?***

Risky Behaviors

Alcohol impacts a person's ability to process information. This means that people who consume alcohol have trouble planning, using judgment, and thinking about the consequences of behavior. For this reason, people who have been drinking alcohol are more likely to engage in risky behaviors. Risky behaviors associated with alcohol use include sexual activity and violence.

People who have been drinking alcohol are more likely to engage in risky sexual behaviors, including unprotected sexual activity and sex with different partners. These behaviors can result in unintended pregnancy, sexually transmitted infections (STIs), and HIV. People who have been drinking also have a higher risk of committing and experiencing sexual violence. Sexually risky behaviors can cause feelings of guilt, fear of being caught, and fear of earning a bad reputation.

People who have been drinking alcohol are more likely to behave violently than those who have not (**Figure 12.11**). Alcohol use is also associated with family violence, including child abuse and neglect and violence between romantic partners. Teens who drink alcohol are more likely to die by suicide or commit homicide.

Accidents

Alcohol slows down the central nervous system, lengthening reaction time and disrupting coordination. This makes tasks such as driving dangerous and increases a person's likelihood of accidents.

Some of the most serious consequences of alcohol use result from people driving after drinking alcohol. In the US, more than 1.4 million drivers are arrested for driving after using alcohol or drugs every year. More than 10,000 people die each year in alcohol-related motor vehicle crashes. Driving after drinking alcohol is extremely dangerous and can hurt or kill not only you, but also your passengers and other people in your community (**Figure 12.12**).

How Does Drinking Alcohol Make It Unsafe to Drive?

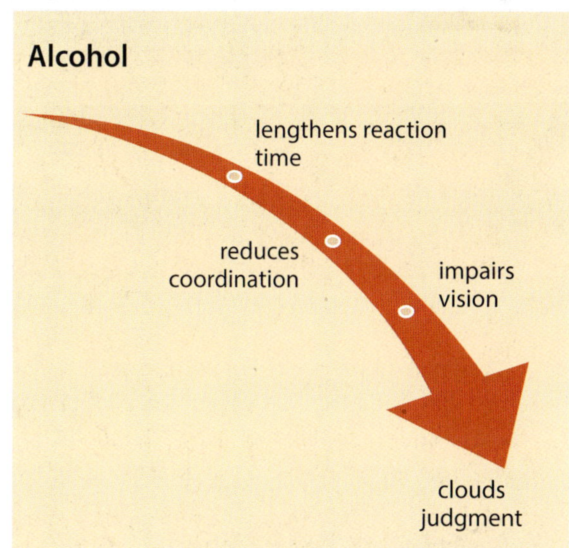

rawf8/Shutterstock.com

Figure 12.12 Drinking alcohol and driving is always unsafe to yourself and others. It is also unsafe to ride with a driver who has been drinking alcohol. ***What is the legal BAC limit for driving for people 21 years of age and older?***

driving under the influence (DUI) operating a motor vehicle with a blood alcohol concentration at or over 0.08% for adults; for teens, this level is lower and varies by state; also known as *driving while intoxicated (DWI)* or *drunk driving*

For people 21 years of age and older, the legal BAC limit for driving is 0.08%. Adults who drive with a BAC of 0.08% or higher can be charged with **driving under the influence (DUI)** or *driving while intoxicated (DWI)*. Drivers who receive a DUI or DWI may have their licenses suspended or revoked and be required to perform community service, pay fines, or serve jail time. Penalties typically increase for repeat offenders, and someone with a revoked license may not be given the license back, even after reapplying.

For people under 21 years of age, the legal BAC limit for driving is lower. This limit varies by state, and many states follow a *zero-tolerance policy*. Under zero-tolerance laws, the only acceptable BAC level for people younger than 21 years of age is 0%. Penalties for violating a zero-tolerance policy vary from state to state.

Alcohol use is also associated with other accidents and injuries. Consuming alcohol increases a person's risk of falls, burns, homicides, suicides, unintentional firearm injuries, electrical shocks, and incidents of near drowning. Alcohol use also increases the likelihood of death while bicycling and swimming.

Mental Health Effects

People may drink alcohol because it makes them feel more relaxed and calm or less self-conscious. These feelings of calm result from alcohol acting as a depressant and slowing down the central nervous system.

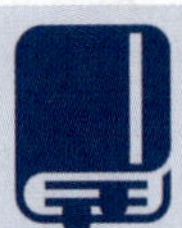

Case Study

The Impact of Alcohol

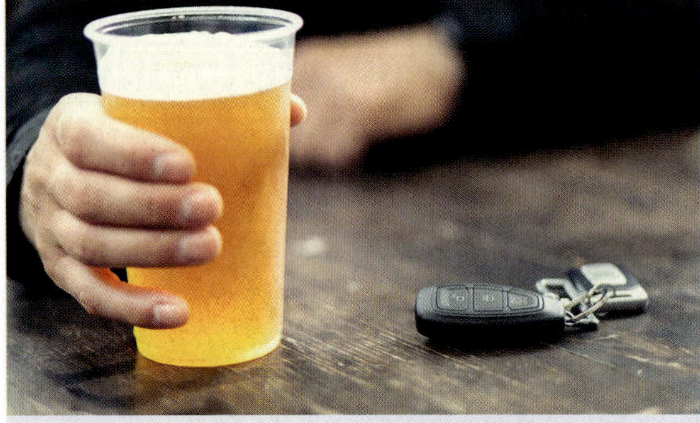

rzoze19/iStock/Getty Images Plus/Getty Images

Casey is 14 years old. For as long as Casey can remember, her father has consumed a lot of alcohol. He has a couple shots of whiskey after he returns home from work and drinks several beers with dinner. Casey has stopped having friends over in the evenings because she is embarrassed by her father's behavior. He speaks loudly and is clumsy when he helps clear the table. Casey's parents have been arguing more often, especially since he was fired from his job because of his drinking.

Cole thought he was just going to a casual hangout with his friends, until some of his friends there started drinking. At the hangout, Cole gets concerned when he notices Diego, who drove him to the hangout, is one of the people drinking. By the end of the night, Cole does not feel comfortable letting Diego drive him home. Cole would drive them home himself, but he does not have his driver's license yet. Cole does not want to call his parents because he knows they will freak out if he tells them what is happening.

Practice Your Skills

Practice Health-Enhancing Behaviors

Based on their situations, how could Casey and Cole respond? What resources could help Casey manage the situation at home? What could Cole do to make sure Diego does not drive while under the influence of alcohol? Working in a small group, brainstorm different actions or responses Casey and Cole could use to help them handle or solve their situations. Then take turns role-playing the scenarios. Demonstrate steps both teens could take.

The calm associated with alcohol use does not last, however. Once alcohol leaves the body, the feelings that were present before a person used alcohol will return. In addition, alcohol can lead to behaviors a person later regrets and increase feelings of depression or tiredness. In this way, alcohol can worsen the symptoms and severity of mental health conditions and negative feelings.

Alcohol use can also lead to mental health conditions. Consuming alcohol can lead to an alcohol use disorder (AUD), which you learned about earlier in this lesson. Like other types of substance use disorders, AUD makes existing mental health conditions worse, harms a person's relationships, and compromises a person's goals.

Sometimes, heavy drinking can lead people to develop certain types of mental illnesses. People who drink heavily may develop an *alcohol-induced disorder*, or a health condition caused by the effects of alcohol. Common alcohol-induced disorders include anxiety disorders, mood disorders, sexual dysfunction, and sleep disorders.

Social Consequences

Alcohol use affects a person's relationships among family and peers and in the community. Consuming alcohol can cause strained relationships with family and friends. Feelings of guilt and fear may result from disappointing loved ones, and friends may become distant if they do not want to drink alcohol. Engaging in risky behaviors can threaten personal and community safety and harm relationships among community members.

Teens who consume alcohol may experience consequences that can negatively impact future educational plans and school relationships (**Figure 12.13**). It may also result in people missing work, behaving poorly, or being disciplined for alcohol use on the job.

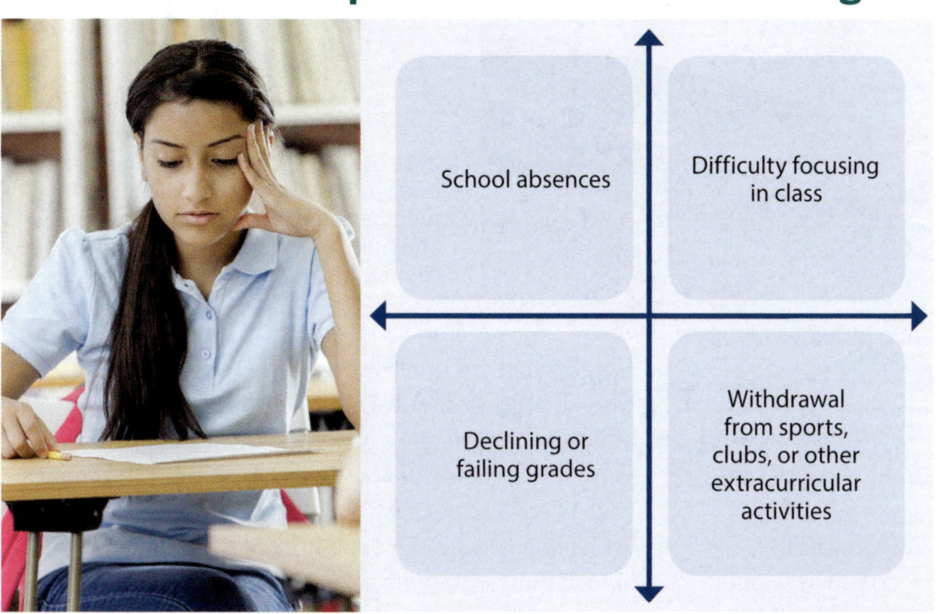

Figure 12.13 Drinking alcohol can disrupt teens' success in school in many ways.

Health Across the Life Span

The Consequences of Drunk Driving Do Not Go Away

Teens often think about the immediate consequences of their behavior—about what will happen right now. In the short-term, alcohol reduces inhibitions and causes impairment. Driving after drinking might seem like no big deal. Driving under the influence is a behavior that has long-term consequences, however. A DUI or motor vehicle accident can change a community and each person's life.

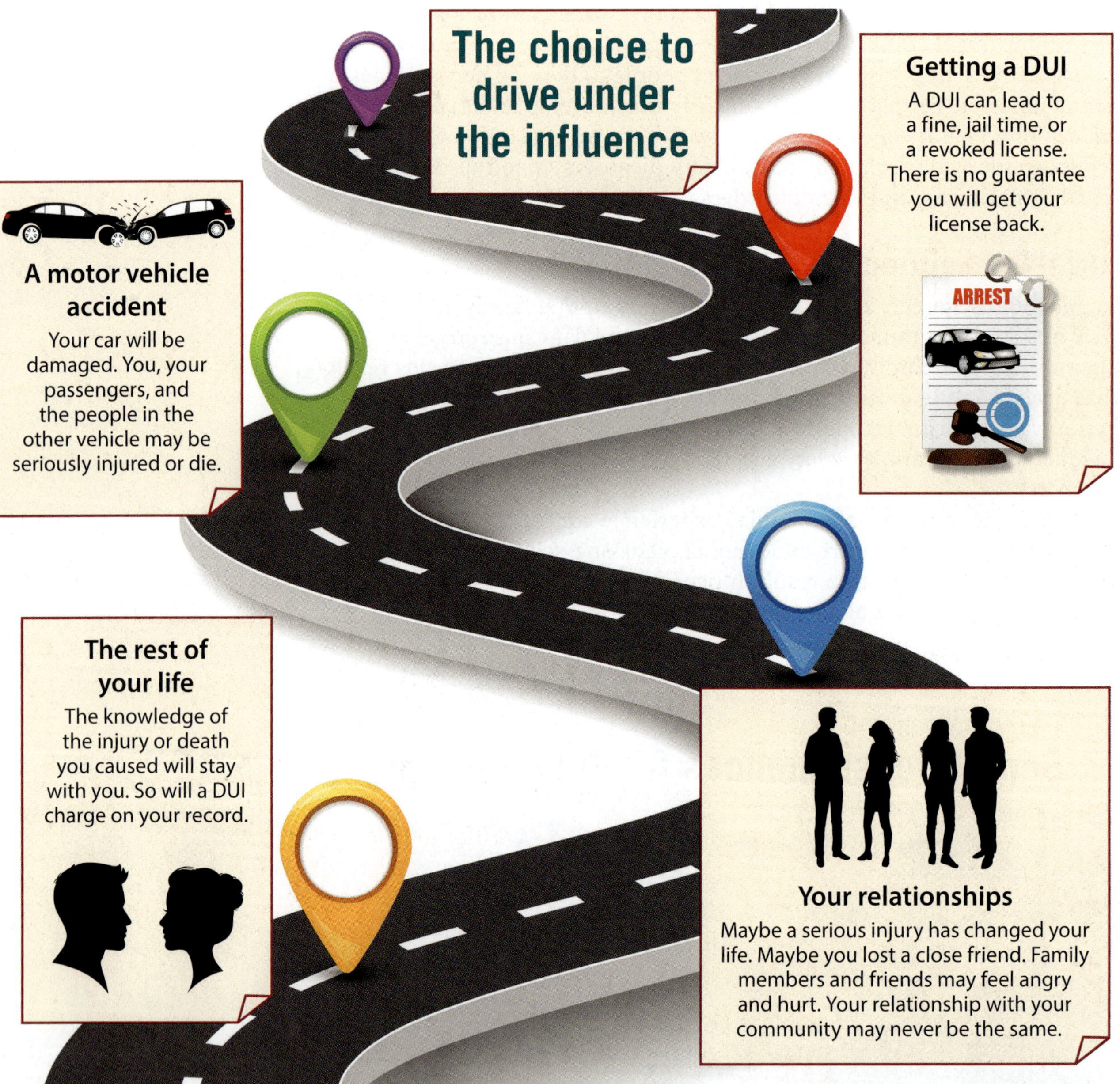

Practice Your Skills

Advocate for Health

On your own, list all of the potential consequences a teen could face for driving under the influence, getting a DUI, and getting into a motor vehicle accident. Then share your list with a partner. Discuss why some teens drink alcohol and drive, despite the very serious consequences. What strategies do you think would help teens make better choices and not drive under the influence? Think about steps you could take to encourage teens in your school and community to avoid driving under the influence. Commit to act on one of these ideas with your partner.

Road: Kolonko/Shutterstock.com; Icons clockwise from top left: PanicAttack/Shutterstock.com; Iarionova Olga 1 1/Shutterstock.com; Pavlo S/Shutterstock.com; Chipmunk131/Shutterstock.com

Legal Consequences

Alcohol use is illegal for anyone younger than 21 years of age. If teens are caught using alcohol, this can lead to legal consequences. Teens may be required to pay a fine (as much as $500), take a class about alcohol use, and perform community service. Teens' driver's licenses may be suspended so they cannot drive. Teens can also face legal consequences for trying to purchase alcohol, using a fake identification, or sharing alcohol with another underage person. Teens can face additional consequences for driving with any level of alcohol in their bodies.

Lesson 12.1 Review

Know and Understand

1. What BAC indicates that a person is legally impaired?
2. Why do males typically feel the effects of alcohol more slowly than females?
3. How is binge drinking different from moderate drinking?
4. Choose one symptom of a hangover and explain how excessive alcohol use causes it.
5. Why does alcohol use increase a person's risk of being in an accident?

Think Critically

6. With a partner, give some examples of inhibitions. How would your behavior change if alcohol lessened these inhibitions?
7. Review what you learned about substance use disorders in Chapter 7. What are the stages of substance use? What might each stage look like for someone who is using alcohol?
8. Write two case studies in which people use alcohol to cope with negative feelings or a mental health condition. How does alcohol influence each person's feelings? Trade case studies with a partner and list healthier strategies each person could use to cope.
9. Search online for stories about people who have a family member with an AUD. How has alcohol use impacted the relationships in these families? How has alcohol use impacted the communities around these families?
10. Using reliable resources, research the laws about alcohol consumption, purchase, and possession in your state. What penalties could a teen who drinks or buys alcohol or uses a fake identification face?

REAL WORLD Health Skills

Communicate with Others Imagine you write an advice column for your school newspaper. It is your job to maturely answer all questions submitted to the newspaper. Suppose you receive the following message from a sophomore.

> My brother is in college. Ever since he turned 21, he has been drinking heavily every weekend. When I ask him why, he says because it is legal. I'm really worried about his health. Can you please tell me how alcohol affects the body, especially the brain?
> *Signed, Sophomore Sister*

Write a response to this message that you would publish in your column. Use effective communication skills and show empathy, keeping in mind your target audience.

Lesson 12.2

Preventing and Treating Alcohol Abuse

Essential Question?

What skills can you use to prevent alcohol use and help those who abuse alcohol?

Learning Outcomes

After studying this lesson, you will be able to

- analyze influences on alcohol use, including genetic makeup, mental health conditions, and environment;
- list government approaches to reducing alcohol use;
- describe strategies for preventing alcohol use and refusing offers of alcohol;
- explain the treatment options available to people with an alcohol use disorder (AUD); and
- assess how you can help someone with an AUD.

Key Terms

Alcoholics Anonymous (AA)
detoxification
enabling

Warm-Up Activity

Agree or Disagree

Access Information Before reading this lesson, record whether you agree or disagree with each statement in the chart shown. Using valid and reliable websites, search for evidence that either proves or disproves each statement. Write down the website and a concise answer. After reading the lesson, consider the statements again based on any new information you read. Then, record again whether you agree or disagree, and check to see whether your opinion changed based on new evidence.

Statements
1. Alcohol use in teens can cause issues with brain development.
2. Learning effective refusal skills can help you avoid alcohol if your peers offer it to you.
3. One of the most effective ways a government tries to decrease alcohol use is by setting a drinking age.
4. Increasing the cost of alcohol by 10 percent led to a 50 percent decrease in deaths caused by alcohol use.
5. The first step in recovering from an alcohol use disorder is detoxification.
6. Alcoholics Anonymous (AA) has 10 distinct steps a person must follow to recover from an alcohol use disorder.
7. Figuring out why a person drinks is an essential step for giving up alcohol.
8. Covering up someone's drinking is called *enabling*.

The effects of alcohol can change a person's life. In the moment, they can change your feelings and thoughts and lead you to behave in ways that embarrass you later. If you drink and drive, you can injure yourself and others and may face long-lasting legal consequences. Analyzing influences on alcohol use and using skills to prevent alcohol use can help you protect your health. Learning about treatment will prepare you to help others in your life who might have a dependence on alcohol.

Factors Affecting Alcohol Use

Think about the exposure to alcohol in your life. Do your parents or guardians occasionally drink alcohol? How many movies and shows have you seen that featured characters drinking alcohol? Does your family have a history of heavy drinking? All of these factors contribute to your decisions about alcohol. Risk and protective factors for alcohol use include the following.

Individual Factors

Individual factors related to identity and behaviors influence risk for alcohol use. These factors include genetic makeup and mental health.

Research has shown that genetic factors contribute to alcohol use (**Figure 12.14**). Some research suggests that people with specific genes have a greater risk of developing an AUD. For example, people with a particular gene may be less sensitive to the effects of alcohol, which usually act as a signal to stop drinking. People who feel less influenced by alcohol may drink even more. This pattern can lead to dependence and an AUD.

Genetic Impact on AUD

If one twin drinks heavily or has an AUD, this person's identical twin is **twice** as likely as a fraternal twin to have similar issues.

Left to right: New Africa/Shutterstock.com; kate_sept2004/E+/Getty Images

Figure 12.14 Alcohol use is more commonly linked among identical twins than fraternal twins, which indicates that genetic factors play a role.

Research in Action

Co-Occurring Disorders: Substance Use and Mental Health

A person's mental health has a significant effect on risk for consuming alcohol and developing an AUD. To examine the link between mental health and substance use, researchers at Binghamton University recruited more than 500 college students across the US to complete an anonymous survey. The survey asked about students' academic performance, substance use, and mental health conditions.

The results of this study revealed major differences between students. Students who reported low levels of mental health conditions had positive attitudes about learning, high academic effort, a high GPA (above a 3.0), and no substance use. Students experiencing severe mental health conditions reported a poor academic attitude, low GPA, and excessive alcohol use.

These findings suggest that there is a strong link between mental health conditions and the use of substances such as alcohol. Using substances can lead to a substance use disorder. When a substance use disorder occurs alongside another mental health condition, it is called a co-occurring disorder.

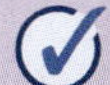

Practice Your Skills

Set Goals

With a partner, discuss the different factors that could explain the link between mental health and substance use. What evidence would you need to test which factors best explain this relationship? Do you think the same link between mental health and substance use would be found in high school students? Why or why not? With your partner, set five SMART goals related to maintaining mental health and preventing substance use. Consider the goals you set in the Unit 2 *Health Management Plan* and try to choose goals that have been effective for you in the past. Explain how each goal reduces your risk for using a substance.

People with mental health conditions also have a greater risk of using alcohol and developing an AUD. People may use alcohol to cope with negative feelings, such as anxiety and depression. They may also use alcohol to cheer themselves up or sleep. Using alcohol to handle these issues is called *self-medication*. This association between mental health conditions and alcohol use is complex. Alcohol use can also cause mental health conditions or make existing conditions worse.

Influence of Family on Alcohol Use

Children whose family members have accepting attitudes toward alcohol are more likely to engage in heavy drinking.

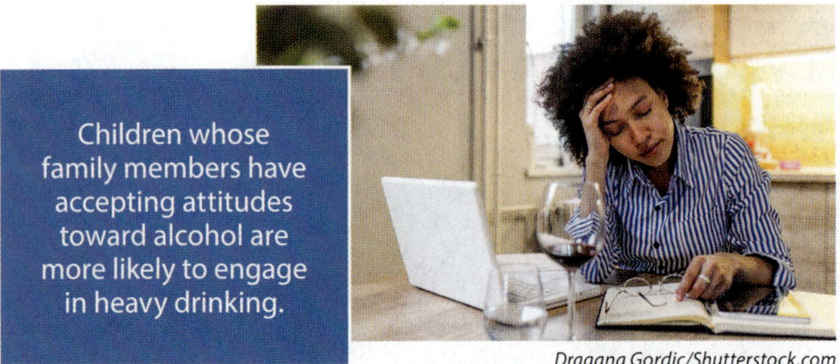

Dragana Gordic/Shutterstock.com

Figure 12.15 People inherit many behavioral habits from what they witness throughout childhood and adolescence. Drinking alcohol, especially in times of stress or celebration, is among them. ***What is the term for using alcohol to cope with negative feelings or difficulty sleeping?***

Environment

Environment includes a person's family, culture, peers, community, and the media. All of these factors influence alcohol use.

Families and cultures have their own attitudes, beliefs, and rules about alcohol use (**Figure 12.15**). Children learn about occasions for drinking, such as stressful days or celebrations, by watching their family members' drinking habits. Through these examples, they can learn that people drink alcohol to cope with negative emotions and enhance positive emotions.

Health in the Media

The Impact of Alcohol Advertisements

Think about the last time you saw an advertisement for alcohol. What images did the advertisement include? Alcohol advertisements are designed to show young, attractive people drinking in appealing settings and having a good time. Advertisements do not show the consequences of excessive alcohol use, including engaging in embarrassing and risky behavior, feeling sick, and getting in trouble with the law.

Alcohol advertisements on social media are especially likely to increase interest in drinking if they include pro-drinking comments from other people. Researchers at the University of Connecticut School of Medicine showed people online advertisements that included pro-drinking or anti-drinking comments. Some advertisements had many responses (likes, shares, and comments), and others had a small number. People who saw advertisements with pro-drinking comments reported more desire to drink alcohol than people who saw advertisements with anti-drinking comments. These findings show the negative effects of alcohol advertisements on social media and how quickly these advertisements can spread.

Practice Your Skills

Analyze Influences

With a partner, discuss what this study shows about the link between alcohol advertisements and people's attitudes toward alcohol. What alcohol advertisements have you seen on social media or elsewhere? How have these advertisements influenced your perceptions of alcohol? How does alcohol use in these advertisements compare to the reality of alcohol use? With a partner, discuss how you think alcohol advertisements impact students at your school. What rules or regulations do you think should be put into place regarding social media advertisements for alcohol? How could you work toward pushing for these changes? What impact would these changes have on how advertisements influence alcohol use among teens?

People tend to drink more alcohol when they have friends who drink. Watching peers drink alcohol creates the belief that alcohol use is appropriate and desirable. People also drink more when they are part of a group than when they are alone. Teens are often mistaken about how much other people actually drink. In fact, many teens are uncomfortable with drinking alcohol. Even most college students believe that there is *too* much alcohol use on campus.

Alcohol use is frequently shown in TV shows and films, even those marketed to children. People who see drinking in movies tend to view alcohol use more positively. In one study, more than 6,000 teens completed surveys about their drinking behavior, movies they had seen, and their home environment. Teens who had seen the most movies including alcohol use were twice as likely to report drinking alcohol. Researchers in another study found that teens whose friends posted photos of themselves consuming alcohol on social media sites were likely to drink themselves. Viewing photos of peers drinking alcohol on social media is an indirect form of virtual peer pressure.

The decisions you make about alcohol today will impact the rest of your life. Avoiding alcohol during adolescence is especially important because drinking alcohol can lead to changes in brain development and long-term dependence on alcohol later in life. Fortunately, there are strategies you can use to avoid alcohol use and keep yourself safe.

Preventing Alcohol Use

Most people know about the harmful effects of alcohol. For this reason, national, state, and local governments regulate alcohol in several ways (**Figure 12.16**). Following are some strategies you can take in your own life to avoid alcohol use.

Pay Attention to Mental Health

Paying attention to your mental health and managing negative feelings and stress is an important part of avoiding alcohol use. Often, people drink alcohol in an attempt to feel better. Alcohol may temporarily distract people from the issues they are facing, but it does not make those issues go away. In fact, it can cause even bigger issues.

If you are struggling with negative feelings, stress, or mental health conditions, take steps to build your self-esteem, express emotions, adopt a positive mind-set, and manage stress. Some healthy ways of managing stress might include getting physical activity, writing in a journal, or spending time with friends. These approaches will help you reduce stress instead of causing more stress. You can also think about stress in a new way. Try to reframe negative events as challenges and opportunities.

Government Regulations on Alcohol Use

Type of Regulation	Description
Legal drinking age of 21	Forbidding people who are younger than 21 years of age from purchasing alcohol makes it more difficult for teens to access alcohol. It is also illegal to use a fake identification to purchase alcohol. People under the age of 21 are also not allowed to possess alcohol, accept it from others, or share it with others. Some states restrict people who are under 21 from entering businesses, such as bars, where the primary purpose is to serve alcohol.
Limits on when, where, and to whom alcohol is sold	In some states, alcohol is not sold on Sundays or in grocery and convenience stores. This limits people's ability to purchase alcohol, which helps reduce heavy drinking. Many states ban serving alcohol to pregnant people or to people who appear intoxicated.
Sales taxes on alcohol	Raising the sales tax on alcohol makes buying alcohol more expensive and discourages the use of alcohol.
Limits on alcohol advertising	Some public policies place limits on alcohol advertisements, including the hours such ads can appear and what they can include.

Figure 12.16 To protect people from the harmful effects of alcohol, governments do their best to discourage its use through various restrictions.

Resist Peer Pressure

Many teens find it hard to resist peer pressure to drink alcohol. That is why it is so important to develop strategies for standing up to peer pressure before it happens. Some strategies you could use include the following:

- Avoid situations in which you think alcohol might be available.
- Surround yourself with friends who encourage and support your healthy decisions. Avoid friends who will pressure you to drink.
- Remind yourself of the negative consequences of drinking alcohol.
- Drink something besides alcohol. If someone offers you an alcoholic drink, you can say you already have something to drink. Always get your drink yourself. If someone hands you a drink, you have no idea if there is alcohol or some other drug in it.
- Never get into a car with a driver who has been drinking alcohol, even if the person claims to feel able to drive. Drinking while under the influence may lead to accidents or fatalities. Get a ride from someone who has not been drinking, or call a parent, guardian, or other trusted adult.

Develop Refusal Skills

Even if you have made the decision not to drink, alcohol may still be present in your environment. Developing and practicing refusal skills can help when others offer you alcohol (**Figure 12.17**).

Participate in Education and Prevention Programs

Education and prevention programs can help stop alcohol use among teens. Many high schools and colleges offer education programs to decrease risky drinking, especially in underage people. These programs include information about the short- and long-term consequences of alcohol use. Other prevention programs focus on the negative effects of alcohol use. You have probably seen ads that portray the negative consequences of drunk driving.

Some prevention programs focus on helping teens feel better about themselves. Teens who lack self-confidence may choose to drink alcohol because they do not have the skills to stand up to peer pressure. Prevention programs may build teens' self-esteem and teach strategies for resisting pressure to drink.

Effective Strategies for Refusing Alcohol
Just say *no*.
No, I don't drink.
I don't have to drink to have fun.
Make a pact with friends to resist pressure together.
No, none of us like to drink.
Leave them alone, they don't want a drink.
Blame not drinking on a health condition.
Drinking makes me sick.
My medication doesn't mix well with alcohol.
Mention other responsibilities you have.
I can't be hungover for work.
I can't let the team down at the game tomorrow.
If you have your license, offer to be the designated driver.
No thanks, I have to drive.
I can't, I'm the DD tonight.
Blame not drinking on another person.
My coach would be so mad.
My parents will say I can't go to parties again.

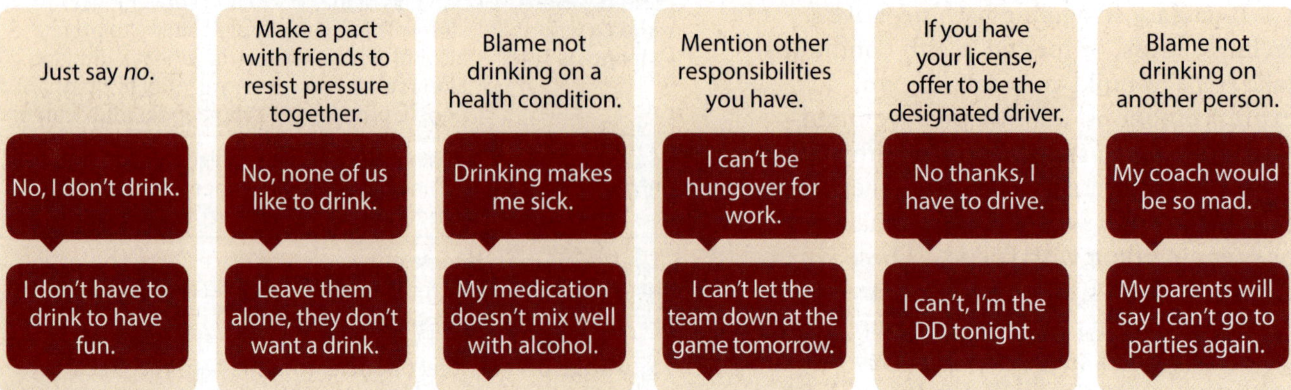

Figure 12.17 To help you refuse alcohol, make a list of reasons you think it is a good idea not to drink alcohol. Practice what you could say to resist pressure to drink alcohol.

Prevention programs may also correct teens' perceptions regarding how others feel about alcohol use. Many teens think other students feel more positively about drinking and drink more than they actually do. Correcting these errors can help teens understand many of their peers actually share their own beliefs about the hazards of alcohol use.

If you are interested in participating in a prevention program, talk to your health teacher. See if you could join a program that already exists. You could also talk to your teacher about starting a new program to advocate for less alcohol use in your school. Talk to your friends or classmates to see if they are interested in working together to reduce alcohol use and improve health in your community.

Treating an Alcohol Use Disorder (AUD)

People with an AUD are physically and psychologically dependent on alcohol. Physically, this means, their bodies require alcohol to function normally. Not drinking alcohol can lead to negative withdrawal symptoms for them. Psychologically, people with an AUD feel like they need alcohol to feel normal. An AUD is a mental illness, and people with it need professional treatment.

detoxification process that allows the body to clear itself of all alcohol or drugs

Detoxification

Often, the first step in treating an AUD is **detoxification**, a process that allows the body to clear itself of all alcohol. During this time, a person does not drink any alcohol and experiences the negative symptoms of withdrawal. Sometimes, withdrawal from alcohol can be severe and include intense anxiety, tremors, and hallucinations. Some doctors prescribe medications to lessen these symptoms. Many people choose to go through detoxification in an inpatient setting. Detoxification from alcohol usually takes two to seven days, but may take up to one month.

Medications and Therapy

Following detoxification, treatment involves methods to help a person not consume more alcohol. These methods include medications and counseling.

Doctors prescribe various medications to help people with an AUD avoid drinking alcohol (**Figure 12.18**). In addition to medications, people with an AUD may receive therapy to break the habit of consuming alcohol and address underlying feelings that lead to alcohol use. A therapist can help people with an AUD learn skills that help them stop drinking. These skills can include identifying behaviors that trigger drinking, managing stress, building a support system, and working toward goals.

Individual therapy can help people develop new skills and strategies for avoiding alcohol use. Sometimes people with an AUD also participate in couples or family therapy to help others in their lives understand how to provide support.

Medications to Treat an AUD

Naltrexone

Reduces the pleasant feelings of alcohol

Antabuse®

Makes people feel extreme nausea or other unpleasant side effects if they consume alcohol

Acamprosate

Decreases alcohol cravings

science photo/Shutterstock.com

Figure 12.18 Medications can help people avoid drinking alcohol by altering how their bodies respond to the use of alcohol. ***What process allows the body to clear itself of all alcohol?***

Support Groups

People with an AUD benefit from continued support. One form of support is community support groups. *Support groups* are groups of people with a common struggle who share the obstacles they face and examples of overcoming them. **Alcoholics Anonymous (AA)** is the most well-known and widely used support group for people with an AUD. The goal of AA is to help people change how they think about drinking alcohol using 12 distinct steps.

Alcoholics Anonymous (AA) support group and program for people with an alcohol use disorder (AUD); outlines 12 steps for overcoming alcohol addiction

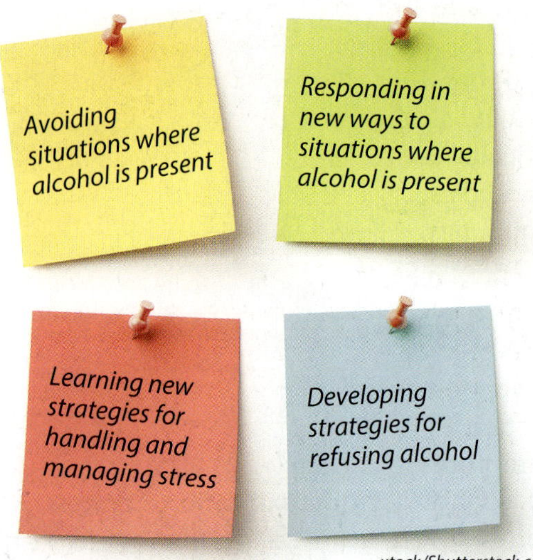

xtock/Shutterstock.com

Figure 12.19 Learning how to manage their own behaviors in situations where alcohol is present can help people with an AUD avoid alcohol.

During AA meetings, group members share alcohol-related struggles, which may help them stop drinking. People who are trying to stop drinking alcohol attend frequent AA meetings, sometimes daily when they are first trying to stop. They may work with a *sponsor*, who provides support, empathy, and accountability.

People who have a family member or friend with an AUD can also benefit from support groups. These groups can help people learn how to cope and can be comforting as family members see other people facing the same challenges. Support groups for family members of people with an AUD include Al-Anon and Alateen.

Self-Management Strategies

Many programs that help people with an AUD also teach self-management strategies. First, these programs focus on helping people become aware of why they consume alcohol. Understanding the motivation to drink alcohol is an important first step in learning how to avoid alcohol.

Next, people develop skills for managing situations in which they want to consume alcohol (**Figure 12.19**).

Skills for Health and Wellness

Reporting Substance Use

Many people who have an AUD believe they can simply stop drinking whenever they want. Unfortunately, this is rarely the case. Treating an AUD requires help from a trained professional. If you care about someone who has an AUD or another substance use disorder, you need to share your concern with a trusted adult to get this person help. For example, you could talk to your parents or guardians. You could also talk to another supportive and understanding adult, such as a teacher, school counselor, other family member, or community leader.

Practice Your Skills

Communicate with Others

Imagine that a close friend of yours has started drinking alcohol. At first, your friend only drank alcohol at parties. Now, your friend drinks alcohol to cope with the stress of school. Your friend's grades are falling, and you barely see your friend at social events anymore. When you told your friend you were worried, your friend laughed it off. Partner with a classmate to role-play how you could talk to a trusted adult to get your friend help. During the discussion, follow these steps:

1. Express how you feel about the person who is using alcohol. You might say, "I care about my friend and worry my friend is going to get hurt."
2. Be specific about the behaviors you have observed. You might share how alcohol use is affecting the person's schoolwork or relationships with friends. You might share the consequences the person has already experienced, such as trouble with the law.
3. State your desire for the person to get help. Your goal in talking to an adult is not to get the person in trouble, but to get the person help to stop using alcohol.

Rotate roles in the role-play and practice each of these steps. Practicing will help you feel comfortable having this conversation and give you confidence. Remember that your motivation for talking to an adult is to get the person help with a serious condition that could have lifelong consequences.

People can use self-management strategies in combination with other treatment methods, such as attending AA meetings or taking medications.

Helping Someone with an AUD

Watching a friend or family member with an AUD can be very challenging. You may worry about that person and probably want that person to be happy and healthy. Many people who care about someone with an AUD experience varied emotions, including shame, anger, fear, and guilt. Other people feel so overwhelmed by their loved one's behavior that they deny the problem and pretend nothing is wrong.

If you care about someone who has an AUD, the first step you need to take is to get the support you need. Find an adult you can talk with openly and honestly, such as a family member, school counselor, or coach.

Some people who know a person with an AUD feel they should try to solve or fix the situation. They may try to punish, threaten, beg, or bribe the person to stop drinking alcohol. They may also cover up the effects of the person's drinking and help the person avoid the natural consequences of this behavior. Encouraging the unhealthy behaviors of a person with an AUD, either intentionally or unintentionally, is called **enabling**. To get treatment, however, the person with an AUD needs to recognize the problem and want to change. No one can force a person to stop drinking alcohol.

enabling protecting a person from the negative consequences of chosen behaviors

Lesson 12.2 Review

Know and Understand

1. What places in your community might you want to avoid if you do not want to be pressured to drink alcohol?
2. List two phrases you could use to say *no* if someone offers you alcohol.
3. What happens during detoxification?
4. How do medications and therapy work together to treat an AUD?
5. Name two support groups for people who have a family member with an AUD.

Think Critically

6. Talk with a parent, guardian, or trusted adult about whether your family has a history of AUD. How does your family history influence your risk?
7. Think about the attitudes your family members and friends have toward alcohol. How have these attitudes shaped your own views about alcohol use?
8. With a partner, discuss the following statement: *Alcohol may temporarily distract people from the issues they are facing, but it does make those issues go away.* Create an engaging PSA that communicates this message and share it with the class.
9. What are some examples of enabling?

REAL WORLD Health Skills

Make Decisions More alcohol-related deaths than usual occur on holidays. Brainstorm as many reasons as you can to explain this connection. Consider the issues of heavy drinking, binge drinking, and alcohol use disorder, which you read about in this lesson. Afterward, make a list of healthy decisions you can make on holidays to avoid the risk factors you researched. Show the decision-making process behind each decision on your list.

Chapter 12 Review and Assessment

Chapter Summary

Alcohol is an addictive drug that alters brain function and has effects on the body and a person's thinking and behavior. The active ingredient in alcohol is ethanol, which is also known as pure alcohol. Blood alcohol concentration (BAC) indicates the amount of alcohol in a person's blood.

Consuming alcohol has immediate and long-term effects on the brain. Alcohol is a depressant, which slows down the central nervous system, including the brain. Consuming alcohol can cause changes in the brain that lead to physical and psychological dependence. People who are dependent on alcohol can develop an alcohol use disorder (AUD).

Excessive alcohol use over time can have negative effects on the brain and cognitive functioning. People who begin drinking early in life experience changes in brain development. People who drink heavily or binge-drink on a regular basis can experience neurological conditions such as dementia, stroke, difficulty remembering, disorientation, and drowsiness.

Alcohol use over time and during pregnancy can lead to the development of chronic health conditions, including liver damage, cardiovascular conditions, reproductive health conditions, and fetal alcohol spectrum disorders (FASD). Alcohol also affects mental, emotional, and social health and can lead to legal consequences that follow a person throughout life.

Individual factors related to identity and behaviors, as well as a person's environment, influence risk for alcohol use. National, state, and local governments regulate alcohol by setting a legal drinking age; limiting when, where, and to whom alcohol is sold; taxing alcohol sales; and placing limits on alcohol advertising.

Making the decision now not to drink alcohol is the best way to protect your brain, body, and mental and emotional health from alcohol's effects. Paying attention to your mental health and managing negative feelings and stress is an important part of avoiding alcohol use. Developing and practicing refusal skills can help when others offer you alcohol. Education and prevention programs can help stop alcohol use among teens.

An AUD is a mental illness and requires professional treatment. Treatment often includes detoxification, medication, and counseling. People with an AUD benefit from continued support from community support groups and programs that teach self-management strategies.

The first step in helping someone with an AUD is to get the support of a trusted adult with whom you can talk openly and honestly. To get treatment, however, the person with an AUD needs to recognize the problem and want to change.

Vocabulary Activity

Analyze a social media post, online article, or website that could potentially encourage teens to try drinking alcohol. Write a short paragraph about how this post, article, or website could negatively affect a teen's behavior or health. Use all the key terms from this chapter in your paragraph and share your paragraph with the class. Include the post, article, or website for the class to view during your presentation.

alcohol	*cirrhosis*	*enabling*
alcohol poisoning	*depressant*	*fetal alcohol spectrum disorders (FASD)*
alcohol use disorder (AUD)	*detoxification*	*hangover*
Alcoholics Anonymous (AA)	*driving under the influence (DUI)*	*inhibition*
blood alcohol concentration (BAC)		

Review and Recall

Review the information in this chapter by answering the following questions.

1. What is the active chemical compound in alcohol?
2. Why is alcohol not measured by the amount of liquid in one drink?
3. What is one factor that contributes to the way alcohol affects different people?
4. How does eating shortly before or while consuming alcohol impact alcoho's effect on a person?
5. Consuming how many drinks qualifies as binge drinking?
6. What type of drug is alcohol?
   A. vasopressin
   B. stimulant
   C. depressant
   D. hormone
7. Name one area of the brain that is affected by alcohol consumption and describe alcohol's immediate effects on that part of the brain.
8. What is cirrhosis, and how does it develop?
9. Which of the following is a possible symptom of a fetal alcohol spectrum disorder?
   A. decreased muscle tone and poor coordination
   B. delayed development
   C. heart conditions
   D. All of the above.
10. What is a zero-tolerance policy in relation to underage drinking and driving?
11. The use of alcohol to handle issues such as negative feelings or difficulty sleeping is called
    A. a co-occurring disorder.
    B. self-medication.
    C. enabling.
    D. inhibition.
12. What is one strategy the government uses to reduce alcohol use?
13. The process of completely withdrawing from alcohol is called
    A. enabling.
    B. disabling.
    C. withdrawal.
    D. detoxification.

Standardized Test Prep

Math Practice

The following results are from a study of alcohol-related deaths among people under age 21. Review the results of this study and then answer the questions that follow.

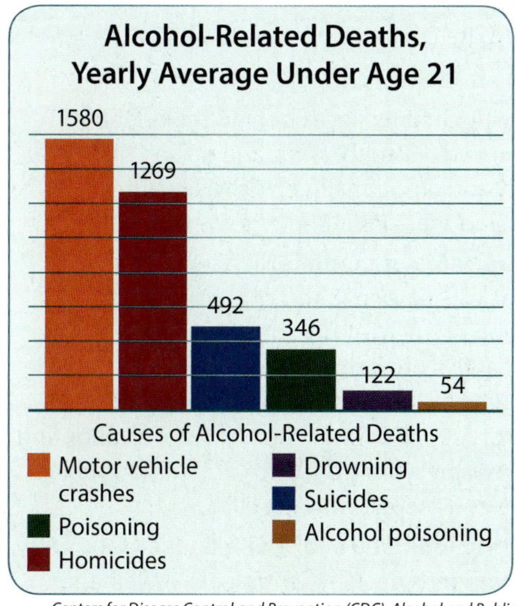

Centers for Disease Control and Prevention (CDC). Alcohol and Public Health: Alcohol-Related Disease Impact (ARDI). Atlanta, GA: CDC, 2016.

14. Motor vehicle crashes accounted for 36 percent of the total number of alcohol-related deaths among people under age 21. What was the total number of alcohol-related deaths among people under age 21 in this study? Round to the nearest hundred.
15. Which cause accounted for about 11 percent of alcohol-related deaths among people under age 21? (Use the total number of deaths you calculated in question 14.)
    A. alcohol poisoning
    B. poisoning
    C. suicides
    D. homicides
16. How many more alcohol-related deaths did drowning cause compared to alcohol poisoning?

Chapter 12 Skills Assessment

Critical Thinking Skills

Answer the following questions to assess your knowledge of what you learned in this chapter.

1. Two people drank the same amount of alcohol at a party; however, one seems more intoxicated than the other. What are some of the possible causes of this difference?
2. How can alcohol, a liquid, dehydrate the body?
3. What are some examples of poor judgment that may result from alcohol consumption?
4. Why might teens who drink alcohol be more likely to have conflicts with their parents or guardians than other teens?
5. In the US, companies are not allowed to advertise tobacco products on TV, radio stations, or billboards. Such advertising is allowed, however, for alcoholic beverages. Why do you think this is the case? Do you think this policy should change? Explain your answer.
6. Are some alcoholic beverages more likely than others to encourage teens to try drinking? Why might teens find these beverages more appealing than others? What are some strategies you could use to resist the temptations of these beverages?
7. Describe the possible effects of an alcohol use disorder on a person's family and friends.
8. Explain how refusal skills can help you turn down alcohol in a social situation. Give at least one example of how you could respond to an offer of alcohol.
9. During what age range are people most likely to develop an alcohol use disorder? Use reliable sources to check your answer. Then create a list of risk factors that may be specific to this age range.
10. With a few classmates, brainstorm ideas for an alcohol education and prevention campaign at your school.
11. Why do you think trying to fix a friend's alcohol issue on your own is not an effective strategy? What are some steps you could take to assist someone with getting the right kind of help?
12. What are some barriers a person might face to getting help for an alcohol use disorder?
13. Research community support groups in your area. How easy or difficult was it to find them? What are some steps these groups could take to make their presence better known in the community?

Health and Wellness Skills

Complete the following activities to assess your skills related to health and wellness.

14. **Analyze Influences.** Find a print or online advertisement for an alcoholic product or drink. Analyze the advertisement and describe it to your class. Explain why you think the advertisement would or would not persuade teens to buy this product. What strategies does the advertisement use? What skills can teens use to see through these strategies and resist the advertising influence?
15. **Access Information.** Choose one celebrity who died due to alcohol-related reasons and research this person using reliable resources. In your research, find out about the celebrity's history of using alcohol and other drugs. Describe key facts, such as when the person started drinking or using drugs and what specific substances the person used. Also find out the specific circumstances behind the celebrity's death. How did alcohol affect the person physically, mentally and emotionally, and socially? Cite your sources and share your findings with the class.
16. **Communicate with Others.** In a small group, use what you learned in this chapter to develop a 10-line rap or poem about the effects of alcohol use and abuse on society. The rap or poem must be appropriate for your target audience and discuss different types of alcohol, the effects of alcohol, and reasons to stay away from alcohol. Record your rap or poem and share it with the class.
17. **Make Decisions.** You and your friends are at a party, and your friends decide they want to drive home. You know they have been drinking heavily all night.

What should you do? Explain how you would use the decision-making process to address this situation. Write and act out a skit describing the scenario and your actions.

18. **Set Goals.** Having clear goals throughout life can help you stay focused on what is important to you and avoid risky behaviors such as drinking alcohol underage. Write a SMART goal that can help you stay alcohol free until you are 21 years old. This goal should be something you would like to accomplish and something drinking alcohol would make difficult to do. Create a written or audio journal entry about how and why this goal will help you remain alcohol free.
19. **Practice Health-Enhancing Behaviors.** Imagine you have received a DUI, and it is now your job to provide the news report about your DUI for a local news show. In your news report, describe all of the facts about the incident, including your BAC. Was anyone hurt in the accident you caused? When will you go to trial? Get a quote from the arresting officer about what happened. After recording the story, write a personal reflection about how this imagined incident and report would affect you. Include at least three researched facts about a DUI arrest in your reflection. Also include strategies you could have used to prevent this incident in the first place.
20. **Advocate for Health.** As an advocate, you have a very important job and can make real change with your peers. Using what you learned in this chapter, design a poster advocating against alcohol use. Your target audience is the students in your school. On the backside of the poster, write a specific, intended age range for your audience. Show some creativity and make sure your poster will apply to the intended age group. On the poster, include the specific consequences of using alcohol at this age, healthy alternatives, and catchy slogans or sayings. Make sure your poster captures the attention of its intended audience.

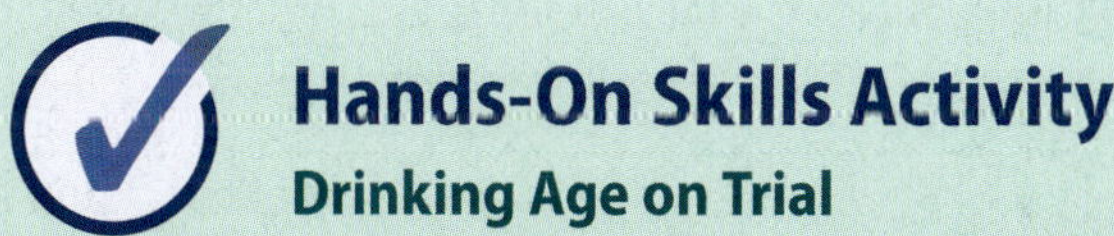

Hands-On Skills Activity

Drinking Age on Trial

In the US, one of the government's methods for reducing alcohol use is setting a minimum legal drinking age of 21. This makes it difficult for teens to access alcohol, reducing alcohol use among minors. Still, some people think the drinking age should be changed. This activity will simulate a courtroom environment where you can argue the case for changing the drinking age.

Steps for This Activity

1. Your teacher will divide the class into two groups. One group will be the *prosecution* in a court trial to convince the jury to change the legal drinking age. The other group will represent the *defense*, which wants to keep the drinking age at 21.
2. In your group, pick a lead prosecutor or lead defense attorney, depending on your side, and then pick three assistant attorneys. The remaining members of the group will be expert witnesses.
3. **Access Information.** The assistant attorneys will conduct research to find as much evidence as possible to support their cases. This research should include interviewing the expert witnesses—who will be acting as local politicians, students, and adults—to get their opinions. Expert witnesses should "become" these people by researching what their assigned people might think. Expert witnesses will be expected to testify on the day of the trial.
4. **Communicate with Others.** The prosecutor and defense attorneys will lead the investigations and present the team's findings to the jury. Using the research gathered, they should write persuasive opening arguments and be prepared to deliver them in class.
5. On the day of the trial, eight jurors will be chosen at random by the teacher from the pool of expert witnesses. These expert witnesses will turn over all of their research to their fellow team members and take their places on the jury as the trial begins.
6. **Advocate for Health.** After the trial, each side should create a poster advocating for that side's position. The poster should be interesting and accessible for teens and present the side's research to the school.

Chapter 13

Medications and Drugs

Look for the skills icon throughout this chapter for opportunities to practice your health skills.

Check Your Health and Wellness Skills

In this chapter, you will learn skills for protecting your health from medication and drug abuse. To understand the skills you currently use, take the following inventory of your behaviors. Indicate how well you think you use each skill. Use a scale of 1–5, *1* meaning you do not use the skill and *5* meaning you feel completely comfortable using it.

Skill	How Well Do You Use Each Skill?
I see a doctor when I think I'm sick.	
I follow the instructions on medication labels.	
I only use medications for their stated, intended use.	
I manage stress in healthy ways by using relaxation techniques or being active.	
I stay away from places where people are using drugs.	
I know what I'd say if someone offered me drugs.	
I feel confident saying *no* when people invite me to abuse medications.	
I encourage others not to abuse medications or drugs.	
I know whom I'd talk to if a friend was abusing medications or drugs.	
I can locate resources in my community that help people with substance use disorders.	
	Total:

Add up your responses to each statement. The higher your score, the more comfortable you feel avoiding medication and drug abuse. Which skill do you think is most important for you? Which skill is the most challenging for you? Which skill would you most like to improve? In this chapter, you will learn how to perform these skills better and more often.

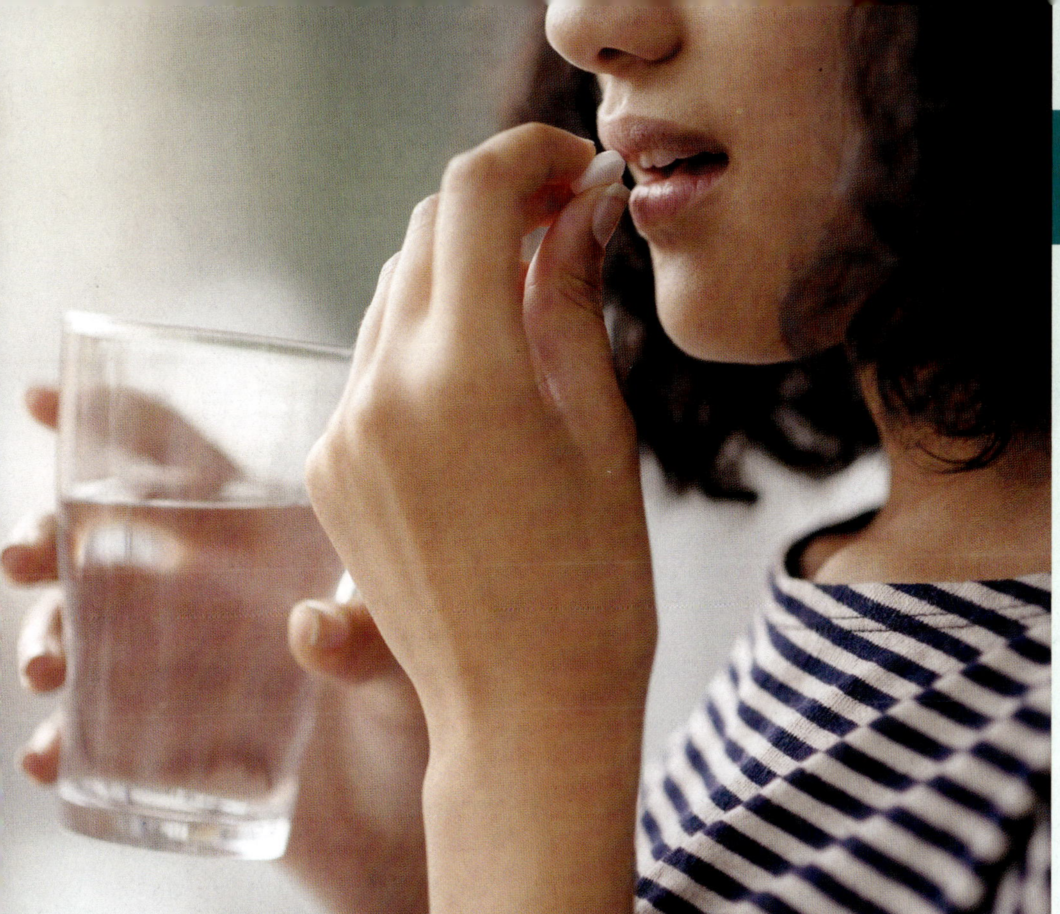
Tassii/E+/Getty Images

Reading and Notetaking

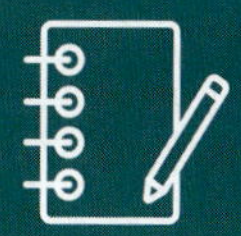

Working in a small group, skim this chapter for key terms and write them on a separate piece of paper. Look up these terms in the dictionary or online. Then, write definitions for each term using your own words. Also write the term's phonetic spelling. Underneath each definition, write an example of the term's meaning in action. After listening to your teacher present this chapter, update your examples and review them with a partner. Practice pronouncing the terms by taking turns reading them aloud and correcting each other's pronunciations.

Term	Phonetic Spelling	Definition and Meaning in Action

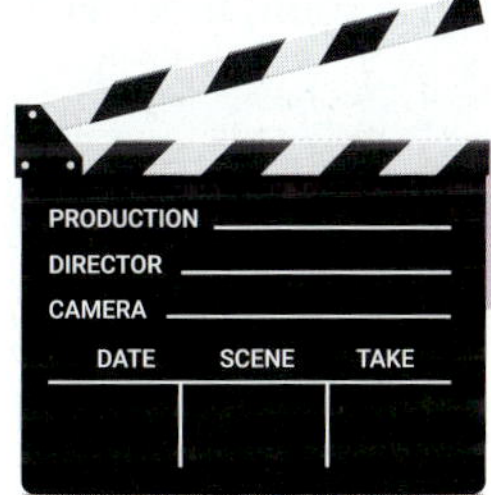

Setting the Scene

The Reality of Medication Abuse

At 16 years old, your life is full of exciting changes. You are a junior in high school, and between all of your schoolwork, you enjoy hanging out with friends and going to parties on the weekends. Most of your friends think using drugs is a bad idea. A few of your friends have started taking Vicodin® to get high though. They say Vicodin® is a prescription medication, so it is not the same as using drugs. Your own experience seems to say something else: You know a lot of people are getting treatment for opioid addiction in your community. A friend of yours lost a sibling to opioid overdose just last year.

One day, after a long and frustrating afternoon at school, you walk into your friend's home to find your friend and another friend getting high. Your friend asks if you want to join.

Thinking Critically

1. What are some factors that might have led your friends to try Vicodin®?
2. Is it true that taking Vicodin® is safer than using drugs? Why or why not?
3. What are some strategies you can use to avoid the temptation or pressure to abuse medications and drugs?

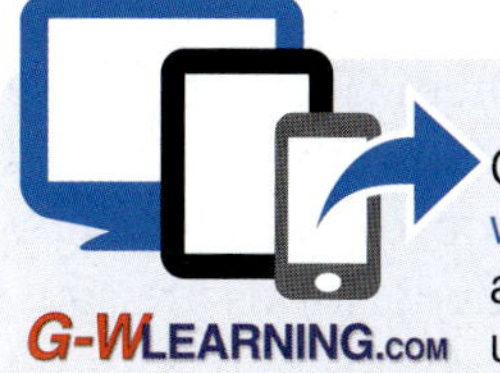

Click on the activity icon or visit www.g-wlearning.com/health/4095 to access online vocabulary activities using key terms from the chapter.

Lesson 13.1

Safe Medication Use

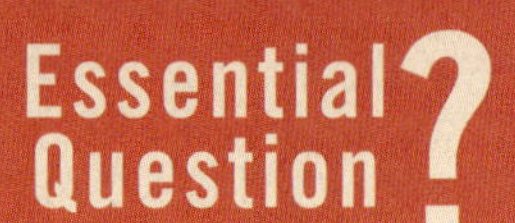

What steps do you need to follow to use medications safely?

Learning Outcomes

After studying this lesson, you will be able to

- identify the main reasons people use medications;
- differentiate between over-the-counter and prescription medications;
- describe different ways to take medications;
- summarize common health risks associated with taking medications;
- list safe strategies for choosing and using medications; and
- define *medication misuse*.

Key Terms

analgesics
drug allergy
drug sensitivity
medication
medication misuse
over-the-counter (OTC) medications
prescription medications
side effects

Warm-Up Activity

Understanding Medications

Comprehend Concepts With a partner, brainstorm as many reasons as you can think of why someone would need to take a medication. What medication would the person need to take? For what reasons have you taken medications? Next, discuss what you know about the health risks of taking medications. Have you ever experienced an unpleasant side effect from a medication? Then, list some strategies you know help people use medications safely and effectively. After reading this lesson, revisit the notes from your discussion and revise them to reflect what you learned.

Reasons for Taking Medications	Health Risks	Safe and Effective Strategies

medication substance that treats disease or relieves symptoms

A **medication** (also called *medicine*) is a substance that treats disease or relieves symptoms such as pain. The four main reasons people use medications are to cure, manage, prevent, or treat symptoms of a disease.

In the United States, companies developing new medications must run tests to prove the medications are safe and effective before selling them. These tests are called *clinical trials*. After a company tests a new medication, the *Food and Drug Administration (FDA)* decides whether to approve it. The FDA is the government agency responsible for making sure medications are safe to use, effective, and secure from tampering.

Types of Medications

In addition to approving medications as safe, the FDA also decides whether a medication requires a doctor's prescription. This determines whether a medication is considered over-the-counter or prescription. People take over-the-counter and prescription medications in different ways depending on their needs (**Figure 13.1**).

Over-the-Counter (OTC) Medications

People can buy **over-the-counter (OTC) medications** without a doctor's prescription. This is because OTC medications are generally considered safe to use without specific instructions from a doctor or pharmacist. These medications still need to be taken according to instructions and warnings on the label, however. People can easily purchase these medications at local stores and pharmacies, though some OTC medications may have age restrictions.

over-the-counter (OTC) medications substances that can legally be sold without permission from a healthcare professional in a particular country

OTC medications treat the symptoms of many relatively minor health conditions. The most commonly used OTC medications are mild **analgesics** (pain relievers), such as aspirin, acetaminophen, and ibuprofen. Other common OTC medications are *antihistamines*, which reduce allergy symptoms; *antitussives*, which suppress coughing; *decongestants*, which relieve nasal and chest congestion; and *antacids*, which relieve heartburn and indigestion.

analgesics medications that relieve pain

Prescription Medications

People can purchase **prescription medications** only with a prescription from a doctor or other licensed healthcare professional. The doctor will determine how much of the medication a patient needs. The patient then purchases the prescribed medication through a licensed pharmacist. A person cannot get more of the prescribed medication unless refills are authorized. Different types of prescription medications have different functions (**Figure 13.2**).

prescription medications substances that can legally be sold only with permission from a doctor or other qualified healthcare professional

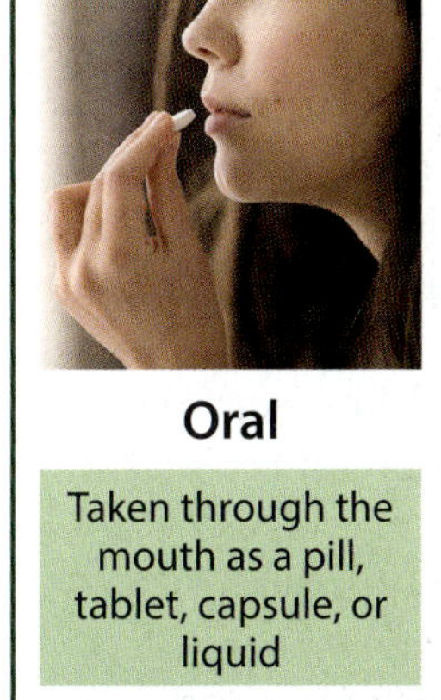

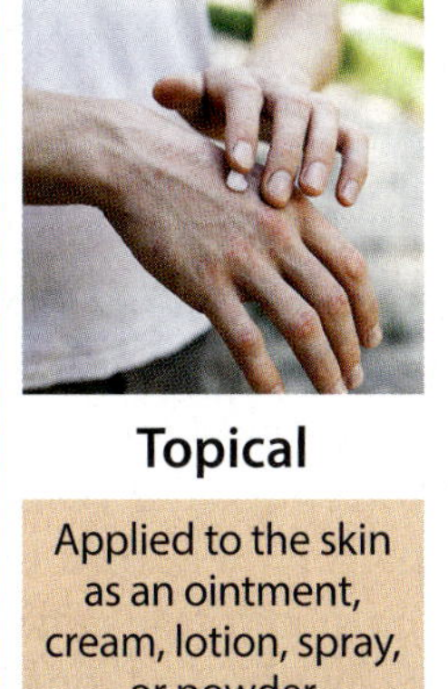

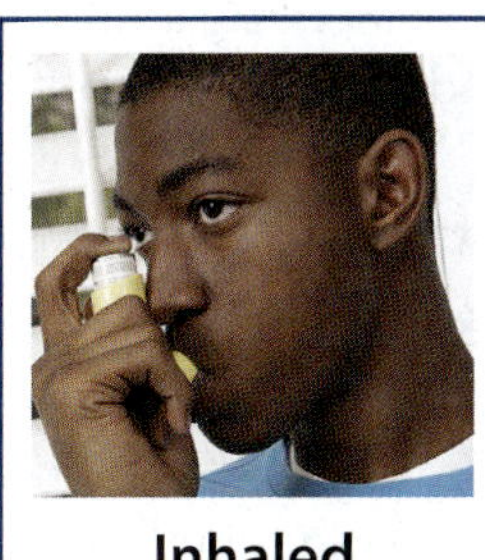

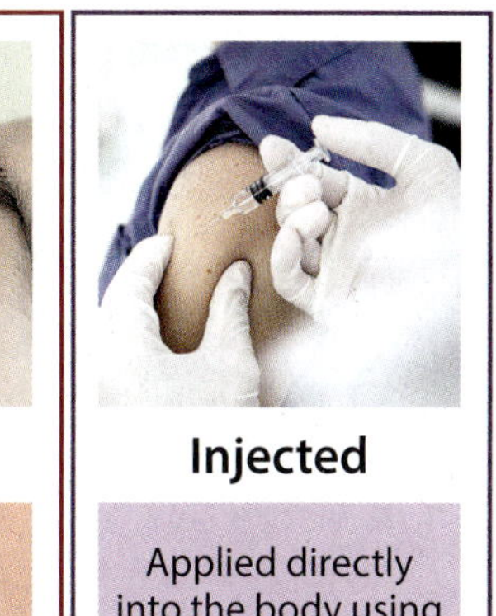

Left to right: fizkes/Shutterstock.com; Ternavskaia Olga Alibec/Shutterstock.com; sirtravelalot/Shutterstock.com; life-literacy/Shutterstock.com; Image Point Fr/Shutterstock.com

Figure 13.1 No matter the method of delivery, medications treat or relieve symptoms of disease to improve health. ***Which government agency ensures medications are safe and effective to use?***

Types of Prescription Medications

Antibiotics
• Kill or slow the growth of bacteria to prevent or cure an infection
Antivirals or Antifungals
• Reduce the effects of viral and fungal infections
Anesthetics
• Eliminate or reduce pain
Antidepressants or Antipsychotics
• Regulate mood and affect brain chemistry to help relieve the symptoms of some mental health conditions

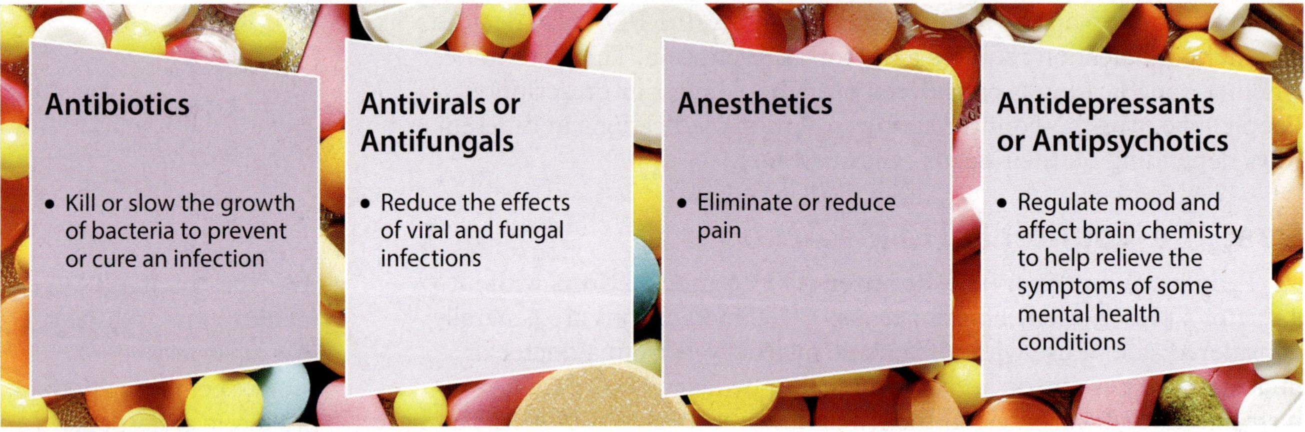

Pavel Kubarkov/Shutterstock.com

Figure 13.2 Some examples of prescription medications are shown. A doctor will prescribe a specific type of medication to treat different symptoms or diseases.

Health Risks of Taking Medications

Taking OTC and prescription medications can benefit your health. Using these medications, however, also carries some risks.

Side Effects

side effects unintended changes that develop in response to a medication

Medications affect the processes at work inside your body. As a result, all medications can have **side effects**. For example, many medications for treating cold symptoms cause drowsiness. Some medications have more serious side effects, such as hallucinations, dizziness, and stomach bleeding and ulcers.

Some OTC medications can cause life-threatening conditions. *Reye's syndrome* is a rare but potentially fatal disease in children. Because some evidence suggests that aspirin can trigger this disease, people under 18 years of age should never take aspirin or medications that contain aspirin, unless specifically ordered by a doctor.

Prescription medication labels list the potential side effects associated with use. Warnings on medication labels also alert consumers to the possible dangers of taking a medication. Reading these side effects and warnings can help you identify what side effects are normal and be alert to more serious issues.

Medication Interactions

Sometimes a medication may cause an *interaction* with other substances at work in the body. These interactions may impact the effectiveness of a medication. Some medication interactions are positive, such as two medications working together to treat a health condition. For example, a person may take one medication to reduce high blood pressure and another medication to strengthen that medication's effectiveness.

Medication interactions with other medications, dietary supplements, foods, or drinks can also pose serious health risks. For example, people should not take acetaminophen, a common OTC pain medication, with some prescription pain and OTC medications. If two medications work together to increase overall effect (called *synergism*), the effect on the body can be too strong. For example, taking sleep medications and pain medications together can lead to serious health risks, including death.

Most medication labels contain guidelines about substances a person should or should not take with a medication. You can learn more about medication interactions by accessing reliable medical resources or talking with your doctor or pharmacist.

Sensitivities and Allergic Reactions

Sometimes the same medication can have different effects on different people, which can cause further health risks. For example, a person who has a **drug sensitivity** is more likely to experience negative side effects using a specific medication. The person might want to avoid that medication and find other ways to manage symptoms.

People can be allergic to some medications. If a person has a **drug allergy**, the immune system responds to a certain medication as if it is harmful to the body. People are most often allergic to antibiotics. Allergic reactions from a drug allergy can range from rashes and itching to swelling, breathing issues, and even death. If you have a history of drug allergies, you should always tell your doctor and pharmacist and read labels carefully when choosing OTC medications.

drug sensitivity increased likelihood of developing negative side effects in response to a particular substance

drug allergy immune response in which the body treats a particular substance as if it is harmful to the body; causes an allergic reaction if the person consumes the substance

Medication Tolerance and Withdrawal

Long-term use of a medication can lead to the body needing more of the medication to achieve the same effect. This is called *tolerance*. As tolerance builds, the body needs larger and larger amounts of the medication, increasing the risk for overdose. In an overdose, the medication's effects become extreme and toxic and can cause death. Ceasing to take a medication after a long time can lead to *withdrawal*. During withdrawal, the body craves the medication, leading to potentially painful and serious symptoms, including depression, anxiety, severe fatigue, sleeplessness, seizures, and hallucinations (**Figure 13.3**). The best way to avoid these health risks is to use medications safely and take them only as directed.

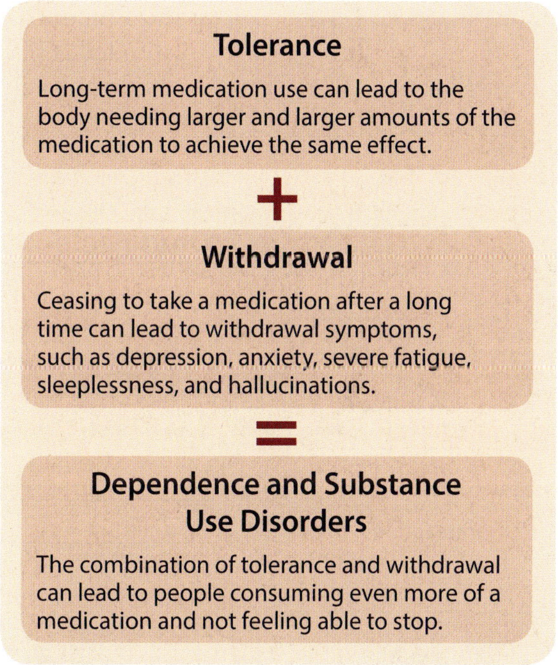

Tolerance

Long-term medication use can lead to the body needing larger and larger amounts of the medication to achieve the same effect.

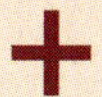

Withdrawal

Ceasing to take a medication after a long time can lead to withdrawal symptoms, such as depression, anxiety, severe fatigue, sleeplessness, and hallucinations.

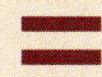

Dependence and Substance Use Disorders

The combination of tolerance and withdrawal can lead to people consuming even more of a medication and not feeling able to stop.

Figure 13.3 Together, medication tolerance and withdrawal can lead to people consuming more of a medication and not feeling able to stop. This can result in dependence and substance use disorders.

Safe Strategies for Using Medications

Medications can benefit the body, but only if people use them safely. Choosing and taking medications carefully can help people avoid the health risks associated with medication use.

See a Healthcare Professional

Medications usually treat a health condition or relieve its symptoms. Sometimes symptoms clearly indicate the cause of a health condition. Other times, the cause of a symptom is uncertain, and using OTC medications may not treat the underlying cause. Only a healthcare professional can examine a person's symptoms and make an accurate diagnosis.

Talking to your doctor or pharmacist will help you understand the appropriate way to take a medication. To start this conversation, use the following steps:

1. Make an appointment with your doctor. Ask a parent or guardian if you need help.
2. List your health concerns or symptoms and bring this list to your appointment.
3. Tell your doctor about any drug allergies or sensitivities. Also tell your doctor about any medications or drugs you are taking.
4. If the doctor prescribes a medication, ask about directions for taking the medication, warnings, and medication side effects. Write these details down. You can also ask if a generic, less-expensive version of the medication is available.
5. Fill the medication prescription at a pharmacy. If you have more questions, you can talk to the pharmacist working there without an appointment.

Use Medications as Intended

Medications are powerful substances that alter the body's chemistry and functions. Because of this, it is important to use medications as intended. This means following medication instructions, using medications responsibly, and avoiding medication misuse.

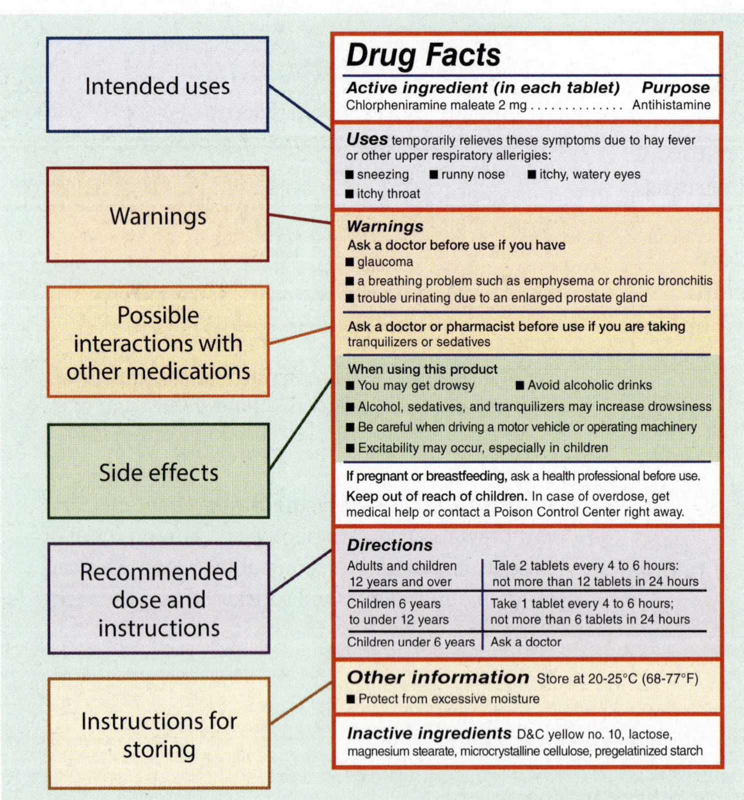

Courtesy of the US Department of Health and Human Services

Figure 13.4 Labels on OTC medications include information about proper and safe use of the medication. ***What should you do if your health condition does not go away after you use an OTC medication?***

Reading and Following Medication Label Instructions

Carefully reading and following medication usage instructions maximizes the effect of a medication and reduces health risks. Medication labels, boxes, and containers include usage instructions. Labels also state other important information about safe and effective usage (**Figure 13.4**).

If you are taking a prescription medication, you will receive instructions from your doctor about how long you should take the medication. This information will also be on the medication's label. Always follow these instructions, even if you start to feel better. If you are taking antibiotics, stopping too soon may not destroy the bacteria causing the infection.

Using Medications Responsibly

Medications treat symptoms or health conditions. If used for any other reason, medications can be dangerous to the body.

To use medications responsibly, follow these guidelines:

- Only take medications that are prescribed for you and appropriate for your symptoms. Never use a medication prescribed for someone else or let someone else use a medication prescribed for you.
- Do not give OTC medications intended for adults to infants or children.
- Store medications safely in their original containers.
- Keep medications out of reach of pets or children.
- Before taking a medication, check its expiration date and discard any expired medications.
- Dispose of medications by dropping them off at a *drug take-back location*. Follow the instructions on the medication label or prescription to dispose of medications at home.

If a health condition does not go away, see a healthcare professional. Let your doctor know right away if you feel worse or develop symptoms such as a rash, vomiting, or difficulty breathing.

Avoiding Medication Misuse

Not following a medication's instructions is **medication misuse**. Misused medications may not be effective; can increase health risks, such as unpleasant side effects; and may result in serious illness, even death. To avoid medication misuse, ensure you understand the directions for taking the medication.

medication misuse act of unintentionally not following the instructions for taking a medication

If a person intentionally misuses a medication or uses a medication for any purpose other than its intended one, this is *medication abuse*, which is a type of substance abuse. You will learn more about medication abuse in the next lesson.

Lesson 13.1 Review

Know and Understand

1. Describe the difference between OTC and prescription medications.
2. In your own words, define *withdrawal*.
3. What should you do if taking OTC medications does not solve your health issue?
4. With a partner, list three examples of medication misuse.

Think Critically

5. Why should you tell your doctor and pharmacist about any medications or drugs you are taking? What factors may discourage teens from doing this? What would you say to a teen who wanted to keep this information from a doctor or pharmacist?
6. Write a story about how tolerance leads to addiction in a teen. Include the signs of each stage of substance use in your story.

REAL WORLD Health Skills

Make Decisions Sadie's grandmother has had some serious health conditions lately, including a broken hip and pneumonia. While visiting her grandmother one Saturday, Sadie found a lot of prescription pain medications in her grandmother's bathroom closet. Sadie knows these medications sell for a lot of money and desperately wants to see her favorite band in concert. She has no money, and her family cannot afford to get her a ticket. Using the decision-making process, help Sadie make a health-enhancing decision.

Lesson

13.2

Medication Abuse

Essential Question?

Why is medication abuse a serious public health issue?

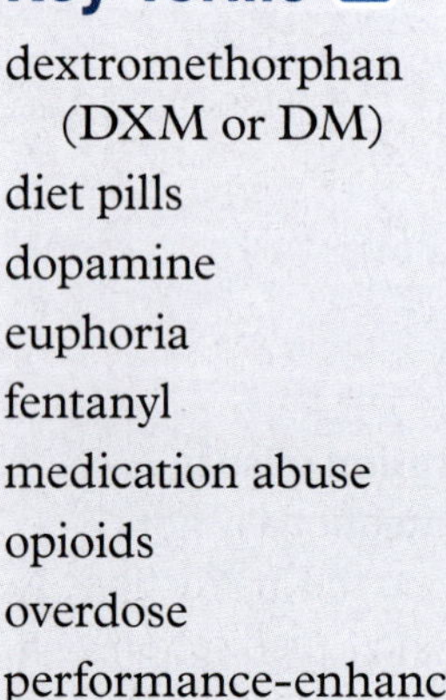

Key Terms

dextromethorphan (DXM or DM)
diet pills
dopamine
euphoria
fentanyl
medication abuse
opioids
overdose
performance-enhancing drugs (PEDs)
stimulants

Learning Outcomes

After studying this lesson, you will be able to

- give examples of medication abuse;
- describe how abusing medications impacts the brain and body;
- analyze the mental, social, and legal consequences of medication abuse;
- explain the health consequences of abusing depressants;
- identify the life-threatening effects of opioid abuse;
- assess the consequences of abusing stimulants;
- explain why some people abuse cold medications;
- analyze the risks of abusing diet pills; and
- summarize why performance-enhancing drugs (PEDs) are dangerous.

Warm-Up Activity

Concerned About Addiction

Access Information Martin has learned a lot about prescription medication abuse in health class. Everything he has learned has made him extremely concerned. He is having an invasive surgery next week and is worried about taking pain medications afterward. Help Martin write a list of questions he can ask the surgeon about his post-operation pain management plan. Include questions Martin can ask about reducing the risks of abuse and addiction.

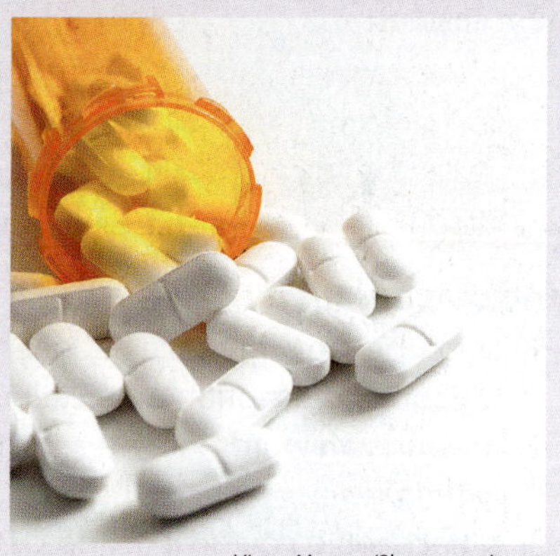

Victor Moussa/Shutterstock.com

When you think of substance abuse, you probably think of illegal drugs and alcohol. The reality is that, after marijuana, prescription and OTC medications are the most commonly abused substances among teens.

Medication abuse is the use of medication in an unintended or harmful way. It includes

- using medications for purposes that are not prescribed or stated on the label;
- sharing a prescription medication with someone else;
- selling a prescription medication;
- taking more than the prescribed or recommended amount of a medication; and
- combining medications without a doctor's approval.

medication abuse use of a medication in an unintended or harmful way; includes using medications for unintended purposes, sharing or selling medications, taking too much of a medication, or combining medications without a doctor's approval

Abusing prescription and OTC medications can have serious consequences, including death (**Figure 13.5**). In this lesson, you will learn about the serious consequences of medication abuse. You will also learn about the most commonly abused medications: depressants, opioids, and stimulants.

More people die each year from the abuse of prescription medications than from illegal drug use.

Krisana Antharith/Shutterstock.com

Figure 13.5 Using prescription medications correctly can effectively treat diseases. Misusing or abusing medications, however, can be extremely harmful to health. ***What is the difference between medication misuse and medication abuse?***

Effects of Medication Abuse

If used correctly, medications can improve health conditions by relieving symptoms. Following instructions and using medications safely can help guard against medication tolerance and withdrawal, which you learned about in the previous lesson. The fact that medications are legal substances and not illegal drugs does not make abusing them less dangerous, however. Medications cause changes in the brain and body. When abused, medications can cause health conditions, long-lasting disabilities, and death. In addition, medication abuse can lead to addiction and serious mental, social, and legal consequences.

Medications and the Brain

Medications contain synthetic and natural chemicals that control how brain cells send, receive, and process information.

Some medications stimulate the brain to release **dopamine**, a major chemical in the brain's reward center (**Figure 13.6**). Naturally, the brain releases this chemical to reinforce the body's fundamental and important

dopamine chemical in the brain that causes feelings of pleasure; motivates behaviors like eating and drinking

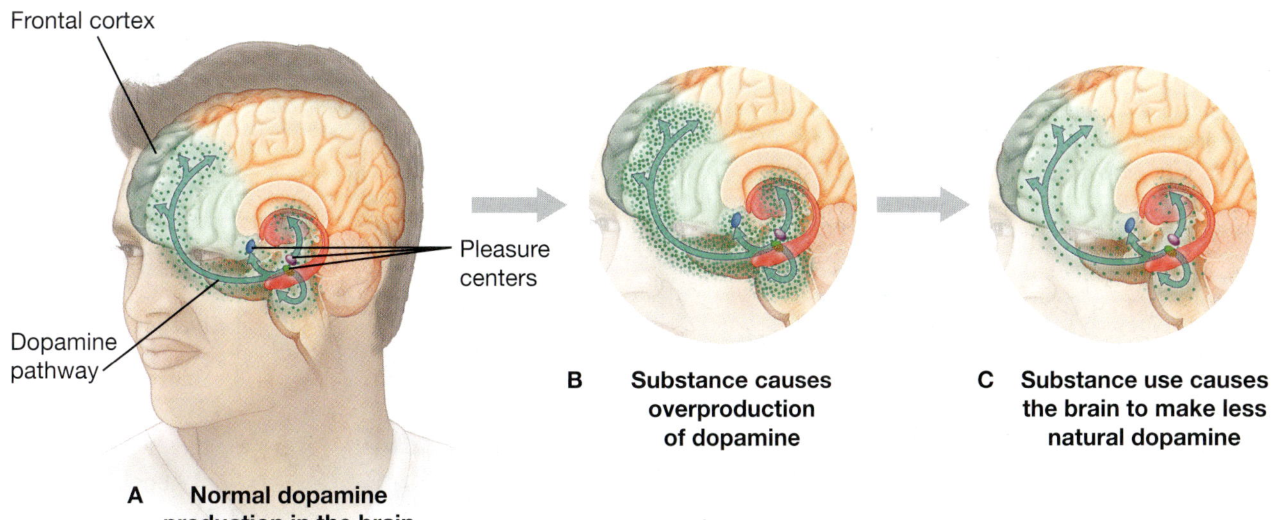

© Body Scientific International

Figure 13.6 Just as you turn down the volume when your headphones are too loud, the brain of someone who abuses medications responds by reducing its production of dopamine. ***What is the name of the intense high that can be caused by the rush of dopamine from medication abuse?***

activities such as eating, drinking, and nurturing behaviors. A small amount of dopamine causes a person to feel good after being physically active, eating chocolate, or listening to music.

euphoria intense pleasurable feeling

Some medications, such as prescription opioids, cause a rush of dopamine and endorphins. When used correctly, this rush relieves severe pain. It can also lead to **euphoria**, or an intense high. As a person abuses a medication, the brain develops a *tolerance* and needs larger and larger amounts of the medication to achieve the same good feelings. When a medication causes the brain to overproduce dopamine, the brain also responds by making *less* natural dopamine, decreasing motivation and pleasure. Without the same natural level of dopamine, the brain becomes dependent on the medication for these feelings. This leads to continued medication abuse. It can also lead to the development of a *substance use disorder*, a serious mental illness you learned about in Chapter 7.

Other Health Effects

The brain is not the only part of the body medication abuse harms. People who abuse medications may experience changes in appetite, diarrhea, weight loss or gain, and vomiting. They may also experience insomnia, sleepiness, fatigue, and muscle and joint pain. Issues with blood clotting and weak immunity are other changes associated with medication abuse.

Medication abuse can harm the liver, especially when medications are combined with alcohol. Severe and permanent liver damage is called *cirrhosis*. A liver with cirrhosis cannot remove harmful substances from the blood. Cirrhosis is a disease that causes toxins to build up and damage the brain and body, eventually leading to death. The only "cure" for this disease is a liver transplant.

overdose act of taking more of a substance than the body can break down at one time; can lead to serious health consequences and death

In addition to these effects, medication abuse can lead to a fatal overdose. An **overdose** occurs when a person takes in more of a medication than the body can properly break down at one time. A person who overdoses may do so intentionally or accidentally (**Figure 13.7**). An overdose can happen in minutes and lead to death within hours. Overdoses that do not lead to death can cause severe, permanent brain damage and other health complications.

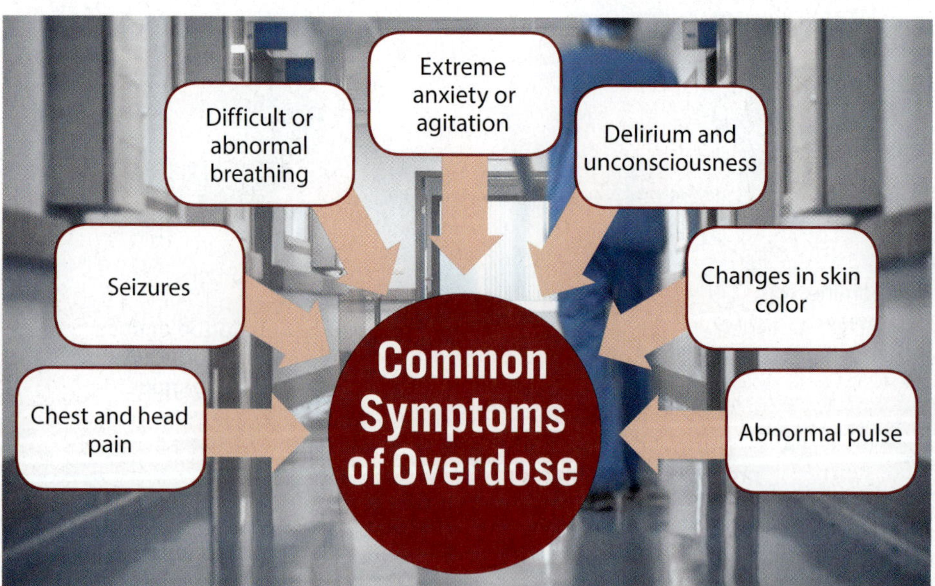

sfam_photo/Shutterstock.com

Figure 13.7 The symptoms of an overdose depend on the medication abused. ***When does an overdose occur?***

Mental, Social, and Legal Consequences

Alterations in the brain due to medication abuse can lead to many mental changes. People who abuse medications may become agitated, anxious, or depressed and are more likely to attempt suicide. They may experience *hyperactivity* (extremely high energy), irrational fear, and mood swings. Medication abuse also distracts people from their goals and makes them more likely to engage in risky behaviors (**Figure 13.8**).

Medication abuse makes teens more likely to
contract STIs
get into motor vehicle accidents
become pregnant
engage in violence
commit crimes
have multiple sexual partners

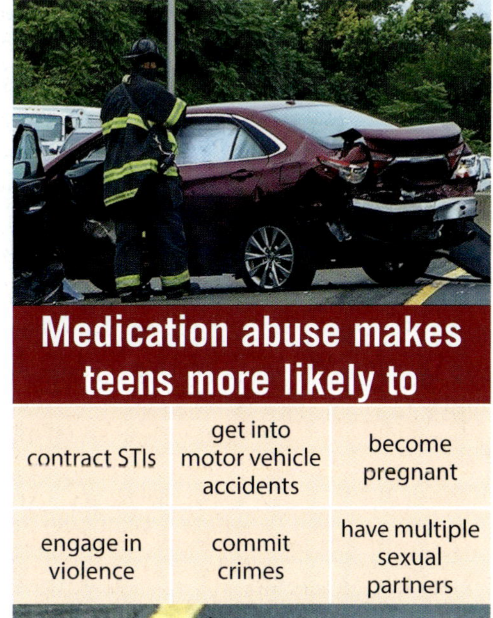

Raymond Deleon/Shutterstock.com

Figure 13.8 The risks increased by medication abuse endanger the health of teens, as well as their families, dating partners, friends, and communities.

Socially, medication abuse can harm relationships. People who abuse medications may lose the trust of family members and feel like others are disappointed in them. The addiction that comes with medication abuse can cause more broken trust. Medication abuse often leads to poor work and school performance, sometimes resulting in job loss or expulsion. As people who abuse medications try to feed their addiction, they may experience violence or commit crimes. The result of these behaviors is social isolation that only fuels a person's negative feelings.

Federal and local laws prohibit prescription medication abuse. At the federal level, the 1970 *Controlled Substances Act* limits the possession, sale, and use of several kinds of medications and drugs. In 1973, the federal *Drug Enforcement Agency (DEA)* formed to enforce federal laws regarding medications and drugs. Most states also have laws about prescription medication abuse. Breaking these laws has severe penalties, including jail time, fines, and loss of driving privileges.

Most schools and employers have rules about abusing medications. Schools may expel students or report students to the police for selling or abusing medications. Employers may fire employees, and a criminal drug record can make it hard to find a job.

Commonly Abused Medications

Commonly abused medications include both prescription and OTC medications. Examples include depressants, opioids, stimulants, cold medications, diet pills, and performance-enhancing drugs (PEDs).

Depressants

Depressants, which are also called *sedatives* or *tranquilizers*, stimulate the brain to release chemicals that slow nerve activity. This reduces anxiety and helps a person relax, stay calm, or sleep. These medications work by slowing the nervous system, breathing, and heart rate. For this reason, combining depressants with alcohol can slow the nervous system to the point of death. Some depressants also stimulate the brain to release dopamine, which contributes to addiction. Abused prescription depressants are often called *downers*. Examples of depressants include the following:

- **Barbiturates:** Barbiturates slow down the nervous system. Though not commonly used, doctors may prescribe them for headaches, seizures, or insomnia. Some commonly prescribed barbiturates are *Luminal*®, *Brevital*®, and *Seconal*®. Abusing barbiturates can lead to difficulty breathing, increased risk of respiratory diseases, anxiety or panic, hallucinations, and death.

- **Benzodiazepines:** Benzodiazepines relieve the symptoms of anxiety disorders, panic disorders, and seizures. Commonly prescribed anti-anxiety medications, such as *Xanax*® and *Valium*®, are benzodiazepines. Abusing these medications can cause digestive issues, memory and attention disorders, emotional numbness, and depression. People who abuse benzodiazepines also have a high risk of overdose and death, especially if they mix them with alcohol or other depressants.
- **Sleeping medications:** Doctors usually prescribe sleeping medications, such as *Ambien*® and *Sonata*®, to treat insomnia. In most cases, doctors prescribe these medications for short-term use. Long-term use can quickly lead to addiction and withdrawal. Abuse of sleeping medications can lead to slurred speech, difficulty focusing, impaired memory, lack of coordination, seizures, and death by overdose.

Opioids

opioids prescription medications that relieve severe or long-lasting pain

Throughout history, people have used *opium*, a chemical in the poppy plant, to relieve pain. Today, many strong pain medications are **opioids**, or prescription medications that contain a synthetic version of opium. Doctors prescribe these medications to relieve severe or long-lasting pain.

Opioids relieve pain by turning off the nerves that send pain signals and stimulating the brain to release endorphins and dopamine. Endorphins are natural painkillers. As you know, dopamine causes euphoria, a pleasurable sensation. These effects explain why opioids are addictive. When a person uses opioids regularly, nerve cells in the brain stop producing endorphins and dopamine on their own. This causes the person to become physically dependent on opioids.

Types of prescription opioids include the following (**Figure 13.9**):

- **Codeine:** Doctors typically prescribe codeine to treat pain and coughing. Some prescription-strength cough medications also contain codeine. Over time, taking codeine can lead to tolerance and dependence. Because codeine produces euphoria, some people abuse it.
- **Morphine:** Morphine is a powerful prescription opioid for pain. Doctors often prescribe it after surgery, for cancer-related pain, or at the end of a person's life. Morphine produces a strong sense of euphoria, which can lead to abuse and addiction.
- **Methadone:** Methadone is a prescription opioid for severe pain, including painful withdrawal symptoms. Unlike other opioids, it does not cause euphoria. For these reasons, doctors often use methadone to treat people with addictions to other opioids.

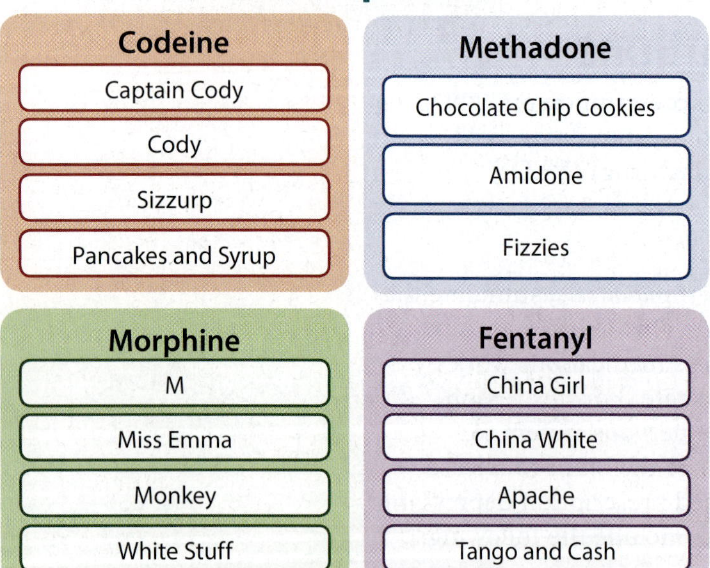

Figure 13.9 People who sell and buy opioids illegally use code names for these drugs. ***What does the nature of these street names indicate about the target audience for illegally sold opioids?***

- **Fentanyl: Fentanyl** is a prescription opioid 50 to 100 times more powerful than morphine. Doctors typically prescribe it for post-surgical or cancer-related pain, including pain other opioids cannot control. Because it is so powerful, it is extremely dangerous. In fact, more than 50 percent of opioid-related deaths in 2017 involved fentanyl abuse.

fentanyl prescription opioid 50 to 100 times more powerful than morphine; prescribed for pain other opioids cannot control

Prescription opioids go by many different names. Some common opioid medications are *Oxycontin*®, *Percocet*®, *Vicodin*®, *Lortab*®, and *Lorcet*®. Some people who abuse opioids get them in these forms from a doctor. Other people buy opioids from criminals who sell them without a prescription.

Local and Global Health

The Opioid Epidemic

In recent years, there has been an alarming increase in opioid overdoses in the US. In fact, approximately one in three people in the US has been personally affected by opioid abuse and knows someone who has overdosed or has an opioid addiction. Opioid overdose has become the 10th leading cause of death, killing more people than suicide. This has been called the *opioid epidemic*.

The opioid epidemic is not evenly spread across the US. In 2016–2017, the majority of fatal overdoses occurred in large cities. More than 70 percent occurred in the Midwest. More and more illegally sold opioids account for these fatal overdoses. The introduction of fentanyl, which is 50 to 100 times more powerful than morphine, now contributes to more than 50 percent of opioid overdose deaths.

According to a study by the United Nations Office on Drugs and Crime, opioid use is growing around the world too. So far, other countries do not have comparable epidemics. Still, widespread use may lead to abuse and addiction.

In the United States and around the world, opioid abuse has serious social, medical, and economic consequences. As opioid abuse spreads, countries see

- more people living with hepatitis and HIV;
- more people turning to illegal drugs as prescription opioids become harder to acquire;
- more babies born with opioid addictions acquired from their mothers;
- more children in foster care after losing parents to overdose;
- fewer people in the country's workforce;
- more people who are homeless; and
- more people living with mental health conditions related to opioid abuse.

Global Opioid Use, 2017

Selected Regions	Number of People Using Opioids	Percentage of Regional Population
North America	12,830,000	3.96
South America	580,000	0.20
Africa	6,080,000	0.87
Asia	29,460,000	0.98
Europe	3,570,000	0.66
Global	53,350,000	1.08

Source: United Nations Office on Drugs and Crime unodc.org

Practice Your Skills

Advocate for Health

Reflect on what you have learned and review the data about opioid use in different regions of the world. Form a small group and discuss possible answers to these questions:

1. Which world region had the highest rate of opioid use? Compare this to rates of opioid use in other regions. Why do you think this region had the highest rate?
2. What factors may explain why opioid overdoses are concentrated in large US cities?

In your group, research the steps US communities are taking to reduce opioid use and prevent opioid overdoses. Using this information, brainstorm strategies for reducing opioid abuse in your community. Identify three different strategies and consider their strengths and weaknesses. Create a promotional flyer describing how your community could make one of these ideas a reality.

Opioid abuse has serious health consequences. Side effects of opioid abuse include drowsiness, dizziness, weakness, nausea, lack of coordination, confusion, sweating, and constipation. Opioids slow a person's breathing and decrease pulse and blood pressure. Therefore, people who abuse opioids can very easily lose consciousness and die from overdose (**Figure 13.10**). Combining opioids with alcohol or other depressants increases the risk of fatal drug overdose.

Stimulants

stimulants substances that cause the brain to release adrenaline, increasing energy, alertness, and attention

Stimulants are substances that cause the brain to release *adrenaline*, which increases energy, alertness, and attention. Doctors often prescribe stimulants such as *Adderall®* and *Ritalin®* to treat attention-deficit hyperactivity disorder (ADHD) and narcolepsy. Slang terms for illegally sold prescription stimulants include *speed*, *uppers*, and *vitamin R*. These medications typically include amphetamine and methylphenidate. Some stimulants, such as energy pills and appetite suppressants, are also available OTC. Caffeine and energy drinks are examples of stimulant supplements people can find in retail settings.

Abusing stimulants, including OTC stimulants, or stimulant supplements can be dangerous and life threatening. Amphetamines rapidly increase levels of dopamine in the brain, producing euphoria and increasing the chance of addiction. Other effects of stimulant abuse include cognitive impairment, depression, delusions, hallucinations, paranoia, and physical health issues. Abusing stimulant supplements like caffeine and energy drinks can lead to addiction, dehydration, hallucinations, heart rhythm abnormalities, heart attack, insomnia, and stroke.

Cold Medications

dextromethorphan (DXM or DM) type of opioid-like medication that suppresses coughing; found in many OTC cough and cold medications

Cold medications help reduce coughing and relieve congestion. Many cold medications are available OTC and benefit people when used properly. If abused, however, cold medications can have serious negative health consequences.

Many OTC cold medications, including cough syrups, contain **dextromethorphan (DXM or DM)**, a type of opioid-like drug that does not relieve pain. In normal doses, DXM suppresses coughing.

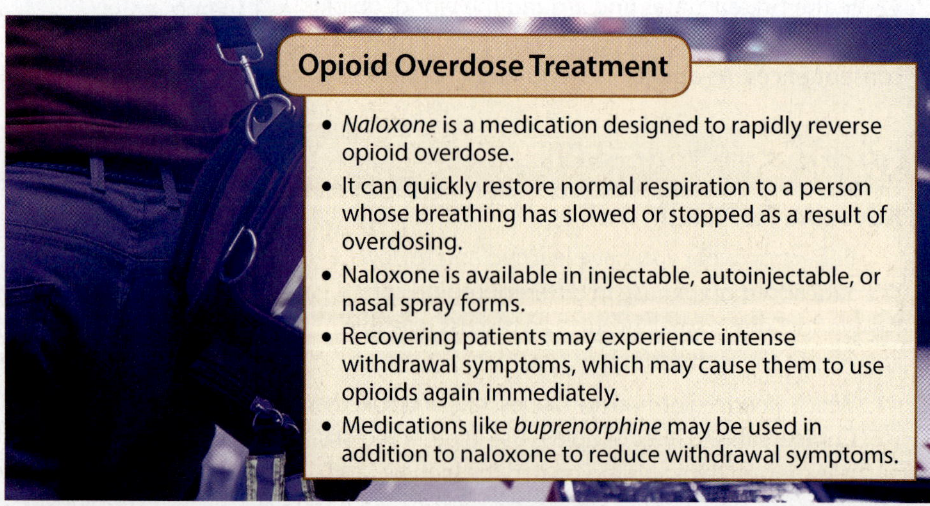

zoff/Shutterstock.com

Figure 13.10 If you witness what you believe to be an opioid overdose, take immediate action and call 911. Your quick action may save that person's life.

In high doses, it can cause temporary euphoria. For this reason, some people abuse DXM medications by swallowing them in high doses or mixing them in drinks such as soda (called *robotripping* or *skittling*). High doses of DXM can cause hallucinations, panic, and aggression. Abusing DXM can lead to addiction.

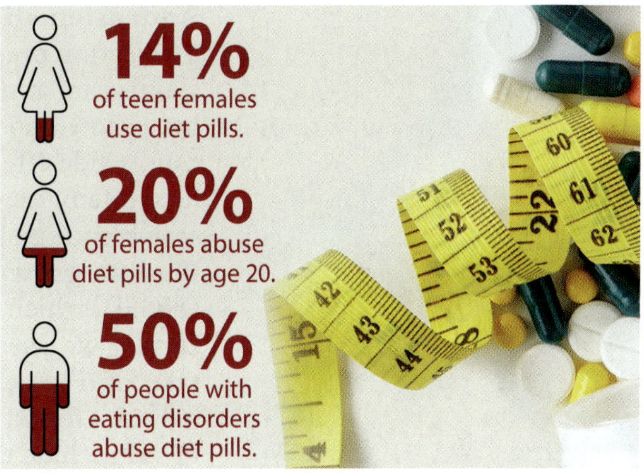

14%
of teen females use diet pills.

20%
of females abuse diet pills by age 20.

50%
of people with eating disorders abuse diet pills.

People: tatianasun/Shutterstock.com; Medication: Stas Malyarevsky/Shutterstock.com

Figure 13.11 Many people with eating disorders and females abuse diet pills in an effort to reduce their weight. This method can have many health consequences. ***What are some emotional side effects of abusing diet pills?***

Diet Pills

Images in the media and advertising present an unrealistic image of the ideal body. As you have learned, this leads to poor body image for many people and may cause some people to try or abuse diet pills (**Figure 13.11**). **Diet pills** are medications that claim to help reduce a person's weight. Examples include *Belviq*®, *Contrave*®, and *Orlistat*®.

Some diet pills work by suppressing appetite. Other diet pills increase metabolism. Diet pill abuse has harmful side effects. Physically, it can lead to an altered menstrual cycle, digestive issues, headaches and dizziness, heart failure, hyperactivity, insomnia, and respiratory failure. Diet pill abuse can also lead to anxiety and panic attacks, mood swings, depression, and unhealthy body image. People who abuse diet pills can easily develop addictions. For all these reasons, people should seek a doctor's supervision if taking diet pills.

diet pills medications that claim to help reduce a person's weight

Performance-Enhancing Drugs (PEDs)

Athletes in competitive sports and students at school often feel pressure to excel and win. This can lead some people to take **performance-enhancing drugs (PEDs)**. PEDs include prescription and OTC medications and artificial drugs made in labs. Many teens who use PEDs acquire them through illegal sales—either in person or online. Types of PEDs include the following:

performance-enhancing drugs (PEDs) medications that people abuse in hopes of improving strength, speed, and stamina

- **Anabolic steroids:** Anabolic steroids are medications that promote growth. Doctors typically prescribe them to treat cancer, HIV, and other diseases. These steroids are different from inhaled steroids, like those found in asthma medications. People who abuse anabolic steroids take them to enhance muscle growth, strength, and physical appearance (**Figure 13.12**). Abusing anabolic steroids—including illegal, synthetic designer steroids—is dangerous. Effects include permanent disability or infertility, liver disease, aggression, depression and paranoia, and addiction.

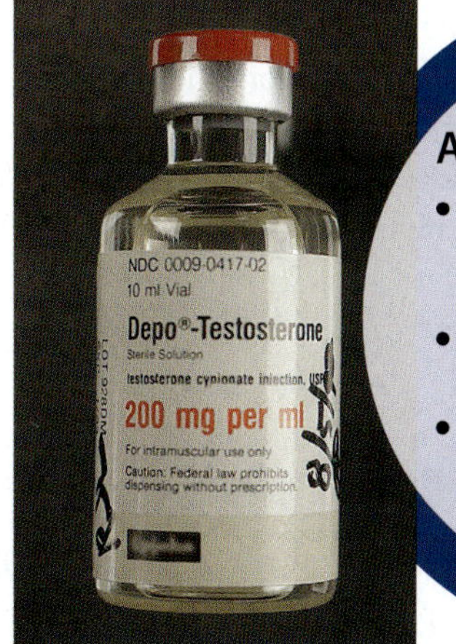

Anabolic Steroids

- It is estimated that 1–2% of teens have used anabolic steroids by 12th grade.
- Most users are males in their 20s and 30s.
- Athletes in particular are known users of anabolic steroids.

Courtesy of the Department of Justice, Drug Enforcement Administration

Figure 13.12 Anabolic steroids are designed to promote growth to treat serious diseases. Abusing steroids can cause serious side effects.

- **Androstenedione:** Androstenedione, also called *andro*, is a medication prescribed to promote growth. Advertisements make claims that andro improves athletic performance, but scientific studies have shown no effect on muscle strength or mass. Abusing andro causes side effects such as infertility, breast development in males, hair loss in females, cardiovascular damage, and increased risk of heart attack and stroke.
- **Human growth hormone (HGH):** Human growth hormone (HGH), which helps build muscle, is prescribed for people with certain diseases that lead to delayed or poor growth. Some athletes take HGH to gain muscle mass and strength, but scientific studies have not found evidence to support this use. Side effects of abusing HGH include diabetes, heart failure, hypertension, muscle pain or weakness, and vision conditions.

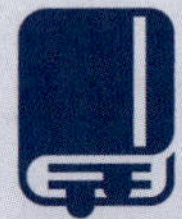

Case Study

Prescription Problems

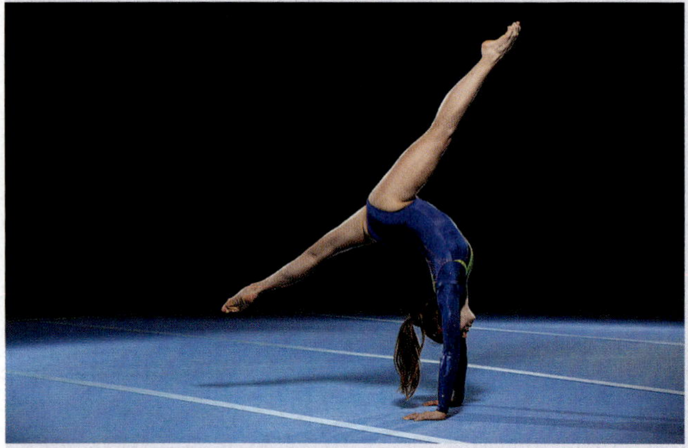

ITALO/Shutterstock.com

Raul has several tests this week, but has found it hard to focus on studying. When Raul confides in his friend Paula, she offers him some of the Ritalin her brother takes for ADHD. She says it really helps her focus on studying and is harmless since a doctor prescribed it. Raul is not sure he should take medication prescribed to someone else and refuses. When he gets his test results back and compares them with Paula's scores, though, he wonders if he should take the medication next time. After all, he really needs help focusing, and it does seem to help Paula.

Conor is best friends with his older sister, Saoirse, and looks up to her. He knows that his sister steals the codeine their dad takes for his migraines. Saoirse tells Conor she just uses them for fun with her friends and makes him promise not to tell anyone. When Saoirse takes the codeine, she comes home drowsy, sweaty, and confused, and Conor has to sneak her up to her bedroom so their dad does not notice. Lately, Conor has been thinking about telling his dad what Saoirse is doing. He does not want to get her in trouble, but he worries she will get hurt if he stays silent.

Amulya is a gymnast who practices almost every day, but she thinks that all of her thinner teammates do much better at their floor routines than she does. Her friend recommends trying diuretics because they helped him go down a weight bracket in wrestling. Amulya tries the diuretics and starts losing weight, but soon feels dizzy and uncoordinated at practice. Her coach says he might have to remove Amulya from the upcoming competition if her performance does not improve. Amulya suspects her performance worsened as soon as she started taking the diuretics, but she wants to keep losing weight. She is not sure what to do.

Practice Your Skills

Set Goals

Brainstorm goals Raul, Conor, and Amulya can set to navigate their different situations. Make a list of at least three possible SMART goals for each scenario. With a partner, evaluate how each possible goal would affect each person's health and the health of friends and family. Also identify any obstacles that might prevent them from reaching their goals. Select one goal for each person and explain to the class why it is the best goal. Break the goal into smaller, short-term goals the person can act on immediately.

- **Erythropoietin:** The hormone erythropoietin causes the body to make more oxygen-rich red blood cells and helps treat people with kidney disease or anemia. Some distance runners and cyclists abuse synthetic erythropoietin, or *epoetin*. Even if epoetin gives athletes a small competitive edge, abuse has dangerous risks, including death, stroke, heart attack, and disability.
- **Diuretics:** Diuretics cause the body to pass water and salts in the urine. Doctors often prescribe them to treat cardiovascular disease and high blood pressure. Some mild diuretics are also available OTC. Some athletes, such as wrestlers, abuse diuretics to lose water weight. Abusing diuretics can lead to dehydration, dizziness, lack of coordination, low blood pressure (which can cause shock and death), muscle cramps, and heart failure.
- **Creatine:** Creatine is a substance muscles naturally use during short, intense muscle activity. Some athletes take OTC creatine to help them train and compete. Creatine supplements may help somewhat for activities such as weight lifting, but do not help muscle activity that requires endurance or increase muscle mass. Side effects of taking creatine include muscle or stomach cramps, dehydration, and weight gain.

People can develop psychological addictions to PEDs. Without access to them, people with psychological addictions to PEDs may feel anxiety and an intense urge to use them during training and competition. As a result, they may continue to use PEDs in spite of serious consequences.

Lesson 13.2 Review

Know and Understand

1. Give two examples of medication abuse.
2. How does the brain respond when medications stimulate it to make dopamine?
3. What happens in an overdose?
4. Which type of medication reduces anxiety?
5. Which opioid is found in some OTC cough syrups?
6. How do diet pills assist with weight loss?

Think Critically

7. How does medication abuse impact relationships?
8. Explain why opioids are so addictive.
9. Why is it dangerous to abuse OTC stimulant supplements like energy drinks?
10. Why do people continue to use PEDs, even when they cause harm?

REAL WORLD Health Skills

Access Information In the US, many people die each day from opioid overdose. In small groups, visit the website of the Centers for Disease Control and Prevention (CDC) to read about opioid overdoses. What are the most common types of opioids abused? What factors lead to overdose, and how have these factors changed over time? What can people do to prevent opioid overdose deaths? What programs and resources exist to battle opioid overdose? After conducting your research, discuss your findings in class.

Lesson

13.3 Drug Abuse

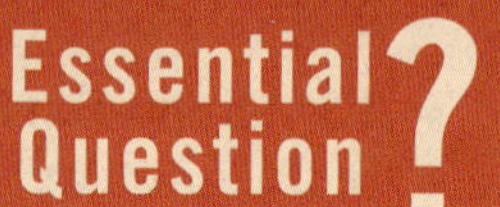

What are the health consequences of drug abuse?

Learning Outcomes

After studying this lesson, you will be able to

- analyze the role of physical and psychological addiction in drug abuse;
- describe the impact of drugs on the brain and other body systems;
- explain the mental, social, and legal consequences of drug abuse;
- summarize how drug abuse impacts families, friends, and society; and
- assess how different types of drugs endanger health.

Key Terms

bath salts
cocaine
crystal meth
drug abuse
drugs
edible
hallucinogens
heroin
hypoxia
inhalants
marijuana
MDMA
methamphetamine
roofies

Warm-Up Activity

Media Versus Reality

Analyze Influences Take a few minutes to think about how the media portrays drugs and what you know about drugs from your environment. Pick three or four examples from both the media and your environment and describe them briefly in a chart like the one shown. Do not mention names or places in your descriptions of real drug use. Compare your examples and form a conclusion about whether the media realistically portrays drug use. How might media depictions like your examples influence teens' behavior? Create a written or audio journal entry stating your conclusion. Include specific examples from your chart that support your conclusion.

Media Examples
Realistic Examples

drugs substances that cause physical or psychological changes in the body; may have medical or nonmedical purposes

drug abuse act of consuming addictive, illegal substances

Like medications, **drugs** are substances that cause physical or psychological changes in the body. Unlike medications, drugs are not always intended for medical purposes. Instead, some drugs cause nonmedical changes that some people find desirable. Drugs that are illegal can be very dangerous. They alter the body's chemistry in ways that can cause serious health consequences, including death.

Drug abuse occurs when a person uses addictive, illegal drugs. In many cases, these drugs have no medical use. People take them to experience the associated high, to fit in with friends, or because they want to escape from reality or negative feelings. Drug abuse can lead to *substance use disorders*, which you learned about in Chapter 7. The more a person uses a drug, the more the person is at risk of developing a dependence on the drug. A person with a substance use disorder continues to use a drug regardless of any harmful or negative consequences.

Effects of Drug Abuse

People who abuse drugs experience many negative health consequences. They also experience mental, social, and legal consequences that can permanently alter their lives.

The Impact of Drugs on the Brain

People often think it is harmless to experiment with drugs, but this is untrue. Experimentation can lead to regular use. Many drugs, just like many medications, stimulate the brain to release *dopamine*, which causes *euphoria*, or a *high*. After being stimulated to overproduce dopamine, however, the brain actually starts releasing less dopamine on its own. Less dopamine leads to less motivation and pleasure, and the person needs to take the drug to experience these feelings.

As people develop a tolerance for a drug through continued use, they often become dependent on the drug. This means their bodies require that drug to function normally. If they reduce the amount they take, they experience *withdrawal*, or unpleasant physical and psychological side effects (**Figure 13.13**).

Unfortunately, many illegal drugs also alter the brain region that regulates self-control. This region normally restrains impulses and behaviors. Think of the self-control region like the brakes on a car. Now think of dopamine as the brain's accelerator, motivating a person to pursue pleasurable behaviors. An addictive drug presses the accelerator (dopamine) and turns off the brakes (the self-control region).

The self-control region plays a role in decision-making. Therefore, people who abuse drugs and certain medications have difficulty thinking clearly and carefully. They are more likely to make risky decisions and engage in unsafe behaviors such as unprotected sexual activity. Drug abuse also impairs a person's ability to drive safely, causing more crashes.

Symptoms of Withdrawal
Physical
• Vision issues
• Digestive issues
• Difficulty concentrating
• Sleeplessness
• Seizures
• Fatigue
• Hallucinations
• Aches and pains
• Muscle tremors
• Decreased appetite
Psychological
• Strong need or desire for that drug
• Intense cravings
• Irritability
• Restlessness
• Anxiety or depression
• Obsession over getting and using that drug

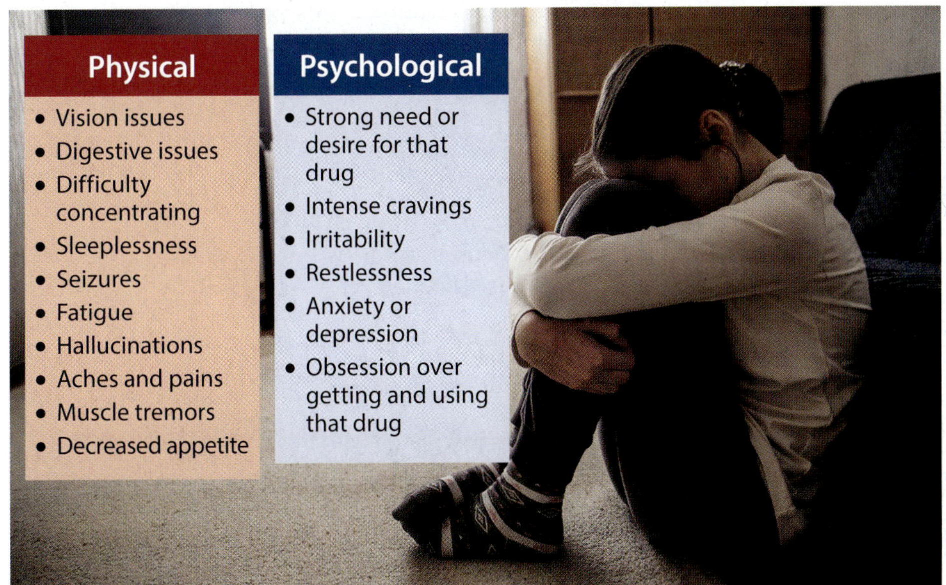

ljubaphoto/E+/Getty Images

Figure 13.13 Often, withdrawal symptoms are so unpleasant that people continue to take drugs or medications to stop them.

Research in Action

Your Brain on Drugs

Did you know that, using positron emission tomography (PET) scans, scientists can visualize the brain as it is working? X-rays and related methods visualize the brain's structures. In contrast, PET scans show these structures at work. From PET scans, scientists have learned that drug abuse causes long-term changes in the brain. The effects of drug abuse are like rewiring electrical circuits or rewriting computer software. Drug abuse can permanently change how the brain works:

- **Opioid abuse:** Opioids rewire the brain's reward centers, making the brain dependent on opioids for sensations of pleasure and happiness. Opioid abuse also causes the brain to swell, which can permanently impair memory and thinking skills.
- **Stimulant abuse:** The damage caused by abusing stimulants can remain for years, even after drug abuse stops. Certain nerve pathways lose their ability to use dopamine, reducing a person's ability to feel motivation, pleasure, and happiness. These changes occur very soon after a person begins using stimulants.
- **Nicotine abuse:** Nicotine abuse causes long-lasting rewiring in the hippocampus, a brain region responsible for forming memories and learning. These effects are most harmful during adolescence and before birth when the brain is developing and maturing. Changes in the hippocampus during adolescence remain through adulthood.
- **Alcohol abuse:** Soon after a person begins abusing alcohol, the brain loses the ability to focus and make responsible decisions. With dependence and addiction, these issues grow worse and become permanent. Severe brain damage can lead to *dementia*, the permanent loss of thinking and memory abilities.
- **Depressant abuse:** Long-term depressant abuse causes brain *atrophy* (degeneration). Depressant abuse also harms the brain regions controlling emotions, anger, and mood. Damage to the brain regions that control breathing reduces the brain's oxygen supply and harms thinking and memory.

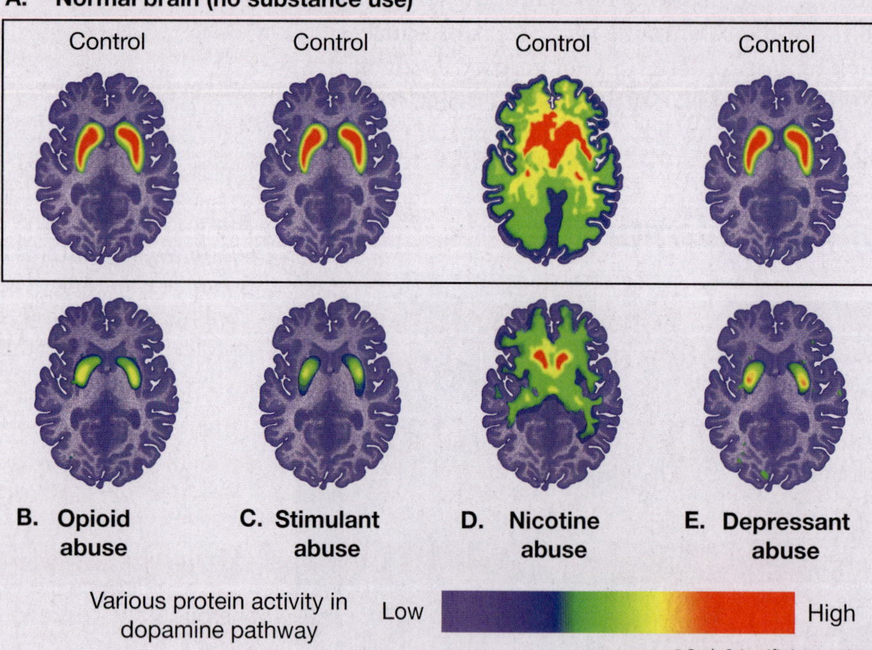

In these PET scans, normal metabolic activity is indicated by bright red and yellow. This is significantly reduced in the brains of people who use these substances, even 100 days after use.

Practice Your Skills

Comprehend Concepts

Choose one type of drug abuse discussed and focus on its long-term effects on the brain. How do the brain changes associated with this type of abuse affect a person's daily life? How will these changes affect a person's future opportunities? Suppose your friend begins using drugs. How would you explain to your friend why it is important to stop using drugs as soon as possible?

Communicable Diseases and Long-Term Damage

Many drugs cloud thinking and judgment and lower inhibitions, which leads to risky behavior. For this reason, people who abuse drugs are more likely to contract *communicable diseases*, or diseases that spread through contact with an organism or object. For example, *human immunodeficiency virus (HIV)* and *hepatitis* are diseases contracted through needle injection or sexual activity. These infections, once acquired, can stay with people throughout their lifetimes. Over time, hepatitis can cause severe, permanent liver damage. HIV can progress to *acquired immunodeficiency syndrome (AIDS)* and suppress the immune system to the point of death.

Vaping drugs can lead to lung damage, since e-liquids for vaping devices contain harmful chemicals and carcinogens. You learned about these chemicals and the dangers of vaping in Chapter 11.

Drug abuse also causes long-term damage to several organs. Some damage may be severe and permanent and can cause death. The organs affected and the severity of the damage depend on the type of drug and how long a person abuses it. In general, the damage builds over time, but there are dangers to using these drugs even once.

Overdose

People who abuse drugs have a high risk of overdosing, which can lead to serious health impairments and often death. As you learned in the previous lesson, overdosing happens when a person takes in more of a drug than the body can properly break down at one time. This can be intentional or accidental. Often, the very changes drugs cause to the brain's thought processes can lead to an overdose. A person may, for example, have trouble paying attention or desire more of a drug to get a certain effect.

Overdoses are extremely dangerous and can kill someone within hours or minutes. Even if they do not kill someone, they can cause irreversible brain damage and other health issues. Many drugs are so powerful they lead to overdose even if people think they are in control (**Figure 13.14**). Because people who abuse drugs usually buy them illegally, they also may not know exactly what is in the drugs they use. People who sell drugs may mix or "cut" drugs with other, stronger drugs or dangerous substances.

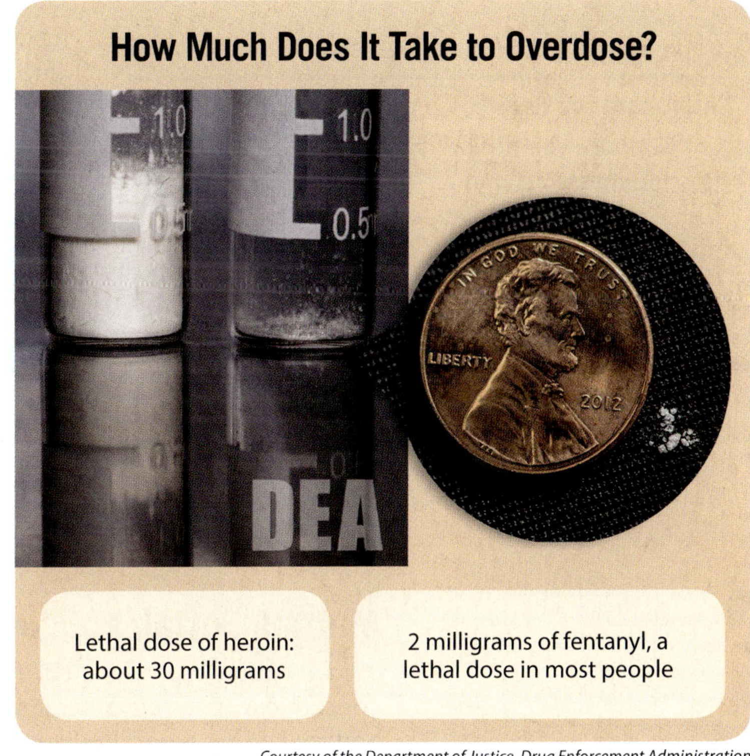

Courtesy of the Department of Justice, Drug Enforcement Administration

Figure 13.14 The two doses shown, of heroin and fentanyl, would kill the average person. Many people accidentally overdose on drugs and medications because the lethal dose is so small. ***What can happen if people who sell drugs "cut" their drugs with more powerful drugs?***

Health in the Media

Drugs and Your Digital Footprint

You probably have heard the advice *always think before you post online*. What you share on social media affects your reputation, tells others about who you are, and forms your *digital footprint*, or the record of your activities online. Now, recall how medications and drugs affect the brain. Medication and drug abuse cloud people's thinking and judgment, reduce inhibition, and increase impulsive behavior. Medications and drugs also affect memory. How would you feel if you posted something insulting about your friend while you were high? if you shared a photo of yourself using drugs and your parents or siblings saw it? Would you want friends, teachers, and future employers to see a video in which you were high?

Under the influence of medications or drugs, people act in ways they normally would not. They might post content harmful to themselves and others. They might share embarrassing or abusive pictures and attract the attention of law enforcement. People who abuse medications and drugs do not always remember what they posted and may not remember posting anything.

What you share online reaches far and wide and may remain on the internet forever. Down the road, college admissions and scholarship officials may check your social media. Potential employers who learn of your post might not want to risk hiring you. People might question your judgment. If you post something that suggests illegal activity, law enforcement may need to investigate. To avoid sharing embarrassing or harmful content, think before you post, and before that, avoid behavior that interferes with your ability to think.

Practice Your Skills

Advocate for Health

Suppose you notice your sister has begun posting messages that are out of character on social media. Some posts are crude comments, and others include embarrassing details about your sister's personal life. You know your sister has been hanging out with a new crowd at school. Now you are concerned something is wrong. Choose a partner to role-play a conversation with your sister. One of you will play the role of the concerned sibling. The other will assume the role of the sister who has started abusing drugs and is posting troubling messages to social media. As the concerned party, try to find out why your sister is behaving strangely on social media and help your sister get help to stop abusing drugs.

In the year 2017, more than 70,000 people died from drug overdose, the highest number of overdose deaths recorded in the US. Approximately the same number of overdoses were recorded in 2018.

Mental, Social, and Legal Consequences

Like medications, drugs affect the brain in ways that have mental consequences. Drug abuse impairs thinking, interrupts people's goals, and makes people more likely to engage in other risky behaviors that can further harm health. Addiction can change the way people who abuse drugs think, making the drug seem more important than everything else. Drug abuse also makes many mental health conditions and mental illnesses worse. When people use drugs to relieve the symptoms of mental illnesses, they are not treating the underlying issue. Lack of treatment and the consequences associated with drug abuse cause more distress and symptoms.

In addition to issues with mental health, people who abuse drugs may also experience

- legal consequences, such as getting arrested;
- academic trouble, such as being suspended or expelled from school;
- work trouble, such as absenteeism, failing drug tests, and getting fired;
- financial difficulty; and
- social consequences, such as losing friends, having conflict with family, or experiencing violence due to criminal activity.

Drug abuse is costly for society. The National Institute on Drug Abuse estimates drug abuse costs US society approximately $700 billion each year. This cost includes the expenses of health services for people who abuse drugs and people hurt by accidents and criminal activities. It also includes the cost of lost work productivity. The criminal justice system spends time and resources tracking down, prosecuting, and jailing people involved in drug-related crimes. Businesses also suffer as a result of productivity loss, absenteeism, and theft. Unemployment and homelessness are other potential issues that stem from drug abuse.

Commonly Abused Drugs

Commonly abused drugs affect the body in different ways. Examples of commonly abused drugs include marijuana, cocaine, methamphetamines, bath salts, hallucinogens, heroin, club drugs, and inhalants.

Marijuana

Marijuana is a mind altering, addictive drug made up of dried parts of the cannabis plant (**Figure 13.15**). It is the most commonly used drug in the US, according to the National Survey on Drug Use and Health.

marijuana mind-altering, addictive drug made up of dried parts of the cannabis plant

Marijuana
Drug Profile
Street names: weed, pot, dope, ganja, hash, herb, Mary Jane, Aunt Mary, grass, skunk
Methods of consumption: smoked (joints, blunts, pipes, bongs), vaped, brewed into tea, eaten as edibles, or a concentrated extract smoked or vaped (dabbing)

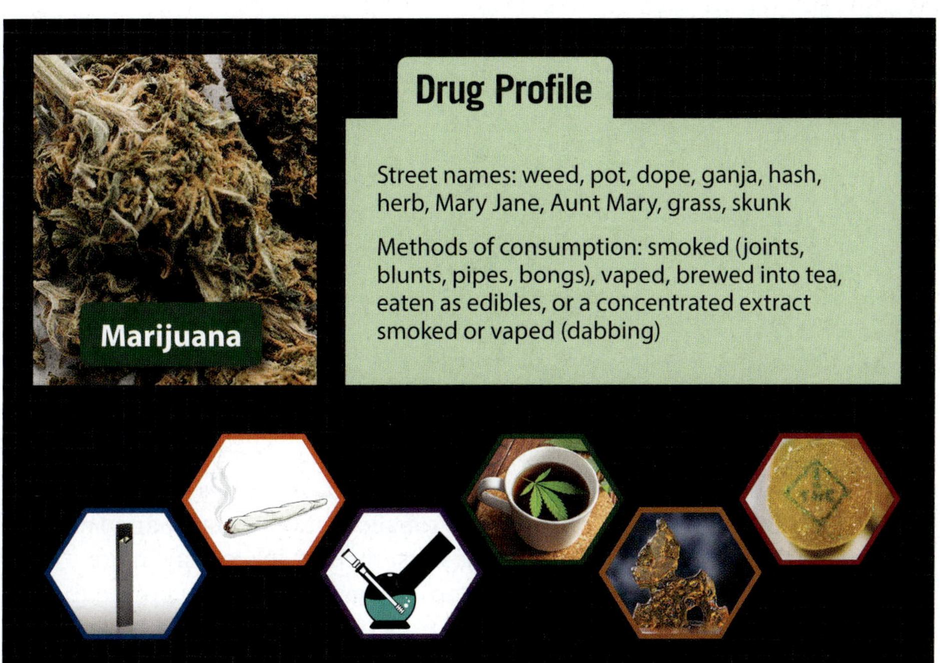

Marijuana: Courtesy of the Department of Justice, Drug Enforcement Administration; Icons from left to right: United States Food and Drug Administration; MSSA/Shutterstock.com; Cartoon Based Lifeforms/Shutterstock.com; FabrikaSimf/Shutterstock.com; Roxana Gonzalez/Shutterstock.com; Israel Patterson/Shutterstock.com

Figure 13.15 Marijuana is known by many street names and is consumed in many different ways. ***What is an edible?***

Misleadingly called *synthetic marijuana*, *synthetic cannabinoids* do not come from the cannabis plant. These mind-altering, manmade drugs have a similar effect to marijuana, but are even more dangerous.

Marijuana can be vaped or smoked using vaping devices, cigar paper (*blunt*), cigarette paper (*joint*), a water pipe (*bowl*), or a portable water hookah (*bong*). It can also be brewed into tea or consumed as an **edible** (a food mixed with marijuana or its active ingredient).

edible food mixed with a drug or a drug's active ingredients

Marijuana affects the brain fastest when inhaled. Some people smoke or vape marijuana extracts or concentrates (called *dabbing*). This practice is hazardous because it delivers a large amount of the drug to the brain quickly. Taking marijuana in food or tea delivers the drug to the brain more slowly. It may take 30–60 minutes for ingested marijuana to affect the brain. As a result, people may take much more of the drug than they realize.

The active ingredient in marijuana is a chemical called *delta-9-tetrahydrocannabinol (THC)*. THC is responsible for marijuana's high. Upon entering the bloodstream, this chemical travels to the brain and other organs. THC affects the parts of the brain that control pleasure, memory, thinking, concentration, sensory and time perception, and movement. THC also causes the brain to release dopamine. Another chemical in the marijuana plant is *cannabidiol (CBD)*. CBD is chemically similar to THC, but does not affect a person's thinking abilities or cause a high. Scientists are studying potential medical uses for CBD, but so far, the FDA has only approved CBD for treating a rare type of seizure in children.

Negative Health Effects

Marijuana is an addictive drug. Using it may lead to addiction and a substance use disorder. Marijuana is commonly called a *gateway drug* because people who use it are more likely to abuse other, more powerful and dangerous illegal drugs. Studies show marijuana is the first drug tried by most people who abuse other drugs.

People who use marijuana experience a number of health effects, including distorted perceptions, poor coordination, difficulty thinking and solving problems, and issues with learning and memory. For this reason, performing certain tasks, like driving, can be very dangerous while a person is under the influence of marijuana. The effects of marijuana on learning and memory can last for days or weeks after the acute effects of the drug wear off.

Marijuana use can also lead to cardiovascular issues. People who use marijuana show a substantial increase in heart rate. Research has shown that a person's risk of experiencing a heart attack in the first hour after smoking marijuana is five times higher than usual.

People who smoke or vape marijuana may experience the same respiratory conditions as people who smoke or vape nicotine. Minor respiratory issues include a daily cough, more frequent chest illnesses, and an increased risk of lung infection. Like tobacco smoke, marijuana smoke contains *carcinogens*, or cancer-causing substances. Marijuana smoke damages people's DNA (genetic makeup) in ways that may increase the risk of developing cancer (**Figure 13.16**).

Myths and Facts About Marijuana

Myth	Fact
Marijuana does not have negative health consequences.	Marijuana harms brain development, thinking, problem solving, mood, and memory. It also causes breathing issues.
Marijuana is not addictive.	Up to 30 percent of marijuana users become dependent and develop a substance use disorder. Using marijuana before age 18 greatly increases one's risk for becoming dependent.
Using marijuana will not affect me long-term.	Using marijuana has long-term effects on brain development, learning, and memory, especially if use begins as a teen.
It is safe to drive after using marijuana.	Marijuana makes driving dangerous by slowing reflexes, clouding thinking, and affecting the senses.
Some people use medical marijuana, so marijuana must be safe.	Using medical marijuana is different from using it without a prescription. Medical use occurs under controlled conditions and a doctor's supervision.
I will not get in trouble for using marijuana.	Even in places where marijuana is legal or approved for medical use, people must be 21 years of age or older to use it. Schools, colleges, and employers often prohibit use and impose serious consequences for using marijuana.
Marijuana helps me deal with anxiety and depression.	Marijuana does not treat underlying causes of anxiety or depression, which can worsen without appropriate treatment.
Consuming marijuana edibles is safer than smoking marijuana.	Marijuana has the same effects on the brain, regardless of how people take it. When taking edibles, people may take much more than expected.

A-spring/Shutterstock.com

Figure 13.16 Due to the widespread use of marijuana, many people believe that it does not have negative health consequences.

Legalization of Marijuana

Until recently, marijuana has been illegal to sell, buy, and use across the US. Today, a majority of states and the District of Columbia allow adults with a doctor's prescription to legally buy and use marijuana. THC, the active ingredient in marijuana and an FDA-approved medication, helps ease the symptoms of various medical conditions, including the nausea patients with cancer experience during chemotherapy.

Although marijuana use is still illegal according to the federal government, 11 states and the District of Columbia have legalized marijuana for recreational use for adults over the age of 21. Several conditions still limit use in these states. Some states regulate the amount of marijuana people can possess at one time. In some states, using marijuana is legal for residents, but not for nonresidents.

There is much debate on both federal and state levels of government about whether marijuana should be legal. Scientists continue to conduct research about medicinal uses for marijuana. The majority of people in the US who use marijuana do so illegally.

Cocaine

cocaine highly addictive stimulant that comes from the leaves of a coca plant

Cocaine, a highly addictive stimulant, is a white powder that comes from the leaves of a coca plant. People who abuse cocaine snort it through the nose, dissolve it in water and inject it, or smoke or vape it. Some people also process this illegal drug into a solid substance known as *crack cocaine*, which they smoke, vape, or inject (**Figure 13.17**).

Cocaine stimulates the central nervous system by raising levels of dopamine in the brain. This causes feelings of pleasure and a fast, intense high that makes users feel more energetic and mentally alert and less fatigued. Once the high wears off, the person feels nervous and depressed and intensely craves more cocaine.

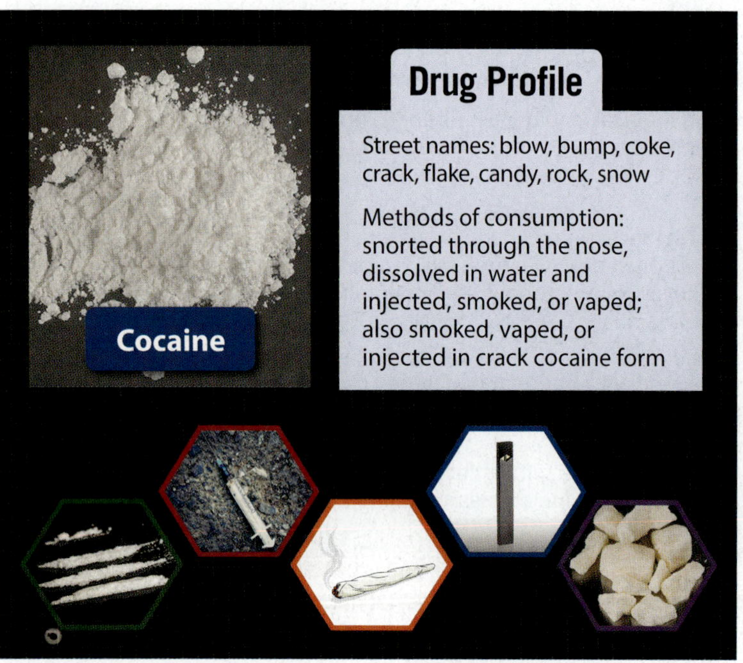

Cocaine: Courtesy of the Department of Justice, Drug Enforcement Administration; Icons from left to right: Cyber Kristiyan/Shutterstock.com; Mettus/Shutterstock.com; MSSA/Shutterstock.com; United States Food and Drug Administration; Courtesy of the Department of Justice, Drug Enforcement Administration

Figure 13.17 Cocaine causes an intense high that, when it wears off, leaves a person feeling nervous and depressed. ***What is the solid processed form of cocaine called?***

Part of what makes cocaine so addictive is that the high it causes does not last long. A person is likely to use cocaine more than once to achieve that intense high again, and tolerance and addiction develop quickly, sometimes after just one use. The more a person uses cocaine, the more dangerous it becomes.

Cocaine has short- and long-term negative effects on many different body systems. These effects include increased body temperature, heart rate, and blood pressure; headaches; hallucinations; abdominal pain and nausea; paranoia and hostility; and loss of sense of smell. Over time, cocaine can cause permanent damage to the body's organs, including the heart, brain, kidneys, and lungs. It can also cause disorientation and severe depression. Using cocaine even once can lead to sudden death due to a heart attack or stroke, respiratory failure, or seizures.

Methamphetamine

methamphetamine extremely addictive, synthetic stimulant; is powerful enough a person can develop an addiction on first use

crystal meth form of methamphetamine that consists of clear crystal chunks

Methamphetamine is a powerful and extremely addictive illegal stimulant. Like cocaine, it raises levels of dopamine in the brain. In the moment, this synthetic drug causes an intense, pleasurable high. Once the high wears off, a person craves the drug intensely. Some people develop addictions the first time they use this drug.

Some people take methamphetamine in powder or pill form. One of the most common forms of methamphetamine is **crystal meth**, which consists of clear crystal chunks (**Figure 13.18**). People who abuse crystal meth usually smoke or vape it, but may also snort it into the nose, inject it directly into the bloodstream, or swallow it.

When people use methamphetamine, they feel energized. They can often engage in continuous activity without stopping for sleep. Users also experience irregular heartbeats, high blood pressure, loss of appetite, sweating, blurred vision, and dizziness. Methamphetamine has many

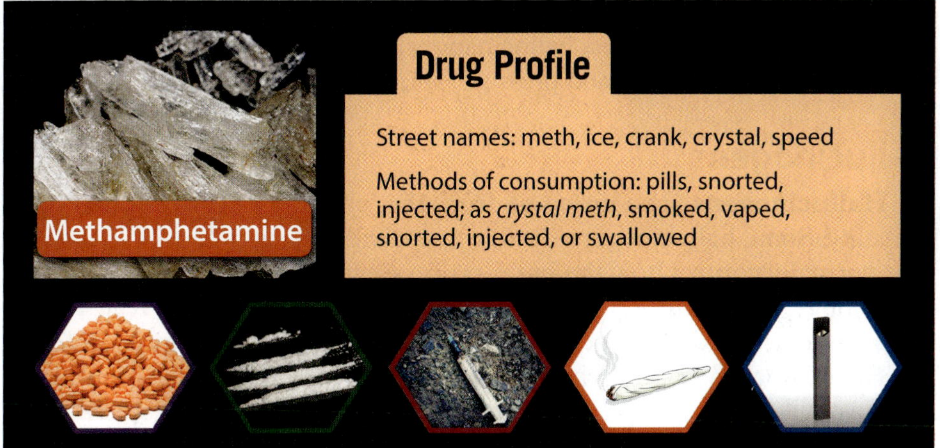

Methamphetamine: Courtesy of the Department of Justice, Drug Enforcement Administration; Icons from left to right: Fahroni/Shutterstock.com; Cyber Kristiyan/Shutterstock.com; Mettus/Shutterstock.com; MSSA/Shutterstock.com; United States Food and Drug Administration

Figure 13.18 Meth is highly addictive because, even after one use, a person craves the drug intensely once the high wears off.

short- and long-term negative health effects, which are similar to those of cocaine. These include violent and unpredictable behavior, mood swings, homicidal or suicidal thoughts, difficulty thinking, hallucinations, memory issues, and severe anxiety and paranoia. Users sometimes develop a condition known as *meth mouth*, which consists of broken or rotten teeth (**Figure 13.19**).

Long-term use of crystal meth can lead to brain damage, malnutrition, tooth decay and cracked teeth, skin sores, coma, stroke, and death. Using too much methamphetamine at one time can also result in brain damage, coma, stroke, and death.

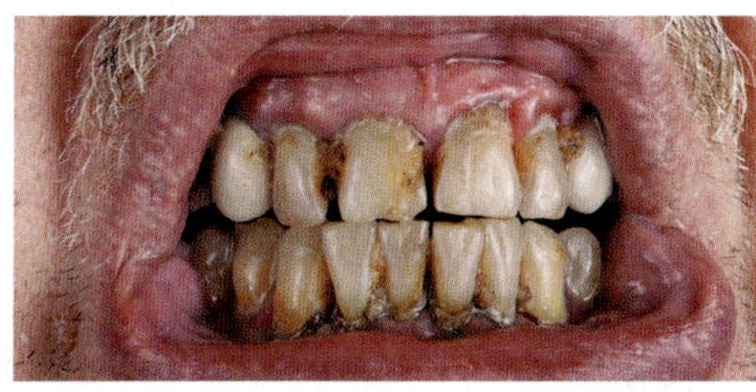

vilax/Shutterstock.com

Figure 13.19 Meth mouth has been linked to causes such as grinding teeth, neglecting to brush or floss regularly, and having a dry mouth without protective saliva. These causes are common side effects of methamphetamine and crystal meth use.

Bath Salts

Bath salts are synthetic drugs that contain a stimulant called *methylenedioxypyrovalerone (MDPV)*. Despite their name and appearance, these addictive, dangerous drugs are not bathing products. Bath salts are chemically similar to *cathinone*, a stimulant that comes from the khat plant. Because bath salts are synthetic, they are extremely powerful—in fact, 10 times stronger than cocaine. Bath salts often come in a white or brown crystalline powder (**Figure 13.20**). Sellers often market them as different products, such as incense, plant feeder, or insect repellent.

bath salts synthetic drugs that contain the stimulant methylenedioxypyrovalerone (MDPV); are often marketed as household products

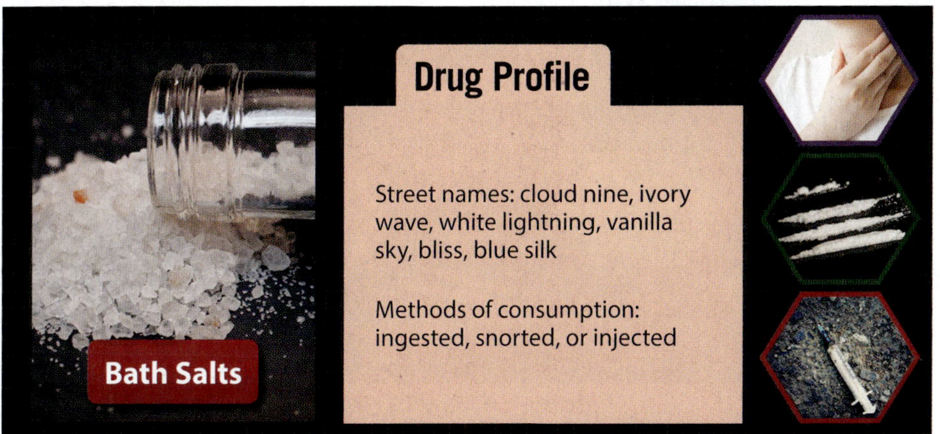

Bath salts: Courtesy of the Department of Justice, Drug Enforcement Administration; Icons from left to right: Orawan Pattarawimonchai/Shutterstock.com; Cyber Kristiyan/Shutterstock.com; Mettus/Shutterstock.com

Figure 13.20 Bath salts are synthetic drugs with dangerous side effects, including paranoia, hallucinations, and violent behavior. ***How much stronger are bath salts than cocaine?***

Using bath salts can lead to serious side effects, including paranoia, chest pains, headaches and nausea, hallucinations, panic attacks, violent behavior, increased heart rate and blood pressure, suicidal thoughts, and death.

Hallucinogens

hallucinogens drugs that change a person's perception of reality; can cause hallucinations, affect mood, and alter a person's sense of time

Hallucinogens are a group of drugs that change a person's perception of reality. Some hallucinogens do this by interfering with chemicals that normally control how the brain processes information. After taking hallucinogens, people see, hear, or feel experiences that are not real. These drugs affect a person's mood and alter perception of time (**Figure 13.21**).

Hallucinogens can be synthetic or derived from plants. People swallow them as pills or capsules, apply them to absorbent paper and dissolve them in the mouth, and consume them in foods or beverages. Some people also snort, smoke, or vape hallucinogens.

Common hallucinogens include the following:

- **DMT:** This drug, also called *Dimitri*, can be synthetic or made from plants. Some people brew it in a tea called *ayahuasca*.
- **Ketamine:** Originally an anesthetic, ketamine is also called *K* or *special K*.
- **LSD:** LSD comes from a fungus. Some people call it *acid*, *blotter*, *dots*, or *yellow sunshine*.
- **Mescaline:** Created from the peyote cactus, mescaline is also called *buttons*, *cactus*, or *mesc*.
- **Psilocybin:** This drug comes from certain types of mushrooms. It is sometimes called *magic mushrooms* or *little smoke*.
- **PCP:** This drug was initially developed for use as an anesthetic. It comes in tablets or capsules, powder, or liquid and is sometimes called *angel dust*, *hog*, and *peace pill*.

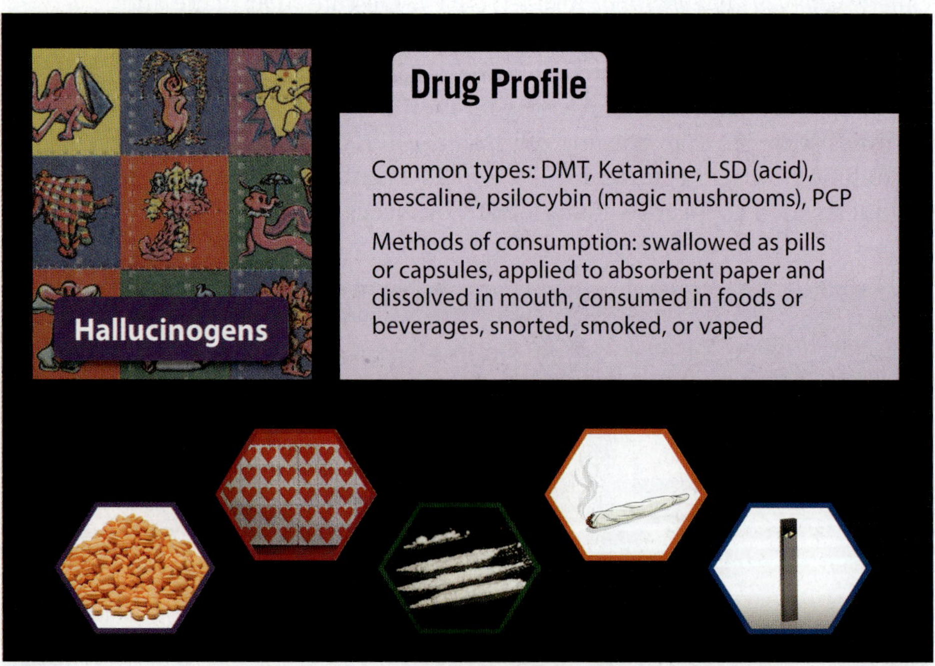

Hallucinogens: Courtesy of the Department of Justice, Drug Enforcement Administration; Icons from left to right: Fahroni/Shutterstock.com; BakalaeroZz Photography/Shutterstock.com; Cyber Kristiyan/Shutterstock.com; MSSA/Shutterstock.com; United States Food and Drug Administration

Figure 13.21 Hallucinogens can be plant-based or synthetic, but all cause people to see, hear, or feel experiences that are not real.

People who use hallucinogens experience many negative health effects, including increased heart rate and blood pressure, sweating and uncoordinated movements, trouble sleeping, nausea, extreme anxiety and depression, and panic reactions and paranoia. Long-term abuse of hallucinogens can lead to memory loss, speech and thinking issues, and anxiety and depression. Using hallucinogens can also lead to *flashbacks*, or recurrences of certain effects of the drugs days or months later. In some cases, even a single use of a hallucinogen can lead to a heart attack, stroke, seizure, or death.

Heroin

The drug known as **heroin** comes from *morphine*, a naturally occurring opioid. Pure heroin is a white powder, but people often mix or "cut" it with other substances (**Figure 13.22**). Some substances used to cut heroin may be toxic or poisonous, and people may not know exactly what is in the heroin they use. For example, heroin cut with fentanyl can cause sudden death due to an accidental overdose.

heroin naturally occurring, illegal opioid; comes as a white powder often mixed with other substances

People usually inject, snort, vape, or smoke heroin. Some people mix heroin with crack cocaine, called *speedballing*. By mixing heroin, an opioid, with crack cocaine, which is a stimulant, people hope to achieve a more intense high and avoid the negative effects of the drugs. In reality, speedballing is extremely dangerous and often leads to fatal overdose.

Once a user takes heroin, the drug rapidly enters the brain. Users feel a sudden, intense high that quickly wears off. Many negative short-term health effects soon follow the high. These include dry mouth, flushed skin, nausea and vomiting, severe itching, difficulty thinking, and semiconsciousness. Heroin is highly addictive, and people experience constant cravings for the drug, making it difficult to stop using heroin.

People with addictions who try to stop using heroin experience severe withdrawal symptoms. These symptoms can begin within a few hours after taking the drug. Symptoms may include vomiting, cold flashes, uncontrollable leg movements, muscle aches, sleep issues, and severe cravings for the drug.

If a person takes too much heroin, death can occur immediately. This is because heroin causes a person's breathing to slow or stop. The lack of oxygen to the brain can cause a coma, permanent brain damage, or death. Long-term effects of heroin use include heart infection, liver and kidney conditions, pneumonia, depression, and HIV or hepatitis from using an infected needle.

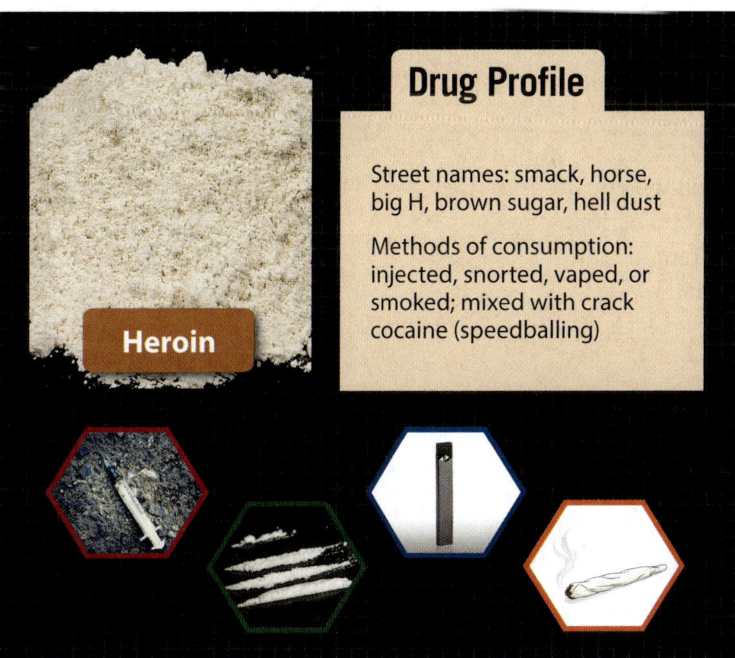

Heroin: Courtesy of the Department of Justice, Drug Enforcement Administration; Icons from left to right: Mettus/Shutterstock.com; Cyber Kristiyan/Shutterstock.com; United States Food and Drug Administration; MSSA/Shutterstock.com

Figure 13.22 Heroin addiction is associated with severe withdrawal symptoms, which coax people to continue using the drug. ***Out of what naturally occurring opioid do people make heroin?***

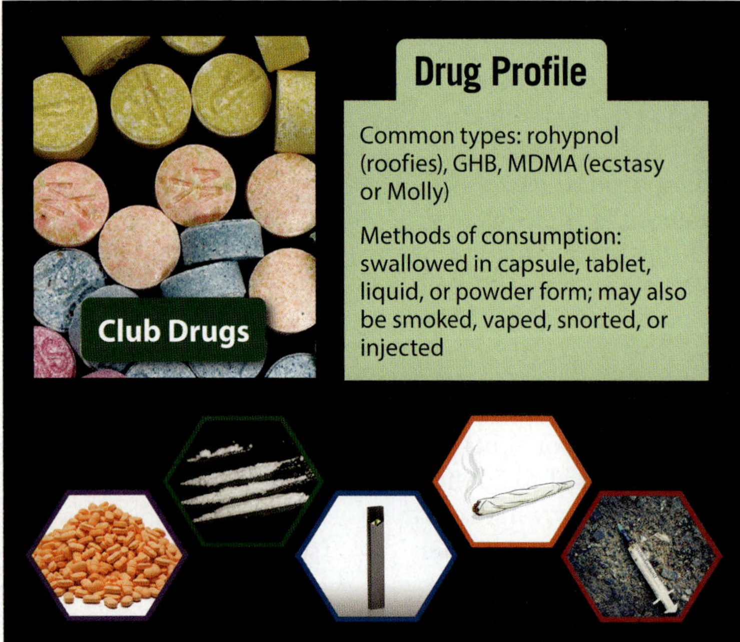

Club drugs: Courtesy of the Department of Justice, Drug Enforcement Administration; Icons from left to right: Fahroni/Shutterstock.com; Cyber Kristiyan/Shutterstock.com; United States Food and Drug Administration; MSSA/Shutterstock.com; Mettus/Shutterstock.com

Figure 13.23 Club drugs are commonly used by young people in party environments, such as at bars, festivals, and concerts. ***Why are some club drugs known as date rape drugs?***

Club Drugs

The term *club drugs* refers to several different types of drugs young people may abuse at parties, bars, festivals, and concerts (**Figure 13.23**). Some club drugs work like hallucinogens by interfering with the brain's ability to make sense of and respond to surroundings. Club drugs often come in capsule, tablet, liquid, or powder form. Some types may also be ground and inhaled or injected into the body. Common examples of club drugs include the following:

- **Rohypnol®:** Rohypnol®, commonly called **roofies**, makes people unable to move or respond to events. After this addictive drug wears off hours later, the person cannot remember what happened. Short-term health effects include headaches, nausea, dizziness, and confusion. Long-term effects may include breathing issues and depression.
- **GHB:** GHB (gamma hydroxybutyrate) slows the processes in the brain, causing an intense high and hallucinations. Short-term health effects include dizziness, nausea, and vomiting. GHB can also lead to unconsciousness and death.
- **MDMA:** **MDMA**, also called *ecstasy* or *Molly*, is a synthetic drug that increases the activity of dopamine, norepinephrine, and serotonin in the brain. Short-term side effects include increased heart rate and blood pressure, muscle tension, nausea, elevated mood, and false feelings of closeness. MDMA can be addictive and lead to permanent brain damage, organ failure, or death.

roofies club drug made of Rohypnol® that makes a person unable to move or respond to events

MDMA synthetic club drug that increases the activity of dopamine, norepinephrine, and serotonin in the brain; also called *ecstasy* or *Molly*

Club drugs often have no smell or taste. Sometimes, people slip these drugs into someone else's food or drink without the person knowing. This can lead to highly dangerous situations. Some of these drugs are known as *date rape drugs* because criminals use them to commit sexual assaults.

Inhalants

Inhalants are chemicals that people breathe to experience some type of high. Common inhalants are often substances found in the home (**Figure 13.24**). People inhale these chemicals into the nose or mouth in several ways. Chemical fumes may be sniffed or snorted from a container, which is called *huffing*. Chemicals may also be sprayed directly into the nose or mouth.

Inhalants cause a high that lasts just a few minutes, so people tend to use inhalants repeatedly to maintain this feeling. When inhaled, these chemicals enter the lungs and can cause **hypoxia**, a condition in which the body does not receive the oxygen it needs. This results in widespread cell

inhalants chemicals that people breathe to experience some type of high; often take the form of household substances

hypoxia condition in which the body does not receive the oxygen it needs, resulting in widespread cell damage

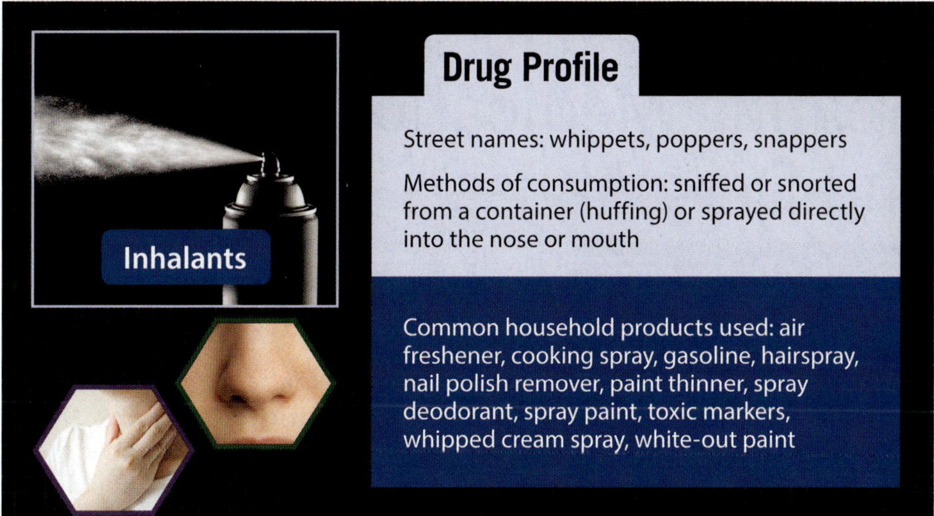

Inhalants: Joe Belanger/Shutterstock.com; Icons from left to right: Orawan Pattarawimonchai/Shutterstock.com; Asier Romero/Shutterstock.com

Figure 13.24 Common inhalants are often substances found in the home, such as hairspray or paint thinner. ***What is the condition in which the body does not receive enough oxygen?***

damage, especially to brain cells. Over time, inhalants reduce the ability of nerve fibers to carry messages throughout the body. Other health effects of using inhalants include slurred speech, memory conditions, lack of coordination, muscle spasms and tremors, dizziness, and hallucinations.

Inhalant use can cause serious, permanent side effects. These include hearing loss and damage to the brain, central nervous system, liver, and kidneys. Using inhalants—even once—can cause death due to heart failure or suffocation.

Lesson 13.3 Review

Know and Understand

1. Why does drug abuse increase the risk of contracting HIV?
2. Explain why drug abuse makes mental health conditions and mental illnesses worse.
3. Explain to a partner why cocaine is so addictive.
4. What does crystal meth look like?
5. What are two health risks of using bath salts?
6. What kind of drug is LSD?
7. Which club drug causes false feelings of closeness? Why are these feelings dangerous?
8. How does using inhalants lead to hypoxia?

Think Critically

9. Why is drug abuse associated with other high-risk behaviors?
10. Explain the dangers of consuming marijuana edibles.
11. How does taking too much heroin lead to death?

REAL WORLD Health Skills

Communicate with Others Imagine that, while driving under the influence of marijuana, you caused a severe, life-altering injury to a close friend who was a passenger in your vehicle. Your counselor suggests you write a letter to your friend expressing how you feel about what happened. Think about your reasons for using marijuana and why you chose to drive with impaired judgment and reflexes. Also think about how the accident has affected your friend's hopes, dreams, and goals for the future, as well as your own. Then write your letter showing effective communication skills and empathy.

Lesson

13.4

Preventing and Treating Medication and Drug Abuse

Essential Question?

How can you protect yourself and others from the negative consequences of medication and drug abuse?

Learning Outcomes

After studying this lesson, you will be able to

- describe risk factors for medication and drug abuse and addiction;
- assess methods of preventing medication and drug abuse;
- identify strategies for refusing medication abuse and drugs;
- describe ways to treat medication and drug abuse and addiction; and
- determine how to help someone with an addiction to medications or drugs.

Key Terms

medication-assisted treatment (MAT)
rehabilitation program
relapse
self-medicate

Warm-Up Activity

Reaching Out for Help

Communicate with Others Aparna is worried her friend Dillon may be in trouble with his pain medication. She talks to Dillon, and he agrees. He is also worried he may be abusing the medication and starting to develop an addiction. Aparna encourages Dillon to talk with his guardian, but Dillon says he does not know how to bring this topic up. Write a letter Dillon could read to his guardian to express his concern and get the help he needs before the problem gets worse. Use effective communication skills and be sure you express Dillon's message clearly.

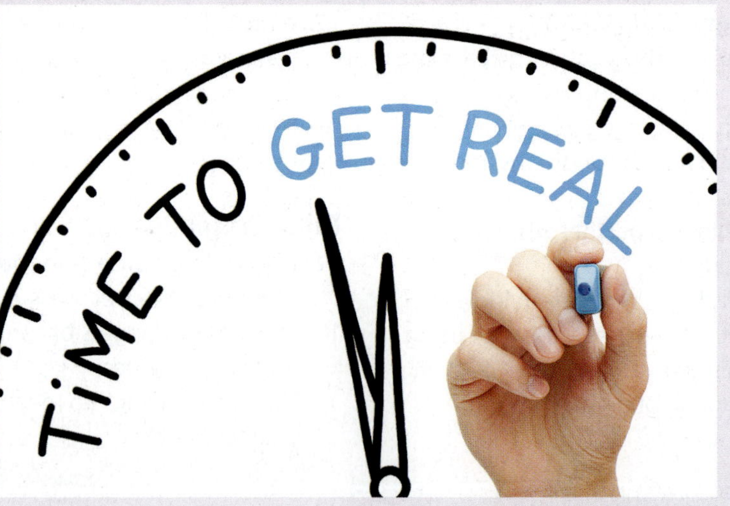

Ivelin Radkov/Shutterstock.com

No one who abuses medications or drugs plans to develop an addiction. Unfortunately, many people who abuse medications and drugs develop addictions and spend years trying to break their habit. In this lesson, you will learn what people can do to avoid developing addictions to medications and drugs. You will also learn how people can get help to treat substance use disorders.

Factors Affecting Medication and Drug Abuse

Although anyone can abuse and develop an addiction to a medication or drug, experts point to certain factors that increase or decrease a person's chances of developing a substance use disorder. Risk and protective factors for medication and drug abuse include the following.

Individual Factors

Factors related to identity and behaviors influence risk for medication and drug abuse. These factors include genetic makeup, mental health, and stage of development.

A person's genetic makeup influences the risk for that person developing a substance use disorder (**Figure 13.25**). People whose biological family members have experienced addiction are at greater risk of developing an addiction themselves. A person's genetic makeup can also influence personality. Some people have a cautious personality and are averse to risk taking. Other people are more curious and likely to take risks.

Experts believe that people's genes account for about
50%
of their risk of developing a drug addiction.

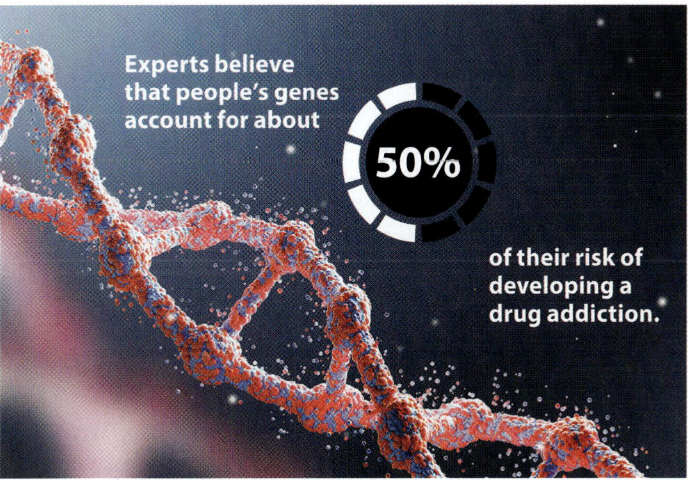

Background: ImageFlow/Shutterstock.com; Progress icon: Zoart Studio/Shutterstock.com

Figure 13.25 Genetic makeup can impact a person's likelihood for developing an addiction or having a risk-taking personality.

Mental health also affects risk for abusing medications and drugs. Having healthy self-esteem and coping strategies can help you handle stress and avoid turning to medications or drugs to feel better. Mental health conditions increase a person's risk of abusing medications or drugs (**Figure 13.26**). People who have mental illnesses, such as depression or anxiety, may **self-medicate**, or abuse medications or drugs to cope with their symptoms. When substance use disorders and other mental illnesses occur together, they are called *co-occurring disorders*. Abusing medications and drugs does not treat the underlying condition of a mental illness and puts people at risk of developing substance use disorders and more severe symptoms.

self-medicate to abuse medications or drugs to cope with symptoms of a health condition

The Complex Relationship Between Mental Health and Drug Abuse

50% of people who abuse drugs also have a mental illness.

- Drug abuse alters the brain and makes it more likely for a person to develop a mental illness, such as anxiety or depression.

50% of people who have a mental illness also abuse drugs.

- People living with anxiety or depression have a higher risk for abusing drugs.

Figure 13.26 Drug abuse and mental illnesses are often co-occurring disorders. Drug abuse makes it more likely for a person to develop a mental illness or for an existing mental illness to get worse, and living with a mental illness makes a person more likely to abuse drugs. ***What is it called when people abuse medications or drugs to cope with the symptoms of an illness?***

In addition, stage of development influences risk for medication and drug abuse. The earlier a person begins abusing a medication or drug, the more likely that person is to develop an addiction. Teens are at particular risk of developing addictions because their brains are still developing in the areas that govern decision-making, judgment, and self-control.

Environment

Your environment includes your family, culture, peers, community, and the media. All of these components affect your risk for abusing drugs and medications.

Family members' attitudes about drug use influence whether teens use drugs or abuse medications. Teens are much less likely to abuse drugs and medications if their families or cultures express strong opposition to medication or drug abuse.

Teens with friends who use drugs are much more likely to use drugs. Peer pressure is an important factor that influences teens' decisions to use drugs. Teens might see drug use as a way to gain acceptance from peers. Other teens might know that using drugs will strain their relationships with peers. Teens might fear they will lose friends if they do or do not use drugs themselves.

The community in which teens live also influences risk. Teens are much less likely to abuse drugs if drugs are not available or being abused in the community. In communities where many illegal drugs are sold, teens are more likely to encounter and use illegal drugs. Communities with violence, less education, and financial struggles often show higher rates of drug abuse.

The media that teens view is an important part of environment. Some movies, TV programs, and music videos glamorize drug use and downplay its harmful consequences. Teens might adopt the values and habits of celebrities and other people they admire in the media. For example, some celebrities are open about their struggles with addiction, which can help teens understand the risks of using drugs. Teens are also influenced by the behaviors of their peers and influencers or celebrities on social media. Drug use might appear harmless or even cool on social media, but teens cannot see the full story about drug use. Social media does not always show the serious, negative consequences.

Choosing to live a drug-free lifestyle can be challenging for teens, especially when teens' environments expose them to medication and drug abuse. There are strategies, however, that teens can use to prevent substance abuse and refuse medications and drugs.

Preventing Medication and Drug Abuse

Medication and drug abuse are risk factors that you can control. People who never try drugs cannot abuse them and develop addictions to them. Using medications properly helps prevent the negative effects of medication abuse. Unfortunately, many people do not understand how quickly medication and drug abuse can lead to addiction. You can help prevent medication and drug abuse by protecting yourself, using refusal skills, and educating others.

Take Care of Your Mental Health

One way to guard against medication and drug abuse is to care for your mental and emotional health. Unmanaged stress can lead to anxiety, depression, and other health conditions. Mental health conditions, mental illnesses, and stress increase a person's risk for medication and drug abuse (**Figure 13.27**). When people abuse medication or drugs to deal with mental health conditions, they only make these issues worse.

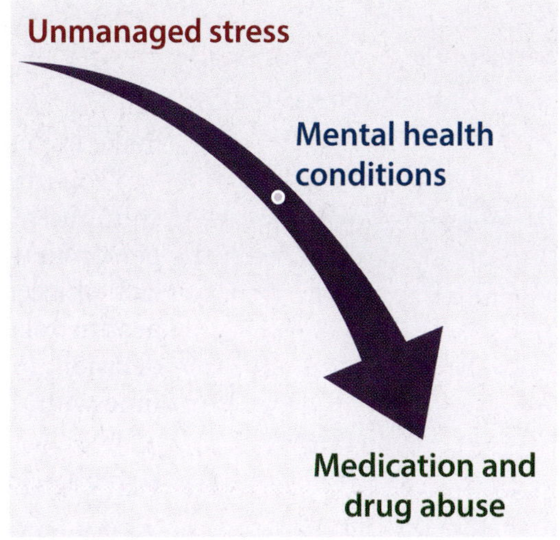

Figure 13.27 It is important to manage stress and get treatment for mental illnesses, since these increase a person's risk for medication and drug abuse.

Avoid Risky Situations

Certain situations can increase your risk for abusing medications or drugs. For example, people sometimes use illegal drugs at parties and clubs. Spending time with someone who abuses medications or drugs can also put you at risk. Avoiding these situations can be as simple as choosing not to go to parties where people are using drugs. If you do go to a party where people are abusing medications or drugs, reduce your risk by having a plan or going with a friend who shares your values about drugs. Having fun with friends who respect your decisions can discourage others from trying to offer you drugs.

You may feel pressured to abuse medications or drugs because it seems like everyone is doing it, but this is not true. Many teens have never tried drugs and have committed to living a drug-free lifestyle. A good rule is to make friends with people who share your values. You may want to make new friends by getting involved in activities that promote health and wellness.

Plan Ahead

Sometimes it can be hard to make a decision and say *no* when someone offers you drugs unexpectedly. In a surprise situation, you might panic or forget what you want to say. You might make a decision you regret. Planning ahead can reduce this risk and help you make decisions that maintain your health.

Before you get into a situation where someone invites you to abuse a medication or try a drug, plan how you will say *no*. What will you say? What will you do if the person keeps asking you? What will you do to get out of the situation? Talking through this plan with a trusted adult or friend can help you feel comfortable acting on your plan.

As you think ahead, consider how you can protect yourself from unintentional exposure to medication and drugs. Do not accept medications from anyone other than your parent or guardian, doctor, or pharmacist. If you have a headache and an acquaintance offers you a pain pill you do not recognize, that pill may be harmless or an illegal, addictive drug. At parties, do not let someone else pour you a drink or leave your drink alone. Sometimes criminals drop drugs into people's drinks to sedate people and commit crimes. At home, store medications in their original, closed containers so you will not accidentally take the wrong medication.

Just Say *No*

If someone offers you drugs or invites you to abuse a medication, you can just say *no* (**Figure 13.28**). When you state your refusal, stand tall and make eye contact with the person.

You may need to say *no* repeatedly in several different ways. If people continue to pressure you, you might ask why it is so important to the person that you use drugs. After all, you have already expressed your lack of interest. Remember that people respect each other's choices in healthy relationships. Let people know that you need them to respect your decision. If a person refuses to accept this, you may need to stop spending time with that person.

Participate in Prevention Programs

Many schools have substance abuse prevention programs to help educate students about the dangers of abusing tobacco, alcohol, medications, and drugs. Studies show that drug abuse is less common among students who participate in school-based substance-abuse prevention programs. These programs explain the short- and long-term effects of drug abuse. In addition, school policies and regulations help eliminate medication and drug abuse on school property.

Certain government groups and programs increase public awareness about medication and drug abuse. For example, the Centers for Disease Control and Prevention (CDC) and the National Institute on Drug Abuse (NIDA) create public service announcements (PSAs) for TV, radio, and the internet.

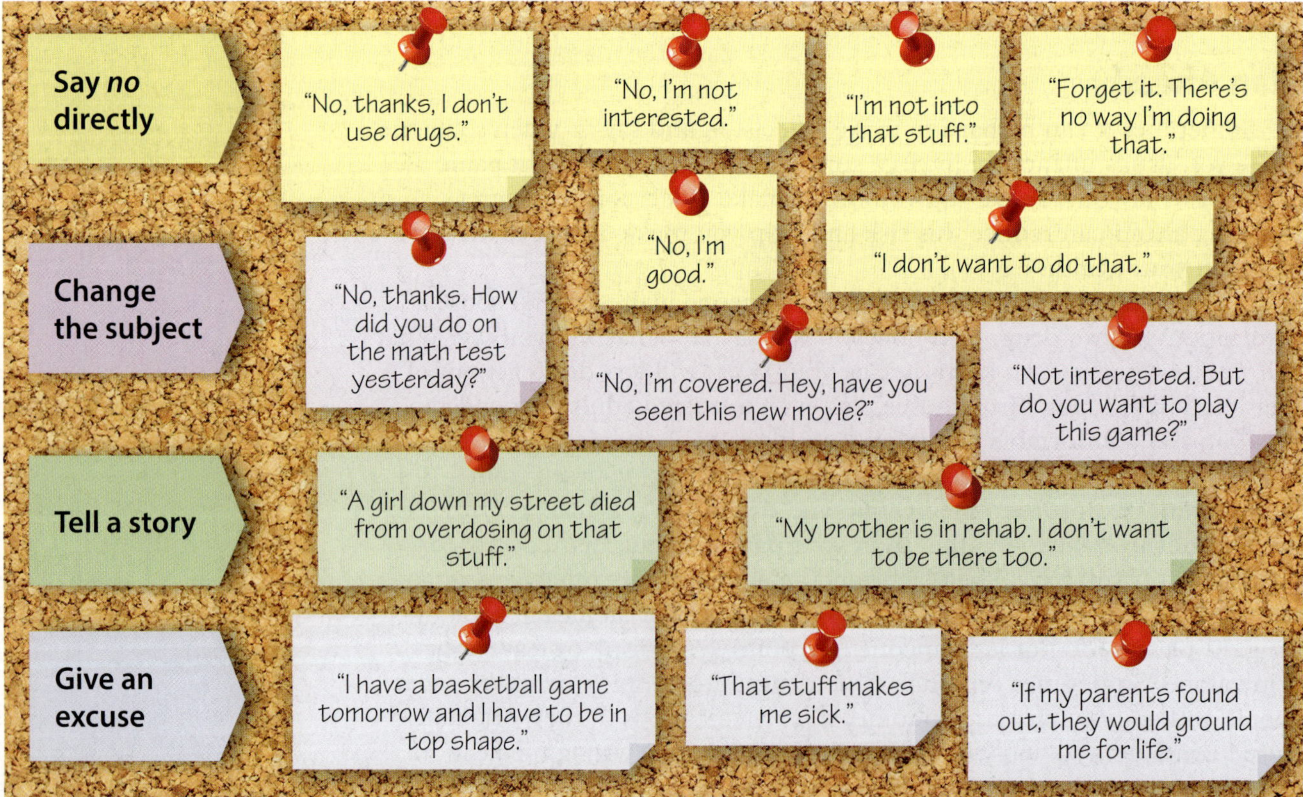

Background: taviphoto/Shutterstock.com; Push pins: Lyudmyla Kharlamova/Shutterstock.com

Figure 13.28 You do not need to offer anyone an excuse for refusing drugs, but sometimes providing an explanation can help.

The *AWARxE Prescription Drug Safety Program* spreads awareness about the growing issue of prescription medication abuse. The program teaches people valuable skills, such as how to use, store, and dispose of medications safely. If followed, the tips in this program can help keep prescription medications away from people who might abuse them.

Media campaigns also help prevent medication and drug abuse. The "Above the Influence" campaign seeks to help young people stand up to peer pressure and other influences that may lead them to abuse medications or drugs. This campaign reaches young people through TV commercials, internet advertising, and social media. "Above the Influence" encourages young people to stay true to themselves and stand up to those who may want them to try drugs.

Hospitals and police departments can provide information about drug prevention programs and how you can participate in them. To bring these programs to your school, you can talk with your teachers or school administration.

Treating Substance Use Disorders

As you learned in Chapter 7, a substance use disorder is a serious mental illness. People with a substance use disorder cannot just fix themselves. They need the help of family, friends, and professionals, such as counselors, to end their dependence on drugs and return to their normal lives. Even after breaking an addiction to medications or drugs, many people need support managing their addiction throughout their lives.

Often, the first step in treating a substance use disorder is getting help from a **rehabilitation program** (**Figure 13.29**). In these programs, healthcare professionals may begin treatment by overseeing the process of *detoxification* (which clears all medications or drugs from a person's body). Healthcare professionals typically use two types of treatment for substance use disorders: medicinal and behavioral. *Medicinal treatment* may include medications that help lessen withdrawal symptoms.

rehabilitation program treatment for a substance use disorder in which a healthcare professional oversees recovery; may involve a combination of medicinal and behavioral treatment

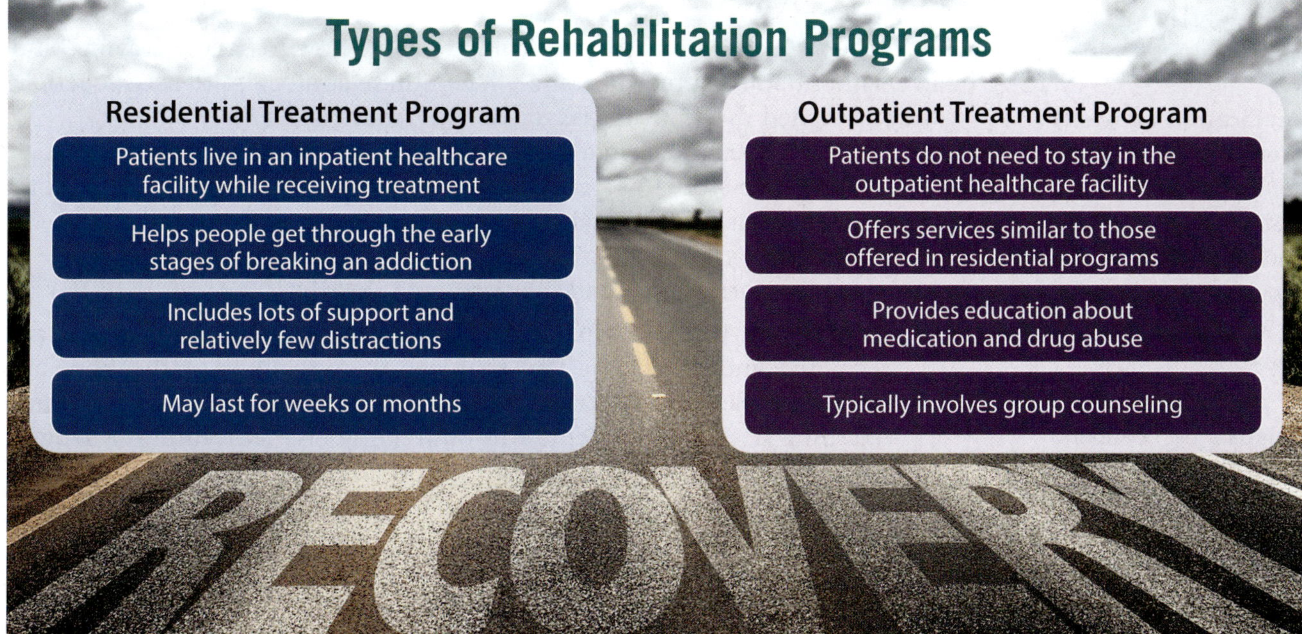

ESB Professional/Shutterstock.com

Figure 13.29 Different types of rehabilitation programs help people treat their substance use disorders in different ways. ***What is the combination of medication and teaching coping strategies called?***

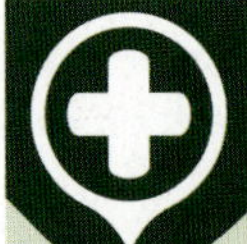

Spotlight on Health and Wellness Careers

Substance Abuse Counselor: Maryann Davis

As a certified substance abuse counselor (also called a *drug counselor* or *addiction counselor*), I work with people who have substance and alcohol use disorders. I also work with people who have another mental illness coupled with a substance use disorder. I originally chose this field as a stepping stone to becoming a marriage and family therapist. Once I began working with clients, however, I knew I had found my career.

To become a certified substance abuse counselor, you must attend an at least two-year, state-accredited program. These requirements vary from state to state. Some of the courses taken include group and family counseling, diverse populations, law and ethics, pharmacology, co-occurring disorders, recovery support, and supervised field work and internships. Counselors may also obtain bachelor's and master's degrees or specialize in specific areas or populations.

Working with clients is a rewarding experience, where one can make a large impact. As a substance abuse counselor, I teach clients skills for coping, self-exploration, and managing relationships. I also run education and process groups to encourage connection, support, and feedback between clients and their peers. As a counselor, I rely on both my education and intuition to navigate clients' progress from addiction and dishonesty through recovery and self-growth. I work with social workers, case managers, psychiatrists, and therapists.

Some of the challenges I face include handling clients' relapses and sometimes the death of a client. Self-care is essential to help me stay healthy and avoid burnout. As a whole, my career is both highly fulfilling and challenging. It requires a strong and solid core, but is an intensely rewarding experience that allows me to literally save lives on a daily basis.

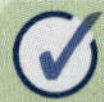

Practice Your Skills

Access Information

Think about your own interests, strengths, and weaknesses. What parts of being a substance abuse counselor do you think would interest you? Which elements would be challenging? Using reliable resources like the US Bureau of Labor Statistics' *Occupational Outlook Handbook*, research substance abuse treatment and related careers. Is the demand for substance abuse counselors growing? What are the educational requirements? Are there related careers that might also interest you? Write a blog post summarizing your thoughts.

Behavioral treatment focuses on teaching people how to handle cravings and live without abusing the substance. When these strategies are used together, they are called **medication-assisted treatment (MAT)**.

medication-assisted treatment (MAT) strategy for treating substance use disorders that involves using medications and teaching a person how to handle cravings and avoid abusing the substance again

relapse act of taking a substance again after deciding to stop

A **relapse** occurs when a person takes a medication or drug again after deciding to stop. It is important for someone to have a strong support system, as well as professional help, if a relapse occurs. People who are recovering from substance use disorders can take advantage of several programs to avoid relapse and move on with their lives:

- **Skills-training programs:** Skills-training programs help people recognize and avoid situations that lead them to abuse medications or drugs. People learn alternative ways of dealing with peer pressure and handling stressful life events without relying on medications or drugs.
- **Support groups:** People who are trying to overcome a substance use disorder come together and discuss the challenges they face. Narcotics Anonymous is an example of a support group for drug abuse.
- **Sober living communities:** Sober living communities are alcohol- and drug-free living environments for people who are trying to abstain from substance use. These environments reduce some of the temptation and pressure to use alcohol and drugs and provide social support for abstaining.

Skills for Health and Wellness

Helping Someone with a Substance Use Disorder

People who have an addiction to a medication or drug are going down a dangerous road. To stop, these people must admit they have a problem, want to break their addiction, and be willing to make the effort to do so. Someone's addiction is never anyone else's problem. Others should not take responsibility for a friend's or family member's medication or drug abuse. If people have a family member or friend with a substance use disorder, they can attend support groups to find help and encouragement. Fortunately, if you know someone who has a substance use disorder, there are some positive ways you can help that person.

Practice Your Skills

Communicate with Others

Imagine that you have a friend who is abusing medications or drugs. Your friend has hidden his behavior well, but you are starting to notice your friend prioritizing the drug over his schoolwork and relationships. Because your friend is spending all his money on drugs, he keeps cancelling plans with you. When he runs out of the drug, he gets irritable and angry. People are talking about how your friend has started trying drugs that are more and more dangerous. You know, as his friend, you have to say something.

With a partner, role-play a conversation with your friend using these steps to help your friend get help:

1. Express your concern about your friend's health. Knowing that you care and are concerned can help your friend understand the seriousness of the issue. Explain why you are concerned and what behaviors worry you.
2. Assure your friend that you care and will be available when help is needed.
3. Offer to help your friend find someone to talk with. For example, you might offer to go with your friend to a meeting with a counselor. You could also give your friend the number of a hotline to call. Try to find a solution with which your friend is comfortable.

Trade roles so you and your partner play both people. Then discuss which strategies were or were not effective for helping your friend. Create a poster with five tips for having difficult conversations about addiction. Share these posters with the class.

Lesson 13.4 Review

Know and Understand

1. How can you protect yourself at a party where people are abusing drugs?
2. Explain why you should not leave your drink alone at a party or restaurant.
3. What is medication-assisted treatment (MAT)?
4. Explain the value of sober living communities.

Think Critically

5. Explain the relationship between mental health conditions and drug abuse.
6. Give one example of a way you could say *no* to drug abuse.

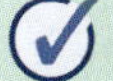

REAL WORLD Health Skills

Practice Health-Enhancing Behaviors In this chapter, you learned about the negative effects of medication and drug abuse on health. Now, consider the positive effects of abstaining from medication and drug abuse. With a partner, share your career goals, important relationships, personal aspirations, and desires. Predict how abstaining from medication and drug abuse will benefit your future lifestyle and research school and community resources that can help you abstain. Film a short video in which you explain the benefits of abstaining from medication and drug abuse and possible community resources. Keep this video to watch later if you ever feel tempted to abuse medications or drugs.

Chapter 13

Review and Assessment

Chapter Summary

A medication is a substance that treats a disease or relieves symptoms such as pain. Over-the-counter (OTC) medications can be purchased without a prescription, but prescription medications require a prescription from a doctor or other licensed healthcare professional.

Using medications carries some risks, such as side effects, medication interactions, complications due to sensitivities and allergic reactions, and medication tolerance and withdrawal. Choosing and taking medications carefully can help people avoid these health risks. Not following a medication's instructions, or medication misuse, can cause serious health consequences.

Medication abuse is the use of medication in an unintended or harmful way. It includes using medications for purposes that are not prescribed or stated on the label, sharing a prescription medication with someone else, selling a prescription medication, taking more than the prescribed or recommended amount of a medication, and combining medications without a doctor's approval.

When abused, medications can cause health conditions, long-lasting disabilities, and death. Medication abuse can also lead to addiction and serious mental, social, and legal consequences. Examples of commonly abused medications include depressants, opioids, stimulants, cold medications, diet pills, and performance-enhancing drugs (PEDs).

Drug abuse occurs when a person uses drugs, which are often addictive and illegal. People who abuse drugs experience many negative health consequences, as well as mental, social, and legal consequences that can permanently alter their lives. Commonly abused drugs include marijuana, cocaine, methamphetamine, bath salts, hallucinogens, heroin, club drugs, and inhalants.

Although anyone can develop an addiction to a medication or drug, certain individual and environmental factors can increase or decrease a person's chances of abusing drugs and developing a substance use disorder. You can help prevent medication and drug abuse by protecting yourself, using refusal skills, and educating others. Strategies for refusing medication abuse and drugs include planning ahead and just saying *no*.

People with a substance use disorder need the help of family, friends, and professionals, such as counselors, to end their dependence on drugs and return to their normal lives. Often, the first step in treating a substance use disorder is getting help from a rehabilitation program. People who are recovering from substance use disorders can take advantage of skills-training programs, support groups, and sober living communities.

Vocabulary Activity

The spelling of English words often follows set rules or patterns. Applying these rules will result in words being spelled correctly. Write three paragraphs about how medication and drug abuse affect the brain and body and all dimensions of health. Use as many key terms as you can from this chapter. Make an effort to spell each word correctly.

analgesics	*drug sensitivity*	*medication abuse*	*prescription medications*
bath salts	*edible*	*medication-assisted treatment (MAT)*	*rehabilitation program*
cocaine	*euphoria*	*medication misuse*	*relapse*
crystal meth	*fentanyl*	*methamphetamine*	*roofies*
dextromethorphan (DXM or DM)	*hallucinogens*	*opioids*	*self-medicate*
diet pills	*heroin*	*overdose*	*side effects*
dopamine	*hypoxia*	*over-the-counter (OTC) medications*	*stimulants*
drug abuse	*inhalants*	*performance-enhancing drugs (PEDs)*	
drug allergy	*marijuana*		
drugs	*MDMA*		
	medication		

Review and Recall

Review the information in this chapter by answering the following questions.

1. What are the four main purposes of medications?
2. Which government agency is responsible for making sure medications are safe to use?
3. What is *synergism*?
4. Which opioid is often used to treat people with addictions to other opioids?
   A. codeine
   B. morphine
   C. methadone
   D. fentanyl
5. Why is fentanyl so dangerous?
6. Which of the following is *not* a slang term for illegally sold prescription stimulants?
   A. speed
   B. uppers
   C. vitamin R
   D. ecstasy
7. Which drug in OTC cold medications can lead to addiction?
   A. androstenedione
   B. dextromethorphan
   C. ibuprofen
   D. acetaminophen
8. What is the difference between medications and drugs?
9. What is a *gateway drug*?
10. What are three symptoms of heroin withdrawal?
11. Which of the following makes people unable to move or respond to events?
    A. heroin
    B. Rohypnol®
    C. yellow sunshine
    D. crack cocaine
12. What is it called when people abuse drugs or medications to cope with symptoms of mental health conditions?
13. How does stage of development influence a person's risk for medication and drug abuse?
14. What is the process of clearing all drugs from a person's body?

Standardized Test Prep

Reading and Writing Practice

Read the passage below and then answer the following questions.

Driving under the influence does not just describe driving after drinking alcohol. It also describes driving under the influence of medications and drugs that impair judgment, reaction time, and coordination. This is sometimes called *drugged driving*. Some examples of these drugs include marijuana, cocaine, methamphetamine, and opioids.

In 2016, according to the Governors Highway Association, 43.6 percent of fatally injured drivers had drugs in their system. More than one-half of these had more than one drug in their system. People with THC, the active ingredient in marijuana, in their blood are about twice as likely to be involved in a deadly motor vehicle accident.

15. Driving under the influence of a medication or drug is sometimes called what?
16. Would it be true or false to say that driving under the influence of prescription medications is safe? Explain.
17. Which statement best summarizes the main point of this passage?
    A. Drugged driving is more serious than drunk driving.
    B. A lot of people are fatally injured due to drugged driving.
    C. Marijuana impairs judgment and reaction time.
    D. Driving under the influence of medications and drugs is dangerous.

Chapter 13 Skills Assessment

Critical Thinking Skills

Answer the following questions to assess your knowledge of what you learned in this chapter.

1. Think of an example of a common medication for each medication delivery method. Why do you think each medication is most effective when a person uses its corresponding delivery method?
2. In your medicine cabinet at home, do you have any prescription medications you no longer use? Are any of them expired? What should you do with these medications?
3. What are some OTC medications you occasionally use? What are the possible side effects of these medications? What are some possible consequences of misusing these medications?
4. Do you think consumers should be skeptical about ads promoting prescription medications? Explain your answer.
5. What are some programs and resources in your community that can help battle the opioid epidemic?
6. What are some of the pros and cons of legalizing marijuana? Discuss these with a partner.
7. Compare physical and psychological dependence. How do they relate to each other? Is it possible for one to cause the other?
8. Aside from the effects of the drugs themselves, why is purchasing illegal drugs dangerous?
9. How do drug abuse and addiction affect success in school? What could happen if a student gets in trouble for abusing drugs at school? How do drug abuse and addiction impact school safety?
10. Why might people use drugs like crystal meth, even if they know they are very dangerous?
11. Imagine a friend tries to convince you to try an illegal drug by saying, "It's only one time." How could you respond?
12. With a partner, create a scenario in which you might have to make a tough decision to refuse medication abuse or drugs.
13. Research your school's drug and alcohol policy. Then create a poster that highlights the consequences of violating the policy.

Health and Wellness Skills

Complete the following activities to assess your skills related to health and wellness.

14. **Analyze Influences.** No one sets out intending to develop an addiction to a medication. In a small group, brainstorm factors that influence people to go from using a medication correctly to abusing it. How do these factors affect a person's life and lead to addiction? For each risk factor, identify a protective factor a person could increase to combat the risk factor.
15. **Access Information.** Go to your school's website and find your school's policies about drugs and alcohol. What are the penalties for possessing, using, or selling illegal substances at school? for being under the influence of an illegal substance on school grounds? Do the penalties change for a second or third violation? Write a reflection about why a student might resort to using or selling drugs at school. What consequences would this student face?
16. **Communicate with Others.** Take the survey on the right for yourself and a friend. This survey will help you assess whether you or your friend is abusing a substance.

Question	Yes	No
Have you missed school due to drinking alcohol or using a substance?		
Do you use a substance to feel more comfortable, forget about worries, or build self-confidence?		
Have you used a substance alone?		
Do you ever feel guilty about your substance use?		
Have you ever been in trouble at home or school for substance use?		
Have you ever borrowed money to get a substance?		
Do you feel a sense of power when using a substance?		
Have you lost friends due to substance use?		
Are you hanging out with a substance-using crowd?		

After taking the survey, talk with your friend: Do you think you or your friend should discuss your responses with a teacher, counselor, or parent or guardian? Why or why not? Use effective communication and negotiation skills during your discussion.

17. **Make Decisions.** Suppose you are invited to a party. When you show up, you see a bowl of pills on the table, and someone tells you to take a handful. The person next to you does. You must make a decision: join the crowd or refuse the risk. Use the decision-making process to determine what you will do, then explain and compare your reasoning with your classmates' ideas.
18. **Set Goals.** Dee Dee has made some unhealthy decisions related to her prescription medications. These decisions have led to an illegal drug addiction. She has just checked into rehab. Her new counselor wants her to set a goal that will help her live a drug-free life. Help Dee Dee write a SMART goal that will help her achieve this.
19. **Practice Health-Enhancing Behaviors.** Review the information in this chapter about using medications safely. Then, create a visual or digital illustration showing strategies students can use to make sure they take medications only for their intended use. Be creative with your illustration so it is visually interesting for your peers and share it with the class.
20. **Advocate for Health.** In a small group, create a rap, song, or podcast episode about finding healthy alternatives to medication and drug abuse. Your rap, song, or episode should suggest healthy behaviors, like effective stress management, positive mental and emotional health strategies, refusal skills, and healthy ways of relaxing and having fun. Explain how each behavior enhances health and is a solution to medication and drug abuse among teens. Keep in mind your target audience: other students. Then share your rap, song, or episode with the class.

Hands-On Skills Activity

Consequences of Medication and Drug Abuse

Medication and drug abuse negatively impact physical health. They cause changes in the brain and can lead to many health conditions and even overdose and death. In addition, medication and drug abuse have mental, social, and legal consequences. Some examples include substance use disorders, trouble with the law, loss of a job, financial difficulty, and strained relationships with loved ones. Follow the steps in this activity to create a scenario in which an individual who is abusing medications or drugs deals with these consequences.

Steps for This Activity

1. Create a story about a fictional teen who abuses a medication or drug. You will tell the story of how medication and drug abuse affect this teen's life and future.
2. **Access Information.** Use the information in this chapter and from valid and reliable resources to identify how abusing medications and drugs impacts the teen's life. Address how abusing this medication or drug affects the teen's relationships (with dating partners, friends, or family members), living situation (due to trouble with the law or financial difficulties), mental and emotional health, physical health (overdose or death), and ability to pursue goals and dreams. Be sure to evaluate and cite all of your sources.
3. Use your research to establish the details of your story. Outline your story and then present your story in storyboard-style comic. Your story should have two endings: one in which the teen gets help and one in which the teen does not. Include images, drawn or taken from other sources, in your comic.
4. In one or two paragraphs, briefly explain what is happening in your comic. How does your story warn teens about the dangers of medication and drug abuse?
5. **Advocate for Health.** Using your comic, create a public service announcement (PSA) about the dangers of medication and drug abuse. Your PSA might take the form of an audio recording or short film. In your PSA, summarize the story of your fictional teen and identify the consequences this teen experienced. Share information about how teens can avoid medication and drug abuse and get help if they need it.

Unit 5

Establishing Healthy Relationships

Big Ideas

- Relationships are the connections you have with other people. Healthy relationships are characterized by honesty; trust; mutual respect; care, commitment, and support; emotional control; understanding; safety; and interpersonal skills. These relationships benefit health. Relationships without these qualities can harm health.
- Healthy relationships with family members can provide support and meet physical, mental and emotional, and social needs. While changes can be hard for families, families can grow stronger by coping together.
- Healthy community relationships help a person feel connected and supported. Some community relationships require professional communication.
- Peer relationships are extremely important during the teen years. Maintaining healthy friendships, in-person or online, provides companionship and can help people gain new perspectives.
- On top of the healthy qualities of all relationships, healthy romantic relationships are characterized by attraction, closeness, and commitment; individuality; balance; love; and physical intimacy. Many teens choose sexual abstinence, which has many benefits. Skills for maintaining sexual abstinence can help teens achieve their goals and build healthy relationships.
- Violent behavior causes or threatens to cause harm to others and has many negative consequences. One type of violence many teens face is bullying, which can be physical, mental and emotional, or social. Cyberbullying occurs online. Teens can help prevent bullying by being upstanders and engaging in healthy behaviors.
- Sexual harassment and assault are sexual attention and activity that occur without affirmative consent. These types of violence have serious consequences and are illegal.
- Abuse is the violent mistreatment of another person. Abuse can be physical, emotional, sexual, or financial and follows a repeating cycle. Stopping abuse requires breaking this cycle and getting help and treatment.
- Examples of community violence include school violence, gang violence, human trafficking, hate crimes, homicide, and terrorism. Learning to recognize and prevent these types of violence can help protect your health.

oscarhdez/Shutterstock.com ▶

Health Management Plan How Are Your Relationships?

Throughout your life, you will form a variety of relationships. These can include close or extended family members, friends from school or extracurricular activities, and romantic relationships. You may also form relationships with coworkers, teachers, or groups within the community. The relationships you form can help you grow as an individual.

It is important not only to recognize the types of relationships in your life, but also to recognize how healthy these relationships are. In healthy relationships, people feel connected and safe and can rely on others for support. Unhealthy relationships make people feel unsafe, withdrawn, and depressed.

As you read this unit, think about the health of your relationships. Use the list you will create to evaluate the health of the relationships you form throughout your life. Open your health management plan. Start a new entry and label it "My Relationships."

1. Begin by creating a list of qualities you want in a healthy relationship.
2. Next, create a second list that includes each type of relationship you have: family relationships, friendships, community relationships, and romantic relationships. For example, you could list each family member you feel close to or each friend you have.
3. As you read the unit, record what you believe makes each relationship you have with each person healthy.
4. Once you have completed this list, compare it to your first list. Do the items in your first list appear in your second list? How would you improve each relationship?
5. If a relationship becomes unhealthy or abusive, how would you recognize the signs? Create a plan of how you would fix or get out of an unhealthy relationship.

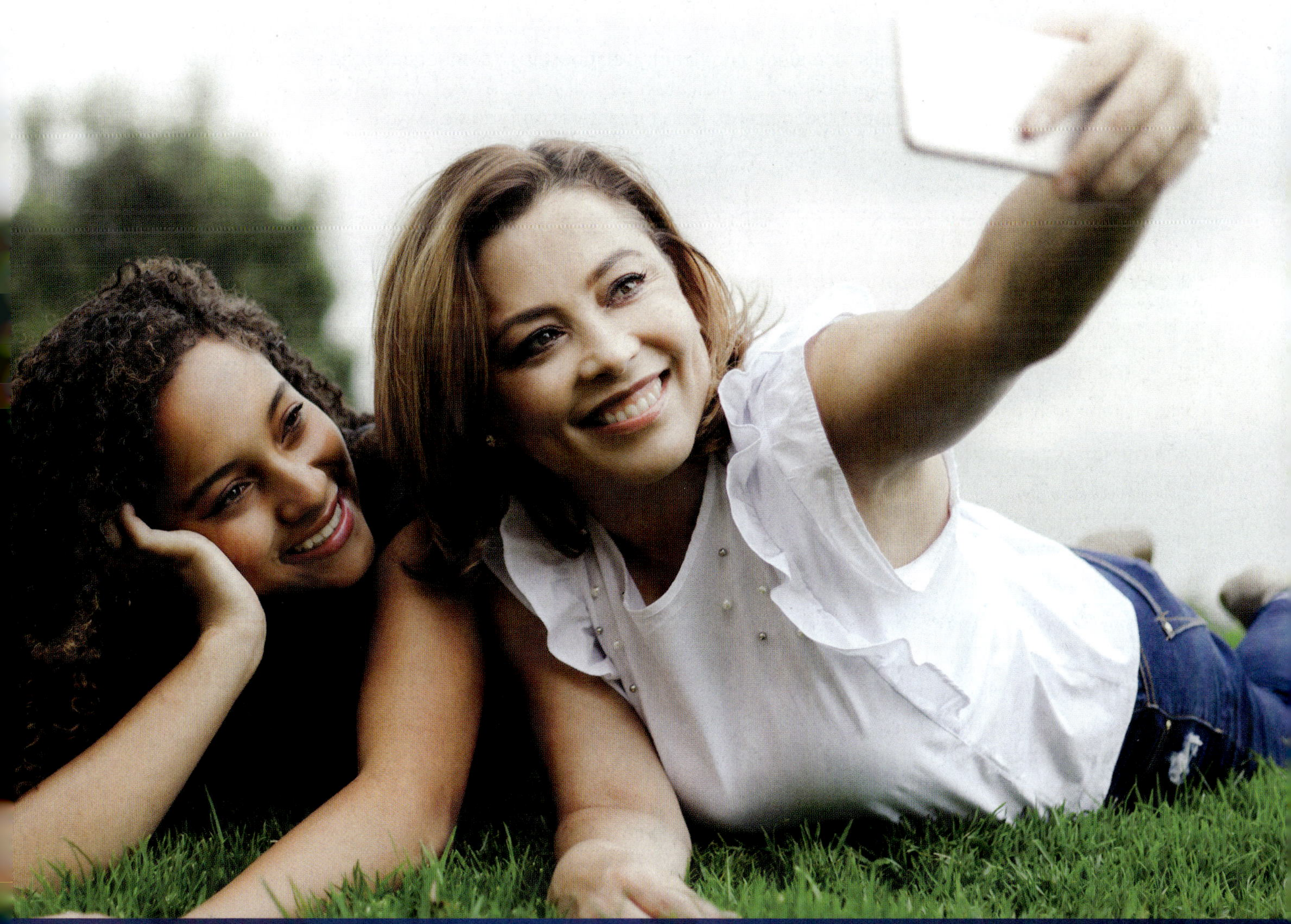

Chapter 14 Maintaining Healthy Relationships

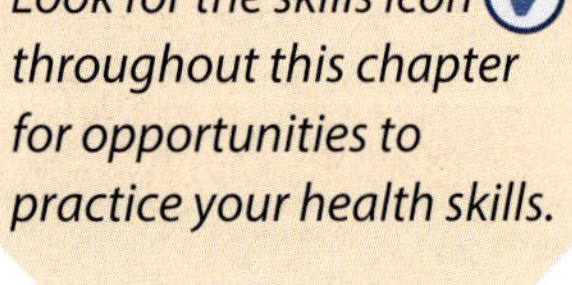

Check Your Health and Wellness Skills

In this chapter, you will learn skills for maintaining healthy relationships. To understand the skills you currently use, take the following inventory of your behaviors. Indicate how well you think you use each skill. Use a scale of 1–5, *1* meaning you do not use the skill and *5* meaning you feel completely comfortable using it.

Skill	How Well Do You Use Each Skill?
I'm honest about my feelings in a relationship.	
I know whom I'd talk to if I felt unsafe in a relationship.	
I follow my family's rules, even if I disagree with them.	
I speak up if I hear people making fun of someone who's different.	
I listen carefully when my friend is speaking and don't judge what my friend is saying.	
I avoid groups of people who exclude others.	
I spend time with several family members and friends—not just a dating partner or one friend.	
When I agree or disagree to do something, I say so directly and verbally.	
I discuss my boundaries with friends or dating partners before those boundaries are challenged.	
I know several ways to say *no* if people try to pressure me into something.	
	Total:

Add up your responses to each statement. The higher your score, the more comfortable you feel maintaining healthy relationships. Which skill do you think is most important for you? Which skill is the most challenging for you? Which skill would you most like to improve? In this chapter, you will learn how to perform these skills better and more often.

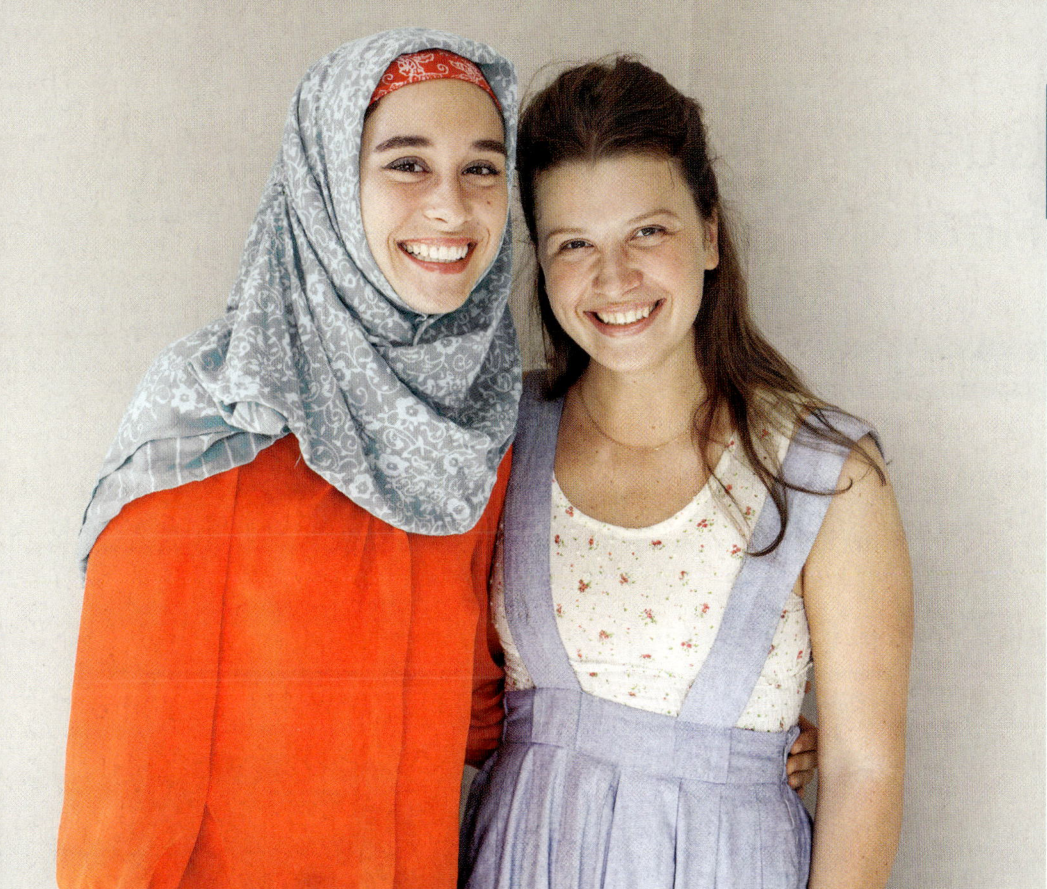

Mila Supinskaya Glashchenko/Shutterstock.com

Reading and Notetaking

In groups of three, arrange a study session to read the chapter aloud with your partners. Take care to speak clearly and pronounce the words in the chapter correctly, looking up pronunciations as needed. Stop at the end of each lesson and work together to identify the main points. Write down these main points and organize them by section. After reading this chapter, draw connections between the types of relationships as a group. Share your notes with the class.

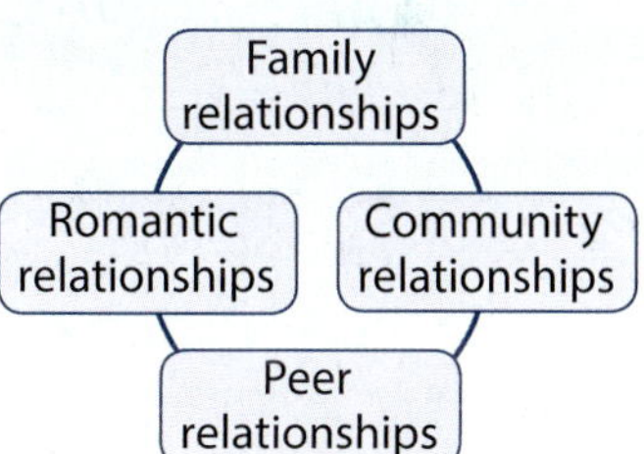

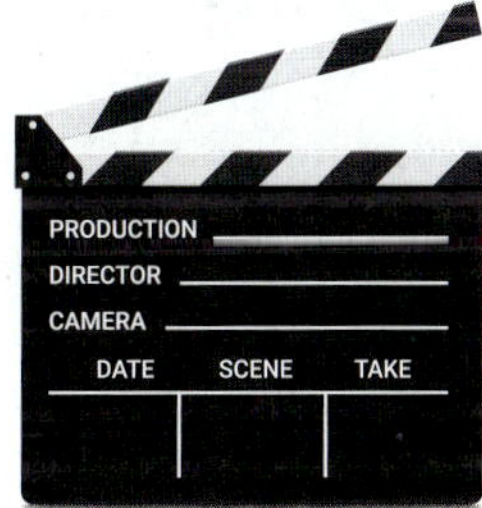

Setting the Scene

Making the Decision to Wait

Your senior year of high school, you are eager to start the next phase of your life. You have a lot of work in all of your classes, plus managing a part-time job after school and staying active in several school clubs. You also enjoy spending time with your dating partner, and the two of you have been dating for nearly a year.

Lately, some of your friends who are dating have started talking about becoming sexually active. They say that everyone in a serious dating relationship has sex. When they talk about sex, you feel uncertain. You care a lot about your dating partner, but also know you are not ready for all the intensity that comes with a sexual relationship. You have seen other couples break up after high school and know having sex would make you feel terrible if your dating relationship ends. You have also talked with some friends online who became sexually active in high school and now regret it.

Still, you and your partner sometimes feel awkward when other people talk about sex. Both of you feel pressure from your peers, even though you know you are making a healthy choice.

Thinking Critically

1. What are some factors that might lead some high school students to choose to be sexually active?
2. What are some strategies you can use to resist peer pressure in this scenario?

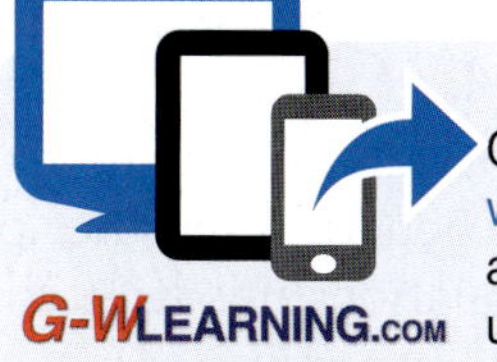

Click on the activity icon or visit www.g-wlearning.com/health/4095 to access online vocabulary activities using key terms from the chapter.

Lesson

14.1 Qualities of a Healthy Relationship

Essential Question?

How do you know if a relationship is healthy?

Learning Outcomes

After studying this lesson, you will be able to

- analyze the impact of relationships on social health;
- identify the characteristics of a healthy relationship; and
- explain what signs point to an unhealthy relationship.

Key Terms

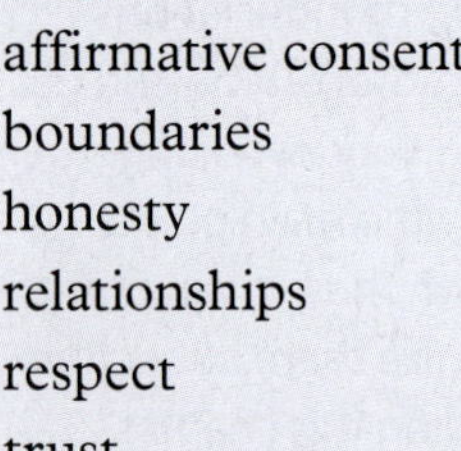

affirmative consent
boundaries
honesty
relationships
respect
trust

Warm-Up Activity

The Interview

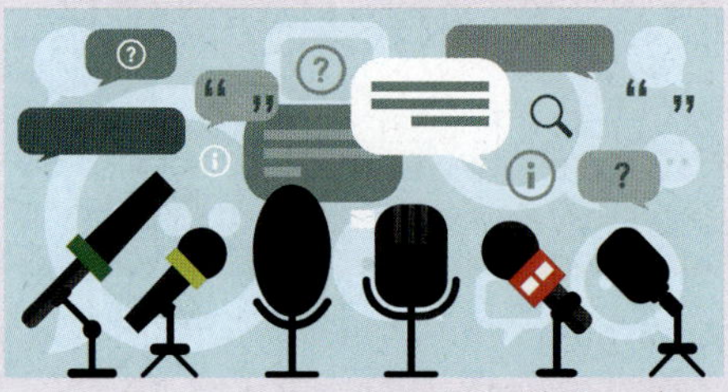

magic pictures/Shutterstock.com

Practice Health-Enhancing Behaviors Your school newspaper is publishing an article about different best friends and couples at your high school. The reporter, knowing you have been with your best friend or dating partner for several years, asks to interview you. First, the reporter asks what has made your relationship so successful and long-lasting. The reporter wants to know what characteristics make your relationship healthy. Next, the reporter asks if anything bothers you about the relationship. The reporter wants to know what characteristics might signal your relationship is unhealthy. Write a script or record a video in which you answer the reporter's questions about a close friendship or dating relationship in your life.

Relationships are the bonds you have with other people. Think about the many ways you are connected to other people and how they are connected to you. Your social network includes family members, friends, classmates, community members, and sometimes dating partners. All of the **relationships**, or connections you form and maintain with other people, affect your *social health*. Enjoyable, healthy, supportive relationships that make you feel good about yourself lead to positive social health.

relationships
connections that people form and maintain with others

Why Are Relationships Important?

At every age, people live in social groups that influence their health. Many people have families and rely on friends and partners for support. In addition, children and teens have relationships with fellow students, teachers, and other peers and adults. As you grow up, you may also have relationships with coworkers, dating partners, and groups within the community.

Some relationships meet basic human needs, such as the needs for nutrition and shelter. Most of these relationships are in families. Your physical health depends on these needs being met. Even if other relationships do not directly meet your physical needs, they also affect your physical health (**Figure 14.1**).

Relationships also impact other areas of your health. For example, relationships meet the need to belong to a group and to feel connected with and loved by other people. Your relationships also impact you emotionally. An argument with a friend can make you feel angry or sad. A smile or a compliment from a friend or classmate can lift your spirits. Socially, relationships give you the opportunity to learn about yourself, receive and provide emotional support, and gain skills related to communication and conflict resolution.

People with social support
• are less likely to get sick
• recover from disease faster
• live longer
than people who lack social support.
Relationships filled with
• conflict
• stress
• tension
can have the opposite effect.

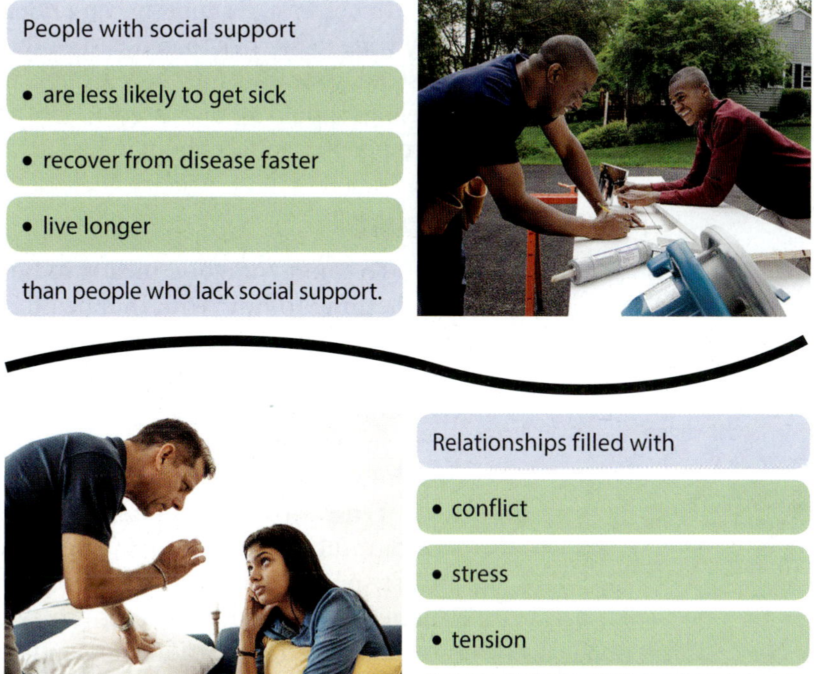

Top to bottom: David Sacks/DigitalVision/Getty Images; Pollyana Ventura/E+/Getty Images

Figure 14.1 Social support can greatly increase people's physical health, while unhealthy relationships can have the opposite effect.

Characteristics of Healthy Relationships

How do you know if a relationship is affecting you in a positive or negative way? One way to know is to assess the health of a relationship. Healthy relationships are likely to improve your health, while unhealthy relationships can hurt you. For example, in healthy relationships, people encourage healthy behaviors and receive support from family members and friends when they go through hard times. This support gives people the strength they need to recover from challenges. On the other hand, people in unhealthy relationships often do not receive the support they need, which can harm physical, mental, and emotional health.

Healthy relationships can improve all aspects of health and wellness. You can judge a relationship's health by examining several key characteristics. A healthy relationship is characterized by honesty; trust; mutual respect; care, commitment, and support; emotional control; understanding; safety; and interpersonal skills.

Honesty

Honesty involves being truthful about what you have done, what you want, and how you feel. In an honest relationship, both people feel comfortable expressing their likes, dislikes, goals, values, priorities, and thoughts. They can discuss these topics openly, honestly, and with respect.

honesty truthfulness about one's actions, desires, and feelings

In contrast, dishonesty can undermine a relationship. For example, if you say you are too sick to come to work, but your boss finds out you went shopping instead, your boss may have trouble trusting you again. In these situations, hurt feelings should be discussed openly and honestly. If the relationship is healthy, two people can talk about the issue and work together to resolve the conflict.

Trust

trust belief in another person's reliability and good intentions

To **trust** someone means to believe the person is not going to do or say something to hurt you. In a healthy relationship, trust is necessary. People need to be comfortable sharing their thoughts, feelings, and ideas without fear of being hurt. For example, in a trusting relationship, you can tell a parent or guardian how you feel without being mocked or insulted. You can tell your friend something personal and expect your friend not to gossip about it to other classmates.

Trust is broken in a relationship if someone is dishonest, disloyal, or unfaithful. All of these behaviors are hurtful, and it can be very hard to trust someone again after trust is broken. Some relationships become unhealthy or end after trust is broken. In other cases, after trust is reestablished, a relationship can grow stronger (**Figure 14.2**).

Mutual Respect

respect acknowledgment that each person has worth and deserves to have needs met; is shown through kindness and considerate behavior

Respect is knowing that each person has worth as a human being and has a right to have personal feelings and desires recognized. Showing kindness and being considerate to others also shows respect.

Figure 14.2 Some people blame themselves when another person violates their trust. They assume they could have done something to prevent the person's behavior, such as being a better person or trusting the person less. In reality, no one is ever to blame for someone else's choices. ***What can happen in a relationship when trust is broken?***

Handling Broken Trust in a Relationship

When deciding whether to maintain a relationship after trust has been broken, think about whether the other person deserves your trust. These questions will help you figure out if trusting the person again is a good idea:

- Is the person apologetic?
- Has the person shown genuine remorse?
- Are there circumstances that explain the person's behavior?
- Do you have reason to believe this person's actions will change in the future?

Some types of broken trust should signal the end of a relationship. For example, if a relationship involves any violence or neglect, leaving the relationship is a better strategy than rebuilding trust. Talk to a trusted adult if you have experienced any kind of violence in a relationship. You could also reach out to a local talk or text help line.

If trust has been broken and both people want to save the relationship, forgiveness is necessary. If you want to restore a relationship after breaking someone's trust, start by forgiving yourself. If someone has broken your trust, remember that it is impossible to move on in a relationship if you cannot forgive the other person. Forgiveness can be very difficult and may take time, but you can try to move on by recognizing that all people make mistakes. Try to focus on that person's positive qualities, even if the person did disappoint you.

In a relationship, respect also means recognizing that each person in a relationship has unique experiences, opinions, and values. Respect should be *mutual*, or go both ways.

Relationships with mutual respect have distinct features. In a respectful relationship, people do not repeatedly call or text to check whom the other person is with or go through each other's belongings without permission. If people are concerned about something in the relationship, they discuss it directly. People in a respectful relationship openly communicate with each another. They do not expect the other person to be a mind reader or withdraw from difficult conversations. People also show respect by making and keeping plans and commitments. When people make a promise, they follow through. These actions show respect for the other person.

Care, Commitment, and Support

People demonstrate care and commitment when they show concern for another person and work to make the relationship better. Working through conflicts is an example of showing commitment to a relationship. In a healthy relationship, both people are invested in resolving disagreements and maintaining the relationship.

Showing care and commitment can also include providing support (**Figure 14.3**). If your friend or dating partner does well in an audition for the school play, you can be supportive by celebrating and being happy. You can also support a sibling or classmate who is sad or hurt. Helping each other through tough times can bring you closer together and strengthen your relationship.

Emotional Control

Controlling your emotions is an important part of building a healthy relationship. If you cannot control your emotions, you might hurt the other person, leading to broken trust. Learning to express your emotions clearly and respectfully can improve a relationship.

For example, controlling your anger can help you work through conflict in a positive way. When you get angry, instead of yelling at another person, you can walk away from the situation to cool down and take a few deep breaths. After doing an activity to calm down (such as being physically active, writing in a journal, or listening to music), you can state your feelings to the other person calmly.

People in healthy relationships should support each other in their
• successes
• failures
• goals
• interests
• happiness
• anxiety
• sadness
• talents
• struggles
• actions
GCShutter/E+/Getty Images

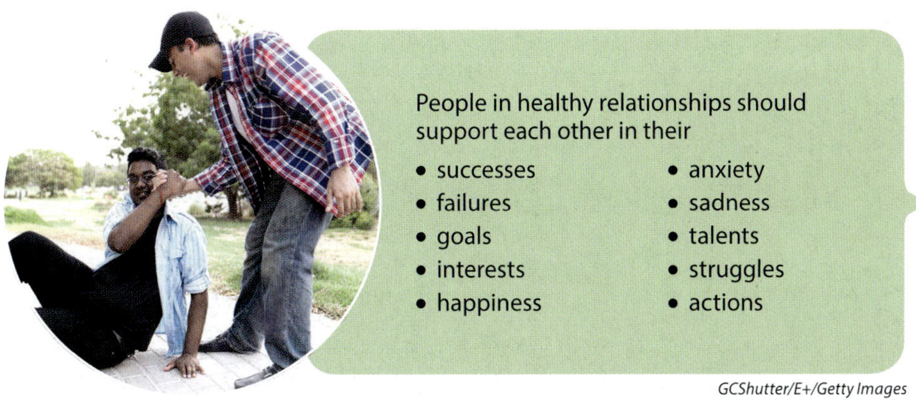

Figure 14.3 One of the most important aspects of a healthy relationship is that each person supports the other person in fun times and in hard times.

Understanding

When you show understanding, you acknowledge and relate to the feelings and thoughts of another person. You use empathy to put yourself in the other person's shoes. For example, if your friend does something you would never do, showing understanding could mean accepting your friend's behavior instead of criticizing it. It could mean acknowledging your friend's feelings instead of saying a situation is not a big deal.

Safety

In a healthy relationship, each person feels safe with the other person. The people in your life—family members, friends, dating partners, teachers and students, and community members included—should never make you feel unsafe. If you feel unsafe, the relationship is unhealthy, and you should speak with a trusted adult or reach out to community resources for support.

In a healthy relationship, people care about each other's well-being. Each person respects the other's personal **boundaries**, or rules about behavior. Part of respecting boundaries is giving and receiving **affirmative consent**, which is a direct, verbal, freely given agreement that occurs when someone clearly says *yes* (**Figure 14.4**). For example, you should ask before touching another person's body. If you tell someone not to call you at a certain time, this person should agree to call you at a different time. You will learn more about affirmative consent in Chapter 15.

boundaries rules about what behaviors are acceptable or unacceptable

affirmative consent direct, verbal, freely given agreement that occurs when someone clearly says *yes*

Interpersonal Skills

Interpersonal skills are the skills used to maintain relationships. You learned about these skills in Chapter 3. They help people communicate and resolve conflicts in positive ways. Healthy relationships are built using interpersonal skills such as communication, active listening, teamwork, leadership, and conflict resolution. Poor interpersonal skills can lead to misunderstandings, unnecessary conflict, and hurt feelings.

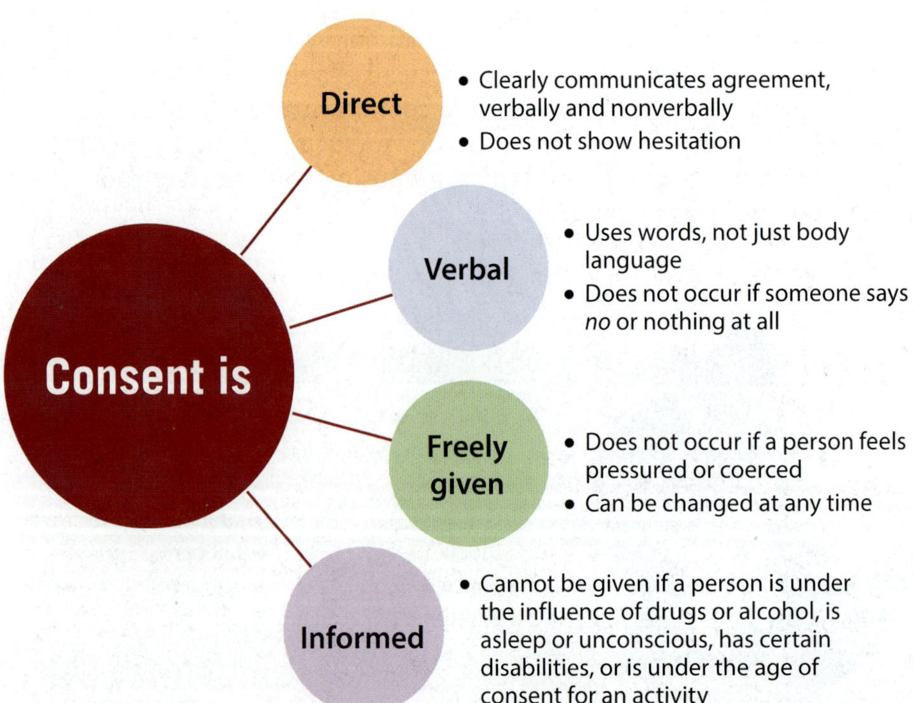

Figure 14.4 Understanding consent is an important part of respecting and communicating boundaries. You will learn more about what consent is and is not in Chapter 15. ***What situations indicate that a person cannot give informed consent?***

Signs of an Unhealthy Relationship

If the characteristics of a healthy relationship are missing from a relationship in your life, then that relationship is unhealthy and needs to change. While you are in a relationship, you may have trouble seeing the signs of an unhealthy relationship. This is especially true for people who were raised in an environment where a lack of respect, kindness, and trust was considered normal and where anger and verbal or physical abuse were present.

Learning to recognize an unhealthy relationship is important (**Figure 14.5**). Once you know a relationship is unhealthy, you can take action to change or leave the relationship and get help from a trusted adult or community resource.

If you have experienced or been threatened with violence, or if you feel unsafe, you should tell someone you trust and get out of that relationship as soon as possible. Some teens make excuses for others' abusive behavior, but there is never an excuse for hurting others—mentally, physically, or emotionally.

Health in the Media

Media Relationships: Healthy or Unhealthy?

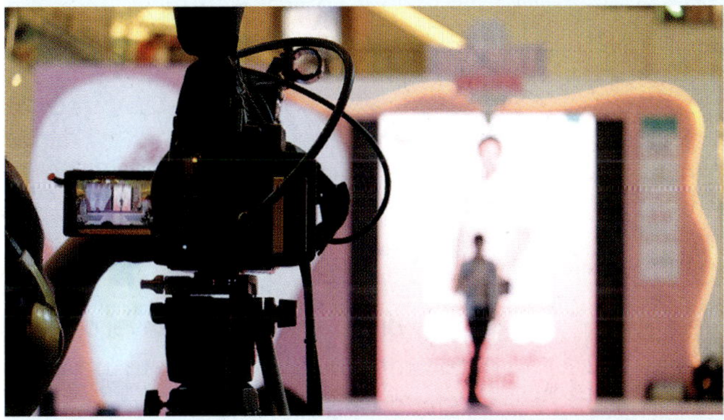

Phawat/Shutterstock.com

Think about the relationships you see portrayed in movies, books, and shows. What are these relationships like? Many teens learn about relationships from representations in the media and social media, but in many cases, the media does not present realistic or healthy examples.

Sometimes friendships in the media rely on aggressive or passive behavior. Relationships may be full of poorly managed conflict or have no conflict at all, and only certain aspects of relationships may be shown. Other times, heroic figures in the media seem detached from friendships or family relationships.

Media depictions of romantic relationships are often glamorous and fast moving with few consequences. For example, many movies, shows, and books portray an overly romantic view of love. Couples appear to fall in love very quickly, rarely have any serious conflicts to resolve, and may be totally dependent on each other. In the real world, love often happens gradually as people get to know each other on a deeper level, which takes time. Conflict is an important component of all healthy relationships and helps people develop communication skills and grow closer. Healthy relationships should include respect for each person's goals and interests.

Practice Your Skills

Analyze Influences

Think about the relationships you have seen portrayed in the media. What media representations have you seen of family relationships? friendships? romantic and community relationships? What are the features of these relationships? Are these relationships healthy? Choose one relationship you have seen portrayed in the media. List the features of this relationship and then compare this list to the features of a healthy and unhealthy relationship. What qualities of a healthy relationship are missing? Does the relationship show any signs of being unhealthy? Does the media recognize that the relationship is unhealthy? Why or why not? Share your thoughts with a partner and discuss how the relationships portrayed in the media could affect teens' expectations for their own relationships.

Figure 14.5 One or both people may contribute these unhealthy behaviors or responses to a relationship. Recognizing these signs is the first step toward improving or leaving an unhealthy relationship.

Unhealthy Relationship Signs

Behaviors

- angry outbursts
- constant fighting
- mocking, making fun of, or criticizing
- extreme jealousy
- telling the other person to stay away from friends or family
- discouraging activities with others
- threats of violence or any acts of violence
- pressuring the other person into activities that make that person uncomfortable
- showing more or less interest in maintaining the relationship than the other person
- constantly excusing the other person's behavior
- not respecting boundaries and consent
- encouraging risky or unhealthy behaviors

Responses

- feeling unsafe or pressured
- feeling used, ignored, or unappreciated
- feeling angry, sad, or anxious about the relationship
- feeling one can never say anything right
- feeling isolated from friends and family
- feeling overwhelmed or smothered

Lesson 14.1 Review

Know and Understand

1. Give one example of how relationships affect health.
2. What does it mean to be honest in a relationship?
3. In your own words, define *mutual respect*.
4. Why is emotional control important for resolving conflicts?
5. With a partner, discuss the signs that a relationship is safe or unsafe.
6. Choose one sign of an unhealthy relationship and explain what qualities of a healthy relationship are missing if this sign is present.

Think Critically

7. With a partner, discuss signs that indicate whether trust should or should not be rebuilt in a relationship.
8. How do you know what level of commitment is appropriate in a relationship?
9. Think of a time a friend or family member showed you understanding. How did it make you feel?

REAL WORLD Health Skills

Communicate with Others Maybe you have heard the common saying "You can't understand someone until you've walked a mile in their shoes." This saying is about *understanding*, one healthy relationship characteristic. Think of a time someone you know caused a conflict or did something you did not like. How did you react? Were you understanding? Did you become angry or judgmental about the situation? On a piece of paper, draw that person's shoes. Imagine yourself in those shoes. How do you feel? Do you feel differently in that person's shoes, as compared to your own shoes? Do you see things differently? Record your notes on the person's shoes. Think back on the same situation. Do you have a new perspective? Why or why not? Would you change the way you reacted if you could? If so, how? Draw your own shoes next to the other person's shoes and write your notes on them.

Supporting Family and Community Relationships

Essential Question?

What can you do to promote the health of your family and community?

Lesson 14.2

Learning Outcomes

After studying this lesson, you will be able to

- analyze the functions of the family;
- utilize strategies to promote healthy relationships with parents or guardians, siblings, and grandparents;
- explain ways to cope with various changes that occur within families;
- give examples of community relationships; and
- demonstrate skills for maintaining healthy community relationships.

Key Terms

coworkers
extended family
immediate family
law enforcement
mentors
professional communication
sibling rivalry
socialize
supervisor
traditions

Warm-Up Activity

Family Village

Analyze Influences One common saying is that "it takes a village to raise a child." Create and decorate your own family village. In your village, list people who have been influential in your childhood. This list might include family members, neighbors, school or community members, or other trusted adults or peers. Next to each person, briefly explain your relationship, why the person holds a place in your village, and how the person has influenced you.

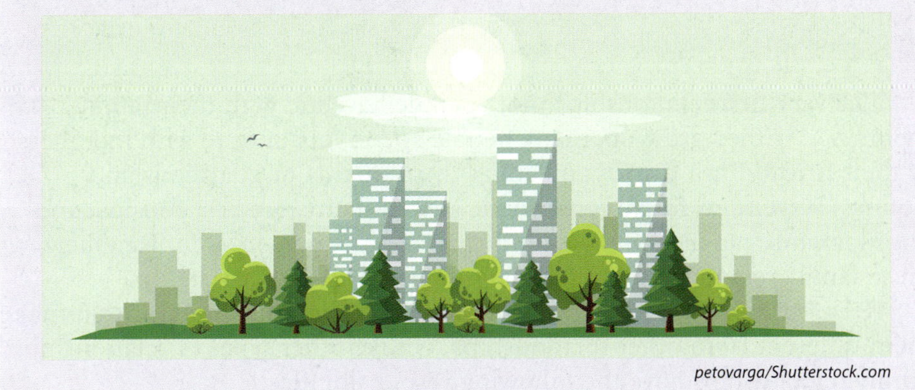

petovarga/Shutterstock.com

Relationships are the bonds and connections you have with other people, including family members, friends, classmates, people in your community, and dating partners. In this lesson, you will learn how to build healthier relationships within your family and community.

Family Relationships

The word *family* has several definitions and may include relatives, partners, and diverse members. There are many different types of families (**Figure 14.6**). No matter the type of family, family relationships are important.

Figure 14.6 Parents and children may be various ages and any marital status. For example, a family may include a single parent and adult children. Parents and children may also be of any gender identity and sexual orientation.

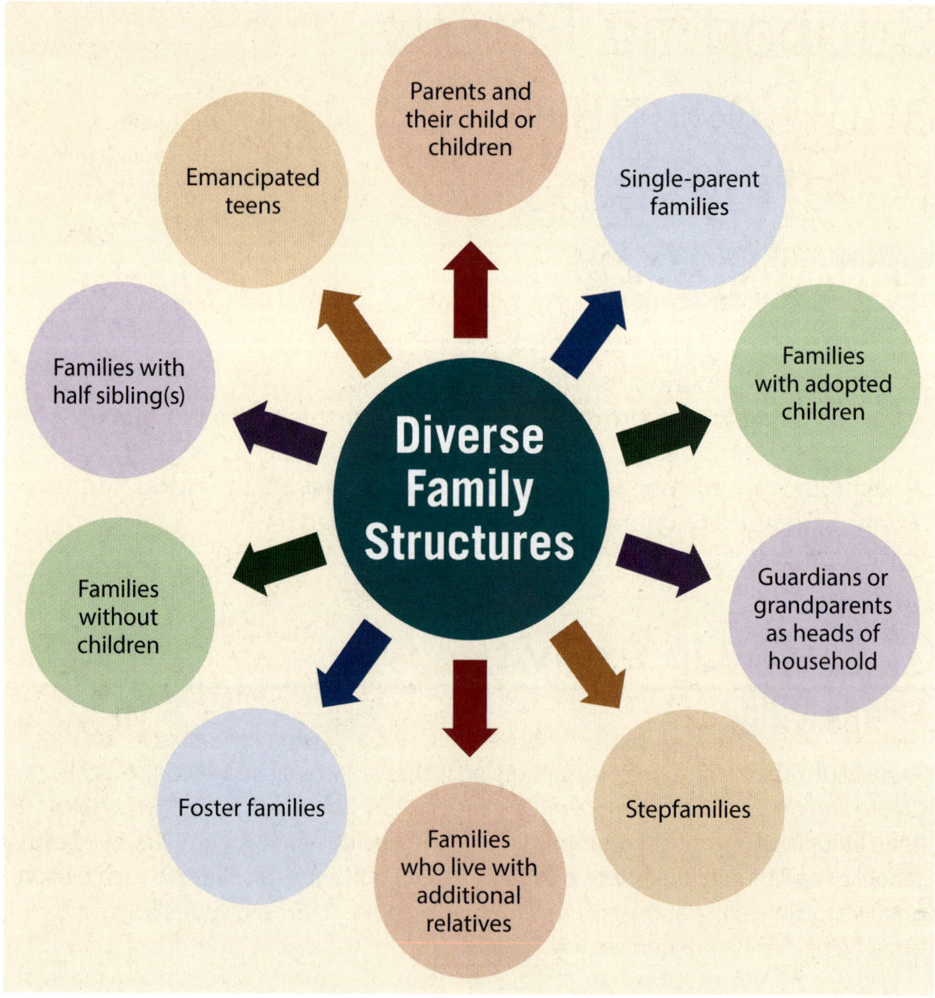

immediate family close relatives, including parents or guardians, children, and siblings

extended family distant relatives, including aunts, uncles, cousins, and grandparents

The very first relationships most people have are with their family members. As they grow up, many people spend lots of time with members of their **immediate family**, meaning their parents or guardians and siblings. **Extended family** members, such as aunts, uncles, cousins, and grandparents, can also play a significant role in a person's life. Together, these family relationships are often among a person's closest.

Relationships within the family have several unique functions that make them different from other relationships. Unlike other types of relationships, family relationships have the following responsibilities:

- **Provide for physical needs:** Families provide for their members' physical needs, including food, clothing, and housing. Healthy families also ensure that members are healthy and safe. For example, your parents or guardians may take you to the doctor and dentist on a regular basis. They may set rules—even rules you do not like—with the goal of keeping you safe and healthy. As children and teens grow older, they take on tasks to help meet the family's physical needs. For example, doing some cleaning chores helps keep the home a healthy place to live.
- **Meet mental and emotional needs:** The goal in a healthy family is to meet members' mental and emotional needs, such as the needs for love, acceptance, self-esteem, and emotional comfort. The support and love people receive from their family members make them feel secure and good about themselves.

- **Educate and socialize:** Families educate children and teens by teaching them about the world and sending them to school or homeschooling. They also **socialize** children and teens by teaching them to behave in socially acceptable ways. Through their families, people learn about culture, values, and **traditions** (specific patterns of behavior). They also learn language from their families, as well as information about culture and religion.

socialize to teach to behave in ways society accepts

traditions patterns of behavior passed down in a culture

Skills for Healthy Family Relationships

If the relationships within a family are healthy, the family is healthy. Building and maintaining family relationships requires many of the same interpersonal skills you need for all relationships. There are also specific strategies you can use to build healthy relationships with family members such as parents or guardians, siblings, and grandparents.

Relationships with Parents and Guardians

The teen years are a time of self-exploration. During this time, teens naturally push for more freedom, independence, and responsibility. They want to figure out who they are as unique individuals. At the same time, parents and guardians want to keep teens safe and healthy and teach them how to function well in society. To do this, parents and guardians set rules and limits that teens sometimes find restrictive. Parents and guardians can also offer valuable advice and help teens navigate difficult situations. Using certain strategies can help you strengthen your relationship with your parent or guardian (**Figure 14.7**).

Teens who have healthy relationships with their parents and guardians can communicate with them about their thoughts and feelings. This helps teens navigate the challenges they face and make healthy decisions. Unfortunately, some teens may feel their relationship with a parent or guardian is unhealthy.

Strategies for Strengthening Relationships with Parents or Guardians

Share your plans with your parent or guardian ahead of time.

- Make sure to get approval before you make a commitment. Revise the plan, if needed, and answer any questions your parent or guardian has.

Discuss family rules with your parent or guardian.

- If you disagree with a rule, calmly explain why you think it should be changed. Your parent or guardian may agree to reconsider the rule.

Follow your family's rules, even if you disagree with them.

- Remember, these rules may be relaxed or disappear if you show responsible behavior and a willingness to follow the limits set for you.

Remain calm.

- When you have a disagreement, do not resort to yelling and do not walk away. Show your parent or guardian that you are capable of having a mature discussion and that you can be responsible.

Spend time doing enjoyable activities with your family.

- You might suggest having a special family dinner one night a week or planning a trip. These types of activities can bring families together.

Figure 14.7 If you find yourself frequently fighting with your parents or guardians or wish your relationship were closer, these strategies can help you see events from another perspective and resolve conflicts.

They may have frequent disagreements or feel misunderstood. They may also experience neglect or abuse. If you do not have a healthy relationship with a parent or guardian, do what you can to improve the relationship and talk to other adults you trust, such as a teacher, school counselor, or school nurse. You can also reach out to community resources.

Relationships with Siblings

Sibling relationships are often the earliest family relationships people have. Even when siblings are biologically related or raised in the same household, however, they may not share interests. Siblings may have different personalities, find different activities interesting, or have different ways of handling major life events. These differences can create conflict, especially when siblings spend a lot of time together.

A common source of conflict among siblings is competition. Competing with a sibling for material and nonmaterial items is **sibling rivalry**. Examples of sibling rivalry include competing for a parent's attention or fighting over use of the family car. When teasing is involved, feelings of competition may increase. Sibling rivalry may encourage negative feelings, such as resentment, anger, or jealousy.

sibling rivalry
competitive feelings between siblings; siblings may compete for material or nonmaterial items

Despite these challenges, sibling relationships can be strong, healthy, and powerful. Some sibling relationships may even become close friendships. **Figure 14.8** shows some effective strategies for managing sibling relationships.

Figure 14.8 These strategies can apply to any type of sibling at any age. ***What is a common source of conflict among siblings?***

Strategies for Managing Sibling Relationships

Express how you feel to your sibling.

- Try to communicate with your sibling to find solutions to disagreements and show respect for your sibling's ideas.

Get away from tense situations and cool down.

- Taking a break from a heated situation can avoid making a conflict worse.

Respect your sibling's space and privacy.

- Do not enter a sibling's room without knocking. If you share a room, respect your sibling's private space within that room.

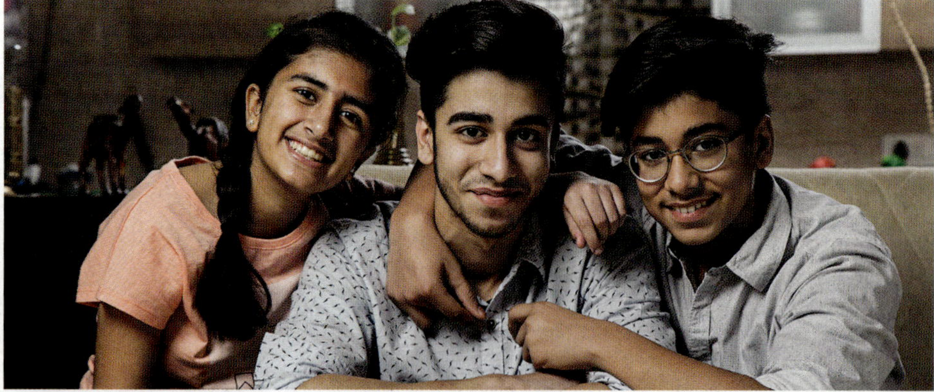

Compromise when you experience recurring issues.

- Try to work out a solution you both think is fair. Together, you can develop specific rules for handling ongoing sources of conflict.

Designate personal space for each person.

- For example, if you share a bedroom with a sibling, talk about designating areas for each of you.

Talk to your parent or guardian about sibling conflicts.

- See if your parent or guardian has advice about how to avoid or solve conflicts with your sibling.

Deepak Sethi/iStock/Getty Images Plus/Getty Images

Maintaining healthy sibling relationships is important today and for the rest of your life. Try to find enjoyable ways of spending time with your siblings. This could include going for a bike ride or having a family game night.

Relationships with Grandparents

Many teens benefit from relationships with grandparents. Grandparents can share wisdom they have learned over the years and give valuable advice. They may help teens better understand their parents by sharing stories about their parents as children and provide support.

At the same time, it is natural to sometimes have conflicts with grandparents. When teens criticize their parents, this can put grandparents in an awkward position. Grandparents may have different rules and expectations about how you dress, what time you go to bed, or how much time you spend on your computer or phone. It is important to respect these rules, even if they are different from the ones at home (**Figure 14.9**).

Skills for Relationships with Grandparents

Be mindful of what you share. Tell your grandparents if you do not want them to share what you tell them with others.

Ask grandparents questions about their lives. Grandparents can talk about how different life was with no cell phones or internet and can tell stories about historical events.

Learn a skill that your grandparent knows, such as how to fish, cook from scratch, or play an instrument.

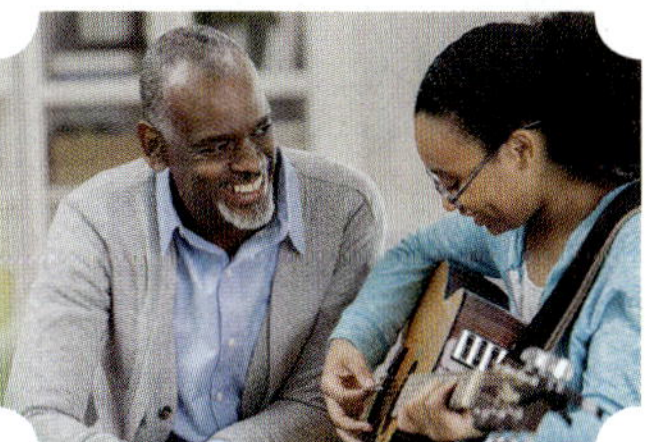

Offer to provide help with household tasks such as moving furniture, planting a garden, or using new technology.

Stay in touch. Visit when you can and find ways to communicate if you live far away. Try sending photos of big events in your life to show your grandparent what you are doing.

SDI Productions/E+/Getty Images

Figure 14.9 Relationships with grandparents can be rewarding, but may not come easily to all teens.

Local and Global Health

Parents and Children Around the World

All around the world, parents and guardians love and want the best for their children, including teens. What this looks like often differs, however. Differences in cultural values and practices influence how parents and guardians interact and communicate with children and teens.

Cultural values and norms impact how much independence parents give their children. For example, in France, parents tend to encourage more independence at younger ages. In the United States, this emphasis would be unusual. Culture and background also influence how much control parents have to influence children and teens. In some Asian countries, parents expect children to respect their authority and show obedience. In contrast, parents and children in the US may have a more collaborative approach.

Whatever cultural norms and values influence your family, all parent-and-child relationships benefit from interpersonal skills. This includes showing respect, honesty, and trust.

Practice Your Skills

Access Information

Work with a small group to examine how different cultures approach parenting. Each person should choose a country or world region and then use reliable resources to find information about parents and teens in that culture. Each person should report to the group with information learned. Think about how each culture approaches parenting and what factors influence that approach. What are some similarities between different cultures? What are some differences? Finally, think about the ways in which each culture's approach to parenting influences health-related behavior.

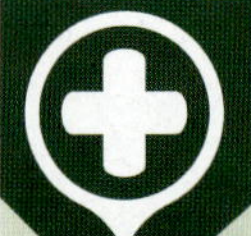

Spotlight on Health and Wellness Careers

Marriage and Family Therapist: Ileana Ungureanu

Marriage and family therapy is my second career, and I discovered my passion for it while practicing as a family physician. As a physician, I liked helping families with their physical health, but found I was more interested in the psychological and social aspects of their lives. I am still fascinated by how stress and emotional and mental health impact physical health.

As a marriage and family therapist, I work with couples and families. I help couples handle conflict, repair their relationships after difficult situations, and strengthen their emotional bond. I also help families through life transitions, such as the birth of a new child, challenges with adolescence, and children leaving home. I help families navigate issues such as grieving, trauma, a chronic illness, and academic or behavioral issues with a child.

I believe that when stress happens with one family member, the entire family is affected. My approach is *systemic*, meaning I work with the entire family system. Sometimes, taking in people's stories of pain and sadness can be difficult and have an impact on me. While it is not always easy to witness the less happy parts of people's lives, I am amazed by human resilience and all the victories I can help families achieve through therapy.

Practice Your Skills

Access Information

Think about your own interests, strengths, and weaknesses. What parts of being a marriage and family therapist do you think would interest you? Which elements would be challenging? Using reliable resources like the US Bureau of Labor Statistics' *Occupational Outlook Handbook*, research marriage and family therapy and related careers. Is the demand for marriage and family therapists growing? What are the educational requirements? Are there related careers that might also interest you? Write a blog post summarizing your thoughts.

Changes in the Family

All families encounter changes over time, such as a physical or mental health condition, loss of a job, or relocation to a new community. These changes can create stress and disrupt family relationships. Even positive changes can create stress. This is because new events can lead to changes in how family members interact in daily life.

Some of the most challenging changes families experience are changes in family structure—the addition or loss of a family member. These changes include the birth or adoption of a new family member, separation or divorce, remarriage, serious illness, and death. Although these events can be difficult, healthy families can work through them together. Sometimes families even grow closer when dealing with changes.

Fortunately, there are strategies you and your family members can use to cope with changes and maintain healthy family relationships, even during challenging times:

- **Acknowledge your emotions:** It is normal to feel upset during difficult times, and change is hard for people of all ages. When faced with family changes, you might feel angry, sad, anxious, or afraid. Do not hold these feelings in. Share them with friends or adults who support you or journal about them.
- **Reflect on other transitions:** In the midst of change, it can seem like you will never feel better. Try reflecting back on other times of change you experienced and worked through. This can remind you it will get better over time and help you recall strategies for coping.

- **Shift your focus:** It is easy to focus entirely on the negative parts of change. Try to balance these negative thoughts by considering what may be positive. Perhaps, following a divorce that causes you to move, your parents or guardians will be happier and fight less. Remind yourself that changes, even hard ones, can lead to some benefits. This is part of developing *resilience*, which you learned about in Chapter 5.
- **Take care of yourself:** During difficult circumstances, treat yourself with care and compassion. Do not beat yourself up for feeling worried and anxious. Instead, do activities that make you feel better. Talk to a friend, watch funny movies, or go for a jog. Treat yourself with kindness, just like you would for a good friend.
- **Use community resources:** Many communities have resources to help families struggling with change. If your family has trouble adjusting, you might suggest talking with a therapist, finding a support group, or getting financial support through a government program.

Relationships in Your Community

As you grow up, you will have more and more relationships outside your family. Some of these will be with adults and others in your community. As you learned in Chapter 2, a *community* is a group of people who live in the same area and interact with one another (**Figure 14.10**).

Teens have relationships with people they see frequently, such as teachers, neighbors, and other students. Other relationships are with people teens see less frequently, but who play an important role in the community, such as doctors, dentists, firefighters, and **law enforcement**.

Some teens have relationships with trusted adults or **mentors**, who can help guide them in positive ways. A mentor could be a teacher, coach, or school counselor. Sometimes teens find it easier to take advice from mentors, who care about them, but are more removed from their daily lives than parents and guardians.

law enforcement community workers who make sure laws are followed

mentors people who guide others in positive ways

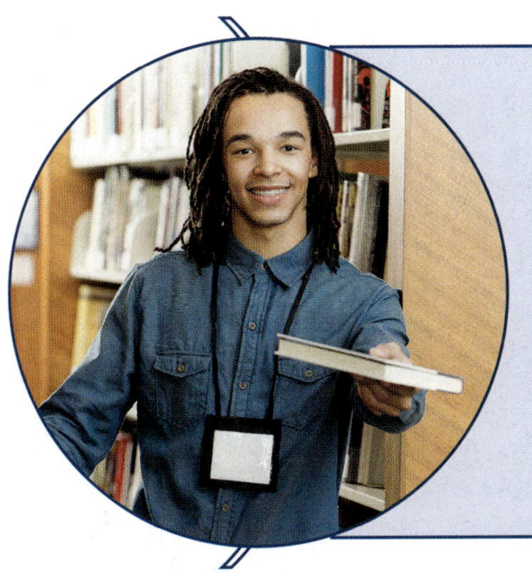

Feeling like you are part of a community can help you
- care about others and be cared for
- develop a sense of belonging and support
- explore different interests and goals
- develop a sense of identity
- build social skills
- learn compassion for other people
- learn skills for making decisions and resolving conflicts

kali9/E+/Getty Images

Figure 14.10 Actively interacting with a community, by volunteering or working at organizations, may help you feel like part of the community. ***Who are community members you interact with regularly?***

Skills for Healthy Community Relationships

All community relationships should have the qualities of a healthy relationship. There are skills you can use to build and maintain these relationships and feel like part of your community.

Advocate for Diversity

Most communities represent greater diversity than other groups, such as a school or family. People in a community have different ages, providing generational diversity. They may also vary in ethnic background, education, beliefs, political attitudes, income or social class, gender identity, and sexual orientation.

Interacting with people from diverse backgrounds gives you an opportunity to learn more about the world from another perspective. This can increase your ability to understand and appreciate people's views and why they hold them.

When interacting with people from different backgrounds, remember to stay curious, not judgmental. When people judge others for having different beliefs and values, this creates a barrier and makes it harder to form and maintain healthy relationships. Ask questions to learn more about other people's perspectives and try to keep an open and flexible mind. If others in your community do not appreciate diversity, urge them to see different perspectives. You can help set the standard for respect by speaking up if people mock others and challenging biased or unfair beliefs.

Communicate Effectively

You learned about effective communication skills in Chapter 3. These skills apply to all relationships, including those in your community. Communication can be difficult if you do not know someone well. In these situations, be sure to speak clearly and concisely. Listen closely, ask questions, and be open-minded. Make sure your body language matches your message and tell a trusted adult if something makes you uncomfortable.

One new type of relationship you may have as a teen is in the workplace. A workplace can include a store, office, factory, farm, or any other setting where work is performed. In the workplace, you will report to a **supervisor**, who has authority over you. You might also have **coworkers**, who engage in similar work. When you are interacting with these people, you need to use **professional communication**, which is more formal than communication with friends and family members. This includes skills in speaking, listening, and writing, in person or electronically (**Figure 14.11**).

supervisor person who oversees one's work in an organization

coworkers people who work for the same employer or do the same kind of work

professional communication process of sending and receiving messages in a formal environment, such as a workplace or school

Strategies for Professional Communication
Show respect.
Demonstrate confidence.
Be receptive to feedback.
Acknowledge others.
Proofread communication.

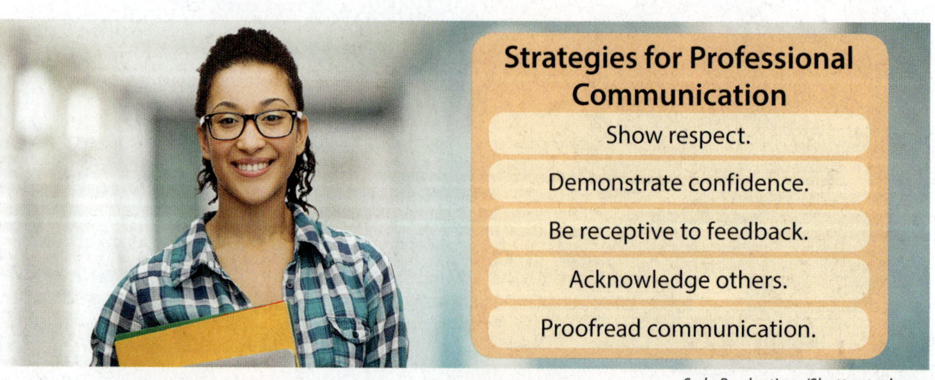

Syda Productions/Shutterstock.com

Figure 14.11 Using these professional communication strategies will strengthen your relationships with customers, coworkers, and supervisors. ***Who has authority over you in a professional setting?***

Some strategies you can use to communicate effectively in the workplace include the following:

- **Show respect:** Simple actions, such as using a person's name and looking that person in the eye, signal respect. Focus on the conversation you are having and use active listening techniques. It is important to be polite when interacting with people in a professional setting.
- **Demonstrate confidence:** Use a friendly but firm tone. This illustrates you believe what you are saying. Avoid making statements that sound like questions, which shows a lack of confidence. Avoid being overly confident, which may come across as aggressive and arrogant.
- **Be receptive to feedback:** All employees receive feedback about how they are doing. Listen thoughtfully to the suggestions you are given and ask questions. Avoid being defensive. Remember that receiving constructive feedback is an important part of improving work performance.
- **Acknowledge other people:** Small gestures that show appreciation help foster a good working environment. Say *please* and *thank you*. Let your coworkers know if they have performed a task well. Tell your supervisor you appreciate the time spent training you and answering questions.
- **Proofread communication:** Emails should be clear, correct, free of errors, and sent from a professional-sounding email address. Take the time to read and review all emails before they go out. Remember that emails can be forwarded. Do not write something in an email that you would not feel comfortable with other people reading.

One of the hardest parts of using professional communication for many teens is managing social media. Remember that whatever you post online may stay forever, and current or future employers might see it. Be very careful what you post, as it could have consequences even years later.

Maintain Healthy Boundaries

Part of having healthy relationships in your community is setting boundaries. Boundaries establish what is and is not acceptable in a given setting. They also help people understand their roles and responsibilities. Examples of boundaries include physical boundaries, such as not touching someone in an inappropriate way. Other types of boundaries include how long you have for a break at work and whether you are allowed to use technology in a teacher's class.

To maintain healthy boundaries in the workplace, learn and follow the rules set by your employer to avoid violating policies. It is also important to maintain healthy boundaries in other community relationships, such as those at school.

Be Involved in Your Community

A great way for many teens to build healthy community relationships is to volunteer in some way. Many schools have clubs focused on community service. Community organizations also provide opportunities to participate in volunteer projects (**Figure 14.12**).

Where Can I Volunteer?

- Find a nonprofit in your area that works with an issue you care about, such as the environment, animal cruelty, poverty, or homelessness.
- Your hometown may have a soup kitchen, food pantry, community garden, homeless shelter, or public library where you can volunteer.
- See what is available in your area from nationwide volunteer organizations like Meals on Wheels, Habitat for Humanity, Junior Red Cross, or Boys and Girls Club.
- Healthcare facilities like hospitals, nursing homes, and assisted living facilities almost always have volunteer opportunities.
- Check your school and public library for programs in mentorship, tutoring, or teaching languages.
- If you know a family or person in need in your community, you can volunteer to help individually: offer to cook meals, babysit, or mow the lawn.
- Volunteer for a crisis support network to help peers.

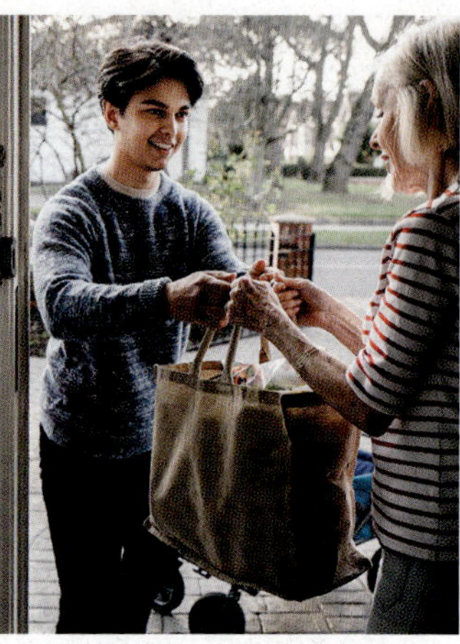

DGLimages/iStock/Getty Images Plus/Getty Images

Figure 14.12 Volunteer opportunities may vary depending on your geographic location and the age requirements for each organization. Search online for opportunities in your neighborhood.

Volunteering in community service projects you care about is a great way to give to others. It can make you feel good about yourself and develop resilience and empathy. It can also teach you valuable skills related to leadership, communication, time management, responsibility, and dependability and highlight different career pathways. These skills can all be useful when you are applying for jobs, colleges, and scholarships. Teens who volunteer also tend to perform better at school.

Lesson 14.2 Review

Know and Understand

1. Identify one strategy for maintaining a healthy relationship with a parent or guardian and explain how you could use it.
2. What is an example of sibling rivalry in a family?
3. Give one example of a community relationship.
4. Explain how you can respect diversity in your community.
5. What kind of communication should you use with coworkers and supervisors? Why?
6. What skills can you learn from community service?

Think Critically

7. How are family relationships different from other types of relationships?
8. Explain why relationships with grandparents are valuable.
9. Why is it helpful to reflect on other periods of change during a difficult family adjustment?
10. How is professional communication more formal than other types of communication?
11. Choose one community relationship you have and explain your boundaries.

REAL WORLD Health Skills

Make Decisions What you post on social media can influence your community relationships. In fact, employers sometimes access social media pages before interviewing or employing candidates. List the social media accounts you have. Evaluate each account and decide if the information posted to it would be appropriate for a present or future employer. Would you be comfortable if other members of your community, including employers, saw your posted content? Is there any content you would want to delete or change? Why or why not? Discuss your findings with a classmate.

Developing Peer Relationships

Essential Question?

What skills do you need to form healthy friendships with your peers?

Lesson 14.3

Learning Outcomes

After studying this lesson, you will be able to

- assess the value of friendships;
- compare and contrast different types of friendships;
- describe skills for building and maintaining healthy friendships; and
- evaluate the impact of common issues in friendships, such as cliques, jealousy, and changes over time.

Key Terms

acquaintances
clique
friendship
jealousy
reciprocal

Warm-Up Activity

My Best Friend

Comprehend Concepts Write a short paragraph identifying whom you consider your best friend and why. Identify the characteristics that make your friendship close, healthy, and enjoyable. Also identify any unhealthy characteristics or conflicts you sometimes have. How did this friendship develop? What skills did you both use to grow closer? Create a journal entry summarizing your thoughts.

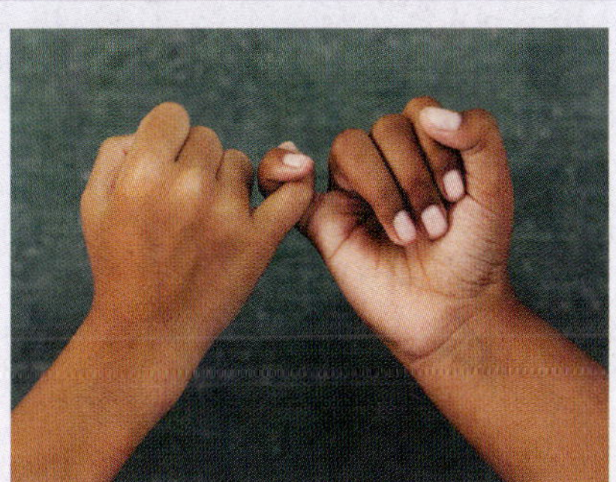

Cat Act Art/Shutterstock.com

Friendships are some of the most important relationships in your life and develop because of mutual respect, care, trust, and affection. Friendships are especially important during the teen years when relationships with *peers* (people of the same age range or status) are often the center of your world. Friendships allow you to learn more about yourself, receive and provide emotional support, and gain skills for communicating and resolving conflicts. Different friendships satisfy different needs.

Types of Friendships

The term **friendship** describes many different types of relationships (**Figure 14.13**). For example, you probably know the difference between your very closest friends and your more casual friends. Perhaps you have a single friend whom you consider your best friend. You may also have **acquaintances**—people you know and interact with, but may not consider friends.

Many people make friends by interacting with people who live in their neighborhood or community or attend their school. This is because common experiences and interests are often a basis for friendship, at least at the start of a relationship. For example, you probably have friends and acquaintances in your classes at school, in the clubs you attend, or in your neighborhood.

friendship relationship between two or more people who share common interests, values, and goals and support each other

acquaintances people in a person's social circle who may not be close enough to be friends

Types of Friendships

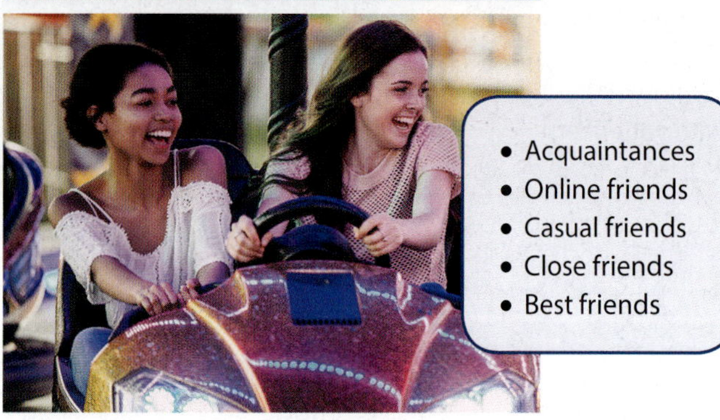

SolStock/E+/Getty Images

Figure 14.13 Friendships can differ in closeness: from acquaintances or casual friends to close or best friends. Online friends can be at any of these levels of closeness. ***How are online friends different from other kinds of friends?***

When friendships based on common interests deepen to include trust, respect, and support, they become stronger and more long-lasting. Because of technology and social media, friends can communicate more now than ever before. This constant communication can enhance friendships and make them especially intense.

Today, many people also have friends who live farther away. In addition to your friends at school and nearby, you may also have *online friends*, or people you met through social media, chat rooms, websites, or gaming. Despite the lack of in-person interaction, close friendships can sometimes develop between online friends. When getting to know an online friend, be careful about sharing information about yourself. Unless you have met a person, you cannot know if the person is being truthful online.

Research in Action

How Close Are Online Friendships?

Many teens spend a lot of time online—posting on social media, playing video games, and messaging others. The connections teens make with people online can sometimes lead to or enhance friendships. A report from the Pew Research Center found that 57 percent of teens have made a friend online, and 29 percent have made more than five friends online. In some cases, online friendships can become in-person friendships. About 20 percent of teens have met a friend they made online face-to-face.

Researchers at the University of California, Irvine, conducted a study comparing teens' online and in-person friendships. First, they identified six key characteristics of in-person friendships: self-disclosure, validation, companionship, support, conflict, and conflict resolution. Then they examined how online friendships meet these same characteristics. Interestingly, they found that online friendships are even stronger than in-person friendships in some ways.

Online communication plays a part in strengthening these relationships. Online communication can allow for more companionship, since friends can communicate day and night. This makes friends feel more connected, and they can receive support during hard times. Friends can also calmly express their thoughts and feelings because they have a chance to calm down before responding to a hurtful or upsetting situation.

In addition to benefits, online friendships also have some downsides. Online, teens can learn about events or activities they were not invited to, which can lead to hurt feelings. Gossip and rumors also spread very quickly online. The ability to communicate day and night can make some online friendships feel overwhelming, and lack of nonverbal cues can lead to misunderstandings. Perhaps the biggest challenge with online friendships is distorted comparisons. Many teens mostly post content that makes them look good, and this can make teens who do not know the whole story feel worse about their own lives.

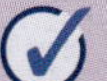

Practice Your Skills

Advocate for Health

Think about your online friendships and how you communicate with your online friends. What strategies do you use to make and maintain online friendships? Make a list of the benefits these friendships provide to you. Next, think about the challenges you have experienced in your online friendships. What strategies could you use to minimize these challenges? Consider how you could share strategies for healthy online friendships with other students at your school. In a small group, create a social media campaign focused on best practices for online friendships. Keep your target audience in mind when crafting each post.

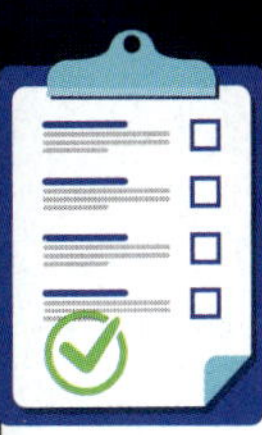

Quiz How Healthy Is Your Friendship?

Think about one of your close friendships. How healthy do you think it is? To assess the health of one of your friendships, read each of the following statements. Indicate the choice that best describes your relationship with someone you would consider a close friend.

Statement				
I enjoy spending time with my friend.	Strongly disagree	Disagree	Agree	Strongly agree
I feel comfortable and safe with my friend.	Strongly disagree	Disagree	Agree	Strongly agree
My friend does not get upset or angry if I am unable to hang out.	Strongly disagree	Disagree	Agree	Strongly agree
I can share personal thoughts and feelings with my friend without fear of being teased.	Strongly disagree	Disagree	Agree	Strongly agree
My friend does not post hurtful comments, images, or posts on social media.	Strongly disagree	Disagree	Agree	Strongly agree
My friend does not judge or criticize me for who I am.	Strongly disagree	Disagree	Agree	Strongly agree
My friend offers support when I am upset.	Strongly disagree	Disagree	Agree	Strongly agree
My friend actively listens to me when I have something to say.	Strongly disagree	Disagree	Agree	Strongly agree
My friend does not pressure me into doing anything that makes me uncomfortable.	Strongly disagree	Disagree	Agree	Strongly agree
I would describe my friend as dependable.	Strongly disagree	Disagree	Agree	Strongly agree
When exciting or positive things happen to me, my friend shares my excitement.	Strongly disagree	Disagree	Agree	Strongly agree
When my friend and I are angry, we take time to cool off before talking.	Strongly disagree	Disagree	Agree	Strongly agree
If my friend and I get into a disagreement, we work through the conflict together.	Strongly disagree	Disagree	Agree	Strongly agree
If I apologize for accidentally hurting or offending my friend, my friend is forgiving.	Strongly disagree	Disagree	Agree	Strongly agree
No matter the situation, I know my friend is always there for me.	Strongly disagree	Disagree	Agree	Strongly agree

Add up the total number for each response.

If you answered mostly *strongly agree*, you have a very healthy friendship. This is a friendship that supports your health! Keep using interpersonal skills to maintain the health of this friendship.

If you answered mostly *agree*, you have a healthy friendship. This friendship enriches your life. Try practicing more healthy relationship skills.

If you answered mostly *disagree*, you have an unhealthy friendship. You might want to have a discussion with your friend about improving your relationship.

If you answered mostly *strongly disagree*, you have a very unhealthy friendship. You should probably talk with a trusted adult, like your parent or guardian or a teacher, about this relationship. Without some changes, this relationship could be harmful to your health.

Practice Your Skills

Communicate with Others

Now that you have assessed the health of your friendship, have a conversation with your friend or a trusted adult. Talk about each statement and whether you both strongly disagree, disagree, agree, or strongly agree. What parts of the relationship can you improve? Are there any behaviors or attitudes getting in the way of the friendship being healthy? Be sure to listen well and respect your friend's thoughts and feelings. Having conversations like this regularly can help you check in and maintain or improve the health of this relationship.

Skills for Healthy Friendships

Healthy friendships provide emotional and social support and companionship during the teen years. They can also help you learn more about yourself and others. Sometimes it can be hard to make and keep friends. Determining whether someone shares your core values and beliefs can take time, especially if you are still trying to figure out what you believe. Even when conflicts arise, however, there are ways to maintain healthy friendships over time.

Get to Know Others

To make friends, first you need to interact with other people and learn about them. You cannot know if you want to be someone's friend until you get to know that other person. If you are shy or anxious around new people, this can be difficult, but there are several strategies you can use to start conversations and learn more about your peers (**Figure 14.14**).

Make Time for Relationships

Maintaining close relationships with friends takes time and energy. Even when you are busy with homework, sports, or a job, try to find time to connect and spend time with your acquaintances and friends. As you build new friendships, you will need time to get to know other people and understand how their values and beliefs align with yours. If you want to get to know someone, try spending time in a group, doing an activity together, or talking and messaging throughout the day. If you have trouble finding time for relationships, plan ahead and set dates to get together with friends.

Getting to Know Other People

Meet new people at new activities.
- Get involved in sports, music, school clubs, or volunteer opportunities to find people with common interests.

Discuss a fun topic or common interest.
- Before you start a conversation, think of a topic to discuss. If you love video games, describe your favorite game or ask what the other person plays.

Compliment the other person.
- Pick something you notice about this person, such as a piece of clothing, jewelry, or the person's skill in a certain activity or class.

Ask follow-up questions.
- After you offer the common interest or compliment, use additional questions to start a positive conversation.

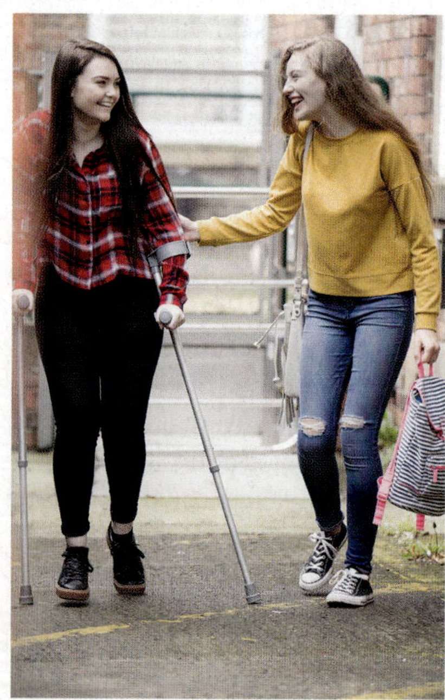

SolStock/E+/Getty Images

Figure 14.14 If you feel as if everyone has their friends set already, remember that people continue to make friends throughout life. This means that most people are open to new friendships, and friend groups may shift or grow.

Committing to time with a friend in advance can help you set aside the needed time, even when you are busy.

Meet Friends Face-to-Face

Online communication is a great way to connect with friends and get to know people, but it is also important to form and maintain friendships through face-to-face interactions. While online communication such as social media, texting, and video games makes it easier to stay in touch, do not rely on these types of interactions alone. Remember that these conversations lack important aspects of nonverbal communication. One of the best ways to keep a relationship strong is to step away from the screen and make time to be physically present with someone (**Figure 14.15**).

If you decide to meet an online friend face-to-face, take precautions to protect your safety. Sometimes people online pretend to be someone they are not, so it is important to be careful. Talk with a parent or guardian about your desire to meet anyone online. You might try to set up a video call with your online friend and include your parent or guardian to keep you safe. Bring your parent or guardian with you if you decide to meet an online friend and meet in a public place.

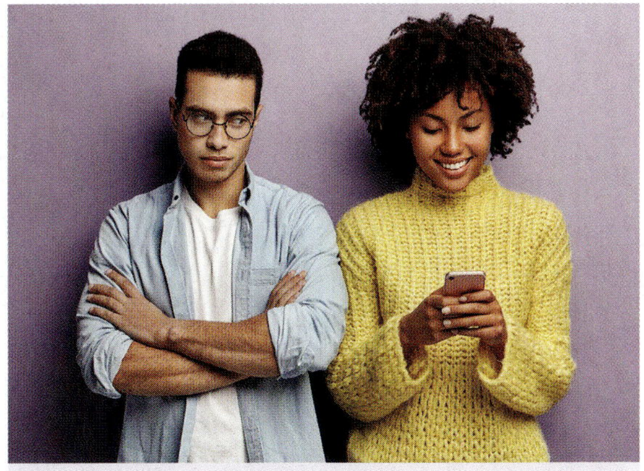

Being Physically Present

- Checking your phone while spending time with someone can leave the other person feeling ignored, annoyed, or pushed away.
- Giving people your undivided attention, listening to what they have to say, and providing responses of your own are essential to building a friendship.
- Even simply having a phone nearby can divert your attention from your current environment, getting in the way of connecting with the people right next to you.

WAYHOME studio/Shutterstock.com

Figure 14.15 Having your phone in front of you while spending time with someone, whether you check it or not, can prevent you from forming a meaningful friendship.

Be Supportive

Caring and support are signs of a healthy relationship. In the best relationships, care and support are **reciprocal**, meaning each person contributes them equally to the relationship. There are many ways you can show care and support for your friends. Some of these ways include the following:

reciprocal shared or exhibited by both sides

- Listen carefully to what your friends say and do not interrupt, judge, or criticize your friends when they talk. Try to empathize with how your friend feels.
- Encourage your friends and celebrate their successes.
- Avoid teasing or criticizing your friends.
- Work with your friends to solve disagreements and collaborate to reach an agreement.
- Express your feelings openly during conflicts and listen carefully to your friend's perspective.
- Apologize if you hurt your friend and try to find ways to make amends.

Handle Common Issues

As with all relationships, certain issues can sometimes complicate friendships. The way you handle these can either strengthen or weaken your friendships. Some of these issues include cliques, jealousy, and changes over time.

Cliques

clique small group of friends who deliberately exclude other people from joining or being a part of their group

Many high school students enjoy spending time with groups of friends. Sometimes these groups of friends exclude other people, which can lead to hurt feelings. A **clique** is a small group of friends who deliberately exclude other people from joining or being a part of their group (**Figure 14.16**).

People who are part of a clique can experience challenging social dynamics, such as feeling pressured to act a certain way. Sometimes cliques pressure group members to act in ways that endanger their health and wellness. For example, a group may encourage vaping. In this way, cliques can reduce each person's individuality and compromise well-being, which is unhealthy.

Cliques are a part of life in some high schools, but you can handle cliques by being true to yourself. If you are in a clique, think about whether being part of the group feels good or not. Do group members support each other? Do they share your values? Use refusal skills to resist peer pressure. Make sure to spend time with people who make you feel good about yourself and respect you for who you are. Do not limit yourself to only making friends with people in one group. You might miss out on some great friendships.

Jealousy

jealousy emotion characterized by wanting or being unhappy about another person's positive experiences or circumstances

Jealousy is an intense emotion that sometimes occurs in a friendship. When people feel jealous, they want what someone else has, often to the point of being angry. You may feel jealous of your friend's achievement in a particular area, such as schoolwork, athletics, or music. You may also feel jealous of other aspects of a friend's life, such as your friend's home, dating relationship, or family life. Feelings of jealousy are normal if they occur once in a while, but continuous jealous feelings can harm a relationship over time.

How Do You Know if Your Friend Group Is a Clique?

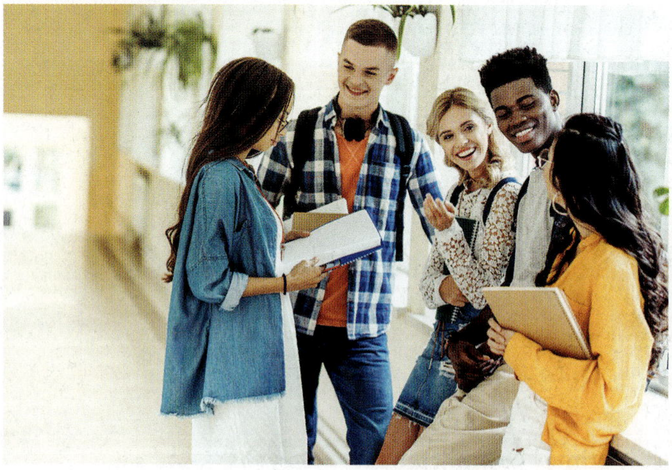

Cliques

- make it clear to people outside the group that not just anyone can be friends with them
- place a high importance on popularity
- exclude or leave other people out on purpose to demonstrate power
- control members of the group by giving unwanted makeovers, dictating clothing choices, or telling members how to act
- discourage individuality
- seek attention through gossip and making fun of others
- do not allow members to socialize outside the group

LightField Studios/Shutterstock.com

Figure 14.16 If a friendship prevents you from being yourself or making new friends, it can be harmful to your health. ***How can being part of a clique increase peer pressure?***

Honestly expressing your emotions, including jealousy, can prevent negative thoughts from building up over time and hurting your friendship. If you value your friendship and want to maintain it, try to move beyond feelings of jealousy.

If you feel stuck in feelings of jealousy, take action. Identify what is going well for your friend and try to make changes in your own life to create positive outcomes. For example, you might study harder, build a bigger social network, or get involved in a new club or activity. In the meantime, try to be happy for your friend. Soon enough, your friend will feel happy for you.

Changes Over Time

Friendships evolve as people change over time. For example, experiencing physical, emotional, and social changes can lead to changes in your friendships. This is particularly true if you and a friend change in different ways. As you get older, you may no longer share common interests with your childhood friends.

Just because you and your friend change does not mean your friendship has to end. If you want to maintain an old friendship, invest time and energy in that friendship. Make a point of connecting with that friend, either online or in person, so you can stay up-to-date on each other's lives. Share events that happen to you and ask about how your friend is doing. These check-ins will help you stay connected.

If you feel as though you and a friend are drifting apart, start a conversation with your friend. If both of you are interested in maintaining the friendship, you can work together to find ways of remaining close.

Lesson 14.3 Review

Know and Understand

1. Why should you be careful meeting an online friend in person?
2. What can you do to maintain friendships, even when you are busy?
3. What steps can you take to overcome feelings of jealousy in a friendship?

Think Critically

4. In your opinion, what is the foundation of a healthy friendship?
5. Why is it important that care and support are reciprocal in a friendship?

REAL WORLD Health Skills

Set Goals If you had the opportunity to form a brand-new, healthy friendship, describe what your friend would be like. What type of person would you want as a friend? What characteristics would you prefer in a friend? What would you bring to the friendship? Think about a friendship you have now. How are the perfect friendship you described and your real friendship different? What changes could you make to your real friendship to make it healthier? Set two SMART goals that could help you make this relationship stronger.

Lesson 14.4

Understanding Romantic Relationships

Essential Question

How do you know if a romantic relationship is healthy or unhealthy?

Learning Outcomes

After studying this lesson, you will be able to

- analyze how attraction, closeness, and commitment impact a relationship;
- assess the importance of maintaining individuality and balance in a romantic relationship;
- compare and contrast love, infatuation, and passion;
- describe how to set boundaries regarding physical intimacy;
- recognize the signs of an unhealthy romantic relationship;
- develop strategies for forming healthy romantic relationships; and
- identify healthy ways to handle a breakup.

Key Terms

attraction
breakup
dating
exclusive
group dating
infatuation
love
passion

Warm-Up Activity

Similarities and Differences

Comprehend Concepts In this chapter, you have learned about several types of healthy relationships. What are some qualities healthy dating relationships have in common with healthy friendships and family and community relationships? What are some qualities unique to each type of relationship? Create a poster that displays the qualities of healthy dating relationships and share it with the class.

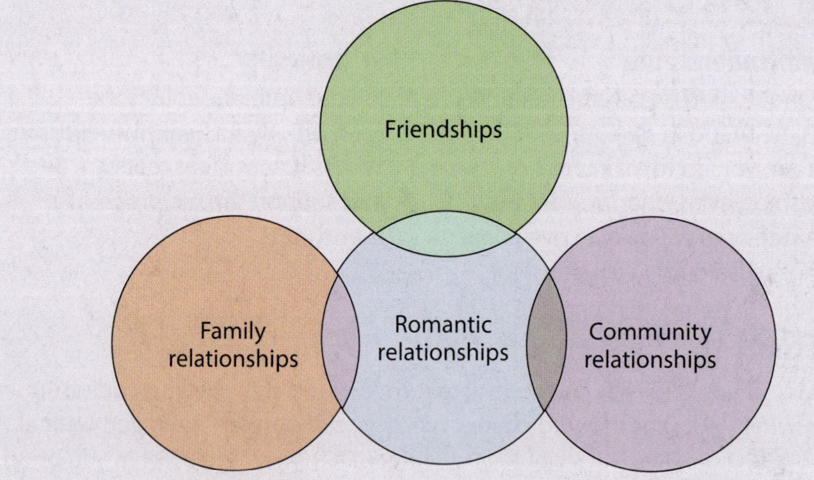

Romantic relationships—and in particular, dating relationships—are a new type of relationship for many teens. When teens begin **dating**, they regularly spend time or communicate with someone whom they are interested in romantically. The intensity of a dating relationship varies depending on the people involved, and the decision to begin dating is personal.

dating regularly spending time or communicating with someone whom a person is interested in romantically

Different people feel ready to begin dating at different times. Some teens are interested in and ready for dating earlier than their peers. These teens may feel attracted to a person in a romantic way and decide to act on those feelings. Other teens may not feel this type of attraction. Some teens may be unsure about their preferences for a romantic relationship as they learn more about their identity and sexual orientation. Some families also have rules that limit or forbid dating, often until a certain age.

Dating relationships can be exciting and can be a positive way to build your social skills, learn about yourself and your values, and practice being in a romantic relationship. As with all relationships, only healthy dating relationships will have a positive effect on your health and well-being.

Characteristics of Healthy Romantic Relationships

All types of healthy relationships share similar qualities, such as honesty, trust, mutual respect, care, commitment, support, emotional control, understanding, safety, and interpersonal skills (**Figure 14.17**). In addition to these, healthy romantic relationships also have other qualities.

Attraction, Closeness, and Commitment

Romantic relationships are driven by a combination of attraction, closeness, and commitment. **Attraction** refers to a physical and emotional connection, or the "chemistry" that draws people together. Being attracted to someone means you find it exciting to be with that person. What you find attractive depends on your preferences, values and interests, and sexual orientation.

attraction physical and emotional connection, or chemistry, that draws people together

Closeness develops when two people share special feelings and thoughts they do not share with others. When they share with each other, these two people develop a bond. Closeness is seen between friends, but friends may not share attraction for each other. Attraction without closeness is called a *crush*.

As healthy romantic relationships deepen, they grow to include *commitment*. Sometimes commitment means promising to be **exclusive**, or romantically involved only with your dating partner. Commitment also means that you agree to try to maintain a relationship over time and work through conflict. The type of romantic relationship affects the level of commitment that is appropriate. For example, a long-term relationship or marriage involves more commitment than a new dating relationship.

exclusive romantically involved only with a dating partner

Individuality

Some people think that being in a romantic relationship means your life should revolve around the relationship. In a healthy romantic relationship, however, each person maintains a unique identity. The romantic relationship does not redefine either person.

If you decide to start dating, stay true to yourself and assert your individuality. You and your partner should respect each other's separate identities. Remember that your partner's personality and individuality is what formed your attraction in the first place. As you get to know your partner, continue meeting your own responsibilities and doing activities you enjoy as an individual.

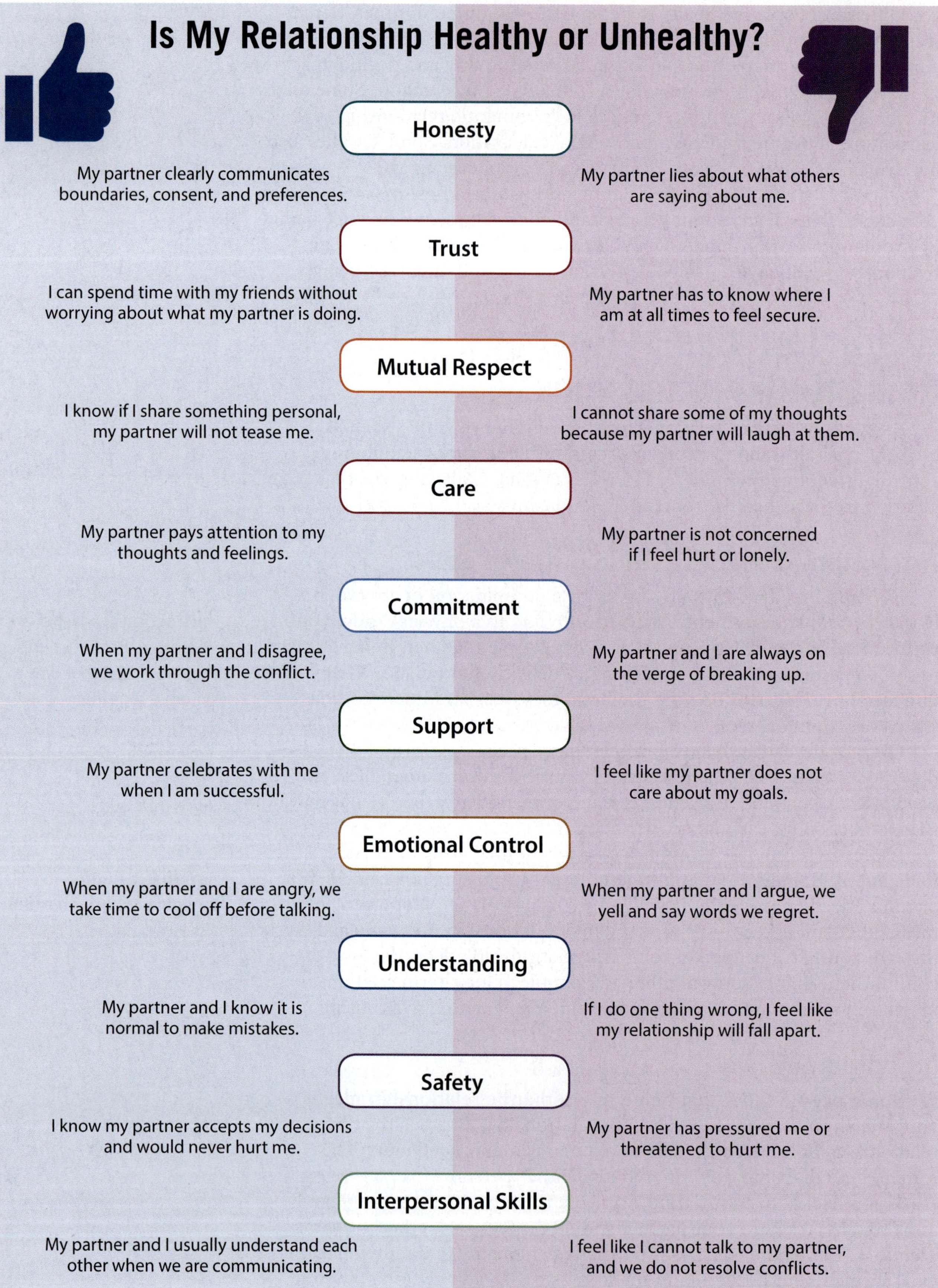

Pavlo S/Shutterstock.com

Figure 14.17 A healthy relationship should demonstrate positive characteristics in each category.

Balance

People in romantic relationships usually want to see or talk with their partners regularly. Making time for friends and family members, however, is also important. In a healthy romantic relationship, both partners balance the different relationships in their lives and do not prioritize one relationship over all others (**Figure 14.18**).

People in a healthy romantic relationship trust each other to spend time with friends and be alone. Your partner should not get angry with you for talking to other people or spending time with family and friends. You and your partner have the right to enjoy time with other people and spend time on your own.

Balance

Your partner's decisions and opinions

Your decisions and opinions

Spending time together

Spending time apart

Time spent with dating partner

Time spent with others

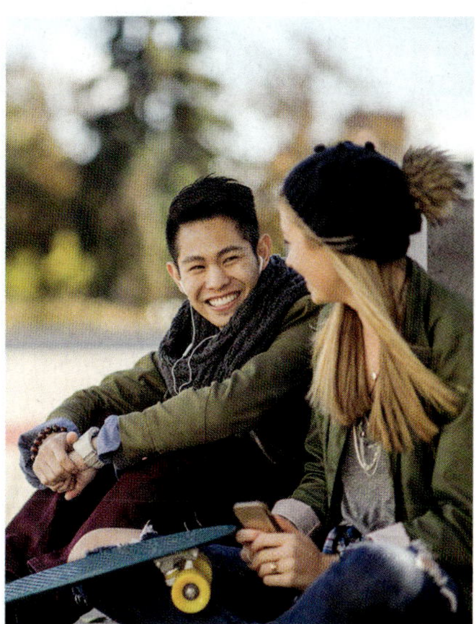

FatCamera/E+/Getty Images Plus

Figure 14.18 People in dating relationships should spend time with their dating partners, hear their opinions, and let them make some decisions. Healthy dating relationships do not, however, overshadow a person's own opinions and decisions, time spent alone and with friends, or other responsibilities.

In a healthy relationship, there is also a balance of power. A relationship is unbalanced and thus unhealthy if one person makes all the decisions without consulting the other person. In a healthy romantic relationship, each partner gets the chance to choose activities and decide how to spend time together. To maintain a healthy romantic relationship, share your thoughts and feelings openly and encourage your partner to do the same.

Love

Over time, love may develop in a dating relationship. **Love** describes an intense affection for and attachment to another person. Love develops gradually as people get to know each other on a more intimate level.

Feelings of love are often confused with infatuation. **Infatuation** describes intense romantic feelings for another person that develop suddenly and are usually based on physical attraction. The other person often does not return these feelings. The person experiencing infatuation may not know the other person very well or at all. A *crush* is an example of an intense, but short-lived, infatuation.

Love may also be confused with feelings of **passion**. Romantic relationships often begin because two people feel attracted to each other. Passion can be very powerful and exciting, especially when it is a new feeling for teens. Passion is typically short-lived, however, partly because it is based on physical attraction rather than a deeper, longer-lasting emotional connection.

love intense affection for and attachment to another person

infatuation intense romantic feelings for another person that develop suddenly and are usually based on physical attraction

passion typically short-lived attraction, based on physical attraction rather than a deeper, longer-lasting emotional connection

Physical Intimacy

Unlike other types of relationships, romantic relationships often include some type of physical intimacy, such as holding hands and kissing. These are ways for people in close romantic relationships to express affection for each other. Physical intimacy does not require sexual activity. People can express affection for each other in many other ways than sexual activity.

Health Across the Life Span

Building a Road Map for Healthy Relationships

Dating gives people the chance to practice the relationship skills needed for a happy, healthy marriage or long-term relationship. This includes skills for communicating thoughts and feelings, receiving and providing support, and working through conflicts. Help Avery and Bailey navigate their relationship. The choices they make throughout their journey will affect whether they have a healthy relationship in the future. Read each scenario and make a decision based on the choices given. At the end, add up how many red signs and green signs you encountered.

Avery and Bailey have been hanging out with a group of friends for several weeks. Avery thinks they have a lot in common and asks Bailey to see the newest superhero movie. Bailey thinks Avery is cute, but does not like superheroes.

Bailey agrees to go to the movie anyway and lies about loving superhero movies.

Bailey is honest with Avery. They agree to go see another movie they both find interesting.

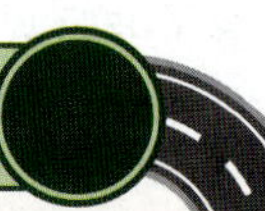

Avery and Bailey start sitting together at lunch. Avery notices Bailey gets jealous around their other friends. Avery does not want to stop hanging out with other people, but Bailey is important too.

When Avery talks to Bailey, Bailey gets angry. Why does Avery have to always want to hang out with other people?

Avery talks to Bailey. Bailey agrees to work on controlling feelings of jealousy, since they are both their own people with other friends.

Avery and Bailey decide to enter an exclusive relationship. Bailey thinks Avery wants to move too fast. Avery wants to go everywhere together and hang out all the time. Bailey just wants some time alone.

Bailey and Avery set boundaries in their relationship so they both have time for themselves.

Bailey starts ignoring Avery's texts. This hurts Avery's feelings. Avery does not understand why Bailey does not respond.

Bailey wants to attend the same college as Avery, but Avery's college does not offer the right major. Bailey worries about attending school several hours away.

Bailey knows their relationship is strong enough to handle being apart.

Bailey decides to change majors to stay close to Avery.

Avery joins several new clubs while at college, and Bailey joins a fraternity. Avery does not like hanging out with Bailey's new friends.

Avery talks to Bailey, and Bailey arranges an outing for Avery to get to know these new friends better. Avery finds they are actually nice people.

Bailey cannot understand Avery's feelings and gets mad. Bailey starts ignoring Avery around these new friends. Avery feels hurt and rejected.

Avery has big plans for the future and wants to become a lawyer, but worries Bailey will not support that. When Avery describes those plans, Bailey says Avery will not have time to be a lawyer when they are married.

Avery explains that these future goals are just as important as their relationship. Bailey decides to be more considerate of Avery's goals.

Bailey does not understand why Avery is mad. Bailey had a stay-at-home parent, so assumes Avery will be one as well.

The more green roads you helped Avery and Bailey take, the stronger their relationship becomes. Relationships take hard work and communication skills to succeed. The skills the pair used during their dating relationship will help them in a long-term relationship or marriage.

Taking multiple red roads will not lead to a healthy relationship. Avery and Bailey do not seem to have similar goals, respect for each other, or communication skills, which are essential to a successful long-term relationship or marriage.

Practice Your Skills

Access Information

Look back at the roads you took in this activity. Why did you make the decisions you did? What factors influenced the decisions you made? Next, choose one scenario from the activity that you would struggle to solve. Explain why the scenario is difficult and then research possible solutions to the scenario using valid and reliable resources. Make a list of strategies you could use to handle this scenario. Then, identify the strategy you think is healthiest and most realistic for you. Be sure to explain your choice.

MicroOne/Shutterstock.com

Before you start dating, consider and decide how you feel about being physically close to another person (**Figure 14.19**). It is better to know your limits before you are in a situation that requires a quick decision. Practice communicating your limits and affirmative consent to your partner. In healthy romantic relationships, each person is open about limits, and each person always accepts and respects these limits. Your partner may even feel relieved that you are clear and honest about your limits and consent. Remember that pressure to engage in physically intimate behavior is *not* part of a healthy romantic relationship and shows a lack of consent.

Questions to Ask About Physical Intimacy and Consent

- Am I comfortable hugging?
- Am I comfortable holding hands?
- Am I comfortable putting my arm around my partner? with my partner putting an arm around me?
- Am I comfortable sitting on my partner's lap? with my partner sitting on my lap?
- Am I comfortable being alone with my partner?
- Am I comfortable kissing?

Figure 14.19 You may feel comfortable in one area and uncomfortable in another. You may also feel comfortable with all or none of the categories of physical intimacy. ***What are sudden romantic feelings based in physical attraction called?***

Skills for Healthy Romantic Relationships

Perhaps you have either already had or are interested in someday having a romantic relationship. Strategies you can use for forming a healthy relationship include the following.

Learn About Your Partner (and Yourself)

Before you begin dating someone, get to know that person. Talk to this person at school, during an activity, or on a phone or video call before going out. The strategies in **Figure 14.20** can help you get to know a potential dating partner and understand your own interests.

Getting to Know a Dating Partner

Ask yourself questions.	Ask your dating partner questions.	Listen well.	Open up.
Think about what you want in a dating partner. Is it important that the person is funny? smart? nice to others?	Think of some questions you can ask your dating partner. What does the person like to do for fun? What activities does the person like?	When the other person is talking, pay attention. Make eye contact and do not interrupt.	Share your own values, goals, and interests honestly. It is important to let the other person know who you really are.
Different people value different qualities in a dating relationship. Consider your own priorities.	Ask questions to get to know another person and figure out if you have interests in common.	Put down your phone and concentrate on the conversation.	Express your own priorities and needs about what you want to do or not do on a date.

Figure 14.20 Talking to a person before going out will help you figure out if you share common interests. ***What method of getting to know someone includes going out with several people along with the person you like?***

group dating spending time in a group that includes someone a person is interested in romantically

Another easy way to get to know someone is to go out with a group that includes the person you like. This is called **group dating**. Being with a group reduces the pressure of having to keep a conversation going with someone you are just getting to know. Group dating is also a way to stay safe, especially if you do not know the person very well.

Enforcing Your Boundaries

Decide on Your Boundaries

- Consider your values, beliefs, and goals.
- Talk with trusted adults.
- Write down your boundaries.

Communicate Your Boundaries

- Tell your partner what your boundaries are.
- Tell your partner you will enforce your boundaries.

Avoid Risky Situations

- Stay clear of situations that might compromise your boundaries.
- Leave situations that threaten your boundaries.

Act on Your Boundaries

- Provide consent for activities you agree to.
- Say *no* to activities that violate your boundaries.
- Repeat your decision, if necessary.
- Know that someone who loves you will respect your boundaries and consent.

Figure 14.21 You have the right to make up your own mind about your personal boundaries and consent. A dating partner who questions, teases, or pressures you about your decision does not love or respect you.

Cope with Nerves

You may feel nervous about talking to or meeting with the person you want to date. These feelings are normal, and the other person will probably be nervous, too. As you begin dating, find ways to cope with your nerves. If talking makes you nervous, plan activities that do not require much conversation, such as playing miniature golf or bowling, or going to a sporting event or a school dance.

Enjoy Common Interests

Many teens enjoy dating someone who shares some of their interests. Dating partners can also find additional common interests by trying new activities. If you have an interest in photography, for example, you can introduce this activity to see if your dating partner might share this interest. If neither of you has tried rock climbing, you can try it together for the first time.

While common interests are important, it is also important for each person in a dating relationship to enjoy time apart and with family and other friends. You can demonstrate care for your dating partner by supporting that person's goals and not expecting your dating partner to sacrifice those goals for the dating relationship.

Enforce Your Boundaries

In healthy dating relationships, partners treat each other with respect and value each other. They understand that each person has boundaries, limits, and preferences. They respect those boundaries, communicate consent, and do not try to change or shift what the other person has consented to do. To maintain a healthy dating relationship, decide on boundaries before the relationship begins and then communicate and enforce those boundaries by providing or not providing consent (**Figure 14.21**).

Ask for Help

Many teens find it helpful to ask parents, guardians, or other trusted adults for advice about healthy dating relationships. These adults are often helpful since they have had their own experiences navigating dating. For example, you might want advice about communicating honestly with a dating partner, balancing a dating relationship with other priorities, and setting and maintaining personal boundaries.

It is especially important to get advice and ask for help when a dating relationship is unhealthy or abusive. A dating relationship is not healthy if one person

- makes all of the decisions and controls the other person;
- is hostile, picks fights, or lies;
- fails to respect the other person's boundaries, ridicules the person's decisions, or pushes the person to change;
- is completely reliant on the other person and does not maintain an independent identity; or
- uses fear tactics, threats, force, or violence of any kind.

If you recognize any of these signs, talk to an adult you trust for advice. A trusted adult can help you think about the relationship, decide what to do, and leave the relationship safely.

The End of a Dating Relationship

Many high school dating relationships eventually end in a **breakup**. Teens' goals and beliefs are still forming and changing as they try to figure out their own identities. This means it can be hard to maintain a dating relationship during high school.

breakup end of a romantic relationship

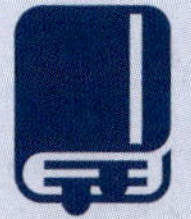

Case Study

Dating Dilemmas

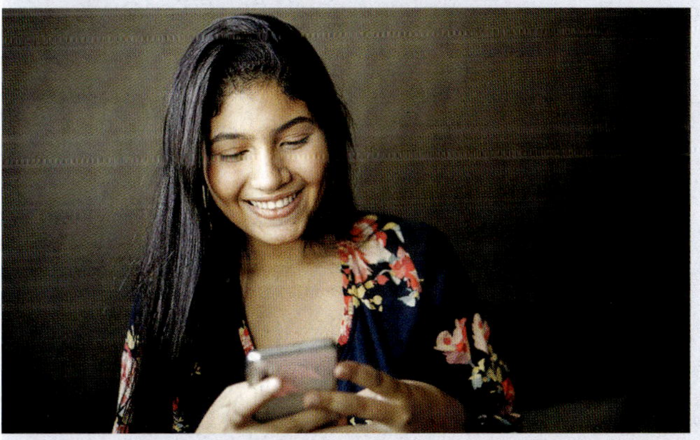

Capuski/E+/Getty Images

Paxson has been dating Jayla for six months now. Everything was going great between them, but lately Paxson has started feeling distant. Paxson has been having a rough time in his math class and wants to be able to talk to Jayla about it. While he talks, she mostly scrolls through her phone or starts talking about her day. Sometimes Jayla even teases him about his grades in math.

Thea recently started talking to her online friend Chaniece, who commented on a post she shared online. Thea really enjoys talking to Chaniece. They share many similar interests, such as action movies and playing volleyball. Thea would like to date Chaniece, but their only form of communication has been through social media and text messages. Thea's friends warn her about the dangers of meeting someone online in-person, but Thea tells Chaniece they can meet at the mall on Friday night.

Jorge's best friend Zoe really wants Jorge to have a girlfriend so they can go on double dates together. Jorge is not interested in dating anyone and feels uncomfortable when Zoe offers to set him up. He has noticed that his other friends are available to hang out less often when they are in relationships, and he would rather spend time with all of his friends than just one person.

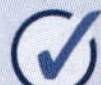

Practice Your Skills

Set Goals

In small groups, talk about the possible actions Paxson, Thea, and Jorge might take and how these choices will impact their health and wellness. Consider the advice friends and family members might provide these three to help them. In your small groups, create a series of SMART goals Paxson, Thea, and Jorge could use to handle each situation in a healthy way. Be sure to break long-term SMART goals into several short-term ones.

Coping with a Breakup

Be kind to yourself.
- Get enough sleep, eat nutritious foods, and get physical activity.
- Remind yourself it is normal to feel sad, hurt, embarrassed, or guilty after a breakup and it will get better with time.
- Remember your positive characteristics. If you find this difficult, ask your friends to remind you.

Share your feelings.
- Find someone to talk to. The people who love you can cheer you up.
- Friends, siblings, and particularly trusted adults have probably been through breakups of their own. They can remind you that your feelings are normal and will not last forever.

Keep yourself busy.
- Fill your time and thoughts with activities you normally enjoy.
- Find a new hobby by joining an after-school club, trying a new physical activity, or volunteering.

Give your ex space.
- No matter who initiated the breakup, exes may feel tempted to stay in each other's lives. Former dating partners can remain friends, but each person needs to allow the other space and time to heal.

Limit how much you see or hear about your ex.
- Block your ex on social media and tell your friends you do not want to hear about your ex. Hearing about or seeing what your ex is doing hurts your ability to move on.

Focus on the good.
- Try to find at least one reason to be grateful every day. This reminder will help shift your attention, even briefly, away from the bad onto what is good.

Figure 14.22 If you have thoughts about self-harm or suicide after a breakup, even just once or every so often, tell a trusted adult. ***What is the end of a relationship called?***

Breakups can be emotionally painful, especially if one person does not want to end the relationship. It is important, however, to recognize when a relationship is not working. People may grow apart, find that their interests or values do not match, or change their minds. Common feelings following the end of a relationship include sadness, anger, physical illness, and loneliness. These feelings are a normal reaction to the end of a relationship and will heal over time.

Some people try to cope with the loss of a dating relationship by quickly beginning a new relationship. By doing this, however, they do not allow themselves time to process their feelings about the end of their previous relationship. Some of these feelings can spill over into the new relationship, which is unfair to new dating partners. **Figure 14.22** lists some healthy strategies for coping with the end of a dating relationship.

Lesson 14.4 Review

Know and Understand

1. Describe the difference between attraction and closeness.
2. Distinguish between love, infatuation, and passion. How would you explain the differences to someone else?
3. What is the advantage of group dating?
4. Explain how to enforce a specific boundary you have and communicate consent.
5. List one sign that a dating relationship is not healthy.

Think Critically

6. Explain what it means to feel safe in a dating relationship.
7. Why is balance of power important in a romantic relationship?
8. Why can it be helpful to cut off contact with a person after a breakup?

REAL WORLD Health Skills

Advocate for Health To advocate for your health and the health of a current or future dating partner, create your own "Dating Bill of Rights." Include your own rights and responsibilities, as well as the rights and responsibilities of your dating partner. Explain the reasoning behind each right and responsibility and share your list with the class.

Practicing Sexual Abstinence

Essential Question?

What are the benefits of choosing sexual abstinence?

Lesson 14.5

Learning Outcomes

After studying this lesson, you will be able to

- discuss why abstinence is a healthy sexual choice for teens;
- list factors that can challenge a person's commitment to abstinence; and
- employ strategies for practicing abstinence.

Key Terms

oxytocin
sexual abstinence
sexual activity
sexual intercourse

Warm-Up Activity

Remaining Abstinent

Practice Health-Enhancing Behaviors In your own words, define what you think *sexual abstinence* means. List five reasons why it might be important for you to remain sexually abstinent. Put your reasons in order, from the strongest to the weakest. If faced with pressure to have sex, would these reasons help you remain abstinent? Why or why not? Are there additional protective factors you could increase in your life to help you remain abstinent?

Reasons to Remain Sexually Abstinent	
1	
2	
3	
4	
5	

During adolescence, you may start to think more about dating relationships and sexuality. This is normal and can get stronger from pressure around you. You might hear your friends talking about sexual topics or encounter people online who seem to know about sex. You have probably even seen sexual content in the media, which might make you curious.

sexual abstinence decision to refrain from sexual activity for physical, social, or emotional reasons

sexual activity actions that involve contact with a person's reproductive organs; can include sexual intercourse and other activities

sexual intercourse sexual activity that involves penetration, or insertion of a body part or object into another body part

Many factors, including your values, beliefs, and judgment, will influence the decisions you make about physical intimacy and sexual feelings. For teens, a responsible decision for handling these feelings is **sexual abstinence**, or the decision to refrain from sexual activity. **Sexual activity** describes actions that involve contact with a person's reproductive organs and may include sexual touching and sexual intercourse. **Sexual intercourse** involves *penetration*, or the insertion of a body part or object into another body part. It is possible to maintain a rewarding, fun, healthy dating relationship without engaging in sexual activity (**Figure 14.23**).

Reasons to Choose Abstinence

Sexual activity can bring intense emotion and stress to romantic relationships and can complicate lives in ways for which teens are unprepared. Many teens choose to be abstinent for these reasons and still experience closeness and intimacy in their dating relationships. The reasons to choose abstinence are physical, social, and emotional. These reasons include the following:

- **Abstinence prevents pregnancy:** Most teens do not want to carry a child or become a parent at their age. Only continuous abstinence works 100 percent of the time to prevent pregnancy. Unplanned teen pregnancies can hurt young people's goals for the future, cause conflict and stress, and lead to negative health consequences.

Effects of Sexual Abstinence

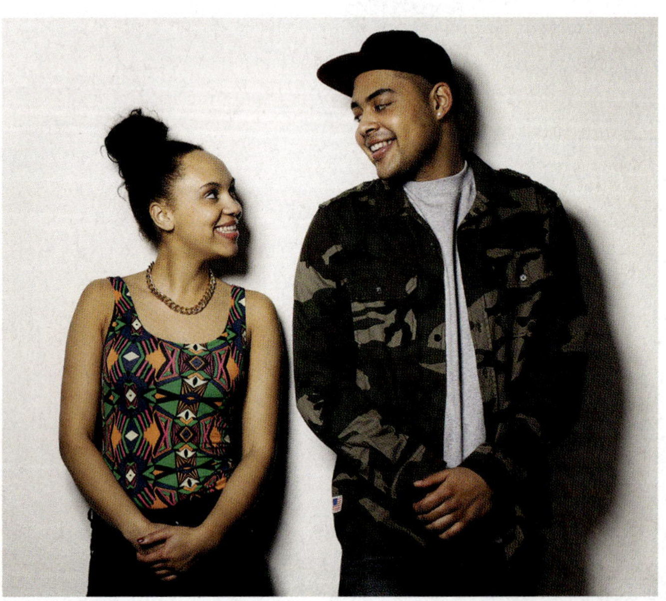

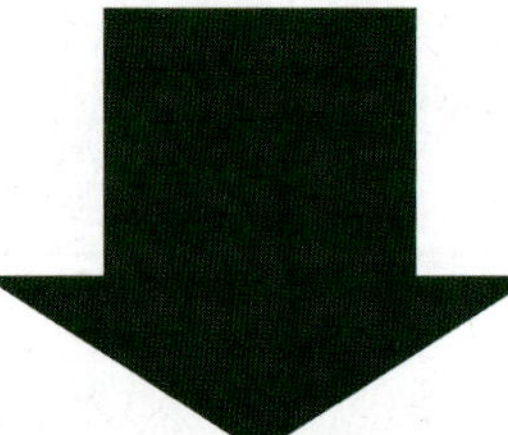

Decreases

- risk of sexually transmitted infections (STIs) and HIV/AIDS
- risk of pregnancy
- pain following a breakup

Increases

- enjoyment of nonsexual activities in a dating relationship
- time for growth in other parts of life

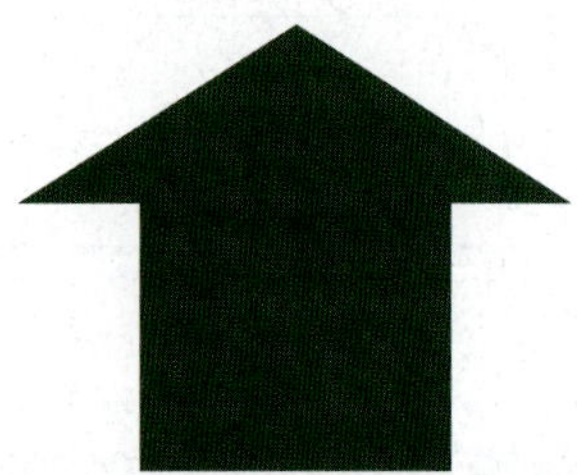

Jacob Lund/Shutterstock.com

Figure 14.23 Abstaining from sexual activity improves the physical, mental and emotional, and social health of teens. ***Is sexual activity the same as sexual intercourse?***

- **Abstinence prevents STIs:** Sexual activity of any type puts people at risk for STIs and HIV. STIs can cause health conditions, be incurable, and lead to infertility. Some STIs, such as HIV, can lead to health conditions that can threaten a person's life. Abstinence is the only method that is 100-percent effective in preventing STIs.
- **Abstinence can increase enjoyment of nonsexual activities:** Abstinence allows teens to enjoy a dating relationship, which can become complicated by sexual activity.
- **Abstinence avoids emotional consequences of sexual activity:** When people engage in sexual activity, their bodies release **oxytocin**, a hormone that promotes bonding and connection. This closer connection brings intensity for which teens are unprepared. Teens may be overwhelmed, feel more pain after a breakup, and have to cope with the stress of pregnancy or an STI.
- **Abstinence allows time for growth and other parts of life:** Sexual activity can create an intensity in teen relationships that makes it difficult to focus on individual growth. Abstinence helps teens fully commit to important goals like their education, career, and other personal interests.

oxytocin hormone released during sexual activity that promotes bonding and connection

Abstinence also encourages emotional growth and maturity. Healthy sexual relationships include emotional maturity, intimacy, closeness, and trust. Many teens feel they are not emotionally ready to handle a sexual relationship or the possibility of becoming a parent. For example, imagine that after having sex with her boyfriend, Winnie finds out that he told his friends. She feels betrayed that he shared something so private with others, and this breach in trust ends the relationship. As another example, after Miko began having sex with her boyfriend, she noticed a change in herself. She became possessive and jealous and got upset if her boyfriend was out with friends. The more she pushes, the more her boyfriend withdraws, and the more unstable the relationship becomes.

Teen dating relationships can be fun and rewarding without sex. Knowing the reasons you want to abstain from sex can help you stick to your decision. Being clear in your own mind about your reasons will help you explain your decision to your partner and remain confident.

Challenges to Abstinence

You may encounter challenges to your decision to practice abstinence. Some of these challenges include pressure from a partner, fear of rejection from a partner or peers, societal and commercial media influences, alcohol or drug use, and a desire for intimacy. Remember that feeling pressured to do something you have not consented to do is a sign of an unhealthy relationship. If your dating partner pressures you to have sex when you have said *no*, the relationship is unhealthy.

Teens may encounter many conflicting messages about sex. Their friends and peers may tell them "everyone is doing it." This is not true. In reality, many teens are not having sex (**Figure 14.24**).

Many of these messages come from the media. Advertisements, films, and other media often portray teens and young adults involved in sexual relationships. The implied message is that sex is a common part of teen relationships. In the media, sexual relationships seem casual, involving little or no responsibility, risk, or emotional fallout. While these scenes create interesting storylines, the messages they convey are not realistic.

Another challenge to abstinence is alcohol and drug use. Alcohol and drug use increase the possibility of engaging in sexual activity. Alcohol and drugs impair judgment and *inhibition* (feelings of restraint), so their use can lead to early and unwanted sexual activity. By avoiding risky situations that may include drugs and alcohol, a person can make responsible decisions involving the choice to maintain abstinence.

Strategies for Practicing Abstinence

There are several strategies you can use to remain sexually abstinent. These include discussing your decision to remain abstinent, avoiding risky situations, using refusal skills, and talking with a trusted adult. A person who has been sexually active in the past can always choose not to have sex in a current or future relationship.

Discuss Your Decision

Healthy dating relationships should include honest communication about physical intimacy, including sexual activity. When a person makes a commitment to sexual abstinence, the person must be ready to explain this commitment to a dating partner. A commitment to abstinence becomes easier when a person's dating partner understands and respects the decision. Communicating your decisions to avoid alcohol and drugs and other risky situations can also help you stick to your decision to practice abstinence. It is best to have this conversation early in the relationship, before there is any pressure.

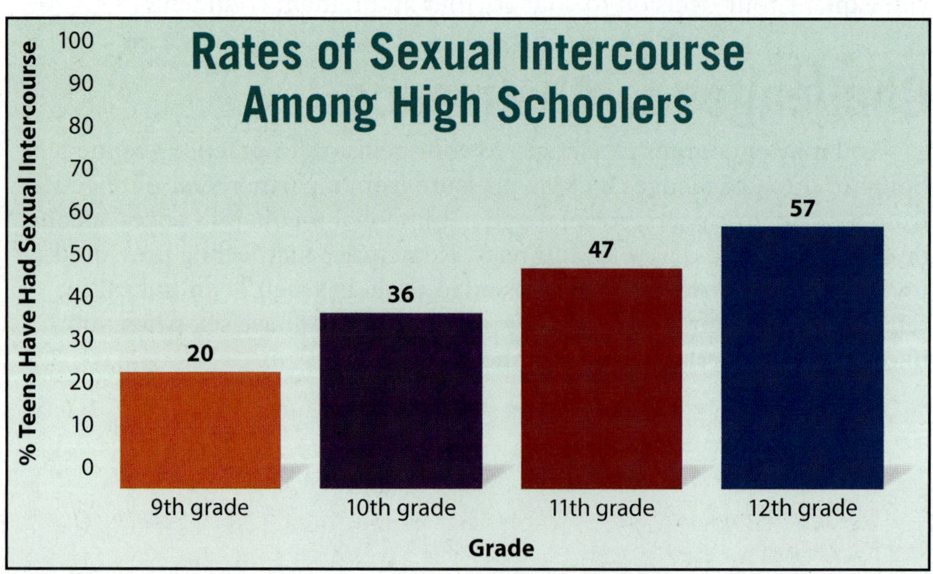

Figure 14.24 Rates of sexual intercourse increase throughout high school. Even by the time they graduate, however, only 57 percent of teens report having ever had sexual intercourse.

Your first major challenge may be if your dating partner disagrees with the commitment to abstinence. In that case, you should be prepared to avoid risky situations and refuse sexual advances. You may need to reevaluate your dating relationship if your partner continues to apply unwanted pressure to engage in sexual activities. If you have made a decision to be abstinent, you need to clearly communicate this to your dating partner (**Figure 14.25**).

Some teens feel pressured by their dating partners to engage in physically intimate or sexual behavior. It is important to remember that this type of pressure does *not* exist in healthy dating relationships. Healthy relationships include respect and safety. Your partner should never tease you when you refuse to do something that makes you uncomfortable. Your partner should also never force you or pressure you into sexual activity. If your partner forces, threatens, or pressures you into any kind of sexual activity, this is a type of violence called *sexual assault*. You will learn more about sexual assault and abuse in Chapter 15.

Avoid Risky Situations

Certain situations can make abstinence difficult. These situations include events with alcohol or drug use and unsupervised parties. Considering what situations are risky ahead of time can help you avoid them. Be prepared to avoid situations in which

- someone does not respect your boundaries and consent;
- there is a lack of adult supervision;
- people are using alcohol or drugs;
- you are in unfamiliar surroundings with people you do not know; or
- you feel unsafe or uncomfortable.

Strategies for Communicating Your Decision About Abstinence

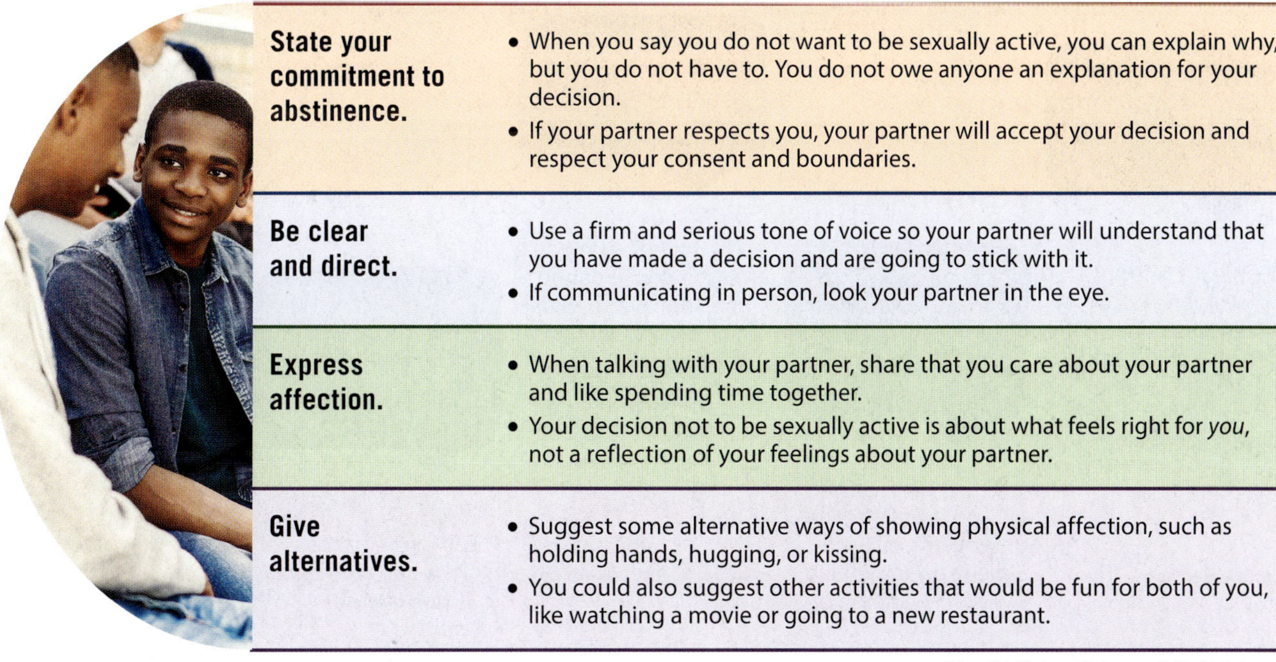

State your commitment to abstinence.	• When you say you do not want to be sexually active, you can explain why, but you do not have to. You do not owe anyone an explanation for your decision. • If your partner respects you, your partner will accept your decision and respect your consent and boundaries.
Be clear and direct.	• Use a firm and serious tone of voice so your partner will understand that you have made a decision and are going to stick with it. • If communicating in person, look your partner in the eye.
Express affection.	• When talking with your partner, share that you care about your partner and like spending time together. • Your decision not to be sexually active is about what feels right for *you*, not a reflection of your feelings about your partner.
Give alternatives.	• Suggest some alternative ways of showing physical affection, such as holding hands, hugging, or kissing. • You could also suggest other activities that would be fun for both of you, like watching a movie or going to a new restaurant.

Stígur Már Karlsson/Heimsmyndir/E+/Getty Images

Figure 14.25 Communicating your decision to be sexually abstinent helps your dating partner respect your boundaries. ***If your partner pressures you into sexual activity, what is this called?***

If you find yourself in any of these situations, take action and leave. It is better to walk away from a dangerous situation than to risk your health and safety. People who care about you will respect your decision and help you enforce your boundaries.

Practice Refusal Skills

Planning and even practicing skills for refusing sex, drugs, and alcohol can help you become familiar with words and actions you can use if risky situations do occur. For example, consider the words you might use if you find yourself at an unsupervised party, or if you are invited to an event where alcohol or drugs may be present, and your dating partner is pressuring you to have sex. How would you respond? **Figure 14.26** shows some approaches you can try in different situations that involve sexual pressure.

Sometimes verbally refusing may not be enough. You may need to physically leave or walk away from the situation. You do not need to face this stress and pressure alone. You might talk to a friend, parent or guardian, teacher, counselor, or other trusted adult for guidance about specific situations.

Talk with a Trusted Adult

If you feel confused about how to make a decision about a sexual relationship, talk to a trusted adult—a parent or guardian, adult sibling, doctor, or teacher. You might also reach out to a community resource. These people and resources can help you understand your concerns so that you can make a well-reasoned decision. Your decision to abstain from sex is entirely your own and is a sign that you are strong, in control of your body, and focused on your goals and the future.

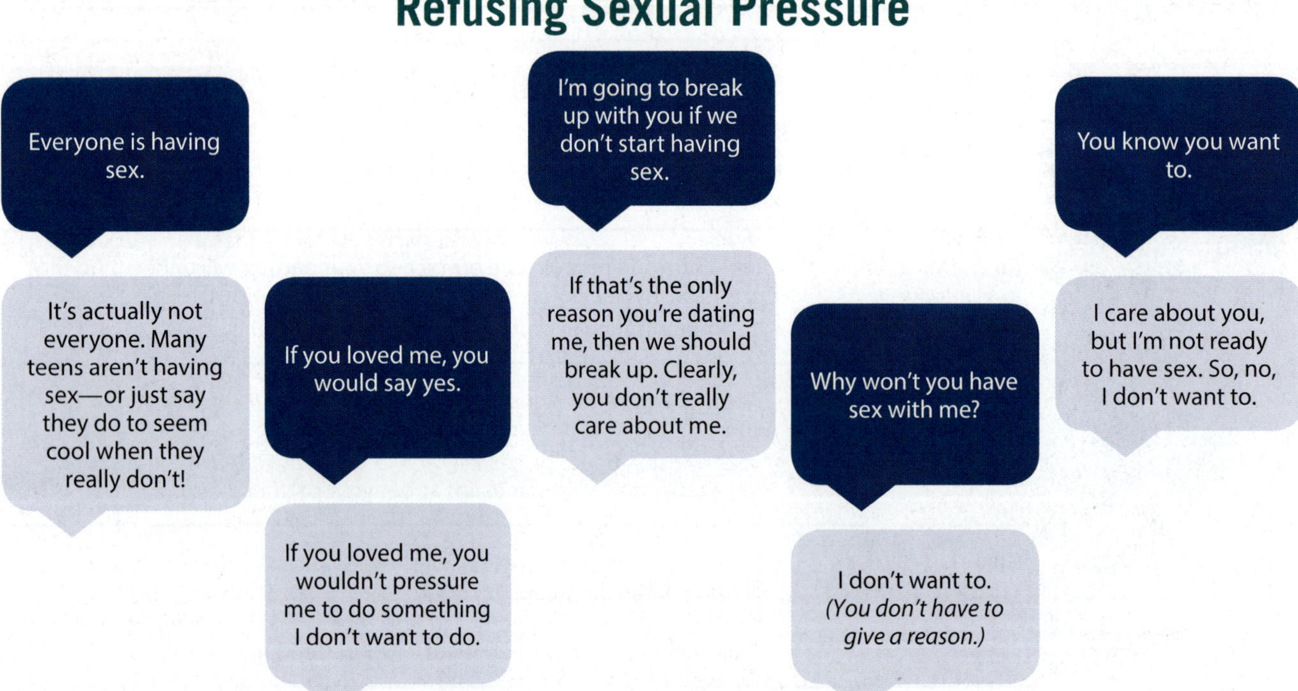

Figure 14.26 Make sure you practice these approaches ahead of time so you feel more confident using them if you face any of these situations. ***What may you need to do if verbally refusing is not enough?***

Skills for Health and Wellness

Abstinence: Words, Action, and Preparation

When you make a commitment to abstain from sexual activity, you may receive challenges to your decision. These may come from your dating partner or friends in various risky situations. Knowing what words to use, what actions to take, and how to prepare can help in these situations.

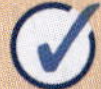

Practice Your Skills

Communicate with Others

Partner with two of your classmates to form a group of three. Then, in your group, write scripts based on the three situations that follow. In each script, one person should write about the person feeling pressure, one person should write about the individual exerting the pressure, and the third person should separately write down any key phrases used to refuse sexual activity.

1. Imagine you are meeting your dating partner of three months at your friend's house for a party. Even though your friend's parents are home, your dating partner arrives at the party drunk. Your dating partner asks you to have sex, and when you say *no*, offers you a drink. Your dating partner suggests going to another party where a friend's parents are not home. What do you say?
2. You are over at your crush's house with some friends playing games, and everything seems to be going well. After a few hours, your friends leave, but your crush asks you to stay and watch a movie. During the movie, your crush starts trying to kiss you and touch you sexually. What do you do?
3. You just started dating someone you have been friends with for a while. You and your partner seem to be on the same page about most issues, but you have not talked about sex. On your last date, you and your partner got closer than you wanted. You call your partner because you want to make your boundaries clear. How do you start the conversation?

After writing the three scripts, review the phrases used to refuse sexual activity. Which approaches were most effective? least effective? Write a guide for yourself with phrases you can use to resist sexual pressure and refuse sexual activity.

Lesson 14.5 Review

Know and Understand

1. Choose one benefit of abstinence and explain how it would affect your long-term goals.
2. Explain one strategy for discussing your decision to remain abstinent with a dating partner.
3. If a partner forces, threatens, or pressures you into any kind of sexual activity, what is this called?

Think Critically

4. In a small group, discuss media messages about teen sexual activity. What examples can you cite? Are these examples realistic? Why or why not?
5. With a partner, discuss the statements in Figure 14.26. What other common statements have you heard people use to apply sexual pressure? Brainstorm responses to each statement.

REAL WORLD Health Skills

Make Decisions Imagine that you write articles for an online teen relationship blog. Write a blog post that discusses why abstinence is a healthy decision for teens. In your post, explain the reasoning for this conclusion using the decision-making process. Be sure to identify why alternatives to sexual abstinence may still hold risks. Use information from this lesson to help support your reasons that teens should remain sexually abstinent.

Chapter 14 Review and Assessment

Chapter Summary

Relationships are the connections you have with other people. Healthy relationships improve all dimensions of health. Unhealthy relationships can harm health. Healthy relationships have several key characteristics.

Healthy relationships have honesty. This means people are truthful about their feelings and thoughts. Healthy relationships also have trust, mutual respect, care, commitment, and support. In healthy relationships, people control their emotions and show understanding. People should feel safe in relationships, set boundaries, and give and receive affirmative consent. Interpersonal skills related to communication and conflict resolution help people maintain healthy relationships. Any lack of these qualities signals an unhealthy relationship.

Family relationships provide for physical needs, meet mental and emotional needs, and educate and socialize. To have healthy family relationships, you can resolve conflicts constructively with parents and guardians and follow rules. You can negotiate with siblings and respect each other's space. You can also seek to understand grandparents and involve them in your life. You can talk with a trusted adult or reach out to community resources to get help for unhealthy family relationships or difficult family changes.

Community relationships are connections with the people around you in your community. To build healthy community relationships, you can advocate for diversity, use professional communication, set healthy boundaries, and get involved in the community.

Friendships are a type of peer relationship. These relationships provide support, whether in-person or online. To build healthy friendships, you can get to know others, make time for relationships, meet face-to-face, be supportive, and handle issues in healthy ways.

Romantic relationships need all the same qualities that other healthy relationships need. In addition, healthy romantic relationships are characterized by attraction, closeness, commitment, individuality, balance, love, and physical intimacy. To build these relationships, you can learn about yourself and your partner, cope with nerves, enjoy common interests, and enforce boundaries. Do not be afraid to ask for help, if needed.

Physical intimacy can lead to sexual activity as teens become more curious about sex. Sexual abstinence, the decision to refrain from sexual activity, has many benefits, including no risk of pregnancy or STIs. Sexual abstinence also benefits mental and emotional and social health. To maintain sexual abstinence, people need to identify and overcome challenges. They should also discuss the decision with a dating partner, avoid risky situations, use refusal skills, and reach out for help, if needed.

Vocabulary Activity

Interview a trusted older adult about healthy relationships. Using the key terms in this chapter, develop at least five questions about relationships that interest you and ask them, using proper vocabulary and maturity. During the interview, ask for clarification on any words or explanations you do not understand. Using all of the key terms in this chapter, write an essay reflecting on the conversation and the information you heard. Before turning your essay in to your teacher, be sure to have the person you interviewed review it and check your essay for proper grammar and spelling.

acquaintances	*extended family*	*mentors*	*sexual activity*
affirmative consent	*friendship*	*oxytocin*	*sexual intercourse*
attraction	*group dating*	*passion*	*sibling rivalry*
boundaries	*honesty*	*professional communication*	*socialize*
breakup	*immediate family*	*reciprocal*	*supervisor*
clique	*infatuation*	*relationships*	*traditions*
coworkers	*jealousy*	*respect*	*trust*
dating	*law enforcement*	*sexual abstinence*	
exclusive	*love*		

Review and Recall

Review the information in this chapter by answering the following questions.

1. If you fear that your friend will mock or insult you for sharing your feelings, which of the following is missing from your relationship?
   A. trust
   B. honesty
   C. commitment
   D. admiration
2. What does it mean that affirmative consent is freely given?
3. Which of the following is a sign of an unhealthy relationship?
   A. disagreements
   B. different interests and goals
   C. accountability for behavior
   D. isolation from family and friends
4. How can teens get help if they have an unhealthy relationship with a parent or guardian?
5. Explain how you can demonstrate confidence in professional communication.
6. What does it mean for caring and support in a friendship to be reciprocal?
7. What is the name for a small group of friends that deliberatly excludes others?
8. Which of the following is *not* part of a healthy romantic relationship?
   A. safety
   B. affirmative consent
   C. balance
   D. loss of individuality
9. When should you start thinking about your boundaries related to physical intimacy?
10. If a dating partner does not respect the boundaries you set, what does this mean about the relationship?
11. List three benefits of sexual abstinence.
12. What role does the hormone oxytocin play in sexual activity?
13. What are two risky situations you might want to avoid to remain sexually abstinent?

Standardized Test Prep

Reading and Writing Practice

Read the passage below and then answer the following questions.

You have probably seen movies or shows about teens who never seem to study for class or take out the garbage. These teens are too busy spending time with the partners of their dreams. Teen dating relationships in the media are often unrealistic portrayals. Dating relationships in real life can be confusing and complicated. Teens sometimes feel rejected by those they want to date. They can have conflicts with their dating partners, such as feeling pressured to engage in behaviors that make them uncomfortable.

Depictions of teen dating may make some people feel pressured to start dating before they are ready. Because of pressure, some teens may begin dating before they feel real affection for someone. Although it may seem like most teens in the media are dating, many teens in real life are not in dating relationships.

14. Which statement best summarizes the main point of this passage?
    A. Most teens are not ready to date.
    B. Most teens are not dating.
    C. Media depictions can give teens unrealistic ideas about teen dating.
    D. Dating is dangerous for teens.
15. In what ways are media portrayals of teen dating unrealistic?
16. Think of a teen dating relationship you recently encountered in the media or social media. How does that relationship relate to this passage? Is the relationship portrayed realistic? Write a short essay describing why or why not.

Chapter 14 Skills Assessment

Critical Thinking Skills

Answer the following questions to assess your knowledge of what you learned in this chapter.

1. How do you know if respect in a relationship is mutual? With a partner, make a list of criteria you could use to determine this.
2. Safety in a relationship does not just refer to physical safety. What does it mean to be emotionally and socially safe in a relationship?
3. Choose one sign of an unhealthy relationship and write a story in which a teen recognizes this sign in a relationship and does something to change the relationship or get help.
4. What conflicts do you most commonly have with your parent or guardian? Why do you think these conflicts occur? How do these conflicts affect the relationship?
5. Are boundaries in community relationships different from boundaries in family or peer relationships? Explain your answer.
6. What factors do you think affect whether online friends become very close friends or remain acquaintances? How do online friendships compare to in-person friendships?
7. How common do you think jealousy is in friendships? Why does jealousy develop, and how can friendships survive and grow deeper even when jealousy is present?
8. With a partner, discuss the following question: *When one person in a friendship changes, does the friendship have to change?* Explain the reasons for your answer and share with another pair.
9. Is attraction, or chemistry, necessary in a healthy romantic relationship? Defend your answer using information from this chapter. Find someone with an opposing view and discuss.
10. What resources are available in your school or community to help people navigating romantic relationships? If you were in an unhealthy romantic relationship, where would you turn for help? Why?
11. Why do you think both people, no matter how the relationship ends, find it difficult to cope after the end of a dating relationship?
12. What challenges to abstinence are most common in your school and community? Why do these challenges exist, and how can you overcome them?
13. Discussing decisions about sexual abstinence does not have to be scary or awkward. With a partner, make a list of strategies for having this conversation in a mature, clear way. Keep this list for your future reference.

Health and Wellness Skills

Complete the following activities to assess your skills related to health and wellness.

14. **Analyze Influences.** Write a story about a teen who did not have a plan for remaining sexually abstinent and ended up having sex. What situation might have led this teen to have sex, despite deciding to be sexually abstinent? What behaviors, situations, or pressures might have led the teen to have sex? List all of the possible physical, social, and emotional consequences the teen may experience because of this decision. What influences could the teen have managed better to prevent this situation?
15. **Access Information.** In this chapter, you learned about several different types of relationships. Choose one type you want to learn more about. Then, gather more information about this type of relationship using reliable and valid online resources. Remember to evaluate each resource you use. You can use the guidelines in Chapter 2 to do this. Create a "Helpful Websites" page for the type of relationship you chose. Include at least five websites that contain beneficial information. Along with each website, include two or three new pieces of advice or information the resource provided.
16. **Communicate with Others.** Professional communication is a skill needed in the workplace. Imagine a coworker at your workplace has accused you of something you did not do. Your supervisor is out of the office for several days, and you are very upset. Write an email to your supervisor explaining your side of the story. Keep in mind that emails can be forwarded and might be viewed by someone other than the intended recipient.

17. **Make Decisions.** Imagine that Marie and Craig have been dating for a while. After a concert, they go to Craig's house, and Craig tells Marie he wants to have sex. Marie does not want to have sex, and she is not sure what to say. Write the ending of this story, using all of the knowledge and skills you have learned so far regarding healthy relationships for teens. Add a definite ending in which Marie and Craig make a healthy decision about whether to have sex or remain abstinent.
18. **Set Goals.** List three SMART goals you have for your future. These can relate to any part of your life, from additional education to a future career or hobby. Next to each goal, identify how the relationships in your life are helping or preventing you from meeting the goal. Predict how each relationship might affect your goal in the future. Are there any changes you need to make to your relationships to help you meet your goals?
19. **Practice Health-Enhancing Behaviors.** Suppose you and your friends are playing ball when some new students at your school ask to join. These new students recently moved to the area and have an ethnic and cultural background uncommon in your community. Two of your friends start making fun of them and act like the new students cannot hear them. What would be your personal plan of action in this type of situation? What could you say or do to speak up, show respect for diversity, and encourage your friends to behave in a healthier way? Write a short paragraph or script explaining what you would do and how these actions would affect your health and the health of others.
20. **Advocate for Health.** In each community, city, or state, different resources exist to help people who have experienced or are in unhealthy relationships. Research these types of resources within your own community or area. After gathering your information, create an advocacy campaign with information that might help a teen in an unhealthy relationship. Formats for this campaign might include a presentation, email blast, social media post, or infographic.

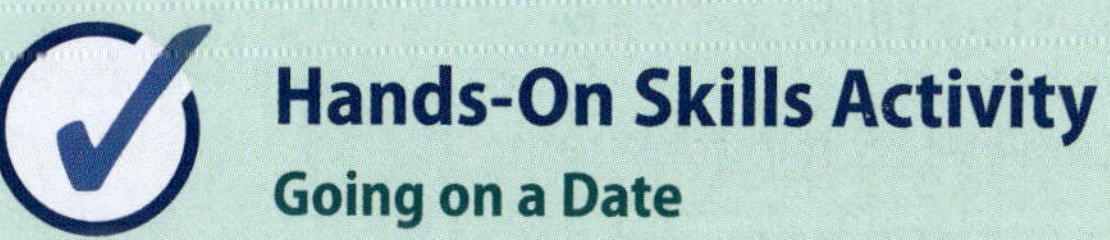

Hands-On Skills Activity

Going on a Date

Dating relationships are a new type of relationship for many teens. Regardless of level of experience, teens benefit from having a plan going into a dating or romantic relationship. In this activity, you will create a character who is going on a date. This character can be whatever you choose to create—an avatar, superhero, cartoon figure, or anime figure, for example. As you create your character, follow the steps in the activity to ensure your character has a sound plan going into the date.

Steps for This Activity

1. **Set Goals.** Draw your character using art supplies or a digital program. Then, think about the goals your character has set for the future. Illustrate two SMART goals your character can set related to balancing a new dating relationship with the effort of meeting future goals.
2. Show the characteristics your character would find attractive and want in a healthy dating relationship. These characteristics might include physical traits, but should also include personality traits and behaviors. Consider your character's preferences and values.
3. **Make Decisions.** Determine where your character will go on the date. Take into consideration how these dating partners met and how well they know each other. Also determine what personal boundaries or limitations your character will set. What will your character be comfortable with early on and then later in this dating relationship? How will your character end the date or relationship if it does not work out?
4. **Communicate with Others.** Make a plan for how your character will communicate personal boundaries and consent. If a situation is uncomfortable or unsafe, how will the character leave that situation? Will the character text a code word to a family member or friend, for example?
5. **Analyze Influences.** Illustrate the people and resources in your character's support network that can provide advice or help.
6. **Advocate for Health.** Your character might like to share information about this date with other characters. Once you have created your character and illustrated the components of the character's date, share your illustration with the class.

Chapter **15**

Violence Prevention and Response

Look for the skills icon ✓ throughout this chapter for opportunities to practice your health skills.

Check Your Health and Wellness Skills

In this chapter, you will learn skills for preventing and responding to violence. To understand the skills you currently use, take the following inventory of your behaviors. Indicate how well you think you use each skill. Use a scale of 1–5, *1* meaning you do not use the skill and *5* meaning you feel completely comfortable using it.

Skill	How Well Do You Use Each Skill?
If someone is intimidating or spreading rumors about me, I assertively tell the person to stop.	
I report any cyberbullying I see online.	
I focus on building my own self-esteem and strengths instead of putting down others.	
I know when affirmative consent has or has not been given.	
When people catcall or make sexist jokes, I tell them to stop.	
I know where I'd get help if I or a friend experienced sexual assault.	
I don't make excuses for violent behavior.	
I know how to report abuse so a person can get help.	
I don't try to change people who show abusive behavior.	
I follow all school rules and policies.	
If meeting someone I don't know well, I meet in a public place with other people.	
	Total:

Add up your responses to each statement. The higher your score, the more comfortable you feel preventing and responding to violence. Which skill do you think is most important for you? Which skill is the most challenging for you? Which skill would you most like to improve? In this chapter, you will learn how to perform these skills better and more often.

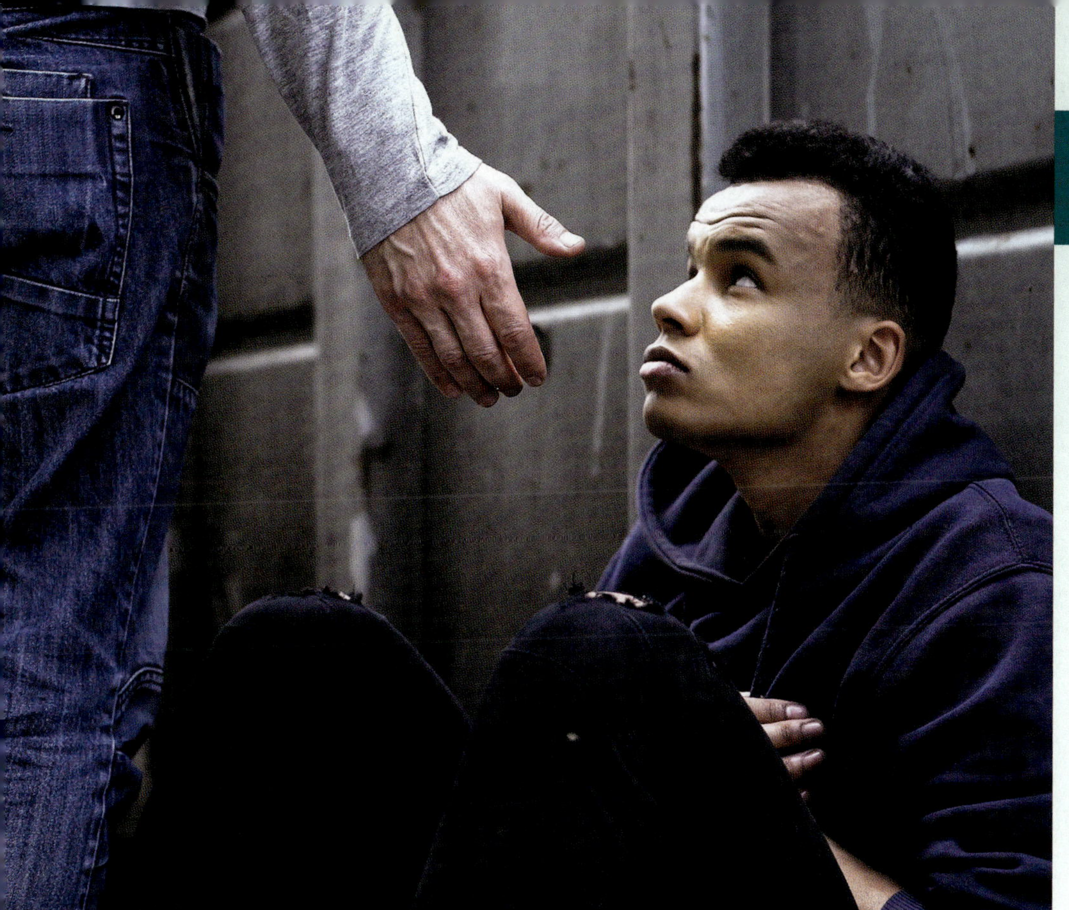

Motortion Films/Shutterstock.com

Reading and Notetaking

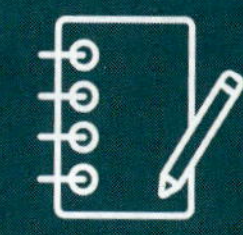

Write the Learning Outcomes for this chapter on a piece of paper. Then, beneath each outcome, rewrite it as a question. While reading the chapter, take detailed notes about information relating to these outcomes and use your questions to organize your notetaking. After reading, refer to your notes and write two or three sentences answering each outcome's question.

Outcome	Question	Answer

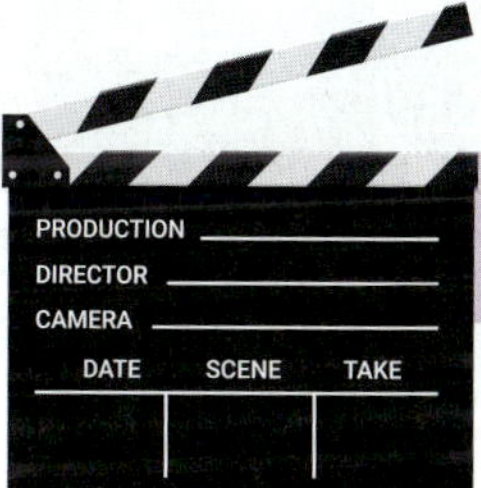

Setting the Scene

A Stressful Start to the Year

At the beginning of this year, you looked forward to starting a new year of high school and meeting new people in your extracurricular activities. A few months into the year, however, school causes you more stress than you imagined. Several people at school started making fun of your best friend since elementary school. They started by gossiping about your friend, but recently, they also took embarrassing videos of your friend and posted them online. Now, your friend checks social media to find dozens of insults and negative comments. These people even started a website centered around humiliating your friend and created fake social media accounts to impersonate your friend.

Ever since the cyberbullying started, your friend has been anxious, upset, and hesitant to hang out with you. You want to help your friend, but fear standing up to the people responsible will make the situation worse. You also fear getting involved would mean being cyberbullied yourself.

Thinking Critically

1. What factors do you think have allowed the cyberbullying of your friend to continue and escalate unchecked? What consequences could occur if someone does not intervene?
2. What would you do if your best friend was being cyberbullied? What actions, if any, should you counsel your friend to take? What options might help your friend get out of this situation?

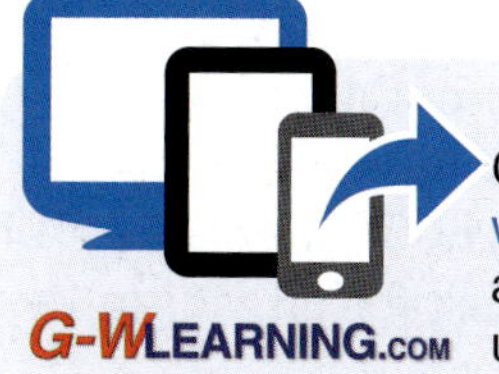

Click on the activity icon or visit www.g-wlearning.com/health/4095 to access online vocabulary activities using key terms from the chapter.

Lesson

15.1

Bullying and Cyberbullying

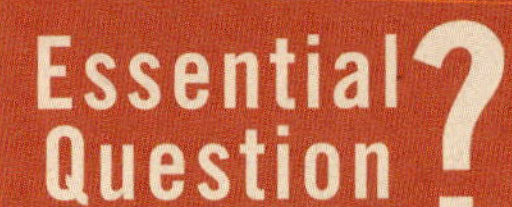

How can you stand up to bullying and cyberbullying?

Learning Outcomes

After studying this lesson, you will be able to

- define *violent behavior*;
- analyze the factors that contribute to violent behavior;
- explain how bullying affects the health of people and their community;
- describe ways to respond to bullying and be an upstander and ally;
- give examples of cyberbullying;
- list steps for responding to cyberbullying; and
- assess strategies for preventing bullying and cyberbullying.

Key Terms

bullying
bystander effect
bystanders
catfishing
cyberbullying
cyberstalking
gossip
harassment
hazing
impersonation
safe zones
stalking
upstander
violent behavior

Warm-Up Activity

Change the Conversation

Communicate with Others Think about your last few days and analyze the conversations or remarks you overheard or participated in. Also analyze the social media posts you saw or posted yourself. List five examples of remarks or posts you think might be considered bullying or cyberbullying. For each remark or post, how could you have spoken up or taken action to stop the bullying? Write a short script in which you change the conversation, challenge the remark, or respond to the social media post.

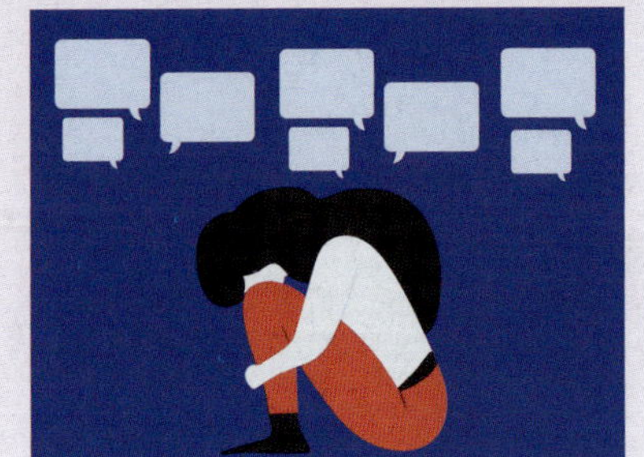

mmstudiodesign/Shutterstock.com

When you think of the word *violence*, you may not think of deliberately excluding someone or spreading rumors about a classmate. Both of these actions, however, are examples of violent behavior. **Violent behavior** is the intentional use of actions or words that cause or threaten to cause harm to someone or something. An example of violent behavior might be hitting someone, forcing someone to do something, or destroying someone's belongings. Although violent behavior often involves the use of physical force, it is not always physical. Violent behavior can also refer to behavior that results in *psychological injury*, or injury to a person's social, mental, or emotional health. There are many factors that can increase a person's risk for engaging in violent behavior (**Figure 15.1**).

violent behavior
intentional use of actions or words that cause or threaten to cause harm to a person or object

Risk Factors for Violent Behavior

Individual	Family	Peer and Social Interactions	Community
• Mental or emotional state, such as frustration or low self-esteem • Lack of control over behavior and anger • Desire for gain or retaliation • Exposure to violence, abuse, and conflict in-person, online, or in the media • Use of tobacco, alcohol, or drugs • Rejection of social values and institutions • Immaturity • *Prejudice* (unfair negative beliefs about a group of people) • Discrimination and bias • Stressful life events • Physical or mental health condition	• Overly strict, overly lenient, or inconsistent discipline at home • Violent behavior in the home • Poor supervision from adults • Low level of involvement from parents and guardians • Lack of attachment to parents and guardians • Use of tobacco, alcohol, or drugs in the family • Criminal activity in the family • Availability of weapons in the home	• Rejection by peers • Bullying • Violent behavior among peers • Peer pressure • Little interest or involvement in school activities • Participation in gangs • Poor academic performance	• Lack of economic opportunities • Poverty • Lack of community groups and social services • Lack of recreational opportunities • Violent behavior in the community • High crime and unemployment rates • Availability of weapons in the community • Lack of healthy families in the community • High rate of families leaving the community

Figure 15.1 Risk factors for violent behavior stem from the individual, family, peer and social interactions, and community.

Violent behavior among peers often happens in schools, but can last 24 hours a day due to the influence of technology. In this lesson, you will learn about the effects and ways of preventing and responding to bullying and cyberbullying.

Bullying

Bullying, also called *peer abuse*, is a type of aggressive behavior toward someone that causes the person injury or discomfort. Bullying involves a *power imbalance*, which means a person uses physical strength or social influence to control or harm others. Bullying is always the fault of the person bullying others. Usually, negative experiences, feelings, or insecurities motivate people to bully others. Regardless, there is never a good reason to bully others, even if a person acts or looks different from you.

bullying aggressive behavior toward someone that causes the person injury or discomfort; can be physical or psychological; also called *peer abuse*

Types of Bullying

Bullying can take many different forms, all of which have severe consequences on health (**Figure 15.2**). People commonly think of bullying as physical. For example, a person might hit, push, corner, or shove someone. Bullying can also be emotional and involve ridiculing or mocking a person, making fun of someone, or taking someone's belongings. Spreading **gossip**, or hurtful rumors that may or may not be true, is a form of social bullying. Social bullying also includes excluding someone from a group, sharing someone's secrets, or making someone feel isolated or rejected.

gossip hurtful rumors about a person that may or may not be true

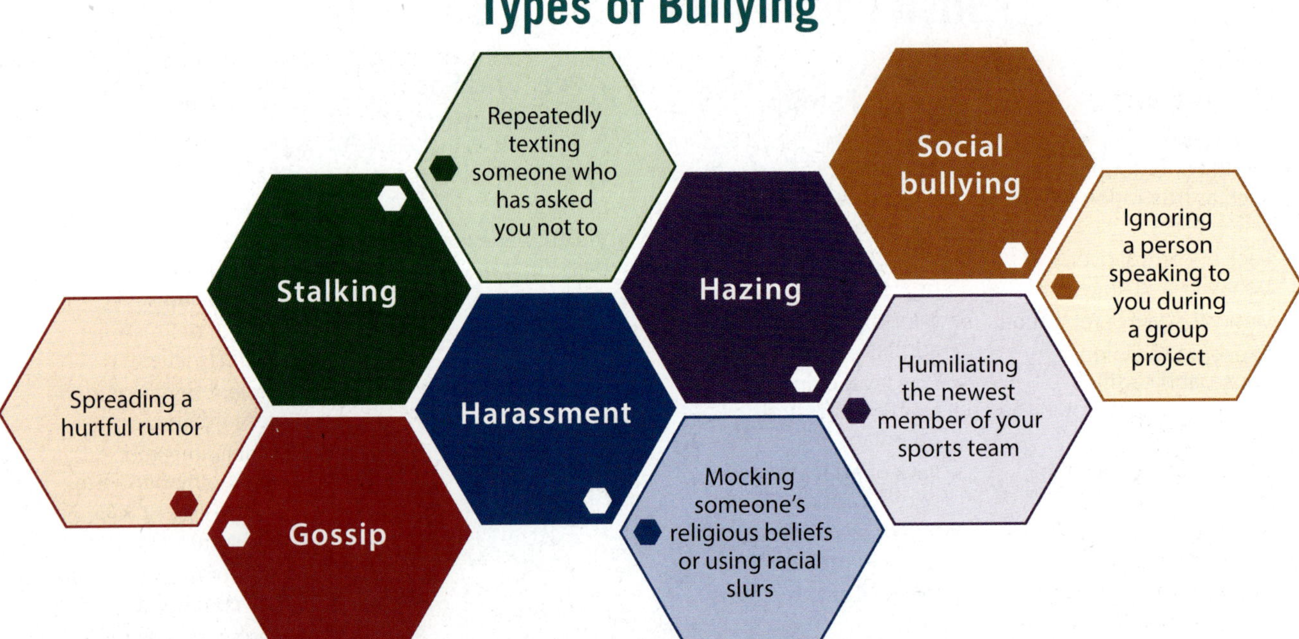

Figure 15.2 Bullying does not always involve physical violence and can take many different forms. ***Which type of bullying involves following someone and making the person feel threatened or nervous?***

harassment aggressive behavior that targets and hurts another person because of a particular part of the person's identity, such as race, religious beliefs, and sex

stalking following and repeatedly contacting someone in a way that causes the person to feel scared, nervous, or threatened

hazing type of bullying that uses group pressure to make someone do an embarrassing or dangerous activity to be accepted in a group

Other forms of bullying include harassment, stalking, and hazing. **Harassment** is aggressive behavior that targets and hurts another person because of a particular part of the person's identity. Harassment may target a person's race, religious beliefs, or sex, for example. It may also target a person's gender identity or sexual orientation. Harassment is a form of discrimination and is therefore illegal. Examples of harassment include using racial slurs or displaying symbols or words that communicate hatred toward a group of people. Excluding or making fun of someone because of the person's religious beliefs, sex, or sexual orientation is also harassment. You will learn more about sexual harassment, which targets a person's appearance, sex, or gender, later in this chapter.

Stalking is a type of bullying that involves following and repeatedly contacting someone. Stalking aims to control or intimidate someone and makes the person being stalked feel nervous, afraid, or threatened. For example, if a former dating partner shows up at places this person knows you visit after you say you do not want to talk, this is stalking. Stalking is a crime and can also occur online.

Hazing is a type of bullying that uses group pressure to make someone do an embarrassing or hazardous activity to be accepted in a group. Hazing can be dangerous, which is why most states have laws against it. Hazing includes forcing someone to do something risky, uncomfortable, or illegal to fit in. Humiliating a new member of a group and making someone endure physical violence to become part of a club are also examples of hazing.

Effects of Bullying

Bullying is dangerous and can have severe and lasting consequences. Physically, teens who are bullied can experience injury. They may also develop stress-related symptoms such as headaches, muscle pain, difficulty sleeping, and digestive conditions. Bullying can even lead to longer-term health conditions, such as reduced immunity to disease and increased risk of heart disease.

Bullying can harm a person's mental and emotional health (**Figure 15.3**). Teens who are bullied have a greater risk of becoming anxious and depressed. Some research shows that bullying can have lasting effects on mental and emotional health, even years later. One study found that children and teens who were bullied had higher rates of emotional distress and mental health conditions into their twenties.

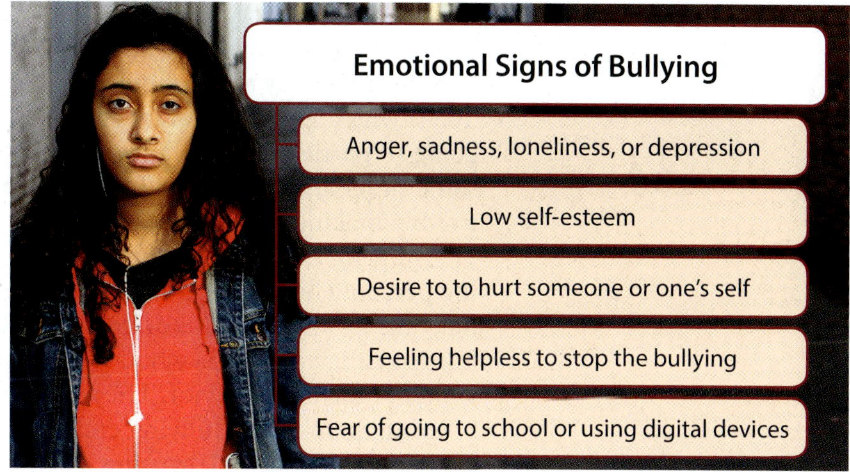

AJR_photo/Shutterstock.com

Figure 15.3 These characteristics may indicate a teen is experiencing bullying.

Research in Action

Do Violent Video Games Cause Violence?

Do you think playing violent video games increases the likelihood that a person will behave aggressively? Researchers have used video games to examine how exposure to violence in the media contributes to aggression.

In one study, researchers randomly assigned participants to play either a violent or nonviolent video game. After playing one of these games for 10 minutes, study participants performed a task with a partner. The task gave participants the ability to punish their partners by blasting their ears with loud levels of noise through headphones. Receiving these blasts was very unpleasant. The researchers wanted to know which group would give their partners louder blasts of noise—those who played the violent game or those who played the nonviolent game.

They found that people who played the violent game chose to send higher levels of noise to their partners than those who played the nonviolent game. Gender also played a role. Men who played the violent game blasted their partners with higher levels of noise more often than women who played the violent game.

In another study, researchers from Ohio State University examined whether playing violent video games increased the risk of gun violence. Children ages 8–12 played either a violent video game—involving a gun or sword—or a nonviolent video game. Afterward, children played in a room with toys and games, as well as a gun in an unlocked cabinet. Can you predict how playing the violent video game influenced children's behavior? Children who played the violent video game were more likely to touch the gun, spent more time holding the gun, and were more likely to point the gun at someone else. Even more seriously, these children were more likely to pull the trigger.

These studies show that exposure to violence in video games can cause people to behave more aggressively in their daily lives.

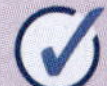

Practice Your Skills

Comprehend Concepts

With a partner, discuss the different factors that may link playing violent video games with engaging in violent behavior. Examine how environmental and social factors may also influence people who play violent video games to show more violent behavior. What strategies could help reduce the prevalence of violent video games? Are there any strategies that could reduce the effects of violent video games on aggression? What do you think families, schools, and communities can and should do to reduce the negative effect of violent video games? Do you think there should be new laws or regulations about violent video games? If so, what laws and regulations? If not, why not?

Socially and academically, teens who are bullied may change their behavior, worry about going to school, or have trouble concentrating. As a result, they may skip school, which can hurt their grades and test scores. Teens who are bullied might stop hanging out with friends after school or going to parties. They might even quit playing a sport or participating in some other activity to avoid the bullying. Some teens who are bullied have trouble making friends.

Bullying does not just hurt the person being bullied. It also hurts the person who bullies others and people who witness the bullying. By bullying, a person does not deal with the deeper issues that are motivating hurtful behavior. Teens who are not being bullied also do not like seeing violent, bullying behavior. They may worry that the person will start bullying them next. Bullying creates an environment in which stress and violence seem normal, causing harm to everyone involved.

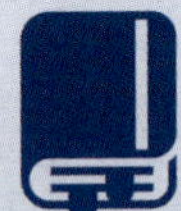

Case Study

Rumors: A Harmless Story?

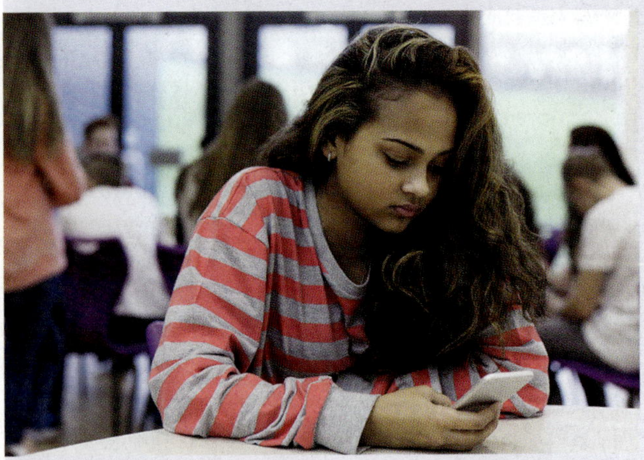

DGLimages/Shutterstock.com

At lunch, one of Jonathan's friends brought up something embarrassing he did earlier in the week, and Jonathan felt self-conscious all over again. He decided to distract them with a story about Gia, a girl in their class. Gia was at a party, he said, and got so drunk that an ambulance came to take her to the hospital. Jonathan knew his story was not true, but it worked as a distraction, and his friends stopped teasing him. Now, they were all talking about Gia. Jonathan did not think telling his friends this rumor was a big deal; after all, nobody gets hurt from a few words.

Gia felt humiliated by the rumors spreading around school about her. Between classes, Gia noticed the side glances and hushed laughter of her classmates when she walked by. Some teachers even pulled her aside after class to offer their assistance. Gia wanted to escape from everything at home, but comments followed her through social media where people posted jokes about her. Gia did not know why someone would be so cruel to start the rumor about her. She felt trapped. What if the rumors never stopped?

When Matias first heard Jonathan tell the story about Gia, he did not believe it was true. Matias felt bad for Gia, but did not want to call Jonathan a liar. At first, he hoped someone else would stick up for her or that the story would die out on its own. It had been a few weeks, though, and everyone was still talking about it. Matias decided that enough was enough and confronted Jonathan, who confessed he made up the whole story about Gia. Matias asked Jonathan to tell the truth on social media, where everyone could see it, and apologize to Gia.

Practice Your Skills

Practice Health-Enhancing Behaviors

Write an action plan outlining what you would do if a harmful rumor was spreading at your school. Identify how you would stop the rumor if you witnessed others spreading it. Also explain what you would do if the rumor were about you. Are there similarities or differences between the actions? How does this plan apply to physical violence, cyberbullying, or hazing? Add more details, if needed, to make your action plan applicable to all kinds of bullying.

Responding to Bullying

Bullying is never the fault of the person being bullied. You and others have a right to feel safe at school and in the community. You can use the following strategies to respond to and stop bullying behavior:

- **Know what bullying is and what causes it:** Pay attention to yourself and your behaviors to recognize if you are engaging in bullying behavior. Often, bullying arises from people's insecurities. Address your insecurities by building self-esteem and healthy relationships. Practice empathy for others and get help if you find yourself acting aggressively toward others.
- **Choose not to respond to anyone who bullies you:** People who bully others feel more powerful when people react to their meanness. Acting like you do not even notice or care can discourage bullying behavior. You can also leave the situation and go to a safe place if the bullying continues.
- **Be assertive:** People who bully others often pick on people who seem scared or weak. Sometimes, simply standing up to someone can get the person to stop the violent behavior. Tell the person to leave you alone calmly and assertively. Then, just walk away.
- **Avoid bullying back:** Even if you are angry, do not respond by hitting, yelling at, or gossiping about the person. This can encourage the person to continue the violent behavior. It can also get you in trouble.
- **Tell an adult if you or someone you know is being bullied:** Teachers, principals, school nurses, and other adults can help stop bullying. This helps keep you and other people safe.

When others are being bullied around you, you may feel tempted to ignore the behavior and not get involved. People who witness a violent event without intervening or getting help are called **bystanders**. Often, bystanders are waiting for someone else to intervene and end the violent behavior. Bystanders may think others besides themselves are responsible for speaking up. This perception of not having any responsibility to intervene is called the **bystander effect**.

When bystanders do not speak up, bullying can continue indefinitely. Instead of being a bystander, it is better to be an upstander (**Figure 15.4**). When you are an **upstander**, or *ally*, you recognize wrong or violent behavior and do something to stop the behavior, help the person being hurt, and promote positive change. Depending on the situation, an upstander might tell the person bullying others to stop or help the person being bullied get out and find help. An upstander might also alert an adult to the bullying.

bystanders people who are present at a situation, but do not participate or intervene

bystander effect situation in which a bystander is less likely to intervene and stop violent, harmful, or unsafe behavior because the person thinks someone else will

upstander person who recognizes when a behavior is wrong, takes steps to intervene and stop the behavior, and promotes positive change; also called an *ally*

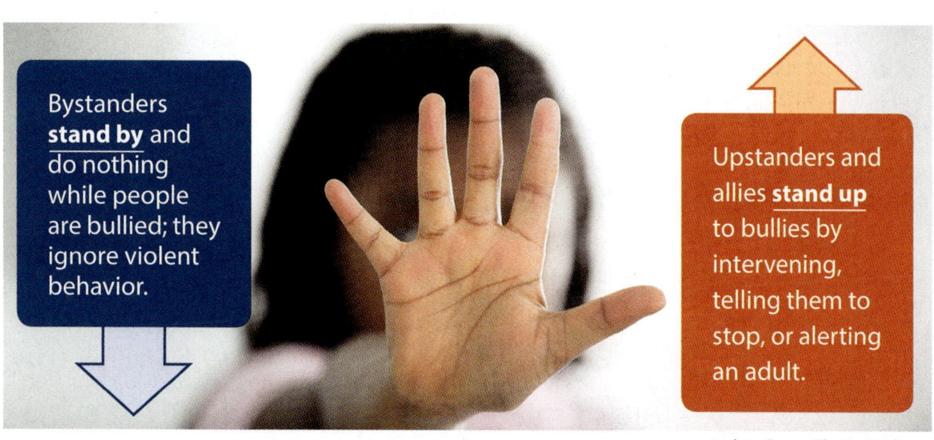

Andrey_Popov/Shutterstock.com

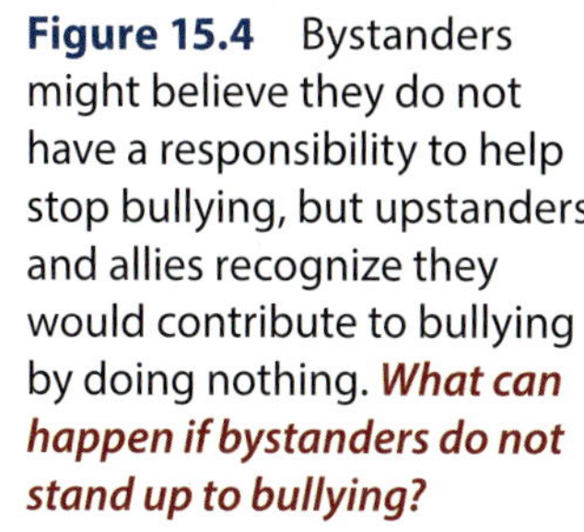

Figure 15.4 Bystanders might believe they do not have a responsibility to help stop bullying, but upstanders and allies recognize they would contribute to bullying by doing nothing. ***What can happen if bystanders do not stand up to bullying?***

Cyberbullying

cyberbullying use of the internet or electronic communication to mistreat or frighten someone

Cyberbullying is a form of bullying that uses electronic communication. In some ways, cyberbullying is similar to traditional bullying. Both cause emotional harm to the person being bullied. In other ways, cyberbullying is worse. Electronic communication can spread words, pictures, and other media far and quickly. Because people can hide behind screen names online, they can say words they would not say in-person.

Sometimes, cyberbullying happens unintentionally. Someone might post an embarrassing photo of a friend and not realize it was hurtful. Cyberbullying that happens repeatedly over time, however, is not accidental. Cyberbullying involves embarrassing, harassing, or threatening peers. It makes the person being cyberbullied feel nervous, intimidated, or humiliated.

Types of Cyberbullying

There are many different kinds of cyberbullying (**Figure 15.5**). Most cyberbullying is mental and emotional or social. Cyberbullying often involves mocking, criticizing, or embarrassing someone—through online messages, in group chats, or on global forums, for example. Socially, cyberbullying can include keeping people out of online groups, forming online groups centered around dislike of a person, or continuously ignoring someone. As it is in-person, harassment that occurs online is still an illegal form of discrimination.

cyberstalking following and repeatedly contacting someone using electronic communication or the internet; causes the person to feel scared, nervous, or threatened

One type of cyberbullying is **cyberstalking**, or stalking that occurs using electronic communication. Cyberstalking involves using the internet, email, texting, phone calls, or social media to hurt, scare, or control another person. A person continues to contact someone after being asked to stop and sends inappropriate, often disturbing content.

impersonation act of pretending to be another person online

catfishing luring someone into a relationship online by creating a fake profile

Another type of cyberbullying is **impersonation**, or pretending to be someone else online. Examples of impersonation include

- creating a fake profile pretending to be another person;
- stealing a person's password and using the account to share hurtful and offensive content;
- posing as another person in chat rooms;
- posting someone's personal information and encouraging others to contact the person; and
- **catfishing**, or pretending to be someone else to trick someone into a fake relationship.

Figure 15.5 Some of the boxes here are examples of cyberbullying, and some are not. ***Which examples shown are examples of cyberbullying? Why?***

A
You post a happy photo of your friends that one friend does not like.

B
Some of Jeff's classmates create a group chat named "Reasons We Hate Jeff."

C
You send a text to ask your crush on a date, and your crush says *no*.

D
Your friends make a fake social media account of you and use it to write mean comments on various posts.

E
Your sibling publicly comments on the selfies you post to say you look ugly.

F
On your video game chat, people gang up on you and tell others you are toxic.

Effects of Cyberbullying

Cyberbullying can have serious and lasting consequences. Many of the consequences of traditional bullying also apply to cyberbullying. The stress from cyberbullying can lead to physical symptoms such as headaches, little appetite, and digestive conditions. Mentally and emotionally, cyberbullying can cause anxiety and depression, loneliness, low self-esteem, and aggression. Cyberbullying can also cause people to withdraw from friends, social activities, and school. People who are cyberbullied may be anxious before, during, or after using digital devices. They may also avoid these devices.

The unique setting of cyberbullying makes it difficult to escape. Most teens spend a lot of time using their phones, computers, or tablets. This means cyberbullying can happen anywhere at anytime of day or night. Teens who are cyberbullied may feel unable to escape the cyberbullying even at home. Humiliating or insulting content posted online can spread.

Skills for Health and Wellness

Being an Upstander and Ally

Upstanders and allies play a crucial role in stopping violent behavior. It is far easier for upstanders to step up and stop bullying than for the person being bullied. Most high school students think bullying is a bad idea, but may not speak up to stop it. You can reduce bullying in your school by being an effective upstander and ally. Some ways you can intervene and stop the violent behavior include the following:

- **Disrupt the situation:** When you see someone being bullied, threatened, or harassed, interrupt in some way. Try distracting the person who is bullying others (say, "Hey, do we have homework due today in math?") or help the person being bullied escape the situation (say, "Let's get out of here. Want to go have lunch?").
- **Confront the person bullying others:** Tell the person bullying others to stop, using a direct, assertive, respectful, and clear voice. Point out that the violent behavior is not appropriate. Talking openly about violent behavior clearly conveys what is not acceptable.
- **Recruit allies:** There is power in numbers. Get support from people around you. The more people willing to stand up to the violent behavior, the better. Talk to friends around you and confront the person bullying others together. This reinforces the idea that bullying is not okay with most students at your school.
- **Support the person being bullied:** Make sure the person being bullied knows the violent behavior is the fault of the person who was bullying. Lend the person being bullied social support and assist the person in getting help, if needed. Many schools and communities have resources and counselors to help put an end to bullying.

Practice Your Skills

Communicate with Others

Partner with two of your classmates to form a group of three. In your group, role-play the four situations that follow. In each situation, a person should play the person bullying others, the person being bullied, and the upstander or ally. Rotate roles so each person has the opportunity to play each role.

1. Walking down a hall in your school, you see one student push another student up against a locker.
2. In the cafeteria, you hear someone say, "No, you can't sit here. We don't eat lunch with losers."
3. You hear one student making fun of another student's body in the locker room at school.
4. Someone is spreading hurtful rumors about your friend online.

After role-playing all four situations, consider which responses were most effective at ending the violent behavior. Keeping these responses in mind will help you stand up to bullying if you are ever in these situations.

As a result, teens who are cyberbullied may feel powerless and angry and think about retaliating. Teens who are cyberbullied may also think about hurting themselves or even have suicidal thoughts.

Responding to Cyberbullying

Sometimes, teens who experience cyberbullying do not want to tell anyone. They may feel embarrassed about the messages, videos, or photos others have shared about them. They may also worry that their parents, guardians, or other adults will take away their phones, tablets, or computers. In all cases of cyberbullying, it is important to remember that cyberbullying is the fault of the person behaving aggressively. Cyberbullying is never the fault of the person being bullied.

If you are being cyberbullied, you can take several steps to protect yourself and discourage the bullying:

1. Block the person's ability to contact you. Do not respond to the person's messages, videos, or photos in any way. Responding will reinforce the person's behavior.
2. Save or screenshot the person's messages, videos, or photos. Also screenshot any hurtful content posted online. This evidence can help prove you are being cyberbullied, even if the person deletes or takes down the content.
3. Report the cyberbullying behavior. Communicate with a trusted adult about the cyberbullying. The adult can intervene and help stop this behavior. Sometimes, the adult may involve law enforcement or your school. You can also report cyberbullying behavior by flagging content as inappropriate on social media or contacting your internet service provider (**Figure 15.6**).

What content should you report on social media?

- Photos or videos that do not belong to the poster
- Photos or videos that contain nudity
- Posts that support crime, such as terrorism, gang activity, or activity related to illegal drugs
- Posts that contain threats or hate speech
- Posts or accounts that target private individuals to insult or shame them
- Personal information meant to blackmail or harass someone
- Images of graphic violence

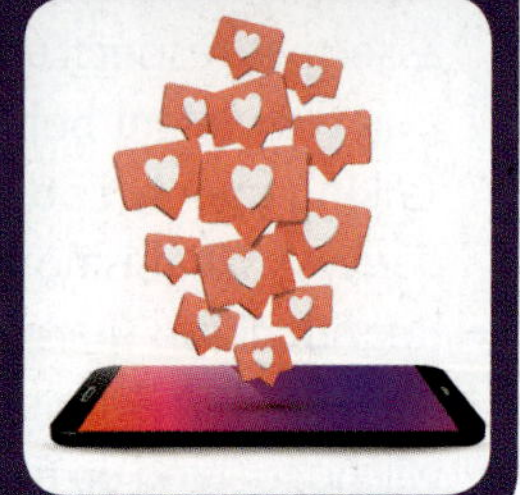

olegback/iStock/Getty Images Plus/Getty Images

Figure 15.6 Many social media platforms are increasing automatic flagging for inappropriate content, but individual users can help by reporting hateful or illegal posts or accounts.

If you see someone being cyberbullied, do not participate. Instead, be an upstander and ally and ask how you can help the person being bullied. Remember that many school districts have rules about cyberbullying. Students who engage in this behavior can be suspended or kicked off sports teams or other activities. Certain types of cyberbullying are even against the law, especially if the cyberbullying results in self-harm.

Ways to Prevent Bullying and Cyberbullying

Bullying and cyberbullying are serious issues in many schools. Schools often have programs for preventing bullying and cyberbullying. Participating in these programs can help you learn about aggressive behavior and ways to respond. You can also take action on your own to prevent bullying and cyberbullying among your peers.

Build Your Self-Esteem

People who bully others sometimes target people who seem weak or insecure. You can help reduce the risk of being bullied by developing your own self-confidence (**Figure 15.7**). Being confident in yourself can keep away people who bully others and help you stand up if you see others being bullied.

Avoid Bullying Behavior

Understand the signs of bullying, such as using words or actions to hurt other people. If you notice yourself being mean to other people, stop and think. If you feel like hurting someone else, find another activity you can do to vent your feelings. For example, you could watch silly videos, talk to a friend, or go for a run. If you recognize you are bullying someone, stop and think about why. Talk to a trusted adult about your feelings and make a plan to deal with them. If you recognize you have bullied someone in the past, apologize to that person.

Developing Self-Confidence

Participate in activities you enjoy or seek out new hobbies.
Appreciate your successes and talents and view mistakes as learning opportunities.
Build healthy relationships and address or leave unhealthy relationships.

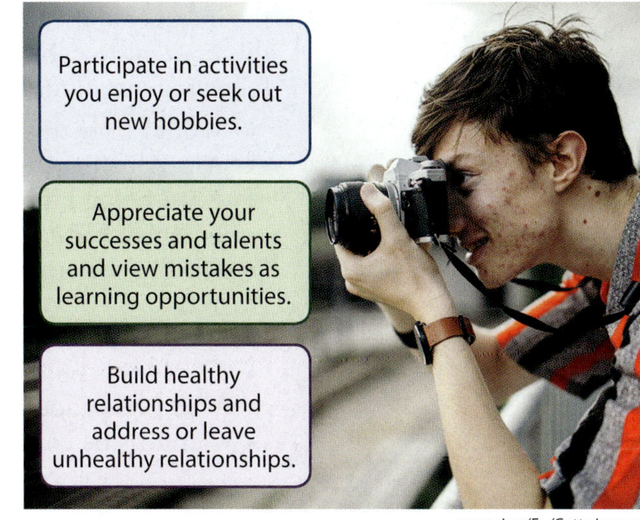

supersizer/E+/Getty Images

Figure 15.7 Building your self-confidence can help you stand up to bullying and avoid being bullied yourself. ***What are some other ways to build self-confidence and decrease your risk of bullying?***

Celebrate Differences

Bullying and harassment often target people because of their differences. To prevent this behavior, recognize that people differ in their backgrounds, interests, and experiences. Appreciating differences and diversity can create a positive environment and help people feel better about themselves.

Some schools have created **safe zones**, where students know they can feel safe and supported, no matter what. A safe zone can be a specific space, such as an office or classroom, or a particular person (for example, a "safe adult"). Students can go to a safe zone to eat lunch, study, or spend time with friends. If your school has not set up a safe zone program, you could take steps to start one.

safe zones spaces where students can go to feel safe and supported, no matter what

Invest in Positive Relationships

Building relationships with people who share your values and beliefs and treat all students with respect can help prevent bullying. Develop friendships with people who like you for who you are. Treat others how you would want someone to treat you or your best friend.

As you build a positive support system, avoid people who bully others. If someone who bullies others is nearby, sit in a different part of the cafeteria or hang out in a different place after school. Using the buddy system might also prevent someone from acting aggressively.

Be Safe Online

To help prevent cyberbullying, never share your passwords with anyone. Sharing passwords increases the risk that someone will be able to impersonate you online and post harmful content. Change your password often to keep it secure.

When using electronic communication, do not share or post anything you would not want shared with others. Content can spread rapidly on the internet and end up in other people's hands. Sometimes, people use this content to cyberbully others. Before posting, you can ask yourself the following questions:

- Would I say this to this person's face?
- Am I posting this to try to get attention or to make people like me?
- Am I being kind? How would this make the person involved feel?
- Is it private? Is it *actually* private? Will it stay private?
- Do I have permission to share this?
- Will this embarrass or humiliate the person involved?
- Will it ruin the reputation of the person involved?
- Could this be interpreted in a way other than how I intend?
- Will I feel good about posting this later?
- Can this be considered hate speech or threats of violence?

Communicate with Trusted Adults

Communicating regularly with a trusted adult can help protect you from bullying behavior. If you tell an adult about your relationships at school and online, that adult can help you with difficult situations. The adult can also advocate for you if bullying does occur. A trusted adult can help address the situation before it gets worse.

Lesson 15.1 Review

Know and Understand

1. With a partner, answer the following question: Can saying something that makes someone scared, anxious, or upset be an example of violent behavior?
2. What usually motivates bullying behavior?
3. Give two examples of social bullying behavior and explain how they cause harm.
4. How is harassment different from bullying?
5. With a partner, list as many examples of cyberstalking as you can. Then explain how cyberstalking hurts others.
6. If someone is being cyberbullied, what steps can the person take to stop the behavior?

Think Critically

7. Choose one risk factor for violent behavior and explain why it increases the likelihood of violence.
8. Think of a situation in which you witnessed the bystander effect. In a small group, discuss the situation and list ways you or someone else could have been an upstander or ally.

REAL WORLD Health Skills

Access Information Using reliable and valid resources, research existing and potential safe zones at your school and within your community. These should be spaces where violence, harassment, and hate are not tolerated. They can also be places teens can get help. Be sure to explain the reasons you consider each place safe. Using the information you found, create a one-page infographic sharing information about these safe zones. Be sure to cite your sources with your infographic.

Sexual Harassment and Assault

Essential Question?

What steps can you take to create a culture free from sexual harassment and assault?

Lesson 15.2

Learning Outcomes

After studying this lesson, you will be able to

- explain the meaning of affirmative consent;
- describe types of sexual harassment;
- summarize ways to respond to sexual harassment;
- recognize types of sexual assault; and
- identify ways to prevent and respond to sexual assault.

Key Terms

age of consent
rape
sexual assault
sexual harassment
sexual violence
statutory rape

Warm-Up Activity

What Is Affirmative Consent?

Comprehend Concepts How do you know if someone is giving consent? Saying *yes* in a strong, clear manner is an obvious, verbal example of consent, just as saying *no* shows an obvious lack of consent. Working with a partner, brainstorm other examples of consent and lack of consent. List your examples in the appropriate columns of a chart like the one shown. Be sure to include examples that use verbal, nonverbal, and online communication.

Ways to Consent	Ways to Not Consent
Saying *yes*	Saying *no*

How would you feel if, every day in math class, one of your classmates asked you to go on a date? Maybe you have said *no* repeatedly and hoped the first few times that your classmate would take the hint. Still, your classmate continues to corner you and ask you—again and again—in front of the entire class. How would you feel if someone you hardly know messaged you on social media, asking for a nude picture even after you refused to send one? How would you feel if a classmate called you every other night and made you uncomfortable by describing sexual acts? Think about what all of these situations have in common. How are these situations different from deciding with a romantic partner to hold hands in public or kiss?

The first three situations are examples of sexual harassment, or repeated unwanted sexual attention. This is different from deciding together to hold hands or kiss because the attention is *unwanted*. The key to separating sexual harassment and violence from normal romantic behavior is *consent*.

What Is Consent?

What do you think of when you hear the word *consent*? Maybe you think of the way characters in movies kiss after coming home drunk or keep asking each other on a date until one partner gives in. In reality, neither of these situations is an example of consent in a healthy relationship. *Affirmative consent* is a direct, verbal, freely given agreement that occurs when someone clearly says *yes* (**Figure 15.8**).

Consent is direct. This means it clearly communicates agreement and does not show hesitation. An example of consent is saying "Yes, I want to do that" or "That sounds nice" while making eye contact and smiling. Consent is verbal. This means it uses words, not just body language. Consent does *not* occur if someone says *no* or nothing at all. People cannot assume a person agrees to a behavior unless the person specifically, verbally expresses a willingness to do so. Giving consent in one activity or relationship does not mean a person gives consent in any other activity or relationship.

Consent is freely given. This means consent does *not* occur if a person feels pressured or coerced into saying *yes*. It also means consent can be changed at any time. A person can agree to an activity and then withdraw consent by saying *no*.

Some people are not legally capable of giving consent to sexual activity. Only people who are *informed*, or who fully understand what they are agreeing to do, can give consent. People cannot consent to engage in sexual activity if they

- feel pressured or coerced;
- are under the influence of drugs or alcohol;
- have certain disabilities or disorders, such as a cognitive disability;
- are asleep or unconscious; or
- are younger than the **age of consent**—16, 17, or 18 years of age, depending on the state.

age of consent age at which a person can legally agree to engage in sexual activity

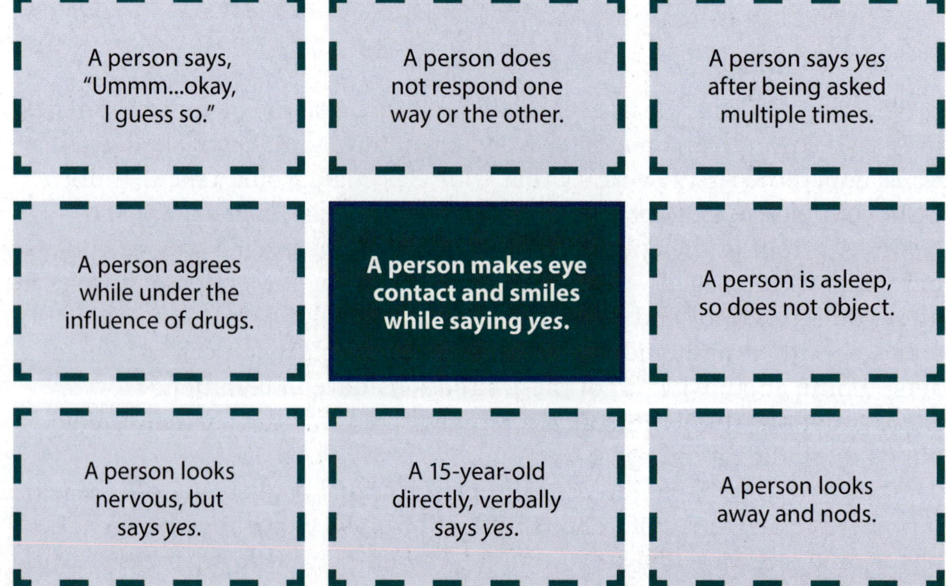

Figure 15.8 Scenarios without a direct, verbal, freely given agreement from someone older than the age of consent are *not* consent. ***Which rectangles include scenarios of affirmative consent?***

Some people believe harmful myths about consent (**Figure 15.9**). They believe that if two people are in a romantic relationship, any kind of sexual activity must be consensual. This is false. No one, not even a long-term romantic partner, has the right to pressure or coerce someone to engage in sexual activity. If sexual activity occurs without consent, the person who committed the sexual assault is entirely to blame. The person who endured the violence is *never* to blame. Without *mutual consent*, or consent by both people, sexual attention is sexual harassment, and sexual activity is sexual assault.

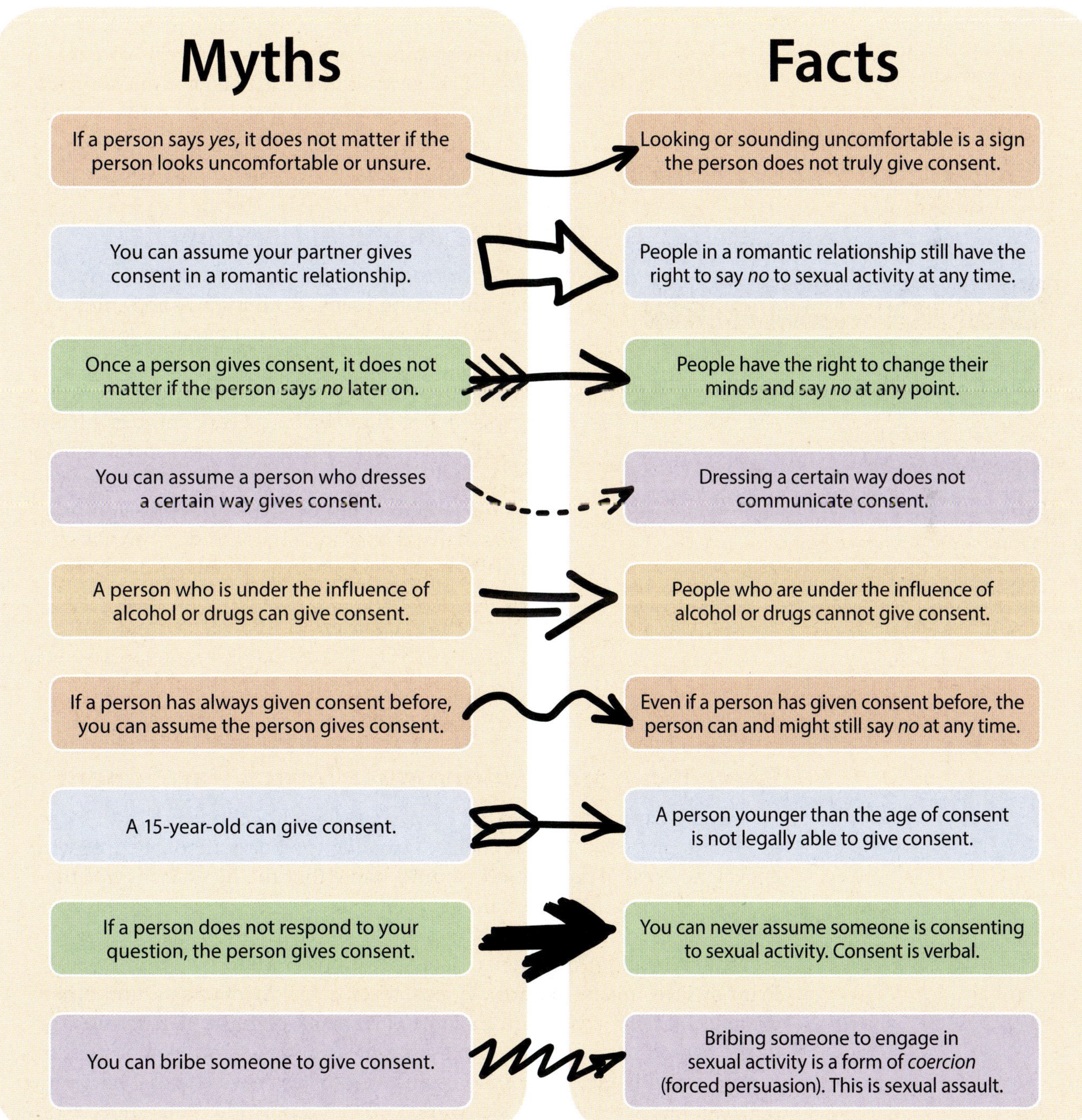

Feuerbach/Shutterstock.com

Figure 15.9 Consent must be given each time and can never be assumed or coerced. ***What is the age of consent in your state?***

Sexual Harassment

sexual harassment
verbal or nonverbal sexual attention that occurs without consent

Sexual harassment is sexual attention that occurs without consent (**Figure 15.10**). When you ask a person on a date, you may not be sure if the person will say *yes*. This is not sexual harassment. Badgering the person to say *yes* after the person has said *no* is sexual harassment. Complimenting a classmate's appearance is not necessarily sexual harassment, but giving an explicit compliment that makes the person uncomfortable is. Sexual harassment does not have to be directed at one person. It can also include sexual comments just spoken in the presence of a person uncomfortable with the comments.

Sometimes, it may be unclear whether someone's behavior counts as sexual harassment. If you are unsure, ask yourself how the behavior makes you feel and whether you want the behavior to stop. If the behavior makes you feel bad and you want the person to stop, you are experiencing sexual harassment.

Verbal Sexual Harassment

- Making sexual statements, questions, or threats
- Spreading sexual rumors or gossip
- Making inappropriate or intimidating comments, including catcalling
- Sharing sexual comments that make people uncomfortable
- Making sexist or sexual jokes
- Making sexual comments about a person's body
- Repeatedly asking a person on a date after the person has said *no*

Nonverbal Sexual Harassment

- Making sexual gestures
- Pinching, rubbing, or brushing up against someone in an inappropriate way
- Staring at a person's body
- Exposing a person's body (for example, pantsing)
- Sharing sexual ideas or images
- Making sexual sounds such as catcalling whistles or kissing noises

Figure 15.10 Sexual harassment can be verbal or nonverbal.

Effects of Sexual Harassment

Unfortunately, sexual harassment is fairly common among teens. Both males and females can commit and experience sexual harassment.

Sexual harassment can be devastating. Teens who experience sexual harassment can become depressed and anxious, lose sleep, withdraw from normal activities, and hate going to school. Changes in behavior, such as avoiding usual activities and missing school, could be signs of depression or anxiety caused by sexual harassment. Sexual harassment can also increase the risk of serious long-term consequences, including drug and alcohol abuse, eating disorders, and post-traumatic stress disorder (PTSD). Sexual harassment can also lead to a stressful environment, in which students fear they will be harassed.

Preventing and Responding to Sexual Harassment

People experiencing sexual harassment often feel powerless to stop it. Others may even accuse them of causing the harassment. People who experience sexual harassment should know that the behavior is not their fault. No one deserves to be sexually harassed.

If you are being sexually harassed, document your experiences by recording details of the events, dates, locations, and possible witnesses. Print or save emails, pictures, videos, texts, social media posts, and other evidence of the harassment. In some cases, you might try talking directly to the person harassing you and asking the person to stop. Sometimes, this can be intimidating. Most schools and workplaces have a sexual harassment policy. If harassment occurs at work, you can report it to your supervisor or someone in human resources. At school, you can speak with your teachers, counselors, or principal to ask for help. If you are ever sexually harassed and are not sure what to do, reach out to a trusted adult or community resource.

If you observe someone being sexually harassed, you can take steps to be an upstander or ally and help. Speak up and tell the person to stop (**Figure 15.11**). Saying nothing tells the person harassing others—and people witnessing the situation—that you do not have a problem with the person's behavior. Do not reinforce the person's behavior by laughing or nodding. Upstanders and allies play an important role in stopping sexual harassment. It is often easier for those not directly targeted to confront the bad behavior.

If you feel unsafe or uncomfortable getting involved, tell a teacher, school counselor, or principal. Remember that harassment is wrong, painful, and criminal. Notifying someone who can stop it is the right thing to do. Reporting behavior is not snitching or tattling. It is standing up for what is right.

Standing Up to Sexual Harassment

"Don't whistle at me, don't you know that's sexual harassment?"

"Please stop touching me."

"Stop harassing people. I don't like it. No one likes it."

"It makes me feel uncomfortable when you do that."

"You're standing too close to me. Take two steps back."

"I can't believe you said that, that's so gross."

Left to right: yongyuan/E+/Getty Images; jacoblund/iStock/Getty Images Plus/Getty Images

Figure 15.11 Standing up to sexual harassment sets the standard that this behavior is not okay. Saying nothing communicates that you do not have a problem with the behavior.

In addition to being an upstander, you can create greater awareness of what sexual harassment is. Some people who catcall or make sexist jokes may not understand that what they are doing is offensive and can negatively affect others. Another strategy is to encourage all people in a community to maintain a safe and respectful environment. This shared accountability for creating a safe environment can go a long way toward reducing harassment.

Sexual Assault

Threatening or forcing someone into sexual activity is **sexual assault**. Sexual assault is a type of **sexual violence**, or sexual behaviors that occur without consent. Other examples of sexual violence are intimate partner violence, sexual abuse, and stalking. Sexual assault is illegal and occurs whenever there is sexual activity without consent. Examples of sexual assault include the following nonconsensual situations:

- **rape**, or nonconsensual sexual intercourse
- attempted rape, even if penetration does not occur
- kissing without consent
- unwanted sexual touching, including the touching or fondling of body parts through a person's clothing
- *flashing*, or exposing one's genitals to another person
- photographing a person who is nude
- exposing someone to pornography

sexual assault act of threatening, pressuring, or forcing someone into sexual activity

sexual violence sexual behaviors that occur without consent

rape sexual intercourse that occurs without consent

Sexual assault includes sexual activity between children or teens and family members (called *incest*) and nonconsensual sexual activity between romantic partners. It also includes rape by a stranger, *date rape* (rape by someone on a date), and *acquaintance rape* (rape by someone the person knows). The crime of **statutory rape** occurs when anyone under the age of consent (including teens) engages in sex. A person can be charged with statutory rape even if the child or teen consents to having sex. This is because the child or teen has not developed the maturity and decision-making abilities to fully consent to sexual activity.

statutory rape sexual intercourse between an adult and anyone under the age of consent

Consequences of Sexual Assault

Physical Health

- Bruises, burns, and broken bones
- Pelvic pain
- Digestive disorders
- Migraines and other frequent headaches
- Back pain
- Unwanted pregnancy
- Sexually transmitted infections (STIs)

Mental and Emotional Health

- Shock or denial
- Fear and anxiety
- Shame or guilt
- Confusion
- Post-traumatic stress disorder (PTSD)
- Depression

Social Health

- Hesitation to trust other people
- Conflict in intimate relationships
- Alienation from friends and family members

Figure 15.12 Sexual assault can impact people's physical, mental and emotional, and social health both short-term and long-term.

Although sexual assault involves violence of a sexual nature, experts say that it is not an act of sex, but an act of power and aggression. People who commit sexual assault may use force, violence, weapons, or alcohol and drugs to make people submit. More males than females carry out sexual assault, and more females than males experience sexual assault. Both males and females, however, can commit sexual assault or be sexually assaulted.

Effects of Sexual Assault

Sexual assault can impact people's health and well-being in lasting and destructive ways (**Figure 15.12**). Sexual assault can also have lasting and harmful effects on a person's family, friends, and community.

Sometimes people scold those who have experienced sexual assault for dressing a certain way or having too much to drink. People who experience sexual assault are never to blame. If they blame themselves or receive blame from others, they may feel shame and guilt, their self-esteem can suffer, and they may withdraw from friends and family. Many people who experience sexual assault fear being blamed, so they do not report the crime to law enforcement, friends, or family members.

Preventing Sexual Assault

Sexual assault causes severe harm to a person's physical, mental and emotional, and social well-being. It also hurts relationships and negatively affects the health of a community. Many high schools and colleges have programs that educate students about consent and sexual assault. These programs also help teach students about the importance of stepping in if they believe an assault might occur (**Figure 15.13**). If your school does not offer one of these programs, you could work to bring one to your school. Talk to your health teacher or other teachers about what steps you could take to make this happen.

There are also steps you can take on an individual level to help prevent sexual assault. Knowing how to prevent and respond to sexual assault can help protect the health and safety of yourself and others.

Understand Consent

The best way to prevent sexual assault is to understand consent and treat others with respect. In your relationships, express consent clearly by stating *yes* or *no* and matching your nonverbal communication to your message. Encourage people around you to also treat others with respect. If you witness or hear people talking about sexual activity without consent, be an upstander and ally and speak up. By intervening, you can help create a culture that respects people and their consent.

Remember that other people get to decide what types of physical contact they feel comfortable having. Actively listen to others to understand if they are clearly giving consent. If you care about someone, you will respect these boundaries.

Sexual Assault Prevention Programs	
Program	**Description**
Green Dot	This program focuses on teaching students how to identify potentially harmful situations and take direct action to prevent harm. The Green Dot program focuses on three intervention strategies: • Create a distraction, such as interrupting the people involved in a potentially harmful situation. • Ask someone else to intervene, such as another friend. • Step up and directly confront the people involved. High schools that have implemented Green Dot training show a 50 percent reduction in rates of sexual violence.
One Love	This program aims to teach people about the signs of healthy and unhealthy relationships. Knowing these signs empowers people to avoid abuse and build relationships that are healthy.
Safe Dates	Safe Dates is a program designed to prevent emotional, physical, and sexual abuse in high school dating relationships. The goals of this program are to • change norms about violence between romantic partners; • improve skills for resolving conflicts; • promote awareness of the importance of getting help if violence occurs; and • decrease rates of violence in dating relationships. Teens who participate in this program report fewer incidents of physical and sexual violence in dating relationships.
Shifting Boundaries	This program focuses on the consequences of violence and harassment, impact of gender roles, and importance of having healthy relationships. Students are taught to identify inappropriate behaviors and report these behaviors to teachers, guidance counselors, or principals.

Figure 15.13 Participation in sexual assault prevention programs has been shown to reduce rates of sexual violence, including sexual assault. ***Does your school have a program designed to create awareness about sexual assault?***

Be sure to respect people's personal space and accept that a person's *no* means *no*. If someone asks you to stop saying or doing something, stop immediately. Ask permission before touching someone else and understand that the absence of a *no* is not the same as a *yes*.

If you think about engaging in sexual activity without consent, or consider any type of violent behavior, talk to an adult you trust. This may be a sign that you need help managing your thoughts, feelings, or past experiences to avoid hurting yourself or someone else.

Avoid Risky Situations

Avoiding situations with an increased risk of sexual assault is another method of prevention. One example of a risky situation is a party or location with drugs or alcohol. Using alcohol and drugs impairs a person's ability to sense danger, resist sexual activity, and make good decisions. Under the influence of alcohol or drugs, a person might be more likely to assume consent or engage in sexual activity without consent. A person under the influence of drugs or alcohol might not be able to effectively refuse the sexual activity or get away. If you see someone in this risky situation, help this person leave safely.

Another risky situation is being alone with someone in an unfamiliar place or without adult supervision, whether you know the person or not. In group settings, stay among friends who can watch out for you. Never go alone to unfamiliar, isolated places with people you do not know very well (for example, a dating partner you met online). If a situation makes you nervous or uncomfortable or if anyone pressures you to do something you do not want to do, leave the situation. After leaving, call a friend, parent or guardian, or other trusted adult immediately.

Some other guidelines for avoiding risky situations are outlined in **Figure 15.14**. Remember that the person who commits the sexual assault is always to blame. The person who is sexually assaulted is *never* to blame, no matter the situation.

Responding to Sexual Assault

If people experience or are threatened with sexual assault, they can try to fight back. Fighting and struggling may give them time to get help by stalling the person committing the assault. Making it physically difficult for the person committing the assault may increase the likelihood that the person will give up. People might also be able to scare away the attacker by yelling "Fire!" and making a lot of noise. People react differently to sexual assault. Sometimes, a person may freeze during a sexual assault and may not feel able to fight back. Other times, a person's body will react in certain ways that resemble sexual arousal. These are normal responses that aim to reduce injury from the sexual assault. No matter how a person reacts to a sexual assault, the person committing the assault is always to blame.

Get Treatment

In the event of a sexual assault, a person should immediately get to a safe place and call 911 or the National Sexual Assault Hotline (800-656-4673) for help. It is important to get medical attention right away at a hospital or clinic. The person will receive an examination, treatment for physical injuries, and tests for STIs. Certain medications can decrease the person's chances of developing an STI or becoming pregnant.

Sexual assault is a crime—even if the person who was assaulted knows the person who committed the assault—and should be reported to law enforcement. Police officers can only arrest the person who committed the assault if they know what occurred, including the time, location, and people involved, and can collect evidence. As a result, a person who experiences sexual assault should not change clothes or shower before going to the police station or hospital. Professionals can gather evidence from clothes and hair.

Avoiding Dangerous Situations

Be aware of your surroundings and avoid walking alone, especially at night.	If you must walk alone at night, stay in well-lit areas and avoid alleys and bushes where someone might hide.	If you are walking alone, have your keys out before you get to your car. Examine the inside of your car *before* you get in. Lock your doors immediately after you get inside.
Never accept a ride from or give a ride to a stranger, no matter how nice that person may appear.	Do not leave a drink unattended or accept a drink from someone you do not know or trust.	The first few times you hang out with someone, make sure you are with friends or in a public place.
Let adults know where you will be and with whom. Do not go to unsupervised parties or leave a party with someone you do not know well.	If someone is following you or attacks you, yell *stop* or *stay back* to attract attention from other people.	If riding in a taxi or rideshare, message or video-call a friend or trusted adult regularly and let that person know when you get to your destination.

Figure 15.14 Certain dangerous situations can increase your risk of experiencing sexual assault, but simple precautions can help you avoid this risk. ***Who is to blame for a sexual assault?***

Health in the Media

The Hazards of Rape Culture

The term *rape culture* describes an environment in which the media and pop culture make sexual violence against women seem normal. While sexual violence against men does occur, it is not normalized in the same way as sexual violence against women. Sometimes, depictions of sexual violence and sexual harassment against women are subtle. For example, songs may use language that is *derogatory* (disrespectful) toward women, or magazines may emphasize women's bodies or body parts. Movies and shows may portray nonconsensual kissing or sexual activity.

Rape culture can influence people to minimize the seriousness and effects of sexual violence. As a result of rape culture, people may

- blame people who have experienced sexual violence by saying, "She asked for it by dressing like that";
- make excuses for violent behavior like "Boys will be boys";
- dismiss some types of sexual violence or sexual harassment because they are not "as bad as rape";
- joke about sexual violence;
- assume reports of rape are false; and
- discuss the consequences for those who commit sexual assault more than the health effects for those who have experienced sexual assault.

Rape culture exists around the world, although specific views differ from country to country. The following are some strategies you can use to help stop the spread of rape culture:

- Reflect on the effects of rape culture and your reactions to sexual violence.
- Avoid using language that degrades women or treats them as sexual objects.
- Do not tell or laugh at jokes about rape or sexual violence.
- Speak up if you hear someone else using sexist or degrading language.
- If people tell you they have experienced sexual violence, take them seriously. Never blame people who have been assaulted or imply they were somehow responsible.
- Respect people's personal space.
- Be aware of the importance of consent in your own relationships.

Practice Your Skills

Advocate for Health

In a small group, list all of the different examples of rape culture you see or hear in the media. Include examples in music, books, news stories, social media, movies, magazines, and shows. How do these examples normalize sexual violence? What are the consequences of normalizing sexual violence? Now, think about steps you could take to reduce the prevalence of rape culture in your community. What strategies could you use to create awareness of this problem? What approaches could you take to change how sexual violence is portrayed and discussed—locally, nationally, and globally? Develop some specific steps you could take to reduce rape culture in your community. For example, write to a local government representative, talk to students at your high school, or join an organization that works to combat rape culture. As a group, choose three specific steps and put them into action.

Many people who have been sexually assaulted find it helpful to talk to specially trained mental health professionals. Therapists can create a safe place for people to express feelings about the assault and teach skills for coping with difficult emotions. Therapists can also provide strategies for developing happy and heathy relationships in the future. Research shows that people who seek help more quickly following an assault recover faster. Survivors of sexual assault may also find support by talking with others who have been through this type of trauma. A school nurse, doctor, or local rape crisis center can provide information about therapists and local support groups. People might also find it useful to talk to other adults they trust, such as parents or guardians, doctors, community leaders, and school counselors.

I'm glad you're alive.
It's not your fault. You didn't deserve this.
I believe you. I'm sorry this happened.
You did the best you could.
You're not alone. I'm here if you need to talk.

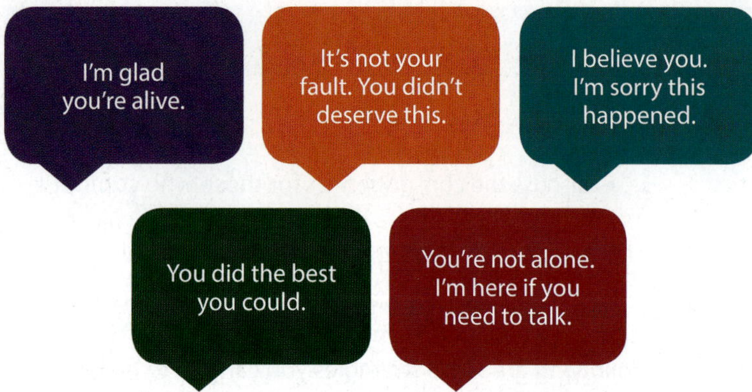

Figure 15.15 If you do not know what to say to help a survivor of sexual assault, these examples show how to incorporate active listening, empathy, trust, and support into the conversation.

Support Survivors of Sexual Assault

If you know someone who has been sexually assaulted, that person may or may not want to talk about the assault. Follow the person's lead and do not ask too many questions. Try to be a good listener and do not judge or blame the person for what happened. To offer support, you can show the person you care and go with the person to get help, if appropriate. Be sure to show empathy, believe the person's story, and check in to see how the person is doing (**Figure 15.15**).

Lesson 15.2 Review

Know and Understand

1. What is affirmative consent?
2. Give two examples of sexual harassment.
3. In a small group, review strategies for preventing sexual harassment. Identify which strategies each of you prefers to use.
4. What is sexual assault?
5. Choose one area of health and explain how sexual assault affects it.

Think Critically

6. Research the age of consent in your state. Do you agree with this age of consent? Why or why not?
7. Experts say that sexual assault is not an act of sex, but an act of power and aggression. Why do you think experts say this? Do you agree? Why or why not?
8. Choose one strategy for preventing sexual assault and create a sheet of 10 tips for using the strategy in daily life.
9. No matter how a person is assaulted or reacts to an assault, the person committing the assault is always to blame. With a partner, list five myths about factors that affect who is responsible for sexual assault. Create a video or podcast explaining how each myth hurts people who have experienced sexual assault and correcting the myth.

REAL WORLD Health Skills

Set Goals Discuss the following questions with a partner to identify goals you can set to enhance your health and the health of others. Set a SMART goal related to each strategy you identify.

- Are there some protective factors you could increase in your life or community to protect yourself and others from sexual harassment? Explain.
- If you experience sexual harassment, what goals could you set to take action and make the harassment stop? Whom could you talk to? How would you get help in this situation, when harassment starts and if the harassment continues?
- What can you do to help others who experience sexual harassment? What concrete goals can you set to discourage harassment and assist others in getting help?

Abuse and Neglect

Essential Question

Why is it important to break the cycle of abuse?

Lesson 15.3

Learning Outcomes

After studying this lesson, you will be able to

- analyze the steps in the cycle of abuse;
- identify forms of abuse;
- describe intimate partner violence;
- assess the consequences of child abuse and neglect;
- explain sibling abuse;
- discuss the meaning of elder abuse; and
- take steps to prevent and respond to abuse.

Key Terms

abuse
child abuse
cycle of abuse
elder abuse
emotional abuse
financial abuse
intimate partner violence
mandated reporters
neglect
physical abuse
sexual abuse
sibling abuse

Warm-Up Activity

How Can You Help?

Make Decisions Imagine you find one of your friends crying outside the school cafeteria. When you get your friend to talk, you find out your friend's parent hits your friend after bad days at work and screams at your friend repeatedly. Your friend has a bruise on the cheek and is obviously shaken up. You want your friend to tell the school counselor, but your friend does not want to tell anyone.

Consider what decisions you could make in this situation to help your friend. Use the decision-making process and then share your decision and alternatives with a partner. Discuss which alternatives are best and why and negotiate to make a final decision.

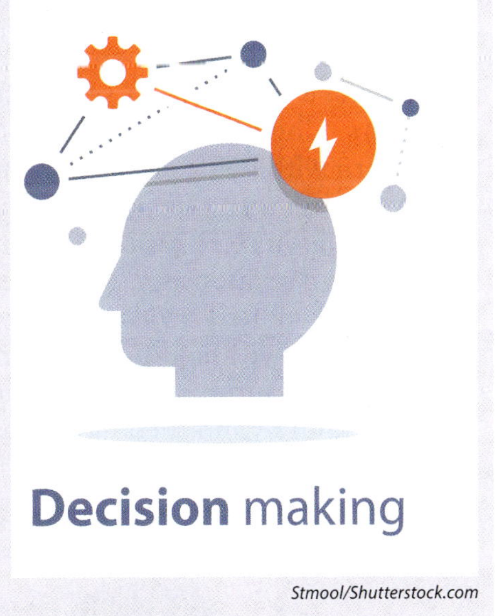

Stmool/Shutterstock.com

Violent behavior has no place in a healthy relationship, where people feel safe and respect and trust each other. You have already learned about some types of violent behavior, such as bullying and cyberbullying and sexual harassment and assault. In this lesson, you will learn about abuse and neglect, which can occur in several types of relationships.

What Is Abuse?

abuse violent behaviors that cause physical, emotional, sexual, or financial harm to another person

Abuse is the violent mistreatment of another person. It can occur in families, between friends, among classmates, or between romantic partners.

Types of Abuse

Like violent behavior, there are many types of abuse. While abuse can be physical, it can also cause psychological injuries, such as low self-esteem, fear, and anxiety. Some major types of abuse include the following:

physical abuse behaviors that cause bodily harm to another person

emotional abuse attitudes, controlling behaviors, or words that harm a person's mental and emotional health; also called *mental*, *verbal*, or *psychological abuse*

sexual abuse behaviors that involve sexual activity to which one person does not or cannot consent

financial abuse behaviors that involve using money to exert power in a relationship; may include controlling finances and using money to make others act in certain ways

- **Physical abuse: Physical abuse** is behaviors that cause physical harm to another person. Physical abuse may involve hitting, kicking, choking, slapping, biting, shaking, or burning someone. Signs of physical abuse can include bruises, black eyes, welts, burns, cuts, broken bones, fear or anxiety, and changes in behavior.
- **Emotional abuse: Emotional abuse** (also called *mental*, *verbal*, or *psychological abuse*) involves attitudes, controlling behaviors, or words that harm a person's mental and emotional health (**Figure 15.16**). Signs of emotional abuse include nervousness around certain people, extreme upset, and withdrawal from relationships and social activities.
- **Sexual abuse: Sexual abuse** is characterized by sexual violence, including sexual assault, or sexual harassment. It can involve physical behaviors such as fondling and sexual intercourse. Sexual abuse can also, however, involve nonphysical behaviors, such as taking nude pictures, exposing one's self, or forcing someone to watch sexual activity. Children who are sexually abused may show excessive anxiety, concern with being alone at night, nightmares, bedwetting, and fear of being alone with certain people.
- **Financial abuse: Financial abuse** is the use of money to exert power in a relationship. Examples of financial abuse include stealing a person's money, giving gifts or money and expecting something in return, and withholding money needed to buy necessities. This type of abuse most commonly occurs between romantic partners and between adult children and their aging parents or guardians.

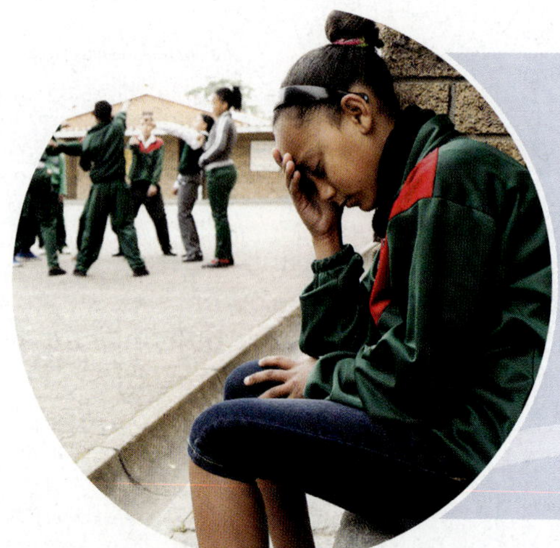

- Using threats or insults
- Withholding love to control behavior
- Ridiculing a person's identity
- Calling a person names
- Isolating a person from supportive relationships

GeorgiaCourt/E+/Getty Images

Figure 15.16 Emotional abuse can occur in-person, online, or over the phone. ***What are other terms for emotional abuse?***

Cycle of Abuse

Abusive behavior usually follows a cycle of four stages: tension building, incident, reconciliation, and calm. This **cycle of abuse** repeats as long as the abuse continues and does not stop unless someone acts to break the cycle (**Figure 15.17**).

cycle of abuse four stages of abuse (tension building, incident, reconciliation, and calm) that repeat as long as the abuse continues

Abuse has serious physical, mental and emotional, and social consequences and can sometimes be a crime. Some consequences are short-term. Immediate physical injuries, such as cuts, bruises, and broken bones, heal with time. In the aftermath of abuse, a person may experience anxiety, depression, and social difficulties. Other consequences last longer. People abused during childhood may develop issues with learning and memory, substance use disorders, and post-traumatic stress disorder (PTSD). They are also more likely to experience violence in other relationships.

Often, a person who abuses others tries to make another person feel responsible for the abuse. This is *never* the case. No matter the situation, the person committing the abuse is *always* responsible for the abuse.

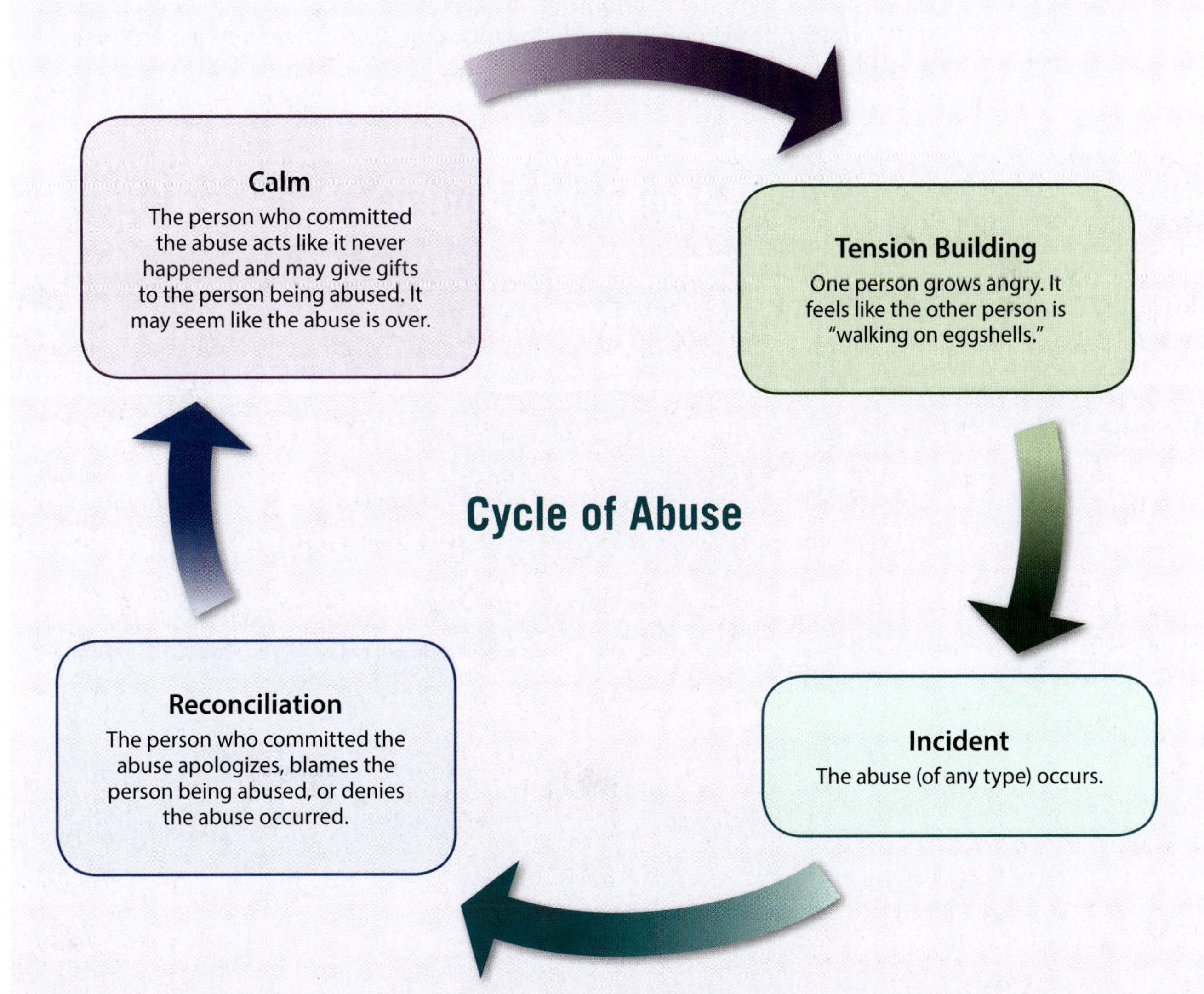

Figure 15.17 Abuse continues unless someone acts to break the cycle.

Intimate Partner Violence

intimate partner violence violent behaviors between two people who are or were married, dating, or in a romantic relationship

Intimate partner violence is abuse between two people who are or were married, dating, or in a romantic relationship. This type of abuse occurs when one or both partners try to dominate or control each other through physical, emotional, sexual, or financial abuse. Threatening a partner is also intimate partner violence. Intimate partner violence is also called *domestic violence*, *spousal violence*, or *dating violence*. Intimate partner violence can occur in person or electronically and may occur between current or former partners.

Intimate partner violence often starts with threats, harmful words, manipulation, and other types of emotional abuse. Over time, this behavior escalates to physical attacks. People who have experienced intimate partner violence may have physical injuries, such as bruises or broken bones. They may also experience depression or feel anxiety, fear, and shame. People who experience intimate partner violence may feel socially isolated and alone, partly because they do not want to tell anyone about the abuse.

Abuse and violence are not part of a healthy relationship. If a partner behaves violently even once, no matter the reason given, the other person should leave the relationship and seek help. There is no good excuse for violent behavior in a healthy relationship. It is essential to get out of a relationship the *very first time* violence occurs (**Figure 15.18**).

Figure 15.18 Some behaviors may not immediately seem like abuse, but patterns like these aim to dominate, manipulate, and control people. ***In what types of relationships does intimate partner violence occur?***

Subtle Examples of Intimate Partner Violence

Gets upset when you spend time with anyone else	Frequently contacts you throughout the day to keep tabs on you and know where you are at all times	Does not take your concerns seriously and does not empathize with your emotions
Becomes insulted easily or has a "short fuse"	Does not take responsibility for personal shortcomings	Questions whom you talk to and wrongfully accuses you of flirting
Puts down your accomplishments	In a conflict, blames you or says it is no big deal	Beats or strikes objects to scare you during conflicts
Asks friends to keep an eye on you	Uses emotions to manipulate you	Encourages spending less time with friends or family members
Calls the use of force "playful"	Equates jealousy with love	Drops by unexpectedly to check up on you

Child Neglect and Abuse

Each year in the United States, nearly 700,000 children experience some form of abuse or neglect. Nearly 1,700 children die from abuse or neglect each year. **Child abuse** is any intentional act committed by an adult that harms or threatens to harm anyone under 18 years of age, including children and teens.

child abuse any intentional physical, emotional, or sexual act committed by an adult that harms or threatens to harm a child

Types of Child Neglect and Abuse

Child abuse includes physical, emotional, and sexual abuse (**Figure 15.19**). Physical abuse includes physical violence or the threat of violence, and emotional abuse includes controlling and harmful behaviors. Child sexual abuse is a specific type of abuse in which an adult involves a child or teen in any sexual activity. This type of abuse may involve the use of pressure, force, or deception and can occur in person, often by someone the child or teen knows, or through electronic communication. Sexual activity with a child or teen is *always* sexual assault. This is because children and teens are not old enough to consent to sexual activity.

Neglect is a form of child abuse that occurs when an adult does not meet the basic physical, emotional, medical, or educational needs of a child or teen. Neglect may be intentional or unintentional. It also occurs when an adult fails to protect a child or teen from harm—for example, through inadequate supervision or a dangerous living situation.

neglect form of child abuse that occurs when an adult intentionally or unintentionally does not meet a child's basic physical, emotional, medical, or educational needs

Effects of Child Neglect and Abuse

People's sense of well-being comes from knowing they have the love, support, and respect of family members, including parents or guardians. When children or teens experience abuse or neglect, this shatters their sense of well-being. Not surprisingly, abuse and neglect do serious short- and long-term harm to a person's health.

Physical child abuse

- Hitting or shaking children or teens
- Pulling hair or biting children or teens
- Forbidding children or teens from eating or sleeping
- Abandoning children or teens in an unfamiliar place

Emotional child abuse

- Withholding love from children or teens
- Isolating or ignoring children or teens
- Constantly criticizing children or teens
- Restricting children or teens from seeing friends and family members
- Threatening to hurt children or teens

Child sexual abuse

- Any sexual activity with a child or teen
- Intimate kissing or sexual touching with children or teens
- Having children or teens view sexual images
- Looking at children or teens sexually (*voyeurism*)

Figure 15.19 Child abuse takes many forms, but all of these actions threaten or harm children or teens. People who commit child abuse can face serious legal consequences.

Physical consequences of abuse may include injuries, brain damage, blindness, motor impairments, and cognitive impairments. Children or teens who have been abused are more likely than others to develop health conditions and diseases as adults, including cardiovascular disease, cancer, liver disease, and obesity. Children or teens who are abused are also more likely than others to behave in ways that can harm their health, such as

- smoking or vaping;
- abusing alcohol and drugs;
- engaging in high-risk sexual behaviors;
- doing poorly in school and failing to graduate from high school; and
- being arrested as juveniles and adults.

Children or teens who are abused or neglected also have a greater risk of experiencing mental health conditions, such as depression, anxiety, eating disorders, and PTSD. The stress of ongoing abuse may also cause learning, attention, and memory issues. These difficulties increase the likelihood of struggling in school.

Long-term, child abuse can interfere with a person's ability to establish and maintain healthy relationships in adulthood. People who do not experience love, trust, and support in their early relationships may have trouble building healthy relationships with others later. Fortunately, children or teens who have been abused can get help to feel better about themselves and others and live fulfilling lives.

Sibling Abuse

sibling abuse chronic physical, emotional, or sexual mistreatment of one sibling by another

Sibling abuse is the mistreatment of one sibling by another. Sibling abuse can be physical, emotional, or sexual and has serious health consequences. According to some studies, sibling abuse is one of the most common types of family abuse (**Figure 15.20**). Sibling abuse most often occurs in families where other unhealthy relationships exist.

Some conflict or rivalry is normal between siblings, but abuse is not. Sibling abuse is typically one-sided and aims to dominate the person being abused. A healthy sibling relationship involves some conflict or rivalry, but does not involve patterns of fear, pain, or control.

Parents or guardians may
• overlook signs of sibling abuse
• dismiss reports of abuse as exaggerated sibling rivalry
• deny that their child is engaging in abusive behavior
• avoid reporting abusive behavior to protect their child
Daisy-Daisy/iStock/Getty Images Plus/Getty Images

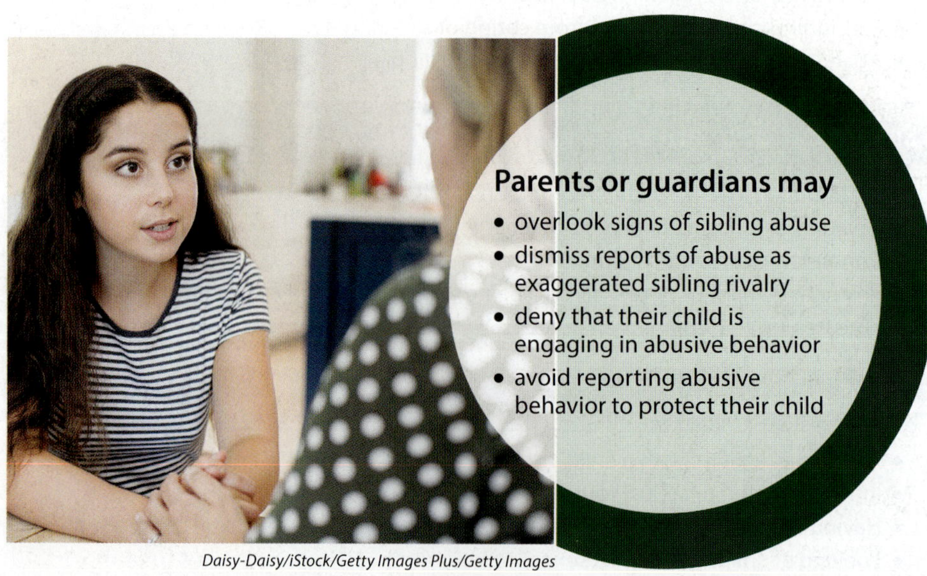

Figure 15.20 Parents and guardians are likely to overlook or dismiss signs of abuse. If you think you are experiencing sibling abuse, explain your situation very clearly to your parent or guardian.

Elder Abuse

Elder abuse is the abuse of an older adult. Elder abuse occurs in older adults' homes, nursing homes, or other living situations. People who commit elder abuse are typically family members or paid caregivers. Elder abuse can take the following forms:

elder abuse behaviors or neglect that cause harm to someone 60 years of age or older

- physical abuse, such as the inappropriate use of medications or restraints
- verbal abuse, such as saying cruel words
- emotional abuse, including ignoring calls for help
- sexual abuse
- *financial abuse*, including the theft of money or property
- neglect, including failure to provide food, water, medications, and basic hygiene

Many cases of elder abuse go unreported. Older adults who experience abuse and neglect feel helpless, lonely, and distressed. They tend to die earlier than older adults who have not experienced abuse.

Preventing and Responding to Abuse

Abuse happens for many reasons, and all of these reasons are the responsibility of the person committing the abuse. Numerous factors can influence whether a person chooses to abuse others. For example, a person who has experienced abuse is more likely to commit abuse in the future (**Figure 15.21**).

Factors Affecting Abuse

Risk Factors

- History of abuse (experiencing or witnessing abuse)
- Mental health conditions or illnesses
- Emotional immaturity and lack of interpersonal skills
- Substance use
- Social isolation and lack of support or unhealthy relationships
- Social environment that tolerates violence
- Negative beliefs about others (gender stereotypes and inequality)
- Marriage difficulties and unplanned pregnancy
- Economic insecurity and unemployment
- Young age and lack of education
- Lack of knowledge about caregiving (for children and older adults)
- Lack of community support and resources
- Expensive or unavailable healthcare

Protective Factors

- Interpersonal skills
- Emotional maturity
- Mental health treatment and resources
- Respect for others
- Stable, healthy relationships
- Education
- Adequate income, access to healthcare, and housing
- Safe, respectful community
- Culture that values diversity
- Knowledge about community support and resources

Figure 15.21 Risk factors make a person more likely to abuse others, while protective factors make a person less likely to do so.

Many communities take steps to help prevent abuse. For example, educational programs give people the facts about abuse and help them recognize when abuse is happening. Some schools hold campaigns to educate students about and prevent peer abuse. Online resources and government agencies also share information about abusive situations and behaviors. You can also help prevent abuse using the following strategies.

Increase Protective Factors

Many factors affecting abuse relate to your mental, emotional, and social health. One way to help prevent abuse is to promote health for yourself, your family, and your community. Improving your mental, emotional, and social health will help you avoid and recognize abuse. You can do this in the following ways:

- If you have experienced abuse, seek help from a mental health professional in processing your experience. People who have experienced abuse can sometimes abuse others themselves.
- Develop your skills in communicating effectively and resolving conflicts.
- Surround yourself with healthy relationships.
- If you have negative beliefs about a group of people, challenge these and encourage others in your family and community to do the same.
- Find ways to value diversity and show respect for others. Be an example to your community.
- Take steps to improve your mental and emotional health and seek treatment for mental health conditions and illnesses, including substance use disorders.
- Educate yourself and your family about the needs of others and effective caregiving.
- Build supportive relationships in your community and use community resources.

Recognize and Report Abusive Behavior

Sometimes people have trouble recognizing when they are being abused. The person who is abusing them might justify the abusive actions and deny what is happening. People who are being abused may blame themselves or be afraid of telling others.

Recognizing abuse is the first step to stopping it. Some laws require children and teens to be educated about signs of abuse. For example, Erin's Law requires that children and teens be taught about body safety to recognize sexual abuse. To recognize abuse, learn about abusive behavior and the cycle of abuse. If you know what abuse is, you can keep yourself from acting abusively and know when others are being abusive. Tell others about the definition of abusive behavior and the signs of abuse (**Figure 15.22**).

Signs of Abuse and Neglect

Physical Abuse
- Injuries, such as broken bones or severe bruises
- Many injuries on different parts of the body
- Several injuries that occurred at different times
- Changes in behavior, including withdrawal, aggression, and depression

Sexual Abuse
- Bruises in the pelvic area
- Difficulty or pain when walking or sitting
- Torn clothing
- Inappropriate sexual behavior

Emotional Abuse
- Withdrawn attitude and unwillingness to talk to others
- Anxiety and worry
- Difficulty sleeping
- Aggressive or inappropriate behavior

Neglect
- Underweight
- Poor physical development
- Lack of cleanliness
- Educational delays

Figure 15.22 Telling others about the signs of abuse and neglect will help more people recognize, report, and avoid abuse and neglect. ***What is the first step to stopping abuse?***

Reporting abuse can get authorities and people in the community involved to stop the abuse. Anyone who suspects that a person is being abused should report this concern to an authority (for example, a police officer or organization) or other trusted adult. Catching abusive behavior early can help prevent abuse from continuing or getting worse.

Several hotlines provide support for people trying to report abuse and leave abusive situations (**Figure 15.23**). People can also report abuse through local or state departments of human services, law enforcement, and state hotlines. Some professionals are required by law to report abuse. These workers, called **mandated reporters**, include teachers and other school personnel, social workers and child welfare workers, and healthcare professionals. Mandated reporters do not have the responsibility to prove that abuse is occurring. They are not penalized if abuse charges are dropped, unless there is evidence abuse was willfully misreported. Mandated reporters can be charged with a criminal offense if they do not report signs of abuse. Typically, the personal information of the person who reported the abuse is kept confidential.

mandated reporters individuals required by law to report signs of abuse

Once abuse is reported, a state organization, such as a child welfare agency or law enforcement, looks into the matter. Investigators will talk with anyone who might have relevant information. If the organization finds that abuse has occurred, it may make arrests. In the case of child abuse, it may take the child away from the parents or guardians and place the child in *foster care* (in which adults agree to care for children who are not their own).

Those who commit abuse may be required to receive therapy and treatment. They may be prosecuted and, if found guilty, sent to prison.

Abuse Hotlines

Childhelp National Child Abuse Hotline

- Call 1-800-422-4453

National Domestic Violence Hotline

- Call 1-800-799-SAFE (7233)
- Visit www.thehotline.org

National Teen Dating Abuse Hotline

- Call 1-866-331-9474
- Text *loveis* to 22522
- Visit www.loveisrespect.org

Figure 15.23 Hotlines provide assistance to people experiencing abuse through online chats, phone calls, and texts. ***Where else can people report abuse?***

Break the Cycle of Abuse

As you have learned, abuse follows a cycle of four stages, which repeat continuously. Because of this, even if abuse seems to stop on its own, it might continue once tension begins to build again. The only way to really stop abuse is to break the cycle of abuse. Steps for breaking this cycle include the following:

1. **Recognize** the abusive situation for what it is. Do not make excuses. There is never a good reason for engaging in abusive behavior. Sometimes, it can help to get another opinion on a difficult situation. Talking regularly with a trusted adult about your relationships can help you identify situations that may become abusive if issues are not resolved.
2. **Remember** that abuse may seem to stop during the calm stage in the cycle of abuse. This period of calm might last a long time, even longer than the previous incident period. This does not mean the abuse is over. Do not let this stage convince you that the abuse is not real. Even if the person acting abusively is being nice, the abuse is still unacceptable and needs to be addressed.
3. **Do not try to change** the person committing the abuse. You cannot change another person. People who abuse others need professional help.
4. **Leave** or help someone leave the abusive relationship or situation. Sometimes it may seem unsafe to leave an abusive situation. Talk with a trusted adult or call a hotline about this and try to leave when it is safe. Crisis shelters are available to help some people who have experienced abuse. In some cases, you may need to do more than leave physically. You might also want to block the person who is being abusive from communicating with you.

Get Help and Treatment

If you experience abuse or are helping someone who has been abused, seek medical treatment for any injuries from the abuse. You can seek medical help by going to a hospital or urgent care center. Going to a crisis shelter can provide safety after you leave an abusive situation.

Seeking professional help after escaping an abusive situation is an important part of moving forward. Mental health therapy sessions provide a safe space for survivors to share their feelings, thoughts, and fears. Therapists can help people work through their experiences, manage traumatic memories, and find strategies for coping with anxiety, anger, and fear. This process can help people have healthier relationships in the future. If you or someone you know has experienced abuse, talk to an adult you trust, such as a teacher, school counselor, or nurse. That person can help you find help from a trained professional.

People who commit abuse or neglect also need professional help. Specific types of treatment may benefit these people. In the case of parents or guardians who abuse children, treatment could include education on appropriate parenting techniques. For people who commit sexual abuse, treatment may include training to increase empathy for others and self-control.

Lesson 15.3 Review

Know and Understand

1. What are the steps in the cycle of abuse?
2. What type of abuse occurs between people who are or were married, dating, or in a romantic relationship?
3. How is child neglect different from child abuse?
4. Give two examples of elder abuse.
5. Describe how to report abuse.
6. Why is it important to break the cycle of abuse?

Think Critically

7. Choose one mental or emotional effect of child abuse and write a social media post explaining how the abuse leads to this effect.
8. Identify one protective factor you can increase to prevent abuse in your community. Film a short video explaining how you can increase this factor.

REAL WORLD Health Skills

Access Information As you know, mandated reporters are people required by law to report any suspected cases of abuse and neglect. Using reliable and valid resources, research laws and procedures in your community for reporting abuse and neglect. Cite your sources and explain why they are reliable. Create a colorful fact page of your findings.

Violence in the Community

Essential Question?

How can you reduce other types of violence in your community?

Lesson 15.4

Learning Outcomes

After studying this lesson, you will be able to

- analyze ways to prevent and respond to school violence;
- assess the consequences of gang involvement;
- describe human trafficking and ways to prevent it;
- explain how hate crimes impact a community;
- discuss the lasting consequences of homicide; and
- recognize ways to stop terrorism.

Key Terms

gangs
hate crime
homicide
human trafficking
school violence
terrorism
vandalism

Warm-Up Activity

Your School

Advocate for Health School violence puts students in danger and disrupts learning. Think about some healthy strategies that help or would help reduce violence at your school. For example, does your school run programs about violence prevention? Does your school have rules meant to reduce violence? As a student, do you have any ideas about actions or programs you could start to reduce school violence? Brainstorm these strategies and make a list. Share your ideas with a partner and then share with another pair of students. Finally, share with the class. Together, come up with a formal proposal for your school administration about programs or actions to reduce violence.

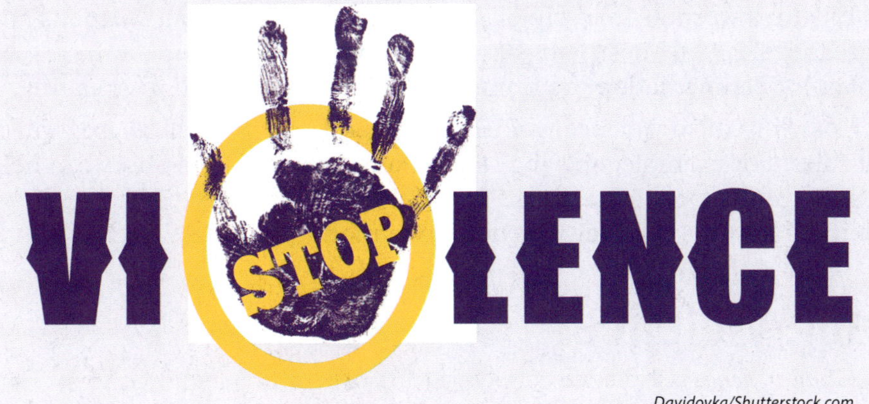

Davidovka/Shutterstock.com

Violence can occur in many places, even in places where people should feel safe. You have already learned about bullying, sexual harassment and assault, and abuse—three types of violence. In this lesson, you will learn about other types of violent behavior and ways to respond to and prevent them.

School Violence

school violence any violent behavior that occurs on school property, at school-sponsored events, or on the way to or from school or school events

School violence is any violent behavior that occurs on school property, at school-sponsored events, or on the way to or from school or school events. School violence can include bullying and cyberbullying. It also includes fighting and the use of weapons at school.

School should be a safe place for all students, but school violence puts students in danger. For example, a fight might seem like it only affects two students. If a fight gets out of control, however, uninvolved students may get hurt. Even if they are not physically injured, students exposed to violence can feel depressed, anxious, and fearful. If a student brings a weapon to school, many people can get hurt or die. Violent behavior in schools can also have serious school and legal consequences. Fighting with another student can lead to detention, suspension, or expulsion. Attacking another student can lead to arrest by the police.

Many schools establish violence-prevention programs to help create a culture that does not tolerate violent behaviors. This means that the school takes violence seriously and seeks to prevent it. Schools often use the following strategies to prevent and reduce violence:

- Select strong, positive, responsible student leaders who act appropriately and are not afraid to speak out against violence.
- Develop positive team-building activities, such as community service work, to forge bonds among students.
- Treat violent behavior as a serious offense. Any acts of violence result in consequences and intervention.
- Have a buddy system, with older students looking out for younger students.
- Encourage students to report any violent acts they observe immediately.
- Enforce rules regarding keeping school doors locked.
- Ensure a weapon-free school. Communicate rules about weapons and search students' belongings as necessary.
- Offer peer mediation programs to prevent conflicts from escalating.

To help reduce violence, students can cooperate with these programs and rules. For example, obeying rules about locking school doors can help keep dangerous people out of the building. Students have an important role in school strategies for violence prevention.

Gang Violence

gangs groups of people who engage in violent and illegal activities

vandalism deliberate destruction of or damage to someone else's property

Gang violence is violence carried out by people in a gang. **Gangs** are groups of people who engage in violent and illegal activities. These activities can include selling drugs; robbing people or businesses; attacking others, especially rival gang members; and **vandalism** (damaging others' property).

Some people join a gang to feel like part of a group and gain a sense of identity. Being part of a gang may make a person feel accepted or important.

Other people join gangs as a result of peer pressure, the desire to make money, or the hope of protecting themselves and their families (**Figure 15.24**).

People who join gangs typically become involved in acts of violence and other crimes. For example, gang members may pressure a teen to commit a violent crime as an initiation into the gang. Because of this, gang members often go to prison or experience violence. They may drop out of school, be unable to find a job, and develop an addiction to drugs. Committing a crime can severely impact a person's future. Many gang members also lose their lives to gang violence.

Communities often use resources to help reduce gang violence. For example, officials in cities often take steps to limit the size and reach of gangs. To be successful, city workers and police officers have to be deeply engaged in the community and build trust. To protect yourself, reduce gang violence, and avoid becoming part of a gang, you can use the following strategies:

- **Be clear that you are not interested in joining a gang:** Tell gang members you are not interested. As much as possible, avoid places where gang members meet and spend time. Develop friendships with people who are not in a gang. Seek help from trusted adults, authority figures, and community resources to resist pressure to join a gang.
- **Focus on your future:** Devote yourself to doing well in school so you will have more options later in life. Many jobs require a high school diploma, additional training, or college. Working hard in school increases your future options.
- **Stay busy:** Find activities that interest you, such as a job, school club, or community organization. These activities can help you feel good about yourself and will not put your safety at risk.
- **Talk to an adult:** Find an adult you trust, such as a parent or guardian, teacher, school counselor, or police officer. Talk to that person if you need advice or are having a hard time feeling accepted or connecting with others. Tell that person if you are pressured to join a gang.

Risk Factors for Gang Involvement

- Environment with widespread gang activity
- Family members, friends, or community role models in gangs
- Low involvement in community
- Alcohol or drug use
- Availability of weapons
- Lack of educational and employment opportunities in the community
- Violence or lack of adult supervision in the home
- Negative self-esteem and feelings of hopelessness

Figure 15.24 Certain environmental risk factors increase a person's likelihood of being involved in a gang. ***Which gang activity involves damaging other people's property?***

Human Trafficking

human trafficking form of modern slavery in which people are forced or pressured to perform labor or sexual acts against their will

Human trafficking is a form of modern slavery in which people are forced or pressured to perform some job or service against their will. In *labor trafficking*, employers use threats of violence, imprisonment, or deportation to force people to work long hours or for very little, if any, money. In *sex trafficking*, people are forced to engage in sexual activity against their will, sometimes for money. Sex trafficking also includes forcing someone to pose for sexually explicit photographs. Traffickers make money off the people they traffic and use threats, violence, drugs, and coercion to make people do what they want.

Human trafficking can begin in many different ways. Sometimes, trafficking begins with kidnapping. More commonly, people trick others by promising better living conditions or a job. For example, a person may post an online ad for a job that is too good to be true or reach out to someone on social media and ask to meet. Once this person pursues these promises and ads, people force them into certain activities. Human trafficking can also begin in a family or relationship. One family member or partner may force another to work or engage in sexual activity (**Figure 15.25**).

People involved in human trafficking make money off those who pay for the services of people being trafficked. Often, people advertise these services online. Human trafficking activity is concentrated in *hot spots*, such as large cities and locations with many transportation options (for example, airports, train stations, and highways). Trafficking is especially common during large events, such as major sporting events or political conventions, which draw many people.

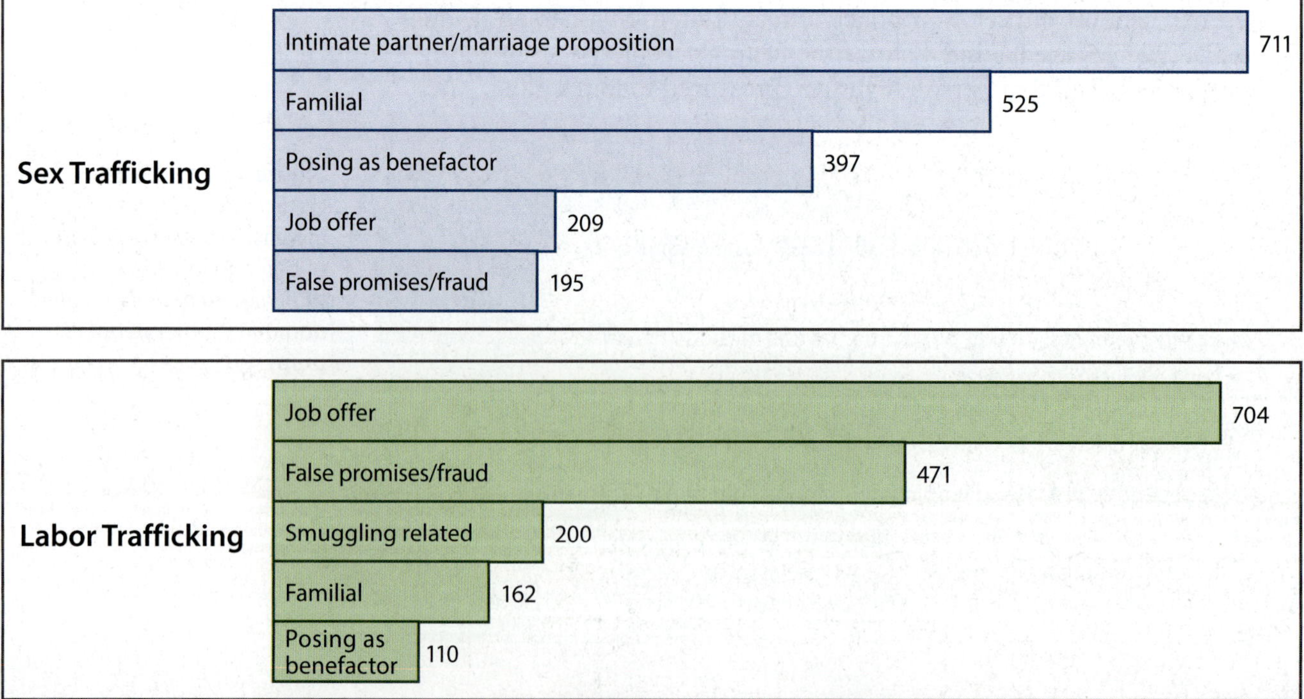

Figure 15.25 Sex trafficking most commonly begins through a false proposition of marriage or intimate partner relationship. Labor trafficking most commonly begins with a fake job offer.

Local and Global Health

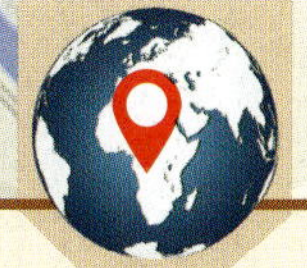

Human Trafficking: A Worldwide Issue

Human trafficking affects countries and people all around the world. A report by the United Nations Office of Drugs and Crime has found that global rates of human trafficking are increasing. Two factors are largely responsible for this increase. First, more women and girls are being forced into trafficking, often for sexual purposes. Second, people who leave their home countries due to violent conditions have an increased risk of being trafficked.

Rates and types of human trafficking differ by country. Labor trafficking is more common in African and Middle Eastern countries than in other countries. In most countries, sex trafficking is the most common form of trafficking. Sex trafficking can affect anyone—men or women, adults or children—but primarily affects women and girls. The region with the largest number of trafficked women and girls is North America, Central America, and the Caribbean.

When people are forced to leave their homes due to violent conflict, they become especially vulnerable to human trafficking. Trafficking may occur through offers to provide jobs, help with travel arrangements, or places to stay. These offers turn out to be fraudulent and instead lead to forced labor, sexual activity, or military service. Children and teens who are separated from their families have an especially high risk of being trafficked.

Detected victims of trafficking in persons by age group and sex, by subregion of detection, 2016 (or most recent)

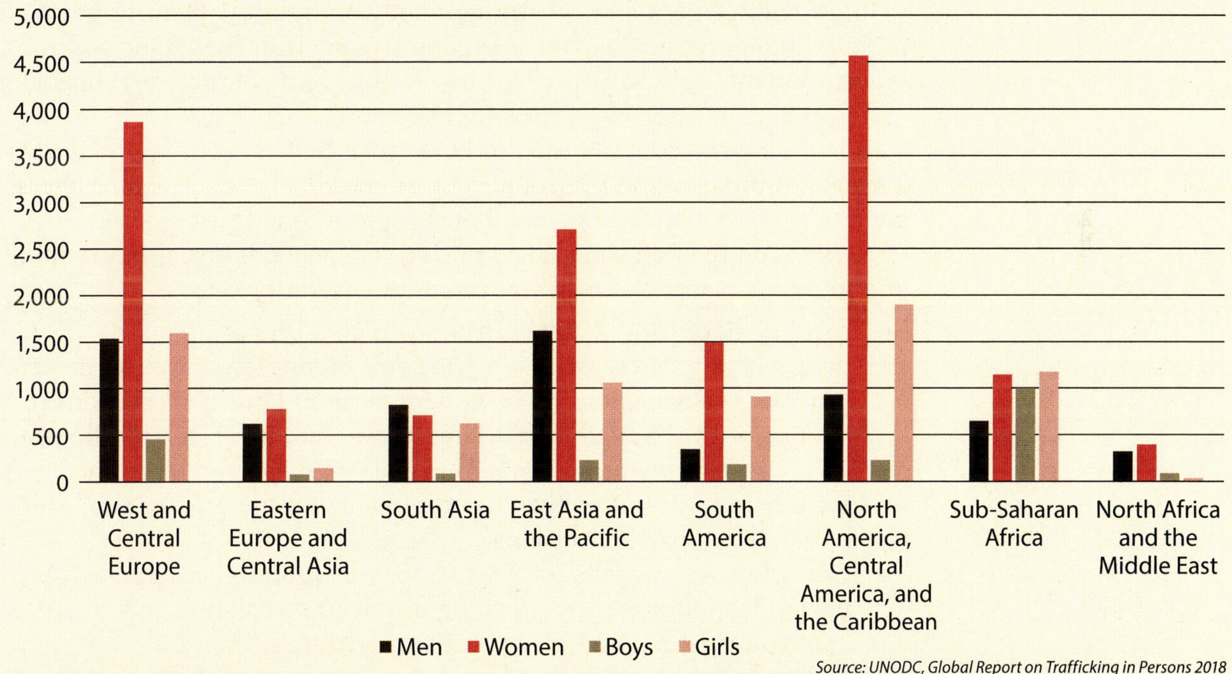

Source: UNODC, Global Report on Trafficking in Persons 2018

Practice Your Skills

Advocate for Health

Think about the varying rates and types of human trafficking in different countries. What are some factors that contribute to these differences? With a partner, list the reasons you think may contribute. Then, compare your reasons with those of another pair. Next, as a class, research the dominant forms of human trafficking in your community. What kind of trafficking is most common? What populations are most affected? Are there any human trafficking hot spots in your community? Also research any organizations in your community that battle human trafficking. As a class, collect your findings and then hold a brainstorming session about ways to reduce human trafficking in your community. What can community officials do? What can each person do? Create an awareness campaign to help other students understand human trafficking and ways to prevent it.

Effects of Human Trafficking

Human trafficking has serious consequences for people who are trafficked and communities. During and even after trafficking, people who are trafficked may experience

- physical symptoms, such as fatigue, headaches, back pain, and weight loss;
- health conditions, such as heat stroke, hypothermia, injuries, frostbite, repetitive-motion injuries, respiratory conditions, skin infections, unwanted pregnancy, and STIs;
- mental health conditions, such as depression, anxiety, substance use disorders, and PTSD; and
- isolation, captivity, and withdrawal from relationships and social activities.

Human trafficking also has negative effects on the community. Kidnappings can lead to grief and loss in families and schools. This loss can also occur if a trafficker takes a person who is being trafficked away from a community. People who have been trafficked may experience lasting physical and mental health conditions. Fear and stress can result if human trafficking is occurring in a community.

Preventing and Responding to Human Trafficking

Law enforcement and government and community organizations work to fight human trafficking and save people being trafficked. One way to prevent human trafficking is to get involved in some of these organizations and promote awareness in your community.

On a personal level, you can prevent human trafficking by opposing violent behavior. If you have thoughts of hurting or controlling others, talk to a trusted adult to get help with feelings and thoughts motivating your behavior.

Practicing the following safety precautions when home alone, online, and in public places can help you avoid human trafficking:

- Lock the doors and windows when you are at home.
- Do not go anywhere with someone you do not know well or meet someone you know online in-person without adult supervision. If meeting with someone you do not know well, meet in a public place.
- Do not give out your personal information, in-person or online.
- Avoid using substances like drugs and alcohol that impair your ability to make responsible decisions.
- If someone offers you a job that seems too good to be true, such as making lots of money by traveling or posing for photos, talk to an adult you trust before having further contact.
- If someone gives you gifts or money or makes a lot of promises, be aware that these behaviors may be *grooming* (building a relationship with the intent of taking advantage of a person).
- If you feel unsafe in a relationship, or are in a relationship with an imbalance of power, leave the relationship, if you can. Reach out to a trusted adult or community resource for help.

Knowing the signs of human trafficking can help you identify if you or others are being trafficked (**Figure 15.26**). If you or someone you know shows signs of being trafficked, talk to a trusted adult, such as a teacher, coach, doctor, or nurse. You can also call the National Human Trafficking Hotline (1-888-373-7888), text *HELP* to BeFree (233733), or visit humantraffickinghotline.org/chat to chat online.

A person who is being trafficked may exhibit

- disconnectedness from family, friends, and the broader community;
- continued absences from school;
- a sudden or dramatic change in behavior;
- a disoriented or confused appearance;
- signs of physical abuse, such as bruises in various stages of healing;
- signs of emotional abuse, such as appearing timid, fearful, or submissive;
- signs of neglect, such as being denied food, water, sleep, or medical care;
- frequent contact with someone who controls what the person says and where the person goes;
- signs of being coached on what to say;
- inability to freely leave home or go places; and
- little sense of location and time of day or year.

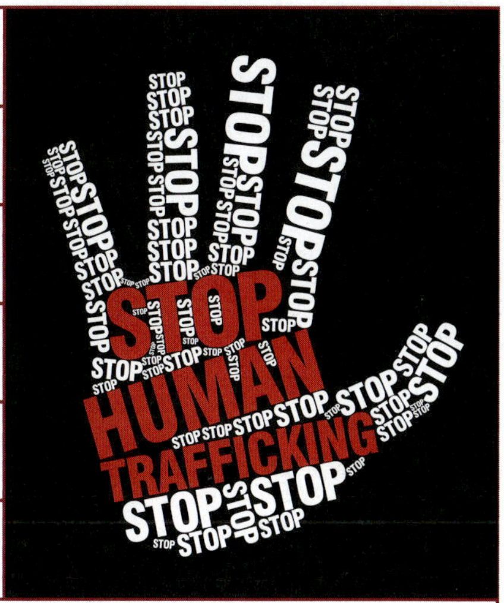

ria_airborne/Shutterstock.com

Figure 15.26 These signs may indicate that a person is being trafficked and needs help. ***What organization are you contacting by texting HELP to BeFree (233733)?***

Hate Crimes

A **hate crime** is any threat or act of violence that targets people because of their race, ethnicity, disability, sexual orientation, gender identity, or religion. Examples of hate crimes include vandalism, offensive graffiti, verbal threats, assaults, and physical or emotional attacks.

hate crime any kind of violence or threat of violence that targets people because of their race, ethnicity, disability, sexual orientation, gender identity, or religion

People who experience hate crimes can suffer injury or loss of property. They may be emotionally scarred by the crime. Hate crimes also tend to have a lasting impact on a person's community. This is because people who commit hate crimes target not just a single person, but also a larger group of people who share an identity. As a result, people often feel unsafe in their community after a hate crime. Most states have laws that increase the punishment for hate crimes, such as personal violence or property damage (**Figure 15.27**).

Appreciating diversity and discouraging violent behavior can help reduce hate crimes. In most cases, people who commit hate crimes are driven by stereotypes, prejudice, and misinformation. These people tend to have low self-esteem, which they try to improve by putting other people down. Do not engage in these behaviors. Instead, celebrate differences and encourage others to do the same.

Committing a hate crime as a teen can result in

- school consequences, such as suspension or expulsion
- legal consequences, such as juvenile criminal charges

Figure 15.27 Hate crimes may be punished within your school or more widely in your state.

Homicide

homicide act of killing a person

Killing someone is an extremely serious crime called a **homicide**. Homicides occur through physical injury. For example, attacking another student and causing death can lead to homicide. So can using a weapon at school. Whether intentional or unintentional, homicides lead to serious, lasting consequences.

Homicide robs another person of life. It devastates families, friends, and communities. No one deserves to be killed, and homicide only makes the problems in a person's life worse. Homicide leads to serious criminal charges. In some states, young people who commit homicide are treated as adults. These young people can be sentenced to life in prison.

The most important step in preventing homicide is reporting violent behavior to trusted adults. If a person threatens to kill someone, take this seriously and tell a school official, teacher, or other adult. You should also immediately report any weapons or violent situations you see at school or in your community. Reporting these situations may allow an adult to intervene before a homicide can occur.

Terrorism

terrorism ideologically motivated use of violence and threats to frighten and control groups of people

Terrorism is the use of violence and threats to frighten and control groups of people. Terrorism is ideologically motivated. This means it aims to punish people for or convince people of certain ideas. Some examples of terrorism are killing or injuring people to promote a political or religious view. Terrorism often leads to the loss of many lives and creates fear in communities. It is a serious crime that does nothing to validate the person's viewpoint.

Most terrorism is a result of *violent extremism*, or beliefs that support the use of violence to promote an idea. For example, a violent extremist view might support hurting people who practice a particular religion. People usually reach the point of violent extremism through *radicalization*, or the process of turning against one's own values and beginning to support terrorism. Someone who is being radicalized may come to believe it is okay to break the law and hurt other people. Often, these views come from people who use social media to reach a wide audience, spread violent and extremist material, and recruit others. Signs that someone is being radicalized include

- sudden changes in appearance, habits, personality, and behaviors;
- extreme statements that do not sound like the person's own ideas;
- attempts to make other people believe hateful ideas; and
- anger if beliefs are questioned.

If you notice these patterns of behavior in yourself or in a friend or classmate, tell a trusted adult. It is important to act quickly and get yourself or your friend needed help. Also be sure to report any suspicious activity to law enforcement (**Figure 15.28**). If you report suspicious activity, you should describe what you saw, when and where you saw it, and why it is suspicious. Another way to prevent terrorism and violent extremism is to celebrate the differences among people and encourage others to do the same.

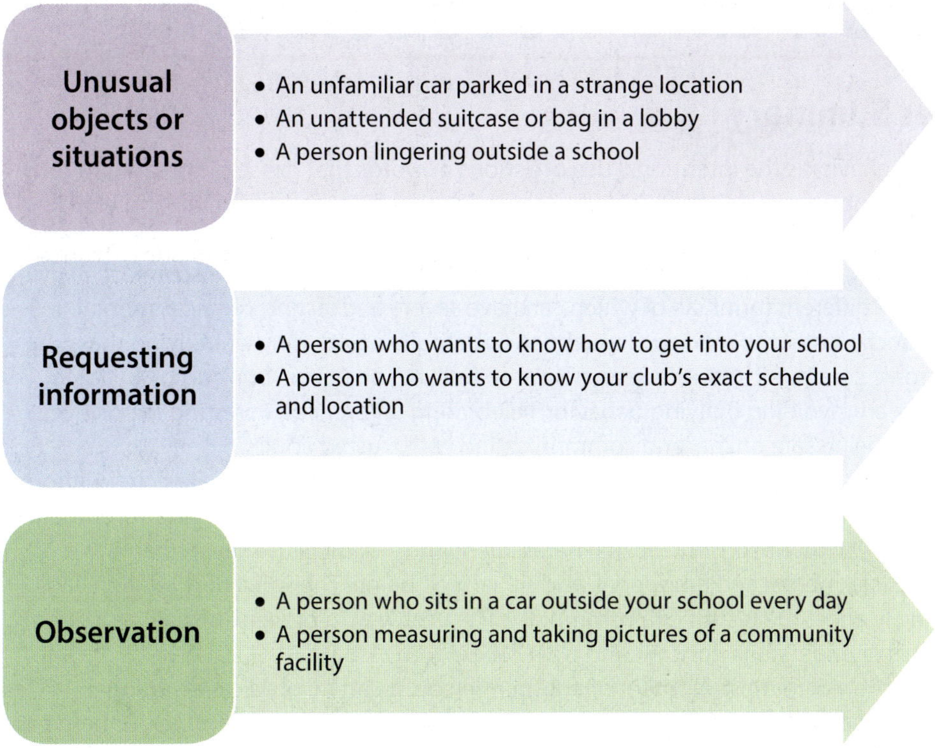

Unusual objects or situations

- An unfamiliar car parked in a strange location
- An unattended suitcase or bag in a lobby
- A person lingering outside a school

Requesting information

- A person who wants to know how to get into your school
- A person who wants to know your club's exact schedule and location

Observation

- A person who sits in a car outside your school every day
- A person measuring and taking pictures of a community facility

Figure 15.28 Unusual objects or situations, requests for specific or personal information, and prolonged observation are examples of suspicious activity.

Lesson 15.4 Review

Know and Understand

1. What are the potential consequences of gang activity?
2. Identify four signs of human trafficking.
3. What aspects of identity do hate crimes target?
4. How does radicalization lead to violent extremism?
5. When reporting suspicious activity, what details should you include?

Think Critically

6. In a small group, list your school's rules and strategies for preventing school violence. Participate in a class discussion about how all students can help prevent violence by following these policies.
7. List activities you could do to feel like part of a group without engaging in gang activity.
8. With a partner, identify a recent hate crime you have heard about and study the crime. Identify who committed the crime, what violence was involved, and what identity the crime targeted. Present strategies you could use to reduce the likelihood of this hate crime in your community.

REAL WORLD Health Skills

Analyze Influences Homicide is the third leading cause of death for teens and young adults. Why do you think this is? Using your local library or reliable internet resources, research this statistic and the most common reasons for these homicides. What individual and environmental factors influence a person's risk for homicide? Write a short blog post describing your findings and suggesting one or two strategies to lower the rate of teen homicide. Include steps teens can take to manage their risk factors and increase protective factors.

Chapter 15 Review and Assessment

Chapter Summary

Violent behavior is the intentional use of actions or words that cause or threaten to cause harm to someone or something. Risk factors for violent behavior stem from the individual, family, peer and social interactions, and community.

Bullying is aggressive behavior toward someone that causes injury or discomfort. Bullying can take many different forms, all of which can have severe and lasting physical, mental, emotional, social, and academic consequences. Cyberbullying is a form of bullying that uses electronic communication. You can help stop bullying and cyberbullying by building your self-esteem, avoiding bullying behavior, celebrating differences, investing in positive relationships, being safe online, and communicating with trusted adults.

Sexual harassment is unwanted sexual attention, or sexual attention that occurs without consent, and can be verbal or nonverbal. Sexual assault is illegal and occurs whenever there is sexual activity without consent. Sexual harassment and assault cause severe harm to a person's physical, mental and emotional, and social well-being. They also hurt relationships and negatively affect the health of a community. The best way to prevent sexual harassment and assault is to understand consent and treat others with respect.

Abuse is the violent mistreatment of another person. It can be physical, emotional, sexual, or financial and can occur in families, between friends, among classmates, or between romantic partners. Abusive behavior usually follows a cycle of four stages: tension building, incident, reconciliation, and calm. This cycle of abuse repeats as long as the abuse continues and does not stop unless someone acts to break the cycle.

Violence in the community can take the form of school violence, gang violence, human trafficking, hate crimes, homicide, and terrorism. Human trafficking is a form of modern slavery in which people are forced or pressured to perform some job or service against their will. A hate crime is any threat or act of violence that targets people because of their race, ethnicity, disability, sexual orientation, gender identity, or religion. Killing someone is an extremely serious crime called a homicide. Whether intentional or unintentional, homicides lead to serious, lasting consequences. Terrorism is the use of violence and threats to frighten and control groups of people. Terrorism often leads to the loss of many lives and creates fear in communities. It is a serious crime that does nothing to validate the person's viewpoint.

Vocabulary Activity

Prepare a presentation about five of the terms from the list. In your presentation, explain each term as it might apply to your own life. Then, provide a more scientific or legal explanation of the term. Answer any questions your classmates may have after your presentation.

abuse	*gangs*	*safe zones*
age of consent	*gossip*	*school violence*
bullying	*harassment*	*sexual abuse*
bystander effect	*hate crime*	*sexual assault*
bystanders	*hazing*	*sexual harassment*
catfishing	*homicide*	*sexual violence*
child abuse	*human trafficking*	*sibling abuse*
cyberbullying	*impersonation*	*stalking*
cyberstalking	*intimate partner violence*	*statutory rape*
cycle of abuse	*mandated reporters*	*terrorism*
elder abuse	*neglect*	*upstander*
emotional abuse	*physical abuse*	*vandalism*
financial abuse	*rape*	*violent behavior*

Review and Recall

Review the information in this chapter by answering the following questions.

1. Which of the following is *not* an example of violent behavior?
   A. hitting someone
   B. destroying someone's belongings
   C. spreading rumors about someone
   D. resolving conflict
2. What is one example of a part of a person's identity that harassment might target?
3. What is *hazing*?
4. Which is an appropriate way to respond to bullying?
   A. fighting back
   B. choosing not to respond to the bullying behavior
   C. being aggressive
   D. keeping the actions a secret
5. What crime occurs when anyone under the age of consent engages in sex?
   A. cyberstalking
   B. date rape
   C. statutory rape
   D. incest
6. Why do many people who experience sexual assault not report the crime?
7. Why should a person who experiences sexual assault not change clothes or shower before going to the police station or hospital?
8. List three physical consequences of child abuse.
9. What is one example of financial abuse?
10. Mandated reporters can be charged with a criminal offense if
    A. they cannot prove that abuse is occurring.
    B. they do not report signs of abuse.
    C. abuse charges are dropped.
    D. they do not agree to publish personal information.
11. What are the possible consequences for teens who commit homicide?
12. Where can school violence occur, other than on school property?
13. Why do people often feel unsafe in their community after a hate crime?

Standardized Test Prep

Math Practice

The following results are from a study of men and women who have experienced intimate partner violence. Review the results of this study and answer the questions that follow.

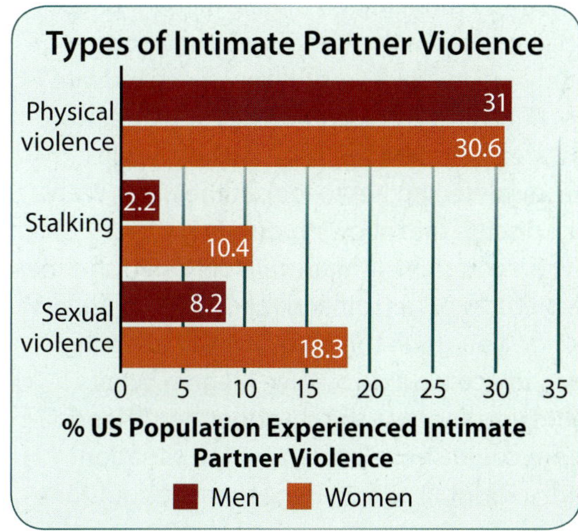

Source: Smith, S.G., Zhang, X., Basile, K.C., Merrick, M.T., Wang, J., Kresnow, M., Chen, J. (2018). The National Intimate Partner and Sexual Violence Survey (NISVS): 2015 Data Brief–Updated Release. Atlanta, GA: National Center for Injury Prevention and Control, Centers for Disease Control and Prevention.

14. Which type of intimate partner violence did more men than women experience?
15. What is the percent difference between men and women who experienced stalking by an intimate partner?
    A. 8.2 percent
    B. 10.1 percent
    C. 4.7 percent
    D. 22 percent
16. This study also found that 43.5 million women, 36.4 percent of women in the US population, experienced psychological aggression from an intimate partner. How many women experienced sexual violence? Round to the nearest whole number.

Chapter 15 Skills Assessment

Critical Thinking Skills

Answer the following questions to assess your knowledge of what you learned in this chapter.

1. Can you think of a time you were a bystander when someone was being bullied? How could you have handled the situation differently?
2. What are some factors that might cause someone to participate in bullying behavior? What can you do if you notice yourself participating in bullying behavior?
3. What are some barriers to being an upstander or ally, and how can you overcome them?
4. What are some situations where you might be vulnerable to violence? For each situation, create a personal safety plan by outlining three to five actions you could take to help keep yourself safe.
5. Why might teens be at greater risk for sexual harassment than adults? What are some steps that you, as a teen, can take to protect yourself from sexual harassment?
6. What are some actions you can take to support a friend or classmate who is a survivor of sexual assault?
7. Why does consent not occur if a person does not respond?
8. What are some of the signs that someone may be experiencing physical or verbal intimate partner violence? How would the signs of verbal and physical abuse be different from each other? How would they be the same?
9. Why might teens who experience violence blame themselves? What are some things you could say to someone who felt that way?
10. How can being abused as a child or teen affect a person's relationships in adulthood?
11. Why might sibling abuse be commonly overlooked or dismissed?
12. What feelings or experiences might make someone more likely to join a gang? What is some advice you could give to a friend who is considering joining a gang?
13. Why is it likely that a person who engages in hate crimes also has low self-esteem?

Health and Wellness Skills

Complete the following activities to assess your skills related to health and wellness.

14. **Analyze Influences.** Like other influences, the media can have a negative or positive effect on how people view violence. Using reliable and valid resources, research three ways the media has a *positive* influence on how people view and respond to violent behavior. Focus on the violent behaviors discussed in this chapter. Outline the three positive influences you found and create a journal entry discussing how these influences affect personal, family, and community health.
15. **Access Information.** In small groups, visit the website of the National Center on Safe Supportive Learning Environments to learn more about human trafficking. With guidance from your instructor, choose one aspect of human trafficking to research (for example, risk factors, ways to identify trafficking, or how to prevent and protect one's self from dangerous situations). Create a digital graphic or animation of your findings to share with your class.
16. **Communicate with Others.** Recently, Megan made friends with a clique of girls at her school. Secretly, these girls created a "Rate Megan" page on social media. On this page, they post pictures of Megan and invite others to view them and rate Megan. Rude and crude comments, as well as low ratings, are posted on the page. Megan begins to get messages telling her to look at the page. With a partner, discuss the following questions:
    - How do you think Megan will feel when she sees the pictures of herself and reads the comments? How do you think this situation will affect her?
    - What advice would you give Megan? What would you suggest she do about her "friends"? Whom could she talk to about the situation? Write a script in which Megan reaches out for help.

17. **Make Decisions.** "What Would You Do?" is a TV show in which hidden cameras film bullying-type situations that require bystanders to intervene or mind their own business. If unfamiliar with the show, you can watch episodes online. In small groups, film a video depicting a bullying-type scenario. Play your video for the class and then lead a discussion about what students would do. As part of the discussion, include alternative actions students might take, either in the moment or after the situation ends. Use the decision-making process to identify the best alternative.
18. **Set Goals.** In this chapter, you learned about types of violence that can happen at home, in school, or in your community. Set three SMART goals related to each of the three areas—home, school, and community—that could help you reduce or respond to violence.
19. **Practice Health-Enhancing Behaviors.** Look through the local news and find a current event that involves one type of violence discussed in this chapter. Make sure you evaluate your news source for credibility. Consider the strategies and prevention methods you learned in this chapter and apply them to the news story you found. Rewrite the article so those involved in the situation use your strategies and reach a different outcome.
20. **Advocate for Health.** Design a pamphlet sharing what people should do if they are in an abusive situation. Include the signs of abuse, some basic steps to take in an abusive situation, and where people can go for help. When designing your pamphlet, be sure to access reliable resources, such as the National Domestic Violence Hotline. Include the names and contact information for local resources that help people who have experienced abuse. Share your pamphlet with members of your school or community.

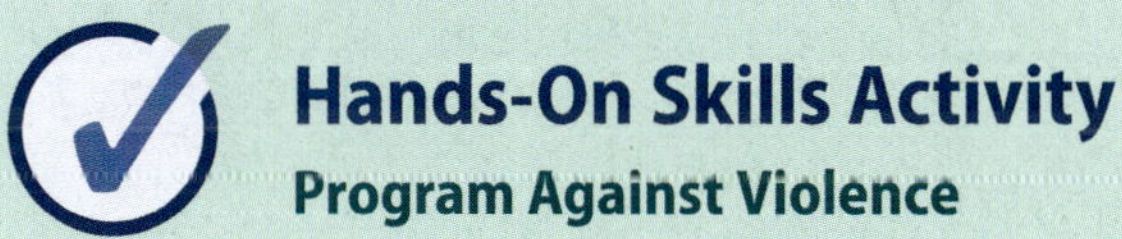

Hands-On Skills Activity

Program Against Violence

Now that you understand more about the different types of violence, the reasons violence occurs, and strategies to prevent violence, design a school- or community-based program to raise awareness about one type of violence.

Steps for This Activity

1. **Access Information.** Study your school or community and identify existing programs that target different types of violence. Organize these programs according to the types of violence discussed in this chapter. This list will show you which types of violence may be insufficiently targeted in your community.
2. As a class, choose one type of violence you want to target. Is there a program that already exists for this type of violence, but is not very successful? Do you, as a student, see a specific need that school or community leaders may not see?
3. **Advocate for Health.** Decide what type of program you want to create. If you are changing an existing program, decide how you will give it new life. Use as many resources as possible, including adults who work in these areas, as you create your program.
4. Once you create your program, obtain any school or community permissions you may need. Assign necessary roles and responsibilities within your program and complete any necessary training. For example, if your program is based on peer mediation, select students and have them trained in peer mediation.
5. Develop a media campaign to advertise your program. Write a creative slogan that highlights your area of focus and communicates information about the services your program offers. This campaign could include advertisements in the local or school paper, brochures or pamphlets, and social media announcements.
6. Put your program into action as a class and observe the results.

Unit

6 Protecting Your Health

Big Ideas

- Staying safe is an important part of protecting your health. One way to stay safe is to take steps to prevent accidents and injuries. This involves preventing falls and avoiding poisonous substances. It also involves reporting the presence of weapons, being safe on the road and in the workplace, and taking precautions around water.
- You can take steps to stay safe in and outside the home. At school, you can follow rules and report dangerous behavior. You can be careful among strangers and in social situations. You can also be prepared for emergencies, such as fire and disasters.
- You probably do a lot of communicating and interacting online. Being safe online is an essential skill. To be safe online, you can follow rules, use good etiquette, and keep personal information private. You can avoid fraud, hacking, viruses, and inappropriate content.
- Using first aid, you can respond to many minor injuries and improve someone's chances of recovery until medical professionals arrive. There are specific procedures you can use to respond to medical emergencies like choking and cardiac arrest.
- Environmental health examines how environmental factors affect health. Humans and the environment affect each other. Factors in the environment also affect health.
- Environmental hazards can harm health. Air pollution can come from natural or human activities. Water pollution can lead to contaminated drinking water. Hazardous chemicals also affect health and the environment. Noise pollution can cause stress and increase risk for health conditions.
- Several regulations help protect the environment. To protect your environment, you can conserve resources, recycle, understand waste treatment and disposal, and contribute to the community.

Dragon Images/Shutterstock.com ▶

Health Management Plan ▸ Making a Plan for Safety

Think of a situation where you felt particularly safe or unsafe. For example, did you feel safe when a friend went with you to a party? Did you feel unsafe during a natural disaster or around contaminated water? Your safety every day has the potential to benefit or harm your health.

Protecting your safety means taking steps to reduce hazards in your environment and lower your risk for accidents, injuries, and health conditions. In this unit, you will learn skills for preventing and responding to accidents, staying safe in social situations and online, and protecting the environment. Open your health management plan. Start a new entry and label it "Protecting My Health."

1. Consider the places you go and situations you face every day. Which places or situations are especially safe? unsafe? List these places and situations and explain your reasoning.
2. For each place or situation you listed, imagine how its safety or lack of safety could influence your health. For example, exposure to air pollution may hurt your health. Strong privacy settings on your social media accounts may benefit your health.
3. For each place or situation, identify what elements that influence safety are within or outside your control. For example, you can control whether you give out personal information online. You cannot control whether you constantly hear trains on the tracks by your home.
4. List three strategies you could use to increase your safety and health in each place or situation. Be specific in these strategies. Keep your list and revisit it after reading this unit. After revisiting the list, turn each strategy into a detailed decision you could make. When creating each decision, think long-term—about your health now and in the future. Keep this list of decisions and act on them to increase your safety.

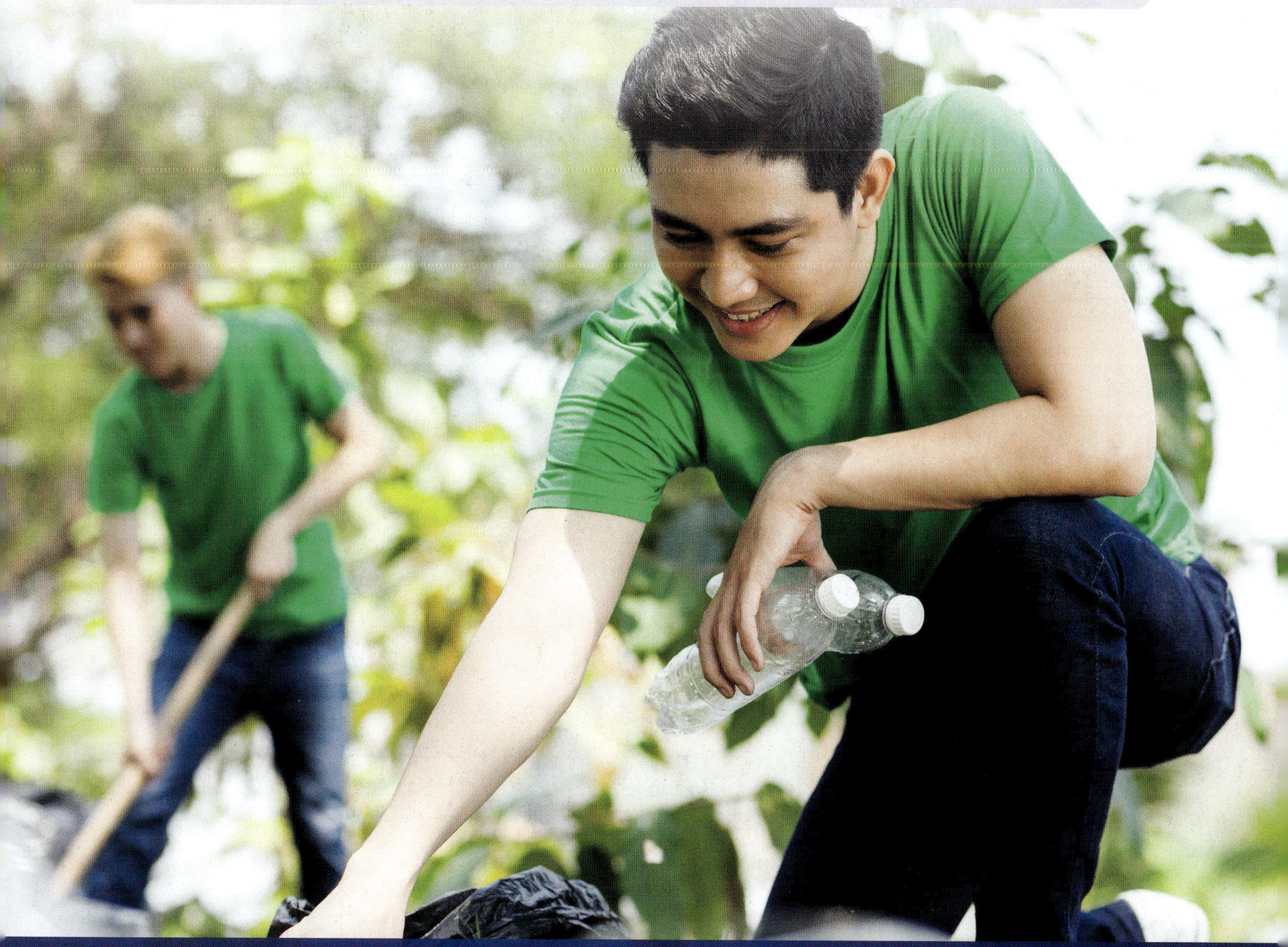

Chapter 16

Personal Safety

Lesson 16.1	Preventing Accidents and Injuries
Lesson 16.2	Handling Dangerous Situations
Lesson 16.3	Being Safe on the Internet
Lesson 16.4	Providing First Aid

Look for the skills icon throughout this chapter for opportunities to practice your health skills.

Check Your Health and Wellness Skills

In this chapter, you will learn skills for protecting your safety. To understand the skills you currently use, take the following inventory of your behaviors. Indicate how well you think you use each skill. Use a scale of 1–5, *1* meaning you do not use the skill and *5* meaning you feel completely comfortable using it.

Skill	How Well Do You Use Each Skill?
I pay attention to my surroundings more than my phone.	
I know whom I'd talk to if I saw a weapon at home or school.	
When driving, I give my full attention to the road.	
I follow all school rules.	
I take a friend with me if going to an unfamiliar place.	
I know my family's escape plan in case of a fire.	
I show respect and am honest online.	
I don't share information, photos, or location settings that might let people I don't know find me.	
I avoid and don't share inappropriate content online.	
I know what information to give if I call 911.	
I can tell if a cut is deep enough I need to see a doctor.	
I know how to use Hands-Only™ CPR.	
	Total:

Add up your responses to each statement. The higher your score, the more comfortable you feel protecting your safety. Which skill do you think is most important for you? Which skill is the most challenging for you? Which skill would you most like to improve? In this chapter, you will learn how to perform these skills better and more often.

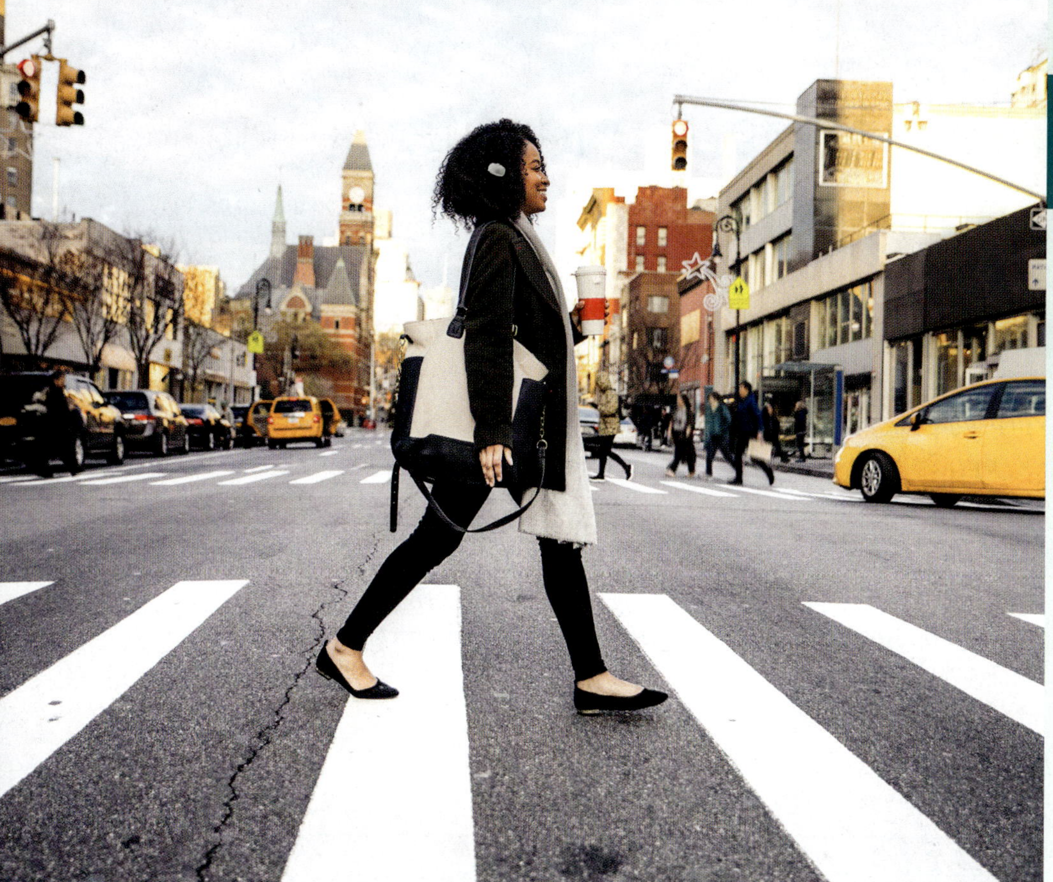

LeoPatrizi/E+/Getty Images

Reading and Notetaking

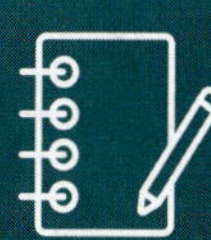

This chapter is about preventing injuries and staying safe. Before reading this chapter, make 10 predictions of safety strategies you think might be included in the chapter. For each prediction, explain why you think this is an important guideline for avoiding injuries and staying safe. Use your previous personal experience, as well as prior personal knowledge, to fill in a table like the one shown. Complete the table from top to bottom, filling in the left column first and then the right column.

Safety Strategies	Why Are They Important?

Setting the Scene

PRODUCTION
DIRECTOR
CAMERA
DATE SCENE TAKE

Staying Safe

You are excited about going to your first big celebration with students from school. The party will kick off the new school year and welcome new students. The party is on the other side of town in an area you do not visit often. One of your friends will drive you to and from the party. You are not familiar with the people hosting the party, and your family will not be home when you come back. Instead, your family has asked that you call or text when you get home safely.

On the way to the party, your friend says you should check in on social media and let everyone know you are coming. Your friend also talks about inviting another student your friend met online. Your friend might give this online friend a ride home too. You feel a little uncomfortable, but you do not know what to say. If your friend wants to give this new friend a ride, too, that is your friend's business, right?

Thinking Critically

1. In this scenario, what factors might impact your safety at the party? Which of these factors can you control? not control?
2. How can you keep you and your friend safe in this situation? What could you say to your friend to express your discomfort and plan for safety?

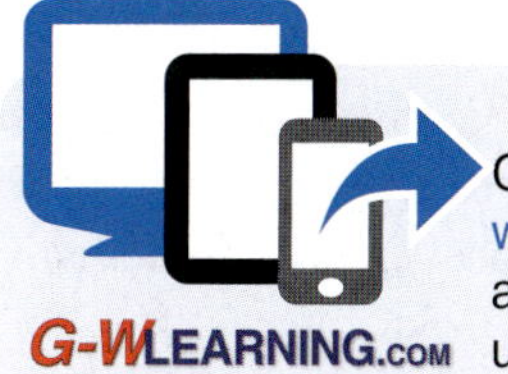

Click on the activity icon or visit www.g-wlearning.com/health/4095 to access online vocabulary activities using key terms from the chapter.

Lesson 16.1

Preventing Accidents and Injuries

Essential Question?

What steps can you take to prevent accidents and injuries?

Learning Outcomes

After studying this lesson, you will be able to

- discuss how to prevent falls inside and outside the home;
- identify poisonous substances and how to respond if someone is poisoned;
- analyze what you should do if you encounter a weapon;
- describe strategies for ensuring safety on the road;
- explain how OSHA requirements and ergonomics promote a safe workplace; and
- summarize ways to stay safe in the water.

Key Terms

ergonomics
pedestrians
poisonous
weapon

Warm-Up Activity

What Do Your Classmates Know?

Comprehend Concepts Recreate the chart shown and then walk around the classroom, trying to find classmates who meet the criteria in each box. Have each classmate explain an answer to the prompt and then sign the box. A different classmate must sign each box. Try to be the first to get a signature in all the boxes. Then, discuss with the class what you and your classmates learned.

I can name three poisonous substances around my home. Signature: ________	I can name three things to stay away from in nature. Signature: ________	I can name three ways to stay safe while in the car. Signature: ________
I can name three dangers of walking, bicycling, or skateboarding to school while wearing my headphones. Signature: ________	I can name three reasons why there are rules to follow at work and school. Signature: ________	I can name three things that should stay locked up and monitored at home or school. Signature: ________

As you gain more independence during the teen years, you will be able to do more activities alone or with friends. You may learn to drive and probably spend part of your day online chatting with friends. All of these activities have benefits and risks. Learning to manage the risks and stay safe will help you maintain your health, grow, and meet your goals for the future. In this lesson, you will learn about skills for preventing accidents and injuries.

Fall Prevention

Did you know that falls cause almost one-half of traumatic brain injuries (such as concussions) in the United States? People can be injured by falls anywhere. In fact, for young people, many fatal falls happen in public places like parks. Falls also happen at home while a person is doing daily activities.

Hazards in the environment cause some falls. Other falls may occur because of a medical condition or the influence of drugs or alcohol. Often, falls occur because a person takes a dangerous risk or is not paying attention. A simple fall can result in a broken bone, traumatic brain injury, or other medical condition. Depending on the severity of the fall, some injuries can even result in death.

One way to prevent falls is to reduce the hazards in your home (**Figure 16.1**). You can also reduce your risk for falls by being aware of your environment, both indoors and outdoors. For example, many falls occur because people text or use social media while walking. Distracted walking can also lead to a motor vehicle accident. Some communities issue tickets to people who text and walk.

The activities you choose to do can also put you at risk for serious accidents and falls. For example, *buildering* (climbing city structures) and *urban exploration* (entering abandoned buildings) can easily result in injuries, paralysis, or death. These activities are often illegal because they are dangerous and involve trespassing on private property.

People can also fall while taking selfies in dangerous locations, such as on a cliff or at a busy intersection. It is tempting to take photos in high places overlooking beautiful landscapes, but people can lose their footing or become distracted. Paying attention to your surroundings, especially in unfamiliar places, can help you stay safe and avoid a fall or other injury.

Reducing Fall Hazards in the Home

- Clear the floors and stairs of clutter.
- Keep electrical cords and telephone lines away from walkways.
- Cover slippery floors with nonslip rugs.
- Install handrails for stairs.
- Install grab bars in bathtubs and near toilets for people with limited mobility.
- Use step stools or ladders to reach high cabinets or shelves.
- Ensure good lighting by replacing burned light bulbs and using night-lights.
- Repair or replace worn carpet edges and seams.

Figure 16.1 Many hazards in the home can increase the risk of a fall.

Poisoning Prevention

At home and in your environment, some substances are dangerous. Some chemicals can cause serious health effects, and some plants can cause severe reactions. A **poisonous** substance can cause illness or death on entering the body. Knowing about these substances can help you avoid them at home and in the community (**Figure 16.2**).

poisonous capable of causing illness or death on entering the body

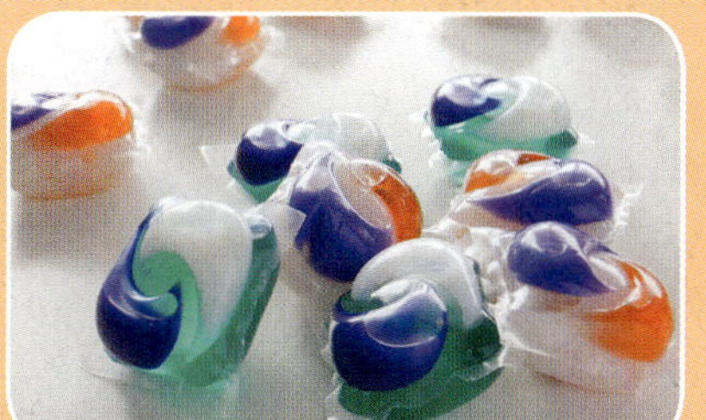

Poisonous Substances Around the Home

- Cleaning products
- Garden and yard products
- Automotive chemicals
- Gasoline
- Carbon monoxide

Stockpot Videos/Shutterstock.com

Figure 16.2 Many of the chemical materials in and around your home contain poisonous substances.

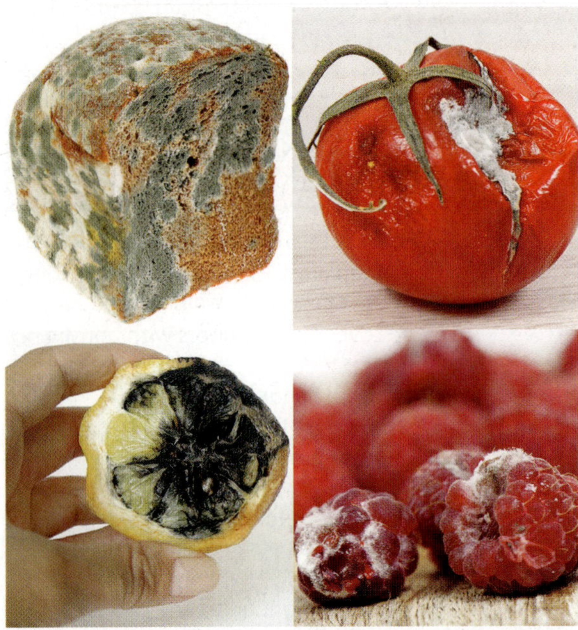

Left to right: ra3rn/Shutterstock.com; ratmaner/Shutterstock.com; Bimolka_gallery/Shutterstock.com; rsooll/Shutterstock.com

Figure 16.3 Certain fungi, such as mold, produce poisons. Molds are microscopic fungi, but may be visible as black, green, or brown fuzz on food. Mold growing on food can cause food poisoning.

To prevent illness or injury from potentially hazardous products, read and follow label directions for safe use. Store all chemicals in original containers in a locked area that children and pets cannot access. When using a chemical, wear protective equipment required by the label directions (for example, goggles, gloves, or a mask). Dispose of chemicals as described on the label.

Natural substances can also be poisonous. For example, certain plants, including some mushrooms and berries, are poisonous if eaten. Unless you are certain about the safety of a plant or plant part, do not eat it. Plant poisoning may cause an upset stomach, vomiting and diarrhea, cramps, convulsions, weakness, confusion, coma, and even death. People should also avoid consuming mold, which may grow on food and cause food poisoning. To prevent mold, store food in the refrigerator and discard it if it appears moldy (**Figure 16.3**).

If poisoning does occur, call the Poison Control Center (800-222-1222) immediately. You may need to seek emergency healthcare at a hospital, urgent care clinic, or emergency room.

Weapons Safety

weapon any object used to cause damage to an object or person

A **weapon** is any object used to cause damage to another object or person. Examples of weapons include firearms, swords, knives, bows and arrows, and bombs. Weapons can be very dangerous, and many federal and state laws govern who can possess them and how they can be used. Some adults may keep a weapon in the home for hunting, personal safety, or a collection. This can pose serious dangers. Accidents involving weapons can seriously injure or kill someone.

To help prevent accidents involving weapons, adults should keep firearms and other weapons locked in a safe place out of reach of other people, especially children. When storing a firearm, adults should remove the ammunition (bullets) and keep it in another locked place away from the firearm.

If you happen to see a weapon such as a firearm, leave the area without touching the firearm. Find a trusted adult to tell right away. It is very important to report any weapon you find, as well as any person who was using or playing with the weapon. It is also important to report if you hear anyone talking about using a weapon or see photos or messages about using a weapon online. These safety rules apply wherever you are—in your own home, at school, and any place you visit.

Road Safety

Did you know that motor vehicle accidents are the leading cause of death among young people? In fact, motor vehicle accidents account for about 70 percent of deaths associated with unintentional injuries. Six teens ages 16–19 die every day because of a motor vehicle accident. Thankfully, there are steps you can take as a pedestrian, passenger, and driver to reduce your risk of accidental injury.

Pedestrian Safety

Pedestrians are people on foot or using methods of transportation with small wheels (for example, bicycles, skateboards, or wheelchairs). Pedestrians have the "right of way" when traveling along a road. This is the legal right of a pedestrian to move before a vehicle moves, in certain situations. For example, if a vehicle comes to a stop sign, and pedestrians are waiting at the corner, the pedestrians have the right of way to cross the street first. The driver must respect that right and allow the pedestrians to cross.

pedestrians people on foot or using methods of transportation with small wheels (for example, bicycles, skateboards, or wheelchairs)

As a pedestrian, you also have responsibilities. To avoid an accident, always assume that drivers cannot see you. Drivers should stop for pedestrians, but that does not mean they always do. Pay attention and make eye contact with drivers at intersections. Be where drivers would expect, which is on sidewalks or in a bike lane. If using the road, travel *facing* traffic, not in the direction of traffic. If using a bike lane, ride in the direction of traffic in single file. Whenever possible, use crosswalks, and always obey traffic signals. If you must travel at night, wear bright or reflective clothing or carry a flashlight.

When bicycling, skateboarding, or rollerblading, always wear the appropriate safety gear, such as a helmet that fits. At intersections, obey pedestrian signals or signal your turns so drivers can anticipate your movements. With your left arm, point left to indicate a left turn and bend your forearm up to indicate a right turn.

Motor Vehicle Safety

Drivers and passengers both play a role in motor vehicle safety. This is because passengers can influence whether a driver is paying attention or obeying traffic laws. The most important safety precaution you can take as a passenger is to wear a seat belt. You can also avoid distracting the driver. Any distractions, such as noisy passengers, can make it difficult for the driver to concentrate. This increases the risk of an accident. Passenger safety is important whether you are in a car or school bus or riding public transportation (**Figure 16.4**).

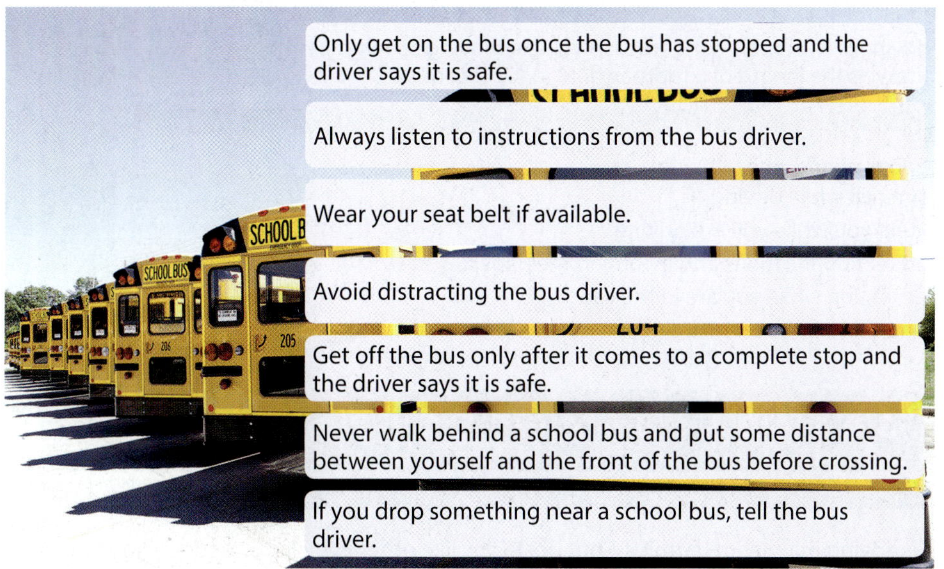

Figure 16.4 Paying attention and following the rules getting on, riding, and getting off school buses can help prevent accidents and injuries.

When you are driving, you are primarily responsible for the safety of yourself and any passengers. Your behaviors directly impact whether you get to your destination safely or experience an accident. Ways of ensuring safety as the driver include the following:

- **Wear your seat belt:** The National Highway Traffic Safety Administration (NHTSA) reports that 47 percent of people who die in motor vehicle accidents are not wearing a seat belt. Wearing a seat belt reduces risk for injury in an accident by 50 percent.
- **Drive defensively:** Aggressive driving and road rage are major factors contributing to motor vehicle crashes. Instead of driving aggressively, drive defensively. Leave distance between yourself and other drivers and focus on getting to your destination safely.
- **Obey traffic laws:** Traffic laws protect the safety of drivers. For example, speed limits reduce the risk for severe injuries. Stop signs and traffic lights promote orderly flow of traffic. Even one driver disobeying a traffic light or speeding can cause a motor vehicle crash. Obey these laws to keep yourself and other drivers safe.
- **Give driving your full attention:** Did you know that about 25 percent of motor vehicle crashes involve talking or messaging on a phone? Distracted driving is a major risk factor for injury. Well-known distractions include talking on the phone, messaging, or using social media (**Figure 16.5**). In some states, using your phone while driving is illegal. Eating, drinking, talking with passengers, and using a vehicle's radio, video equipment, and GPS navigation can also distract drivers.
- **Avoid drowsy driving:** Driving while drowsy causes at least 5,000 deaths in motor vehicle crashes each year. People are three times more likely to have a crash if they drive while drowsy. This is because not getting enough sleep reduces a person's reaction time and alertness. You can avoid drowsy driving by getting enough sleep. If you are tired while driving, pull over in a safe place to take a short nap or call for a ride. Read medication labels and do not drive after taking a medication that causes drowsiness.

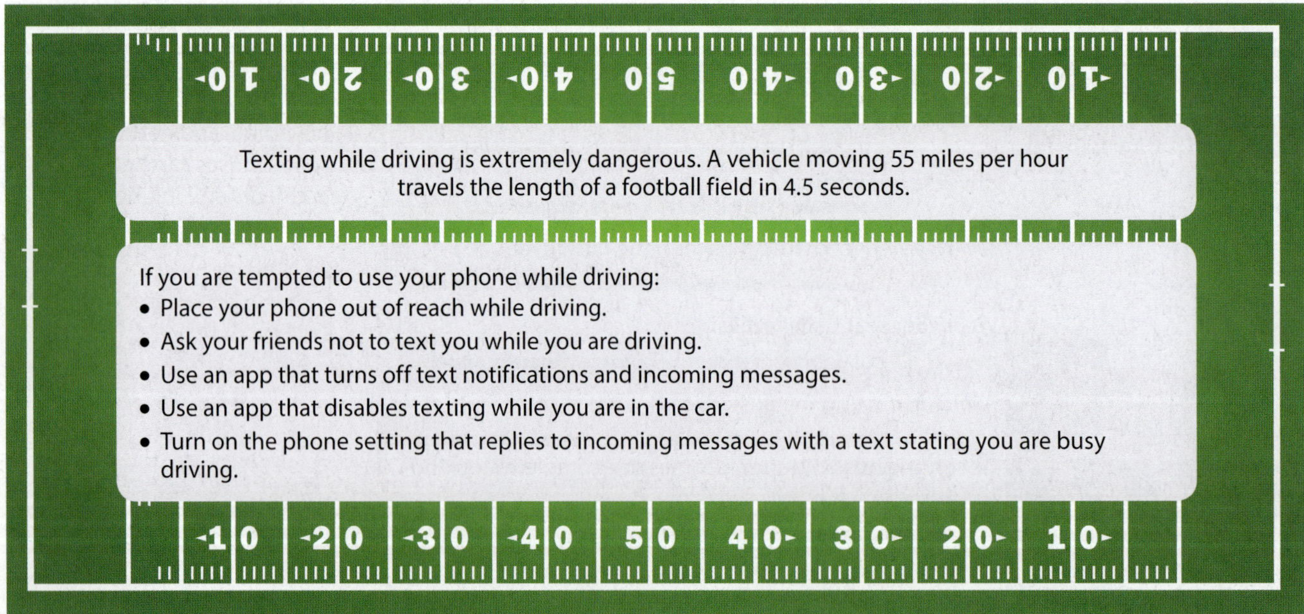

Mr.Timoty/Shutterstock.com

Figure 16.5 Using your phone while driving may seem harmless, but obstacles like other vehicles or pedestrians can enter the path of your vehicle quickly and without warning. ***How many motor vehicle accidents involve phone use?***

- **Do not drive under the influence:** Even a single alcoholic drink significantly reduces a driver's coordination and attention. Alcohol use is involved in about 10,000 deaths in motor vehicle crashes each year. Never drive under the influence of alcohol or any other drug and do not enter a vehicle with a driver who has been drinking alcohol or using drugs. Instead, call a parent or guardian, trusted adult, friend, or rideshare for a ride home.

Workplace Safety

In the US, laws guarantee all workers certain rights to safety in the workplace. Employers are responsible for providing their employees with a working environment free from known dangers and hazards. The law that protects workers and gives them rights is called the *Occupational Safety and Health Act*. This law is enforced by the Occupational Safety and Health Administration (OSHA), a specific branch of the Department of Labor (**Figure 16.6**).

Workers are responsible for following the policies and procedures in place to protect their health and safety. They should ask about any hazards and dangers in the workplace and alert their supervisors to unsafe work practices or working conditions. Workers have the right to refuse to do work that could cause injury or illness. They cannot be fired or disciplined for reporting workplace hazards and dangers.

OSHA Protections for Workers

- If known hazards are present in the workplace, employers must inform workers before they begin their work.
- Employers must train workers in the safe and correct execution of their duties.
- Employers must train workers to handle workplace emergencies and accidents.
- Employers must provide workers with equipment such as helmets, goggles, and earplugs, if needed to work safely.

Figure 16.6 Under the laws enforced by OSHA, workers have the right to a safe working environment.

Health in the Media

Social Media Challenges and Dares

On social media, people can share experiences, ideas, and feelings and communicate instantly with friends and family members. Some people who use social media participate in *social media challenges* or *social media dares*. Some of these challenges or dares are harmless or even health-promoting. Others encourage people to engage in risky, harmful, and potentially deadly activities. Often, people who participate film themselves and share their videos with others. In some cases, one person anonymously coordinates these activities and uses messages or sometimes threats to convince others to carry out the activities.

Social media challenges or dares can take many forms. Some involve dancing or trying certain poses. Examples of dangerous challenges or dares include consuming hazardous substances, stepping out of moving vehicles, drinking alcohol, or posing in dangerous places for "extreme selfies." Participation in dangerous challenges can have negative consequences, such as harm to a person's reputation, injury or death, legal consequences if engaging in activities that break laws, and embarrassment.

Practice Your Skills

Access Information

In a small group, use reliable resources to research one social media challenge or dare that is active right now. How did this challenge or dare start? What does it encourage people to do? Research the potential consequences of participating in this challenge or dare. Would you recommend that teens participate in this challenge or dare? Why or why not? Create a public service announcement (PSA) with this information and share it on social media.

Figure 16.7 Working or playing on the computer with an ergonomic arrangement helps prevent back and neck pain, eyestrain, and headaches. ***Which common injury causes swelling in a nerve in the wrist?***

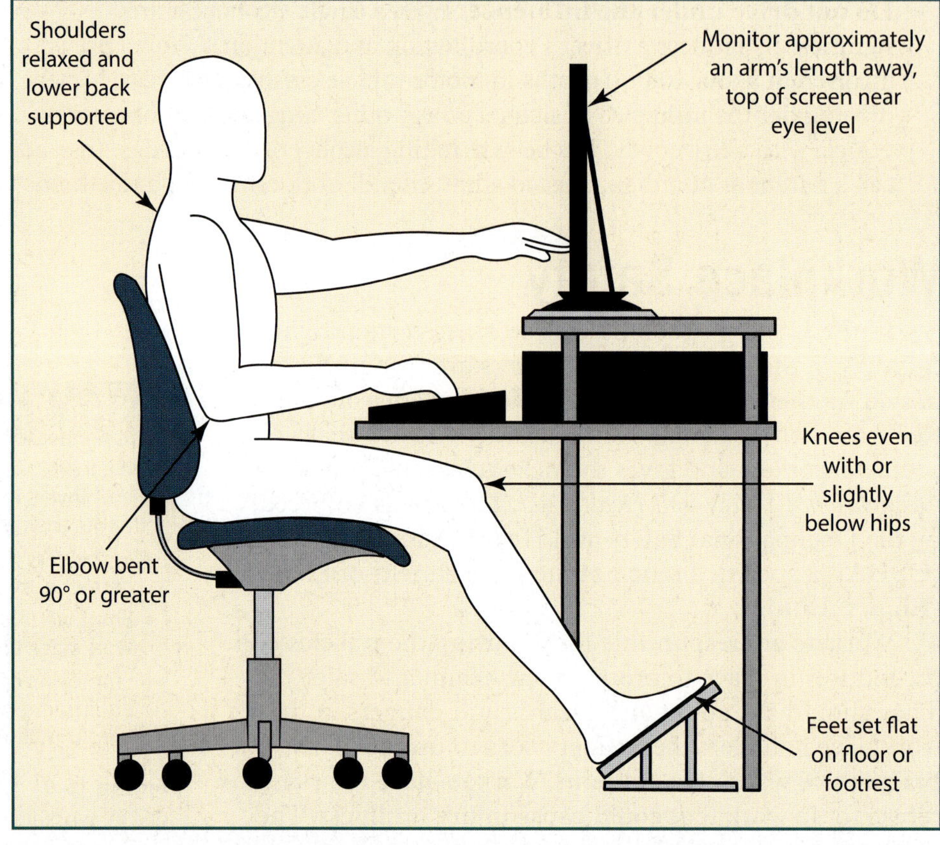

Teens should be aware of labor laws that specifically apply to teen workers. For example, certain types of jobs are too dangerous for teens. Laws describe which jobs teens can and cannot do. These laws also describe acceptable hours for teen workers, on weekends and school days.

ergonomics practices that ensure health and safety during the performance of a task

In addition to following safety rules, you can also protect your health by using **ergonomics**, or practices that ensure health and safety during the performance of a task. Many kinds of work require repeated movements that could cause *repetitive strain injuries (RSIs)*. *Tendinitis*, inflammation of a tendon, is a type of repetitive strain injury. Another common injury is *carpal tunnel syndrome*, a painful swelling of a nerve in the wrist. Practicing ergonomics can help reduce the risk of these injuries (**Figure 16.7**).

Water Safety

When the weather is hot, people often engage in water-related activities such as swimming in the local public swimming pool, sailing, water-skiing, and spending time at the beach. This means that water-related accidents can occur. Whenever you are around water, take precautions for preventing drowning. For example, it is important to never leave children alone in or near water of any kind, even when lifeguards are on duty. This also means never leaving children alone in bathtubs. Drowning can occur in minutes when someone stops paying attention or turns away.

To protect yourself from drowning, wear a life jacket when boating and never swim alone or in unsupervised areas. Do not dive in shallow water. Before getting in the water, check the weather to see if a storm is coming. Do not swim in a river after a storm because currents may be stronger. Also check the water temperature and avoid swimming in very cold water.

If you believe someone is drowning, call 911 or tell someone to call right away. The American Red Cross recommends that untrained rescuers avoid entering the water. Drowning people panic and might push you down, drowning you. Instead, throw the drowning person a flotation device, life jacket, rope, or any object that will float.

Lesson 16.1 Review

Know and Understand

1. What should you do if you suspect a poisoning has occurred?
2. What distractions make driving riskier for students at your school? What steps could you take to reduce these distractions?
3. Why does the American Red Cross recommend that untrained people not enter the water to help someone who is drowning? What does the American Red Cross recommend instead?

Think Critically

4. Research a recent news story about a person who experienced a fall due to distracted walking or another risky behavior. Rewrite the news story to show preventive strategies.
5. With a partner, brainstorm situations involving weapons that you would need to report to your school or a trusted adult. Create a guide for students about what to report.
6. In a small group, research ergonomic guidelines for a task you perform every day. Film a short video explaining proper ergonomics and how they protect safety and health.

REAL WORLD Health Skills

Practice Health-Enhancing Behaviors With a partner, look at each image that follows. Assess how safe each situation is and discuss any risks present in the situation. Then, for each image, identify three safety precautions the person could take to make the situation safer and promote health. Share your precautions with another pair.

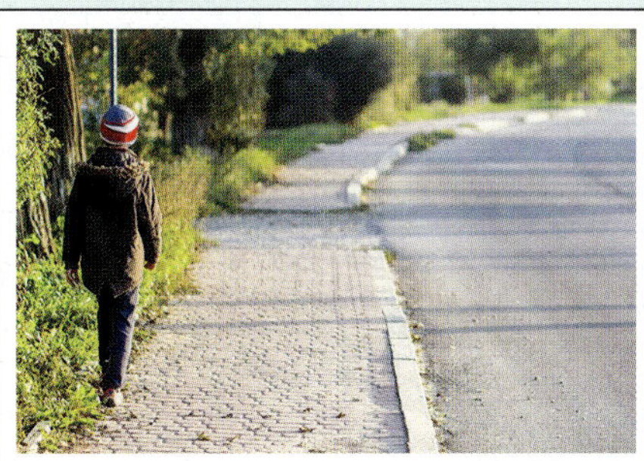

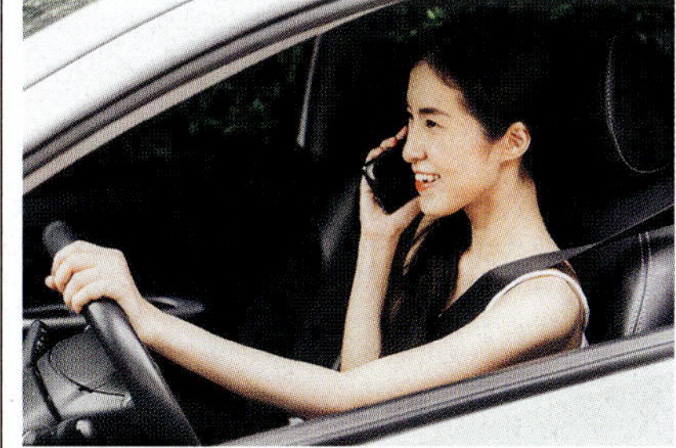

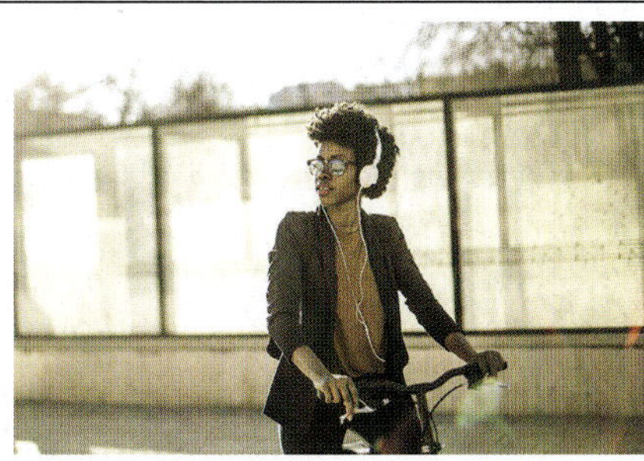

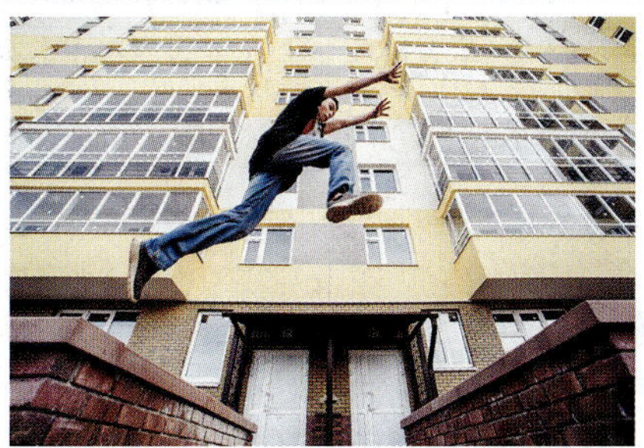

Clockwise from top left: Bilanol/Shutterstock.com; Twinsterphoto/Shutterstock.com; Anna Berdnik/Shutterstock.com; Ollyy/Shutterstock.com

Lesson

16.2

Handling Dangerous Situations

Essential Question?

How can you protect yourself in situations that have the potential to cause harm?

Learning Outcomes

After studying this lesson, you will be able to

- assess strategies for staying safe when home alone;
- explain the importance of following school rules and reporting violent behavior;
- identify safety precautions to take among strangers and in social situations;
- analyze how to prevent and respond to fires; and
- describe how to prepare for an emergency or disaster.

Key Terms

disaster
emergency preparedness
escape plan
fire triangle
natural disasters

Warm-Up Activity

The Truth About Safety

Communicate with Others In small groups, review each statement shown in the table that follows. Before reading this lesson, discuss in your group whether you think each statement is true or false. During your discussion, use effective communication and negotiation skills. Defend your opinions and work together to come to a consensus. Then, revisit your conclusions after reading this lesson. Work as a team to review your answers, if necessary.

Statement	True	False
A fire needs four things to continue burning.		
When you leave and go somewhere, you should not tell anyone where you are going.		
When you are home alone, you should tell a lot of people.		
Schools have rules to keep you and others safe.		
It is okay to accept food and drinks from strangers.		
There is little use in planning how to handle an emergency in the home.		
If someone is doing something dangerous at school, it is best to keep quiet.		
You should know when all natural disasters are coming.		
Practicing what you would do in an emergency promotes safety.		
It is important to remove yourself from uncomfortable situations.		

Practicing safety means protecting yourself from the threats in your environment, such as poisonous substances, water, and falls. It also means avoiding dangerous situations at home, at school, and in your community. To keep yourself safe, you can use caution in situations where you are alone or with other people.

Staying Safe at Home

When you are at home, and especially when you are alone, you can take steps to ensure your safety and avoid a dangerous situation. Your parents or guardian have probably set rules for you to follow when you are home. It is important to follow these rules, which are meant to keep you safe and prevent accidents. If you are home alone after school, your parent or guardian may expect you to call and check in. Other rules may involve whether you can leave to go to a friend's house or have friends come over. There may also be rules about whether you can do any cooking.

In addition to following the rules set by your family, other precautions you can take include the following:

- Know whom you can call if you need help. Make sure this person's phone number and address are easily accessible.
- Tell your parent or guardian if you are having anyone over. When you are home alone, do not invite people you do not know very well.
- Do not leave home without telling your parent or guardian where you are going and when you will return.
- Make sure that all doors and windows are locked.
- Never unlock the door for strangers, including delivery people.
- Do not go outside to check out any unusual noises or situations. If a situation is alarming, call your parent or guardian or the police.
- Do not tell anyone in person, on the phone, or online that you are home alone. Instead, say that your parent or guardian is home, but is busy.

Staying Safe at School

Your school may feel like a very safe place, and it probably is most of the time. At times, however, you might encounter dangerous situations at your school. Someone may try to start a fight. Another student may bring a weapon into the school. You may experience an injury during sports practice or class.

All schools have safety rules and procedures. Principals and school administrators set these rules to protect you from school-related hazards. For example, your school probably has a rule about not letting strangers into the building. This rule is in place to protect students and staff from violence or inappropriate behavior. Your school probably also has rules about behaving safely and wearing safety equipment such as helmets during sporting events or PE classes. Be sure to follow these safety rules and procedures whenever you are on school property.

You should also alert school staff to unsafe conditions, violence or threats of violence, and emergencies that may exist, such as the presence of weapons (**Figure 16.8**). By following these rules and reporting dangerous behavior, you ensure your safety and the safety of others. If you are uncomfortable about anything you see at school or during extracurricular activities, tell a teacher, coach, counselor, dean, or school security officer. Your school may also have an anonymous tip line or app.

Behaviors to Report

- You see a weapon.
- You hear people talking about the presence of a weapon.
- Someone threatens you or others with violence or talks about engaging in violent behavior—in person or online.
- Someone talks about considering or planning suicide.
- You see someone using or selling drugs.
- You see a suspicious person or vehicle.
- Someone intentionally damages classroom, laboratory, athletic, or other school equipment.
- Someone uses classroom chemicals or fire unsupervised or outside the classroom.
- Someone intentionally misuses or damages safety equipment such as fire alarms.

REPORT IT!
KEEP QUIET

iQoncept/Shutterstock.com

Figure 16.8 By alerting appropriate staff to potential risks, you may reduce the risk of an accident or injury occurring.

My Life, My Actions

Throughout your life, there will be many times you have to practice healthy behaviors to stay safe. As you progress through this activity, choose the option that best promotes safety for you and your family. At the end, see whether you are prepared to encounter potentially dangerous situations across your life span.

You arrive at home before your parents every day. Today, you realize you have left part of your school project at a friend's house.

You figure you will just go get it and be back before your parents arrive home, but you end up staying for a couple hours. Your parents are worried and upset when you arrive home.

You message your parents to let them know where you are going and then message again when you arrive at your friend's house. You know telling them where you are keeps them happy and you safe.

You live in an area prone to natural disasters. Your school recently held a disaster-preparedness seminar to raise awareness.

You tell your family about the seminar, but do not act on the information you learned. You and your family are unprepared when a natural disaster occurs.

You tell your family about what you learned, and together you come up with a disaster-preparedness plan. You know exactly what to do when a natural disaster strikes your area.

You have a lot of followers on social media who like your pictures. You are very open about your life and are active on social media. You start receiving messages from strangers asking you personal questions.

You ignore the messages and keep sharing, but since you are not careful about what you share, someone steals your identity and opens credit cards.

You are not comfortable with the messages, so you decide to make your profiles private so only your friends can see what you post. You also take down many old posts that reveal personal information.

You are cleaning your home, and your toddler is helping. You are using some toxic substances that could be harmful if swallowed.

You leave out the cleaning supplies, and your child accidentally ingests some of it. You have to rush your child to the hospital for treatment.

You make sure to put away any toxic substances after use. You also make sure to supervise your child around potentially harmful substances.

Your elderly parents move in with you and your family. They are not as mobile as they used to be and fall easily. You worry about how to make sure they stay safe in your home.

You keep the floor clear of debris, but you do not make any other changes. Your parents have a hard time navigating your home.

You make sure to pick up the floor and secure all the rugs to prevent tripping. You also install handrails in the bathroom.

If you chose mostly green paths, good job! You are being responsible and safe. Keep up the good work!

If you chose mostly red paths, watch out! You are not taking enough precautions when it comes to potentially harmful situations.

Practice Your Skills

Practice Health-Enhancing Behaviors

Think of additional situations where you could practice personal safety in your own life and in the future. How would you react in each situation you describe? Share your situation with a classmate and brainstorm additional safety methods you could use.

Border: Red sun design/Shutterstock.com; Tape: gst/Shutterstock.com

Staying Safe in Public Places

As you get older, you will probably spend more and more time outside the home. You may start working; travel for extracurricular activities; or spend time with friends at the movies, a park, or the mall. Visiting these places and spending time with friends is part of developing independence. You may even gain the ability to drive yourself places and run errands at the local grocery store or library.

Among Strangers

When you are in public places, you are often around people you do not know. These people are *strangers*. To stay safe among strangers, you can take precautions such as the following:

- When you go out, tell your parent or guardian where you are going, how you will get there, who will be with you, and when you will be home.
- Carry identification, only enough money for your needs, and a charged cell phone with you.
- When you are walking, travel in well-lit areas, on main roads, and with other people. Pay attention to your surroundings.
- Do not go anywhere with or accept money or gifts from anyone you do not know. This includes letting a stranger give you a ride somewhere.
- If a stranger asks you for help or directions, do not get too close to the person. If you feel uncomfortable, leave the situation.
- If anyone makes you uncomfortable, get away from that person and tell a trusted adult right away.
- If someone confronts you and tries to steal your purse or phone, hand the items over without fighting. Trying to stop the person will only put you in more danger.

In Social Situations

Even among people you know, it is important to pay attention to your safety. Some social situations can put you at risk for injury, violence, sexual assault, and criminal activity (**Figure 16.9**).

Staying Safe in Social Situations

Tell your parent, guardian, or a trusted adult where you are going, how you are getting there, how long you will be gone, and how the person can contact you.	Do not go to unsupervised parties. Before the party, make sure an adult will be present.	Do not go anywhere with unfamiliar people. If you will be in a social situation where unfamiliar people are present or are going to an unfamiliar place, take a trusted friend or adult with you.
Leave social situations if drugs or alcohol are present. Never use drugs or alcohol in any social situation.	Do not enter a vehicle with a driver who has been using drugs or alcohol. If you cannot drive, call your parent, guardian, or a trusted adult for a ride.	In social situations, do not accept food or drinks from other people. Get your own food and drinks and watch them to make sure others do not put anything else in them.

Figure 16.9 Using certain precautions can help you stay safe in social situations.

Preparing for Emergencies

An emergency is a situation with the potential to cause great harm to people and property. Some examples of emergencies include fires, natural disasters, and violent attacks like terrorism. How you respond in the event of an emergency can determine your level of safety. Before an emergency occurs, you can protect your safety by practicing **emergency preparedness**. This involves knowing how to respond to a specific type of emergency and remaining calm.

emergency preparedness
steps one takes to ensure safety before, during, and after an emergency or natural disaster

fire triangle
representation of the three elements (fuel, heat, and oxygen) needed to start a fire

Fire Prevention and Safety

A fire is a dangerous emergency that can be deadly. There are three elements needed to start a fire: fuel (the material that is burning), heat, and oxygen. The **fire triangle**, also known as the *combustion triangle*, is a model that can help you remember these elements (**Figure 16.10**). When fuel, heat, and oxygen are present in the right amounts, a chemical reaction occurs that can start a fire. To *extinguish* (put out) the fire, you need to remove one element in the fire triangle. For example, putting a fire blanket over flames will remove the oxygen from the fire. When firefighters use water, they remove heat, which cools down the fire and extinguishes it.

To help prevent fires, inspect your surroundings to make sure the environment is safe. Properly installed smoke detectors can reduce your risk of injury and death from fire. It is important to test smoke detectors monthly and replace the batteries at least yearly. Also check for fire hazards such as frayed wires, overloaded outlets, and unattended cooking pans or candles.

Everyone should know the locations of fire extinguishers in a building and learn how to use them. Fire extinguishers can control small fires and prevent them from causing damage or injury. There are different types of fire extinguishers, so be sure to check labels carefully. Fire departments often provide training on how to properly use fire extinguishers.

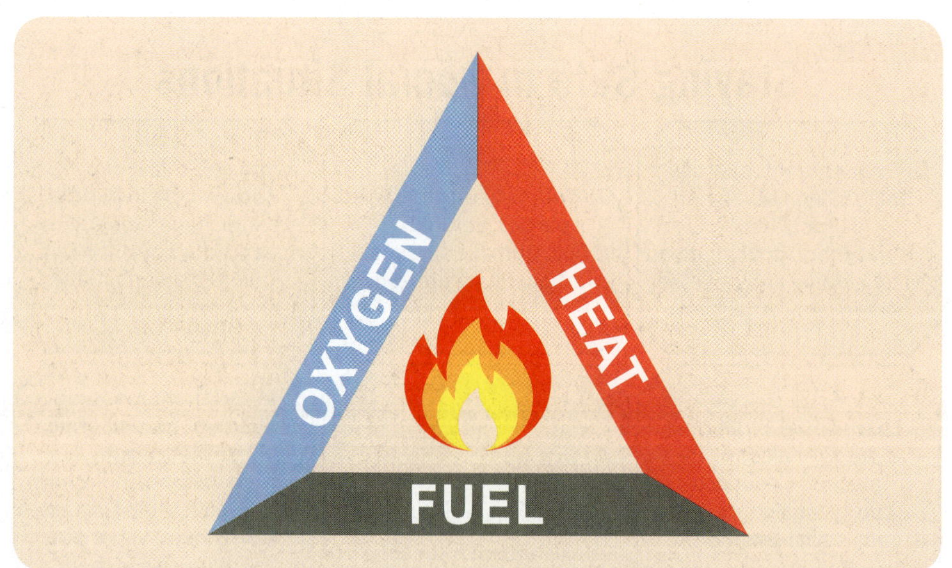

Figure 16.10 The fuel in the fire triangle refers to the material that is burning. Materials that are easily set on fire are *flammable*. Examples of flammable materials include wood, oils, paper, fabrics, and some liquids. When a heat source, such as a match, comes in contact with flammable materials, a fire starts. To burn, the fire needs oxygen.

BALRedaan/Shutterstock.com

Even with prevention efforts, a fire may break out. This is why families, schools, and other organizations should have an escape plan in place. An **escape plan** outlines safe routes and procedures for leaving a building in the event a fire occurs (**Figure 16.11**).

escape plan document that outlines safe routes and procedures for leaving an area or building during an emergency

It is important to practice an escape plan before a fire occurs. Many schools conduct *fire drills* so teachers and students can practice the school's escape plan. You can also practice a fire escape plan with your family. During the practice, make sure everyone knows how to respond to the sound of the smoke alarm. You may want to have a family member time how long it takes everyone to exit the home.

As you leave a building that is on fire, you can follow certain procedures to stay safe. These include the following:

- Identify at least two ways to get out of each room in a fire. During a fire, feel doors with the back of your hand before opening them. If the door is hot, escape another way, such as through a window. If you are trapped in a room, keep the door closed and signal or call for help.
- Make sure that all bedrooms in your home have a window that opens quickly and is easy to unlock.
- If you can, alert people about the fire. Get out of the building and call 911. Take the stairs instead of an elevator.
- Crawl near the floor to escape dangerous smoke, toxic fumes, and heat, which rise toward the ceiling.
- If your clothing catches fire, stop, drop, and roll to put out the flames.
- Once outside, never reenter a burning building.

Disaster Preparedness

Like a fire, a disaster requires you to prepare and act quickly. A **disaster** is a large-scale event that causes harm to people or property.

disaster large-scale event that causes harm to people or property

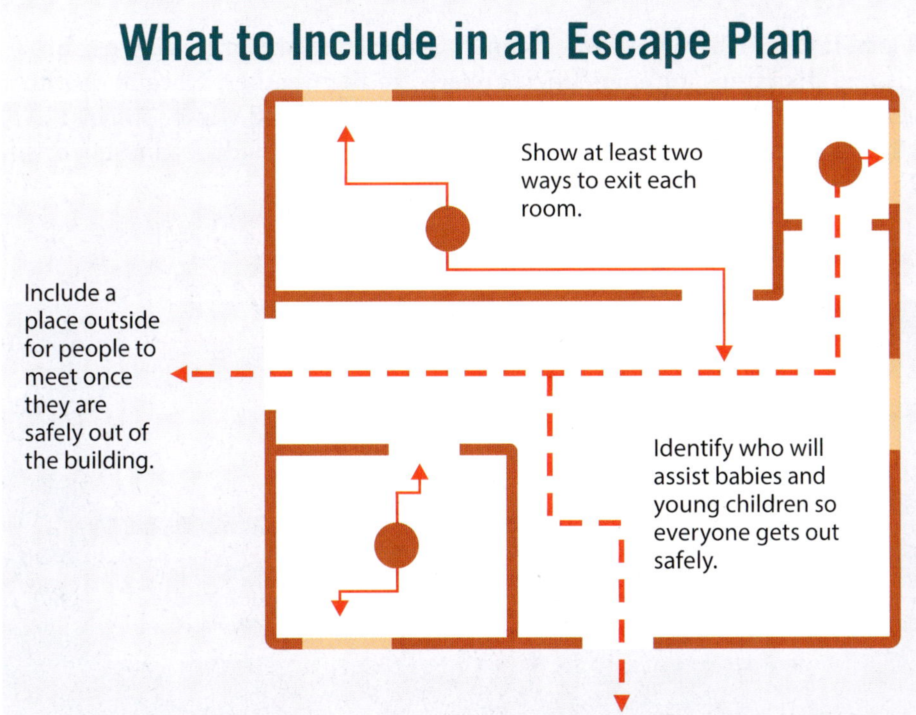

Figure 16.11 An escape plan should include multiple ways to exit each room of the building, an assigned person to assist babies and young children, and a location outside the building for everyone to meet. ***What devices help alert people to the presence of a fire?***

Local and Global Health

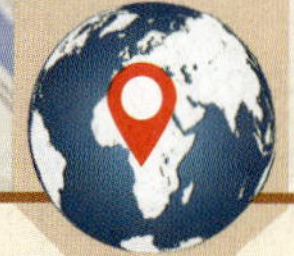

Extreme Weather and a Changing Climate

Did you know that, since the 1960s, the number of weather-related natural disasters around the world has more than tripled? Scientists cite rising average global temperature as one reason the frequency and severity of extreme weather have increased. Every year, weather-related disasters cause more than 60,000 deaths, primarily in low-income countries.

In the US, the National Oceanic and Atmospheric Administration recorded an average of 570 weather-related deaths each year over the last few decades. Floods are the most dangerous element of extreme weather and cause the most deaths. Deaths from floods have increased in recent years. The Union of Concerned Scientists predicts that the increased frequency and intensity of floods, hurricanes, and rainfall will also cause extensive property damage in US coastal communities.

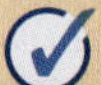

Practice Your Skills

Advocate for Health

If you have not experienced the effects of extreme weather, you might not understand why it is important to prepare. Extreme weather is becoming more common. It is wise to be prepared and make a plan in case of a weather-related disaster or emergency. To advocate for the health of your family and protect your safety, follow these steps:

1. **Meet with your family:** Discuss the types of extreme weather that could occur in your community or region. The National Weather Service and the National Oceanic and Atmospheric Administration are helpful resources for weather and climate information.
2. **Identify the potential weather-related hazards in your area:** What steps could you take to remain safe during extreme weather? How could you prepare for these hazards before they occur?
3. **Write an emergency plan:** In the plan, describe how your family will prepare for extreme weather and how you will remain safe if a weather-related emergency occurs. Share the plan with your family and be sure everyone understands the plan.

natural disasters
emergencies caused by naturally occurring events, such as floods, earthquakes, wildfires, or hurricanes; cause great damage or loss of life

Depending on where you live, you may experience one or more types of **natural disasters**, or emergencies related to the weather. Natural disasters include tornadoes, floods, hurricanes, earthquakes, and winter storms. Other disasters may include power failure, landslide, wildfire, and terrorism (**Figure 16.12**).

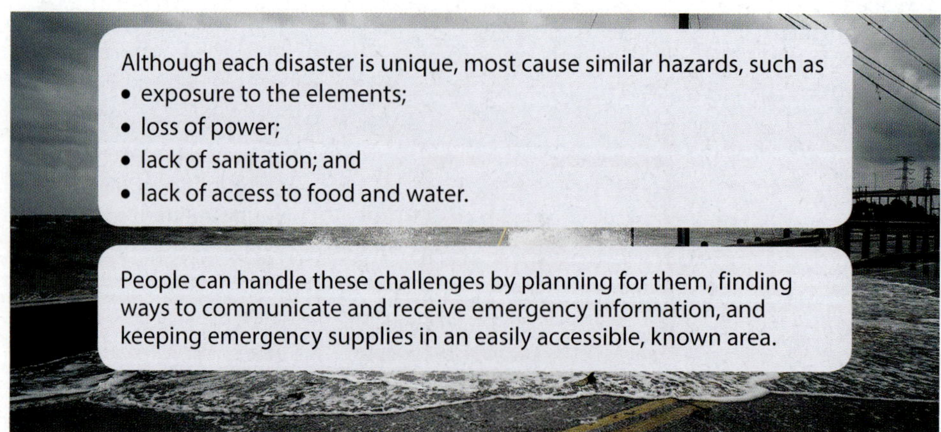

Cire notrevo/Shutterstock.com

Figure 16.12 Different disasters are common in different seasons and locations, but specific strategies can help people plan for any disaster. ***What is the name of a disaster related to the weather?***

To prepare for disasters, people can also write an emergency plan, which will answer the following questions:

- Where will you take shelter? For example, plan to go to a basement or a sturdy inner room, such as a bathroom, during a tornado. If you live in an area affected by hurricanes or floods, know evacuation routes and shelters.
- How will you communicate with your family? Do you know how to reach a parent or guardian at work? Can you designate a contact person who lives outside the area to share information with all family members? How and where will you meet if family members are separated?
- Whom will you contact for emergency assistance, and how will you contact them? For example, know how to contact the police, fire department, and paramedics in an emergency.
- What supplies and equipment will you need? Where will the supplies be located? What do you need to do to make sure these supplies are available?
- How will you learn when the danger has passed?

Lesson 16.2 Review

Know and Understand

1. In your school, what behaviors need to be reported if you see them? How and to whom should you report dangerous behavior?
2. Choose one strategy for staying safe among strangers or in social situations. Rewrite this strategy into a catchy slogan you and your classmates can easily remember. As a class, create your own list of safety slogans.
3. In the event of a fire, why should you crawl near the floor to escape?
4. What precautions can people take to prepare for a disaster?

Think Critically

5. Write a short scenario in which a teen encounters a situation at home that might threaten safety. Pass your scenario to a classmate and complete your classmate's scenario by having the teen respond in a safe way.
6. What disasters have you experienced in your lifetime? What did you and your family do to stay safe during these disasters?

REAL WORLD Health Skills

Make Decisions Find a partner and then create a dialogue or monologue of a situation where a teen might have to make a decision about a conversation with a stranger, time with acquaintances, or another social situation. For example, a stranger might be making the teen uncomfortable, or people may be acting unsafely at a party. In your dialogue or monologue, show how the teen uses the decision-making process to stay safe. Act out your dialogue or monologue for another group and discuss the following questions:

- How did you feel watching the teen handle this situation?
- Did you feel confident or shy about the decision your teen made?
- Can you envision yourself using these skills in the real world? Why or why not?

Lesson
16.3

Being Safe on the Internet

Essential Question?

What skills do you need for interacting safely online?

Learning Outcomes

After studying this lesson, you will be able to

- explain the importance of forming a positive digital footprint;
- list skills for evaluating online information;
- describe strategies for following rules and showing online etiquette;
- analyze the importance of keeping personal information private;
- discuss ways to avoid hacking and viruses; and
- assess the consequences of sharing inappropriate content.

Key Terms

anonymity
copyright
digital citizenship
digital footprint
flaming
hacking
identity theft
internet predators
online etiquette
phishing
privacy settings
sexting
trolling
virus

Warm-Up Activity

My Online Presence

Analyze Influences Before reading this lesson, list all the social media platforms you use. Then, consider the following questions:

- How many different accounts do you have with each social media platform?
- Do you know all the users who can see your social media account? How private are your accounts?
- Are your location settings enabled?
- Do you have some accounts simply because other people have them?
- Do you know exactly what other people can see and access about you online?
- Do you think that, by viewing all your social media accounts, someone could find out where you are and what you are doing? How does that make you feel?

After answering these questions, share them with a partner. Discuss how your answers to these questions influence your safety and health.

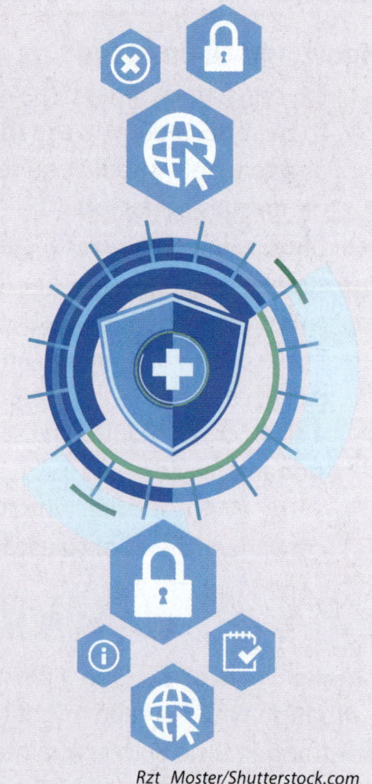

Rzt_Moster/Shutterstock.com

How much time do you spend online—chatting with your friends, playing video games, or sharing pictures and ideas? On average, teens spend about nine hours online each day. Learning to stay safe online can help you protect your health and avoid negative consequences.

The internet plays important roles in how people communicate, spend their free time, and obtain information. Over the course of your life, you have probably grown up knowing how to use the internet and communicate online. Internet use might be so familiar that you do not notice its many benefits, including instant connection and access to resources. At the same time, you might not think about the internet's potential dangers. In this lesson, you will learn skills for maintaining your safety and privacy online. You will also learn how misusing the internet can harm emotional and social health and even put you in physical danger.

Your Digital Footprint

When you walk in sand, your steps leave footprints that show where you were and what route you took. By looking at these footprints, people can learn about you and your location. On a beach, these footprints eventually get washed away. On the internet, however, the actions you take are not so easily erased or forgotten.

When you share a picture, post a message, or communicate with a friend online, these actions are recorded. Others can see your shared picture, screenshot what you sent, or read your post. Your friend can look back at old messages at any time. Even if you delete a picture or post, people can still find it. All of these actions, even those you took a long time ago, make up your **digital footprint** (**Figure 16.13**).

digital footprint all of the content people share, access, or have shared about them online

Your digital footprint can bring many advantages. Creating a positive digital footprint for yourself can bring you opportunities and help you learn about yourself. It can show others your identity, values, and personality, as well as your good qualities, accomplishments, and skills.

All of the strategies you will learn in this lesson can help you create a positive digital footprint. Remember that many people, including employers and college admissions staff, will see your digital footprint. The footprint you leave today will affect your success now and in the future.

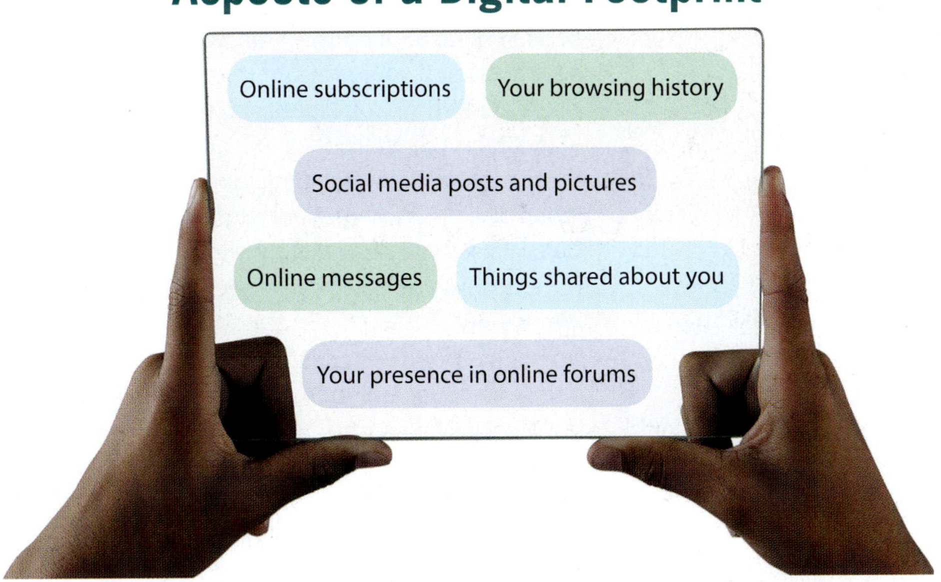

wavebreakmedia/Shutterstock.com

Figure 16.13 Your digital footprint contains information about you and your actions online. ***How can temporary posts online still become part of your digital footprint?***

Positive Online Behavior

anonymity notion that others do not know who a person is online

digital citizenship practice of taking responsible, healthy actions as part of the digital community

Sometimes, the internet can make people more likely to behave poorly. People do not have to see the person with whom they are talking. While they may not yell at a friend in-person, they may say hurtful words online. Some people think they have **anonymity**, or an unknown identity, online. This is rarely the case. Law enforcement, officials, and sometimes employers can usually trace a person's online identity. Poor behavior has consequences online, just as it does in person.

Behaving respectfully online is an important part of safety and your digital footprint. By engaging in positive online behaviors, you can practice **digital citizenship**, or responsible, healthy actions as part of the digital community.

Following the Rules Online

As with any social setting, certain rules govern people's behavior online. You have probably seen these rules when joining a website. The website may have asked you to verify your age or agree to a set of rules about acceptable and unacceptable behavior. Pay attention to rules and do not try to get around them. Do not try to fake your age and do not violate rules by posting violent, hateful, or sexual material. Many websites, including social media, will ban members who engage in these behaviors and may even report the behavior to law enforcement.

Skills for Health and Wellness

Promoting an Online Environment of Respect

As a digital citizen, you contribute to the online environment, which affects all areas of a person's health. This means you can help create a respectful, productive, and enjoyable environment on social media, websites, and chat rooms. This environment will then improve your health and the health of those around you. Skills in communicating respectfully and not tolerating disrespectful behavior can help you encourage this kind of environment.

Practice Your Skills

Set Goals

With a partner, review the following guidelines for promoting a respectful online environment. Choose one guideline and create a SMART goal to help you use it in daily life. Be specific and break your goal into several subgoals. Make a plan for overcoming any obstacles that get in your way. Put your goal into action and evaluate its effects on your life.

- Before posting, identify the topic under discussion. Learn what has been discussed and read any questions and answers already posted. Move the discussion forward and stay on topic.
- Ask questions related to the topic being discussed. To make the conversation easier to follow, post only one question at a time. Before asking another question, wait until others have answered your previous question.
- When answering a question, make sure you understand the question. If you do not, then ask the person to clarify what you do not understand.
- When disagreeing with people, do so respectfully. Do not insult the person with whom you disagree. For example, you could say, "I see it differently. Here's why."
- Do not insult, bully, or lie to others. Think carefully before you post. Do not respond to people who insult or bully you.
- If you observe unacceptable, violent, or threatening behavior, report this to a website administrator. You can usually find procedures for reporting on the website. Leave the website if the behavior continues.

The internet is a great way to share and find original material like music, videos, photos, art, and books. People use the internet to promote themselves and hope people find them online. Original material posted online is protected by copyright. A **copyright** states that the creator exclusively owns the original material and can use it in any way, including selling it. Copyright automatically applies to original materials as soon as they take physical or digital form. For example, a photo is copyrighted as soon as a person takes it. An essay is copyrighted as soon as it is written. Others are *not* allowed to claim to own the work or publish or share the work without permission.

copyright right of a creator to exclusively own original material and use it in any way

Copyright protects creators of original material. Think of a musical artist who writes a song. Copyright permits only the artist to make profits from selling the song. If people download the song without paying for it, they are breaking copyright laws, and the artist is not paid. Just as you would not steal a poster or book from someone's bedroom, you should not steal someone's online property, including images, videos, and words. Using someone's original material without permission is *stealing*.

Breaking copyright laws can lead to legal consequences and is poor online behavior. Digital citizens follow copyright laws and do not support those who break them (**Figure 16.14**). To avoid breaking copyright laws, do not download from or upload to unlicensed websites. If you want to repost or use material you see online, always ask the creator for permission. This can be as easy as asking, "Can I share this?" Once permission is given, credit the creator. On social media, the best way to provide credit is to directly share the original post. You can also link to the original post or creator.

Using Online Etiquette

Online etiquette describes positive online behaviors and effective communication techniques. Online etiquette promotes respectful communication and helps people have informative and positive online experiences. It is especially important in social media.

online etiquette positive behaviors and effective communication techniques that are expected online

The key to using online etiquette is *respect*. Think about how you speak to people face-to-face. If you disagree, do you insult them? Do you change the subject? Do you make fun of their statements and personal qualities?

Copyright Laws	
Action	**Legal or Illegal**
Purchasing and downloading music online	Legal; paying for the music
Recording a new movie in a theater and posting it online	Illegal; breaking copyright law
Using a photographer's photo in a blog post with permission and credit	Legal; creator giving permission for the photo's use and giving credit to the creator
Downloading music from an unlicensed website	Illegal; stealing the artist's work without paying
Watching a TV show on an unlicensed website	Illegal; watching the TV show on a website that stole it
Sending your friend a digital copy of an album you purchased	Illegal; sharing the work without permission from the creator
Downloading a photograph online and selling it as your own	Illegal; claiming to own the work
Reposting content someone else created on your own social media without permission	Illegal; distributing copyrighted material without permission

Figure 16.14 When accessing or sharing content online, including music, videos, photos, and words, make sure to follow copyright laws. ***When is copyright applied to original material?***

The goal of online discussions should be to understand a subject and share points of view. Changing the subject abruptly can be disrespectful. Insults and personal comments are poor etiquette, do not promote discussion, and can hurt people. In fact, some people become depressed and frightened when insulted and harassed online.

trolling drawing others into arguments and disrupting discussions

flaming writing mean and hateful comments with the intention of hurting others

People with online etiquette do not participate in trolling, flaming, or cyberbullying. **Trolling** is an online behavior in which people draw others into arguments and disrupt discussions. Trolls often do this by writing false statements or outrageous opinions. **Flaming** is writing mean and hateful comments with the intention of hurting others. If you encounter these behaviors online, ignore them and report them to the website administrator. *Cyberbullying*, which you learned about in Lesson 15.1, involves abusing or mistreating someone online. This type of abuse can have serious consequences. You should refuse to participate and tell a trusted adult if you see cyberbullying happening.

Online etiquette also requires honesty. You should not pretend to be someone else online or deceive people in other ways. Pretending to be someone else online is called *catfishing* and can hurt others and lead to public embarrassment and violence.

Privacy

Before the internet became widely used for shopping, communication, and social media, people kept much of their personal information private. This helped people keep certain information to themselves and avoid contact with strangers or people who might mean them harm. Today, people share much more information online. Sharing too much information about yourself can be dangerous. Sharing personal information especially can put you in a risky situation.

Keeping Personal Information Private

As you make friends and communicate online, you will probably share a lot of information about yourself. You will want to tell friends about your interests, activities, and plans. You might want to post pictures of your experiences and friends. Sharing information about your favorite books, shows, and activities can be fun and will not put you in danger. There is some personal information, however, that you should not share for your own safety.

Personal Information—What You Should Keep Private

Social Security number
Address
Phone number
Birthday
Hometown
School
Workplace
Current location
Bank account
Credit card number

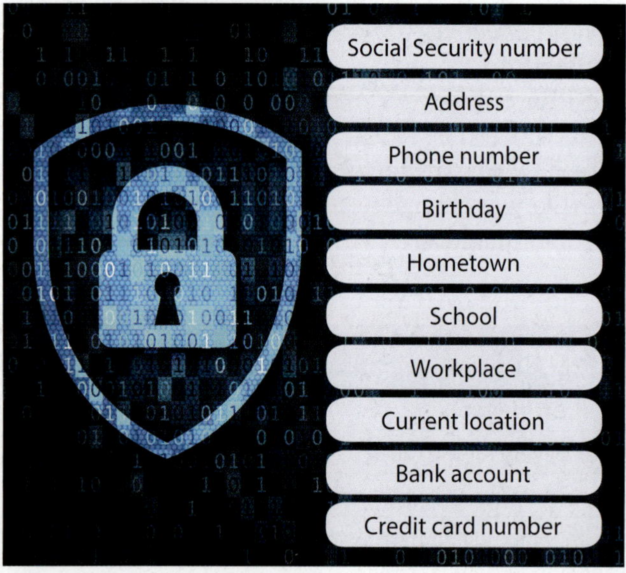

NicoElNino/Shutterstock.com

Figure 16.15 Protect any personal information that could help strangers identify you online.

Some personal information can make it possible for people to identify you or know where you are (**Figure 16.15**). This can lead to issues like **identity theft** (when people use your personal information to pretend to be you), financial theft, and unwanted interactions with people who might be dangerous. It can also put you in great danger from internet predators.

identity theft act of using people's personal information to pretend to be them

Internet predators use personal information to find and harm people or violate their privacy. Some predators pose as other people in chat rooms or social media. They may pretend to be teens and try to build trust by beginning an online relationship through discussions or private chats. Internet predators often ask for personal information, want to video-call, or want to meet in person. They may also use hacking to retrieve personal information or gather information from people's social media accounts and online posts.

internet predators people who use personal information to find and harm people or violate their privacy

To protect yourself from internet predators and other people who might use your personal information to harm you, do not post any personal information on social media or anywhere online. If you want to post this kind of information, talk with a parent or guardian first to make a plan for protecting your privacy. Keep in mind that sometimes the photos you post can also give away your information. Avoid posting photos of your school, home, or other locations that could help someone find you. Avoid tagging yourself at certain locations or indicating you will be at certain public events. In addition, always ask permission before sharing photos of another person. This shows respect for your friends' and classmates' privacy.

When talking with people you met online, *never* share personal information. Do not share photographs of yourself or agree to video-call or meet with someone you met online. A video-call can help an internet predator identify you. Meeting in-person can put you at risk for violence, human trafficking, or kidnapping. If someone you met online asks for your personal information or asks to video-call or meet with you, leave the conversation and tell a trusted adult what happened. If you want to share personal information, video-call, or meet with someone you met online, talk with your parent or guardian first. Your parent or guardian should go with you if you decide to meet.

Using Privacy Settings

Most social media websites have **privacy settings**, or features that allow you to control who can see your personal information (**Figure 16.16**). Using privacy settings, you can post a picture that your friends can see, but others cannot. Privacy settings do not make it safe to share personal information online. Using privacy settings, however, you can feel more comfortable sharing other facts about your life.

privacy settings features for controlling who can see personal information online

Tips for Using Privacy Settings

Try limiting those who can see your posts and accounts to people you know and friends.	Be careful about accepting social media requests or connecting with people you do not know well.	Check your privacy settings regularly and update them for maximum security.

Figure 16.16 Many social media websites default to minimal privacy settings. Check your accounts to make sure only people you know can see your personal information and the content you share. ***What personal information is connected to your social media accounts?***

Avoiding Fraud

Some people try to get personal information using *fraud*, or deception. For example, an internet predator might pretend to be someone your age. Someone might create a fake website to steal people's information (called *pharming*). When people pretend to be representatives of companies or government agencies and ask for personal information, this is called **phishing**. Phishing is an example of a *cybercrime*, or a crime that uses digital devices or the internet.

phishing pretending to represent companies or government agencies and asking for personal information

In phishing, a criminal tricks a person into opening a message, file, or link. The message might ask for personal information. The link might corrupt a digital device's files. Phishing is also called vishing or smishing.

Case Study

Navigating Life Online

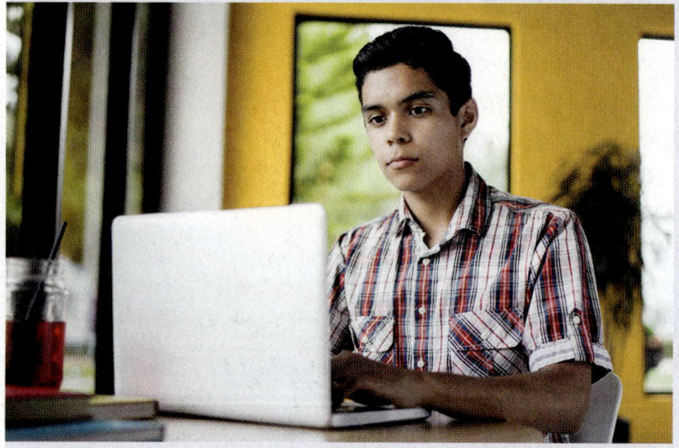

aldomurillo/E+/Getty Images

When Brooklyn was in high school, she never gave much thought to what she posted on social media. She would post rude comments about customers at her part-time job, complain about bad days, and share controversial articles and videos. Recently, Brooklyn graduated from college and is struggling to find a full-time job. At a recent interview, a potential employer advised Brooklyn to clean up her social media accounts because her posts from high school reflect poorly on her character.

Max follows a lot of celebrity athletes on social media. Lately, he has noticed the comments on their posts quickly get out of hand. People leave hateful comments, and trolls use outrageous statements to create arguments with friendly people. Max does not understand why people act this way online. He has never seen anyone act like this in real life! Max becomes overwhelmed when he looks at these posts, so he tries to limit how much he scrolls through celebrity content.

Iyanna is concerned for her friend, Summer. Summer's social media account is public. Iyanna has noticed Summer posts photos of herself and tags her locations to gain more likes and followers. Summer also shares information about her hometown and activities in school. Iyanna is worried someone may use this information to steal Summer's identity. Iyanna recently talked to Summer about switching her accounts to private.

Over the years, Jose has posted his animations on social media. A few of his animations have gone viral, and he is always both excited and frustrated. Jose knows the best way to make a career as an artist is for people to show an interest online. When people share his animations, however, only a few tag him as the original creator. He worked really hard on these animations and does not want others taking credit for his art.

Practice Your Skills

Advocate for Health

Make a list of tips for being safe and appropriate on the internet, including social media. In small groups, compare your lists. Choose one tip you think would help students at your school make better decisions online. Create an advocacy campaign for safe and appropriate internet use focused on this tip. Come up with a catchy slogan to help people remember your tip. Make a poster to hang in your school hallway or post on the school's website.

Vishing tricks a person using a telephone call or voice message. *Smishing* involves sending harmful links or videos.

To avoid phishing attempts, do not answer calls from unfamiliar numbers or open emails or messages from unknown senders. If a message contains a link, do not open it. Just delete the message. Do not respond to an email, message, or telephone call that asks for your personal information.

Hacking and Viruses

Even if you do not share your personal information, it may still be stored on devices such as phones and laptops. Personal information might also be stored on websites used for shopping, social media, or other activities. This personal information is vulnerable to **hacking**, a cybercrime in which someone uses computer code to open and read files on computers, websites, or other digital locations. The person does not need to use the device where a file is stored. If a device is connected to the internet, the person can hack it from distant locations. In addition to stealing personal information, the person can take over social media accounts and pretend to be someone else.

hacking cybercrime that uses computer code to open and read files on computers, websites, or other digital locations

Passwords help protect your personal information from hacking. A *password* is a code that acts like a key to files and information. A strong password is hard to guess, but easy to remember. Weak passwords include your name, a pet's name, simple words, or a predictable sequence of letters or numbers (**Figure 16.17**). To protect your privacy, do not share passwords with others or use the same password for different devices or websites. Change your password occasionally to keep anyone from guessing it. You can use a password manager app if you have trouble remembering or creating strong passwords.

A **virus** can change the way a digital device works. It works like a miniature software program and can allow someone to steal passwords and personal information. A virus can also disrupt or destroy a device's files. To avoid viruses, install a virus protection program on your device. Avoid visiting unfamiliar or unlicensed websites, clicking on advertisements, downloading unfamiliar files, or opening messages from unknown senders.

virus piece of computer code that changes the way a digital device works to disrupt functions or steal personal information

Facial recognition and fingerprinting software are not the most secure way to protect your accounts. Use a strong password to maintain your privacy.

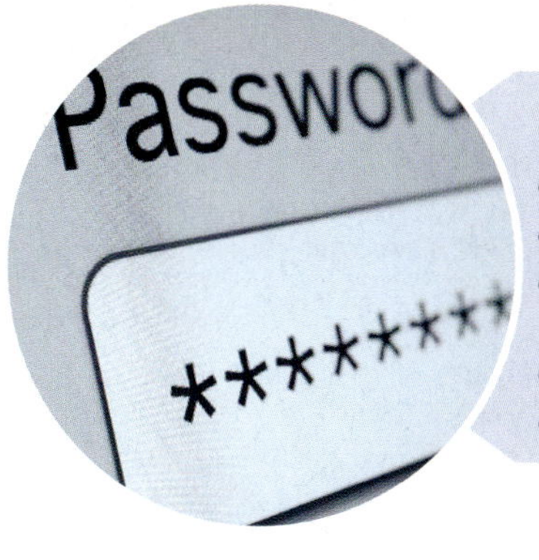

A strong password has

- 8–12 characters
- both letters and numbers
- no obvious personal information (like your birthday or pet's name) or full words
- a mix of uppercase and lowercase
- other keyboard characters (such as @ # $!)

JMiks/Shutterstock.com

Figure 16.17 Try not to use the same password for multiple accounts. If your password becomes compromised, this can endanger your information in all of the other sites used.

Inappropriate Content

The internet is a platform where many people can share their ideas, which means you will likely encounter content on the internet you will not find elsewhere. Some of this content will enrich your life and motivate you. Consuming and sharing some content, however, can lead to long-term consequences and health risks.

Avoiding Harmful Websites

Anyone can make a website on the internet. As a result, some websites can be harmful to people's health and well-being. Even if you are not looking for these websites, you may find them accidentally through an online search or advertisement.

Illegal websites include those that advertise illegal drugs, weapons, and stolen goods. Do not buy illegal or stolen items from these websites. There are severe penalties for selling or buying stolen goods, as well as weapons and drugs.

Websites with violent or hateful content can pose threats to your health and the health of others. Posting violent content on these websites can lead to serious legal consequences. Being around violent and hateful ideas can make people more likely to engage in violence.

Some websites contain *sexually explicit media*, such as sexual photos and videos. If you see sexually explicit media, it is important to remember that it does not represent realistic, healthy relationships. Sometimes sexually explicit media can even be violent and disturbing.

To protect yourself from harmful websites, use the strategies in **Figure 16.18**.

Figure 16.18 Websites can contain violent, hateful, or sexual content. Fortunately, you are in control of where you go online.

Navigating Websites Safely

01 Do not click on a website link in an email or message from someone you do not know or trust.

02 Do not visit unfamiliar websites or websites unrelated to the subject you are researching.

03 Avoid viewing websites with lots of advertisements.

04 If you accidentally visit a website with inappropriate or harmful content, do not navigate any further. Instead, close the website and talk to a trusted adult.

05 Talk to a trusted adult if you find yourself spending time on violent, hateful, or sexually explicit websites.

06 Use internet search settings to filter out websites with sexual, violent, or adult-only content.

Ollie The Designer/Shutterstock.com

Thinking Before You Post

It is easy to think that what you share online is temporary, that everyone will forget about it in a few days, or that no one is paying attention to what you post. You might not remember everything you post. Your friends might not either. Everything you post or share, however, remains part of the internet for someone to discover at a later date. Even if no one notices now, people in your future may care about what you share today.

On the internet, people can read and share what you post. They can screenshot your words or pictures and store them even after you have deleted them. Thus, everything you share can become part of your digital footprint. You may not be able to take words and pictures back. What you share online reflects on you and your reputation. Thoughtful posts can lead to a positive network and strong relationships. Violent, hateful, and sexual posts can lead to serious legal consequences, public embarrassment, and broken relationships. They can also attract the attention of dangerous people.

When communicating online, consider whether you want everyone to see what you are saying now and in the future. Violent, sexual, or hateful posts can lead to legal consequences such as criminal charges and can also hurt others and promote a hostile environment. Posts that promote bullying or illegal activity may become problematic when you apply for schools or jobs or if you face legal consequences. Posts with sexual content can be shared with anyone and remain on the internet for a long time.

Before you post online, take a moment to think about what you are sharing and whether you will regret it later (**Figure 16.19**). In-person, the presence of a listener may slow your impulse to say the first words you think. Online, you may feel more comfortable saying some things because you have no face-to-face audience. If you are unsure about a post, read your draft out loud or show the photo or video you are sharing to a trusted friend or adult.

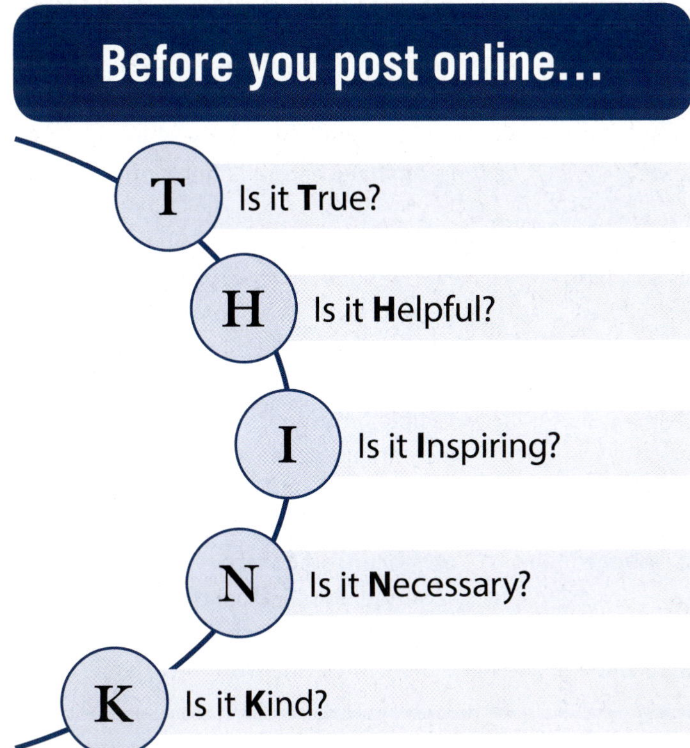

Figure 16.19 T.H.I.N.K. about what you say before you send a message or post content to social media. Often, just taking a second look at a message can help you see that it is hurtful or inappropriate.

Even if you think before you post, you might see posts from others that contain dangerous or disturbing content. If you receive any message or see any content related to suicide, gang activity, substance use, bullying, threats of violence, sexual activity, or violent behavior, tell a trusted adult immediately.

Dealing with Sexting

sexting sending sexual content in the form of digital text, pictures, or videos

As teens learn more about themselves and sexual relationships, they may be tempted to send online messages with sexual content. This behavior, called **sexting**, may involve sending sexual content in the form of actual text, pictures, or videos. Sometimes adult partners in romantic relationships send messages like these. Among teens, sexting is risky, harmful, and illegal. It is sometimes used to harass, frighten, threaten, or bully others.

Sexting has many potentially serious consequences. Legally, sexting can be seen as harassment and lead to jail time and fines. In some cases, people who sext can be charged with child pornography.

Research in Action

Sexting and Mental Health

Did you know that sexting can have an influence on mental health? Sexting involves sending or receiving messages or pictures containing sexual content. Recently, doctors and scientists have been studying the effects of sexting on the behavior and mental health of teens and young adults.

Researchers at Deakin University in Australia examined sexting behaviors and the number of people who received or sent sexts without wanting to. They found that 36 percent of the people surveyed had received unwanted sexts. Twenty-three percent of participants had sent sexts because they felt pressured to do so. Researchers then examined levels of anxiety, depression, and stress among participants.

Can you guess what they found? Participants who received unwanted sexts or felt pressured to sext reported lower self-esteem and more symptoms of depression, anxiety, and stress. Interestingly, receiving an unwanted sext affected males more negatively than females. This study shows that nonconsensual sexting can have harmful effects on mental health.

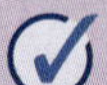

Practice Your Skills

Practice Health-Enhancing Behaviors

With a partner, discuss the reasons some teens sext and the impact sexting has on teen relationships. How do you think sexting during the teen years is different from sexting between adults? How is consensual sexting different from nonconsensual sexting? What are the risks of sexting? Then, working with your partner, develop a plan for how to respond to an unwanted sext.

1. Suppose you have received an unwanted sext. You want the sender not to sext you again. With your partner, brainstorm what you could say to tell the sender to stop. What should you do with the sext the person sent you?
2. Imagine that the sender keeps sending you unwanted sexts. You have told the sender multiple times to stop. What can you do to get help and put an end to this behavior?
3. The sender has stopped sexting you, but you still feel nervous every time you get a notification. You feel uncomfortable whenever you are around the sender at school, and you know the sender is making fun of you. Whom could you talk with to get help and cope with these issues?

Sexting carries the risk of exploitation. Once sexual photos have been sent, they can be posted online and end up on inappropriate or illegal websites. These photos will not go away and can affect a person's chances of employment or college admission. A person can also share sexts with friends and classmates. This can happen if a relationship ends or even within a trusting relationship and can lead to embarrassment, emotional distress, social isolation, depression, and anxiety. It can also lead to criminal charges for the person who shared the sext.

Not sexting is the best way to avoid these consequences (**Figure 16.20**). If someone sends you a sext, do not share it with others. If you do this, you can be charged with child pornography and have to register as a sex offender. Immediately delete the sext and tell a trusted adult. If someone asks for a sext, use refusal skills to say *no*. You might say, "I don't want pictures like that online" or "We could get in trouble for that." Remember that, if someone really cares about you, that person will not pressure you.

Before You Send a Message, Ask...

- Will your message harm or harass someone?
- Does your message contain inappropriate or illegal content?
- Are you sending an inappropriate message to a child or underage person?
- Will someone be embarrassed or harmed if others view the message?
- Will you regret sending the message someday?
- Are you sending the message to someone who has asked you not to send such messages?

Figure 16.20 To avoid sexting, ask yourself these questions before sending a message with sexual content.

Lesson 16.3 Review

Know and Understand

1. What is included in a person's digital footprint?
2. How do you know if material posted online is copyrighted? If you want to share copyrighted material, what should you do?
3. Why is it best to avoid posting photos of your school or home?
4. If you come across a website that contains violent, hateful, or sexual content, what should you do?
5. Explain the risks of sexting.

Think Critically

6. How do you think anonymity affects how people behave online?
7. With a partner, create a list of dos and don'ts for online etiquette. Record a podcast introducing and explaining these tips to your classmates.
8. Review the list of personal information you should keep private in Figure 16.15. For each piece of information, explain why it is important to keep it private.
9. With a partner, develop a list of specific questions to ask before posting online. These questions should help you determine if what you are posting is helpful, appropriate, and respectful.
10. What do you think are the mental and emotional consequences of accessing violent, hateful, or sexual websites?

REAL WORLD Health Skills

Advocate for Health Create an app you think could help someone be safer in the digital world. Be sure to draw what the app icon would look like, what kind of service the app would provide, and how you would advertise it. Pitch the idea to your classmates, as if you were trying to sell them your app. Explain the benefits of the app during your pitch and keep your target audience in mind.

Lesson

16.4

Providing First Aid

Essential Question?

What skills do you need to provide first aid for injuries and medical emergencies?

Learning Outcomes

After studying this lesson, you will be able to

- list what should be in a first-aid kit;
- describe the first steps a person should take to provide first aid;
- explain how to provide first aid for wounds such as cuts, scrapes, puncture wounds, bites, stings, and burns; and
- identify the steps for responding to a medical emergency.

Key Terms 

anaphylaxis
automated external defibrillator (AED)
cardiopulmonary resuscitation (CPR)
first aid
first-aid kit
five-and-five method
medical emergency
shock
standard precautions

Warm-Up Activity

Injury List

Comprehend Concepts Find a partner, and before reading this lesson, list all the injuries you can think of that start with each letter shown. You will have 30 seconds to list as many of these injuries as you can. After the 30 seconds, share your injuries with the class. For each injury, briefly discuss how it might affect health.

B	C	F	H	S

The first line of defense against accidents and injuries is prevention. Even if you take safety precautions, however, accidents, injuries, and dangerous situations can still occur. If they do, skills related to first aid can help you reduce the damage and protect your long-term health. **First aid** is treatment given in the first moments after an accident or injury, usually before medical professionals arrive to help. In an emergency situation, the first-aid treatment you give in those first moments can help save a life.

first aid treatment given in the first moments after an accident or injury, usually before medical professionals arrive

Have a First-Aid Kit Ready

Certain supplies, such as bandages and cold packs, can help you administer first aid after an accident or injury. Many people collect these supplies in a **first-aid kit**, which contains the necessary items to treat minor injuries (**Figure 16.21**). You can put together your own kit and enclose it in a waterproof bag or clearly labeled box. You can also purchase a ready-made kit at most drugstores or from the American Red Cross.

first-aid kit collection of necessary items to treat minor injuries

Figure 16.21 A first-aid kit should include the essentials shown here and any additional supplies you need for yourself or your family.

First-Aid Kit Essentials

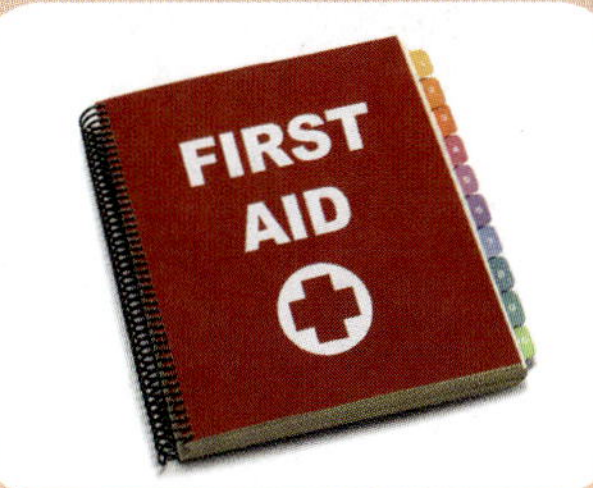

Resources

- First-aid manual
- Phone numbers for the Poison Control Center, family doctor, police department, and fire department

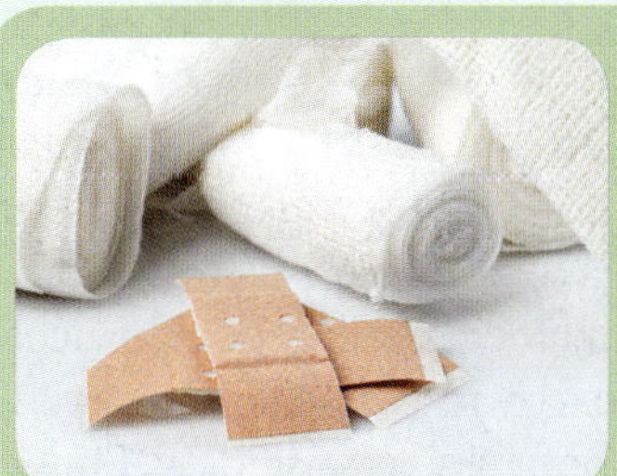

Supplies for Treating Wounds

- Gauze pads and assorted bandages
- Medical tape
- Cotton balls and cotton swabs
- Scissors

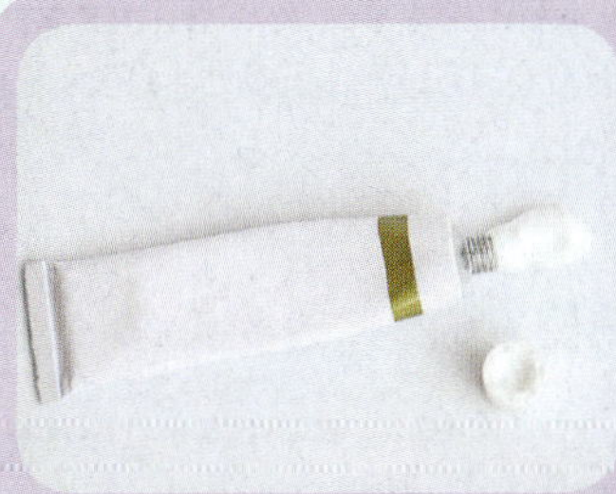

Supplies for Preventing Infections

- Antibiotic ointment (cream)
- Antiseptic wipes
- Hand sanitizer
- Disposable latex or synthetic gloves

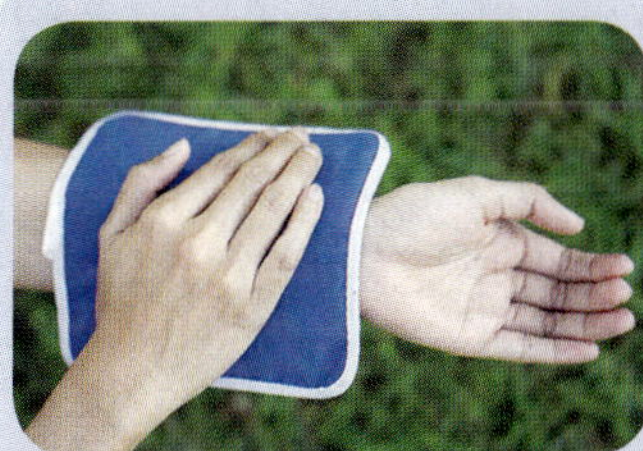

Supplies for Treating Various Injuries

- Elastic wrap
- Instant cold packs
- Tweezers
- Sterile eyedrops or eyewash solution
- Oral thermometer (nonmercury/nonglass)

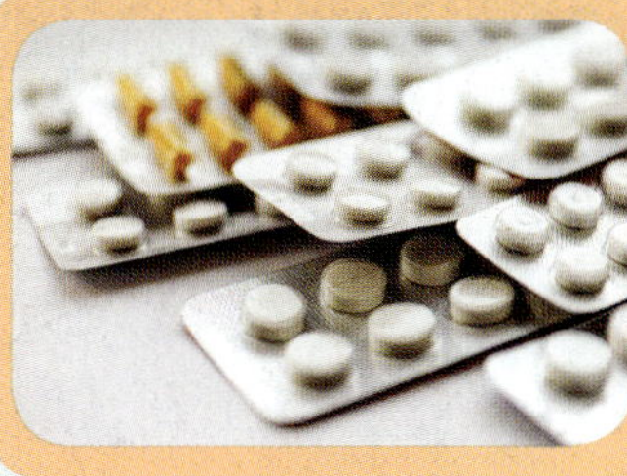

Over-the-Counter Medications

- Pain relievers such as ibuprofen or acetaminophen
- Hydrocortisone cream
- Antihistamine medications

Top to bottom: Mega Pixel/Shutterstock.com; Henrik Dolle/Shutterstock.com; nokwalai/Shutterstock.com; Chutima Chaochaiya/Shutterstock.com; DedMityay/Shutterstock.com

The American Red Cross suggests keeping a first-aid kit in the home and in vehicles. When spending time doing outdoor activities, such as hiking or camping, carry a first-aid kit with you. Be sure to keep the first-aid kit out of reach and out of sight of small children and away from family pets.

Assess the Situation and Call 911

Accidents and injuries can cause dangerous situations, both for the person injured and anyone trying to help. In an emergency situation, it is important to call 911 before trying to help by administering first aid. To protect yourself and respond appropriately, begin by checking the scene. If you cannot safely get to the injured person, call 911 immediately. Do not risk becoming injured yourself. If you can safely provide help, then stay calm and follow these steps:

1. **Check the injured person's condition:** Begin by quickly assessing the situation. Is the person awake and responsive or unresponsive? Does the injury appear to be life threatening? Signs of a life-threatening injury include severe bleeding and labored or no breathing. Other signs include **shock**, a life-threatening condition in which the vital organs do not receive enough blood and oxygen, and unconsciousness. Do not move the injured person unless you must leave a dangerous situation.
2. **Call 911:** As soon as you can, call 911 or your local emergency services. If you are performing first aid, tell someone nearby to call (**Figure 16.22**). If you are at school, tell a teacher or coach about the emergency. These trusted adults can call 911 or help give first aid while you call 911.
3. **Give first aid:** If possible, ask whether the injured person wants to receive first aid. This is called *obtaining consent*. If the injured person is a child, ask the parent or guardian for consent.

shock life-threatening condition in which the vital organs do not receive enough blood and oxygen

Provide First-Aid Treatment

In the moments after an accident or injury, you can take steps to help an injured person until medical professionals arrive. By learning and practicing first-aid skills, you will be able to remain calm, think clearly, and act rationally during the stress of helping an injured person. By studying Chapter 10, you have already learned how to treat sprains and know what to do if a bone becomes fractured or dislocated. In the following sections, you will learn about standard precautions and basic first-aid treatments for some other common injuries.

Figure 16.22 Communicating appropriately with 911 dispatchers can help them better understand the situation and get aid to you faster.

Calling 911: What They Need to Know

1. Dial 911. State your location and the street address. If you do not know the address, ask a bystander to tell the 911 dispatcher while you begin first aid.
2. Tell the dispatcher why you called. Name the specific type of emergency.
3. Describe the injured person's condition, age, and biological sex.
4. Give any important information about the scene. For example, tell dispatchers about downed power lines, poisons, or anything that might help them understand the emergency.
5. If you have begun first aid, describe what you have already done.
6. Listen to and follow the dispatcher's directions.
7. Stay on the phone with the 911 dispatcher until emergency help arrives.

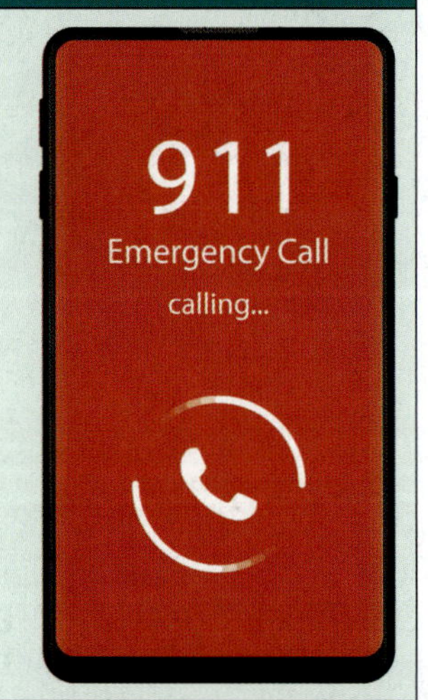

Korosi Francois-Zoltan/Shutterstock.com

Standard Precautions

First-aid procedures often involve contact with an injured person's bodily fluids, such as blood. Because bodily fluids can carry communicable diseases, people should follow standard precautions when giving first aid.

Standard precautions are infection control practices based on universal precautions. Developed by the Centers for Disease Control and Prevention (CDC), standard precautions protect from bloodborne infections, such as HIV, and infections transmitted by respiratory droplets.

standard precautions infection control practices to prevent the spread of disease during first aid

An example of a standard precaution is to wear protective gloves when there is a risk of contact with blood or bodily fluids that may contain blood. Washing hands with soap and water after giving first aid is another example. You cannot know if a person you are helping has a communicable disease. Therefore, you should always assume infection is possible when giving first aid.

Cuts, Scrapes, and Puncture Wounds

People often do not need professional medical treatment for minor cuts or scrapes. Minor cuts and scrapes may cause some bleeding, but the bleeding will often stop on its own. If the bleeding does not stop on its own, follow the steps in **Figure 16.23**. If a cut or scrape is deep, it requires medical attention. A cut or scratch is considered deep if applying gentle pressure does not easily press the edges together. Scrapes require medical attention if they cover a large area.

People with deep cuts, puncture wounds, or scratches need professional medical attention. Puncture wounds—such as penetrating wounds from nails, thorns, or other sharp objects—usually bleed a small amount and close up right away. The object that caused the puncture, however, can introduce bacteria. A doctor needs to clean puncture wounds and deep cuts and scrapes because they are prone to developing dangerous infections.

Deep cuts may require stitches from a medical professional. Some cuts are so deep they expose the dermis or fatty tissue. They may contain debris that can cause a serious infection. People with deep cuts, scrapes, and puncture wounds may need a vaccine to prevent *tetanus*, a serious bacterial infection associated with these types of wounds.

Until you can receive medical attention for a deep cut, scratch, or puncture wound, apply pressure to stop the wound from bleeding and cleanse it with clean water. Remove any debris and cover the wound with a bandage. Then elevate the wound until you receive medical attention.

Treating Minor Injuries

Apply pressure using a sterile bandage. → Flush the wound with clean water. → Apply an antibiotic cream or ointment. → Apply a bandage and change it daily.

Figure 16.23 These steps can help you care for a cut or scrape that does not stop bleeding. If the bleeding does not stop after these steps, or if the cut is deep, seek medical attention.

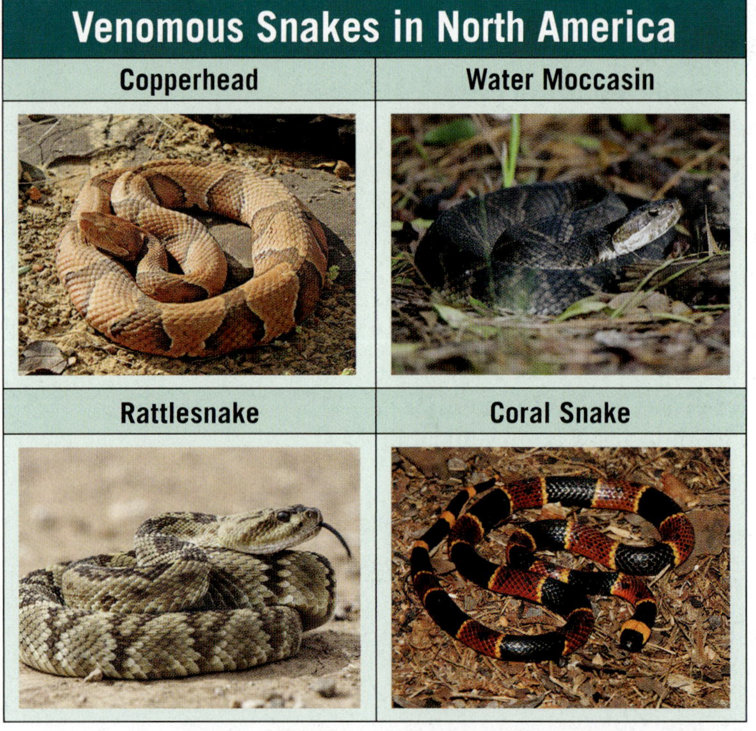

Left to right: Creeping Things/Shutterstock.com; Tony Campbell/Shutterstock.com; Viktor Loki/Shutterstock.com; Jay Ondreicka/Shutterstock.com

Figure 16.24 These snakes have venom, a poison that can seriously damage the bitten area and even be life threatening.

Bites and Stings

Bites and stings from animals and insects can be cause for concern. People may experience bites from domestic animals, such as dogs or cats. Wild animals, such as raccoons, may also bite people. Common biting and stinging insects include bees, wasps, mosquitoes, and some types of ants.

All animal bites require a doctor's attention. Bite wounds that break or puncture the skin carry the risk of infection. The most dangerous of these infections is the *rabies* virus, which infects the nerves, brain, and spinal cord. Rabies is fatal if not treated immediately, before the virus reaches the brain and symptoms begin. To prevent animal bites, stay away from wild animals, animals that act unusually, and unfamiliar cats and dogs, which may not be vaccinated for rabies. If you are bitten, wash the bite wound with soap and water, cover it with a clean bandage, and elevate the affected area until you see a doctor.

Four snakes in North America have poisonous bites (**Figure 16.24**). Nonpoisonous snake bites often look like scratches. A poisonous snake bite looks more like a puncture wound and becomes very painful. Any snake bite requires professional medical treatment, even if the snake is not venomous. If a snake bite occurs, call 911, position the bitten area lower than your heart, and stay calm and still. You can apply a loose, clean bandage, but otherwise leave the bite alone until you can get medical treatment.

Insect bites often cause mild reactions in people, such as swelling or itching at the site of the bite. Treat these reactions with cool cloths, calamine lotion, or over-the-counter hydrocortisone cream if the itching is severe.

Stings from bees, wasps, yellow jackets, and fire ants can cause more severe reactions. The venom from these insects triggers pain, swelling, and redness. Some people develop *hives*, a swollen, fluid-filled skin rash. If you are stung, use tweezers to remove any stingers stuck in the skin, wash the area, and apply hydrocortisone cream to relieve swelling and itching. As you recover, use cold compresses or ice and pain medication, elevate the stung area, and get plenty of rest.

A few people experience extremely severe, life-threatening allergic reactions to insect stings. This reaction is called *anaphylaxis*. **Anaphylaxis** is an allergic response in which fluid fills the lungs and air passages narrow, restricting breathing. Other symptoms of anaphylaxis include nausea and vomiting, swelling, intestinal cramps, fainting, confusion, and a rapid heartbeat. This type of reaction requires immediate emergency

anaphylaxis severe allergic response in which fluid fills the lungs and air passages narrow, restricting breathing

care or the person could die. People who have such severe allergic reactions often carry medication such as the EpiPen® (**Figure 16.25**). To use an EpiPen®, follow the directions on the package.

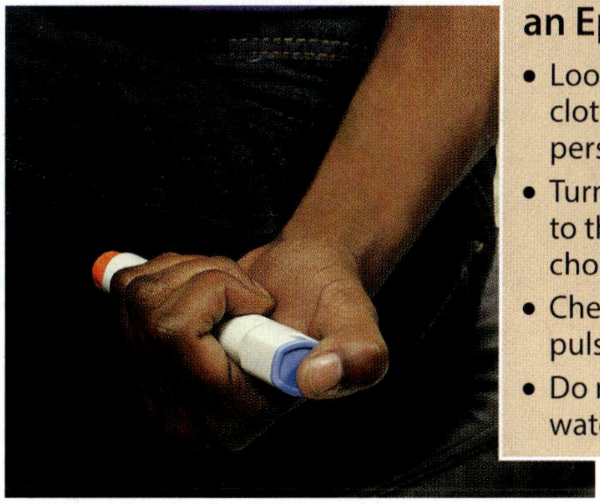

After administering an EpiPen®:

- Loosen a person's clothing and cover the person with a blanket.
- Turn the person's head to the side to prevent choking from vomit.
- Check breathing and pulse.
- Do not give the person water or any other liquid.

Rob Byron/Shutterstock.com

Figure 16.25 An EpiPen® helps treat allergic reactions and are important in emergency situations. ***What is the name of the life-threatening allergic reaction that restricts breathing?***

Burns

Burns are common injuries that range from mild to life threatening. Exposure to any source of heat and energy such as fire, burning or smoldering materials, steam, hot surfaces, or extremely hot gases and liquids can cause burns. Chemicals, electric current, and the sun are also possible causes of burns.

All types of burns can seriously damage skin. Burns can also cause dangerous complications, such as infection, shock, dehydration, pain, and immobility of the affected body part. First aid is essential for all burns. To give appropriate first aid, you need to identify whether the burn is a first-, second-, or third-degree burn (**Figure 16.26**).

Types of Burns

First-Degree Burns	Second-Degree Burns	Third-Degree Burns
• Damage only the outer layer of skin • Cause redness, swelling, and pain • Treatment includes holding the burned skin under cool water, covering the burn, and taking pain reliever	• Affect the second layer of skin • Cause blisters, redness, and swelling • Burns affecting less than 3 inches can be treated like first-degree burns • Burns affecting more than 3 inches are medical emergencies and should be treated like third-degree burns	• Affect all layers of skin and underlying tissue • Are medical emergencies • To respond, call 911 immediately and check the person's breathing and pulse, elevate the burned body part, cover the burn, and treat for shock until help arrives • Do not remove burned clothing or immerse burns in cool water

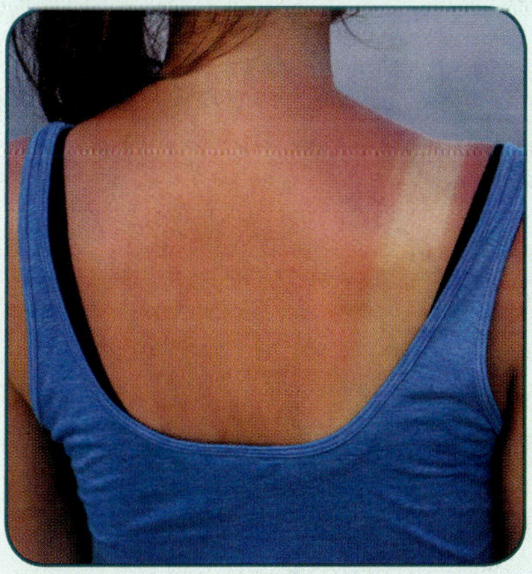

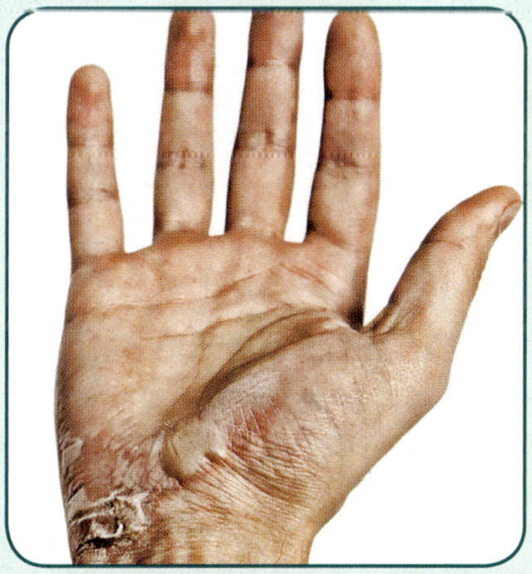

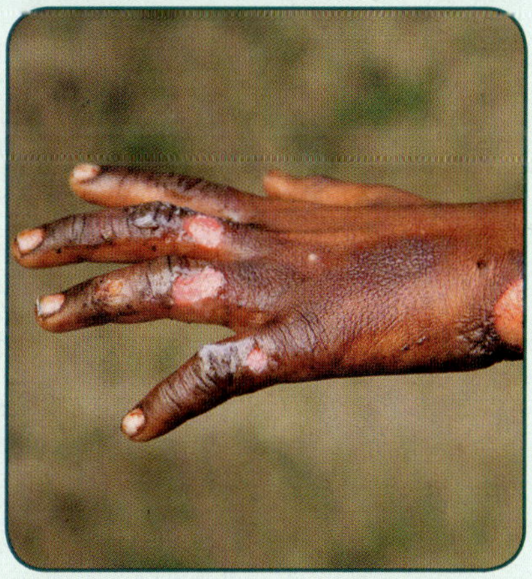

Left to right: yurakrasil/Shutterstock.com; nikkytok/Shutterstock.com; Naiyyer/Shutterstock.com

Figure 16.26 It is important to be able to differentiate between first-, second-, and third-degree burns because each requires different care. ***What can cause burns?***

Respond to Medical Emergencies

medical emergency
urgent, life-threatening situation

A **medical emergency** is an urgent, life-threatening situation. Examples of medical emergencies include third-degree burns, anaphylaxis, severe bleeding, electrical shock, choking, and situations requiring cardiopulmonary resuscitation (CPR). When medical emergencies arise, call 911 right away. Then, follow emergency first-aid treatment until medical professionals arrive. Medical emergencies require an immediate first-aid response. Otherwise, the injured person could die.

Severe Bleeding

Wounds that do not close on their own can result in severe bleeding. Losing too much blood can be extremely dangerous. A person can only lose 20 percent of total blood volume before going into shock. The goal of first aid for severe bleeding is to stop the bleeding by applying pressure and carefully positioning the body. After calling 911, follow these steps to provide first aid to someone experiencing severe bleeding:

1. Apply pressure to the wound, using a sterile bandage if possible.
2. Position the wound higher than the heart, if possible. This will reduce blood flow to the area.
3. Continue applying pressure and cover the wound with gauze and bandages.
4. Keep the injured person calm. Keep applying pressure until medical professionals arrive.
5. Treat the injured person for shock by covering the person with a blanket. Signs and symptoms of shock may include cold, pale skin; rapid pulse and breathing; nausea; weakness and dizziness; and anxiety. Lay the person down, elevate the legs, keep the person still, and turn the head to the side to prevent choking.

Cardiopulmonary Resuscitation (CPR)

Your heart beats and your lungs breathe in and out air to circulate oxygen throughout your body and keep you alive. If a person's heart stops beating or if a person stops breathing, this is a life-threatening emergency. In these situations, first aid and medical care must begin as soon as possible to restore breathing and heartbeat. The main technique used to restore breathing and heartbeat is cardiopulmonary resuscitation, or *CPR*.

cardiopulmonary resuscitation (CPR)
emergency procedure that uses chest compressions and sometimes rescue breathing to restore heartbeat

Cardiopulmonary resuscitation (CPR) is an emergency procedure that uses chest compressions and sometimes rescue breathing to restore heartbeat. Full CPR involves mouth-to-mouth breathing, or *rescue breaths*. You should only use this technique if you have been well trained in performing it. *Hands-Only™ CPR* only involves chest compressions. The American Heart Association (AHA) and the American Red Cross recommend that rescuers use Hands-Only™ CPR for adults in most cases. This is because rescue breaths require training, and almost anyone can perform chest compressions without training.

Hands-Only™ CPR delivers blood circulation to people who suffer *cardiac arrest*, in which the heart stops beating. Hands-Only™ CPR includes two steps:

1. **Call 911:** Call 911 immediately. Have someone else call 911 if you cannot.
2. **Push hard and fast:** Position your hands over the center of the person's chest and push hard and fast using your own body weight (**Figure 16.27**). Push down at a rate of 100 compressions per minute and compress the chest at least 2 inches. Allow the chest to rise completely before each compression.

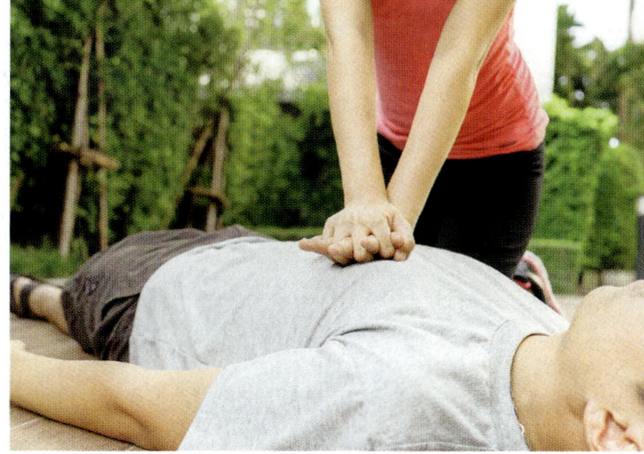

To locate the correct hand position, place two fingers at the tip of the breastbone. Place the heel of the hand right above your fingers and stack your other hand on top.

KittisakJirasittichai/iStock/Getty Images Plus/Getty Images

Figure 16.27 Administering CPR can save a person's life by restoring heartbeat and breathing. Under Good Samaritan laws, if a person makes a mistake while administering CPR, this person cannot be held legally liable for damages in court. ***What technique for CPR should only be provided after full training?***

Do not slow down or stop performing CPR until emergency services arrive, you become too tired to continue, or an **automated external defibrillator (AED)** is available and ready for use. This rescue device delivers a controlled, precise shock to the heart and gives automated instructions (**Figure 16.28**). An AED can restore a person's heartbeat after cardiac arrest. Even people with little or no training can use Hands-Only™ CPR and AEDs.

automated external defibrillator (AED) device that delivers a controlled, precise shock to the heart to restore a person's heartbeat

Using an Automated External Defibrillator (AED)

After calling 911, adults trained in using an AED can use the following steps if an infant, child, or adult is unconscious and not breathing. If the person is an infant or child, obtain parental consent, if possible.

- **Step 1.** Turn on AED.
- **Step 2.** Wipe bare chest dry.
- **Step 3.** Attach pads.
  For infants and children younger than eight years of age: Use *pediatric pads* if possible. Place one pad on the upper-right side of the chest and the other pad on the left side of the chest. If the pads touch (because the infant or child is too small), place one pad in the middle of the chest and one pad in the middle of the back.
  For children older than eight years of age and adults: Place one pad on the upper-right side of the chest and the other pad on the left side of the chest.
- **Step 4.** If necessary, plug in connector.
- **Step 5.** Tell everyone to stand clear.
- **Step 6.** Deliver shock.
- **Step 7.** Perform about five cycles of CPR.

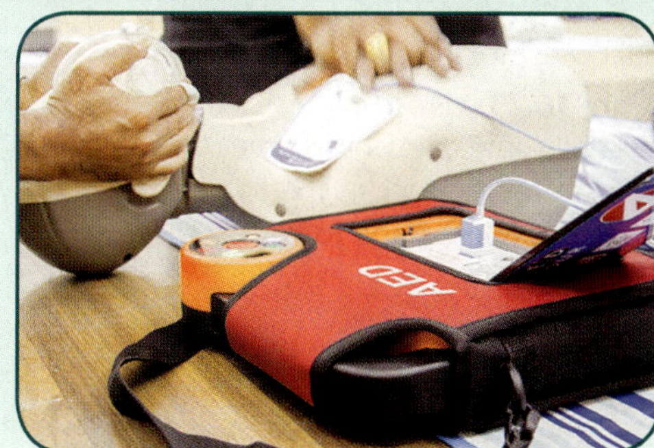

narin phapnam/Shutterstock.com

Figure 16.28 An AED can be found in most public places.

Electrical Shock

Electrical shock occurs when an electrical current comes in contact with the body. A shock could come from fallen power lines due to severe weather or contact with damaged or frayed cords or wiring. People also get shocked when standing in flooded streets or basements. In these situations, water conducts electricity to the body from electrical wires, outlets, or downed power lines.

Electrical shock may cause burns, internal injuries, cardiac arrest, or even death. While you wait for emergency medical help to arrive, use the following steps:

1. Call 911 immediately. Have someone else call 911 if you cannot.
2. Do not touch the person if in contact with electricity. Turn off the electricity source. Move electrical wires with wood, plastic, or cardboard.
3. Check breathing and pulse. Begin CPR, if necessary.
4. Treat the person for shock and apply bandages to burns.

Cold- and Hot-Weather Emergencies

Severe weather, including extremely cold and hot temperatures, can cause emergencies. Learning about how to respond to these emergencies can help you stay safe and help others.

Exposure to extreme cold causes two serious health issues: frostbite and hypothermia. *Frostbite* is a condition in which skin and underlying tissue freeze (**Figure 16.29**). If left untreated, frostbite can kill tissue and cause infection or loss of limbs. If frostbite occurs, people should remove wet clothes, put the frostbitten area in warm (not hot) water, and use a warm blanket to warm affected areas and preserve body heat. They should not rub the area. People should seek medical attention for signs of superficial or deep frostbite; increased pain, swelling, redness, or discharge in the area; and fever.

Figure 16.29 Frostbite especially affects exposed skin and extremities, such as the nose, ears, fingers, and toes.

Signs and Symptoms of Frostbite	
Frostnip	• Mild frostbite • Numbness • Pain and tingling when skin warms • No permanent damage
Superficial frostbite	• Reddened skin that turns white or pale • Skin begins to feel warm, even in the cold • When skin warms, surface of skin may appear mottled and you may notice stinging, burning, and swelling. You may also experience blistering.
Deep (severe) frostbite	• White or bluish-gray skin • Numbness, losing all sensation of cold, pain, or discomfort in the affected area • Joints or muscles may become stiff • Large blisters form after rewarming, then area turns black and hard as tissue dies.

Hypothermia is a medical emergency characterized by dangerously low body temperature and can be fatal. It often occurs when people are wet and exposed to cool air or cold. Symptoms include uncontrollable shivering, slurred speech, loss of coordination, abnormal or slow breathing, extreme fatigue, and confusion or memory issues. To treat hypothermia, move a person indoors and warm the person using dry clothing, blankets, coats, warm drinks, and your own body heat. Seek immediate medical attention and do *not* use heating pads, give the person alcohol, or massage the person's skin.

Exposure to hot weather can tax the body's capacity to regulate temperature. Heat and dehydration can cause *heat cramps*, or the more serious *heatstroke* and *heat exhaustion* (**Figure 16.30**). Infants, young children, older adults, individuals who experience overweight, and people doing physical labor or playing sports outdoors have more risk for these heat-related illnesses.

Choking

Choking is a medical emergency in which an object, such as a piece of food, blocks the airway. This means that a choking person cannot breathe. Choking may occur when people chew their food too quickly or when young children put objects in their mouths.

Heat-Related Illnesses

Heat Cramps

- **Symptoms:** Painful muscle cramps and spasms, especially in the leg
- **Treatment:** Have the person rest, stay hydrated, and avoid vigorous activity for several hours.

Heat Exhaustion

- **Symptoms:** Cool and moist skin; pale, gray, or flushed skin; headache; nausea; dizziness; and weakness or exhaustion
- **Treatment:** Move the person to a cooler place and remove the person's clothing. Apply cold, wet towels to the person's trunk, back of the neck, and forehead. Have the person sip nonalcoholic, uncaffeinated, cool drinks and stretch any cramping muscles.

Heatstroke

- **Symptoms:** High body temperature, red skin, altered consciousness or confusion, seizures, and rapid or weak pulse
- **Treatment:** Call 911 immediately and submerge person's body in cold water. Have the person lie down with feet elevated and cover the skin with towels soaked in cold water or bags of ice. Monitor the person and be prepared to give CPR or treat for shock.

Figure 16.30 Heat cramps can lead to heat exhaustion, and eventually heatstroke.

Many people instinctively grab their throats with both hands when they are choking, but there are other signs as well. If you know these signs, you can quickly recognize when someone is choking and provide help. The following are signs of choking:

- inability to breathe normally
- inability to talk or make noise
- inability to cough or expel air forcefully
- blue skin, lips, and nails

five-and-five method
procedure of responding to choking that involves a series of back blows alternating with abdominal thrusts

The American Red Cross recommends the **five-and-five method** for helping a person who is choking (**Figure 16.31**). This method involves a series of back blows alternating with abdominal thrusts, which force air out of the choking person's lungs. This should help push the stuck object out of the airway. Abdominal thrusts are also called the *Heimlich maneuver*.

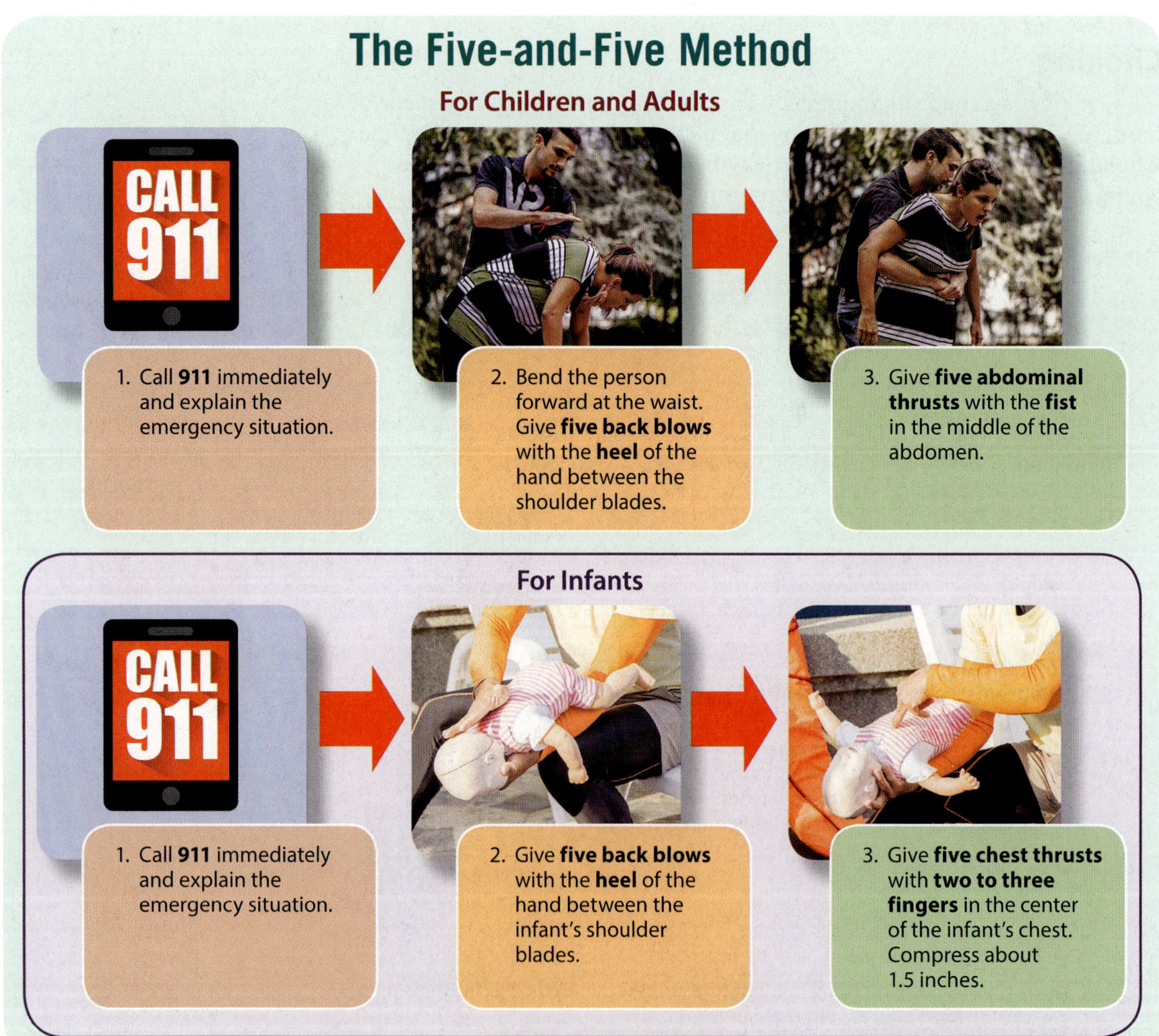

Top left to right: gst/Shutterstock.com; pixelaway/Shutterstock.com; Bottom: narin phapnam/Shutterstock.com

Figure 16.31 If a person is choking, use the five-and-five method to give aid. After you call 911, perform steps 2 and 3 and continue them, if necessary, until help arrives. ***How does the five-and-five method adjust for aid to infants?***

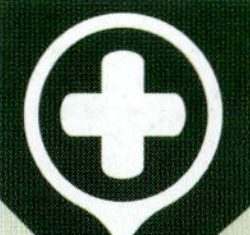

Spotlight on Health and Wellness Careers

Paramedic: Cristian Hinojosa

As a captain in the Dallas Fire Department, I have spent seven of the last 14 years as an active paramedic on an ambulance. Today, I serve in a similar capacity on an advanced life support (ALS) fire engine and use my paramedic skills numerous times each shift.

The field of emergency medicine is an exciting and rewarding one. A successful paramedic adapts to dynamic environments, works irregular hours, and intimately experiences some of the most precious and tragic moments in a person's life. Paramedics undergo extensive training in advanced life support (ALS), perform numerous invasive lifesaving procedures, and can treat a patient using more than 30 different drugs. In many large cities, paramedics work on ambulances and as technicians in emergency departments. A typical shift may include working for up to 24 hours at a time, usually followed by a few days off.

Seasoned paramedics can recount delivering babies and successfully resuscitating lifeless patients, but they also experience inevitable tragedy. They often must make split-second decisions in unfamiliar environments. Being a paramedic requires compassion, critical thinking, physical and mental strength, and an ability not to personalize difficult calls. This career has been extremely rewarding. I rarely have a shift that does not provide a strong sense of making a positive difference in people's lives.

Practice Your Skills

Access Information

Think about your own interests, strengths, and weaknesses. What parts of being a paramedic do you think would interest you? Which elements would be challenging? Using reliable resources like the US Bureau of Labor Statistics' *Occupational Outlook Handbook*, research emergency medicine and related careers. Is the demand for paramedics growing? What are the educational requirements? Are there related careers that might also interest you? Write a blog post summarizing your thoughts.

Lesson 16.4 Review

Know and Understand

1. Examine your family's first-aid kit or look at a first-aid kit you could buy in a store. Are there any supplies the first-aid kit is missing?
2. What are the signs that a condition is life threatening?
3. How do you know if a cut is deep enough to require medical attention?
4. What kind of burn is a medical emergency?
5. Which type of CPR is recommended for rescuers without full training?

Think Critically

6. Choose one animal or insect that is common in your area. Research the potential effects of and treatments for a bite or sting by this animal or insect.
7. Why does positioning a wound higher than the heart reduce blood flow to the area?
8. Choose one hot- or cold-weather emergency. Explain how the condition develops and how it is treated.
9. Review the five-and-five method and create a poster of its steps that you can easily reference and remember.

REAL WORLD Health Skills

Make Decisions Choose one of the injuries or medical emergencies discussed in this lesson. Then, write a case study in which a teen encounters this injury or emergency and has to make a decision about how to respond. Show how the teen goes through the steps of the decision-making process to provide first aid and get medical attention, if needed.

Chapter 16 Review and Assessment

Chapter Summary

Learning to manage risks and stay safe will help you maintain your health, grow, and meet your goals for the future. Practicing safety includes protecting yourself from threats such as falls, poisonous substances, weapons, and water. You can also take steps as a pedestrian, passenger, and driver to reduce your risk of injury on the road. In the US, the Occupational Safety and Health Act protects workers and gives them rights.

Practicing safety also includes avoiding dangerous situations at home, at school, and in your community. In public places, you must be aware of strangers who could be a danger to you. Even among people you know, some social situations can put you at risk for injury, violence, sexual assault, and criminal activity. Emergencies such as fire, natural disasters, or violent attacks can cause great harm to people and property. You can practice emergency preparedness by knowing how to respond to specific types of emergency.

The digital footprint you leave today will affect your success now and in the future. You can practice digital citizenship by engaging in positive online behaviors. Always evaluate online information for truthfulness and reliability. Digital citizens follow copyright laws, which protect creators of original material. Online etiquette promotes respectful communication and helps people have informative and positive online experiences. People with online etiquette do not participate in trolling, flaming, or cyberbullying.

Sharing personal information online can lead to dangers like identity theft, financial theft, and unwanted interactions with people who might be dangerous. You can protect your devices from hacking and viruses by selecting strong passwords, installing virus protection programs, and avoiding unfamiliar or unlicensed websites, advertisements, files, or senders.

First aid is treatment given in the first moments after an accident or injury, usually before medical professionals arrive to help. By learning and practicing first-aid skills, you will be able to remain calm, think clearly, and act rationally during the stress of helping an injured person. Medical emergencies are urgent, life-threatening situations, such as third-degree burns, anaphylaxis, severe bleeding, electrical shock, choking, and situations requiring cardiopulmonary resuscitation (CPR). When medical emergencies arise, call 911 right away. Then, follow emergency first-aid treatment until medical professionals arrive.

Vocabulary Activity

Watch a video or listen to a podcast that shares tips about personal safety. Take notes as you listen to the tips and identify the most important ideas using the vocabulary from this chapter. Then, share the video or podcast with your classmates and use a meme, hashtag, or other online feature to highlight the most important ideas in the story.

anaphylaxis	*escape plan*	*online etiquette*
anonymity	*fire triangle*	*pedestrians*
automated external defibrillator (AED)	*first aid*	*phishing*
cardiopulmonary resuscitation (CPR)	*first-aid kit*	*poisonous*
copyright	*five-and-five method*	*privacy settings*
digital citizenship	*flaming*	*sexting*
digital footprint	*hacking*	*shock*
disaster	*identity theft*	*standard precautions*
emergency preparedness	*internet predators*	*trolling*
ergonomics	*medical emergency*	*virus*
	natural disasters	*weapon*

Review and Recall

Review the information in this chapter by answering the following questions.

1. What is the number for the Poison Control Center?
2. Which of the following is *not* a safe practice for pedestrians?
   A. walking facing traffic, if using the road
   B. assuming drivers can see you while crossing at a crosswalk
   C. wearing bright or reflective clothing when traveling at night
   D. making eye contact with drivers at intersections
3. Why are people more likely to have motor vehicle accidents if they drive while drowsy?
4. Which of the following precautions should you take to stay safe among strangers?
   A. Carry a charged cell phone.
   B. Travel in well-lit areas.
   C. Tell your parent or guardian where you are going.
   D. All of the above.
5. What are the three elements of the fire triangle?
6. What should you do if you are trapped in a room during a fire?
7. Which of the following is an online behavior in which people draw others into arguments and disrupt discussions?
   A. trolling
   B. flaming
   C. cyberbullying
   D. catfishing
8. What is it called when people pretend to represent companies and ask for personal information?
9. What are two characteristics of a strong password?
10. What are standard precautions?
11. List three symptoms of anaphylaxis.
12. Which of the following is a step you should take if a person has hypothermia?
    A. Use heating pads to warm the person.
    B. Give the person alcohol.
    C. Use blankets to warm the person.
    D. Massage the person's skin.
13. Which of the following is *not* a sign of choking?
    A. constant coughing
    B. inability to breathe normally
    C. inability to talk or make noise
    D. blue skin, lips, and nails

Standardized Test Prep

Reading and Writing Practice

Read the passage below and then answer the following questions.

According to the National Highway Traffic Safety Administration, in 2017, 3,166 people were killed in motor vehicle accidents that involved distracted driving. This accounted for 9 percent of all fatal crashes in the US. Distracted driving involves several behaviors, but using a phone while driving is one of the most common.

Using a phone reduces brain activity associated with driving by 37 percent, which explains the large number of crashes that result from distracted driving. Unfortunately, in 2017, nearly 40 percent of high school students reported texting or emailing while driving in the past month.

14. What is the meaning of the word *fatal*?
    A. serious
    B. causing death
    C. digital
    D. distracted
15. Which statement best explains the main point of the second paragraph in this passage?
    A. There are many types of cell phone use.
    B. Phone use causes all deaths due to distracted driving.
    C. Using the phone while driving is extremely dangerous, but some teens still do it.
    D. Many teens use the phone while driving.
16. Why do you think some teens still use their phone while driving, despite the negative consequences? Write a short essay explaining your thoughts.

Chapter 16 Skills Assessment

Critical Thinking Skills

Answer the following questions to assess your knowledge of what you learned in this chapter.

1. What are some actions you can take as a passenger to ensure road safety?
2. Research your state's laws about phone use while driving. Is it legal in your state to talk on a handheld cell phone and drive at the same time? Is it legal to talk with a hands-free device while driving? Is it legal to text and drive? Do you think these laws are adequate? Explain your answer.
3. Analyze your habits and posture when studying or working at a computer. Do you use good posture and ergonomics? What aspects can you improve?
4. Teens are sometimes responsible for the care of younger children at home. What are some additional safety precautions you might need to take when babysitting or caring for younger siblings at home?
5. What are some possible barriers to reporting dangerous situations and behaviors at school? How could you overcome these barriers?
6. Create a floor plan of your school building and outline the fire escape plan. Make sure to include the locations of fire extinguishers and fire escapes.
7. Make a list of the types of natural disasters that might affect the area where you live. Then create an emergency plan for responding to each one.
8. Can you think of an example of something you read online that made you feel uncomfortable? How did you respond?
9. Create a poster promoting digital citizenship. Make sure to include examples of online etiquette and advice on how to think before you post.
10. Evaluate the privacy settings you use on social media. Are privacy settings a fail-safe way of keeping your personal information safe online? Why or why not?
11. Have you ever witnessed a medical emergency? How did you respond? Were you able to stay calm in the situation? Create an illustration of the situation and share your experience with a classmate.
12. Have you ever experienced a medical emergency yourself? How did the people around you respond to help you? How could you apply what you learned from that experience to help someone in a future medical emergency?
13. Select one medical emergency discussed in this chapter and create a poster that lists at least four facts about emergency care for the emergency you have chosen. Include how these actions can slow down or reduce injuries and complications.

Health and Wellness Skills

Complete the following activities to assess your skills related to health and wellness.

14. **Analyze Influences.** Find an interview or news story about someone who experienced a fire in the home. What kinds of emotions did the person express? Could the person have done anything to be safer or more prepared? With a partner, discuss whether you think most teens understand how dangerous fire can be. How do teens' attitudes influence their behavior and health? Do you think teens' attitudes and behaviors would change if they talked with the person in the interview or news story?
15. **Access Information.** Using reliable and valid resources, research resources in your community that offer education and training about the following safety topics: natural disasters, fire safety, first aid, CPR, using an AED, heat exhaustion, and frostbite. Document what services these resources offer and how to access them.
16. **Communicate with Others.** Create a PSA warning your peers about the dangers of not being safe online. Your PSA could be a radio announcement, video, or poster campaign. As you craft your PSA, think about your target audience: other teens. Make your PSA engaging and effective and share it with the class.

17. **Make Decisions.** Write a case study about a teen who did not take personal safety seriously and was injured. Be as detailed as possible and be creative, but also realistic. Switch case studies with a classmate and complete the case study by showing how the teen uses the decision-making process to respond to the injury. Reflect on how the subject of the case study could have avoided injury by making different decisions.
18. **Set Goals.** Think about how safe you are when driving or riding in a car. Then, set three SMART goals that would increase safety. Use the SMART goals to create a contract with yourself. Sign this contract as a promise to yourself that you will do everything you can to stay safe in the car. Share this with your parent or guardian to sign too. Remind yourself of this contract when the time comes to act on your goals.
19. **Practice Health-Enhancing Behaviors.** Meet with your family members to make an emergency preparedness and escape plan for your home. If you already have a plan, review and revise it as needed. Bring in your plan and share it with a partner. Work with your partner to add anything else you think is important to your plan. Bring the plan home and discuss it with your family to have in case of an emergency.
20. **Advocate for Health.** Imagine you have been given the task to donate first-aid kits to places in and around your community that do not have any. You are in charge of deciding what supplies to include, how to find them, and how to raise the funds to get them. Describe how you would get the word out about the need for donations, how you would explain the importance of first aid, and how you would determine which places need the kits.

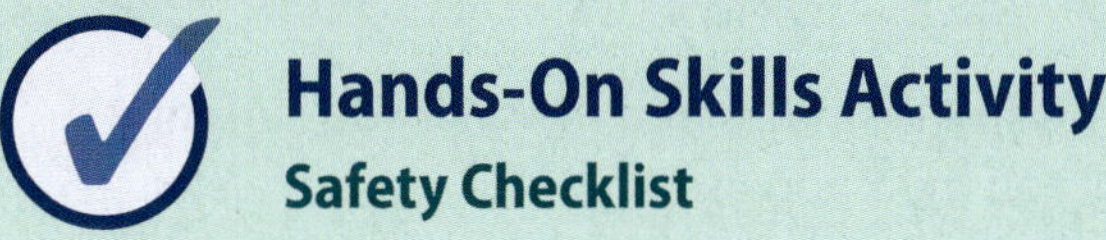

Hands-On Skills Activity

Safety Checklist

In this chapter, you learned about ways to stay safe in many different settings. For this activity, you will assess the safety of a setting in your community, using what you have learned.

Steps for This Activity

1. **Access Information.** In groups of three to five students, choose a setting from the list shown and make a checklist of at least nine items you think should be in the setting to make it safe (for example, signs, locks, directions, or caution labels). Use reliable and valid resources and the information in this chapter to identify these items.

- Kitchen
- Bedroom
- Bathroom
- Garage
- Parking lot
- Chemistry classroom
- Stadium
- Doctor's office
- Veterinarian's office
- School hallway
- A public beach, river, lake, or pool

2. Switch checklists with another group. When you get another group's checklist, review it and add at least one item your group thinks should be included.
3. Switch checklists one more time with another group. When your group gets the checklist, make sure all group members have access. Within three days, take the checklist to the appropriate setting and indicate what items on the list are present.
4. **Practice Health-Enhancing Behaviors.** After three days, discuss the following questions as a group and share your findings with the class:
   A. Which items on the checklist were present? Which were not present?
   B. How should people use the setting, knowing what safety features are and are not present? What precautions should they take?
   C. What could you do to respond safely to an emergency in this setting? What items in the setting would you use?

Chapter

17 Environmental Health

Look for the skills icon throughout this chapter for opportunities to practice your health skills.

Check Your Health and Wellness Skills

In this chapter, you will learn skills for promoting environmental health. To understand the skills you currently use, take the following inventory of your behaviors. Indicate how well you think you use each skill. Use a scale of 1–5, *1* meaning you do not use the skill and *5* meaning you feel completely comfortable using it.

Skill	How Well Do You Use Each Skill?
I check the Air Quality Index (AQI) before going outside.	
I wear ear plugs if using power tools.	
I look for green or biodegradable products when shopping.	
I donate items to charities or resale stores when I no longer use them.	
I only buy as much food as I know I can eat.	
When I leave a room, I turn off the lights.	
I use reusable water bottles and bags.	
I recycle the items I can in my community.	
I know how to find out about disposing of hazardous waste.	
I encourage others to reduce waste and be environmentally friendly.	
	Total:

Add up your responses to each statement. The higher your score, the more comfortable you feel promoting environmental health. Which skill do you think is most important for you? Which skill is the most challenging for you? Which skill would you most like to improve? In this chapter, you will learn how to perform these skills better and more often.

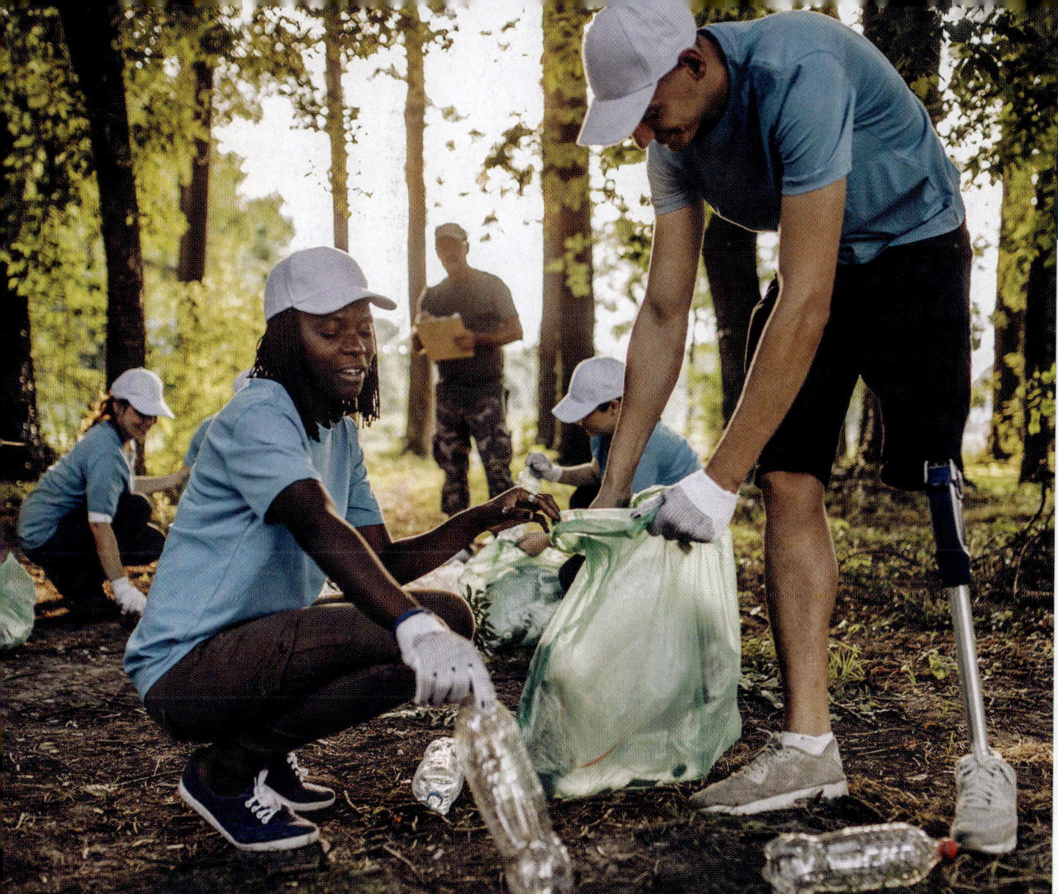

South_agency/E+/Getty Images

Reading and Notetaking

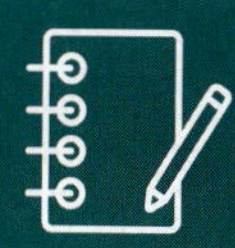

Think about the places you visit every day—for example, your school, your home, or the park. List these places on a piece of paper or electronically. As you listen to the presentation of this lesson, take notes about environmental issues and laws that affect each location and about strategies you can use to preserve the environment in each place you visit. An example is provided for you.

Home	School	Friend's Home
Noise pollution—railroad tracks nearby Use energy-efficient appliances	Issues with chemical pollution from nearby factory Composting program	Lead paint in kitchen Bring a refillable water bottle

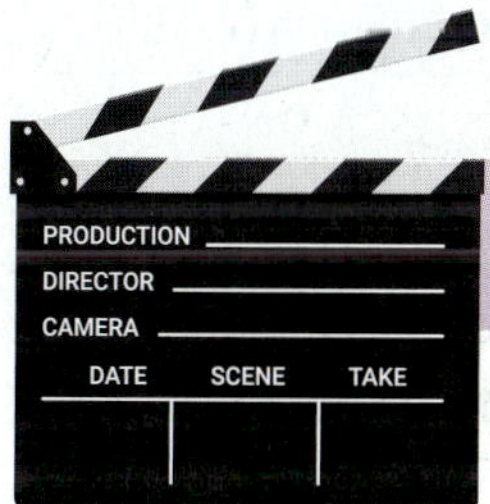

Setting the Scene

Small Changes Count

Lately, you feel like you see an article about the environment every time you browse your social media feed. Articles about polluted communities, contaminated water, and climate change discourage you, and you do not know what you can do. Your actions seem like just a drop in the bucket of the impact human activities have on the environment.

This year, some students started a club focused on sustainability at your school. You have attended several meetings. The club is running campaigns encouraging students to recycle, carpool or use public transportation, and reuse items instead of throwing them away. You are thinking about participating in one of these campaigns. Maybe doing something to protect the environment will make you feel less discouraged.

Thinking Critically

1. Is it true that people's actions are just a drop in the bucket of how human activities impact the environment? Explain.
2. How do recycling, carpooling, using public transportation, and reusing items help protect the environment?
3. Why do you think more teens do not take steps to act more sustainably and protect the environment?

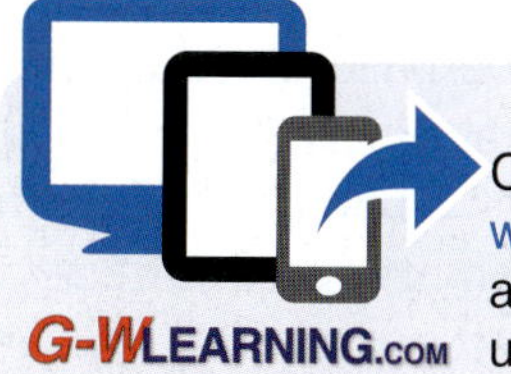

G-WLEARNING.COM

Click on the activity icon or visit www.g-wlearning.com/health/4095 to access online vocabulary activities using key terms from the chapter.

Lesson

17.1

Understanding the Environment

Essential Question?

What is the relationship between people and their environment?

Learning Outcomes

After studying this lesson, you will be able to

- summarize how ecosystems affect the natural environment;
- identify resources in the natural environment;
- explain how human activities, population, and economy impact communities and the environment; and
- identify global environmental issues.

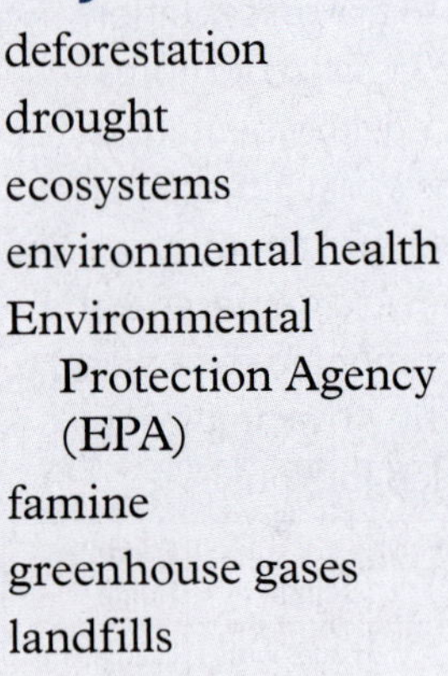

Key Terms

deforestation
drought
ecosystems
environmental health
Environmental Protection Agency (EPA)
famine
greenhouse gases
landfills
natural resources

Warm-Up Activity

Find the Facts

Access Information Before reading this lesson, read the following statements together as a small group. Then, using reliable and valid resources, determine whether each statement is true or false. Be sure to evaluate and cite your sources. After deciding on each statement, read this lesson and then explain why each statement is true or false and rewrite any false statements to make them true.

Statement	True or False	True Statement
Population growth positively affects the usage of natural resources.		
Sunlight is a natural resource that humans use for agriculture and solar power.		
Ecosystems are separate natural systems that do not interact with each other.		
Climate change only affects how hot or cold you are during seasons.		
Clean, running water is available to the whole world.		

When you think about health, you probably think about getting physical activity, eating nutritious foods, and building healthy relationships. You might also think about avoiding risky behaviors. All of these factors influence your health. As you know, another factor that impacts health is the environment in which you live.

The field of **environmental health** examines how factors in the environment affect your health. Factors in the *natural environment* include air, water, and soil. Your health is also affected by your *built environment*, which includes homes, apartments, schools, and offices. People interact

environmental health
field of health that focuses on interactions between different natural systems

with their natural and built environments. The environment can harm or benefit people's health. Human activity can also help or harm the environment.

Understanding the Natural Environment

The natural environment includes multiple natural systems called **ecosystems**, which are made of interrelated living and nonliving parts. The living parts of an ecosystem may include plants, animals, fungi, and microscopic creatures. These are called the *biotic* parts of an ecosystem. Nonliving parts are called *abiotic* and include water, air, sunlight, temperature, and chemicals in the air, water, and soil.

ecosystems natural systems made of interrelated biotic and abiotic parts

Earth has many ecosystems, and each ecosystem is different. For example, a pond ecosystem may have plants, algae, microscopic creatures, insects, fish, frogs, and ducks. The abiotic parts of an ecosystem influence the kinds of life found in the ecosystem. Different lakes may have different living parts. This is because ponds and lakes could have different water temperatures, chemicals, water currents, water depths, and amounts of sunlight.

Ecosystems interact with each other. This is because there is no barrier between ecosystems. Nothing prevents air, water, and living things from moving between ecosystems. Pollution, toxins, and environmental damage can also move between ecosystems. For example, if people harm their surrounding environment, that damage can affect other areas of the environment as well.

Resources in the Natural Environment

Natural resources are materials in the natural environment that people can use. You are probably familiar with many natural resources. They include water, soil, minerals and metals, fossil fuels (oil, natural gas, and coal), timber, and naturally occurring food such as fish or livestock (**Figure 17.1**).

natural resources materials in the natural environment that people can use, such as water, oil, timber, and soil

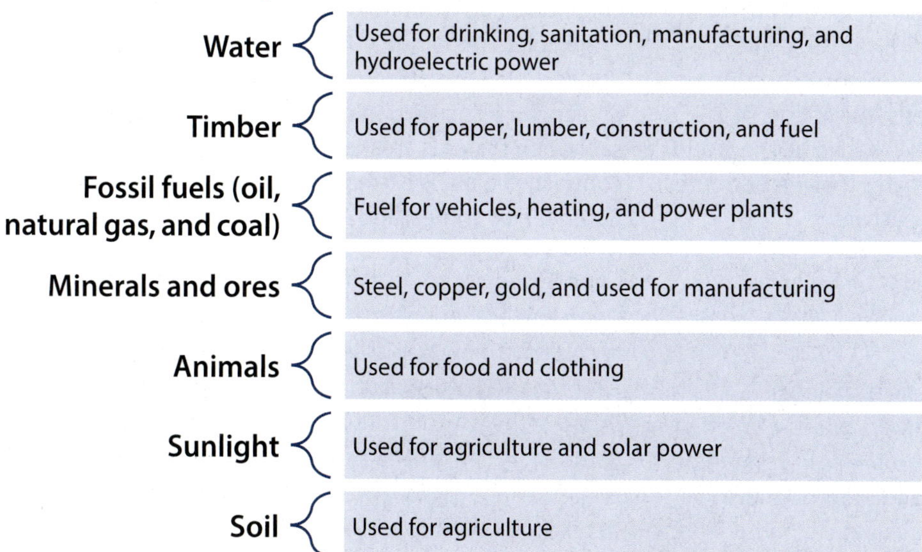

Figure 17.1 Humans use natural resources in a variety of ways.

Humans and the Environment Affect Each Other

In chapters 1 and 2, you learned about some of the ways the environment affects your health. For example, overpopulation can harm the health of communities, and pollution can lead to disease. Just as the environment affects your health, your actions also affect the environment, creating a cycle where humans and the environment affect each other. Around the world, people's actions impact both natural and built environments in diverse ways.

A Growing Human Population

The human population is estimated to be 7.7 billion people. It is difficult to comprehend a number so large. It is even harder to understand how fast the human population is growing. It took until the year 1800 for the human population to reach one billion. It took only 12 years to grow from six billion to seven billion. Scientists estimate that between 9 and

Local and Global Health

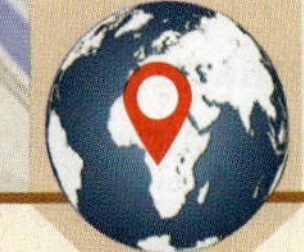

Water and Sanitation

Unlike most people in the US, 2.5 billion people around the world do not have safe drinking water in their homes or within a 30-minute walk. About 580 million people must take untreated water directly from rivers, lakes, ponds, or wells. In regions with poor sanitation systems, these water sources may be contaminated with human waste that carries disease-causing bacteria and viruses.

Drinking unsafe water can cause serious water-borne infections, including typhoid, cholera, dysentery, hepatitis, and polio. Many of these are *diarrheal diseases*, which means they cause severe, life-threatening diarrhea. Most diarrheal diseases occur in young children who cannot resist the effects of severe diarrhea and dehydration. Worldwide, the World Health Organization (WHO) estimates that water-borne infections cause 850,000 deaths each year.

Water-borne infections do not affect all countries equally. Diarrheal diseases are the first or second leading cause of death in many low-income countries, but are not leading causes of death in higher-income countries. Water-borne infections are especially common in low-income countries affected by war and natural disasters. For example, cholera became widespread in Yemen after years of war cut people off from clean drinking water. Following a devastating earthquake that destroyed sanitation systems in Haiti, cholera spread through the country.

Cholera remains a serious threat in some African and southeast Asian countries. In these countries, cholera affects crowded cities and rural areas, where sanitation systems are ineffective or nonexistent. In contrast, cholera is extremely rare in the US, Canada, European countries, and Japan.

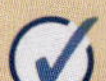

Practice Your Skills

Advocate for Health

Water sanitation is an example of a global environmental issue. In a small group, brainstorm other environmental issues that affect both your community and communities around the world. How do these issues affect the health of individuals and communities?

Choose one environmental issue to research in depth. Use reliable resources to describe the health effects of this issue, how this issue develops, and what steps countries and organizations are taking to correct or improve the issue. Identify one step teens in your community can take to help solve this environmental issue. Create a campaign encouraging your classmates to take this one step with you.

12 billion people can live on planet Earth. This estimate, however, does not take into account people's health and quality of life.

The three most populous countries in the world are China, India, and the United States. More than one-third of the world's people live in just two countries: China and India. In these and many countries, most people live in large, crowded cities.

As a population grows, it consumes more resources and produces more waste. For many years, the human population has been growing rapidly, and many parts of the world have become overpopulated. Overpopulation can lead to shortages of food and water. Without enough food, people can experience undernutrition and develop a variety of diseases, especially infections. A lack of safe drinking water causes infections, other diseases, and dehydration. A shortage of water combined with **drought**, a period with no rainfall, can harm crop production. Without crops and food, **famine**, or widespread hunger and starvation caused by lack of food, can develop.

drought extended period with no rainfall

famine widespread hunger and starvation caused by lack of food

Economic Development and Wealth

The world's countries have different levels of economic development and wealth. In general, higher-income countries make a bigger impact on the environment than low-income countries (**Figure 17.2**).

In low-income countries, people might have few options for making a living. Thus, many people obtain food and income directly from the natural environment. People use land, forests, and water as much as possible to get enough food and income.

Unfortunately, a low-income country might need to choose between feeding its people and preserving its natural resources. In contrast, a higher-income country with greater economic development may be able to feed its people as well as conserve resources.

Waste Management

Every community produces waste. Examples of solid waste include discarded paper, metal, plastic, rubber, fabric, food, and glass. Solid waste takes up space and does not break down naturally in air, water, or soil. Therefore, communities must manage their solid waste. Many communities collect solid waste from homes and businesses and store it in **landfills**.

landfills locations where waste is buried between layers of soil

Higher-Income Countries and Waste

The US has more vehicles than any other country.
For every 10 people in the US, there are about 8 vehicles.
Driving and producing vehicles and building the bridges and roads for traffic use energy and resources and produce waste like pollution and gases.

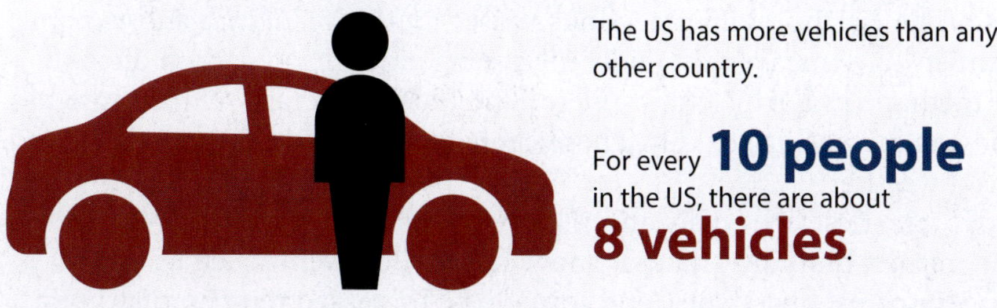

matsabe/Shutterstock.com

Figure 17.2 People in a higher-income society can consume more materials and natural resources, which produces more waste.

Environmental Protection Agency (EPA) US government agency that sets and enforces laws related to protecting the environment and human health

Some landfills are large pits dug in the ground. The bottoms are covered with clay and special liners to prevent harmful chemicals from leaking into soil and water. Solid waste is spread over the landfill surface and covered with layers of soil, followed by more waste and more soil. The US **Environmental Protection Agency (EPA)** sets and enforces laws related to landfills. These laws require safe storage of waste and protect people, water, and soil from any hazards in waste.

Disposing solid waste in a landfill has drawbacks. Landfills have limited storage space. Once full, a landfill must be closed. A full landfill cannot be used again, so people must build new landfills. Unfortunately, it is hard to find suitable land to build landfills. Landfills must be built in certain kinds of soil, and a community might object to the construction of a landfill nearby.

Landfills cannot store hazardous waste. Hazardous waste includes batteries, motor oil, gasoline, and certain household and industrial chemicals. This waste is too dangerous to dispose in a landfill. The EPA requires that communities manage hazardous waste in certain ways. You will learn more about hazardous waste in the next lesson.

Deforestation

deforestation condition in which forests are removed faster than they can grow

Forests can be removed quickly using machines and fire, but cannot quickly regrow. **Deforestation** occurs if forests are removed faster than they regrow. Deforestation harms the environment. Forests are complex ecosystems with many living creatures. Cutting down all or part of a forest threatens the survival of creatures that live in the forest. Scientists estimate tropical forests hold about 80 percent of all the Earth's animal species.

Forests release oxygen into the atmosphere and take in carbon dioxide. They also cool and humidify the surrounding air. Tree and plant roots hold soils in place, which prevents erosion of valuable soil. Several communities make their homes in forests. These people depend on forests for food and shelter.

Greenhouse Gases and Climate Change

greenhouse gases gases in Earth's atmosphere that trap heat, acting like the glass walls and roof of a greenhouse

Greenhouse gases in the Earth's atmosphere act like the glass in the walls and roof of a greenhouse. Greenhouse gases permit sunlight energy to reach the Earth's surface. Some light is absorbed by the Earth, and some light is reflected back to space. Greenhouse gases also trap the sunlight's heat close to Earth. Without greenhouse gases, sunlight's heat would escape back to space. Earth would be as cold as the Moon and Mars without greenhouse gases.

If there are more greenhouse gases, more heat is trapped near the Earth. The Earth's main greenhouse gases are *carbon dioxide* and *methane.* Scientists have measured rapidly increasing amounts of carbon dioxide and methane in Earth's atmosphere. The Earth's average temperature has also been increasing steadily. These changes are expected to continue and impact weather.

Weather describes daily and short-term conditions, such as temperature, humidity, rain, or snow. It includes events such as thunderstorms, hurricanes, and tornadoes. Increased temperature in the atmosphere changes how heat, wind, and weather circulate around the Earth. These changes have caused extreme temperatures, rainfall, droughts, and storms (**Figure 17.3**).

Climate Change Affects Health	
Effect of Climate Change	**Impact on Health**
Air pollution	Warmer air worsens pollution with ozone, smog, and tiny particles. When inhaled, these pollutants cause respiratory conditions such as asthma, severe allergies, and infections. Warmer air also causes longer spring and summer seasons, leading to more pollen in the air.
Extreme heat	Extreme heat causes heat-related conditions such as heatstroke. Heatstroke occurs when the body cannot cool itself. The body overheats to dangerously high temperatures, which can cause death or permanent damage.
Extreme precipitation	Extreme precipitation includes heavy or very little rain and snow. This can lead to flooding, dangerous snowstorms, or drought. Flooding can lead to disasters, mold growth, and water contamination. Drought can lead to famine, dust storms, and wildfires. Snowstorms can lead to cold-weather emergencies and accidents.
More active mosquitoes and ticks	More warm weather can make mosquitoes and ticks more active. Certain mosquitoes and ticks transmit diseases. Ticks carry bacteria that can cause Lyme disease. Some mosquitoes carry viruses that cause West Nile virus, yellow fever, malaria, and other diseases.

Figure 17.3 The impact that climate change has on weather patterns causes various health risks. ***What are the Earth's main greenhouse gases?***

Lesson 17.1 Review

Know and Understand

1. What effect does overpopulation have on the environment?
2. Why does a higher-income country have more of an impact on the environment than a low-income country?
3. How does deforestation affect the people living in an environment?

Think Critically

4. Think about one full day in your life. List all of the Earth's natural resources you consume in one day.
5. Give one example of how two different ecosystems affect each other.
6. Choose one effect of climate change on health. How does this effect impact health in your community?

REAL WORLD Health Skills

Comprehend Concepts Working in a small group, review the chart below. For each resource, identify its uses, how people abuse it, and how *you* use it. Several examples are shown for you. After filling in the chart, discuss ways you could use each natural resource in a more environmentally friendly way.

Resource	Uses	How It Is Abused	How You Use It
Water			*Brush my teeth*
Timber		*Not recycling*	
Natural gas, oil, and coal	*Fuel for cars*		
Minerals and ores	*Steel manufacturing*		
Oceans, lakes, and rivers			*Swim*
Sunlight			*Solar phone charger*
Soils		*Littering*	

Lesson 17.2

Identifying Environmental Hazards

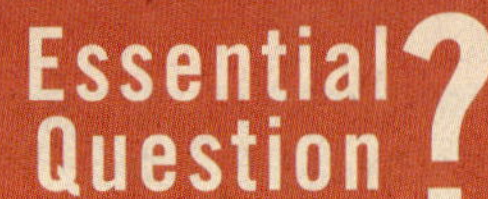

What risk factors in the environment impact health?

Learning Outcomes

After studying this lesson, you will be able to

- identify the natural and human causes of air pollution;
- explain how air pollution affects health, communities, and the environment;
- list ways to reduce air pollution;
- analyze the causes of water pollution, both natural and human;
- summarize the impact of water pollution on health, communities, and the environment;
- explain how to prevent exposure to water pollution;
- identify hazardous chemicals and ways to avoid them; and
- summarize the impact of and ways to reduce noise pollution.

Key Terms

Air Quality Index (AQI)
arsenic
asbestos
bisphenol A (BPA)
fertilizers
fossil fuels
herbicides
lead
mercury
mold
noise pollution
noise-related hearing loss
particulates
Per- and Polyfluoroalkyl Substances (PFAS)
pesticides
pollen
radon
volatile organic compounds (VOCs)

Warm-Up Activity

Identify the Influence

Analyze Influences Before reading this lesson, review the following scenarios about people interacting with their environment. Choose one scenario and write a short reflection analyzing the influence the individual has on the environment. How does this environmental impact affect the health of others? After writing your reflection, share your thoughts with a partner.

While washing dishes, Evan fills up the sink and then turns off the faucet.	Junior class president Rashawn stays after school once a week with some classmates to pick up garbage around campus.	Debbie chooses not to smoke.
Ms. Smith uses a glass water bottle and refills it every day.	A farmer chooses not to use pesticides on crops.	In woodshop, Mr. Scott wears ear protection and provides them to the students working with large power tools.

All communities produce some waste. This waste affects the environment, which then impacts people's health. As you learned in Chapter 2, the presence of waste in the environment is called *pollution*. Pollution can affect the air, water, and level of noise in an environment. Hazardous chemicals can also pollute the environment. In this lesson, you will learn about pollution, its effects on health, and ways of limiting pollution and exposure to it.

Air Pollution

You might not notice the air around you except when the air is very cold or hot, humid, or polluted. Still, the Earth's air is important for the health and survival of all living creatures (**Figure 17.4**).

Air pollution is the presence of harmful amounts of chemicals and other substances in the air. Many of these harm the health of people, other living creatures, and climate. Some types of air pollution are produced naturally, and some air pollution comes from human activities. Both outdoor and indoor air can be polluted.

Natural Sources of Air Pollution

Some air pollution occurs naturally in the environment. This type of pollution comes from natural events and sources.

Smoke and Ash

Smoke and ash produced by natural events can pollute the air. For example, *wildfires* are natural events that release smoke containing harmful **particulates**, or tiny particles suspended in air, made of burnt material and ash. Wildfire smoke can affect entire continents because wind currents carry particulates far and wide. Gases from wildfires include carbon dioxide and poisonous carbon monoxide. Breathing this smoke irritates the throat and lungs and increases the risk of respiratory conditions such as bronchitis and asthma.

particulates tiny particles suspended in the air

Volcanic eruptions also produce air pollution, which can carry across oceans and continents. Volcanos release tiny particles of ash and dust and harmful chemicals such as sulfuric acid and chlorine. These chemicals burn the eyes, skin, and throat.

Radon

Radon is a colorless, odorless, tasteless gas. Soil and rocks that contain uranium naturally produce it. Radon seeps up from the ground and can collect in the basements of buildings. It is the leading cause of lung cancer for people who do not smoke.

radon colorless, odorless, tasteless gas produced naturally from soil and rocks that contain uranium

Gases in the Earth's Air

Gas	Percentage
Nitrogen	78%
Oxygen	21%
Other gases	1%

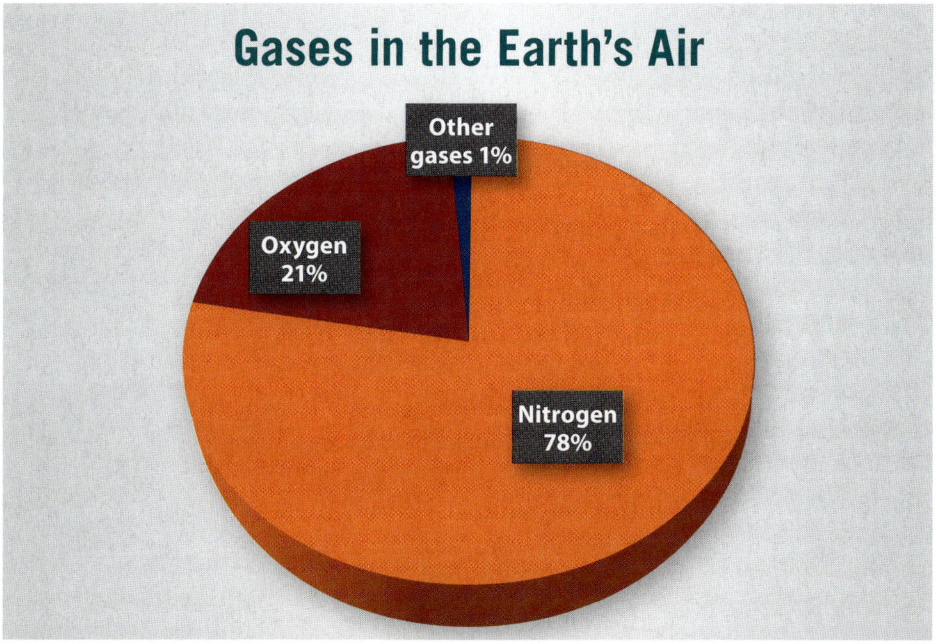

Figure 17.4 The air on Earth contains gases, including nitrogen, oxygen, and small amounts of other gases, such as argon and carbon dioxide. The air also contains water vapor.

Mold

mold fungus that grows in moist areas

Mold is a fungus that grows in moist areas. In homes, mold can grow on wet walls in basements, under sinks, around bathtubs, and in wet carpets. Breathing mold causes allergies, itchy eyes, nasal congestion, coughing, and sore throat. Mold also causes respiratory diseases and infections.

Dust

Breathing in dust may trigger indoor allergy symptoms:

- Runny nose
- Itchy eyes
- Chills and body aches
- Symptoms that linger for days or weeks

Figure 17.5 Dust can trigger indoor allergies. Indoor allergy symptoms are difficult to pinpoint because they often mimic symptoms of the common cold. ***What is the name for dead skin cells and saliva from pets found in dust?***

Dust is made of materials small enough to be carried in air. Household dust can contain mold, fibers from fabrics, and *dander* (dead skin cells and saliva from pets). Dust might contain dried urine and feces from rats, mice, and cockroaches (**Figure 17.5**).

Tiny animals called *dust mites* and their feces may also be in dust. Dust mites live in most pillows, sheets, and blankets. They eat skin cells that rub off the body. Breathing dust mite feces can lead to allergic reactions, itchy eyes, nasal congestion, and sneezing. Scratching mite feces into skin makes skin itchy and swollen.

Pollen

pollen dry, dusty powder made by flowers

Pollen is a dry, dusty powder made by flowers. In spring and warm seasons, many flowers make pollen. Pollen can cause itchy eyes, runny nose, sneezing, nasal congestion, and coughing. This allergy is sometimes called *hay fever*, though the pollen does not cause a fever. Most pollen is in outdoor air and enters homes in air currents.

Air Pollution from Human Activities

Air pollution also occurs through human activities such as industrial burning of fossil fuels, driving, smoking or vaping, and using perfume. Several human activities contribute to air pollution.

Fuel Emissions

fossil fuels natural gas, coal, and oil; are burned to produce energy

Natural gas, oil, and coal are called **fossil fuels** because they were produced over millions of years from decomposed animals and plants. Once these fuels are used, they cannot be replaced during humanity's near future. As fossil fuels are burned for energy to power human activities, they release carbon dioxide, carbon monoxide, and chemicals called *sulfur oxides* and *nitrogen oxides*. These waste products from burning fuels are called *emissions* or exhaust.

Fuel emissions harm health and the environment. For example, carbon dioxide is a greenhouse gas. The Earth grows warmer as carbon dioxide increases in the atmosphere. *Carbon monoxide* is a colorless, odorless gas that, when inhaled, prevents the blood from carrying oxygen. This can lead to headaches, confusion, and unconsciousness and can cause death without emergency treatment.

Sulfur oxide and nitrogen oxide also enter the air when fuels burn. Nitrogen oxide irritates the nose, mouth, throat, and lungs. Sulfur oxide and nitrogen oxide combine with water vapor and make sulfuric acid and nitric acid, which have negative effects on the environment.

How Fuel Emissions Impact the Environment	
Effect	**Description**
Acid rain 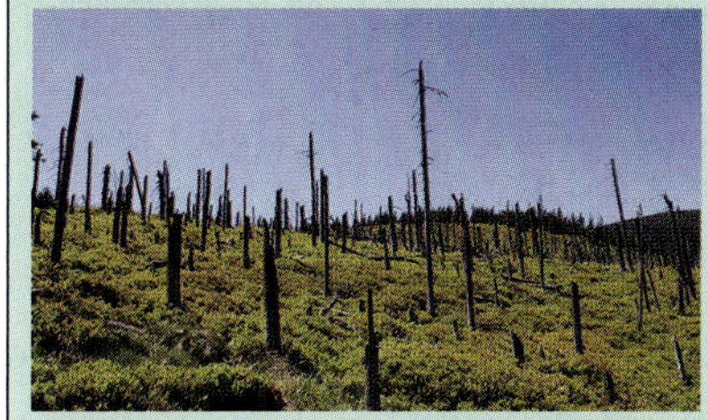	Sulfuric acid and nitric acid in the atmosphere turn water vapor into acid rain. Acid rain damages trees, other plants, and metal and stone structures and can harm creatures that live in the water.
Smog 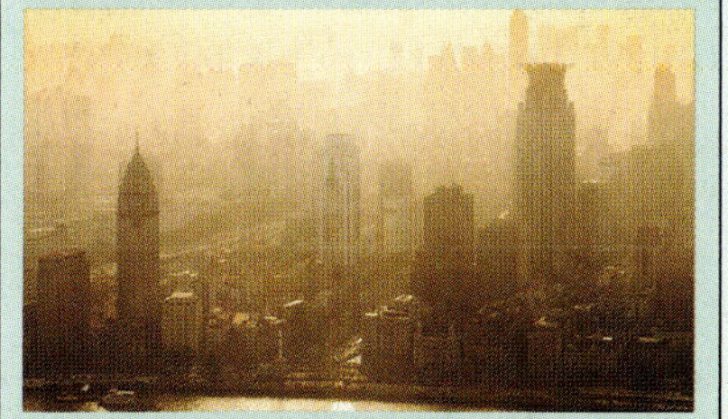	Smog is a hazy cloud made from nitrogen oxide, particulates, sulfur oxide, and carbon monoxide. Sunlight and vehicle emissions react to form smog, which is common around cities where many vehicles produce emissions. Smog irritates the eyes and causes respiratory conditions like asthma, wheezing and coughing, throat irritation, and chest pain.
Ozone 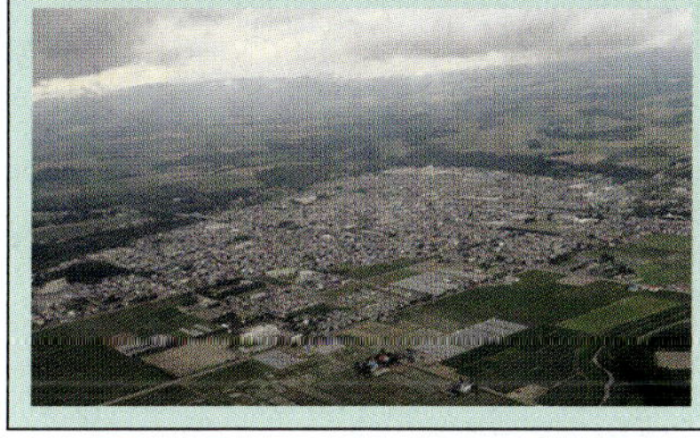	Ozone is a gas that, when high in the atmosphere, benefits human health by blocking some radiation from the sun. Ozone near the Earth's surface is a pollutant. Ozone damages the lungs and causes wheezing and chest pain. It also damages crops and other plants. On days when ground-level ozone levels are high, weather forecasters warn people to stay indoors when possible and to avoid physical activity outdoors.

Top to bottom: Tomasz Bidermann/Shutterstock.com; iamlukyeee/Shutterstock.com; Xi kou/Shutterstock.com

Figure 17.6 Acid rain, smog, and ozone are three of the negative effects that fuel emissions can have on the environment. ***Which chemical fuel emission irritates the nose, throat, and lungs?***

Interactions between these waste products in the air can lead to serious consequences (**Figure 17.6**).

Smoke, Dust, and Aerosols

Smoke and dust from human activities can also pollute the air. For example, burning wood produces particulates, carbon dioxide, and carbon monoxide. Smoke from tobacco products also pollutes the air and harms health. You learned about the dangers of tobacco smoke in Chapter 11.

While dust occurs naturally, tractors and farm machinery can stir up dust as farmers plow fields. Construction of buildings and roads also stirs up dust. Dust irritates the eyes, nose, throat, and lungs. It can cause allergic reactions, coughing, and difficulty breathing.

Another pollutant is *aerosols*, or tiny airborne droplets. Perfumes, spray paints, air fresheners, and scented candles make aerosols. Breathing in these aerosols can be harmful to some people. Coughing and sneezing also produce aerosols containing bacteria and viruses.

Volatile Organic Compounds (VOCs)

Volatile organic compounds (VOCs) are chemicals that come from paint, varnish, cleaning supplies, gasoline, scented candles, perfume, and other sources. These pollutants evaporate in the air and can cause several health issues.

volatile organic compounds (VOCs) chemicals found in paint, varnish, cleaning supplies, and other sources; evaporate in the air

In the past, asbestos was used for insulation and fire protection. In homes, asbestos is sometimes found in the walls of attics, surrounding pipes, around furnaces and fireplaces, and in roof materials and floor tiles.

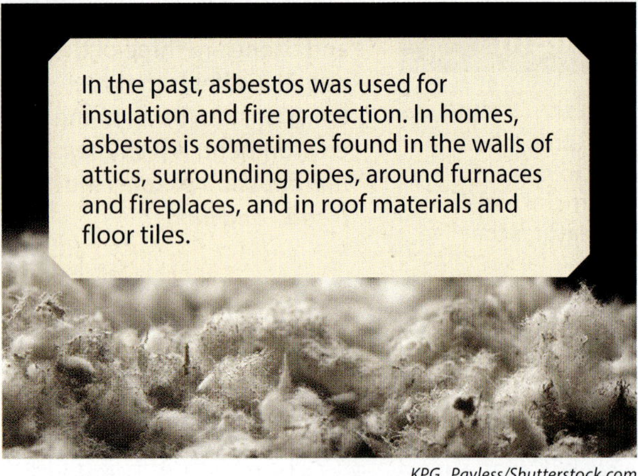

KPG_Payless/Shutterstock.com

Figure 17.7 Breathing asbestos fibers can cause lung disease and lung cancer.

When people first breathe VOCs, their eyes, nose, and throat may be irritated. They may also have difficulty breathing and nausea. VOCs can affect the nervous system and cause dizziness, blurred vision, and confusion. If you are exposed to VOCs and experience these symptoms, get away from the chemicals, move to fresh air outdoors, and call Poison Control (800-222-1222) or 911 for help. Breathing VOCs can damage organs such as the liver, lungs, kidneys, and nervous system. The injured lungs and respiratory system can develop diseases that make breathing difficult. These respiratory diseases include emphysema, asthma, and bronchitis. Scientists are trying to learn if certain VOCs cause cancer in humans.

Asbestos

asbestos natural mineral in soils; was formerly used for insulation and fire protection, but can cause cancer when inhaled

Asbestos is a natural mineral in soils (**Figure 17.7**). You should never touch anything you think has asbestos because it might crumble and release fibers. In fact, it is safer to leave asbestos alone than to try removing it yourself.

Preventing Exposure to Air Pollution

Air Quality Index (AQI) tool for reporting daily air quality and how air quality impacts different health concerns

You can get information about levels of air pollution in your community by checking the **Air Quality Index (AQI)**. The AQI tells you about five major air pollutants, including ozone and particle pollution. This index is available online or by signing up for a free email or app. If air pollution is high in your community one day, try to spend more of your time inside, especially in the afternoon, when ozone levels are typically highest. Staying inside is especially important if you have allergies or asthma (**Figure 17.8**).

Figure 17.8 Other strategies for preventing exposure to air pollution are listed here. ***What is the tool that measures the level of air pollution in different communities?***

Strategies for Avoiding Air Pollution

- Test homes for pollutants such as radon, mold, and asbestos. If radon, mold, or asbestos is detected, get the help of a professional to remove the pollutant.
- Install and regularly replace furnace air filters in the home. You could also try using an air purifier.
- Reduce moisture in the home by fixing leaky faucets, pipes, and roofs.
- Frequently change and wash bedding. Using a bedding cover can reduce exposure to dust mites.
- Dust and vacuum the home regularly.
- Close windows if levels of air pollution outside are high.
- Install and maintain carbon monoxide detectors in sleeping areas and near furnaces, fireplaces, kitchens, basements, garages, and other areas where gas may collect.
- Do not run car engines inside an enclosed garage or a garage attached to the home. Never use a gas or charcoal grill indoors, in garages, or in tents.
- Avoid using aerosol sprays in public. If you are allergic or sensitive to aerosols, stay away from people who are using them.
- Only use paint, varnish, and cleaning supplies in well-ventilated areas. Open windows and doors or use fans to circulate air.
- Always follow label directions when using, storing, and discarding cleaning products.
- Avoid places with lots of motor vehicle traffic. If you are driving in traffic, keep your windows closed.
- Wear a mask if levels of air pollution are high.

Water Pollution

Water covers the majority of the planet's surface. At least 97.5 percent of Earth's water is saltwater, and 2.5 percent is fresh water. Most of this fresh water is in glaciers, permanent fields of snow, or soils and water vapor. As a result, people can only use 1 percent of the Earth's fresh water. This is only 0.025 percent of all of the water on Earth. All of the world's people use this fresh water for drinking, watering crops and livestock, cooking, cleaning, and sanitation.

The quality of water depends not just on water itself, but also on the conditions of surrounding air and land (**Figure 17.9**). In the water cycle, pollutants can spread between the air, water, and land. More than 50 percent of the human population now lives in cities next to water or a short distance from water. Therefore, human activities make a big impact on the world's water.

Chemical Pollution

Chemicals become water pollutants when amounts of them in water harm health. For example, some chemicals normally in water are harmless in small amounts, but harmful in larger amounts. Other chemicals are pollutants because they do not naturally occur in water. Many chemical wastes are produced through manufacturing. The EPA protects water supplies by regulating disposal of these wastes.

Lead, mercury, and arsenic are examples of naturally occurring elements that can enter and pollute water. Each is toxic to humans and animal life. You will learn more about these elements later in this lesson. Sometimes, naturally occurring pollutants enter the water through mining or because acid rain dissolves toxic elements in rocks. For example, some gold mines produce runoff containing mercury.

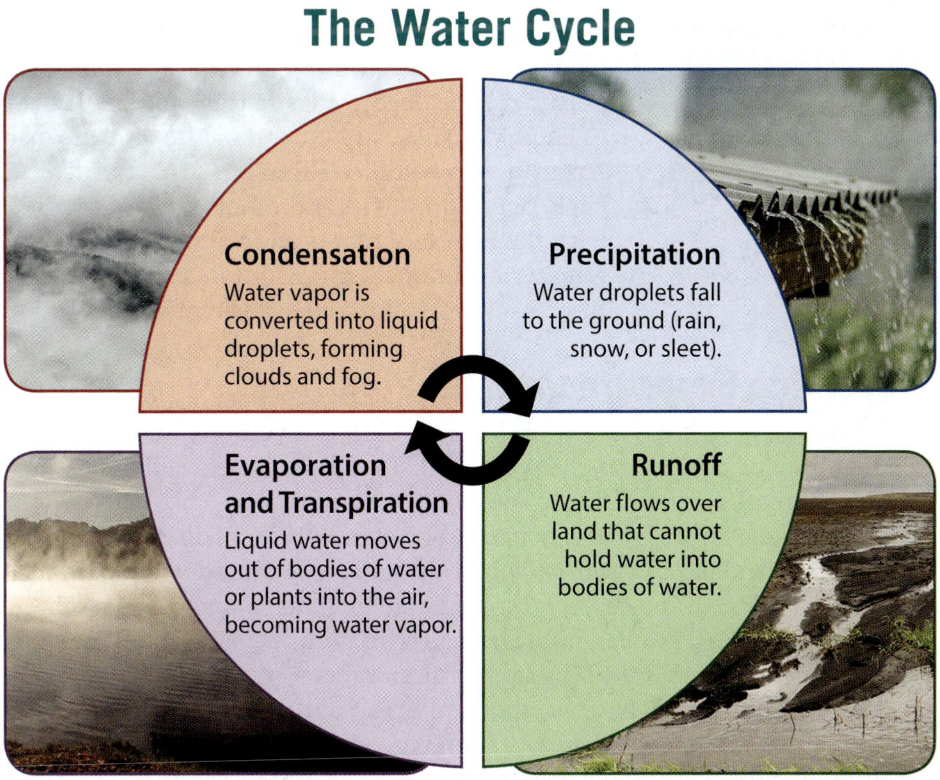

The Water Cycle

Condensation
Water vapor is converted into liquid droplets, forming clouds and fog.

Precipitation
Water droplets fall to the ground (rain, snow, or sleet).

Evaporation and Transpiration
Liquid water moves out of bodies of water or plants into the air, becoming water vapor.

Runoff
Water flows over land that cannot hold water into bodies of water.

Clockwise from top left: Volodymyr Burdiak/Shutterstock.com; Anna Nikonorova/Shutterstock.com; JJ Gouin/Shutterstock.com; Michael Shake/Shutterstock.com

Figure 17.9 The surrounding air and land affect water quality because water follows a cycle and changes between liquid, solid, and vapor forms. ***What percent of the Earth's water is fresh water?***

fertilizers chemicals applied to farmland, gardens, and lawns to promote growth

pesticides chemicals used to destroy insects or other organisms that harm plants or animals

Chemicals used in agriculture can also pollute water. Chemical **fertilizers** are applied to farmland, gardens, and lawns to promote plant growth. Runoff may carry fertilizers to water sources, where they promote overgrowth of algae and other microscopic organisms. This harms water quality and can kill aquatic life. Chemical **pesticides** control mosquitoes and plant pests. Runoff can carry pesticides from plants and soil to water supplies. You will learn more about pesticides and hazardous chemicals later in this lesson.

Oil can pollute water during collection, transport, or conversion into other products such as gasoline. Oil contains many hazardous chemicals. If an *oil spill* (release of oil into the water) occurs, this can endanger living creatures and their ecosystems. People cannot use water contaminated with oil.

A mass of plastic roughly the size of Texas is floating in the southern Pacific Ocean.
Inventors and scientists around the world are racing to figure out how to clean up this huge mass.

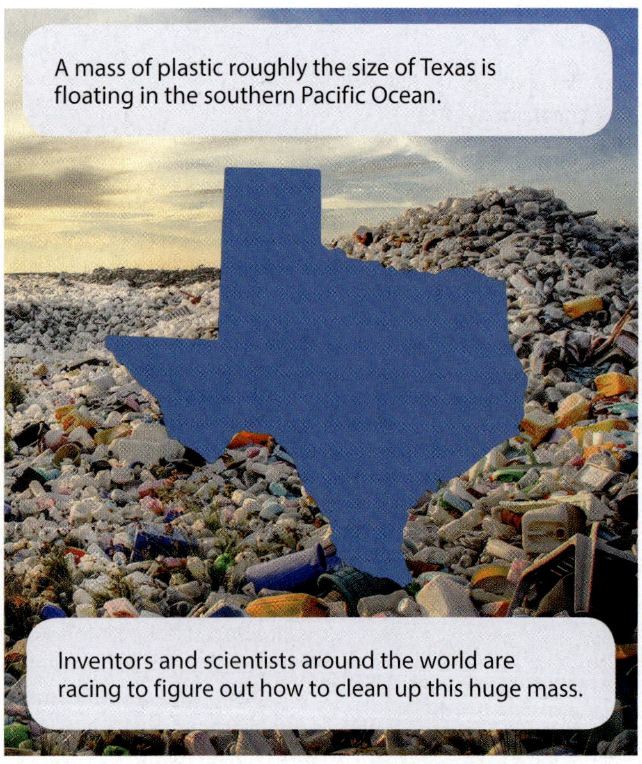

Texas: T. Lesia/Shutterstock.com; Plastic: MOHAMED ABDULRAHEEM/Shutterstock.com

Figure 17.10 As plastic does not break down and is hazardous to the health of plants and wildlife, the mass of plastic floating in the Pacific Ocean raises serious concerns.

Biological Pollution

Biological pollution refers to the presence of dangerous organisms. For example, runoff from farm fields, ranches, or meat-processing businesses can carry pathogens. When floods cause sewers to overflow, *sewage* (human waste) can enter water supplies and cause serious communicable diseases. Toxic algae can grow in polluted water and harm wildlife and people.

Litter

Litter, or waste that is not properly disposed, is another familiar water pollutant. Some litter does not break down and remains in the environment. For example, plastic does not break down and decay. Plastic can fracture into small pieces, which last indefinitely in the environment.

Plastic has been found in the stomachs of birds, whales, and fish. Unfortunately, ingested plastic can be deadly. Plastic rings for six-packs of canned drinks, straws, and fishing line are also hazardous to wildlife (**Figure 17.10**). Bottles, cans, paper products, and other litter interfere with the health of plants and wildlife. Some litter releases harmful chemicals into water, and litter blocks sewers and drains, causing floods.

Preventing Exposure to Water Pollution

To reduce your exposure to water pollution, test your drinking water for the presence of harmful chemicals. Most counties have a soil and water conservation office that will test household water.

If your home floods, avoid touching floodwater with bare skin. Keep children, pets, and food away from floodwater and avoid contact with floodwater outside your home. If you suspect drinking water is contaminated, find another source of water, use a purifier, or boil water for 10 minutes to destroy bacteria and viruses. Wash your skin with soap and clean water if you touch floodwater.

Construction or freezing weather can break underground water pipes. Broken pipes take in contaminants from surrounding soil. Until pipes are repaired, boil drinking water for 10 minutes to ensure its safety.

Hikers and campers should not drink from natural water sources, even if the water looks clear and clean. This water can make you sick if it contains contaminated runoff. Boil the water for 10 minutes or treat it with disinfectant. You can purchase disinfectant tablets or a portable water filter at camping supply and home improvement stores.

Hazardous Chemicals

Chemicals make up you, your food, medications, and the natural environment. In that sense, chemicals are important, valuable, and not necessarily harmful.

Not all naturally occurring chemicals are safe. Not all manufactured chemicals are harmful. Whether a chemical is dangerous depends on the type of chemical, the amount, and type of exposure. For example, some chemicals are dangerous when inhaled or harmful when swallowed. One chemical might be dangerous in small amounts; another could be hazardous only in large amounts. Chemicals that are poisonous to the body are called *poisons* or *toxins*. Chemicals known to cause cancer are *carcinogens*.

Research in Action

Which Substances Are Carcinogens?

The causes of cancer are complex. Damage to DNA is the primary cause, and damaged DNA can develop due to genetic, behavioral, or environmental factors. One factor in the environment that can influence cancer risk is the presence of carcinogens. A *carcinogen* is a substance known to cause cancer. *Probable* or *possible carcinogens* are substances that may cause cancer, but experimental results are incomplete or uncertain. While the presence of a carcinogen will not always lead to cancer, people should treat carcinogenic substances with caution. Some examples of carcinogens are shown in the table.

To study carcinogenic substances, scientists examine them in test tubes with cells and in animals. They also observe humans with cancer to see if a substance is connected. After many experiments, which can take months or years, scientists review the results and decide if the substance should be called a carcinogen. Organizations that decide if experiments show a substance is carcinogenic include the International Agency for Cancer Research (IARC), EPA, and US National Toxicology Program (NTP).

Carcinogen	Type of Cancer
Asbestos	Lung cancer
Tobacco	Lung, mouth, and throat cancer
Alcohol	Breast cancer in females and colon, liver, esophagus, and mouth cancer
Radon	Lung cancer
Ultraviolet radiation	Skin cancer
Human papillomavirus (HPV)	Cervical cancer
Hepatitis C virus (HCV)	Liver cancer

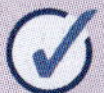

Practice Your Skills

Access Information

In a small group, brainstorm a list of substances you have heard are carcinogens. List as many of these substances as you can. Choose one substance to research in depth. Using reliable resources, research the following information:

- whether the substance is considered a carcinogen
- studies that show the substance is or is not a carcinogen
- where the substance is most often found
- what, if any, cancers the substance causes

Once you have collected all of this information, create a public service announcement (PSA) about the substance chosen. Educate your fellow students about the scientific facts surrounding this substance. If the substance is a carcinogen, share tips for reducing exposure to it.

Hazardous chemicals can move from the natural environment into homes and schools. For example, toxins can enter water and food before you consume them in your home. Fortunately, you can reduce your exposure to hazardous chemicals.

Naturally Occurring Hazardous Chemicals

Many naturally occurring chemicals are hazardous in certain amounts. Examples of these chemicals include mercury, lead, and arsenic.

Mercury

mercury silver metal that is liquid at room temperature; is naturally found in coal, oil, and other fuels

Mercury is a silver metal that is liquid at room temperature. It is extracted from mined rocks and is naturally present in coal, oil, and other fuels.

People have used mercury in industry, chemical research, electrical switches, blood pressure monitors, thermometers, and dental fillings. In the past, some types of vaccines even contained a form of mercury in the preservative *thimerosal*. Most uses of mercury have been discontinued, and mercury has been replaced with other chemicals. Today, mercury is in fluorescent lights, compact fluorescent lights, neon lights, and some batteries.

Mercury in the atmosphere comes mostly from human activities, such as burning coal. Volcanic eruptions and forest fires also release mercury into the air. Airborne mercury can travel far before it enters the water as precipitation. In water, mercury builds up in large fish such as swordfish and tuna. For this reason, people should avoid regularly eating these fish, and pregnant people should not eat them. The EPA and Centers for Disease Control and Prevention (CDC) have guidelines about how much fish you should eat and the kinds to avoid.

Lead

lead soft gray metal mined from the ground; was used in some products and then banned due to its toxicity

Lead is a soft gray metal mined from the ground. It has been used in water pipes, ammunitions, and fishing weights. Lead was once added to gasoline and paint (**Figure 17.11**). In the 1970s, the US banned many uses of lead because of its toxicity. Some soils contain lead from car exhaust produced when gasoline contained lead. For this reason, make sure to wash your hands with soap and water after handling soil. Do not let children put dirt in their mouths or play with paint chips.

Many old water supply pipes contain lead. Over time, lead in damaged or rusted pipes can dissolve and enter drinking water. Many cities have recognized this problem and chemically treat pipes. Some old pipes have been replaced.

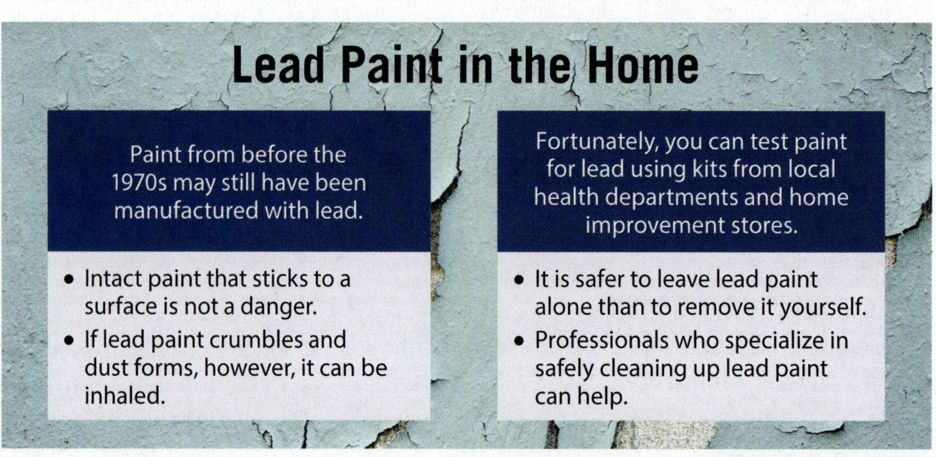

Joyce Vincent/Shutterstock.com

Figure 17.11 Because manufacturers once used lead in paint, many houses still have walls, furniture, and other household items painted with lead.

Ingesting or inhaling lead causes brain damage and issues with learning, attention, and memory. Unfortunately, bones store lead in the body, and the amount of lead in the body can build over time. If you think you have been exposed to lead, see your doctor. You can get your blood tested for lead, and your doctor can give you medical advice.

Arsenic

Arsenic is an element normally found in soils and rocks. Erosion and runoff can carry arsenic into water, and arsenic enters the air when wind picks up small amounts from soil. Volcanic eruptions and forest fires also add arsenic to the air. Arsenic settles to the land and water in precipitation and particulates.

arsenic element normally found in soils and rocks; is poisonous and carcinogenic at high levels

Waste from copper and lead mining often contains arsenic. In the past, some pesticides also contained arsenic. As a result, the soil of farm fields may have arsenic from past pesticide applications. Arsenic has also been used in wood preservatives to make pressure-treated wood.

Arsenic is a poison and carcinogen. Breathing a small amount irritates the throat and causes lung damage. A small amount in food or water irritates the stomach and causes diarrhea and blood abnormalities. Swallowing or breathing a large amount of arsenic causes death. People eat, drink, and breathe some arsenic every day because food, water, and air contain a small amount of arsenic. This amount is not considered harmful. To prevent additional, harmful exposure, test drinking water and never burn pressure-treated wood. Be sure to wash fruit and vegetables and wash your hands after handling soil.

Manufactured Hazardous Chemicals

Manufactured chemicals can also be hazardous in certain amounts. Examples of manufactured hazardous chemicals include household chemicals, pesticides and herbicides, bisphenol A (BPA), and Per- and Polyfluoroalkyl Substances (PFAS).

Household Chemicals

Household chemicals, such as cleaning supplies, paint, and fuels, can pose risks to health if they are not handled properly. For example, getting some chemicals in the eyes can lead to vision loss. Contact between some chemicals and the skin can cause burns.

To avoid harmful exposure to household chemicals, pay attention to the product symbols found on chemical packages. These symbols tell you how the chemical may impact your health and the environment (**Figure 17.12**). Make sure to read warning labels carefully and store and dispose of chemicals according to the instructions. Keep chemicals away from items used in cooking and eating and do not move chemicals into new containers.

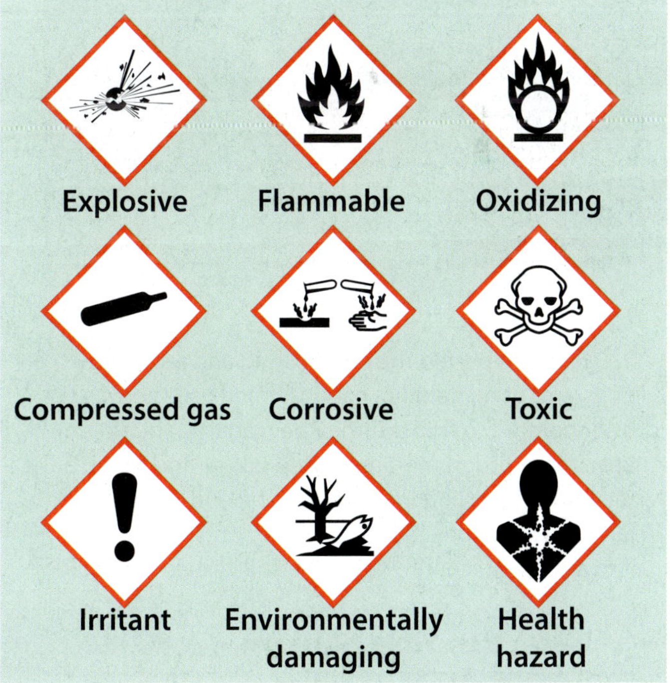

Rainer Lesniewski/Shutterstock.com

Figure 17.12 By recognizing the chemical symbols on packaging, you can understand the warnings about health risks associated with chemicals in different products. ***Look at the packaging of a cleaning product you use regularly. What chemical symbols are on the packaging?***

Be careful about mixing different chemicals. For example, mixing bleach and ammonia (such as in toilet bowl or window cleaning products) together produces a highly toxic gas. When using household chemicals, protect your skin and eyes by wearing gloves, long sleeves, and goggles. Use chemicals in well-ventilated areas and wash your hands with soap and water afterward.

Pesticides and Herbicides

Pesticides are chemicals that kill insects and other living creatures that damage plants or harm people. For example, pesticides kill certain insects that damage crops, fruits, and vegetables. Around homes, people use pesticides to control insects that damage plants. People should use pesticides according to label directions and store them away from children, pets, wildlife, food, and water.

herbicides chemicals used to kill unwanted plants, such as weeds

Herbicides kill plants and weeds and are often applied to protect crops. Herbicides may cause a number of illnesses in humans. People who manufacture and apply herbicides have the highest risk for disease.

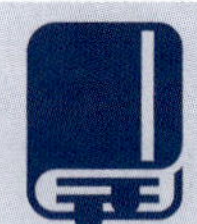

Case Study

Environmental Impact

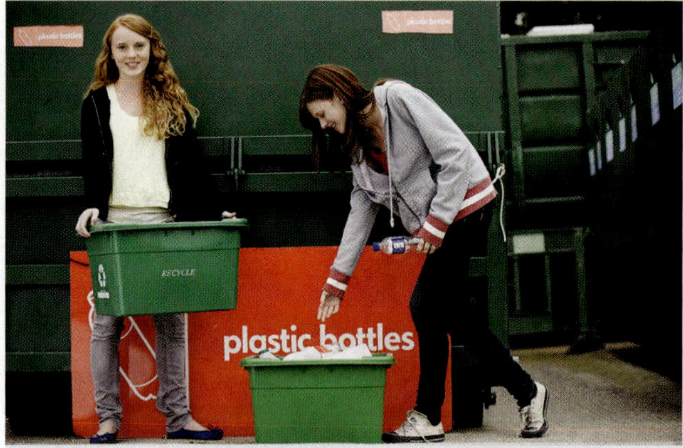

Air Images/Shutterstock.com

Katharine loved the composting and recycling programs at her family's old apartment, so she was disappointed to find out their new apartment did not have these programs. She looked online and found a recycling campaign in her neighborhood. Now, her family saves paper, plastic, and glass waste and takes it to a drop-off center. Katharine still wishes she could compost their food waste. She wonders if she could start a campaign at school to create a small garden with composting bins.

Jesse and his mom recently moved closer to the local airport, where Jesse's mom works as a ground traffic controller. Jesse loves his new home, but is worried about the constant noise from the airplanes. He knows his mom has hearing loss from her job and from attending concerts when she was his age. He is concerned he will start to lose his hearing. When Jesse tells his mom about his concerns, she suggests Jesse wear noise-cancelling headphones at home and at his summer landscaping job to prevent hearing loss.

Samuel's community has been experiencing a long drought season and record-setting high temperatures. There is a shortage of water, and lots of people, including some family members and friends, have gone to the hospital for heatstroke or dehydration. In addition, the lack of rain is increasing the chances of a wildfire in neighboring forests. Samuel is worried for the safety of himself and his family in this environment.

Practice Your Skills

Advocate for Health

Evaluate the green programs that exist in your community (for recycling, composting, community gardens, trash cleanup, renewable energy, or any other environmental initiative). Then, identify programs that are missing from your community. As a class, choose one environmental issue that is not addressed. Create a campaign to implement a new initiative at your school or in your community. Be sure to include any fundraising, volunteer, and upkeep needs in your plan. Prepare a presentation you could give to your city council or school board outlining your ideas.

You can reduce your exposure by washing vegetables and fruit under clean running water. You should use weed killers with care; wear gloves, long sleeves, long pants, and goggles during application; and wash your hands after handling weed killer.

BPA

Bisphenol A (BPA) is a chemical used to make the plastic in water bottles, food packaging, and coatings inside metal food cans. BPA in plastic containers can move into food or water, especially when heated. Swallowing BPA is the main way people are exposed. Studies suggest that most people in the US have BPA in their bodies.

Research with animals suggests BPA can harm humans. Scientists are trying to determine how BPA affects health. Until more research is available, people should avoid storing and heating water and food in plastic containers. People can also purchase plastic cans and bottles labeled *BPA free*.

bisphenol A (BPA) chemical used to make some plastics; may be harmful to humans

PFAS

Per- and Polyfluoroalkyl Substances (PFAS) are chemicals used to make some nonstick coatings on cookware and water- and stain-resistant fabrics. Most people in the US have PFAS in their bodies due to contact with various sources. In humans, PFAS can raise cholesterol, affect the immune system, and may cause cancer.

Although alternatives have replaced PFAS for most uses in the US, fire control foams still contain PFAS. Therefore, PFAS are in soil and water where fire departments and the military practice firefighting. If you are concerned about PFAS in drinking water, consult the EPA for locations that have large amounts of PFAS. Check with the EPA or your area health department for information about testing your water.

Per- and Polyfluoroalkyl Substances (PFAS) chemicals used to make some nonstick coatings on cookware and water- and stain-resistant fabrics

Noise Pollution

Noise can be all around you and feel like a natural, harmless part of your world. A lot of noise, however, is **noise pollution**, or unnatural noise that can harm your health (**Figure 17.13**). Sometimes, you can control the level of noise you experience—by turning down the volume of your music, for example.

noise pollution exposure to unnatural, harmful noise

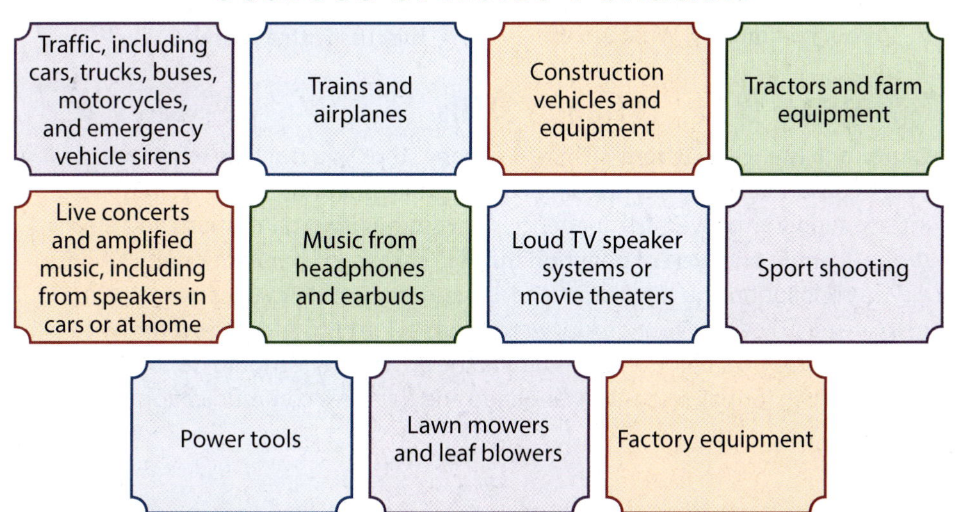

Figure 17.13 High levels of noise or noise over a long period of time becomes noise pollution.

Other times, you cannot control the noise in your environment. For example, people who spend time near railroad tracks, highways, and airports experience a lot of noise pollution.

noise-related hearing loss
condition in which hearing worsens due to exposure to loud or long-lasting sounds

Noise affects physical and emotional health. For example, **noise-related hearing loss** affects 17 percent of US teens. People who experience gradual hearing loss usually do not notice for a long time. Early signs may be difficulty hearing voices through background sounds, difficulty hearing someone speaking from a distance, and *tinnitus* (ringing or buzzing in the ears). There is no cure or treatment for hearing loss, so it is important to protect your hearing.

During the day, noise causes stress, raises blood pressure, and interferes with concentration. Noise at night interferes with sleep, causing daytime tiredness, difficulty learning, and anxiety and depression.

To protect yourself from noise pollution, recognize and try to avoid harmful sources of noise. For example, you could leave the noisy area or use ear protection if you cannot leave. Wear ear plugs or sound-dampening ear coverings when using loud tools such as leaf blowers, lawn mowers, or power drills. Reduce the volume in headphones, earbuds, and car sound systems. Reduce the time you spend listening to loud music.

Lesson 17.2 Review

Know and Understand

1. How do wildfires contribute to air pollution?
2. Explain how fuel emissions in the environment affect human health.
3. What are the symptoms of VOC exposure?
4. How do fertilizers and pesticides enter and pollute the water?
5. In what ways can people be exposed to lead?

Think Critically

6. With a partner, create a list of tips for avoiding exposure to air pollution in your community. What are the most common air pollutants in your community? What steps should students at your school take to avoid them?
7. Choose one manufactured hazardous chemical. Where in your environment is this chemical found? What steps could you take to reduce exposure to it?
8. What are some examples of common chemicals you should not mix?
9. Why do you think noise pollution contributes to stress and reduced mental and emotional health? Discuss with a partner.

REAL WORLD Health Skills

Communicate with Others There are many steps you can take to reduce your exposure to various types of pollution. Some pollution, however, requires intervention from government agencies or community organizations. In a small group, identify one type of pollution that is common in your community. Choose a type of pollution you think your local government could take better steps to help prevent. Then, in your group, write a formal letter to a local government representative explaining what you think the government should do to reduce pollution. Use formal, respectful language and effective communication skills.

Protecting the Environment

Essential Question?

What skills can you use to protect, maintain, and improve your environment?

Lesson 17.3

Learning Outcomes

After studying this lesson, you will be able to

- identify the actions of the environmental protection hierarchy;
- summarize laws that help protect the environment;
- explain how to conserve resources and reduce waste;
- take steps to reuse products and recycle;
- summarize how hazardous waste is treated and disposed of; and
- identify ways to increase environmental awareness in your community.

Key Terms

Clean Air Act
compost
environmental protection hierarchy
green products
recycling
renewable energy
Resource Conservation and Recovery Act
Safe Drinking Water Act
sustainability

Warm-Up Activity

Deciding to Protect the Environment

Make Decisions In a small group, brainstorm strategies you already know help protect the environment. Then, choose one strategy and write a series of social media posts showing a teen using the decision-making process to put the strategy into action. Include specific details in your social media posts and outline each step of the decision-making process. Afterward, share your social media posts with other groups.

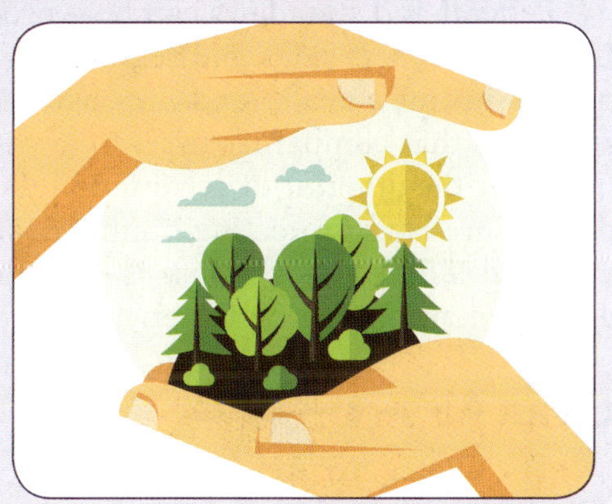

Incomible/Shutterstock.com

The term *environmental protection* describes any type of practice to prevent, eliminate, or reduce harm to the environment. Different strategies are better—or worse—for the environment. The EPA has created a graphic called the **environmental protection hierarchy** (**Figure 17.14**).

As shown in the environmental protection hierarchy, you can take actions in your home, school, workplace, and community to help protect yourself and the environment. Your goal should be to make choices that create **sustainability**, or help maintain the natural resources in your environment.

When you make responsible choices about using and consuming products, you help protect the Earth so these natural resources can last for many years. For example, sustainable gardening is a way to grow plants that reduces any negative impact on the environment. This means growing plants without using chemicals that can pollute the soil and capturing rain to water plants. Making environmentally friendly choices helps to maintain the planet not just for yourself, but for future generations.

environmental protection hierarchy graphic created by the EPA that shows four different ways of protecting the environment: disposal or release, treatment, recycling, and source reduction

sustainability actions that help maintain the natural resources in the environment

Figure 17.14 The environmental protection hierarchy shows different ways of protecting the environment. The higher up in the hierarchy, the better the approach. ***What is the most preferred way of protecting the environment?***

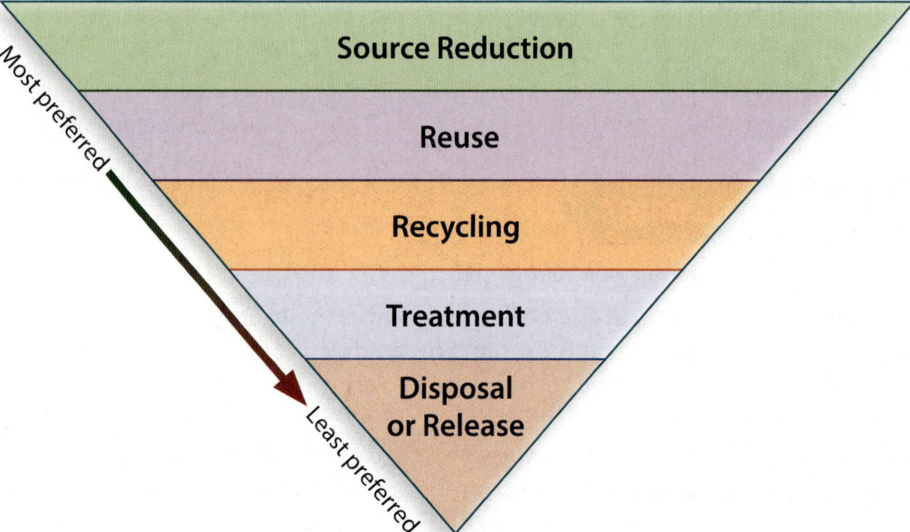

Laws Protecting the Environment

Federal and state laws can help promote a safe environment. In the US, the EPA sets rules and regulations based on scientific research to protect people's health and the environment. For example, the EPA sets rules that companies must follow to limit pollution. These rules set limits for the amount of certain pollutants in air and water. The EPA also makes sure laws protecting human health and the environment are fairly enforced. The EPA's purpose is to protect people from risks related to the environment, including the environment at home, work, and school.

Clean Air Act

Clean Air Act federal law that regulates air pollution levels to protect people's health

The **Clean Air Act** is a federal law that regulates air pollution levels. This law sets specific limits on the amount and type of pollution power plants can release into the air. It also regulates the amount of and type of pollution produced by motor vehicles. This law has helped reduce air pollution.

Safe Drinking Water Act

Safe Drinking Water Act federal law that requires drinking water be tested for more than 90 different pollutants

The **Safe Drinking Water Act** requires that drinking water be tested for more than 90 different pollutants. This includes metals, such as lead. It also includes pollutants that could spread diseases, such as *E. coli* and salmonella. Water systems are continually tested against standards to keep people safe.

Resource Conservation and Recovery Act

Resource Conservation and Recovery Act federal law that provides rules and regulations about the management of hazardous wastes

The **Resource Conservation and Recovery Act** provides rules and regulations for managing hazardous wastes. For example, particular chemicals and toxins could cause harm if they were placed in the trash and then leaked into the ground or water. Instead, specific rules now regulate how this waste is disposed and stored to protect people's health and reduce environmental damage.

Sometimes land contains environmental hazards that can hurt people's health. A *brownfield site* is land that may contain hazardous waste, such as from an old factory or gas station. The EPA's land revitalization program cleans up land that may be contaminated and makes it safe to use.

Conserving Resources

Every person creates small amounts of environmental pollution through daily life activities. These activities include driving (or riding) in a motor vehicle, flying in an airplane, using electricity, and throwing items away. The highest step in the environmental protection hierarchy, *source reduction*, focuses on reducing this pollution. Source reduction is achieved through conserving resources. This includes thinking carefully about what you consume and reducing waste.

Buy Green Products

green products items that have a less harmful impact on the environment than some traditional (nongreen) items

All products require energy to produce. **Green products** are those that have a less harmful impact on the environment than a traditional (nongreen) product (**Figure 17.15**). These include products that are made of recycled materials, made without chemicals, or are *biodegradable* (break down naturally and easily in the environment). Products obtained from local stores or farms are also greener than products shipped from far away. You can assess whether a product is green by examining its label. For example, a product's label will often tell you whether the product is made of recycled materials and where the product was manufactured.

Another measure of whether a product is green is *energy efficiency* (how much energy a product must use to operate). To help people buy products that are environmentally friendly, the EPA created the *Energy Star* symbol. This symbol appears on products that use smaller amounts of energy. These products save people money over time because they require less energy to run. They also lessen energy consumption, which reduces pollution in the environment. Make sure to look for the Energy Star symbol when you are choosing which product to buy.

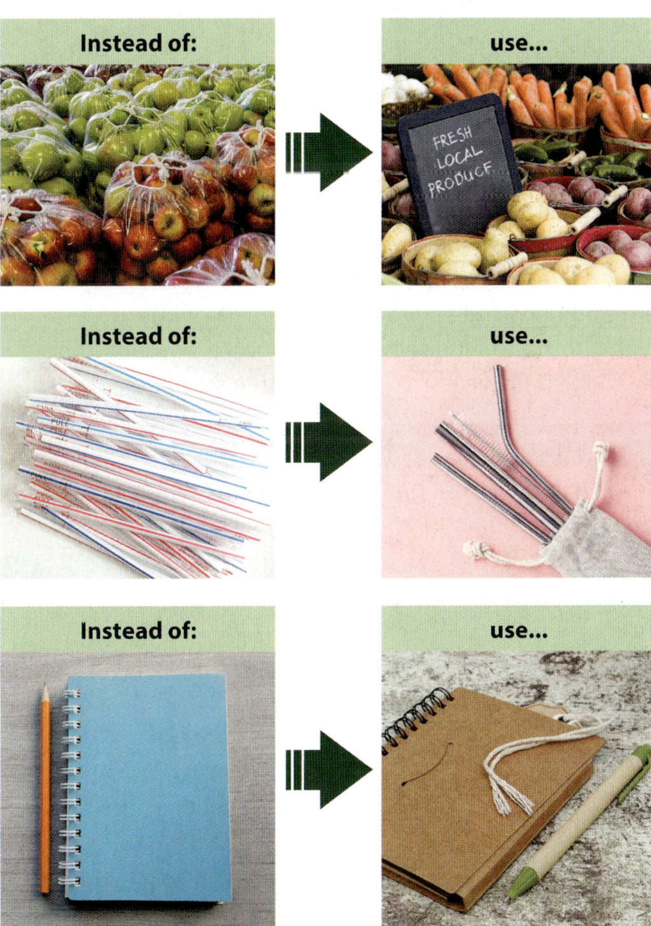

Left to right, top to bottom: UT07/Shutterstock.com; Arina P Habich/Shutterstock.com; Yoyochow23/Shutterstock.com; zakalinka/Shutterstock.com; Orawan Pattarawimonchai/Shutterstock.com; Raihana Asral/Shutterstock.com

Figure 17.15 Local products, reusable items, and recycled materials are examples of green products you can use in your everyday life.

Reduce Waste

When you throw items in the trash, that trash gets taken away. It does not disappear, however. Instead, it ends up in a landfill. Trash people throw away often includes chemicals. When rain falls on a landfill, these chemicals can run out into nearby bodies of water. Garbage rotting in a landfill can release gases into the atmosphere.

Most people probably do not think much about how much waste they produce. The average person in the US, however, produces more than 4 pounds of waste each day. Several strategies can help you reduce the amount of waste you produce.

Before throwing an item away, think about what else you can do with it. For example, if you are discarding old shoes, ask yourself why you are throwing them away. If the shoes are worn or dirty, could you clean them and still wear them for some activities? Could you give the shoes to a friend, family member, neighbor, resale store, charity, or community organization? Could you repurpose the shoes into another type of product?

You can also reduce waste by buying used or reusable materials. For example, instead of buying a brand-new shirt, you could buy a gently used shirt at a local resale store. Instead of buying bottled water, you could carry a refillable water bottle. You can also take care of and repair your belongings so they last longer.

Health in the Media 

The Hidden Costs of Cheap Goods

As you browse social media, websites, and blogs, you probably see dozens of advertisements boasting sales and bargains—the lowest prices anywhere. Low prices appeal to consumers who want to save money. An unusually cheap T-shirt, however, includes hidden costs.

The US has laws that regulate the working conditions and environmental impact of businesses that produce and sell goods. Around the world, some countries have less strict laws. Often, businesses in these countries can sell very cheap goods because they pay workers very little, make them work long hours, and do not pay attention to environmental impact. Some businesses even hire children or people who are being trafficked. These business practices would be considered illegal in the US. Though they produce very cheap goods, they harm people's health and the environment.

Buying unusually cheap goods promotes the unethical practices of businesses that do not protect the health of their workers and the environment. Buying unusually cheap goods can also make people more likely to throw goods away because they are inexpensive to replace. The next time you see an unusually cheap product, take a moment to think about why the price is so low. Often, you can research a company's business practices and sourcing online.

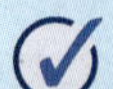

Practice Your Skills

Practice Health-Enhancing Behaviors

Through the purchases you make, you communicate support or lack of support for businesses in your community and world. Learning more about these companies and their business practices can help you make informed decisions that promote individual, community, and environmental health. Choose one business from which you purchase products. Then use reliable resources to answer the following questions:

- Where are the goods sold by this business manufactured? How safe and ethical are working conditions in these factories?
- What, if any, steps has this business taken to produce goods in a sustainable way?

Prepare a podcast reporting on your findings and discuss if there are more environmentally friendly alternatives to purchasing products from this business. Collect your classmates' podcasts into a series and share with the school, encouraging students to support businesses that promote health.

Reducing food waste can have a large impact on the environment. Every year, people in the US throw away more than 38 million tons of food. This includes spoiled food and leftovers. Most of this food ends up in landfills. To reduce your food waste, be mindful about your food choices and only buy food you expect to eat. Store food carefully so it lasts longer. When buying meals, do not take more napkins or utensils than you need. At restaurants, take home food you cannot finish and eat any leftovers you have.

Use Energy Efficiently

Energy and electricity are produced through the consumption of the Earth's natural resources. In many cases, people burn fossil fuels to produce energy. By using energy efficiently, you can help protect the environment.

Be Green at Home

Making small changes in your behavior can help reduce energy consumption and conserve natural resources (**Figure 17.16**).

Use Efficient Transportation

You can reduce energy use and pollution by making greener choices when you travel. For example, walking or biking to school is a greener choice than driving. For longer distances, try to use public transportation, such as a subway, train, or bus. These forms of transportation carry many people and use much less energy than if each person drove.

You can also make simple changes in how you drive. Aggressive driving, such as speeding up and quickly braking, wastes gas. Idling a car also wastes energy. It is better to turn off the engine and restart it than to idle for more than 10 seconds.

Cars differ in how much gas they use. Cars with higher *miles per gallon (MPGs)* use less gas than those with low MPGs. A high-MPG car costs less to drive and reduces pollution. Some cars have features that increase fuel efficiency. Although most cars run on gasoline, some cars use forms of energy that are better for the environment. For example, *electric cars* do not use any gas or produce exhaust. *Hybrid cars* are powered with both gas and electricity.

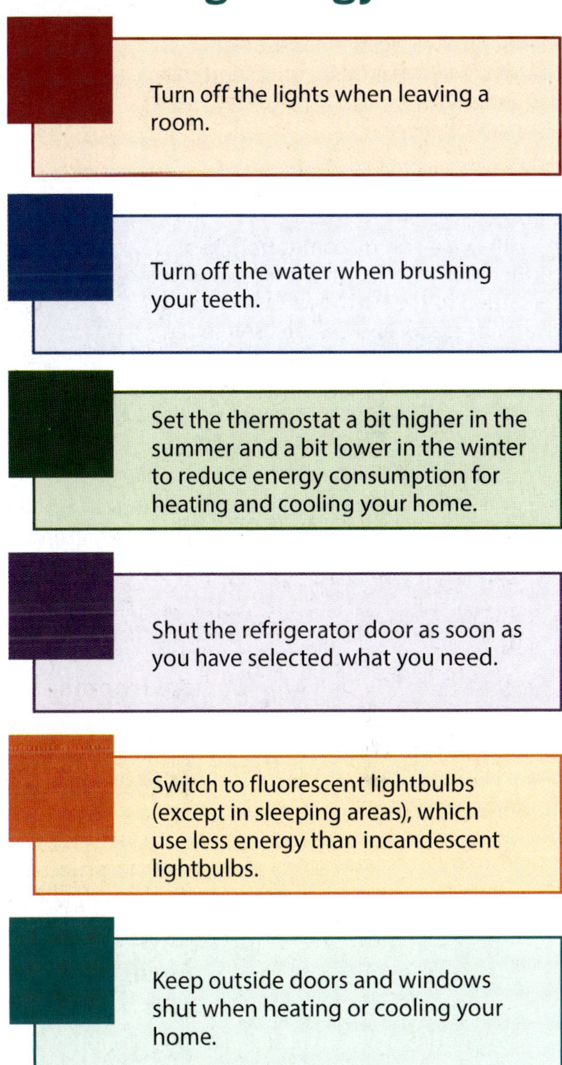

Figure 17.16 Some simple strategies for using less energy in your home are shown here.

Consider Renewable Energy

Many forms of energy use the Earth's natural resources, such as fossil fuels like coal and natural gas. Fossil fuels are not renewable, meaning they cannot be replaced. These fuels also cause pollution.

Using renewable energy is more efficient. **Renewable energy** also comes from the Earth's natural resources. It comes from sources such as wind, water, and sunlight, which do not run out. This type of energy also does not cause pollution and is sometimes called *clean energy*.

renewable energy
energy that comes from the Earth's natural resources, such as wind, water, and sunlight; cannot be used up

Renewable Energy

Solar power

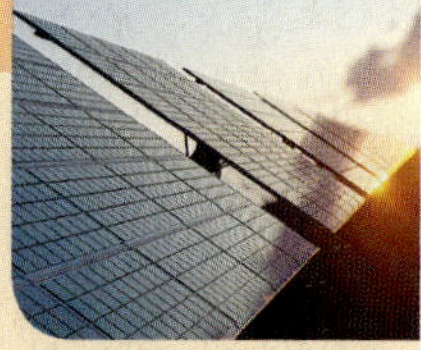

Solar power works by capturing sunlight and turning it into electricity. Homes and businesses with solar panels can get more than one-half of the energy they need from the sun. Solar power cannot be stored over time. Solar panels create electricity on a sunny day, but on a cloudy day, people need other sources of energy.

Wind power

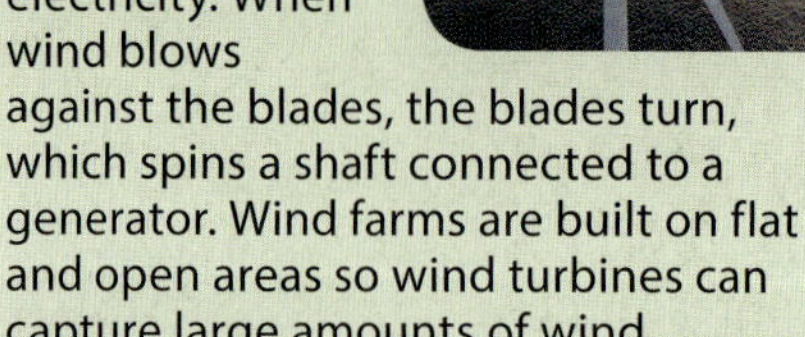

Wind turning the blades on a windmill produces electricity. When wind blows against the blades, the blades turn, which spins a shaft connected to a generator. Wind farms are built on flat and open areas so wind turbines can capture large amounts of wind.

Hydro power

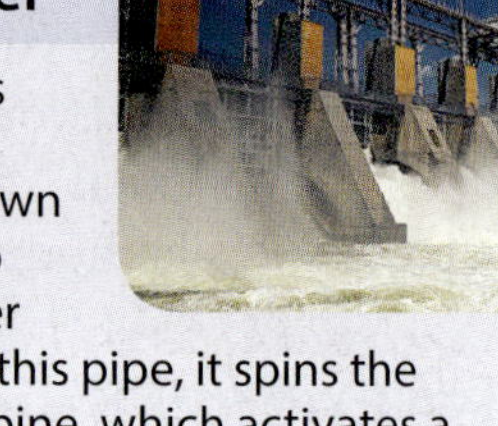

Hydro power is created when water flows down a river and into a pipe. As water flows through this pipe, it spins the blades of a turbine, which activates a generator and produces electricity.

Geothermal energy

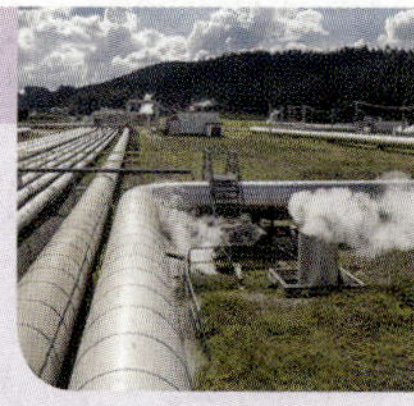

Geothermal energy comes from heat underneath the Earth's surface. This heat is carried to the Earth's surface through water or steam and can be used to generate electricity and provide cooling or heating.

Biomass energy

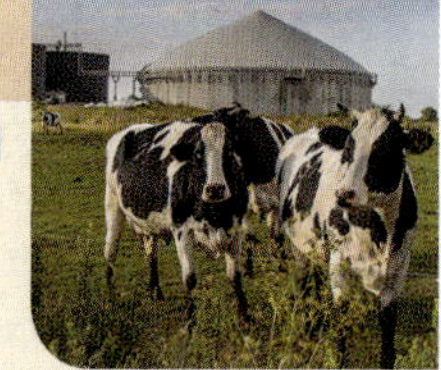

Biomass energy is created using natural materials (like trees and plants). For example, burning wood produces heat. Crops such as corn and sugar can also produce biomass energy. When garbage rots in a landfill, it produces methane gas, which can be turned into natural gas and provide energy. Even cow manure contains methane gas, which can be an energy source.

Left to right, top to bottom: Pixelci/Shutterstock.com; syeols/Shutterstock.com; igorwheeler/Shutterstock.com; Chrispo/Shutterstock.com; Rudmer Zwerver/Shutterstock.com

Figure 17.17 Renewable energy creates power from the sun, wind, water, the Earth's heat, or natural materials like trees and plants.

The more people use renewable energy, the more they protect their environment (**Figure 17.17**).

Reuse and Recycle

Though you can reduce the amount of waste you produce, you may not be able to eliminate waste altogether. How you handle the waste you produce also has an impact on the environment. You may have heard of the three R's: reduce, reuse, and recycle. Once you have reduced your waste as much as possible, focus on reusing and recycling items.

Reusing Products

One easy way to protect the environment is to reuse products when you can. Instead of getting a new plastic or paper bag every time you go shopping, carry a reusable bag. Some cities even enforce taxes to encourage this. Buy rechargeable batteries you can reuse. At school, reuse school supplies from year to year and bring reusable lunch containers.

When you are done using an item, try to donate it so someone else can use it. For example, when you outgrow clothes, you could donate them to a local homeless shelter, resale store, or charitable organization. Donating saves space in landfills and reduces energy, since a new product does not have to be created.

You can also reuse products by converting them to fit your needs. For example, if a piece of clothing goes out of style, you can alter it to be more in style instead of getting rid of it. You could turn broken crayons into candles or repurpose bowls or cans as pots or containers for organizing.

Recycling Items

Recycling is an important part of greener living. Recycling helps conserve natural resources and reduce energy consumption. If possible, recycle bottles, cans, and newspapers in your home and school. Try to buy items made from recycled products.

recycling treating or processing used or waste products to make them suitable for reuse

Certain types of products need to be recycled in particular ways to protect the environment. These include electronics, such as TVs and computers, and appliances, such as microwaves and refrigerators. Although these products contain valuable resources, including metals, plastics, and glass, they can also contain toxic substances. It is important to recycle these products so these substances do not pollute landfills. Many towns have days people can drop these products off for recycling. Some stores also collect these products for recycling.

Skills for Health and Wellness

Donating Used Belongings

Donating used belongings is a great way to reduce the items you purchase, reuse items, and recycle. *Resale stores*, sometimes called *thrift shops* or *secondhand stores*, accept donations and then sell the donated items. Even if resale stores cannot sell all the donations they receive, many work with community organizations to recycle unsold items such as clothes. They may also partner with charitable organizations, which accept their unsold donations.

You can also donate used belongings directly to charitable organizations or other organizations in your community. Many charitable organizations have donation boxes, where people can drop off used items. Other organizations that may accept used items include homeless shelters, schools, and community organizations. If you are unsure how to donate items, research online or call your city government offices.

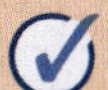

Practice Your Skills

Advocate for Health

The next time you have items that can be donated, where will you go? In a small group, think about the items teens in your community go through most quickly. Some examples might include clothes, books, shoes, or electronics. How do teens usually dispose of these items? What impact does disposing of these items have on the environment? In your group, create a donation campaign using the following steps:

1. Choose one type of item teens use and then discard and research opportunities for donating this item in your community. In your research, identify at least three ways teens can donate this item or recycle it safely.
2. Narrow your list down to the one method you think teens would be most likely to use. Research the organization that accepts the donated item.
3. Create a campaign using several PSAs that inform your fellow classmates. In your PSAs, include the name of the organization that accepts this item, where the organization is located, and how the organization accepts donations. Make sure your PSAs are engaging and relevant to your audience. Provide your classmates with all the information they would need to donate this item on their own.

Composting

compost mixture of food scraps and other organic matter that breaks down in the environment; can be used to fertilize gardens

One great way to reduce waste is to **compost** by throwing food scraps or leaves into a separate bin or pile instead of the trash. This type of natural waste breaks down over time and can then be used as fertilizer for a lawn or garden. Composting reduces waste that would otherwise end up in a landfill.

Some schools have a composting program to help reduce the amount of food waste that is thrown away. If your school has this type of program, dispose of your food scraps properly so they are composted. If your school does not have this type of program, you could work with friends to start one.

Learn About Waste Treatment and Disposal

Sometimes pollutants need to be treated to reduce their harm to the environment. Although treatment helps reduce the effects of pollutants, it requires time, money, and energy.

Some products contain hazardous materials and therefore cannot be treated or recycled. These products need to be disposed very carefully to avoid harming the environment. They cannot be placed in a trash can and then dumped in a landfill. Products that require special disposal include some batteries, full or partially full aerosol cans, tires, household chemicals (such as motor oil and antifreeze), and medical waste. Most communities provide specific instructions for carefully disposing of these products.

Contribute to Your Community

Environmental protection is a community effort. People need to work together to protect the environment and prevent pollution.

Advocating for the Environment

You can take the lead for conserving the environment in your school and neighborhood (**Figure 17.18**). Encourage your friends, family members, teachers, and local business leaders to take steps to conserve the environment. Educating people in your school or community about the benefits of reducing energy consumption can help protect the environment and improve overall health in your community.

Planting a Tree

Another simple way to contribute to your community and protect the environment is to plant a tree. Trees beautify your surroundings and provide shade. Trees also have a number of environmental benefits, including:

- reducing air and soil temperature;
- reducing water runoff from storms by absorbing water, which decreases particulate matter in streams, ponds, lakes, and rivers;
- shading surface areas to reduce heat buildup during the day;
- trapping dust, pollen, and smoke from the air; and
- absorbing carbon dioxide from the air and releasing oxygen.

Ways You Can Advocate for Your Environment

Organize a collection of shoes, clothes, or toys for shelters, charities, and resale stores.

Start an environmental health club at school. The club can help a community garden grow fresh food for the community and food pantries.

Organize litter cleanup in parks, in neighborhoods, and along rivers and lakeshores.

Begin a recycling system at your school.

Work with school or town leaders to create a recycling or food composting system.

Suggest to school or town leaders a switch to energy-efficient lightbulbs in school and town buildings.

Join an Earth Day celebration in your school or community—or start your own! You can find lots of ideas for activities to do in support of Earth Day online.

Figure 17.18 Each person's choices impact the environment, and even small changes can help protect the planet.

Lesson 17.3 Review

Know and Understand

1. Which government agency sets rules and regulations to protect the environment and health?
2. What types of products are green?
3. What items can you recycle at your school? What items have to be recycled specially?
4. In composting, how can the resulting compost be used?

Think Critically

5. How much waste do you produce in one day? List everything you throw away and then identify three ways you can reduce your waste
6. Choose one source of renewable energy and explain how you could use it in your home or community.
7. With a partner, discuss one way your community could be more environmentally friendly. Identify three strategies you could use to advocate for the environment.

REAL WORLD Health Skills

Set Goals After reading this lesson, have a conversation with a partner and discuss the following questions:

- Are your priorities different now compared to when you began reading this lesson? Explain.
- Do you feel more confident in your ability to be more environmentally friendly?
- Are you more motivated to take actions that have a positive impact on the environment?

Once you have discussed these questions, set one SMART goal to live in a more environmentally friendly way. Have your partner verify that your goal is SMART. Put this goal into action and evaluate your results.

Chapter 17 Review and Assessment

Chapter Summary

The field of environmental health examines how factors in the environment affect your health. The natural environment includes multiple natural systems called ecosystems, which are made of interrelated living and nonliving parts. Natural resources are materials in the natural environment that people can use.

Just as the environment affects your health, your actions also affect the environment, creating a cycle where humans and the environment affect each other. As populations grow, they consume more resources and produce more waste. Overpopulation can lead to shortages of food and water. The economic development and wealth of countries also affect the environment. Waste management, deforestation, and greenhouse gases and climate change are global environmental issues that must be considered.

The presence of waste in the environment is called pollution. Pollution can affect the air, water, and level of noise in an environment. Hazardous chemicals can also pollute the environment. Some types of pollution are produced naturally, while others come from human activities.

The environmental protection hierarchy is a graphic created by the Environmental Protection Agency (EPA) to show different ways of protecting the environment. The EPA also sets rules and regulations such as the Clean Air Act, the Safe Drinking Water Act, and the Resource Conservation and Recovery Act to protect people's health and the environment.

The highest step in the environmental protection hierarchy, source reduction, focuses on reducing the pollution created by each person through the activities of daily life. Source reduction is achieved through conserving resources. This includes thinking carefully about what you consume and reducing waste.

While it may not be possible to eliminate waste altogether, how you handle the waste you produce does impact the environment. Reusing and recycling products and composting natural waste are all ways you can responsibly handle waste. Pollutants that cannot be reduced or recycled must be treated to reduce their harm to the environment. Some products contain hazardous materials and therefore cannot be treated or recycled. These products need to be disposed carefully to avoid harming the environment.

Educating people in your school or community about the benefits of reducing energy consumption can help protect the environment and improve overall health in your community. Another simple way to contribute to your community and protect the environment is to plant a tree.

Vocabulary Activity

Think about a time pollution in the environment negatively affected you. What were your symptoms? How did you feel? With a partner, write several paragraphs explaining this experience in detail. Use as many terms from this chapter as you can. Then, identify a few strategies you could use to reduce the pollution that negatively affected you.

Air Quality Index (AQI)
arsenic
asbestos
bisphenol A (BPA)
Clean Air Act
compost
deforestation
drought
ecosystems
environmental health
Environmental Protection Agency (EPA)
environmental protection hierarchy
famine
fertilizers
fossil fuels
greenhouse gases
green products
herbicides
landfills
lead
mercury
mold
natural resources
noise pollution
noise-related hearing loss
particulates
Per- and Polyfluoroalkyl Substances (PFAS)
pesticides
pollen
radon
recycling
renewable energy
Resource Conservation and Recovery Act
Safe Drinking Water Act
sustainability
volatile organic compounds (VOCs)

Review and Recall

Review the information in this chapter by answering the following questions.

1. What are the biotic and abiotic parts of an ecosystem?
2. Which of the following is *not* true of using landfills for disposal of solid waste?
   A. Landfills have limited storage space.
   B. It is hard to find suitable land to build landfills.
   C. Landfills cannot store hazardous waste.
   D. Once full, landfills can be dug up and used again.
3. How do forests benefit the environment?
4. What are Earth's two main greenhouse gases?
5. How do greenhouse gases affect weather?
6. What are *fossil fuels*, and how are they used?
7. What is the purpose of the Air Quality Index (AQI)?
8. Which of the following chemicals can be found in batteries, fluorescent lights, and glass thermometers?
   A. mercury
   B. arsenic
   C. lead
   D. carcinogens
9. Where can the chemical bisphenol A (BPA) commonly be found?
10. Which law provides rules and regulations about managing hazardous waste?
    A. Clean Air Act
    B. Safe Drinking Water Act
    C. Resource Conservation Recovery Act
    D. Energy Independence and Security Act
11. What is the highest step in the environmental protection hierarchy?
12. List three sources of renewable energy.
13. Which of the following products is safe for disposal in a trash can?
    A. car batteries
    B. cellophane wrappers
    C. antifreeze
    D. full aerosol cans

Standardized Test Prep

Math Practice

The following results are from a study of US waste materials. Review the results and answer the following questions.

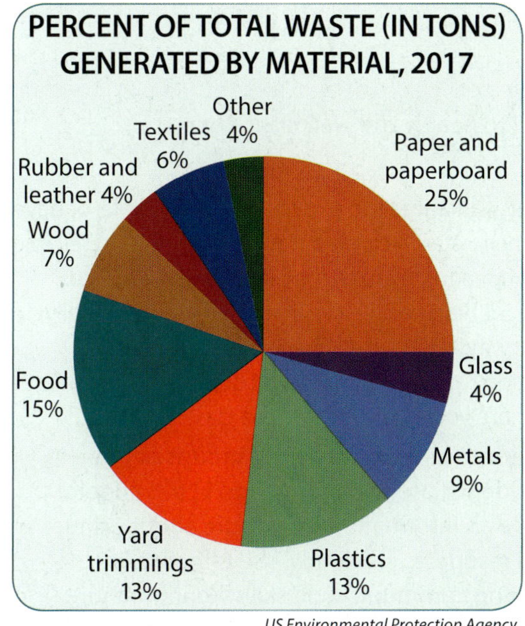

US Environmental Protection Agency

14. Which type of material accounted for the most waste in tons?
15. The total amount of food waste in 2017 was 40,670,000 tons. Calculate the total amount of waste in tons.
16. Which type of material accounted for 13 percent of the total waste in tons?
    A. textiles
    B. yard trimmings
    C. plastics
    D. Both B and C.

Chapter 17 Skills Assessment

Critical Thinking Skills

Answer the following questions to assess your knowledge of what you learned in this chapter.

1. How do your natural environment and your built environment relate to each other?
2. Assess the various efforts to minimize climate change. Which efforts are most and least effective? Why?
3. Assess the following statement from the text: *A low-income country might need to choose between feeding its people and preserving its natural resources.* What are some of the challenges of balancing preservation of the environment with keeping up with the basic needs, growth, and development of a population?
4. Wildfires occur naturally, but they can also occur as a result of human actions. What are some human causes of wildfires? What can be done to prevent them?
5. Choose an example of air pollution, water pollution, hazardous chemical pollution, or noise pollution that affects your community. Create a poster to increase awareness and promote ways citizens can fight it.
6. Analyze this statement from the text: *Not all naturally occurring chemicals are safe. Not all manufactured chemicals are harmful.* What are some examples of this statement in your environment? What factors affect the safety of different chemicals in your environment?
7. What cleaning products in your home contain chemicals that might be harmful to the environment? What are some alternatives to these products?
8. How has technological advancement impacted the environment? What is one example of how technology has helped the environment? harmed the environment?
9. Research your community's recycling program. Make a poster advertising what items can be recycled and how to properly recycle them.
10. Research apps that help promote a greener lifestyle and select one to use throughout the coming week. How did it help you make more environmentally conscious choices? Share your findings with a classmate.
11. Can you think of a product you use regularly that creates excess waste? Write a letter to the manufacturer describing how to protect the environment by reducing the amount of waste produced by the product.
12. What are some obstacles to practicing a green lifestyle? How can they be overcome?
13. With a partner, write down as many ethical issues related to environmental health as you can. Then select one issue to research in depth. What are some possible solutions to the issue you have chosen?

Health and Wellness Skills

Complete the following activities to assess your skills related to health and wellness.

14. **Analyze Influences.** On a scale of 1 to 5 (*1* being not at all and *5* being all the time), rate how often your family uses the following practices. Compare ratings with a partner and then discuss how your family's practices influence your health and the health of others. How would using these practices more often benefit health?
    A. composting
    B. using biodegradable products
    C. donating clothes
    D. recycling
15. **Access Information.** Sometimes people do not feel they have the resources or time to do activities that protect the environment. People may find energy-efficient appliances too expensive, for example, or have little time to start a composting program. Using reliable and valid resources, research community resources that might help people live in more environmentally friendly ways. Also research inexpensive ways of protecting the environment that do not take much time. Share your findings with the class.
16. **Communicate with Others.** In groups of three to four students, use the information in this chapter to create an informational brochure about using natural resources efficiently. Use effective and convincing communication skills. Your brochure should include three sections, address at least

three natural resources, and include three facts about natural resources and three ways human activities affect resources. It should also include one suggestion for making your community more environmentally friendly and one drawing or image.

17. **Make Decisions.** Imagine that, while browsing social media, you see posts that show pollution with the following hashtags. For each set of hashtags, draw the post you imagine accompanies it. Then, using the decision-making process, decide how you would respond to each post. Write your response and explain why you chose it.
    A. #yardcleanup #burningleaves #burningtrash #winterwork
    B. #sistertime #pinkaerosol #sprayit #hairdye
    C. #roadtrip #pack2 #gottasmoke
18. **Practice Health-Enhancing Behaviors.** Think of one habit you have you know negatively affects the environment. Then, create a flowchart showing how that habit affects your health, your environment, your community, and the world. Go back and identify how you could change this habit. Recreate the flowchart showing how your changed habit would affect all these areas.
19. **Set Goals.** Revisit the habit you changed in question 18. Then, work with a partner to create a SMART goal for changing this habit. Ask your partner questions to make the goal as specific as possible. Put your goal into action and hold each other accountable.
20. **Advocate for Health.** Create a mock website or social media account that aims to inform your community about environmental protection. On your page, be sure to include the page's name or title, cover photo, pictures and captions, posts, shared information, and links to additional resources. Keep in mind the target audience of your community members. Publish your website or account for other classmates to see.

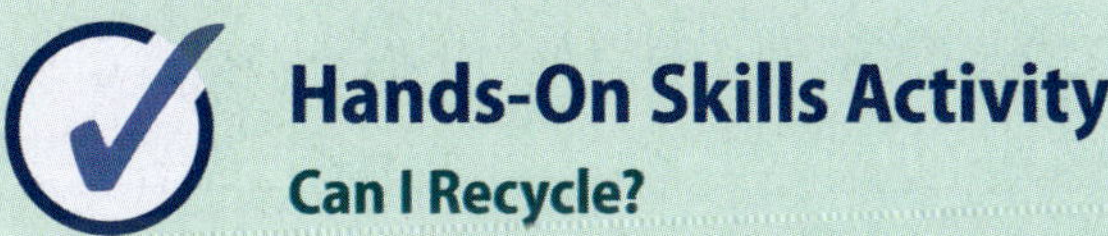

Hands-On Skills Activity

Can I Recycle?

Sometimes it is hard to know what can be recycled and what cannot. In this activity, you will learn about what items around you can be recycled. For this activity, you will need a collection bin and copy of the chart shown.

Steps for This Activity

1. Over the course of three days, when walking around school, keep an eye out for items you think are recyclable. Pick them up; rinse them, if needed; and put them in a class collection bin. Each student must collect at least five different items.
2. **Access Information.** At the end of the collection period, pick five items randomly from the bin and fill in the chart shown. Use reliable and valid resources to verify the information you supply in the chart.
3. **Comprehend Concepts.** After completing your chart, find a partner and discuss the following questions:
    A. Were you surprised by how many items could be recycled? Explain.
    B. Are there items you saw, but did not pick up because you did not know they could be recycled?
    C. Do all recyclable items get treated the same? How much money could you have gotten if you recycled these items? Explain.
    D. Do you think completing this activity will help you recycle in the future?

Item	Recyclable?	Item Classification (i.e., glass, plastic)	Ways of Reusing	Cash Refund Amount

Unit 7

Understanding Diseases and Disorders

Big Ideas

- Communicable diseases spread between living organisms and objects. They are caused by pathogens, which cannot be seen with the naked eye. The body has several defenses against pathogens, including the skin and immune system.
- Some of the most common communicable diseases are respiratory diseases like the common cold and flu. Other common communicable diseases include the stomach flu, athlete's foot, pinkeye, staph infections, mononucleosis, meningitis, hepatitis, and tetanus.
- Emerging infectious diseases are communicable diseases that are growing around the world. Several factors affect the spread of these diseases.
- To prevent communicable diseases, people need to promote resistance to infection and stop the spread of pathogens. Treatments for communicable diseases usually involve medications.
- Sexually transmitted infections (STIs) spread through sexual activity. Some common STIs include chlamydia, gonorrhea, syphilis, trichomoniasis, genital herpes, and human papillomavirus (HPV).
- The most effective way of preventing STIs is sexual abstinence. Condoms also provide some protection. Not all STIs are curable, but medications can help control symptoms and can cure some STIs.
- The human immunodeficiency virus (HIV) is a bloodborne virus that weakens the body's immune system. This virus is found in blood, semen and pre-seminal fluids, vaginal secretions, and breast milk. There are many effective treatments for HIV. HIV can progress to acquired immunodeficiency syndrome (AIDS), in which the body's immune system is severely damaged.
- Noncommunicable diseases do not spread between living organisms and objects. Instead, they develop due to genes, diet, behavior, and other factors.
- Cardiovascular disease is a noncommunicable disease and the first leading cause of death in the United States. Types of cardiovascular disease include diseases of the blood vessels and heart.
- Cancer is a complex noncommunicable disease that occurs when abnormal cells grow uncontrollably. There are many different types of cancer.
- Other examples of noncommunicable diseases include diabetes mellitus, Alzheimer's disease, allergies, asthma, epilepsy, arthritis, and osteoporosis.

SDI Productions/E+/Getty Images ▶

Health Management Plan ▶ Disease Prevention

A *disease* is any condition that disrupts normal function. The common cold and flu are diseases. So are cancer, asthma, and diabetes. Throughout history, diseases have affected the health of many people. Today, scientists understand more about preventing and treating diseases than ever, but diseases are still a personal and community health issue.

In this unit, you will learn about communicable diseases, including sexually transmitted infections (STIs). You will also learn about noncommunicable diseases. Open your health management plan. Create a new entry called "Disease Prevention." Then, work through these steps to make a plan for preventing diseases.

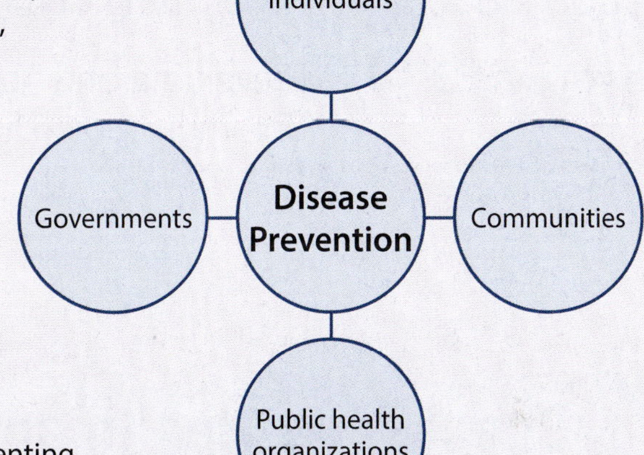

1. The success of disease prevention depends on actions by individuals, communities, public health organizations, and governments. In a graphic like the one shown, brainstorm the role you think each party plays.
2. Next, brainstorm actions you can take to affect how successful each party is. For example, you can take specific steps as an individual to prevent disease. You can also advocate for disease prevention in your community.
3. As you read this unit, take notes about additional actions. Once you have read the unit, revisit the actions you identified and update them. Use them to create 10 personal SMART goals for preventing diseases in your life, community, and world.

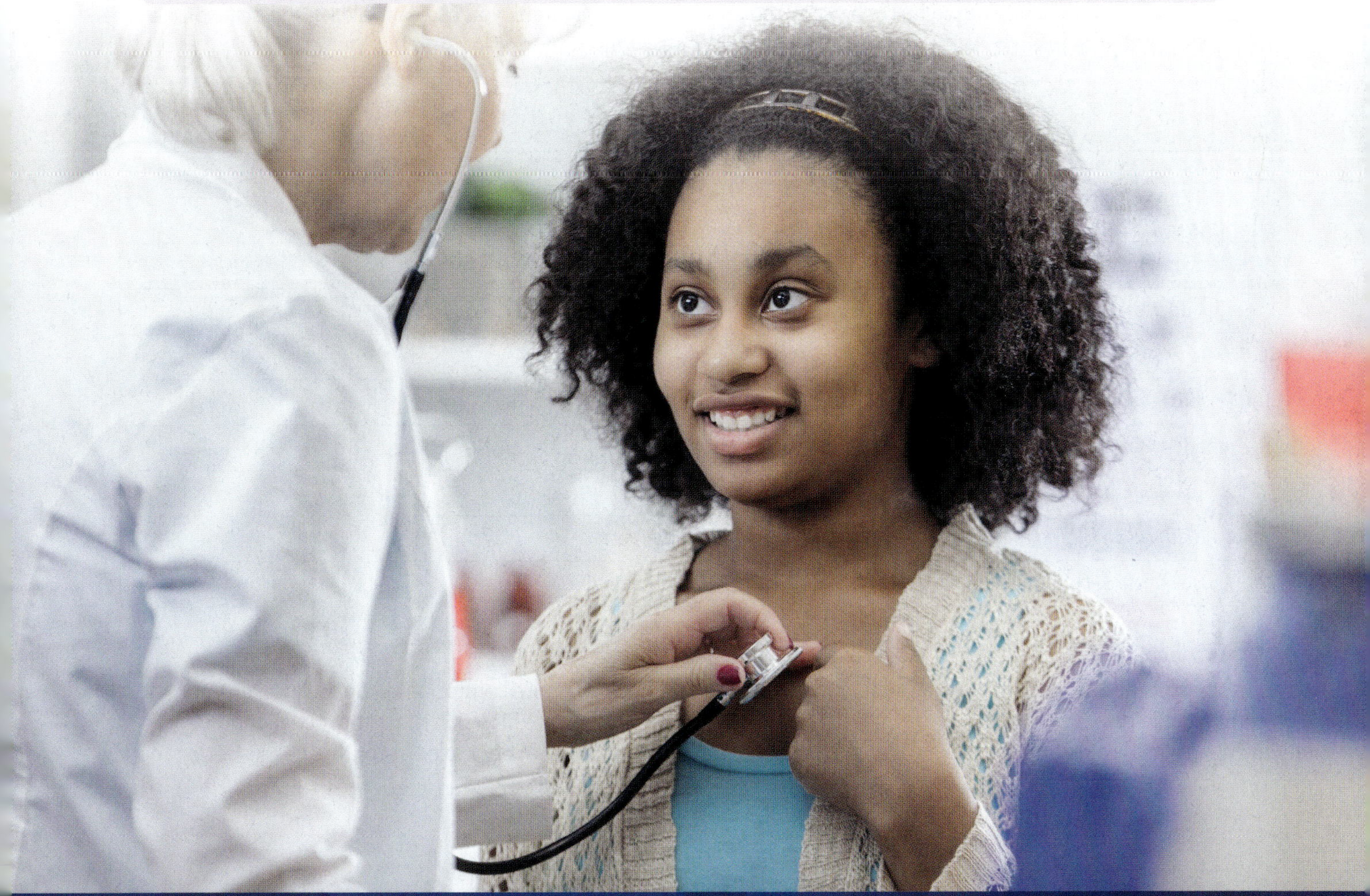

Chapter 18

Communicable Diseases

Look for the skills icon throughout this chapter for opportunities to practice your health skills.

Check Your Health and Wellness Skills

In this chapter, you will learn skills for preventing communicable diseases. To understand the skills you currently use, take the following inventory of your behaviors. Indicate how well you think you use each skill. Use a scale of 1–5, *1* meaning you do not use the skill and *5* meaning you feel completely comfortable using it.

Skill	How Well Do You Use Each Skill?
I eat nutritious foods and get the recommended amount of sleep.	
I see my doctor regularly, at least for an annual checkup.	
After blowing my nose, I always wash my hands.	
I cough into a tissue or my elbow, not into my hands.	
I throw away tissues after one use.	
Before eating fruits and vegetables, I wash them.	
I get needed vaccinations from my doctor.	
I follow the directions for taking a medication exactly.	
I take a medication for the full length of time prescribed, even if I feel better.	
I don't use over-the-counter antibiotics for anything other than bacterial infections.	
	Total:

Add up your responses to each statement. The higher your score, the more comfortable you feel preventing communicable diseases. Which skill do you think is most important for you? Which skill is the most challenging for you? Which skill would you most like to improve? In this chapter, you will learn how to perform these skills better and more often.

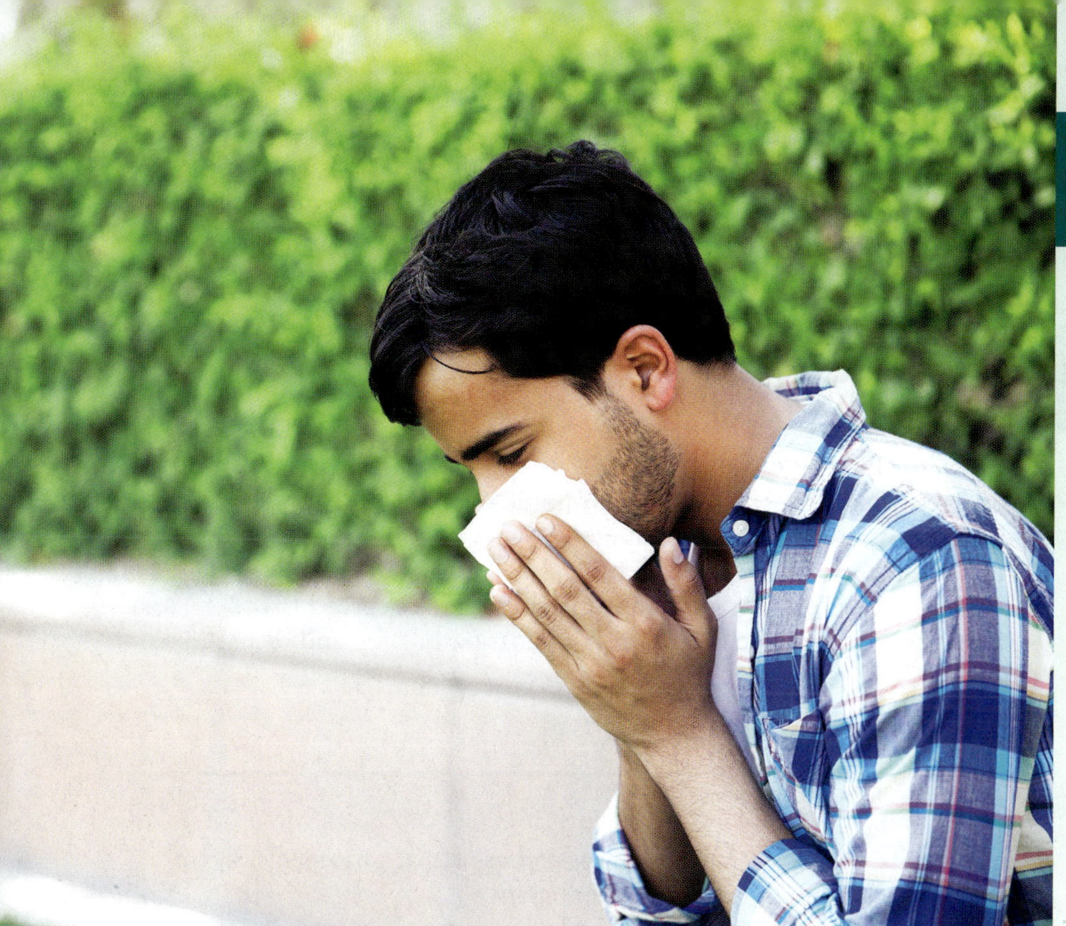
GCShutter/iStock / Getty Images Plus/Getty Images

Reading and Notetaking

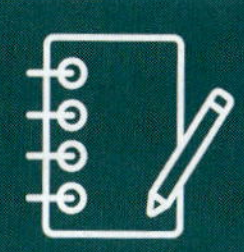

Hearing is a physical process that involves paying attention to the sounds and patterns of spoken language. As your teacher presents the content in this chapter, note when you hear words that are unfamiliar. Listen for familiar sounds that can provide clues about how these words are spelled. After your teacher presents this lesson, review your list of words with a partner to confirm spelling. Then, locate the definition of each new word in the chapter, a dictionary, or the glossary of this text to confirm your spelling.

Unfamiliar Words	Definitions

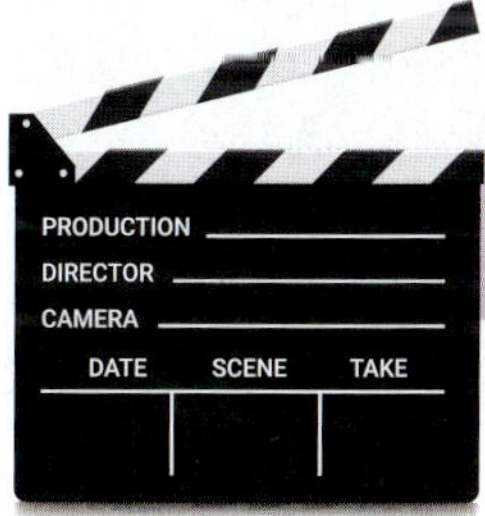

Setting the Scene

Trying Not to Get Sick

A few months into the new school year, you visit the doctor for your annual checkup. Your doctor asks you questions about your behaviors and any symptoms you have had. Your doctor also asks if you have gotten the flu vaccine this year. You say you have not. You had the vaccine last year and you have all of the other vaccines you need to register for school. Your doctor still recommends getting a flu vaccine this year.

After your appointment, you message your friend and say you need the flu vaccine. Your friend is surprised and messages back, *But the flu vaccine can give you the flu!*

Thinking Critically

1. Why do you think your doctor in this scenario recommended getting the flu vaccine this year, even though you got one last year?
2. Is your friend's belief that the flu vaccine causes the flu true or not? What sources could you use to verify or debunk this claim?

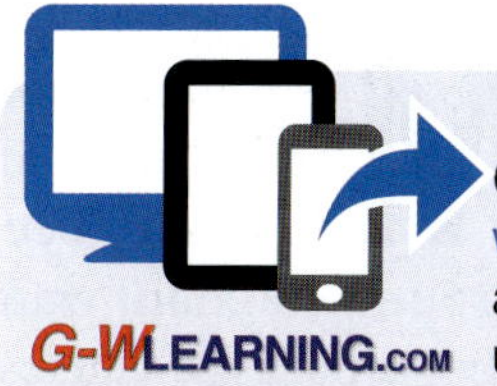

Click on the activity icon or visit www.g-wlearning.com/health/4095 to access online vocabulary activities using key terms from the chapter.

Lesson

18.1

What Are Communicable Diseases?

Essential Question?

What causes communicable diseases?

Learning Outcomes

After studying this lesson, you will be able to

- explain what makes a disease communicable;
- identify different types of pathogens;
- list the stages of infection;
- analyze the different ways communicable diseases spread to others; and
- assess how the body defends itself against pathogens and disease.

Key Terms

antibiotics
antibodies
bacteria
communicable diseases
direct transmission
fever
fungi
germ theory
indirect transmission
inflammation
parasites
pathogens
phagocyte
viruses

Warm-Up Activity

The Body As a Fortress

Comprehend Concepts The body is like a fortress in that it has many ways of defending itself against disease-causing intruders:

A. walls to keep intruders out
B. warriors to fight intruders if they get in
C. substances to dissolve intruders
D. heat to weaken or kill intruders
E. a sticky substance to trap intruders
F. liquids to flush out intruders

With a partner, find an image of the human body with major organs identified or trace the image shown. Determine and label where on the human body each defense (A–F) exists. As a class, compare drawings, making additions or corrections as needed.

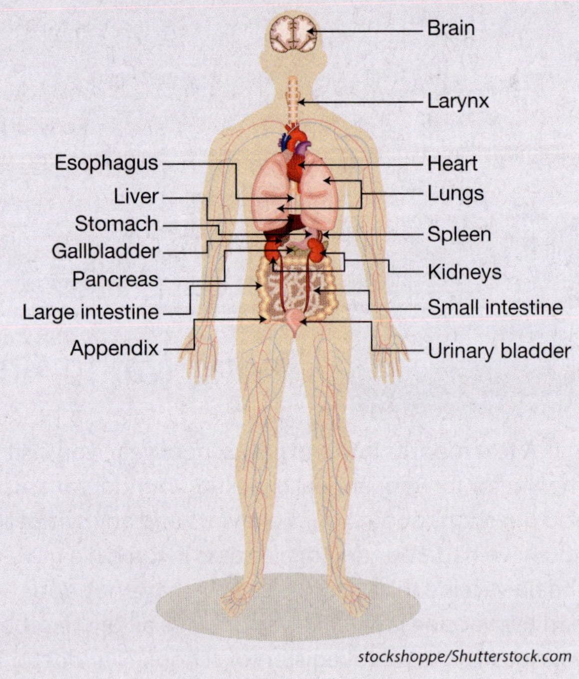

stockshoppe/Shutterstock.com

Malaria, a dreaded illness that causes flu-like symptoms, high fevers, and chills, was once a mystery to people. The word *malaria* means "bad air" because people thought exposure to the still, warm air around stagnant water and swamps caused the disease. People now know that a parasite causes malaria. Mosquitoes, which breed in water, carry this parasite and transmit it to humans.

Today, people know that **communicable diseases** (also called *infectious diseases*) like malaria are caused by organisms too small to see with the naked eye. In the late nineteenth century, scientists used improved microscopes and many experiments to show that these *microorganisms* can cause certain diseases. These discoveries led to the scientific concept of **germ theory**, which states that specific disease-causing microorganisms, called **pathogens**, cause specific diseases. Pathogens can spread between living organisms and objects; therefore, communicable diseases can too.

communicable diseases diseases caused by pathogens that spread through contact among living organisms and objects; also called *infectious diseases*

germ theory scientific theory that specific pathogens cause specific diseases

Types of Pathogens

Pathogens are diverse, specialized, and complex organisms. They are everywhere, though you typically cannot see them. There are four types of pathogens: bacteria, viruses, fungi, and parasites.

pathogens disease-causing microorganisms

Bacteria

Bacteria are single-celled organisms present in nearly every possible place that can sustain life. Most bacteria are helpful and do not cause disease (**Figure 18.1**).

bacteria single-celled microorganisms with no nucleus; are mostly beneficial, but can cause disease

Bacterial cells are 10–100 times smaller than many of your body's cells. They have a relatively simple structure surrounded by a sturdy cell wall and do not have a nucleus. Each kind of bacterial cell has a specific shape, habitat, and nutritional needs.

While most bacteria are beneficial, certain bacteria cause diseases, which range from minor to deadly. The bacterium *E. coli* resides in animal and human intestines and causes food poisoning. Another common bacterium is *Staphylococcus aureus* (*S. aureus*), which causes serious skin infections called *staph infections*, abscesses, pneumonia, bone infections, and other diseases. Most bacterial infections are treated with **antibiotics**, or medications that target and kill disease-causing bacteria.

Of the trillions of cells that make up your body, 90% are bacterial cells.

In fact, large amounts of bacteria live in the body's digestive system, where they:

- hold back the growth of pathogens
- produce vitamin K
- aid in digestion

Figure 18.1 Most bacteria are not dangerous. In fact, most of your body is made up of bacterial cells.

antibiotics medications that target and kill disease-causing bacteria

Viruses

You probably are aware of two well-known viral diseases: the common cold and influenza. Viruses also cause HIV/AIDS, coronavirus, measles, chicken pox, West Nile virus, mumps, and many other diseases.

Viruses do not grow or reproduce independently, have no metabolism, and do not use energy. Instead, viruses depend entirely on other cells, live inside them, and use their resources and energy for reproduction and growth.

Viruses are much smaller than bacteria. They contain only viral genetic material wrapped in a protein coat and sometimes a fatty membrane. Essentially, viruses are made of specially packaged genes that direct cells to make more viruses.

viruses pathogens that invade cells and direct them to create more viruses

Fungi

Fungi are much more complex than bacteria and viruses. A typical fungus contains cells that are specialized for feeding, that anchor the organism to surfaces, and that produce spores for reproduction. Examples of fungi include mushrooms, molds, and yeast.

fungi multicellular organisms that produce spores; are mostly beneficial, but can cause disease

Severe Fungal Infections

Pneumocystis jirovecii	causes pneumonia
Candida auris	infects the skin, mouth, and blood
Cryptococcus neoformans	causes dangerous brain infections

Figure 18.2 Serious fungal infections can cause life-threatening health conditions. ***What are the typical targets of mycosis?***

Like bacteria, few fungi cause disease. In fact, many are beneficial. The mold *Penicillium notatum* makes the life-saving drug *penicillin*, which controls bacterial infections.

Certain fungi, however, damage crops, spoil stored food, and cause disease in humans. When a fungal infection develops, it is called *mycosis*. Mycosis usually affects damaged tissues or people weakened by other infections. People with low immunity are especially susceptible to mycoses.

Athlete's foot is a common fungal infection that takes advantage of some imbalance or damage in the tissues. More serious infections affect individuals with compromised immunity (**Figure 18.2**).

Parasites

parasites microorganisms that live on or inside other organisms (*hosts*)

Parasites are organisms that must live inside or on other living organisms. These parasites cause damage and disease. Worldwide, as many as 1.2 billion people experience infection with the intestinal roundworm *Ascaris lumbricoides*, and about 740 million people have intestinal hookworms. There are two types of infectious parasites: protozoa and worms.

- **Protozoa:** *Protozoa* are single-celled organisms that possess a nucleus and other complex structures and are larger than bacteria. These microorganisms live nearly everywhere, and only a few cause disease. Certain protozoa, however, cause some of the world's most feared diseases, such as malaria and *dysentery*, a severe intestinal infection.
- **Worms:** Parasitic worms are multicellular organisms with specialized tissues and organs. People contract them by having contact with contaminated soils, ingesting food or water contaminated with human waste, or eating undercooked meat and fish. The eggs of the intestinal roundworm *Ascaris lumbricoides*, for example, exist in contaminated water or food. After ingestion, these eggs grow into adult worms that absorb nutrients from the intestine, causing malnutrition and anemia. These worms can grow so large and numerous they block the intestine and even tear holes in it.

Stages of Infection

After pathogens enter the body, they grow, reproduce, and produce toxins. Certain bacterial toxins cause fever, diarrhea, and other symptoms. Pathogens also trigger the immune response and cause inflammation and pain. Infections often follow three stages:

1. **Incubation period:** First, a pathogen enters the body at a specific site and begins to grow and reproduce. For example, influenza enters the respiratory system when a person swallows or inhales infected droplets produced by sneezing or coughing. The incubation period is the time between the pathogen's entrance into the body and the first symptoms. Even with mild or no symptoms, a person may still be contagious. Incubation periods vary from disease to disease.

For example, influenza's incubation period is about two days. The incubation period for salmonella ranges from several hours to two days.

2. **Clinical stage:** During the clinical stage, signs and symptoms of the disease arise. The pathogen produces toxins, and the immune response reaches its height, causing familiar signs of illness. If symptoms worsen, a person may need to see a doctor or other healthcare provider to receive medications that help the immune system fight the pathogen. This stage lasts until the immune system destroys the pathogen responsible for the disease.
3. **Convalescent stage:** If the immune system successfully destroys the pathogen, a person enters the convalescent stage, during which signs and symptoms fade. The length of this stage varies. Usually, a person is no longer contagious during this stage.

Each disease differs in the length of its incubation period, window of contagiousness, and the duration and severity of the clinical stage.

Methods of Transmission

Understanding how diseases spread is the single most important key to prevention. Methods of transmission are direct or indirect, depending on how transmission occurs. The *epidemiological triangle* can help people understand how diseases spread (**Figure 18.3**).

direct transmission
method of disease transmission in which infectious material and pathogens travel from their origin to an individual

Direct Transmission

Direct transmission occurs when infectious material and pathogens travel from their origin to an individual. This transmission can occur through direct contact or droplet spread.

- **Direct contact:** Direct contact occurs when pathogens pass to others through physical contact. Infections transmitted through direct contact between people include sexually transmitted infections (STIs), skin infections, and respiratory diseases.
- **Droplet spread:** Coughing, sneezing, and talking can produce an enormous number of respiratory droplets that contain pathogens. These contaminated droplets can be inhaled or swallowed and can land on hands or other objects. Transmission through these droplets is called *droplet spread* and occurs when an individual is near a person who is coughing, sneezing, or speaking. Respiratory droplets transmit the common cold, influenza, strep throat, meningitis, measles, mumps, pneumonia, and tuberculosis.

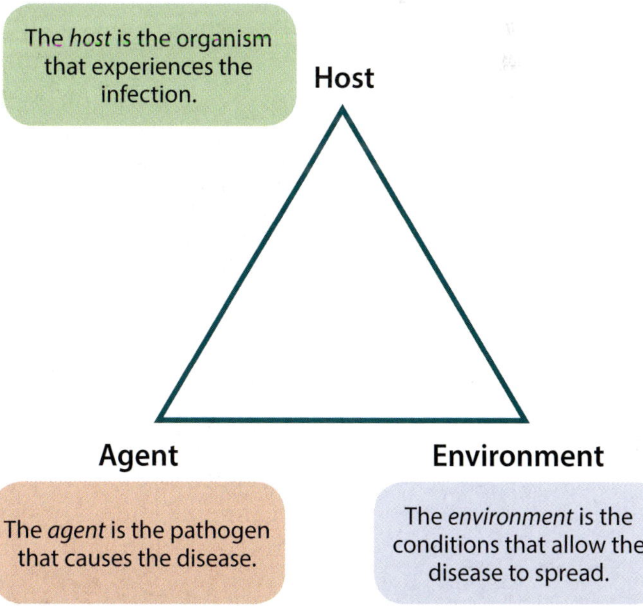

Figure 18.3 In an example of the epidemiological triangle, a virus (agent) causes the common cold in a person (host), and poor respiratory etiquette (environment) may spread the common cold to others.

indirect transmission
method of disease transmission in which infectious material and pathogens pass to a person from a source that acts solely as a carrier

Indirect Transmission

Indirect transmission occurs when infectious material and pathogens pass to a person from a source that acts solely as a carrier. The infectious material does not originate in the carrier. It simply moves the infectious material from one source to another. Forms of indirect transmission include the following:

- **Vector transmission:** Sometimes pathogens travel through *vectors*, or animals and insects such as mosquitoes, flies, ticks, fleas, and lice. For example, Lyme disease is transmitted by ticks, and mosquitoes transmit malaria, West Nile virus, and encephalitis. In *zoonosis*, an animal with an infection transmits the infection to a human, even if the infection is not contagious among humans. A well-known example is the viral disease *rabies*, which is transmitted through bites from warm-blooded animals such as raccoons, foxes, bats, dogs, and cats.
- **Indirect contact:** Some infections spread through contact with contaminated objects (**Figure 18.4**). Food and water are common sources of infection, transmitting some of the world's most well-known pathogens, including the bacterial infection *cholera*. Infected water and waste can contaminate food crops, as can people who handle food during harvest, storage, and processing. Bacteria from animal intestines can contaminate meat during butchering and processing. That is why eating undercooked meat has been linked to diseases such as *E. coli*.
- **Airborne transmission:** Pathogens, such as those that cause tuberculosis and measles, can travel on dust particles or tiny droplets in the air. These particles and droplets can remain suspended in the air for extended periods. When they make contact with a person, a pathogen has found its next opportunity to spread infection.

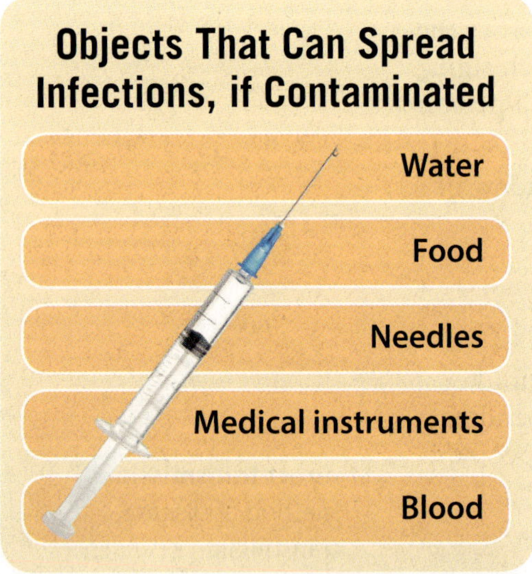

Lipskiy/Shutterstock.com

Figure 18.4 When people come into contact with contaminated objects like water, food, or needles, infections can spread. ***Does infectious material originate in the carrier?***

Immunity: The Body's Defense Against Infection

The immune system continually defends the body against infection. The importance of the immune system becomes obvious when you see what happens if it breaks down. For example, an inherited disease called *severe combined immunodeficiency (SCID)* wipes out a person's immune system. This makes a person vulnerable to attacks from all types of pathogens, results in repeated and serious infections, and is fatal without treatment. The body's immune system has a number of different ways to protect itself from communicable diseases.

The First Line of Defense

The first line of defense against infection includes the internal and external body surfaces, which are always in contact with microorganisms. Several body systems protect the body's surfaces against invasion (**Figure 18.5**).

Body Systems of the First Line of Defense

Integumentary system	Layers of scaly, overlapping cells form the body's outermost skin, a nearly impenetrable physical barrier to pathogens. The skin is also dry, which deters microorganisms. Sweat secreted onto the skin contains salt, which blocks bacterial growth. Oils make the skin acidic, which controls bacterial growth.
Respiratory system	*Mucus* covers the surfaces of the nasal passages, trachea, and inner air passages of the lungs. This thick, watery substance shields the body against pathogens. In addition, the respiratory system includes microscopic *cilia*, or short, hair-like appendages that move mucus up and away from the lungs. This moves pathogens lodged in mucus up to the throat, where they are swallowed and destroyed by the acid in your stomach.
Digestive system	Mucus coats the inner surfaces of the mouth, throat, esophagus, stomach, intestines, and rectum to repel pathogens. Additionally, enzymes in the intestines digest microorganisms not killed by stomach acid. Millions of helpful bacteria normally live in the large intestine and work to stop pathogens.
Urinary system	Normally, a few bacteria make their way into the urinary system through the *urethra*, the small tube that carries urine out of the body. The regular flow of urine usually flushes microorganisms from the urinary system.

Figure 18.5 Different body structures make up the body's first line of defense.

The Second Line of Defense

In spite of the barriers provided by the first line of defense, pathogens sometimes invade the body's tissues. Pathogens entering the blood or tissues face a second line of defense that includes phagocytes, inflammation, and fever.

A **phagocyte** is a white blood cell that specializes in engulfing and destroying pathogens, especially bacteria. A phagocyte surrounds the bacteria, pulls them inside, and digests them (**Figure 18.6**).

A clear indication that the second line of defense is working is **inflammation**, which prepares the body to control and remove pathogens.

phagocyte white blood cell that specializes in engulfing and destroying pathogens, especially bacteria

inflammation immune response characterized by redness, heat, swelling, and pain

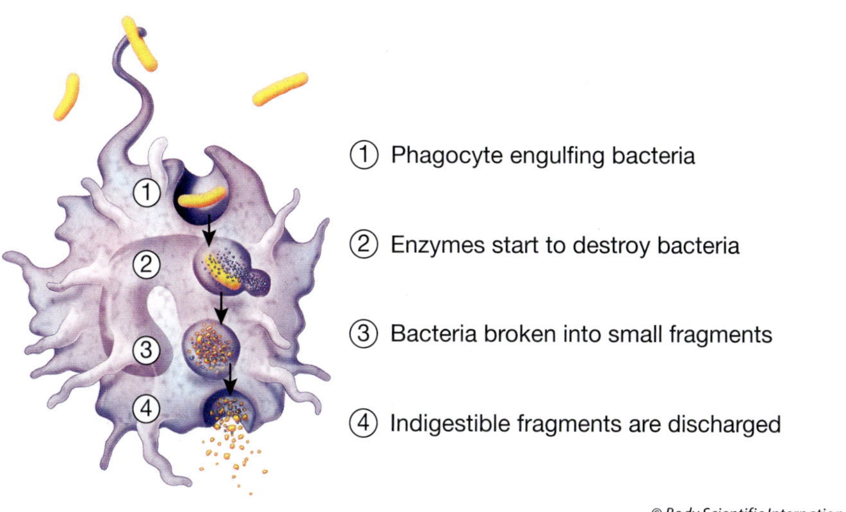

Figure 18.6 Phagocytes engulf foreign bacteria to fight infection and keep the body healthy. ***What type of cell is a phagocyte?***

Inflammation has four key signs: redness, heat, swelling, and pain. During inflammation, chemicals released by injured tissues cause increased blood flow to the site, which causes redness and heat. Increased blood flow also brings more phagocytes to the area. The smallest blood vessels become leaky, and more fluids and phagocytes leave the blood and enter the tissues. As fluids enter the inflamed area, swelling occurs, which may cause pain.

fever body temperature over 98°F (37°C); body temperature rises as part of the immune response

Fever may accompany infection and inflammation. During **fever**, the body's temperature rises above its normal level of about 98°F (37°C). Higher body temperature stimulates phagocytes and other white blood cells important for immunity. It also blocks the growth of bacteria. Although fever is a protective and helpful body function, you should consult a doctor if a fever lasts more than a few days.

Local and Global Health

The Unequal Burden of Communicable Disease

Vaccines prevent an estimated 25 million deaths each year. At the same time, three million people still die each year from vaccine-preventable diseases. The hardest-hit populations reside in countries with limited resources, political instability, and war. In these countries, healthcare systems and vaccination programs are not always equipped to prevent and treat communicable diseases.

One example of this is measles. Low-income countries have more cases of measles, and 95 percent of measles deaths occur in low-income countries. In comparison, the US and other higher-income countries have had more success controlling measles. Before a measles vaccine became available in 1963, the US had 550,000 cases and 500 deaths from measles each year. Vaccination reduced measles cases 99 percent over the following decades. In the year 2000, measles was declared eliminated in the US.

In recent years, the number of measles cases in the US has been increasing. The vast majority of these cases occur when unvaccinated US residents contract measles abroad. After returning, they infect other unvaccinated US residents. Measles spreads rapidly among unvaccinated populations. Protecting people from measles requires 95 percent of a population to be vaccinated. The Centers for Disease Control and Prevention (CDC) reports that some regions of the US are only 90 percent vaccinated.

While the number of measles cases in the US is growing, however, it is still small compared to the burden of this disease in low-income countries. In the year 2019, measles cases in the US accounted for 0.3 percent of cases worldwide.

Number of Measles Cases by Country

Country	Measles Cases
Madagascar	127,520
Ukraine	56,430
India	52,950
Philippines	39,726
Nigeria	26,793
United States	1,243
United Kingdom	698
Japan	685
Germany	472
Netherlands	67

Official data based on monthly data reported to WHO (Geneva) as of October 2019

Practice Your Skills

Access Information

With a partner, choose one communicable disease to research. Using reliable and valid resources, research the number of cases for this disease around the world. You can also research the number of deaths due to this disease. Create a table showing the top 10 countries with the most cases and the 10 countries with the smallest number of cases. Then, research factors that affect the number of cases in these countries. Cite your sources and verify they are reliable. What programs help provide healthcare and vaccination in the countries you identified? What are public health organizations doing to reduce the number of cases? Prepare an illustrated report of your findings and present it to the class. Lead a class discussion about the factors you discovered.

The Third Line of Defense

The third line of defense consists of specialized cells and chemicals that attack and remember specific pathogens. At the heart of this system are T cells, B cells, and chemicals called *antibodies*.

T cells are a type of white blood cell and reside in the blood, lymph nodes, and spleen. One type of T cell, called a *T-helper cell*, coordinates and stimulates the immune response. T-helper cells activate other T cells, B cells, and phagocytes, turning on the immune system. Another type of T cell, the *T-cytotoxic cell*, attacks and kills cells infected with viruses. This stops cells from reproducing viruses and helps control viral infections. Some T cells kill tumor cells and fungi too.

B cells are also white blood cells. These cells make **antibodies**, or chemicals that attach to the part of a pathogen called the *antigen*. Antibodies label pathogens as foreign bodies, making it easier for phagocytes to find and engulf them.

antibodies chemicals that attach to pathogens and label them as foreign bodies to be destroyed

B cells and T cells remember encounters with pathogens and respond more quickly. The first time a pathogen invades your body, you often become sick. During later encounters, however, you may not become ill at all.

The body's defenses benefit from nutrition and physical activity. Some lifestyle choices suppress immunity. For example, smoking interferes with the respiratory system's defenses by paralyzing cilia. Stress produces chemicals that suppress white blood cells. Quitting smoking and reducing stress will help restore immune system resistance to infections.

Lesson 18.1 Review

Know and Understand

1. What makes communicable diseases different from other types of diseases?
2. Would it be true or false to say that all bacteria are harmful? Explain.
3. Choose two pathogens and explain the similarities and differences between them.
4. During which stage of infection do signs and symptoms arise?
5. Which method of disease transmission explains why you can get sick from eating spoiled food?

Think Critically

6. Choose one communicable disease and find out what pathogen causes it. What are the symptoms of this disease? How is it treated?
7. Write a short story in which a teen gets sick with a communicable disease, and the disease spreads to others. Identify each element of the epidemiological triangle.
8. Create a short slogan educating teens about the body's different lines of defense. Share your slogan with a partner.

REAL WORLD Health Skills

Access Information Divide a sheet of paper into four sections. Label each section with the name of a microorganism discussed in this lesson: *bacteria*, *viruses*, *fungi*, or *parasites*. Research each type of microorganism using reliable and valid resources. Be sure to evaluate your sources using the guidelines in Chapter 2. Within each section, draw a general picture of each microorganism and include a short definition. Though some of these microorganisms are generally helpful, they can also cause disease. In each microorganism's section, list two diseases caused by that microorganism, along with the method of treatment for each disease.

Lesson 18.2

Recognizing Communicable Diseases

Essential Question?
What communicable diseases do people commonly encounter?

Learning Outcomes

After studying this lesson, you will be able to

- differentiate between signs and symptoms of disease;
- identify common infections of the respiratory system;
- list the symptoms of common communicable diseases such as the stomach flu, athlete's foot, pinkeye, impetigo and MRSA, mononucleosis, meningitis, hepatitis, and tetanus; and
- describe the impact of emerging infectious diseases.

Key Terms

antibiotic-resistant bacteria
athlete's foot
common cold
emerging infectious diseases
endemic
epidemic
hepatitis
influenza
meningitis
methicillin-resistant *Staphylococcus aureus* (MRSA)
mononucleosis
pandemic
pinkeye
pneumonia
stomach flu
strep throat
tetanus

Warm-Up Activity

Your Signs and Symptoms

Practicing Health-Enhancing Behaviors Common communicable diseases you will learn about in this lesson are the common cold, flu, pneumonia, strep throat, stomach flu, athlete's foot, pinkeye, MRSA, mononucleosis, meningitis, hepatitis, and tetanus. Choose one of these diseases that has directly affected you. Describe how you knew you had this disease and how you felt. What signs and symptoms did you experience? How did you contract the disease, and did you pass it to others? What precautions could you take to avoid being affected again? Write a short reflection about this experience.

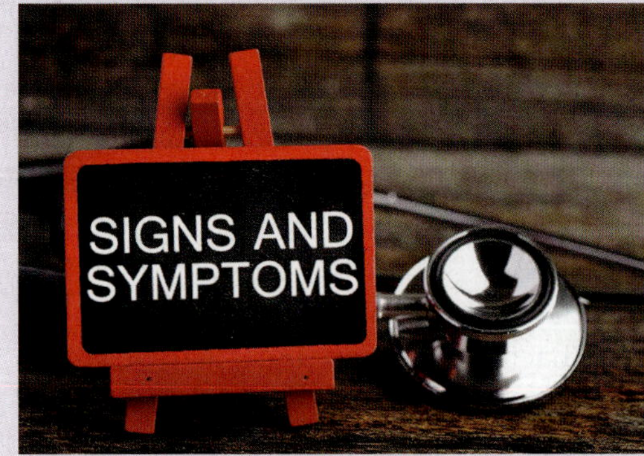

Tuan_Azizi/Shutterstock.com

Specific pathogens cause different communicable diseases. Chances are, you have probably had the common cold, the flu, or an ear infection. Maybe you have heard about people with strep throat or mononucleosis. In this lesson, you will learn about some common communicable diseases. You will also learn about epidemics and emerging diseases around the world.

Common Communicable Diseases

All communicable diseases have distinct signs and symptoms (**Figure 18.7**). In this section, you will learn the signs and symptoms of common communicable diseases.

Signs

Evidence of disease that can be outwardly observed or measured
- Includes fever, abnormal pulse, changes in skin color, or altered breathing rate

Symptoms

Evidence sensed by the person with the disease
- Includes pain, shortness of breath, itching, and headache

Figure 18.7 Though often used synonymously, signs and symptoms have different meanings.

Respiratory Diseases

Respiratory diseases primarily affect the respiratory system. Some symptoms of these diseases include a runny nose, sore throat, and coughing. Common respiratory diseases include the common cold, influenza, pneumonia, and strep throat.

Common Cold

Millions of cases of the common cold affect people each year in the US. A virus called the *rhinovirus* usually causes the **common cold**. There are more than 200 *strains*, or subtypes, of rhinovirus and other cold viruses.

The common cold spreads through tiny droplets released in the air when people cough and sneeze. These droplets land on surfaces such as body parts or furniture. People can contract the cold if the virus comes in contact with their eyes, mouth, or nose.

The common cold primarily affects the nose and throat, causing a sore throat, runny nose, coughing, and sneezing. It can also cause headaches and body aches. Fortunately, most people recover from the common cold in 7–10 days.

common cold viral disease usually caused by the rhinovirus; spreads through droplets in the air and primarily affects the nose and throat

Influenza

Together, **influenza** (the flu) and pneumonia are the eighth leading cause of death in the US. The flu affects people of all ages and is especially dangerous for older people, young children, and people with respiratory conditions such as asthma.

Influenza is caused by two types of influenza virus, called *type A* and *type B*. Every few years, the type A influenza virus causes an unusually large number of infections. This is because it can change dramatically each year, causing few people to be immune. The type B influenza virus causes the majority of infections each flu season. The type B virus changes slightly each year, which is why people need updated flu vaccines each flu season.

The flu spreads through droplets released when people cough, sneeze, or even talk. People can contract the flu if the virus enters the nose, mouth, or lungs. Flu symptoms include a runny nose, sore throat, fever, muscle and headaches, congestion, and weakness or exhaustion.

influenza disease caused by the influenza virus; causes respiratory symptoms and body aches; also called the *flu*

Pneumonia

Pneumonia is a lung infection caused by bacteria or viruses. Around the world, more children under five years of age die from pneumonia than from any other infectious disease.

pneumonia infection in which tiny air sacs in the lungs swell, making breathing difficult

Pneumonia spreads through droplets released during coughing and sneezing. People may also develop pneumonia when they have the flu. Some people get pneumonia during long hospital stays or in long-term healthcare facilities such as nursing homes. People who have weak immune systems or other respiratory diseases such as asthma are more likely to develop pneumonia.

Pneumonia causes the lungs' tiny air sacs to fill with fluid, which makes breathing difficult. Signs and symptoms include chest pain when breathing or coughing, coughing that produces *phlegm* (a thick, sticky fluid), fever, sweating, chills, and fatigue. Pneumonia affects people of all ages and is most serious in young children and older people. A vaccine can protect people from infection with *pneumococcus*, a type of bacteria that commonly causes pneumonia.

Strep Throat

strep throat disease caused by the *Streptococcus* bacterium; characterized by a painful sore throat and swollen, tender tonsils

Each year, millions of cases of strep throat occur in the US. **Strep throat** is an extremely contagious disease spread through droplets released during coughing and sneezing. Strep throat is named for the type of bacteria that causes it: *Streptococcus*. Touching the mouth and nose and sharing food and drinks can also transmit strep throat.

The main symptoms of strep throat are a painful sore throat and swollen, tender tonsils. Other signs and symptoms include fever, aches and pains, nausea in children, and a red skin rash. Red spots and white blotches of pus sometimes appear on the tonsils.

Stomach Flu

stomach flu infection of the intestines (*gastroenteritis*) caused by the norovirus; characterized by vomiting, diarrhea, fever, and stomach cramps

The stomach flu is not related to influenza, which is an infection of the respiratory system. Rather, the **stomach flu** is a common name for *gastroenteritis*, an infection of the intestines. A virus called *norovirus* is the most common cause.

Norovirus spreads through food and water. This virus can stay on the hands following poor hand washing. People can also contract the stomach flu by ingesting contaminated food or water. Signs and symptoms include frequent, watery diarrhea; vomiting; stomach cramps; and a low fever. Most people recover, but may become dehydrated from vomiting.

Athlete's Foot

athlete's foot fungal infection of the skin between the toes or in the groin; causes an itchy, burning rash

Athlete's foot is an infection that commonly affects the skin between the toes or around the groin (called *jock itch*). It is caused by a fungus that lives on moist surfaces. The fungus that causes athlete's foot spreads through skin contact. It can grow on moist floors in showers, gyms, locker rooms, and pool decks. It can also survive on towels and socks. The fungus causes an itchy, burning rash.

Pinkeye

pinkeye infection of the surface of the eye; causes itchy, red, watery eyes and dry crust on the eyelids

Pinkeye, also called *conjunctivitis*, is an infection of the surface of the eye. It is usually caused by bacteria or viruses that infect the surface of the eye and inner lining of the eyelid. Pinkeye is highly contagious and easily transmitted through touch. Its symptoms include red, itchy, and watery eyes. While a person sleeps, tears and fluids form a dry crust on the eyelids, making it hard to open the eyes later.

Impetigo and MRSA

The bacterium *Staphylococcus aureus* (*S. aureus*) causes two well-known infections: impetigo and methicillin-resistant *Staphylococcus aureus* (MRSA). *Impetigo* is a contagious skin infection most common among young children. It can be caused by *S. aureus* or the *Streptococcus* bacterium. In impetigo, bacteria spread through contact with hands or objects such as towels, clothes, or toys. Scratched or injured skin is more likely to become infected. Impetigo usually affects skin around the mouth and nose. It begins with itchy red sores that produce yellow, dry, crusty fluid. Most cases are mild and can be treated at home.

Methicillin-resistant *Staphylococcus aureus* (MRSA) is a dangerous infection caused by antibiotic-resistant bacteria (bacteria that do not respond to treatment with certain antibiotics). Because the bacteria that cause MRSA are resistant to the antibiotic methicillin, MRSA infections are difficult to treat. MRSA can infect the skin, bone, lungs, and bloodstream. It can also cause a rare, dangerous infection called *toxic shock syndrome (TSS)*.

methicillin-resistant *Staphylococcus aureus* (MRSA) dangerous disease caused by a strain of the *Staphylococcus aureus* bacterium that is resistant to the antibiotic methicillin; can infect the skin, bone, lungs, and bloodstream

MRSA grows on skin and in the nose. It can spread through contact with contaminated skin or objects such as bed sheets, clothing, gym mats and equipment, or hospital equipment (**Figure 18.8**). MRSA most often spreads in healthcare facilities through medical equipment and procedures such as surgery.

The signs and symptoms of a MRSA skin infection may begin with a raised red bump that fills with pus. The infected spot may feel warm. The infection causes fever and can quickly spread to deeper tissues and the bloodstream.

Mononucleosis

Mononucleosis, also called *mono* or *kissing disease*, is an infection of a type of white blood cell. The Epstein-Barr virus (EBV), which causes mononucleosis, is found living in many people and usually does not cause disease. The disease mononucleosis usually occurs in teens and young adults. Though not as contagious as other diseases, it spreads through saliva and sometimes other bodily fluids such as semen or blood.

mononucleosis disease caused by the Epstein-Barr virus (EBV); causes fever, sore throat, fatigue, swollen lymph nodes, and a swollen spleen; also called *mono* or *kissing disease*

Signs and symptoms of mononucleosis include fever, sore throat, fatigue, and swollen lymph nodes, especially around the neck and in the armpits. Another sign is a swollen spleen, located on the left side of the stomach.

Reducing Risk of MRSA for Athletes

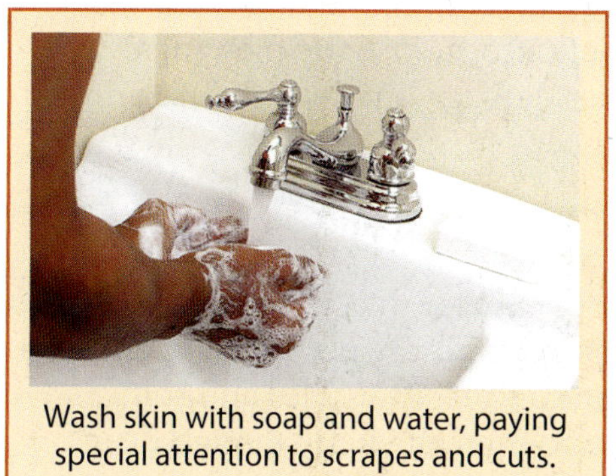

Wash skin with soap and water, paying special attention to scrapes and cuts.

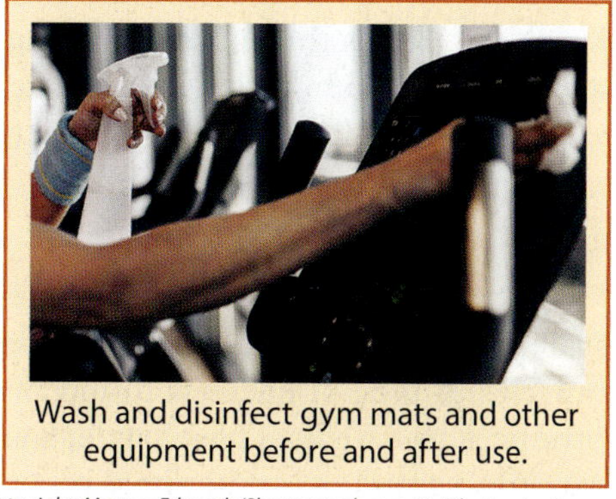

Wash and disinfect gym mats and other equipment before and after use.

Left to right: Margoe Edwards/Shutterstock.com; Xx/Shutterstock.com

Figure 18.8 Athletes may come in contact with MRSA through wrestling mats or other athletes. ***What dangerous infection can be caused by MRSA?***

After people recover from mononucleosis, the spleen can stay swollen for weeks or even months, so people should avoid heavy physical activity and contact sports to prevent injuring or rupturing it. Most people recover from mononucleosis after several weeks, but some remain weak and tired for a month or more.

Meningitis

meningitis inflammation of the membranes around the brain and spinal cord; can cause brain and nerve damage, disability, and death if untreated

Meningitis is inflammation of the *meninges*, the membranes surrounding the brain and spinal cord. This disease is potentially life threatening, and immediate treatment can prevent brain or nerve damage, disability, and even death.

Most cases of meningitis in the US are viral. Certain kinds of bacteria (such as *meningococcus*), fungi, and parasites can also cause meningitis. Meningitis can spread through coughing, sneezing, and sharing utensils, food, and drinks. Teens, young adults, and others who live in close contact have more risk for meningitis. Signs and symptoms include a severe headache, stiff neck, sudden high fever, vomiting, confusion, sleepiness, seizures, and sometimes a rash. Fortunately, a vaccine can reduce one's risk for contracting bacterial meningitis.

hepatitis inflammation of the liver; caused by the hepatitis A, B, or C virus

Signs and Symptoms of Hepatitis

- Loss of appetite
- Weakness and fatigue
- Low fever
- Aches and pains in muscles and joints
- Nausea and vomiting
- Pain in the abdomen
- Dark urine
- Light-colored feces
- *Jaundice* (yellow skin and whites of the eyes)
- Itchy skin
- Mild-to-severe confusion or coma
- Bleeding and bruising

Figure 18.9 All three types of hepatitis cause similar signs and symptoms. ***What organ becomes inflamed from hepatitis?***

Hepatitis

Hepatitis is the inflammation of the liver and ranges from a mild, short-term illness to one that is lifelong and severe. Three common viruses—hepatitis A, B, and C—cause this disease. While they share certain symptoms, the viruses spread differently and have different effects on the body (**Figure 18.9**):

- *Hepatitis A* usually spreads through food and water contaminated with human waste. People with hepatitis A can contaminate food they handle. It is also possible to contract hepatitis A through sexual activity. Symptoms may be mild or severe, and most people recover well. A vaccine can reduce someone's risk of contracting hepatitis A.
- *Hepatitis B* spreads through sexual activity, contaminated needles, and childbirth. The virus is present in a person's blood and bodily fluids such as semen, saliva, and vaginal secretions. Many people do not know they have hepatitis B. This virus can cause liver damage and liver cancer. A vaccine can provide long-lasting protection.
- *Hepatitis C* is present in a person's blood. People can contract hepatitis C through contaminated needles, such as those used for drug use, tattoos, or body piercings. Hepatitis C can cause liver damage and liver failure and increases risk for liver cancer.

Tetanus

tetanus disease caused by a toxin that leads to painful muscle contractions that can interfere with breathing

Tetanus is a life-threatening infectious disease that affects the nervous system. It is caused by a toxin that interferes with the nerves that control muscles. A type of bacteria found in some animal intestines and soil produces this toxin. These bacteria usually enter the body though deep wounds, scratches, and animal bites.

Tetanus causes painful muscle contractions, including strong contractions of the jaw muscles. It is dangerous because it interferes with the muscles used for breathing. While treatment can relieve symptoms, there is no cure for tetanus. Fortunately, a vaccine can prevent tetanus. In the US, most children get tetanus vaccines. Most adults get follow-up vaccines, or *boosters*, every 10 years.

Emerging Infectious Diseases

Communicable diseases can affect small or large populations. For example, an **epidemic** is a disease that occurs in unexpectedly large numbers over a particular area. In some years, influenza is an epidemic. A **pandemic** disease spreads to much of the world. From 1918 to 1919, for example, an influenza pandemic killed about 40 million people around the world. In contrast, an **endemic** infection is one that naturally occurs at low levels in a particular area. The common cold and strep throat are examples of endemic infections in the US. Yellow fever and malaria do not often occur in the US, but are endemic in certain tropical countries.

Emerging infectious diseases are diseases that are new or increasing unexpectedly. These diseases develop and spread for several reasons, including changing environments and climates, antibiotic and drug resistance, and decreasing vaccination rates.

epidemic disease that occurs in unexpectedly large numbers over a particular area

pandemic disease that spreads to much of the world

endemic disease that naturally occurs at low levels in a particular area

emerging infectious diseases communicable diseases that are new or increasing unexpectedly

Changing Environments and Climates

Many insect-borne diseases are growing, partly because insects and ticks are spreading to new regions (**Figure 18.10**). At least three new tick-borne diseases have been discovered, including Heartland virus and Bourbon virus. Scientists are carefully monitoring these diseases. Another new insect-related disease is *alpha-gal*, a potentially severe allergic reaction to red meat. The alpha-gal allergy is triggered by tick bites, and the number of cases is increasing and spreading.

Changing weather conditions have also caused mosquitoes to spread and carry diseases to new regions. For example, areas with increased flooding are experiencing outbreaks of West Nile virus. Scientists are monitoring tropical mosquito-borne diseases that usually do not occur in North America. Fortunately, only a few cases have developed, and most involve people who contracted the diseases abroad. For example, the Zika virus from tropical Africa has spread to South America, and in 2016, it was found in the US. Researchers are trying to determine if Zika virus has become established in certain areas of the US.

Since 2004, total cases of tick-borne disease in the United States have increased from about 22,000 to about 60,000.

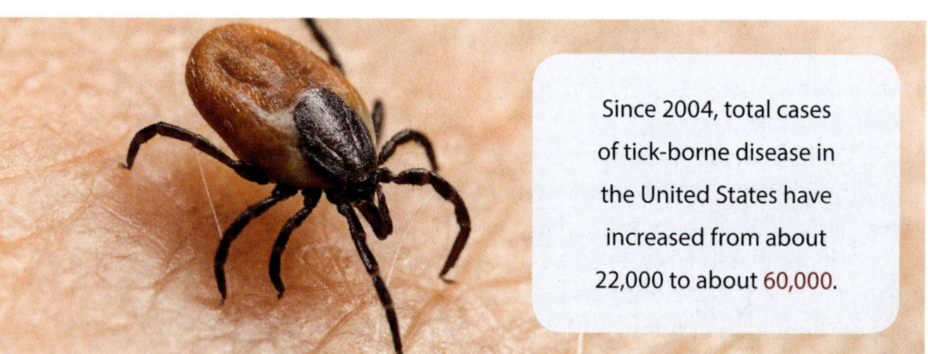

KPixMining/Shutterstock.com

Figure 18.10 As insects spread, they bring new diseases to new areas. ***What is the name for a disease that is new or increasing unexpectedly?***

antibiotic-resistant bacteria bacteria that do not respond to treatment with certain antibiotics

Antibiotic and Drug Resistance

Antibiotic-resistant bacteria, or bacteria that do not respond to certain antibiotics, have also emerged as a major health concern around the world. These bacteria make even mild infections difficult to treat and sometimes life threatening. Some bacteria are even resistant to multiple antibiotics. MRSA is one example of an antibiotic-resistant emerging disease. Antibiotic resistance has also developed in bacteria that cause tuberculosis, pneumonia, gonorrhea, and many other infections.

Though fungi and viruses are not affected by antibiotics, they can still develop resistance to the drugs used to treat them. For example, the fungus *Candida auris* has developed drug resistance. This fungus causes infections in people with weak immune systems, such as patients in hospitals or nursing homes. Untreated, these infections are life threatening.

Decreasing Vaccination Rates

Vaccines are one of the safest and most effective ways to prevent certain communicable diseases. Unfortunately, vaccination rates have been decreasing in the US and around the world. As a result, cases of vaccine-preventable diseases have been increasing. Two examples are measles and *pertussis* (also called *whooping cough*). These diseases, once under control, are reemerging, especially among unvaccinated populations. In the US, for example, lower vaccinations rates have led to rapidly increasing cases of measles. By July 2019, the US had three times more cases of measles than it had in the year 2018.

Lesson 18.2 Review

Know and Understand

1. Is fatigue a sign or symptom of disease? Explain.
2. Why do people need updated flu vaccines each year?
3. What is the difference between the stomach flu and the flu?
4. List all of the common communicable diseases in this lesson and classify them as bacterial, viral, fungal, or parasitic.
5. How does antibiotic resistance contribute to the reemergence of diseases?

Think Critically

6. With a partner, list the different ways respiratory diseases spread. What can people do to reduce the risk of transmission?
7. Write a case study about a teen who has one of the diseases in this lesson. Be sure to describe the teen's signs and symptoms and how the teen seeks treatment.
8. What factors do you think affect vaccination rates in a given country or region?

REAL WORLD Health Skills

Make Decisions Imagine you are a doctor with the CDC specializing in communicable diseases. Several communicable diseases have emerged worldwide, and you need to research and track how they spread. Choose one of the emerging diseases in this lesson or choose another current disease that has emerged or reemerged. Using reliable resources, research the disease to find out where it originated, how it spreads, and where it has spread. Then, formulate a plan consisting of decisions people and communities can make to contain the disease and prevent future outbreaks. Outline a health alert that conveys the information you found, as well as your plan.

Preventing and Treating Communicable Diseases

Essential Question?

What skills can you use to protect yourself and others from communicable diseases?

Lesson 18.3

Learning Outcomes

After studying this lesson, you will be able to

- explain ways to promote resistance to infection;
- describe the importance of washing your hands;
- practice respiratory etiquette;
- analyze how vaccination prevents disease; and
- describe ways of treating bacterial, viral, fungal, and parasitic infections.

Key Terms

hand washing
respiratory etiquette
vaccination
vaccine

Warm-Up Activity

What Do You Touch?

Comprehend Concepts List all the objects you touch each day. Then find a partner and compare lists. Highlight the objects your lists have in common. It is likely others touch these objects as well. As a result, touching these items increases your likelihood of coming in contact with pathogens. With your partner, brainstorm ways to avoid contracting a communicable disease from the objects you touch daily.

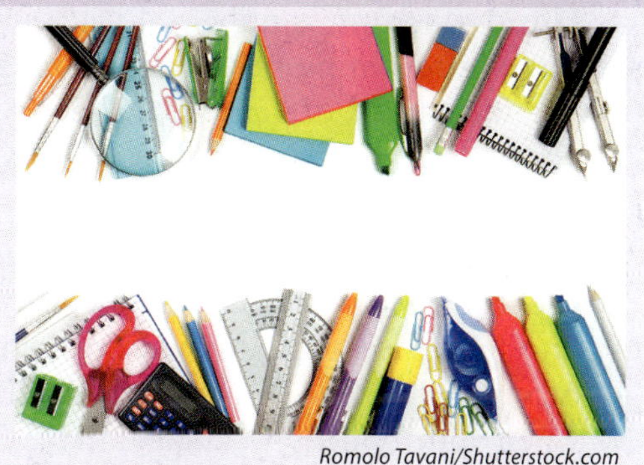

Romolo Tavani/Shutterstock.com

The nature of communicable diseases means that most methods for preventing and treating them focus on destroying the pathogenic cause. Not spreading the pathogens reduces infection in others. Destroying the pathogen or reducing its effects help the body successfully fight the infection and recover. In this lesson, you will learn strategies for preventing and treating communicable diseases.

Preventing Communicable Diseases

During most wars before World War II, infections killed far more people than swords, bullets, and bombs did. Since then, medical science has developed preventive measures to reduce the spread of communicable diseases. One way to prevent the spread of disease is to practice *food safety*, which you learned about in Chapter 8. Other strategies include promoting resistance to infection, washing your hands, using respiratory etiquette, and getting vaccinations.

Promote Resistance of Infection

The *immune system* uses powerful biological processes to resist infection and get rid of pathogens. Like all body systems, the immune system functions well or poorly depending on other aspects of health. Taking care of your body and making healthy lifestyle decisions can keep your immune system in good shape. Some ways to support the work of your immune system include the following:

- Eat a balanced diet with plenty of fruits, vegetables, and fiber.
- Get eight to 10 hours of sleep. A tired body has a weak immune system and is vulnerable to infection.
- Develop strategies for managing stress. Too much stress can suppress the immune system.
- Get plenty of physical activity, which stimulates the immune system.
- Avoid alcohol, tobacco products, and medication and drug abuse. Using alcohol and tobacco products and abusing medications and drugs reduce resistance to infection.
- Get regular checkups with your doctor. Your doctor can help you catch developing diseases early and ensure your vaccinations are up-to-date.

Wash Your Hands

hand washing practice of using soap and water to clean the hands

Hand washing is universally acknowledged to be the most important method of preventing many communicable diseases (**Figure 18.11**). To prevent the spread of pathogens, be sure to wash your hands

- after using the bathroom or changing a diaper;
- before preparing and eating food;
- after blowing your nose or having contact with other bodily fluids, such as when you cough or sneeze;
- after handling trash, waste, or uncooked meat and fish;
- before and after visiting a healthcare facility; and
- when your hands are visibly dirty.

When soap and water are unavailable, try using an alcohol-based hand sanitizer. If hands are visibly dirty, wash them first so the hand sanitizer works. You can often find alcohol-based sanitizer dispensers in stores and other public places.

Hand Washing

Wet hands and apply soap. Begin timing 20 seconds, or hum the "Happy Birthday" song to yourself twice.

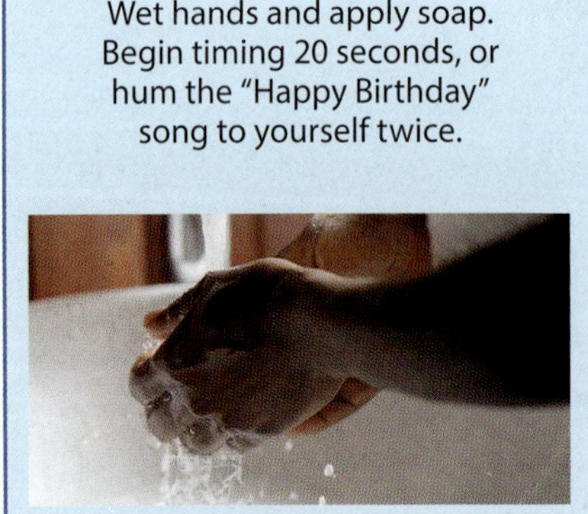

Rub your hands together. Include your palms, the backs of your hands, your fingernails, in between your fingers, the bases of your thumbs, and your wrists.

Rinse your hands and dry them completely. Try to use a reusable towel at home or a hand dryer in public instead of disposable towels.

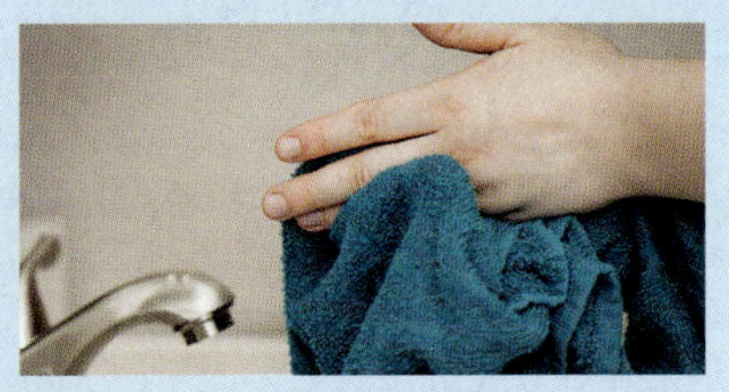

Left to right: fizkes/Shutterstock.com; BonNontawat/Shutterstock.com; Moonborne/Shutterstock.com

Figure 18.11 Practiced regularly and correctly, hand washing dramatically reduces the transmission of diseases through droplets, blood, or direct skin contact.

Use Respiratory Etiquette

From November through March each year, colds and the flu spread rapidly. People who have these diseases disperse the cold and flu viruses in respiratory droplets. Droplets inevitably coat a person's hands and make their way to the nose and mouth of another person, spreading the disease.

Doctors recommend people use **respiratory etiquette** to prevent spreading diseases. To practice respiratory etiquette, cover your nose and mouth with a tissue when coughing or sneezing. Do not reuse or store used tissues. Instead, throw them in the trash after use. If you have no tissues, do not cough or sneeze into your hands. Instead, cough or sneeze into your upper arm, sleeve, or elbow. Wash your hands after using a tissue or sneezing and coughing into your hands.

respiratory etiquette behaviors that prevent the spread of disease through droplets

Get Needed Vaccinations

Vaccination is the only proven method of successfully eliminating a communicable disease. For example, vaccination eliminated the highly contagious, deadly viral infection smallpox. In the next few years, vaccination will probably conquer polio, which has paralyzed many people throughout history. Because vaccination activates the immune system, it is also called *immunization*.

vaccination process of introducing a dead pathogen or nontoxic part of a pathogen into the body to provoke an immune response that prevents a certain disease; also called *immunization*

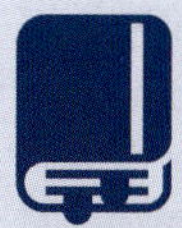

Case Study

Blocking Germs Every Day

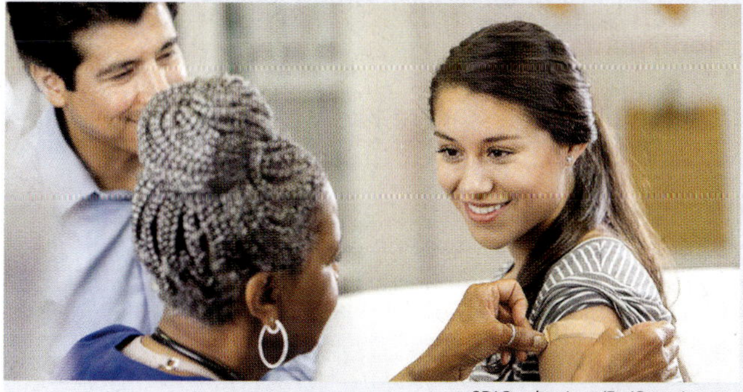

SDI Productions/E+/Getty Images

Tyrone used to catch a cold several times a school year. Tyrone considers himself a healthy person. He has a well-balanced diet and gets physical activity. He does not understand why he always catches colds. Eventually, Tyrone asks his sister how she manages not to get sick as often. His sister points out that Tyrone frequently stays up until 2:00 a.m. on weekdays and gets very little sleep. When Tyrone starts getting more sleep, his cold symptoms pop up less frequently.

Since Nia's dad is a nurse, she knows how easily the flu spreads during flu season. She gets a flu shot every year, but knows this only protects against some types of the flu. Nia washes her hands more frequently when kids at school are getting sick, but she catches the flu anyway. Her dad tells her she has to stay home from school until her fever goes away. Nia wonders if the other kids know that going to school sick gets others sick too.

Abby started noticing a red, itchy rash between her toes this swim season. Her doctor tells her she has athlete's foot. She tells Abby she should wash her feet daily, avoid walking barefoot by the pool, and wear shoes in the locker room and showers. She also tells Abby she should change her towels often and not share them with her teammates.

Practice Your Skills

Set Goals

Select one disease-prevention method discussed in this case study. With a partner, set a SMART goal for preventing the spread of communicable diseases using this method. How can you make sure to use this method consistently? For example, do you need to set a reminder or use an app to track whether you use the method? Do you need someone to hold you accountable? Do you need to learn more information about practicing the skill? Include these details in your goal and then share your SMART goal with the class.

vaccine substance containing a dead pathogen or nontoxic part of a pathogen; introduced into the body to provoke an immune response

During vaccination, a person receives a **vaccine**, usually through injection. The vaccine contains a dead pathogen or a nontoxic part of a pathogen, such as a bacterial cell wall or the coating of a virus. This dead pathogen or pathogen component is *not* capable of causing infection. When injected, the vaccine provokes an immune response, which may cause minor symptoms. A person's body produces white blood cells, proteins, and chemicals that fight the disease associated with the dead pathogen or pathogen component.

Because of this immune response, the immune system will respond strongly and quickly if it encounters the real, live pathogen. It will produce many white blood cells and antibodies, often destroying the pathogen before symptoms of the disease begin. Some vaccines remain effective for nearly a lifetime. Others require follow-up injections called *boosters* to restimulate the immune system.

Health in the Media 

The Health Hazards of Misinformation

Studies suggest that one-third of people in the US consult social media for health information. Some of this information is reliable and valid, but social media can also spread *health misinformation*, which is false. Believing health misinformation can have harmful consequences. For example, people who believe vaccines are not safe and effective risk disability or death from vaccine-preventable diseases. They also risk community health. People who accept questionable health claims about dietary supplements risk dangerous medication interactions, allergic reactions, and ineffective treatment.

Shown below are some criteria for separating health misinformation from credible health information.

It may be health misinformation if it	Health information is more likely to be accurate if it
• is brief and lacks details • includes only positive testimonials • is posted to social media by unverified sources • contains links to a sales website • presents results that seem too good to be true • comes from a celebrity or influencer	• originates with scientists or doctors • is up-to-date • is based on scientific research • includes scientific comparisons with other products or services • includes a statistical analysis of the study's results

You learned about other indicators of credible health information in Chapter 2. If you are unsure about health information you see, ask a trusted adult, doctor, or other healthcare professional about the information. This person can help you determine if the information is true.

 Practice Your Skills

Access Information

Select a topic related to disease prevention you would like to learn about in more detail. Then, use reliable and valid online resources to get more information about this topic. As you conduct your research, follow these steps:

1. Identify one source you think has reliable and valid health information. Explain why you think this.
2. Identify one source you think has health misinformation. Explain why.
3. Explain the harmful consequences people might experience if they accepted and used the health misinformation you found.
4. Explain what search terms or research methods helped you obtain sources with reliable health information. What did you learn from your research?

Skills for Health and Wellness

Help Prevent the Spread of Disease

Effective disease prevention requires cooperation between individuals and the larger community. Taking steps to prevent disease not only protects your health, but the health of those around you. You can apply your knowledge and skills to protect your health as well as the health of people in your community.

Practice Your Skills

Advocate for Health

Suppose you want to teach your classmates effective methods for preventing communicable diseases. Follow these steps in a small group to advocate for disease prevention in your school community.

1. In your group, choose one method of disease prevention you learned about in this lesson. Some examples might include accessing credible information, avoiding alcohol and tobacco, hand washing, and getting vaccinations.
2. Using reliable and valid resources, research answers to the following questions about this method:
   - How exactly does this method prevent communicable diseases from spreading?
   - Is this method effective against some diseases more than others? Explain.
   - What steps and behaviors are part of this disease-prevention method?
   - What behaviors or barriers can lower the effectiveness of this method?
3. With the information you learned, create a how-to video sharing what you learned with your school community. Be creative and adapt your language and approach for your audience: other teens. Be sure to demonstrate the exact steps involved in this method. Make your video engaging and cite your sources in the video.
4. Share your video with the class and collect feedback on the video's effectiveness. Revise the video based on this feedback and share it with your school community.

In the US, children must receive several vaccines before attending school. One example is the *MMR vaccine*, which prevents the viral infections measles, mumps, and rubella. Another is the *DTP vaccine*, which prevents diphtheria, tetanus, and pertussis (whooping cough). You may also have received vaccines for chicken pox, polio, hepatitis B, human papillomavirus (HPV), and hemophilus (for ear infections and meningitis).

People receive other vaccines as needed. Each year, people can receive a vaccine to prevent the flu. Getting this vaccine can help keep you healthy and prevent flu outbreaks. To learn more about vaccinations, talk with your doctor or another healthcare professional.

Treating Communicable Diseases

Sometimes a communicable disease can overwhelm the body's defenses. When this happens, a doctor may prescribe certain medications to kill the invading pathogens. Such medications also shorten a disease's length, reducing the chance of lasting damage. The exact treatment for a communicable disease depends on the type of pathogen involved.

Bacterial Infections

Treatment for communicable diseases caused by bacteria usually includes antibiotics. Naturally made by fungi and helpful bacteria, *antibiotics* are substances that target and kill disease-causing bacteria. Antibiotics are effective against many kinds of bacteria, but are ineffective against viruses, fungi, and parasites.

As you know, antibiotics cannot kill antibiotic-resistant bacteria. These strains of bacteria are extremely difficult, if not impossible, to treat. For example, *MRSA* (methicillin-resistant *Staphylococcus aureus*) is a strain of *S. aureus* that many antibiotics cannot control.

Antibiotic resistance is both a personal and public health issue. To avoid contributing to the issue,

- use antibiotics only when prescribed;
- do not share antibiotics;
- do not take antibiotics for viral infections; and
- take the entire dose for the length of time prescribed by your doctor.

Research in Action

Combating Antibiotic Resistance

Bacteria possess *antibiotic resistance* if certain antibiotics cannot kill them. In any population, some bacteria have mutations that permit them to survive in the presence of antibiotics. Antibiotics kill vulnerable or weak bacteria, leaving behind those with resistance. In this way, a population of bacteria evolves to be antibiotic resistant.

Antibiotic resistance has been observed in gonorrhea, pneumonia, and tuberculosis (TB). Some strains of TB bacteria are resistant to several antibiotics. These strains cause *multidrug-resistant (MDR) tuberculosis*.

To combat antibiotic resistance, doctors prescribe other antibiotics to which bacteria do not have resistance. Sometimes, combinations of two or more antibiotics are effective. Scientists have also found new antibiotics naturally made by bacteria and fungi in soil and water. Scientists use computers and artificial intelligence to rapidly design, make, and test new antibiotics. Another new strategy attacks bacteria with *phages*, or viruses that naturally kill specific bacteria. Research results for this strategy have been promising.

The World Health Organization (WHO) and CDC have made researching and combating antibiotic resistance a top public heath priority.

Practice Your Skills

Communicate with Others

Antibiotic resistance threatens personal and community health. Learning to apply strategies for combating antibiotic resistance can promote your health and the health of others. In a small group, choose one of the scenarios that follow. Then, write a script in which a teen uses effective communication to take steps that combat antibiotic resistance. Use your script to film a video or role-play for the class.

- You see the doctor for what you think is a bacterial infection. During your appointment, you give the doctor a complete and accurate description of your symptoms.
- Your doctor wants to prescribe you an antibiotic, but based on your symptoms, you are not totally convinced your infection is bacterial. You want to ask if your doctor is sure. You know there are still some symptoms you have not shared.
- Your doctor prescribes you an antibiotic. You want certain questions answered, like how many pills you should take, how long you should take them, and any possible side effects.
- You start taking an antibiotic and feel better after a few days. You want to stop taking it, but the directions say to take it for three weeks. You go to the pharmacy to ask for advice.
- A friend who was recently sick says you can use the antibiotics a doctor prescribed your friend. Your friend offers you the medication bottle and says it is no big deal.

Viral Infections

Medications used to treat viral infections usually target the effects of the viral infection and do not attack the virus itself. In many cases, people take medications to treat the signs and symptoms of disease, with the goal of being more comfortable. That is the purpose of medications like acetaminophen, which reduces the fever, aches, and pains associated with influenza.

For infections such as genital herpes, hepatitis, and severe influenza, *antiviral medications* can reduce the severity of the infection and risk of transmission. These medications keep the virus under control while the body fights back. Rest, nutrition, and fluids strengthen the body.

Fungal Infections

Like viral infections, fungal infections cannot be treated with antibiotics. Instead, specialized *antifungal medications* treat fungal infections. Some are prescription medications, and others are over-the-counter. Medications for skin and nail infections include creams applied to affected areas. If these do not work, a doctor may prescribe an oral medication.

Parasitic Infections

Parasitic infections must be treated with prescription medications that target the specific parasite causing the infection. Treating parasitic infections may take longer than treating bacterial infections. Unfortunately, some parasites, including the malaria parasite, have developed resistance to some medications.

Lesson 18.3 Review

Know and Understand

1. What is the universally acknowledged most important method of preventing communicable diseases?
2. Which type of disease transmission does respiratory etiquette most help prevent?
3. How does vaccination protect the body from communicable diseases?
4. Why is it important not to take antibiotics for viral infections?
5. How do antiviral medications work differently from antibiotics?

Think Critically

6. Choose one way of promoting resistance to infection through lifestyle choices. Then, create a one-page tip sheet reminding students of ways to take care of their health in this area.
7. The idea that vaccines cause communicable diseases is a myth. Create a short, clever slogan debunking this myth and share it with the class.

REAL WORLD Health Skills

Analyze Influences In this lesson, you learned about different methods of preventing communicable diseases. With a partner, choose one of these methods and consider the influences that might affect how easily people around the world can put it into practice. What factors might make preventing diseases this way easier? more difficult? In your community, what factors affect whether people use this method? With your partner, present your ideas to the class and discuss how people can manage these influences.

Chapter 18 Review and Assessment

Chapter Summary

Specific disease-causing microorganisms, called pathogens, cause specific diseases. Pathogens can spread between living organisms and objects; therefore, communicable diseases can too. There are four types of pathogens: bacteria, viruses, fungi, and parasites.

Direct transmission occurs when infectious material and pathogens travel from their origin to an individual through direct contact or droplet spread. Indirect transmission occurs when infectious material and pathogens pass to a person from a source that acts solely as a carrier.

The first line of defense against infection includes the internal and external body surfaces. Pathogens entering the blood or tissues face a second line of defense, which includes phagocytes, inflammation, and fever. The third line of defense consists of specialized cells and chemicals that attack and remember specific pathogens.

The common cold, influenza, pneumonia, and strep throat are diseases that primarily affect the respiratory system. Other common communicable diseases include the stomach flu, athlete's foot, pinkeye, impetigo and MRSA, mononucleosis, meningitis, hepatitis, and tetanus.

Emerging infectious diseases are diseases that are new or increasing unexpectedly. These diseases develop and spread for several reasons, including changing environments and climates, antibiotic and drug resistance, and decreasing vaccination rates.

Hand washing is universally acknowledged to be the most important method of preventing many communicable diseases, and doctors recommend people use respiratory etiquette to prevent spreading diseases. Vaccination is the only proven method of successfully eliminating a communicable disease.

Treatment for communicable diseases caused by bacteria usually includes antibiotics. Antibiotics are effective against many kinds of bacteria, but are ineffective against viruses, fungi, and parasites. Antiviral medications target the effects of the viral infection to reduce risk of transmission and keep the virus under control while the body fights back. Specialized antifungal medications treat fungal infections. Parasitic infections must be treated with prescription medications that target the specific parasite causing the infection.

Vocabulary Activity

In this chapter, you learned that antibiotics target and kill bacteria. The word *antibiotic* comes from the word parts *anti-* (meaning "against"), *bio* (meaning "life"), and *-tic* (meaning "pertaining to"). Using reliable resources, look up the meanings of the word parts *demo*, *-ic*, *pan-*, *epi-*, *en-*, *hepat*, *mening*, *-itis*, *path*, *phag*, *-cyte*, *trans-*, and *-gen*. Identify how these word parts (along with *anti-*, *bio*, and *-tic*) relate to the terms in the chapter. Then, with a partner, make a list of other terms that contain these word parts. These terms may be used in everyday language or belong to the health field. You may use a dictionary to locate words.

antibiotic-resistant bacteria	*emerging infectious diseases*	*inflammation*	*phagocyte*
antibiotics	*endemic*	*influenza*	*pinkeye*
antibodies	*epidemic*	*meningitis*	*pneumonia*
athlete's foot	*fever*	*methicillin-resistant* Staphylococcus aureus *(MRSA)*	*respiratory etiquette*
bacteria	*fungi*	*mononucleosis*	*stomach flu*
common cold	*germ theory*	*pandemic*	*strep throat*
communicable diseases	*hand washing*	*parasites*	*tetanus*
direct transmission	*hepatitis*	*pathogens*	*vaccination*
	indirect transmission		*vaccine*
			viruses

Review and Recall

Review the information in this chapter by answering the following questions.

1. What is the scientific concept that states that specific microorganisms cause specific diseases?
2. Which defense is indicated by redness, heat, swelling, and pain?
   A. inflammation
   B. phagocytosis
   C. fever
   D. B cell production
3. How does the integumentary system provide protection against invasion by pathogens?
4. What method of communicable disease prevention relies on the immune system's "memory" to be effective?
5. Which of the following statements is true about protozoa?
   A. Protozoa are parasites.
   B. Protozoa are very similar to bacteria.
   C. Certain protozoa cause dysentery and malaria.
   D. Both A and C are true.
6. What virus is usually the cause of the common cold?
7. For which three groups of people can the flu be particularly dangerous?
8. Explain the differences between hepatitis A, B, and C transmission.
9. A disease that spreads to much of the world is called a(n)
   A. pandemic.
   B. endemic.
   C. epidemic.
   D. emerging infectious disease.
10. Describe how bacteria acquire antibiotic resistance.
11. Which of the following statements is true about vaccines?
    A. Vaccines contain live pathogens.
    B. Vaccines can cause infections.
    C. Vaccines provoke an immune response in the body.
    D. Vaccines are also called antibiotics.
12. List three times when you should wash your hands.
13. What are behaviors that prevent the spread of disease through droplets called?

Standardized Test Prep

Math Practice

The following results are from a survey counting how many people in the US population received a flu vaccine in the last 12 months. Review these results and answer the questions that follow.

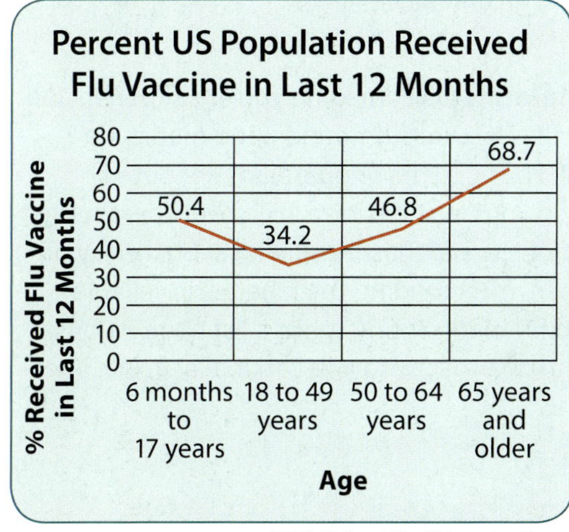

NCHS, National Health Interview Survey

14. Which statement best describes how rates of receiving the flu vaccine changed across age groups?
    A. Rates steadily increased.
    B. Rates increased and then decreased.
    C. Rates steadily decreased.
    D. Rates decreased and then increased.
15. What was the percentage difference between the rate at 65 years and older and the rate at 18–49 years?
16. This survey also found that the rate of flu vaccination at 12–17 years was 44.8 percent. How does this number compare to the rates in other age groups?

Chapter 18 Skills Assessment

Critical Thinking Skills

Answer the following questions to assess your knowledge of what you learned in this chapter.

1. Individuals who are fighting infections often have elevated white blood cell counts. Why do you think this happens?
2. Create a table that lists all five methods of disease transmission mentioned in this chapter (direct contact, droplet spread, vector transmission, indirect contact, and airborne transmission). In one column of the table, give one example of an infection that can be transmitted by each method and in another, provide an example of how it can be spread in that manner.
3. Which disease transmission method do you think would be the hardest to control? easiest? Why?
4. Research a recent outbreak of a communicable disease. What actions were taken to halt the spread? Were they effective or ineffective? How could it have been fought more effectively?
5. Do you think the government should require vaccinations for certain diseases? Why or why not?
6. Select one of the diseases discussed in this chapter and research how it has been treated throughout history. Has treatment for this disease changed over the years? How has new research affected treatment of this disease? How has treatment changed with updated research?
7. Once a type of bacteria has acquired antibiotic resistance, do you think it is possible for the resistance to go away over time? Why or why not?
8. Think about the ways you might encounter various pathogens throughout your day, and make a list of at least five ways that you can avoid catching or transmitting infectious diseases during your typical day at home and at school.
9. With a partner, discuss various myths you have heard about communicable diseases and how they are transmitted. Then, refute these myths using information from this textbook or other reliable sources.
10. Imagine that there is an influenza outbreak at your school. What can you do to protect yourself from contracting the disease? If you contract the disease, what can you to do help stop the spread of infection?
11. What are some of the misgivings people might have about vaccinations? Do you think any of them are accurate? Why or why not?
12. What immunizations have you had? Do any of them require booster shots? Are there any additional vaccinations you think you should consider as you grow older?
13. Do you think it is possible to completely eradicate communicable disease? Why or why not?

Health and Wellness Skills

Complete the following activities to assess your skills related to health and wellness.

14. **Analyze Influences.** Many different factors may influence whether a parent or guardian decides to vaccinate a child. Make a list of factors that influence your decisions about vaccination and decide if you would vaccinate a child or not. Research your arguments using reliable and valid resources. Did any of your research change your mind about vaccinations? Find a classmate with an opposing opinion and debate your reasoning and arguments.
15. **Access Information.** Imagine you are experiencing cold- or flu-like symptoms and need medication for relief. Your parents or guardians are out of town, and you must decide which over-the-counter medications to purchase. Visit a local pharmacy or its website. After reading the labels on available cold and flu medications, make a list of questions to ask the pharmacist so you can make an informed decision.

16. **Communicate with Others.** Imagine it is cold and flu season. You have observed many students at your school do not wash their hands properly or often enough. You want to get the word out about how important hand washing is. Working in small groups, consult the CDC website and gather information about hand washing. With the information your group finds, write a dialogue that emphasizes the importance of hand washing to people who do not wash their hands. Each group will share their dialogue with the rest of the class.
17. **Make Decisions.** If you have experienced strep throat or another bacterial infection, you were probably prescribed some type of antibiotic. Typically, after taking an antibiotic for three to four days, you begin to feel better and might think it is okay to stop taking the medication. Still, it is important to finish a course of antibiotics. Write a script or dialogue that might take place between your doctor and yourself, outlining the importance of finishing all medications prescribed, especially antibiotics.
18. **Set Goals.** In this chapter, you learned about ways to prevent communicable diseases. Using what you learned in this chapter, set five SMART goals that will help you prevent communicable diseases now and in your future. Consider any obstacles you may face and make a plan for overcoming them.
19. **Practice Health-Enhancing Behaviors.** Review the information about food safety in Chapter 8 (Figure 8.23). Then, help prepare a meal at home. While preparing the meal, be observant of proper sanitation to help prevent foodborne illnesses. After helping with the meal, create a digital presentation or poster that reflects the steps you took to avoid foodborne illnesses.
20. **Advocate for Health.** Working in small groups, create a public service announcement (PSA) about the importance of getting a flu vaccine. Your group's PSA can be in the form of a radio, TV, or social media advertisement. Your TV or radio ad should be 60 seconds or less in duration, and your social media ad should be one post. Your message should be engaging, be clear and concise, and include current information that creates emotional awareness in your audience.

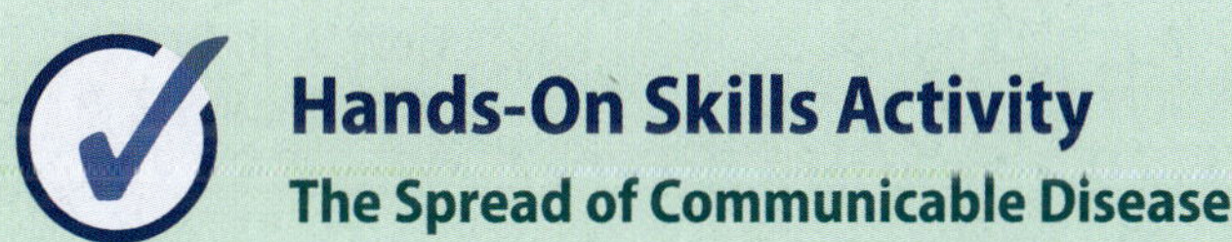

Hands-On Skills Activity

The Spread of Communicable Diseases

This activity will show how communicable diseases can spread through person-to-person contact. The liquid in the cups will simulate respiratory droplets produced by coughing, sneezing, or talking. For this activity, you will need plastic cups, water, lemon juice, and bromothymol blue pH indicator. Do *not* drink the liquid in the cups.

Steps for This Activity

1. Your teacher will give you one cup of water filled halfway. One person in the class will have "infected" water (2 teaspoons of lemon juice for every 2 cups of water).
2. "Interact" with a classmate by "sharing" the liquid in your cup. (Do not drink the liquid.) Pour all of your liquid into your classmate's cup, and then your classmate will pour all the liquid back into yours. You will then pour half of the liquid from your cup back into your classmate's cup.
3. Repeat this process with several other classmates.
4. Form a circle. Your teacher will drop a few drops of bromothymol blue in each student's cup. The liquid in any "infected" cups will turn yellow. The liquid in the cups that are not infected will turn blue.
5. **Practice Health-Enhancing Behaviors.** Consider and discuss the following questions: How many cups were infected? Were you able to tell if your cup was infected just by looking at it? Predict the outcome if more rounds of "interactions" had been done. What does this teach you about the steps you can take to reduce the spread of communicable disease?

Chapter 19

Sexually Transmitted Infections and HIV/AIDS

Look for the skills icon throughout this chapter for opportunities to practice your health skills.

Check Your Health and Wellness Skills

In this chapter, you will learn skills for preventing sexually transmitted infections (STIs). To understand the skills you currently use, take the following inventory of your behaviors. Indicate how well you think you use each skill. Use a scale of 1–5, *1* meaning you do not use the skill and *5* meaning you feel completely comfortable using it.

Skill	How Well Do You Use Each Skill?
I know how sexually transmitted infections (STIs) are spread.	
I understand the importance of getting tested for STIs, even if I have no symptoms.	
I know that sexual abstinence is the only 100-percent effective method of preventing STIs.	
I understand how condoms help prevent STI transmission.	
I encourage peers who are sexually active to get STI testing and treatment.	
I know whom I'd talk to if I thought I had an STI.	
I know which resources in my community offer STI testing and treatment.	
I know what activities can transmit HIV.	
I don't share needles for injection or piercing with anyone else.	
I accept and advocate for those living with HIV.	
	Total:

Add up your responses to each statement. The higher your score, the more comfortable you feel practicing health skills related to preventing STIs. Which skill do you think is most important for you? Which skill is the most challenging for you? Which skill would you most like to improve? In this chapter, you will learn how to perform these skills better and more often.

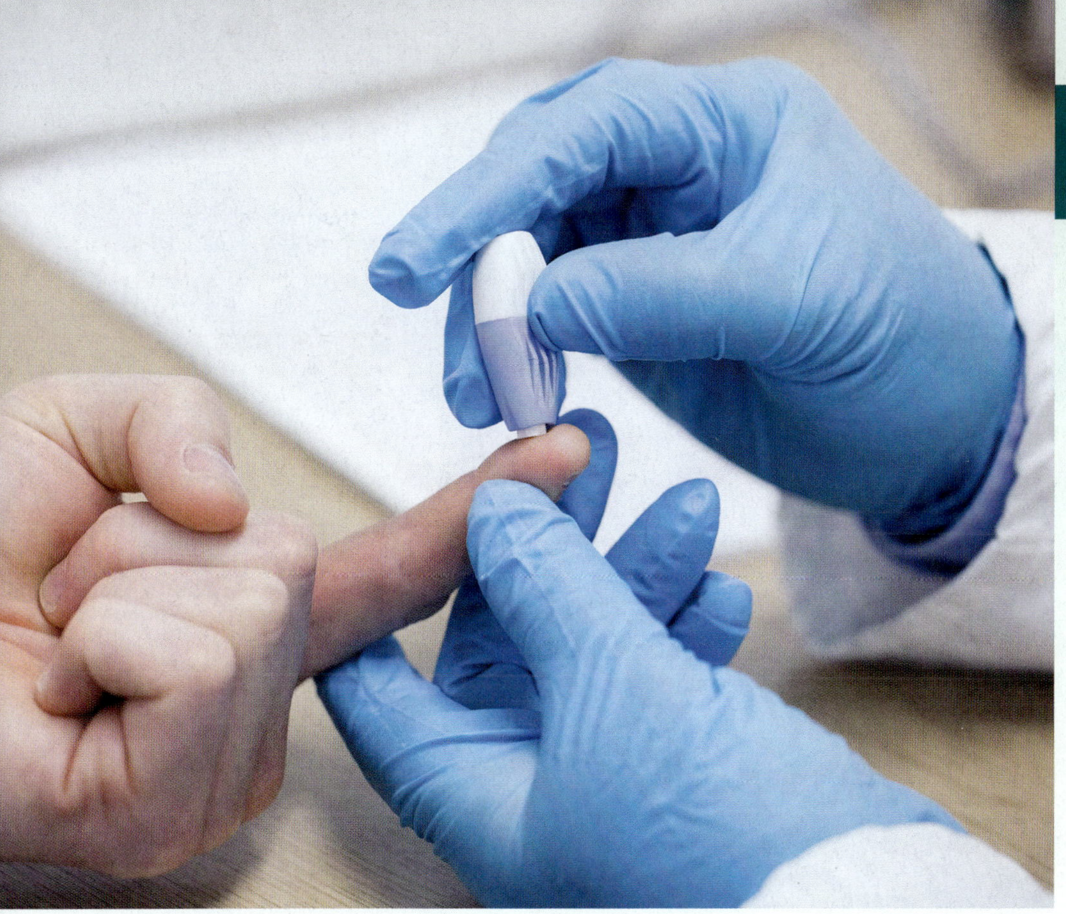

wavebreakmedia/Shutterstock.com

Reading and Notetaking

Before you read the chapter, list any sexually transmitted infections (STIs) you have heard about. Also list what you think you know about HIV/AIDS. As you read, make connections between your prior knowledge and the chapter content by looking for references to the infections and facts you listed. After reading the chapter, review your list of STIs and facts and write two paragraphs reflecting on your list in light of what you learned in this chapter.

STIs	Facts About HIV/AIDS

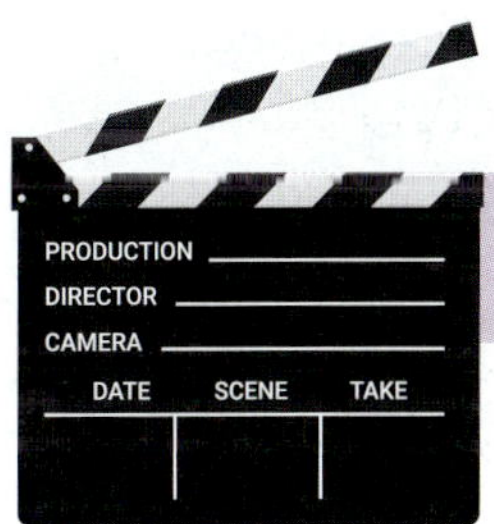

Setting the Scene

STI Concerns

When you and your partner began dating, you agreed to talk regularly about the place physical affection would have in your relationship. So far in your dating relationship, you and your partner have both decided to be sexually abstinent. This is the best decision for you, since you want to focus on your schoolwork and do not want to worry about an unplanned pregnancy.

This month, your partner asks if you still do not want to have sex. You share your reasons for choosing sexual abstinence and also mention the risk of sexually transmitted infections (STIs). Your partner is puzzled by your concern. Frowning, your partner asks, "Why should we be worried about STIs?" As you think of a response, your partner says, "What's the worst that could happen? We're only seeing each other."

Thinking Critically

1. In this scenario, explain why you should be concerned about STIs, even if you and your partner are only seeing each other.
2. How do you think STIs are similar to other communicable diseases? How are they different?
3. What valid and reliable resources could you and your partner use to better understand STIs?

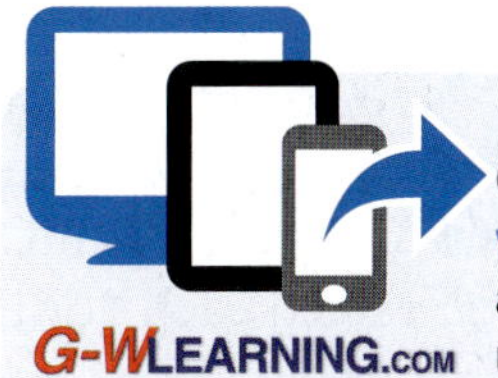

Click on the activity icon or visit www.g-wlearning.com/health/4095 to access online vocabulary activities using key terms from the chapter.

Lesson

19.1

Common STIs

Essential Question

How do sexually transmitted infections (STIs) affect the reproductive system?

Learning Outcomes

After studying this lesson, you will be able to

- analyze how STIs spread and affect the body;
- describe how chlamydia can lead to pelvic inflammatory disease;
- assess the effects of gonorrhea on health;
- explain the stages of syphilis;
- discuss why trichomoniasis often goes untreated;
- describe the symptoms of herpes; and
- summarize the serious health effects of HPV.

Key Terms

asymptomatic
cervical cancer
chlamydia
genital herpes
genital warts
gonorrhea
human papillomavirus (HPV)
oropharyngeal cancer
pelvic inflammatory disease (PID)
sexually transmitted infections (STIs)
syphilis
trichomoniasis

Warm-Up Activity

Agree or Disagree

Access Information Recreate the chart shown on a separate piece of paper. Before reading the lesson, decide whether you agree or disagree with each statement. Using valid and reliable resources, search for evidence that proves or disproves each statement. Be sure to cite your sources. When you have finished reading the lesson, consider the statements again based on any new information. In the final column, record whether you agree or disagree and check to see whether your opinion has changed based on new evidence.

Before Reading	Statements	After Reading
Agree / Disagree	1. Chlamydia is the most reported STI in the United States.	Agree / Disagree
Agree / Disagree	2. Ectopic pregnancies can be fatal.	Agree / Disagree
Agree / Disagree	3. There is no cure for bacterial infections.	Agree / Disagree
Agree / Disagree	4. Syphilis is fatal if not treated.	Agree / Disagree
Agree / Disagree	5. Herpes blisters can appear on the mouth as well as the genitals.	Agree / Disagree
Agree / Disagree	6. Herpes can be cured with antibiotics.	Agree / Disagree
Agree / Disagree	7. Almost all sexually active people carry human papillomavirus (HPV) at one time or another.	Agree / Disagree
Agree / Disagree	8. Human papillomavirus (HPV) can cause cervical cancer in females.	Agree / Disagree

Sexually transmitted infections (STIs) are a type of *communicable disease.* This means they spread from person to person. According to the World Health Organization (WHO), more than one million STIs are contracted each day around the world. In this lesson, you will learn about what causes STIs, how they spread, and common types.

What Are STIs?

Sexually transmitted infections (STIs) are infections spread from one person to another during *sexual activity*, or actions that involve contact with a person's reproductive organs. As you learned in Chapter 14, sexual activity can include sexual touching and *sexual intercourse*, which is any sexual activity that involves penetration. STIs can affect people of all sexes, ages, races, nationalities, sexual orientations, gender identities, and ethnic origins. Sometimes, STIs are also called *sexually transmitted diseases (STDs)*.

sexually transmitted infections (STIs) communicable diseases that spread from one person to another during sexual activity; also called *sexually transmitted diseases (STDs)*

Like other communicable diseases, STIs are caused by *pathogens*, or disease-causing microorganisms, including bacteria, viruses, and protozoa. These pathogens live in and on the surfaces of the reproductive organs, including the penis and vagina. Depending on the type of STI, pathogens may also reside in the mouth or rectum or in a person's blood, semen, vaginal secretions, and other bodily fluids.

When discussing STIs, many young people ask, "Am I at risk of contracting an STI?" The answer is *no* if young people do not engage in sexual activity. The answer is *yes*, however, if young people are sexually active. Engaging in sexual activity one time with just one partner who has an STI is all it takes to contract an STI. People with more sexual partners have greater chances of getting an STI (**Figure 19.1**). Although it is possible for certain oral STIs to spread through kissing, most STIs spread only through sexual activity. Casual contact, such as using the same toilet seat, does not transmit STIs.

When you are *not* sexually active, you are not exposed to risks for STIs.
When you engage in sexual activity, you expose yourself to the risk of STIs from your sexual partner...
any previous sexual partners of your partner...
previous sexual partners of those people...
and their previous sexual partners too.
STIs spread through sexual activity. More sexual partners mean more chances of being exposed to STIs.

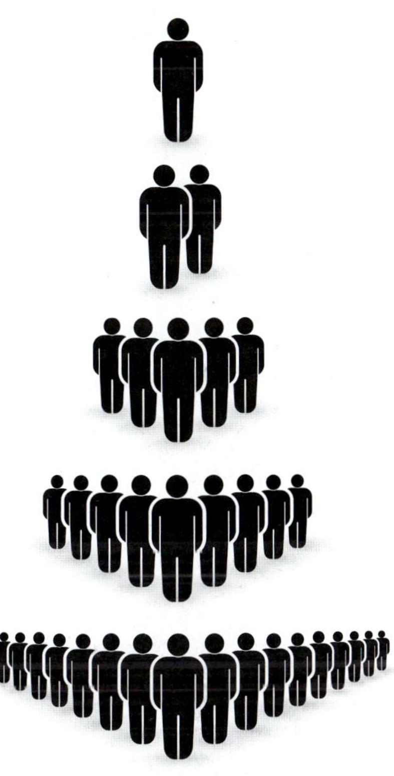

Kovalov Anatolii/Shutterstock.com

Figure 19.1 Each new sexual partner increases your risk of getting an STI.

Some STIs are **asymptomatic**, meaning they show few or no signs of infection. Even so, all STIs are contagious and can cause serious damage to the body. Many STIs trigger *inflammation*, the body's reaction to infection in which body parts become red, warm, swollen, and painful. STIs can damage the reproductive organs and cause *infertility*, the inability to conceive and have children. If left untreated, STIs can also damage the brain, heart, liver, and other internal organs.

asymptomatic showing few or no signs of infection or disease

A few STIs are incurable. Some cause cancer, and some are fatal. Sadly, it is possible for a pregnant person with an STI to transmit the infection to the baby during pregnancy, birth, or breastfeeding. This may cause health conditions for the baby at birth and months or years after birth.

Chlamydia

chlamydia bacterial sexually transmitted infection (STI) with few or no symptoms; can cause pelvic inflammatory disease (PID) and infertility in the female reproductive system

According to the Centers for Disease Control and Prevention (CDC), nearly three million new cases of **chlamydia** (kluh-MID-ee-uh), a bacterial STI, are reported each year in the United States. The CDC also estimates the actual number may be much higher because chlamydia causes few symptoms. For this reason, chlamydia is sometimes called a *silent disease*. The majority of chlamydia infections occur in young people ages 15–24. In fact, experts estimate that 1 in 20 sexually active females ages 14–24 have chlamydia.

pelvic inflammatory disease (PID) infection of the fallopian tubes and pelvic cavity that sometimes leads to infertility

Chlamydia poses a threat to the health of the female reproductive system, especially for young people whose bodies have not fully developed. The "silent" nature of chlamydia allows it to quietly progress to an infection of the fallopian tubes and pelvic cavity. This condition is called **pelvic inflammatory disease (PID)** and can cause infertility (**Figure 19.2**).

A person with PID who becomes pregnant may develop an *ectopic pregnancy*. This is a life-threatening condition in which a fertilized egg implants outside the uterus. A fertilized egg cannot develop properly outside the uterus. If it implants elsewhere, such as in the fallopian tube, the egg could rupture the tube and cause serious bleeding and a dangerous pelvic infection.

Signs and Symptoms

Symptoms of chlamydia are often mild or absent. If symptoms do arise, males may experience burning during urination, itching at the opening of the penis, and watery discharge from the penis. Rectal and oral infections may also occur.

A female may experience abnormal vaginal discharge and a burning sensation during urination. The bacteria associated with chlamydia can infect the cervix, which connects the vagina to the uterus. If the infection spreads past the cervix to the fallopian tubes, a female may still have no symptoms. A female may also experience nausea, abdominal pain, fever, and abnormal bleeding between menstrual periods.

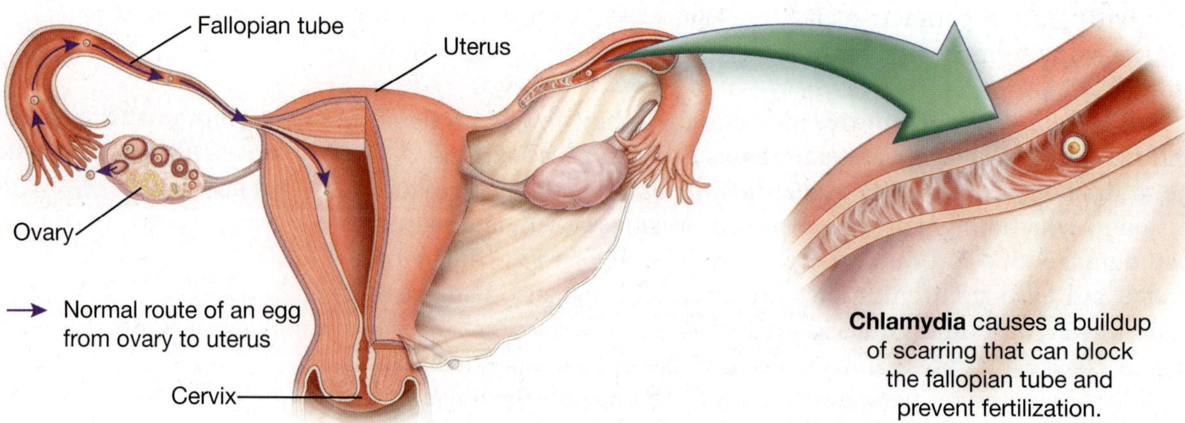

Figure 19.2 Untreated chlamydia can damage the fallopian tubes. ***What is the name of the health condition that affects the fallopian tubes and pelvic cavity and can cause infertility?***

A pregnant person with chlamydia may deliver a baby prematurely (too early). A baby born to a pregnant person with chlamydia can develop pneumonia, pinkeye (conjunctivitis), or *trachoma* (an eye infection that leads to vision loss).

Diagnosis and Treatment

Diagnosing chlamydia is simple, quick, and painless. Two methods include a urine test and a laboratory test of a sample swabbed from an infected site such as the penis or cervix. Test results are often available within one day. If a person tests positive for chlamydia, a doctor can prescribe antibiotics to cure the infection.

Gonorrhea

Gonorrhea (gah-nuh-REE-uh) is a bacterial STI that primarily affects the rectum, throat, and reproductive system, including the *urethra* (tube that carries urine out of the body), cervix, uterus, and fallopian tubes. According to the CDC, an estimated 820,000 people contract gonorrhea each year. Of these, 70 percent are young people ages 15–24.

gonorrhea bacterial sexually transmitted infection (STI) with mild or no symptoms; primarily affects the rectum, throat, and reproductive tract

Signs and Symptoms

Like chlamydia, gonorrhea causes mild or no symptoms in many people. If symptoms do arise, males experience burning in the urethra during urination and yellow or white urethral discharge. Sometimes the testes also swell.

Females with gonorrhea may experience mild burning or itching that seems like a vaginal yeast infection. In addition, females may have pelvic pain, abnormal bleeding between menstrual periods, and abnormal vaginal discharge. Females may also develop chronic pelvic and lower back pain.

If left untreated, gonorrhea can cause PID and infertility. In the rectum or throat, gonorrhea may cause anal itching and bleeding or a sore throat. Gonorrhea can also infect the blood and spread throughout the body in a potentially fatal complication called *disseminated gonococcal infection (DGI)*.

Diagnosis and Treatment

To diagnose gonorrhea, a healthcare provider may swab and examine urethral discharge from the penis. For females, diagnosis may involve a urine test or laboratory analysis of a sample swabbed from an infected body part.

While antibiotics often successfully treat and cure gonorrhea, some gonorrhea bacteria are antibiotic resistant. Treatment is difficult for these infections. Therefore, treatment for gonorrhea often involves two kinds of antibiotics.

Syphilis

Syphilis (SIH-fuh-lus) is a bacterial STI that can be fatal if untreated and can threaten the life of a developing fetus during pregnancy. According to the CDC, the number of syphilis infections has been increasing each year since 2001, when the lowest number of infections was recorded. Between 2016 and 2017, syphilis infections among people ages 15–19 increased by about 10 percent.

syphilis bacterial sexually transmitted infection (STI) that is fatal if untreated and has four stages: primary syphilis, secondary syphilis, latent syphilis, and late-stage syphilis

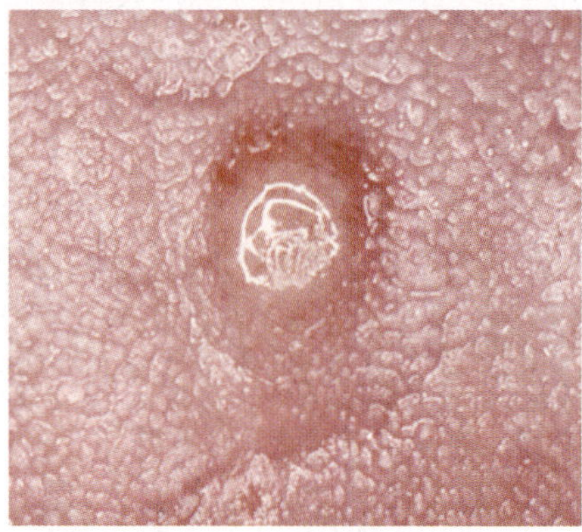

Courtesy of the Centers for Disease Control and Prevention

Figure 19.3 During primary syphilis, painless sores may develop on the genitals, rectum, or mouth. ***What is the name of this syphilis sore?***

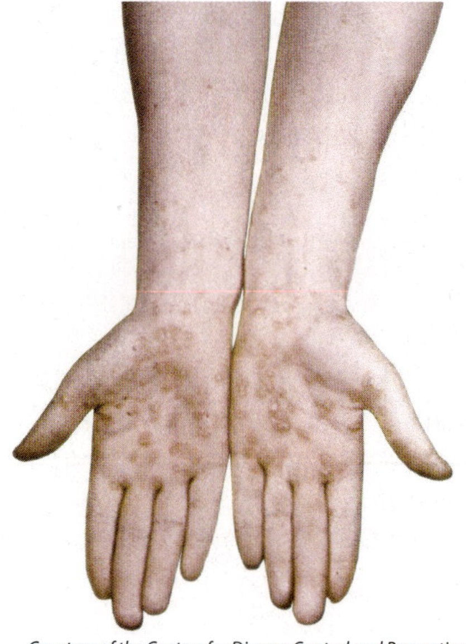

Courtesy of the Centers for Disease Control and Prevention

Figure 19.4 A rash will appear on the palms or soles during secondary syphilis. This rash may be accompanied by fever or fatigue.

Signs and Symptoms

Syphilis is an STI that progresses through four distinct stages. Signs and symptoms depend on the stage of infection. As with all STIs, sexual activity can transmit syphilis bacteria. The four stages are primary syphilis, secondary syphilis, latent syphilis, and late-stage syphilis.

1. **Primary syphilis:** During this first stage, a sore called a *chancre* develops at the site of infection (**Figure 19.3**). Sometimes, only a single sore develops on the penis or in the vagina, mouth, or rectum. This sore can easily be missed or go unrecognized. Chancre sores are not painful, do not itch, and heal after a few weeks. Without treatment, however, the person still has syphilis.
2. **Secondary syphilis:** Secondary syphilis develops days, weeks, or even months after infection. In this stage, a red or copper-colored rash appears, usually on the palms and soles, but sometimes elsewhere (**Figure 19.4**). The rash does not itch, may go unnoticed, and cannot transmit syphilis. Other symptoms include swollen lymph nodes, fatigue, and mild fever. These symptoms resemble those of many other diseases, which is why syphilis is sometimes called the *great imitator*. The rash heals, but the person still has syphilis and enters the next stage.
3. **Latent syphilis:** The latent, or hidden, stage of syphilis is asymptomatic. During this stage, a person experiences no noticeable signs or symptoms. This stage of syphilis can last for years.
4. **Late-stage syphilis:** If left untreated for 10 or more years, syphilis can progress to late-stage syphilis, which is characterized by internal infection. Though late-stage syphilis may not have obvious symptoms, it damages the brain and can lead to *dementia* (deteriorating cognitive function) and paralysis. It also causes fatal damage to the heart, liver, and blood vessels. Children born to a pregnant person with syphilis are often stillborn or die shortly after birth. Children who survive are born with *congenital syphilis*, a condition that causes physical and intellectual disabilities.

Diagnosis and Treatment

To diagnose syphilis, a doctor will examine a sample swabbed from a syphilis sore using a special microscope. Doctors can also use blood tests to detect antibodies the body makes in response to syphilis. Both tests are easy and painless. Because of potential complications, all people who are pregnant should receive a syphilis blood test at the first prenatal visit and receive treatment, if the test is positive.

Early diagnosis is important for treating syphilis. This is because syphilis is most treatable during its early stages. During the primary and secondary stages, antibiotics can cure syphilis. Antibiotics cannot reverse or repair the organ damage caused by late-stage syphilis.

Research in Action

Point-of-Care Testing and Diagnosis for STIs

Technology has evolved so doctors can now test for STIs in their offices during an appointment. This is called *point-of-care testing (POCT)*, which leads to *point-of-care diagnosis (POCD)*. Rapid testing and diagnosis allows early treatment, which can cure certain STIs and reduce the risk of complications.

Doctors use a blood drop, saliva sample, cheek swab, or urine sample to perform POCT and POCD. These tests use portable supplies and small quantities of chemicals and can be done on a countertop without large, expensive lab equipment. During POCT, doctors may test for diseases that frequently occur together. For example, a doctor may test for human immunodeficiency virus (HIV), hepatitis, and liver damage caused by hepatitis. Doctors can also perform POCT and POCD in mobile community clinics, public health clinics, and urgent care facilities.

Today, people can also find and order kits for STI testing online. These kits are then mailed in, and a person receives results online or in the mail. The accuracy of these tests depends on correct sample collection. People who test positive or experience symptoms should see a healthcare provider.

Practice Your Skills

Communicate with Others

Suppose a close friend confides in you about having unprotected sex. Your friend did not plan to have sex and worries about getting an STI. To assist your friend, research where in your community your friend can go to get medical help. What can you say to convince your friend it is important to be tested and treated? Write a short letter to your friend emphasizing the importance of testing and treatment and explaining why it is easier than your friend thinks. Use effective communication skills as you try to convince your friend.

Trichomoniasis

Trichomoniasis (TRIK-uh-muh-NIGH-uh-sus) is an STI caused by a single-celled parasite called a *protozoan*. Trichomoniasis is often asymptomatic and is the most curable common STI (**Figure 19.5**).

trichomoniasis common sexually transmitted infection (STI) caused by a protozoan; is easily treated once diagnosed

Signs and Symptoms

Most males with trichomoniasis have no symptoms, but some experience itching and burning in the urethra and discharge from the penis. In males, these symptoms tend to go away without treatment. Even so, males can still carry the protozoa and infect their sexual partners.

In females, trichomoniasis primarily infects the vagina and causes few symptoms. Trichomoniasis may cause yellow-green vaginal discharge with a foul odor and burning, itching, and pain during urination and sexual intercourse. A pregnant person with trichomoniasis will often have a baby with a low birthweight.

The CDC estimates that almost
4 million
people in the US have trichomoniasis.
Almost 70% of these people do not show any symptoms.
70%

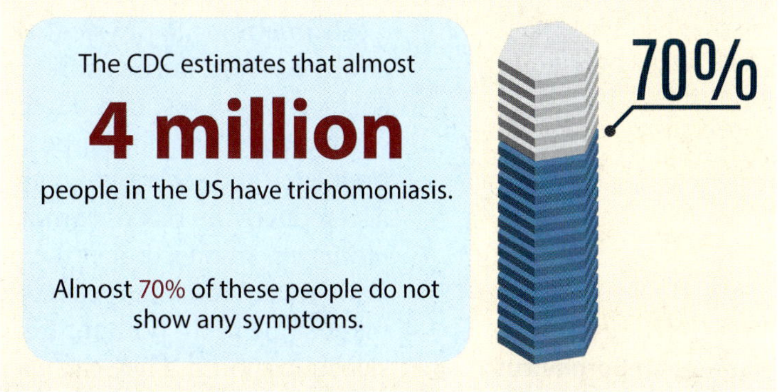

bbgreg/Shutterstock.com

Figure 19.5 Trichomoniasis is a common STI. Despite being the most curable STI, most people do not show symptoms and therefore frequently do not seek treatment.

Diagnosis and Treatment

Trichomoniasis is difficult to diagnose without an examination and laboratory test. To diagnose trichomoniasis, a doctor will examine the vagina and cervix for small red sores and test a sample of vaginal fluid. Trichomoniasis does not cause visible sores on the penis, but a doctor can swab the urethra or test a urine sample in males.

Prescription medications can easily cure trichomoniasis. Because people often have no symptoms, however, the infection may go undiagnosed and untreated, making it easy to infect partners again. Therefore, both partners should seek treatment to control the recurrence of infection.

Genital Herpes

Herpes is a viral infection that can affect almost any part of the body. It is caused by the herpes simplex virus (HSV). There are two types of HSV. HSV type 1 (HSV-1) causes cold sores on the mouth and lips, but can also cause genital infections if saliva has contact with the reproductive organs. Kissing; sharing drinks, lip balms, or eating utensils; and sexual activity can transmit HSV-1. HSV type 2 (HSV-2) causes genital infections exclusively and spreads only through sexual activity.

genital herpes herpes simplex virus (HSV) infection of the reproductive organs, mouth, or rectum

Genital herpes refers to an HSV infection of the *genitals* (reproductive organs), mouth, or rectum. Genital herpes is very common in the US, occurring in about 12 percent of people ages 14–49.

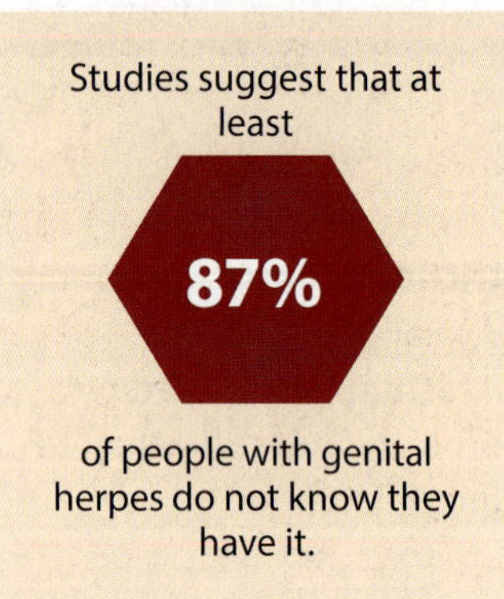

Figure 19.6 Many people do not know they have genital herpes. This increases the chances of unknowingly passing this STI to a sexual partner. ***How many types of HSV are there? Name each type.***

Signs and Symptoms

A person with herpes often has mild or no symptoms (**Figure 19.6**). Blisters develop at the site of infection, burst, and heal after a few weeks. Typically, these blisters return repeatedly, but in a milder form, perhaps with swollen lymph nodes and fever. This recurrence of herpes is called an *outbreak*.

A pregnant person can pass genital herpes to an unborn baby, which can lead to serious illness and even death. Treatment of pregnant people with herpes has improved, and it is now uncommon for a parent to transmit the infection to a developing baby. Still, people should discuss the risk with a doctor during prenatal visits.

Diagnosis and Treatment

Sometimes, a physical examination and laboratory tests of samples swabbed from herpes sores can diagnose herpes. If a person has no visible sores, a blood test can detect antibodies that indicate the presence of HSV.

No cure exists for herpes, but prescription medications can control the frequency and severity of outbreaks and lower risk for transmission. Treatment also reduces the risk of complications resulting from the disease, such as *meningitis*, an infection of the membranes surrounding the brain that can be fatal. Early treatment of herpes reduces the risk of the infection spreading to other parts of the body. Without treatment, people can infect their own eyes, fingers, skin, and mouth. They can also transmit the virus to another person.

human papillomavirus (HPV) common sexually transmitted infection (STI) that infects cells in the skin and membranes, causing them to grow abnormally

Human Papillomavirus (HPV)

With 14 million new infections each year, **human papillomavirus (HPV)** is the most common STI in the US. HPV infects cells in the skin and membranes, causing them to grow abnormally. At least 40 types of HPV cause genital infections, and some types can cause cancer.

genital warts abnormal growths on the skin and membranes around the reproductive organs and anus; caused by some forms of human papillomavirus (HPV)

cervical cancer abnormal cancerous growth of the cervix; often caused by the human papillomavirus (HPV)

oropharyngeal cancer abnormal cancerous growths on the back of the throat, base of the tongue, and tonsils; often caused by the human papillomavirus (HPV)

Signs and Symptoms

Almost all people who are sexually active carry HPV at one time or another. Some types of HPV cause **genital warts**, or abnormal growths on the skin and membranes around the genitals, mouth, and rectum. These growths can range from small, raised bumps to large, cauliflower shapes. New genital wart infections affect 350,000 people each year.

Some types of HPV can also cause cancer. The most common cancer caused by HPV is **cervical cancer**, which is characterized by abnormal cancerous growth of the cervix. Cervical cancer may be asymptomatic until it becomes life threatening. Each year, 12,000 females are diagnosed with cervical cancer, and about 4,000 die from this disease.

HPV can also cause **oropharyngeal cancer**, which affects the back of the throat, base of the tongue, and tonsils. Altogether, every year, new cases of HPV-related cancer affect at least 12,000 males and 19,000 females.

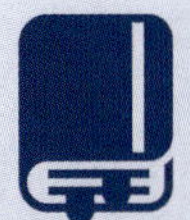

Case Study

A Vaccine for an STI

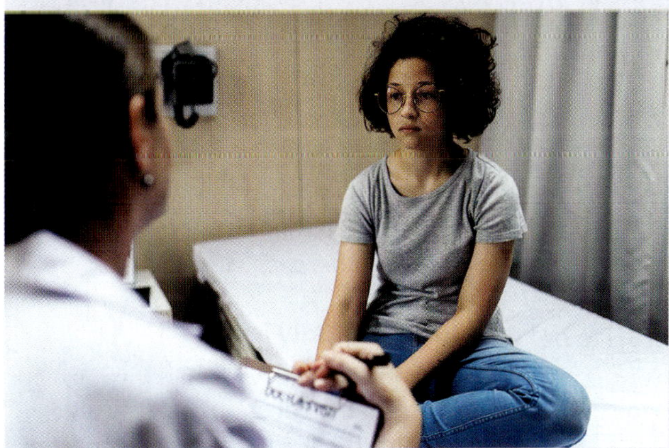

Rawpixel/iStock / Getty Images Plus/Getty Images

In the doctor's waiting room, 14-year-old Carla and her grandmother see a poster about the HPV vaccine. The poster states that HPV is a sexually transmitted infection. Carla's grandmother asks her if she wants to receive this vaccine. Carla tells her grandmother that she is not sexually active, so she does not need the vaccine. Her grandmother explains that getting the vaccine now can help protect her from HPV if she is sexually active later in life.

AJ has been seeing the same doctor many years for regular checkups. He trusts his doctor and feels comfortable asking questions about his health. When his doctor talks about the HPV vaccine, AJ asks why the vaccine is important for him. His doctor explains that the HPV vaccine can help protect against genital warts and HPV-related cancers.

Mikko knows it is important to get all of her vaccines. She just read a brochure about the HPV vaccine, which said the vaccine is recommended for people between the ages of 11 and 12. At 17 years old, Mikko was anxious she missed the window for protecting herself from HPV. She asks the school nurse, who tells her she can still get the HPV vaccine until the age of 26.

Practice Your Skills

Communicate with Others

With a partner, research what facilities, resources, or programs in your community offer HPV vaccine services and create a list of these locations and resources. Then, brainstorm a list of questions you would ask a healthcare professional about the HPV vaccine. With your partner, practice asking these questions using effective communication skills.

Diagnosis and Treatment

For females, a laboratory test can detect an HPV infection and identify the type of HPV. If an HPV infection is present, a doctor will recommend regular follow-up appointments and tests for cervical cancer. Doctors do not routinely perform HPV tests for females under age 30 because many females and males carry HPV. HPV tests are not available for males.

To diagnose genital warts, a doctor will perform a physical examination. Sometimes genital warts are hard to see, so the doctor may apply special droplets to make warts more visible. If a person develops visible genital warts, a doctor may prescribe skin treatments, prescription medications, or surgical removal. These treatments do not cure HPV, but they do reduce symptoms.

Since HPV can lead to cervical cancer, doctors screen for this type of cancer using a *Pap test*, also called a *Pap smear*. In a Pap test, a doctor swabs the cervix. The sample is then examined under a microscope for abnormal cells. Sometimes, the sample is also tested in a laboratory for HPV. Using these methods together is called *HPV/Pap co-testing*. If cancer is present, the doctor and patient will discuss treatment options. Doctors conduct a physical examination to diagnose HPV-related cancers in the mouth and throat. Several treatments are available depending on the characteristics of the cancer.

Receiving an HPV vaccine can reduce a person's risk of contracting HPV. The CDC recommends that all people receive the HPV vaccine between the ages of 11 and 12. The HPV vaccine consists of two shots given over a six-month time period. If people do not get the HPV vaccine at the recommended age, they can still receive it between the ages of 13 and 26.

Lesson 19.1 Review

Know and Understand

1. How are STIs similar to and different from other communicable diseases?
2. What does it mean for an STI to be asymptomatic?
3. How can chlamydia lead to infertility?
4. What challenges do people face in recognizing the symptoms of syphilis?
5. How is trichomoniasis cured?
6. What treatment is available for genital herpes?

Think Critically

7. With a partner, research the prevalence of antibiotic-resistant gonorrhea. What are the dangers of this type of gonorrhea?
8. Before reading this lesson, what did you know about HPV and the HPV vaccine? Did what you learned in this lesson confirm or correct your previous knowledge?

REAL WORLD Health Skills

Comprehend Concepts With a partner, review the information in this lesson. List all the STIs discussed and briefly summarize their effects on the body. Identify the type of infection (bacterial, viral, or parasitic) and methods of transmission for each STI and whether the STI can or cannot be cured. Arrange your notes into a fact sheet to keep and reference.

Preventing and Treating STIs

Essential Question

What skills can you use to prevent and get treatment for STIs?

Lesson 19.2

Learning Outcomes

After studying this lesson, you will be able to

- explain why abstinence is the only 100-percent effective method for preventing STIs;
- practice skills for abstaining from sexual activity;
- analyze the effectiveness of condoms and dental dams for preventing some STIs;
- list the three critical components for effective treatment of an STI;
- identify resources for STI testing and treatment; and
- summarize treatment options for different STIs.

Key Terms

condom
dental dam
external condom
internal condom
reinfection

Warm-Up Activity

Staying STI Free

Practice Health-Enhancing Behaviors Before reading this lesson, brainstorm with a partner strategies for staying STI free. For each strategy, explain how a teen could put it into action. Also explain how the strategy would reduce health risks and enhance health. Share your strategies with the class to create a class list. After reading this lesson, review the strategies on the class list and add to them or revise them.

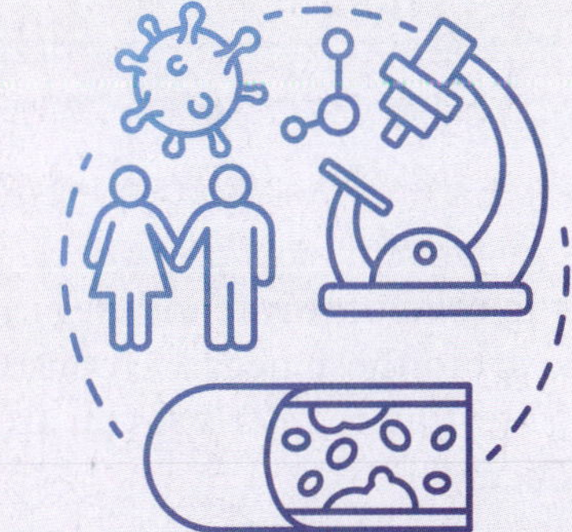

bsd/Shutterstock.com

STIs are communicable diseases caused by pathogens (bacteria, viruses, and protozoa) that spread through sexual activity. Some STIs also spread through certain bodily fluids like blood or saliva. Treatment for an STI depends on the type of STI (for example, bacterial or viral) and whether the STI is curable.

Skills for Health and Wellness

Promoting Awareness About STIs

Many people have misconceptions about STIs. Some people do not know the facts, and others do not understand the importance of prevention, testing, and treatment. You can advocate for the health and well-being of your peers and community by promoting awareness about STIs and sharing reliable resources of STI information. Sharing this information can help prevent the spread of STIs in your community and empower people to protect their health.

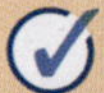

Practice Your Skills

Advocate for Health

In a group, use the following steps to create a campaign advocating for awareness about STIs. In each step, be sure to divide the work among group members and access valid and reliable sources of health information.

1. Research the state of STI prevalence, testing, and treatment in your community. Using valid and reliable sources of information, find answers to the following questions:
    - How common are STIs among people your age in your community? your state?
    - What healthcare facilities provide testing for STIs? What online testing options are available? What is the cost of testing?
    - What healthcare facilities provide STI treatment? How much does treatment cost?
2. Find out how much other students at your school know about STIs. Do students at your school know how common STIs are? Do they know how to find testing and treatment? You could gather this information through a survey or a series of interviews.
3. Identify one area where the knowledge of students at your school could be improved.
4. Create a campaign to educate students at your school about this area of knowledge. For your campaign, you could create a series of public service announcements (PSAs) or social media posts. You could organize an event or club or invite speakers to come in and share information. Choose activities you can realistically complete.
5. Put your campaign into action. After completing the campaign, survey or interview students to see how their understanding of STIs has changed. Use this information to evaluate the effectiveness of your campaign.

STIs can have serious negative effects on your health. They can cause health conditions, conflict in relationships, and negative feelings and thoughts. The best ways to avoid these negative consequences are to avoid getting an STI, receive STI testing regularly if you are sexually active, and seek treatment if an STI occurs.

Preventing STIs

Two methods commonly used to help prevent STIs are practicing sexual abstinence and using condoms or dental dams. Other birth control methods are ineffective. For example, the birth control pill can help prevent pregnancy, but it has no effect on STIs. A person taking birth control pills must abstain from sexual activity or insist on using a condom to prevent STIs.

Sexual Abstinence

The only 100-percent effective method for preventing STIs is *sexual abstinence*, or the decision to refrain from sexual activity. Abstaining from activities that involve contact with a person's reproductive organs prevents STI transmission and also has many other benefits (**Figure 19.7**).

For some people, sexual abstinence can prove challenging in practice. Obstacles may include pressure from a dating partner or peer pressure, fear of rejection, influences from society and the media, alcohol or drug use, or a desire for closeness.

In Chapter 14, you learned about the skills you can use to commit to abstinence and stick to your decision. When you are practicing abstinence, be sure to discuss your decision with your dating partner. Talking about sexual abstinence might seem awkward, but it is good practice for communicating about sensitive topics in relationships.

Certain situations can make it difficult to practice abstinence. For example, maybe you are at an unsupervised party or around people who are using alcohol or drugs. These are high-risk situations that can challenge your decision to be abstinent. To avoid these situations, enforce your boundaries and leave situations that make you uncomfortable.

Refusal skills are a key part of practicing abstinence. If someone asks you to engage in some type of sexual activity, you need to learn and practice how to say *no*. For example, if someone pressures you to have sex, you could say, "No, I don't want to risk getting an STI" or "I'm not ready for that." Sometimes you may need to say *no* several different ways or physically leave a situation. Someone who cares about you will always respect your decision to practice abstinence. Talking with a trusted adult can help you think of ways to stick to your decision.

Condoms

Although abstinence is the only 100-percent effective method for preventing STIs, a correctly used condom can also reduce the chances of contracting some STIs. A **condom** is a birth control device that acts as a barrier against pathogens during sexual activity.

condom device that acts as a barrier against pathogens during sexual activity; also acts as a barrier method of contraception

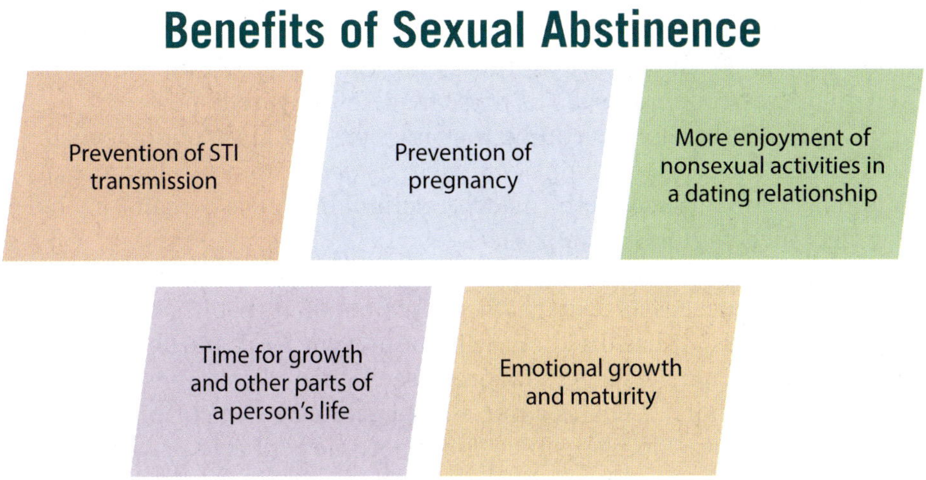

Benefits of Sexual Abstinence

- Prevention of STI transmission
- Prevention of pregnancy
- More enjoyment of nonsexual activities in a dating relationship
- Time for growth and other parts of a person's life
- Emotional growth and maturity

Figure 19.7 There are many benefits of practicing sexual abstinence.

Health in the Media

Conversations About Sexual Activity

Think about the last book you read or the last movie or video you watched. Was there a romantic couple in the story? If so, how did they interact? Did they ever talk about protecting themselves from STIs? Most popular books, movies, videos, and shows are created to entertain audiences, not to educate them. As a result, media portrayals of romantic couples are rarely accurate. In the media, romantic partners rarely communicate consent about their relationship, sexual activity, and STIs.

Media representations give the impression that adults in a romantic relationship do not even discuss *if* they should have sex, not to mention how they will protect themselves from STIs. In reality, partners in a healthy, romantic relationship do discuss these topics. They regularly communicate about consent, what they expect within the relationship, and the role intimacy and sexual activity will play in their relationship. This includes discussing STI testing and methods of preventing STI transmission.

Talking about STIs and your sexual decisions now is helpful practice. To get more comfortable with these topics, you could ask a trusted adult questions about STIs and the importance of prevention. You could have a talk with your dating partner about your commitment to sexual abstinence. Having these conversations will help you learn skills for communicating about these topics in the future.

Practice Your Skills

Analyze Influences

Reflect on how popular books, movies, videos, and shows portray adult relationships and sexual activity. Choose several different examples of romantic relationships in the media. For each portrayal, describe how people would behave in a healthy, realistic relationship. Make a poster or infographic summarizing these facts and fictions and share with your class. Be prepared to tell your classmates how teens can resist the influence of unrealistic portrayals on their relationships and decisions.

external condom device that fits over an erect penis; helps prevent many STIs and can reduce the chance of pregnancy occurring during sexual intercourse

internal condom device that fits inside the vagina or rectum; is less effective than an external condom at preventing some STIs; also reduces the chance of pregnancy occurring during sexual intercourse

dental dam condom-like sheet that fits between one person's mouth and another's reproductive organs; helps prevent the transmission of STIs

Condoms may be external or internal. An **external condom** fits over an erect penis. An **internal condom** fits inside the vagina or rectum. External and internal condoms should *not* be used together. Using them together reduces their effectiveness in preventing STIs. A condom-like **dental dam** can also help prevent STI transmission by forming a barrier between the mouth and a person's reproductive organs.

A condom's material can influence effectiveness. Most condoms are made of latex, which is effective at reducing the risk of STI transmission. Some nonlatex condoms, such as those made of polyurethane or polyisoprene, also help prevent the transmission of STIs. Condoms made of natural materials (for example, *lambskin condoms*) do not help prevent STIs. This is because condoms made of natural materials contain tiny holes through which pathogens can pass.

A condom can be used only once. A new condom must be used each time a person engages in sexual activity. Any condom that has expired, has holes or tears, or has dried out will not prevent STIs and should be discarded. In fact, a person should only use unexpired condoms acquired from a reliable source, such as a nurse at a healthcare clinic. Condoms may be damaged if stored in places they could become very cold or hot (for example, in a car) or be crushed (for example, in a wallet).

Condoms are not as effective as abstinence at preventing STIs (**Figure 19.8**). For example, even if a condom or dental dam is used,

Effectiveness of Methods for Preventing STIs	
Method	**Effectiveness Against STIs**
Abstinence	The only 100-percent effective method of preventing STIs
External condom	Effective against many STIs; less effective against STIs spread through skin-to-skin contact (HPV, genital herpes, and syphilis)
Internal condom	Effective against many STIs; less effective than the external condom and against STIs spread through skin-to-skin contact (HPV, genital herpes, and syphilis)
Dental dam	Effective against many STIs

Figure 19.8 The only methods of pregnancy prevention that help prevent STI transmission are abstinence and using condoms or dental dams. Other methods of pregnancy prevention, such as withdrawal, birth control pills, sterilization, and intrauterine devices (IUDs), do not reduce the risk of contracting an STI. ***Which method of preventing STIs is 100 percent effective?***

STIs can still spread through contact with sores and areas not covered. For a condom to protect against STIs effectively, a person must apply it correctly, use it for the whole duration of sexual activity, and remove it correctly. The condom must fit well and be undamaged. You will learn more about internal and external condoms, including how to apply and remove them, in Chapter 24.

Treating STIs

Treatment is effective for many STIs, especially in the early stages. Even if an infection is not curable, treatment reduces the chance it will spread to other people. Effective treatment of STIs requires three critical components:

1. Treatment from a healthcare provider must begin as soon as possible, and the person with the STI must take all medications exactly as prescribed.
2. All sexual partners of the person must be notified, tested, and treated. Otherwise, **reinfection**, or a recurrence of the STI, can occur.
3. A person with an STI must abstain from sexual activity until a doctor determines the disease is cured and will not spread.

reinfection recurrence of a communicable disease

People who think they might have an STI should see a medical professional as soon as possible. For teens, it can seem embarrassing to talk about STIs, but not getting help can have serious consequences. If you think you have an STI, talking with a trusted adult can help you get the care you need. You might also be able to make a doctor's appointment, visit a public health clinic offering free or reduced-price services, or access testing online. In all 50 states, minors can consent to STI services, including testing and treatment.

Before visiting the doctor or clinic, write a list of symptoms and questions. Be prepared to ask if you want your results kept confidential and know that your doctor might ask you to contact any sexual partners to let them know they should be tested for STIs. Go to an emergency room or urgent care clinic if you have severe pain, abdominal pain, a fever, or skin rashes and sores. You should also seek immediate care if you feel weak or faint or have been sexually assaulted.

Treatment for STIs	
STI	**Treatment**
Chlamydia	Prescribed antibiotics
Gonorrhea	Prescribed antibiotics
Pelvic inflammatory disease (PID)	Prescribed antibiotics; in severe cases, surgery
Syphilis	Prescribed antibiotics or penicillin injection
Trichomoniasis	Prescribed antibiotics
Genital herpes	No cure; antiviral medications can control outbreaks and symptoms
Human papillomavirus (HPV)	No cure; antiviral medications can control symptoms

Figure 19.9 Many STIs are easily treated, especially in their early stages. Some can be cured, but others cannot. ***What is the term for the recurrence of an STI?***

Once an STI is diagnosed, treatment can begin (**Figure 19.9**). For example, bacterial STIs are treatable, even curable, with antibiotics prescribed by a doctor. Exposure to the STI again, however, will result in another infection. Viral infections cannot be treated or cured with antibiotics, but they can be controlled with antiviral medications. Antiviral medications do not cure the infection. They simply control the virus, sometimes greatly reducing the severity and frequency of symptoms.

When handling STI diagnosis and treatment, you may need additional emotional support. Counseling services, helplines, and support groups can help meet this need. Friends and family members can also be a source of support. Getting help when necessary is a good way to promote overall health and well-being.

Lesson 19.2 Review

Know and Understand

1. Explain why sexual abstinence is more effective at preventing STIs than using a condom.
2. How does a condom's material impact its effectiveness at preventing STIs?
3. What are the three critical components of effective treatment for STIs?
4. How is treatment for a viral STI different from treatment for a bacterial STI?

Think Critically

5. With a partner, discuss how you know if someone respects your decisions about sexual activity and STI prevention. Why does someone have to respect these decisions to care about you?
6. With a partner, consider the pros and cons of talking with a trusted adult to get STI treatment or getting treatment on your own.

REAL WORLD Health Skills

Make Decisions After reading this lesson, list 10 reasons you might make the decision to remain sexually abstinent. On the back of that sheet, list 10 strategies you could use to stick to your decision to remain abstinent while dating. Make this list specific to your likes, interests, and the support systems in your life. Then, write a case study in which you have to make the decision to remain abstinent and use your strategies. Show you would use the decision-making process to remain abstinent and protect yourself from STIs.

HIV/AIDS

Essential Question?

How does HIV/AIDS develop?

Lesson 19.3

Learning Outcomes

After studying this lesson, you will be able to

- differentiate between HIV and AIDS;
- explain how HIV is transmitted;
- list signs and symptoms of HIV/AIDS;
- explain how HIV/AIDS is diagnosed; and
- describe treatment methods for HIV/AIDS.

Key Terms

acquired immunodeficiency syndrome (AIDS)
antiretroviral therapy (ART)
human immunodeficiency virus (HIV)
long-term non-progressors
opportunistic infections
post-exposure prophylaxis (PEP)
pre-exposure prophylaxis (PrEP)
viral load

Warm-Up Activity

Staying HIV Free

Set Goals Many factors can distract you from your goals and ideals. This is why an important part of setting goals is identifying situations or factors you might have to avoid to reach those goals. What behaviors, situations, or pressures might prevent a person from remaining HIV free? What strategies could a person use to avoid dangers? Organize your answers in a table like the one shown.

Behaviors, situations, or pressures to avoid	Strategies to help avoid them

Around the world, more than 37 million people are living with HIV/AIDS. Since this epidemic began, the WHO estimates 35 million people have died from AIDS-related causes. HIV/AIDS does not discriminate and knows no national boundaries. It affects people of all sexes, ages, races, nationalities, sexual orientations, gender identities, and ethnic origins. HIV can spread through blood, semen, vaginal secretions, and breast milk. Because of this, sexual activity and other activities that exchange these bodily fluids can transmit HIV. HIV transmission is most common among people ages 13–34. According to the CDC, one in seven people with HIV do not know they have it.

What Are HIV and AIDS?

It is important to distinguish between HIV and AIDS. Where HIV refers to a virus, AIDS refers to a health condition caused by the virus (**Figure 19.10**). The **human immunodeficiency virus (HIV)** is a bloodborne virus that infects and kills the body's immune cells, weakening the body's defense against infections.

human immunodeficiency virus (HIV) bloodborne virus that infects and kills the body's cells, weakening the immune system

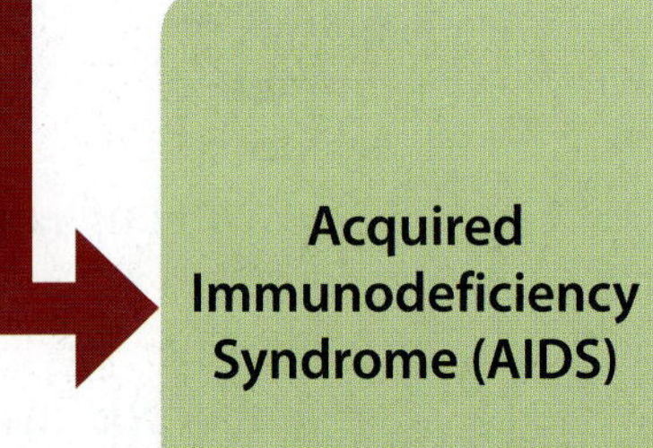

Figure 19.10 HIV is a virus. Sometimes, this virus can develop into a health condition called AIDS.

Like other viruses, HIV cannot grow and reproduce by itself. To survive, HIV uses the resources inside cells of the immune system. HIV targets immune cells called *CD4 cells*, including *T-helper cells*, which activate and coordinate the immune system. CD4 cells reside in the lymph nodes and travel throughout the body in the bloodstream and other bodily fluids.

When HIV comes into the body, it attaches to CD4 cells and enters them. HIV moves into the *nucleus*, or the cell's control center. From there, HIV directs the cell to make copies of the virus. This can kill the cell, and the new viruses attack and kill more CD4 cells.

Because the immune system remains healthy for a while, people may not notice the early stages of an HIV infection. As the number of viruses increases and as more CD4 cells die, however, the immune system will become weak.

acquired immunodeficiency syndrome (AIDS) health condition in which the body can no longer fight infections and disease; caused by the progression of HIV

opportunistic infections diseases that develop by taking advantage of a weakened immune system

If left untreated, HIV infection can progress into a serious health condition in which the body can no longer effectively fight infections and diseases. This health condition is called **acquired immunodeficiency syndrome (AIDS)** and can lead to severe **opportunistic infections**, or diseases that take advantage of a weakened immune system. In people living with AIDS, these opportunistic infections can result in early death. Fortunately, treatment can slow the progression of HIV into AIDS and help people with AIDS live longer. Many people who have HIV/AIDS can live long, healthy lives if they receive regular treatment. Treatment also greatly reduces the risk for transmitting HIV.

Signs and Symptoms of HIV/AIDS

The signs and symptoms of HIV and AIDS depend on how far HIV has progressed and whether it has developed into AIDS. Without treatment, HIV progresses through three stages, the last of which is AIDS.

Stage 1: Acute HIV Infection

The first signs and symptoms of HIV typically develop two to four weeks after a person contracts the virus. Even though there is a large amount of the virus in the blood during this stage, symptoms are usually minor and may not be recognized. Some people may not experience them at all. Early symptoms resemble a flu-like illness with fatigue and swollen, painful lymph nodes. Because of this, many people in this stage do not know they have HIV at all.

Stage 2: Latency

During the second stage of HIV, a person may experience no symptoms at all, and levels of HIV in the blood are low. This stage can last 10 or more years, though some people may progress through the stage more quickly. Some people, called **long-term non-progressors**, pass through this stage very slowly.

long-term non-progressors people living with HIV who progress very slowly through the latency stage of HIV

Treatment can lengthen this stage, sometimes by several decades or indefinitely. At the end of this stage, immunity begins to slowly decrease, leading to AIDS.

Stage 3: Acquired Immunodeficiency Syndrome (AIDS)

The last stage of HIV is AIDS. In AIDS, the immune system is severely damaged and cannot fight off infections that would not normally harm the body. To measure this decline in immunity, blood tests track numbers of CD4 cells.

In AIDS, unusual or normally harmless microorganisms continuously assault the body, causing opportunistic infections. These infections take advantage of the body's weakened immune system and can result in death (**Figure 19.11**).

Other signs and symptoms of AIDS include severe weight loss, diarrhea, fever and chills, and nausea.

HIV damages the immune system, making it vulnerable to opportunistic infections such as

- *pneumocystis pneumonia*, an infection of the lungs that the immune system can usually combat
- yeast infections in the mouth (called *thrush*), throat, lungs, and vagina
- *tuberculosis*, a bacterial lung infection
- infections of the intestines, skin, eyes, and nervous system
- brain infections and *meningitis* (infection of the membranes around the brain and spinal cord)
- blood vessel tumors (*Kaposi's sarcoma*)

Figure 19.11 With AIDS, the body does not have the necessary defenses to fight opportunistic infections.

HIV Transmission

There are many misconceptions about what does and does not transmit HIV. HIV is a bloodborne virus. This means it is found in

- blood;
- semen and pre-seminal fluids;
- vaginal secretions; and
- breast milk.

For HIV to spread, it must come in contact with a mucous membrane (such as those found in the penis, vagina, rectum, and mouth), damaged skin or tissue, or a person's bloodstream. Healthy, intact skin provides an effective barrier against HIV, though HIV can spread through open sores on the skin, in the mouth, or on the genitals. At one time, blood transfusions sometimes transmitted HIV. In the US, however, the blood supply is screened for HIV, so transfusions no longer pose a serious threat (**Figure 19.12**).

Certain factors increase the risk for HIV transmission. For example, people who inject medications or drugs are more likely to share needles and potentially become exposed to HIV.

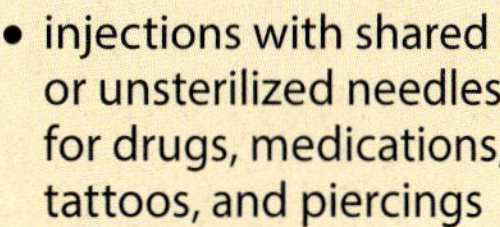

HIV can be transmitted by

- injections with shared or unsterilized needles for drugs, medications, tattoos, and piercings
- sexual activity
- from parent to baby during childbirth or breastfeeding
- exposure of open sores on skin, in the mouth, or on genitals to contaminated blood

HIV *cannot* be transmitted by

- kissing or hugging
- mosquitos
- sharing food or drinks
- shaking hands
- coughing or sneezing
- using the same toilet seat
- spit, sweat, tears, urine, or feces

Figure 19.12 HIV is only found in blood, semen and pre-seminal fluids, vaginal secretions, and breast milk.

Local and Global Health

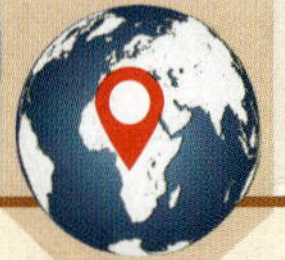

Reducing HIV Transmission in Africa

While HIV transmission is on the decline in the US and other high-income countries, transmission rates are still high in many low-income regions, especially Africa. The WHO reports Africa is home to 25 percent of the world's people living with HIV and about two-thirds of people newly diagnosed with HIV. Most of these people live in eastern and southern Africa. The majority of adults living with HIV in eastern and southern Africa are female.

The US President's Emergency Plan for AIDS Relief (PEPFAR) instituted the DREAMS initiative in 2015. The goal of DREAMS is to help girls in eastern and southern Africa develop into *determined*, *resilient*, *empowered*, *AIDS-free*, *mentored*, and *safe* women.

DREAMS has four core interventions in 15 sub-Saharan African countries that account for the majority of new HIV diagnoses. These interventions address structural issues in the region that drive HIV transmissions in girls and young women. The four core interventions are (1) empower girls and young women, (2) reduce the risk of sexual partners, (3) strengthen families, and (4) mobilize communities for change. DREAMS hopes to reduce HIV transmissions by 40 percent in these regions. Its approach allows it to address the factors that lead to unsafe behavior and social situations with a high risk of HIV transmission. By involving the whole community, DREAMS also engages men and boys in addressing social behaviors that increase the risk of HIV transmission for girls and young women.

The DREAMS program has led to a 25-percent reduction in new diagnoses among girls and young women ages 15–25.

Practice Your Skills

Advocate for Health

The DREAMS program's core interventions focus on structural and community issues that lead to widespread HIV transmission. With a partner, discuss why this approach works better than an approach singularly focused on disease prevention. Using reliable resources, research DREAMS' core interventions and consider how they could be adapted for at-risk communities near you. Which programs would work well? How could some of the ideas be implemented in your area? Create a presentation you could give to a local health group advocating for the implementation of your HIV-prevention ideas.

As you know, sexual activity with just one partner who has an STI can lead to transmission. Therefore, having different sexual partners significantly increases the chance of contracting HIV and other STIs.

Having other STIs also increases the risk of HIV transmission. Intact, healthy skin is a barrier against HIV, but syphilis sores break that barrier. So does the inflammation associated with genital herpes, chlamydia, gonorrhea, trichomoniasis, and genital warts. A person with syphilis is five times more likely to contract HIV than a person without syphilis. The reverse is also true: a person who has HIV and other STIs more easily transmits STIs to sexual partners.

Testing and Diagnosis

HIV testing is critical for personal and community health. It can lead to early diagnosis for someone with HIV and a better chance of long-term health with treatment. It is also the key to controlling HIV transmission within society. In fact, about 40 percent of new HIV transmissions come from people who do not know they have HIV. People who are sexually active should be tested every year and every time they switch sexual partners.

Testing for HIV

Testing for HIV involves a blood test. A doctor will examine a blood sample for the presence of antibodies the body produces in response to HIV. Weeks or months may pass before a person's body develops antibodies following exposure to HIV. Therefore, if people test negative for HIV, but think they were exposed within the past three months, they should repeat the test after three more months have passed. Test results usually become available in a few days.

HIV testing can take place in a doctor's office, hospital, or other healthcare facility. Some community organizations also offer HIV testing. In the US, people can also use a home test approved by the Food and Drug Administration (FDA) to detect HIV. If this test is positive, people should see a healthcare provider for a confirming test.

Confidentiality of Test Results

The *Health Insurance Portability and Accountability Act (HIPAA)* is a federal law that requires confidentiality for medical records, including HIV test results. If a person tests positive for HIV, healthcare providers must report this to the state so the state can track and study the number of HIV cases. Because of HIPAA, these results must contain no identifying personal information and protect the identity of the individual.

It is important that someone who tests positive for HIV notifies any sexual partners. In fact, some cities and states have partner-notification laws that require people with HIV or their doctors to notify sexual or needle-sharing partners.

Minors have some rights pertaining to HIV testing and results. All 50 states in the US allow minors to give consent to receive STI testing and treatment. Thirty-two states clearly include HIV testing in this definition. In some states, there are some specific requirements regarding consent and confidentiality.

It is illegal to discriminate against someone because of the person's HIV status (**Figure 19.13**). Anti-discrimination laws also protect the families of people living with HIV.

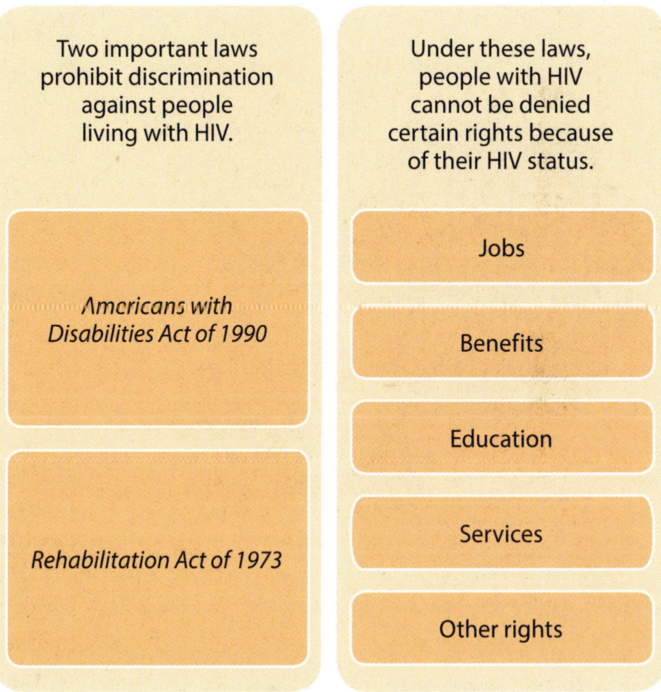

Figure 19.13 The federal government has passed laws to protect the rights of people living with HIV and their families from discrimination. ***Which federal law requires confidentiality for medical records, including HIV test results?***

Treatment for HIV/AIDS

In the 1980s, there was no effective treatment for people living with HIV/AIDS. For several years, treatment focused only on controlling opportunistic infections, and people began to think HIV/AIDS was an untreatable, incurable, fatal disease. Today, this view of HIV/AIDS is outdated and inaccurate. Advances in treatment have significantly improved the health and quality of life for people living with HIV.

antiretroviral therapy (ART) treatment for HIV/AIDS that includes a mixture of three medications, each of which interferes with the reproduction of HIV inside the body

viral load amount of HIV in the blood

The medical treatment for people living with HIV is **antiretroviral therapy (ART)**, which consists of a combination of medications that interfere with the reproduction of HIV. The aim of ART is to reduce a person's **viral load**, or the amount of HIV in the blood. This can help stabilize the number of CD4 cells in a person's body and strengthen the immune system.

People should start ART as soon as possible after an HIV diagnosis. Today, ART can reduce a person's viral load to the point of being undetectable, or so low lab tests cannot measure it. Studies also suggest that people using ART regularly do not transmit HIV. ART has become highly effective against HIV, and some people taking ART never develop AIDS.

HIV Prevention

There are steps you can take to help prevent the transmission of HIV. Some of these steps involve managing activities with a risk of HIV transmission. Certain medications can also reduce a person's risk of contracting HIV.

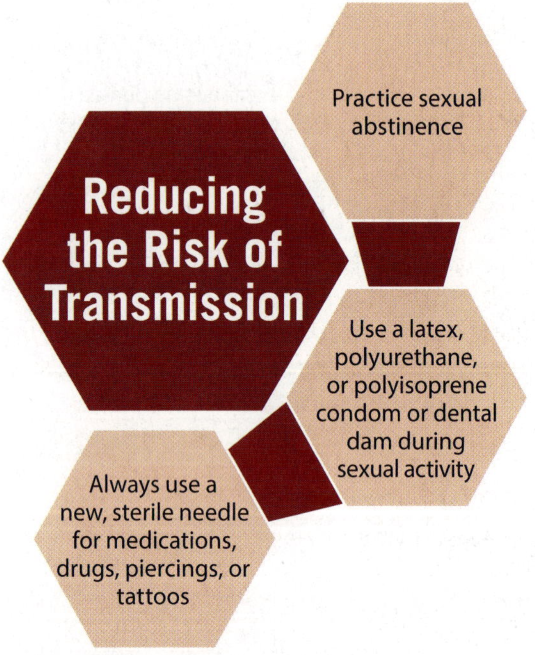

Figure 19.14 Knowing that HIV is most commonly transmitted through sexual activity and sharing needles, you can take steps to protect yourself from this virus.

Precautions to Reduce the Risk of Transmission

Understanding the activities that can cause transmission is the best way to avoid contracting HIV (**Figure 19.14**). These include any activities that involve contact with a person's blood, semen or pre-seminal fluids, vaginal secretions, or breast milk. In the US, HIV is most commonly spread through sexual activity and needle sharing.

Since HIV can spread through sexual activity, methods of preventing other STIs also help prevent HIV. The only 100-percent effective method of preventing HIV transmission through sexual activity is sexual abstinence, the decision to refrain from sexual activity. Using a latex, polyurethane, or polyisoprene condom or dental dam also reduces the risk of HIV transmission.

HIV transmission can also occur if people share needles, such as those used for injections, piercings, or tattoos. If you take a medication you need to inject, never share needles with another person. Be sure to use a new, sterile needle for each injection. If you choose to get a piercing or tattoo, make sure the piercer or tattoo artist is licensed and uses a new, sterile needle and new ink for each customer.

Pre-Exposure Prophylaxis (PrEP)

pre-exposure prophylaxis (PrEP) combination of two medications in one pill taken daily to prevent HIV transmission

Pre-exposure prophylaxis (PrEP) is a course of ART that can protect a person from contracting HIV. PrEP comes as a single pill that contains two ART medications. It is a prescription medication and must be taken every day so its presence in the blood remains steady. Having enough of these ART medications in the blood stops HIV from taking hold and spreading in the body.

PrEP is intended for people who have tested negative for HIV, but have a high risk of contracting HIV. People taking PrEP should be tested for HIV every three months. If they test positive for HIV, they should see a doctor to begin appropriate ART.

PrEP, when taken properly, reduces a person's risk of contracting HIV from sexual activity by more than 90 percent. When combined with other prevention methods, PrEP reduces the risk to near-zero. PrEP also reduces the risk of contracting HIV from shared needles by more than 70 percent. If not taken every day, however, PrEP becomes much less effective. PrEP does not prevent other STIs.

Post-Exposure Prophylaxis (PEP)

Post-exposure prophylaxis (PEP) is a course of ART a person can take within 72 hours of potential exposure to HIV. PEP is intended only for emergency situations of potential exposure and is available in emergency rooms.

post-exposure prophylaxis (PEP) emergency course of ART that a person can take within 72 hours of potential exposure to HIV

There are two kinds of PEP: oPEP and nPEP. *Occupational post-exposure prophylaxis (oPEP)* is used by healthcare professionals after HIV exposure from a needle stick injury or contact with bodily fluids. People can use *nonoccupational post-exposure prophylaxis (nPEP)* after HIV exposure outside the workplace, such as through sexual activity, sexual assault, or shared needles. Both types of PEP reduce the risk of HIV transmission. People who use PEP take it twice daily for 28 days after exposure.

Lesson 19.3 Review

Know and Understand

1. Describe the difference between HIV and AIDS.
2. Why do many people in the first stage of HIV infection not know they have HIV?
3. Explain why opportunistic infections can lead to death in people living with AIDS.
4. Why does having another STI increase a person's risk of contracting HIV?
5. How does ART work to treat HIV/AIDS?
6. Which method of preventing HIV transmission through sexual activity is 100 percent effective?

Think Critically

7. Make a list of activities that involve exchanging the bodily fluids that carry HIV. What do these activities have in common? How do they transmit HIV?
8. What barriers do you think sometimes prevent people living with HIV from seeking treatment?
9. Why is it important for people living with HIV to notify their sexual or needle-sharing partners?
10. Why do you think some people living with HIV experience discrimination? Why is it important to have laws protecting people living with HIV?
11. In what situations would people benefit most from PrEP and PEP? Where in your community could you go to learn more about or receive PrEP or PEP?

REAL WORLD Health Skills

Communicate with Others Imagine that you have just tested positive for HIV. You also recently became involved in a new dating relationship with someone you really like. At what point do you share this personal information with your new dating partner? Working with another class member, take turns role-playing the conversation you would have with your new dating partner, using effective communication skills.

Chapter 19

Review and Assessment

Chapter Summary

Sexually transmitted infections (STIs) are infections spread from person to person during sexual activity. STIs can cause inflammation, damage to the reproductive organs, and infertility. If left untreated, STIs can also damage the brain, heart, liver, and other internal organs. Some cause cancer, and some are fatal. A pregnant person with an STI can transmit the infection to the baby during pregnancy, birth, or breastfeeding. Common STIs include chlamydia, gonorrhea, syphilis, trichomoniasis, herpes, and human papillomavirus (HPV).

The only 100-percent effective method for preventing STIs is sexual abstinence. Correctly used condoms and dental dams can also reduce the chances of contracting some STIs. Other methods of pregnancy prevention do not reduce the risk of contracting an STI.

Effective treatment of STIs requires three critical components. First, treatment from a healthcare provider must begin as soon as possible, and the person with the STI must take all medications exactly as prescribed. Second, all sexual partners must be notified, tested, and treated in order to prevent reinfection. Third, a person with an STI must abstain from sexual activity until a doctor determines the disease is cured and will not spread. Bacterial STIs are treatable, even curable, with antibiotics prescribed by a doctor. Viral infections cannot be treated or cured with antibiotics, but they can be controlled with antiviral medications.

The human immunodeficiency virus (HIV) is a bloodborne virus that infects and kills the body's immune cells, weakening the body's defense against infections. Without treatment, HIV progresses through three stages: acute HIV infection, latency, and a serious health condition called acquired immunodeficiency syndrome (AIDS). With AIDS, the body can no longer effectively fight infections and diseases.

HIV is found in bodily fluids, such as blood, semen and pre-seminal fluids, vaginal secretions, and breast milk. For HIV to spread, it must come in contact with a mucous membrane, damaged skin or tissue, or a person's bloodstream. This can happen through sexual activity, childbirth and breastfeeding, or exposure to contaminated blood through an open sore. HIV transmission can also occur if people share needles, such as those used for injections, piercings, or tattoos.

HIV testing can lead to early diagnosis for someone with HIV and a better chance of long-term health with treatment. It is also the key to controlling HIV transmission within society. The medical treatment for people living with HIV is antiretroviral therapy (ART), which consists of a combination of medications that interfere with the reproduction of HIV. Prevention of the transmission of HIV can involve managing activities with a risk of HIV transmission, taking certain medications, and practicing methods used to prevent other STIs.

Vocabulary Activity

Find a current news story (print or video) from the last six months that discusses rates of STI or HIV transmission. In a presentation to the class, summarize the article and discuss the accuracy of the facts presented. How well were you able to understand the story? What key terms from this chapter did the story use? What can a teen learn from this news story, and what questions may remain? Properly cite the news story.

acquired immunodeficiency syndrome (AIDS)
antiretroviral therapy (ART)
asymptomatic
cervical cancer
chlamydia
condom
dental dam
external condom
genital herpes
genital warts
gonorrhea
human immunodeficiency virus (HIV)
human papillomavirus (HPV)
internal condom
long-term non-progressors
opportunistic infections
oropharyngeal cancer
pelvic inflammatory disease (PID)
post-exposure prophylaxis (PEP)
pre-exposure prophylaxis (PrEP)
reinfection
sexually transmitted infections (STIs)
syphilis
trichomoniasis
viral load

Review and Recall

Review the information in this chapter by answering the following questions.

1. Which STI is also known as a *silent disease*?
   A. chlamydia
   B. syphilis
   C. gonorrhea
   D. herpes
2. Which STI is often treated with two kinds of antibiotics? Why?
3. What occurs during a herpes outbreak?
4. Which of the following STIs is caused by a protozoan?
   A. herpes
   B. gonorrhea
   C. HPV
   D. trichomoniasis
5. What is the most commonly reported STI in the United States?
6. Which STI is often called the *great imitator*?
7. Which type of STI is treatable, even curable, with antibiotics prescribed by a physician?
   A. viral
   B. bacterial
   C. antiviral
   D. retroviral
8. List three methods that are ineffective in preventing STIs.
9. What factors can increase the risk for HIV transmission?
10. When does AIDS develop?
11. What is meant by the term *long-term non-progressors*?
12. How often should sexually active people be tested for HIV?
13. HIV is found in which bodily fluid?
    A. saliva
    B. tears
    C. sweat
    D. blood

Standardized Test Prep

Math Practice

The following results are from a study of new STI diagnoses among people of different ages in the US. Review the results of this study and answer the questions that follow.

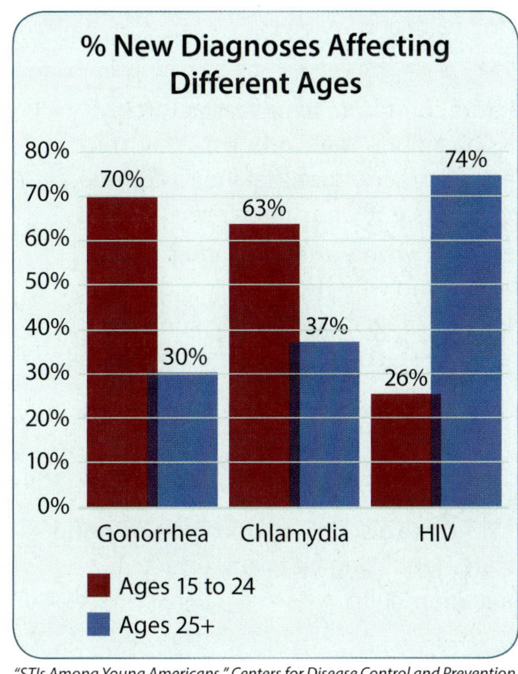

"STIs Among Young Americans." Centers for Disease Control and Prevention.

14. For which STIs were new diagnoses more common among people ages 15–24?
15. In this study, there were 2.9 million new diagnoses of chlamydia among all age groups. How many new diagnoses occurred among people ages 15–24?
    A. 1.1 million
    B. 4.6 million
    C. 1.8 million
    D. 2 million
16. In this study, there were 820,000 new diagnoses of gonorrhea and 47,500 new diagnoses of HIV among all age groups. Which STI showed the largest number of new diagnoses among people ages 15–24?

Chapter 19 Skills Assessment

Critical Thinking Skills

Answer the following questions to assess your knowledge of what you learned in this chapter.

1. What are the possible advantages and disadvantages of point-of-care testing (POCT)? What problems might occur with using POCT at home?
2. Compare and contrast the two kinds of herpes simplex virus (HSV).
3. On which STI do you think research efforts should focus most? Why?
4. Compare and contrast two STIs discussed in this chapter. Include information on signs, symptoms, diagnosis, and treatment.
5. Explain how alcohol and drug use can increase a person's risk for contracting an STI.
6. What are some reasons teens may avoid getting the help they need in preventing and treating STIs? What can be done to ensure teens have access to the information and help they need regarding STIs?
7. With a partner, discuss how culture might affect the likelihood of contracting an STI.
8. Construct a plan to help a young person avoid contracting HIV. Begin with a clearly stated goal and include at least four steps toward meeting that goal. Be sure to consider ways people can and cannot contract HIV, and what activities might put someone at risk for infection.
9. Analyze how having other STIs can increase the risk of HIV transmission.
10. What are the laws in your state regarding consent, confidentiality, and discrimination of people with STIs? Do you think these laws are adequate? Why or why not?
11. With a partner, discuss as many myths about STIs as you can think of. Then discuss why those myths are not true and how you can promote better awareness of how to find accurate information about STIs.
12. With a partner, discuss how living with an STI might affect a person's daily life.
13. What is one thing you learned about STIs from this chapter that surprised you? How can you help make sure others are aware of this information?

Health and Wellness Skills

Complete the following activities to assess your skills related to health and wellness.

14. **Analyze Influences.** Think about your environment and community. Then, consider how your culture, behavior, attitude about sexuality, family, physical environment, technology, and the media might influence your STI status and ability to seek testing and treatment now and in the future. Consider how each influence might have a positive or negative impact and identify at least three ways to manage these influences to protect your health.
15. **Access Information.** Review what you have learned about HIV and AIDS and then use valid and reliable resources to research the populations most affected in the US and around the world. Does HIV affect some populations more than others? What factors contribute to increased rates of transmission among some groups? What steps are countries and organizations taking to address these needs and reduce HIV transmission?
16. **Communicate with Others.** Imagine that you have a friend who has been in a dating relationship for several years. You know your friend recently started being more sexually active and have been encouraging your friend to be careful about not getting an STI. Your friend shrugs and says, "We aren't doing anything that could get us pregnant, so it's fine. I won't get an STI." Write a script in which you respond to this statement using facts and effective communication skills.

17. **Make Decisions.** Think about how you want to live when you are 25 years old. Where do you want to live? What activities do you want to do? Would you like to have a romantic partner or children? What job or career will you have, and what will you have done to get there? What achievements will you have made? Now, consider how contracting an incurable STI would influence this imagined life. Reflect on how the decisions you make now could affect your future.
18. **Set Goals.** Pat and Chris have been dating for six months. Pat feels ready to have sex, but Chris does not feel the timing is right. Chris worries that having sex now could compromise some of their goals for the future. Write two SMART goals that represent Pat's and Chris's goals for the future. Then, write a case study in which Pat and Chris defend these goals and pursue them effectively.
19. **Practice Health-Enhancing Behaviors.** Create a character that interests you and describe the character's appearance, sex, relationships, interests, gender identity, and sexual orientation. Then, construct a plan to help this character avoid contracting an STI or HIV. The plan should have a clearly stated goal, at least four steps toward meeting the goal, and ways of evaluating progress. The plan should consider ways people can and cannot contract STIs and HIV and activities that might put someone at risk for infection.
20. **Advocate for Health.** Now that you know about common STIs and HIV, create an infographic or video that addresses the dangers of sexual activity and other behaviors that transmit STIs and HIV. In your infographic or video, offer positive alternatives to risky behaviors to influence other teens in healthy ways. Your infographic or video should promote sexual abstinence and be inclusive of people with different gender identities and sexual orientations. Keep in your mind your target audience—other teens—as you create your infographic or video. Submit your infographic or video to your teacher and then share with the class.

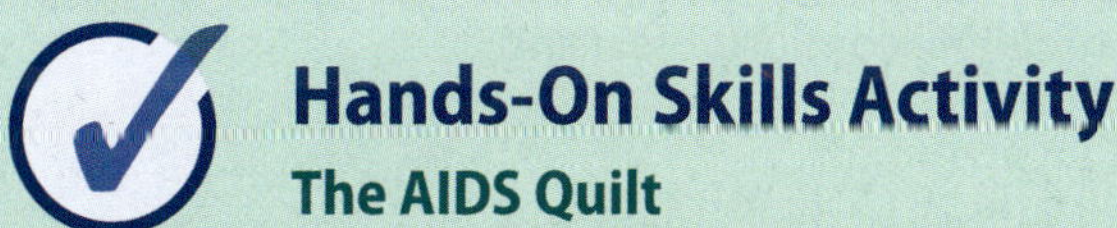

The AIDS quilt was started in San Francisco, California, during June of 1987. The purpose of the quilt is to commemorate the lives of people who died of AIDS. Each panel of the quilt is 3 feet wide and 6 feet tall, the size of a coffin. Each panel is decorated with the date of birth, date of death, photos, and various objects that best represent the person who died of AIDS. In this activity, you and your classmates will each research the AIDS quilt that started in San Francisco and recreate a panel of your choice. For this activity, you will need one sheet of poster board, photos and objects that represent the original quilt, and tape.

Steps for This Activity

1. **Access Information.** Visit the AIDS quilt website and view the panels of at least three people.
2. Create a poster that represents one of the people from the quilt. On your poster, include the person's date of birth and any photos or objects that highlight the person's most important relationships, activities, or experiences. Once everyone in your class has finished, tape your posters together to make one "poster quilt."
3. As a class, reflect on the following questions:
    - What new facts did you learn as you made your poster?
    - Approximately 50 people die each day from complications due to AIDS. What kind of impact do you think this has on society?
    - If your life ended right now, what goals and aspirations of yours would remain unfulfilled?
4. **Comprehend Concepts.** Write a paragraph about your thoughts and feelings after viewing these panels. Does anything about these panels surprise you? Why or why not? How do these panels influence your perception of HIV and AIDS?

Chapter 20

Noncommunicable Diseases

Look for the skills icon throughout this chapter for opportunities to practice your health skills.

Check Your Health and Wellness Skills

In this chapter, you will learn skills for preventing noncommunicable diseases. To understand the skills you currently use, take the following inventory of your behaviors. Indicate how well you think you use each skill. Use a scale of 1–5, *1* meaning you do not use the skill and *5* meaning you feel completely comfortable using it.

Skill	How Well Do You Use Each Skill?
I have talked with my doctor about my family history of disease.	
I know where I'd go for support if I got a scary diagnosis.	
I get at least 60 minutes of physical activity each day.	
I stay away from secondhand smoke as much as possible.	
I use healthy stress-management strategies like relaxation techniques.	
When someone offers me alcohol, I say *no*.	
I eat a diet rich in fruits and vegetables.	
I examine my skin regularly to check for changes.	
I avoid foods with lots of added sugars.	
I participate in weight-bearing activities like walking and jogging.	
	Total:

Add up your responses to each statement. The higher your score, the more comfortable you feel preventing noncommunicable diseases. Which skill do you think is most important for you? Which skill is the most challenging for you? Which skill would you most like to improve? In this chapter, you will learn how to perform these skills better and more often.

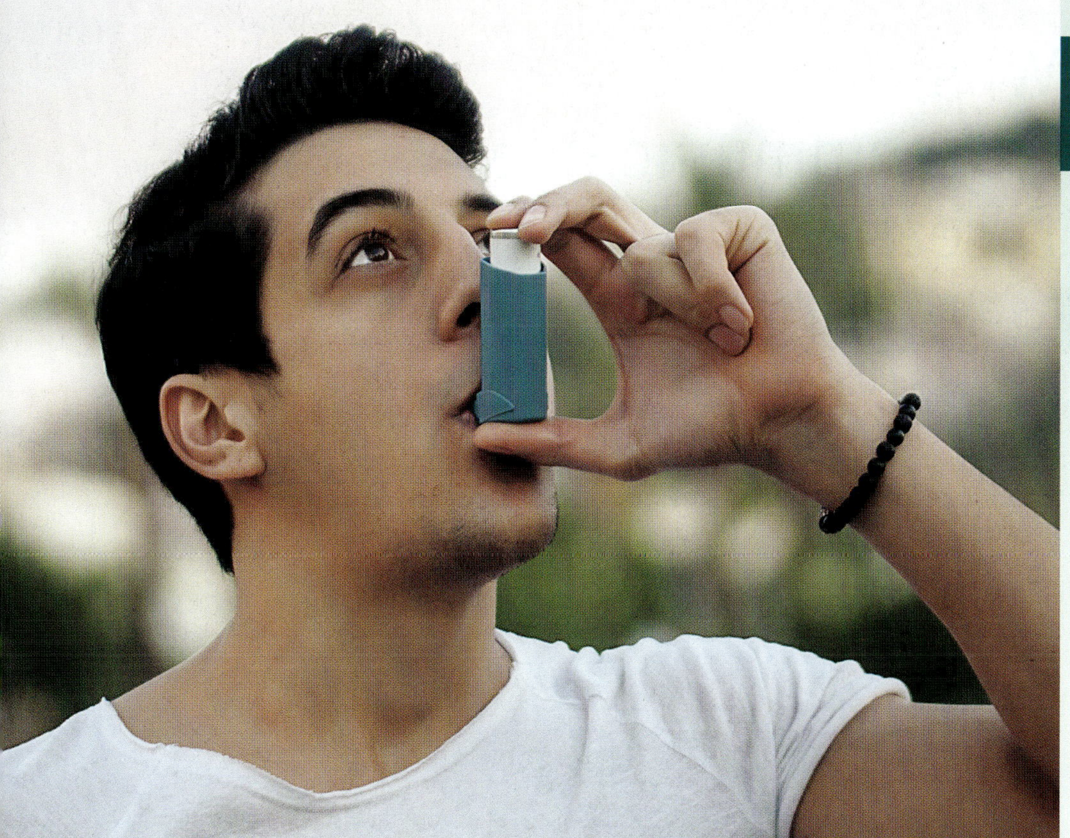

Mehmet Hilmi Barcin/iStock / Getty Images Plus/Getty Images

Reading and Notetaking

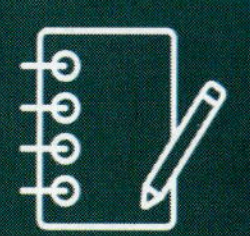

Arrange a study session to read this chapter aloud with a classmate. Take turns reading each lesson. Stop at the end of each lesson and identify its main points. Take detailed notes about your study session to share with the class.

Lesson	Main Points

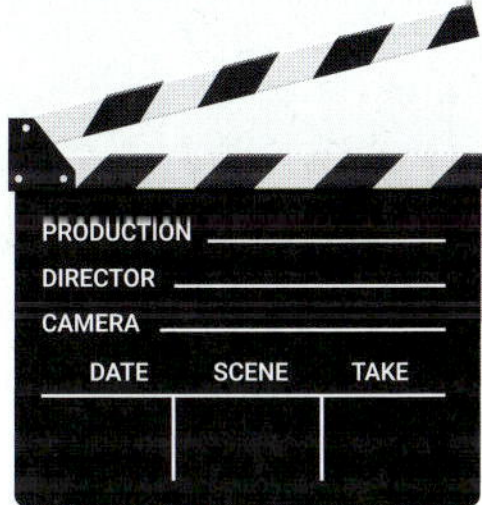

Setting the Scene

Understanding Risk

Before going back to school, you see a doctor for your annual physical exam. This doctor is new to you, and during your exam, the doctor asks if your close family members have had diabetes, heart disease, or cancer. As far as you know, people in your family do not have these diseases. Hopeful, you ask your doctor if that means you also will not have these diseases. You are surprised to hear it is still possible to develop these diseases, even though none of your family members has them.

Your doctor starts to talk about your health habits, like diet and physical activity. The doctor recommends getting more physical activity and eating more fruits and vegetables. You wonder how these behaviors relate to your risk for certain diseases.

Thinking Critically

1. If none of your close relatives has these diseases, but you are still at risk, what other factors might lead to these diseases?
2. If your answer was different and your close family members did have these diseases, would that mean you will develop these diseases in the future? Why or why not?

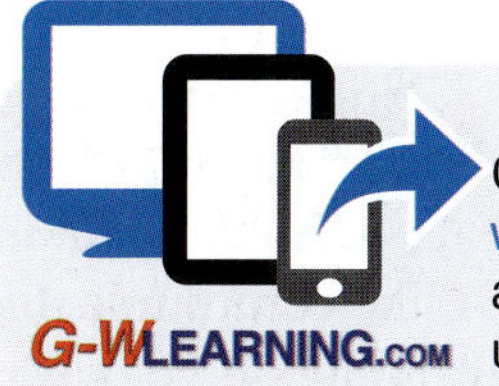

Click on the activity icon or visit www.g-wlearning.com/health/4095 to access online vocabulary activities using key terms from the chapter.

Lesson

20.1

What Are Noncommunicable Diseases?

Essential Question

What factors lead to the development of a noncommunicable disease?

Learning Outcomes

After studying this lesson, you will be able to

- contrast communicable and noncommunicable diseases;
- explain how noncommunicable diseases develop;
- analyze the causes of noncommunicable diseases;
- describe how noncommunicable diseases progress; and
- discuss how doctors diagnose and plan treatment for noncommunicable diseases.

Key Terms

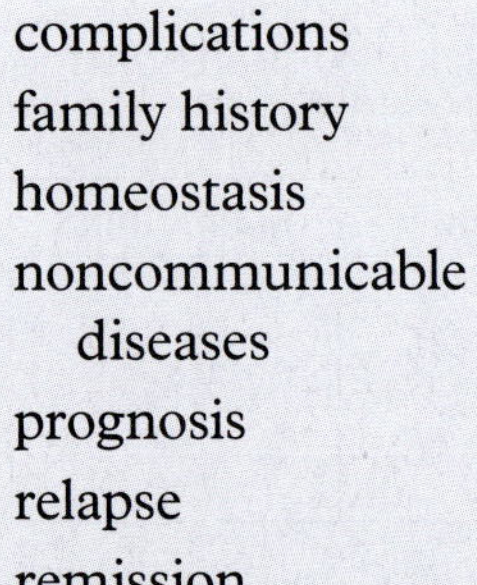

complications
family history
homeostasis
noncommunicable diseases
prognosis
relapse
remission

Warm-Up Activity

What Does It Mean to Be Noncommunicable?

Comprehend Concepts Think about the diseases in your family. Have any of your family members had heart disease, cancer, diabetes, arthritis, dementia, or asthma? Think about your family member's experience. Could you be around this family member without getting sick too? How was this disease different from having the common cold or flu? Discuss these questions with a partner and then share your thoughts with the class. As a class, identify the similarities and differences between communicable and noncommunicable diseases.

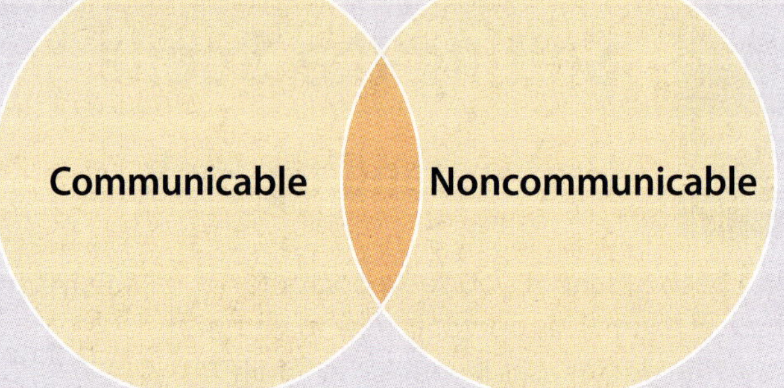

What do you know about cardiovascular diseases and cancer? about diabetes? Maybe these diseases seem distant to you, or maybe you or a family member has one of these diseases. In this lesson, you will learn about what noncommunicable diseases are. You will discover how they are different from communicable diseases.

Noncommunicable diseases are diseases that develop due to genes, diet, behaviors, and other factors. These diseases occur when the body's state of **homeostasis**, or internal balance, is disrupted (**Figure 20.1**). Unlike communicable diseases, noncommunicable diseases do not spread through contact with living organisms or objects. Your choices impact your chances of getting some of these diseases.

noncommunicable diseases health conditions that develop over time as a result of genes, environment, and behaviors; do not spread between living organisms and objects

homeostasis body's internal, steady state of balance; the body maintains homeostasis by regulating body temperature, the amount of sugar in the blood, blood pressure, and oxygen level in tissues

What Causes Noncommunicable Diseases?

Cardiovascular disease, cancer, and diabetes are leading causes of death around the world. In fact, of the approximately 2.8 million deaths in the United States each year, cardiovascular disease and cancer cause nearly one-half. A person's likelihood of developing cardiovascular disease or cancer is not written in stone. Behaviors, habits, diet, and preventive healthcare significantly affect a person's chance of developing these diseases.

The causes of noncommunicable diseases are complex. Genetics have a strong influence on some diseases. Environment and behavior strongly influence others. Though noncommunicable diseases can develop during adolescence, most noncommunicable diseases develop from interactions among these different risk factors over time.

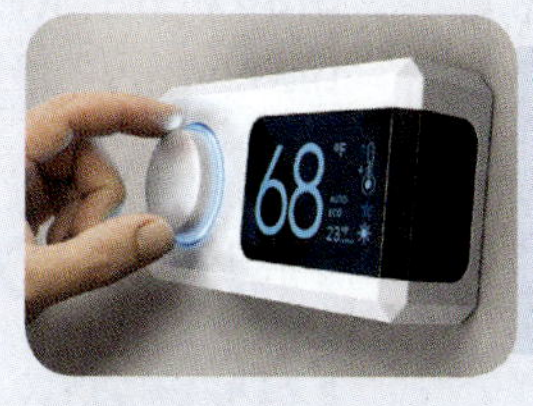

Homeostasis is your body's internal balance. Think of homeostasis like the way your home maintains temperature.

- When your home is in a state of homeostasis, the thermostat signals the furnace to turn on when the home is too cold. When your home is at the correct temperature, the thermostat will signal the furnace to turn off again.
- If the furnace does not turn on during a cold winter, however, the house would become very cold and could cause pipes to freeze and burst. In this situation, your house would have departed from its homeostasis.

Olivier Le Moal/Shutterstock.com

Figure 20.1 When homeostasis is disrupted, your body can become very sick.

Genetic Factors

Genetic factors play several roles in causing noncommunicable diseases. In some cases, genes directly lead to the development of a noncommunicable disease. As you learned in Chapter 1, these diseases are called *genetic disorders*. Genes can also make a person *more likely* to develop a noncommunicable disease (**Figure 20.2**).

One way to assess your genetic factors for noncommunicable diseases is to look at your biological family. **Family history** refers to the record of diseases among close biological relatives, such as parents, grandparents, or siblings. If multiple, close biological relatives have the same noncommunicable disease, for example, you probably have more genetic risk factors for that disease.

family history record of diseases among close biological relatives

Environmental Factors

Factors in the environment also affect risk for noncommunicable diseases. For example, outdoor and indoor air pollution are risk factors for respiratory diseases such as lung cancer and asthma. Exposure to hazardous chemicals in the environment can cause cancer, respiratory diseases, and other illnesses.

Other environmental factors include lack of access to nutritious food or healthcare services. Not getting needed nutrients or healthcare increases risk for many noncommunicable diseases. Unsafe communities, exposure to crime, and frequent and severe weather are also environmental risk factors.

Behavioral Factors

Behavioral, or lifestyle-related, factors have a significant influence on the development of noncommunicable diseases. You have learned about many of these influences throughout this book. For example, smoking or vaping, using alcohol or drugs, being physically inactive, and eating a poor diet can lead to disease. Getting physical activity, managing stress, and using refusal skills reduce the risk of disease.

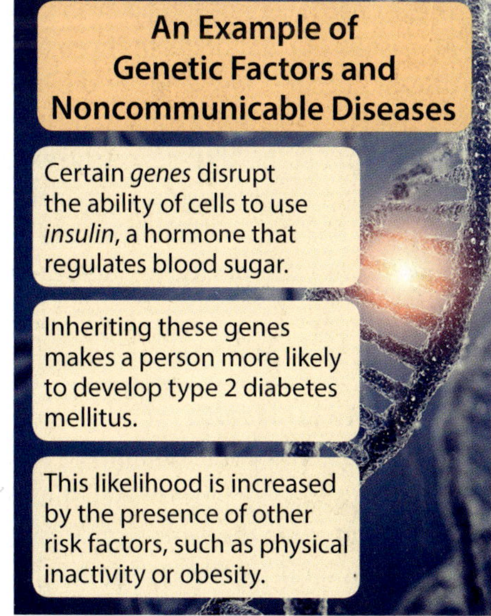

nobeastsofierce/Shutterstock.com

Figure 20.2 Certain genes make it easier for other factors to cause disease.

The behaviors you practice during adolescence are likely to continue into adulthood. This is why engaging in healthy behaviors now is so important. Many noncommunicable diseases in adulthood can be traced to unhealthy habits that began in youth.

How Do Noncommunicable Diseases Progress?

complications health conditions that develop as a result of another disease

remission period of time without signs and symptoms associated with a disease

relapse recurrence of a disease, in which signs and symptoms return after a period of remission

Noncommunicable diseases have different lengths and patterns. If a noncommunicable disease is *acute*, it occurs suddenly and resolves fairly quickly, often without long-lasting effects. Most noncommunicable diseases are *chronic*, meaning they are long-term diseases that may not resolve for years. These diseases can cause permanent disability or health conditions. Noncommunicable diseases can also cause **complications**, or health conditions that develop from the disease.

Noncommunicable diseases can intensify and fade multiple times over the course of a person's life. Sometimes a noncommunicable disease enters **remission**, a period of time without signs and symptoms associated with the disease. Remission may last for weeks, years, or longer. The term **relapse** refers to the recurrence of a disease, in which signs and symptoms return after a period of remission. For example, certain cancers can leave remission and recur in an even more severe way than before.

Local and Global Health

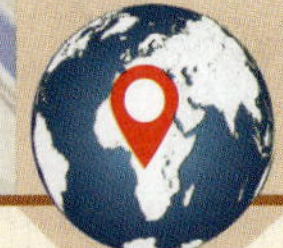

Noncommunicable Diseases in Your Community and World

The World Health Organization (WHO) reports that noncommunicable diseases cause up to 75 percent of all deaths around the world each year. These deaths are not spread evenly around the world. At least 80 percent of deaths from noncommunicable diseases occur in low- and middle-income countries.

Part of the reason for this trend is that treatment for noncommunicable diseases can be expensive. Expensive treatment can reduce people's financial resources, even in higher-income countries, and force people into poverty. Noncommunicable diseases can also reduce productivity and quality of life, keeping people from work and school. In addition, low-income countries may not have the resources to provide expensive healthcare services to all citizens, reducing access to needed care.

Rates of noncommunicable diseases also relate to income and education. As you know, these two factors are related. Lack of income can keep people from getting education and make it more difficult to make healthy decisions. Without education, people may not know the decisions they can make to lower their risk for noncommunicable diseases.

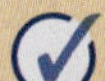

Practice Your Skills

Advocate for Health

Think about your community. What income and education levels are most common in your community? Are there many grocery stores with nutritious foods and opportunities for safe physical activity? How accessible are healthcare services? Can most people afford healthcare services? In a small group, identify one action you can take to advocate for the health of your community. Your action should help people reduce their risk for noncommunicable diseases. Some examples might include donating fresh fruits and vegetables to a food pantry, starting a community garden, serving food at a homeless shelter, or making community members aware of free or low-cost healthcare options. As a group, act on your idea together.

Diagnosis and Treatment for Noncommunicable Diseases

A doctor or other healthcare professional diagnoses a noncommunicable disease and then makes a treatment plan. To diagnose a disease, a doctor uses information from a physical exam, medical history, and tests.

When diagnosing a noncommunicable disease, a doctor will typically provide a **prognosis**, or statement about the likely outcome of the disease. This statement includes the likelihood for full recovery, disability, or death. A prognosis also predicts the length and severity of a disease. Diseases that will end in death are called *terminal*.

prognosis statement about the likely outcome of a disease; made by a medical professional

Treatment for noncommunicable diseases usually involves a combination of methods. Sometimes, treatment requires a person to modify behaviors or make changes in the environment to avoid environmental risk factors. Medications can also help the body return to a state of homeostasis. *Physical therapy* can help a person maintain or improve strength, balance, and mobility. Some people need *occupational therapy*, which helps them learn skills to maintain an active lifestyle at home or work. Mental health therapy can help people understand and cope with stress and challenges related to the disease (**Figure 20.3**).

Some treatments are meant to slow or stop the progression of a disease. Treatment may also work to fix the underlying causes of disease. Sometimes, the goal of treatment is to eliminate or reduce signs and symptoms. For chronic diseases, treatment may allow a person to manage the disease and live a productive, active life for as long as possible.

Promoting Health After a Diagnosis

- Ask questions and work with your doctor to understand the details of treatment and management.
- Remember that no disease defines who you are.
- Accept and express your emotions.
- Keep taking care of your health by engaging in healthy behaviors. Work with your doctor to adjust any habits or activities needed.
- Engage in activities you enjoy and find meaningful.
- Build meaningful, healthy relationships.
- Reach out and talk to friends, family members, and other supportive people.
- Find community resources and support groups for people with your disease.
- Seek professional help, if needed.

Figure 20.3 Receiving a noncommunicable disease diagnosis is hard for many people. Fortunately, people can still promote their health, even with a chronic disease. ***What kind of treatment can help a person maintain or improve strength, balance, and mobility?***

Lesson 20.1 Review

Know and Understand

1. What is the name for the body's internal state of balance?
2. What is the difference between a genetic disorder and a noncommunicable disease for which genes and other factors influence risk?
3. Describe the difference between remission and relapse.

Think Critically

4. What factors in your environment influence risk for noncommunicable diseases?
5. Think about all the activities you do each day. How does each activity affect your risk for noncommunicable diseases?

REAL WORLD Health Skills

Analyze Influences Many different factors affect a person's risk for developing a noncommunicable disease. With a partner, take turns listing factors that affect your risk. Record all of these factors on a piece of paper and then categorize them as genetic, environmental, or behavioral. Also identify whether each factor is modifiable of nonmodifiable. Be sure to include both risk and protective factors. With your partner, discuss ways you could increase protective factors and reduce risk factors.

Lesson

20.2

Cardiovascular Diseases

Essential Question?

How do cardiovascular diseases affect the body, and how can they be prevented?

Learning Outcomes

After studying this lesson, you will be able to

- explain how the heart and blood vessels work together to circulate blood throughout the body;
- differentiate between arteriosclerosis and atherosclerosis;
- analyze the consequences of hypertension;
- discuss how diseases of the blood vessels and hypertension can lead to a stroke or heart attack;
- describe what happens in congestive heart failure;
- identify the symptoms of arrhythmias and mitral valve prolapse; and
- assess steps for preventing and treating cardiovascular diseases.

Key Terms

angina
arrhythmias
arteries
arteriosclerosis
atherosclerosis
blood pressure
capillaries
cardiovascular diseases
congestive heart failure
coronary arteries
heart attack
hypertension
stent
stroke
valves
veins

Warm-Up Activity

Your Heartbeat

Comprehend Concepts Before reading this lesson, stand up and breathe normally, noting how your heartbeat feels in your chest. Next, do 10 jumping jacks. Breathe like normal and note how long it takes for your breathing and heartbeat to decrease back to how they felt before the jumping jacks. Do another 10 jumping jacks. Then, make a fist with your hand and press your fist against your mouth, making a very small space to breathe in and out. Breathe this way for 10 seconds and then breathe normally. How much harder was it to breathe when less oxygen was available to you? How long did it take your heartbeat to return to normal?

In this lesson, you will learn about how cardiovascular diseases affect blood and oxygen flow, making activities like doing jumping jacks and breathing much more difficult.

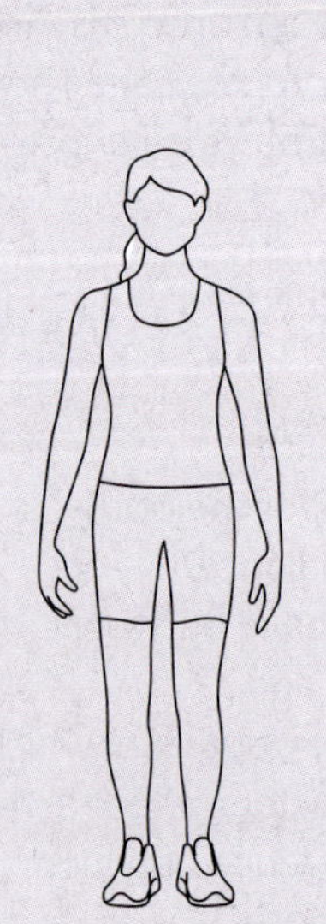

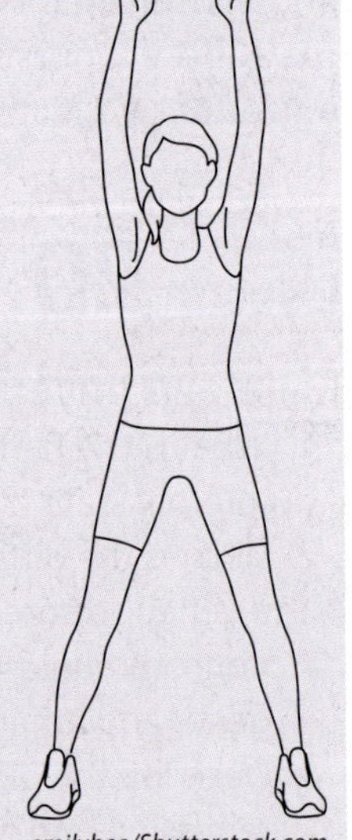

emilybee/Shutterstock.com

The heart and blood vessels make up the body's *cardiovascular system*, sometimes called the *circulatory system*. **Cardiovascular diseases** are noncommunicable diseases that affect the heart and blood vessels in ways that hinder function and cause harm. Harm to this body system can have serious consequences.

cardiovascular diseases health conditions that harm and hinder the function of the heart and blood vessels

How the Cardiovascular System Works

The *heart* is a muscular organ that pumps blood throughout the body. In a state of health, the heart adapts to the body's changing needs, speeding up when your body requires more oxygen and slowing down when your body is at rest. The heart requires its own continuous supply of oxygen and nutrients, delivered by blood vessels called **coronary arteries**. These blood vessels are branches of the largest artery in the body, called the *aorta*. The coronary arteries enter the heart muscle, form increasingly smaller branches, and eventually become microscopic **capillaries**, or tiny blood vessels with thin walls. Because the walls of capillaries are so thin, oxygen can leave the blood and enter the heart's muscle cells.

The heart delivers blood to the rest of the body through blood vessels. In addition to capillaries, there are two different types of blood vessels. **Arteries** are large, muscular blood vessels that carry blood from the heart to the capillaries. **Veins** are blood vessels that return blood from the capillaries to the heart (**Figure 20.4**). Blood vessels work best when their inner walls are smooth and somewhat *elastic*, or capable of stretching and rebounding.

coronary arteries blood vessels that supply the heart muscle with blood containing oxygen and nutrients

capillaries tiny blood vessels with thin walls through which oxygen, nutrients, and waste can pass

arteries large, muscular blood vessels that deliver blood from the heart to the rest of the body

veins blood vessels that deliver blood from the rest of the body back to the heart

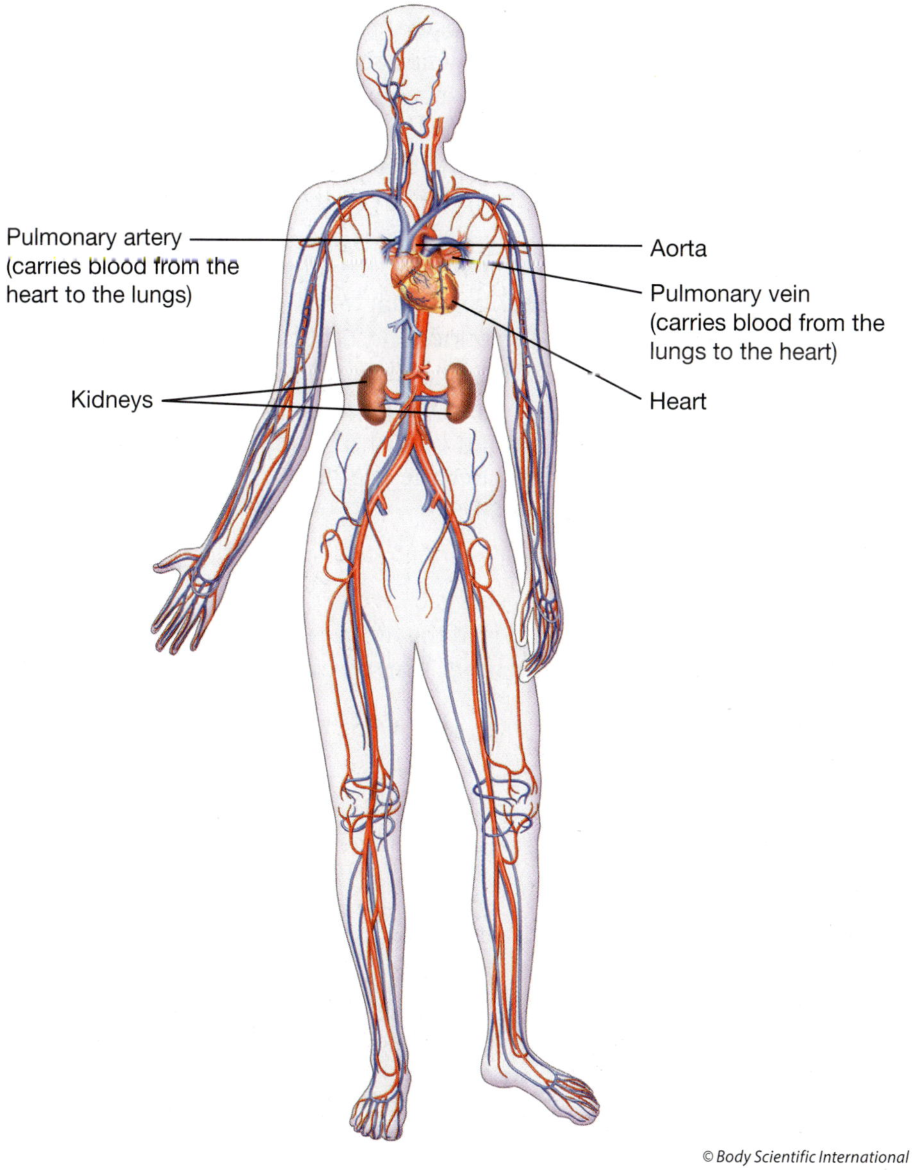

Figure 20.4 In this illustration, arteries are shown in red. These blood vessels carry oxygen-containing blood from the heart to the rest of the body. Veins are shown in blue. These blood vessels carry blood from the rest of the body to the heart, where the heart works with the lungs to fill the blood with more oxygen. ***Which blood vessels return blood from the capillaries to the heart?***

Other muscles in your body can function without oxygen for a period of time, but the cells in the heart muscle cannot. If the heart's supply of oxygen becomes restricted or cut off, the heart's muscle cells die quickly. When its cells die, the heart muscle weakens and stops circulating blood.

Types of Cardiovascular Diseases

Genetics, environment, and behavior all affect the health of the cardiovascular system. When these factors cause harm to the cardiovascular system, cardiovascular diseases result. Cardiovascular diseases affect the blood vessels and heart and can cause medical emergencies. These diseases are the leading cause of death around the world.

Diseases of the Blood Vessels

Many cardiovascular diseases begin with changes in the blood vessels. As you know, healthy blood vessels are smooth and elastic, and blood flows freely through them. Diseases of the blood vessels cause changes that restrict blood flow. When these diseases affect the coronary arteries that supply blood to the heart, they are called *coronary artery disease*. Diseases of the blood vessels include arteriosclerosis and atherosclerosis.

arteriosclerosis disease in which the walls of the arteries thicken, harden, and become inflexible

Arteriosclerosis is a disease in which the walls of the arteries thicken, harden, and become inflexible due to age and family history, other diseases, and lifestyle choices such as physical inactivity and smoking. As a result, arteries lose their elasticity and cannot stretch when the heart pumps blood through them. This inability to stretch leads to high blood pressure and other cardiovascular diseases.

atherosclerosis disease in which fatty deposits collect in the walls of arteries, restricting blood flow

Atherosclerosis is a disease in which fatty deposits called *plaque* collect in the walls of arteries. Behavioral factors such as a high-fat diet and smoking or vaping, genetic background, and other diseases (for example, high blood pressure) also contribute to atherosclerosis. As plaque builds up, it can restrict blood flow to organs such as the heart and brain. Plaque can become unstable, break away, and lodge in smaller arteries, completely blocking blood flow. It also stimulates the production of blood clots, which can block small arteries (**Figure 20.5**).

blood pressure force that blood exerts on the arterial walls; measured in millimeters of mercury (mmHg)

Hypertension

When the heart pumps blood into the arteries, the blood inside the arteries exerts force on the artery walls. This force is called **blood pressure**.

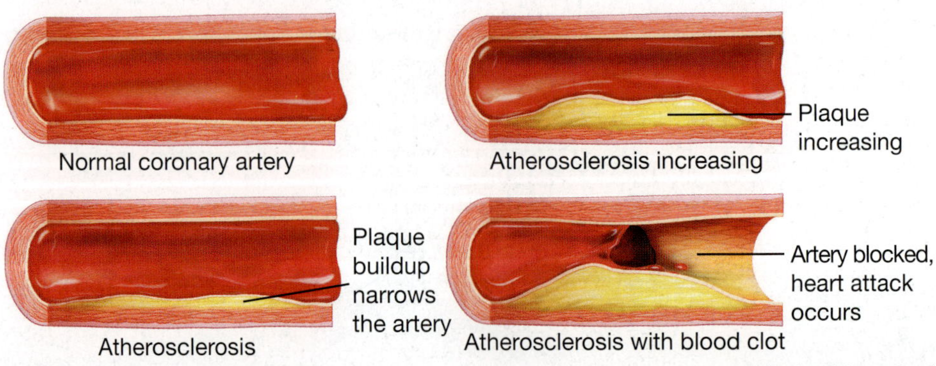

Figure 20.5 The buildup of plaque in atherosclerosis can block an artery and cut off blood flow to a part of the body. If the blocked artery is in the brain, it can lead to a stroke. A blocked artery in the heart can cause a heart attack.

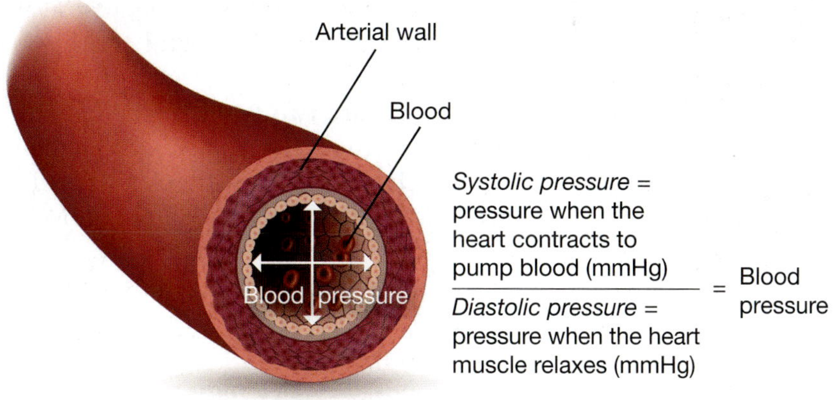

Figure 20.6 Blood pressure has two components: pressure when the heart is contracting (systolic pressure) and pressure when the heart is relaxed (diastolic pressure).

Blood pressure is measured in millimeters of mercury (mmHg) (**Figure 20.6**). The first number of a blood pressure measurement is systolic pressure; the second number is diastolic pressure.

When blood pressure is too high, a person has **hypertension**. Hypertension can occur in people of any age. In fact, the American Heart Association reports almost 50 percent of adults in the US do not know they have hypertension. This is partly because hypertension usually produces few signs and symptoms. Instead, it silently damages blood vessels and organs. For example, hypertension injures blood vessels by causing arteriosclerosis and atherosclerosis, setting the stage for a heart attack or stroke.

hypertension disease characterized by high blood pressure

To prevent damage from hypertension, teens should work with their doctors to monitor their blood pressure. Because different factors, such as sleep, stress, and physical activity, cause changes in blood pressure, measuring blood pressure over a few days will give the most accurate reading. Ranges for blood pressure are shown in **Figure 20.7**.

Stroke

Arteriosclerosis, atherosclerosis, and hypertension can all contribute to arteries becoming blocked, which cuts off blood flow. Blocked blood flow can have serious consequences to organs, which need oxygen to survive. **Stroke** is a cardiovascular disease and medical emergency that occurs when blood flow to a part of the brain is interrupted. A blood clot that develops in the brain or breaks off and travels from a blood clot elsewhere in the body can cause this. Lack of blood flow deprives the brain of oxygen, injuring or killing brain cells.

stroke medical emergency in which blood vessels in the brain become narrow or blocked or burst, disrupting blood flow to a part of the brain

Blood Pressure Ranges

Healthy range	Lower than 120/80 mmHg
Prehypertension	Systolic pressure 121–129 mmHg; diastolic pressure lower than 80 mmHg
Hypertension	Systolic pressure equal to or greater than 130 mmHg; diastolic pressure equal to or greater than 80 mmHg

These ranges indicate an adult's blood pressure level. The ranges for children and teens are calculated differently.

The ranges for healthy blood pressure, prehypertension, and hypertension in children or teens differ depending on the person's age, sex, and weight.

Figure 20.7 Blood pressure is measured using a medical device called a *sphygmomanometer*, which includes a cuff that wraps around the arm. ***What is another name for high blood pressure?***

Symptoms of a Stroke

- Numbness or weakness on one side of the body, face, arm, or leg
- Confusion
- Trouble speaking or understanding speech
- Vision conditions affecting one or both of the eyes
- Dizziness
- Loss of balance or coordination
- Trouble walking
- Severe headache

Figure 20.8 Someone with these symptoms needs immediate medical attention. People nearby should dial 911.

A stroke can cause paralysis, lost abilities, intellectual disabilities, and death (**Figure 20.8**).

There are two types of stroke. The most common type is an *ischemic stroke*, in which narrowed or blocked blood vessels in the brain disrupt the flow of blood. Some people experience *transient ischemic attacks (TIAs)*, or *ministrokes*, in which blood flow to a part of the brain temporarily stops. These strokes suggest that a person has a high risk for an ischemic stroke.

The second, less common type of stroke is a *hemorrhagic stroke*. In a hemorrhagic stroke, a blood vessel in the brain bursts and fails to deliver blood to brain cells. This stroke occurs when blood vessels become weakened after years of hypertension.

Risk factors for stroke include genetics and advanced age. Health conditions such as hypertension and atherosclerosis are also risk factors. Behavioral risk factors include tobacco use, particularly smoking; a high-fat diet; obesity; and an inactive lifestyle.

heart attack medical emergency in which the coronary arteries that supply blood to the heart become narrow or blocked, disrupting blood flow to the heart

angina pain in the chest that often accompanies a heart attack; may feel like pressure or squeezing or a dull or sharp pain

Heart Attack

A **heart attack** occurs when the coronary arteries become blocked due to coronary artery diseases like arteriosclerosis and atherosclerosis. Blocked arteries disrupt blood flow to the heart muscle, causing cells in the heart to die. A heart attack is a medical emergency often accompanied by **angina**, or chest pain. Angina typically feels like pressure or squeezing in the chest or a dull or sharp pain. Chest pain sensations differ among people. Some people say chest pain feels like an elephant sitting on their chest. Heart attack can also cause pain or tingling sensations radiating to the left arm, shoulder, and jaw; sweating; dizziness; nausea; and shortness of breath.

While males and females may have several of these symptoms, some females do not feel chest pain and may not realize they are having a heart attack. Females are more likely to have shortness of breath, and sensations of pressure or pain occur in the lower chest, upper abdomen, or upper back. Females are more likely to feel dizzy, lightheaded, and fatigued. Some females say this fatigue feels like having the flu or completing an extremely challenging exercise.

If a heart attack goes untreated, it can cause severe heart damage and death. Immediate help can save a person's life. If a person experiences symptoms of a heart attack, call 911 right away (**Figure 20.9**). As you learned in Chapter 16, giving *Hands-Only*™ *CPR* can also improve a person's chances of survival while you are waiting for professional medical help.

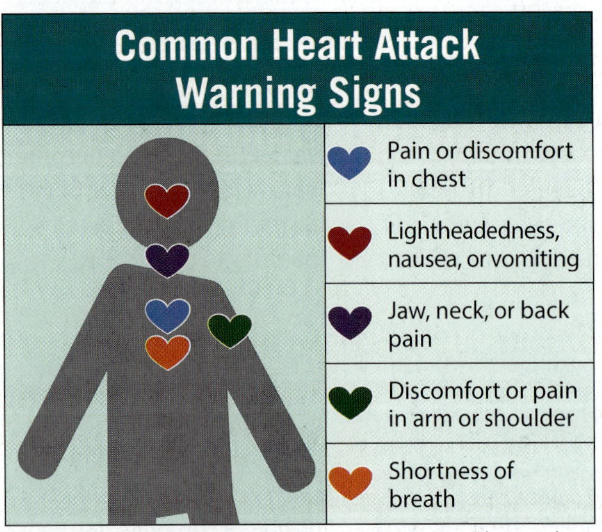

Figure 20.9 The symptoms of a heart attack often vary between males and females. Females are more likely to experience symptoms besides chest pain, such as nausea, shortness of breath, and back or jaw pain. ***What symptom of a heart attack feels like pressure, squeezing, or pain in the chest?***

Congestive Heart Failure

Even if arteriosclerosis and atherosclerosis do not cause an artery to become blocked, they can lead to other cardiovascular diseases. **Congestive heart failure** is a condition in which the heart becomes too weak to pump blood effectively. Heart failure results from chronic strain on the heart. This strain usually comes from pumping blood through narrow, stiff blood vessels. Over time, the heart weakens until it can no longer circulate blood effectively through the body (**Figure 20.10**).

congestive heart failure condition in which the heart becomes too weak to circulate blood effectively through the body

Signs and symptoms of congestive heart failure include ankle swelling, shortness of breath, and fatigue. As the heart weakens, its pumping power lessens, and blood does not move as effectively through the blood vessels. Instead, blood pools within the blood vessels of the feet and hands, causing swelling. Fluid builds up in the lungs, interfering with breathing. People feel short of breath even when resting. At this point, some people develop blue-tinged skin and lips, a condition called *cyanosis*. This happens because blood in the skin's capillaries turns blue when it does not carry oxygen.

Treatment for congestive heart failure can reduce the severity of symptoms and slow the disease's progression. Medications and lifestyle changes can help lower blood pressure, relieve the heart's workload, and strengthen the heart's pumping. Another treatment is a heart transplant. This complicated surgery involves removing the heart and replacing it with a heart donated by another person.

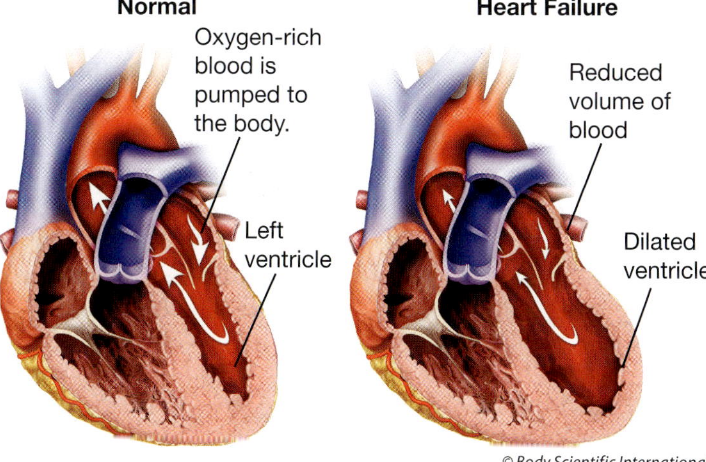

Figure 20.10 In congestive heart failure, the heart weakens and expands, reducing pumping power. This prevents the heart from circulating blood effectively throughout the body.

Arrhythmias

In a healthy state, the heart muscle beats in a coordinated fashion at a regular rate. Uncoordinated or irregular heartbeats pump blood inefficiently and strain the heart. Disorders of heart rhythm are called **arrhythmias** and can arise from abnormal conditions within the heart (**Figure 20.11**). These conditions may result from other cardiovascular diseases, smoking and vaping, or drug use.

arrhythmias abnormal heart rhythms; include fast, slow, and uncoordinated heartbeats

Types of Arrhythmias		
Tachycardia	**Bradycardia**	**Fibrillation**
Tachycardia is an abnormally fast heart rate of more than 100 beats per minute. It causes the heart to feel like it is racing even when the body is resting. Tachycardia raises risk for stroke.	Bradycardia is an abnormally slow heart rate of fewer than 60 beats per minute. The heart fails to keep up with the body's demands for oxygen and nutrients. This can lead to weakness, fatigue, and fainting. Some athletes may have bradycardia, but their strong hearts pump blood more efficiently and can therefore beat more slowly.	Fibrillation is uncoordinated beating of the heart. Atrial fibrillation is the most common type of arrhythmia. Fibrillation raises the risk for stroke, congestive heart failure, and cardiac arrest (in which the heart stops beating).

Figure 20.11 The three main types of arrhythmias are tachycardia, bradycardia, and fibrillation.

People with an arrhythmia have a wide variety of symptoms. In general, they feel like their heart is fluttering, skipping beats, or quivering. Arrhythmia can also make people feel faint, lightheaded, and out of breath due to poor blood circulation.

Some medications can control arrhythmia. If medications are ineffective, doctors can recommend *cardioversion*, which uses electrical voltage to reset the heart's normal rate and rhythm. If cardioversion does not provide relief, *ablation* can selectively destroy the parts of the heart sending abnormal signals. Some people have a pacemaker inserted, which electrically sets the pace of the heart.

Diseases of the Heart Valves

Blood flows in one direction as the heart pumps it to the lungs and the rest of the body. The heart receives blood in the *atria*, the two chambers at the top of the heart. The atria pump blood into the two larger chambers, called *ventricles*, at the bottom of the heart. The ventricles then pump blood out of the heart to the lungs and the rest of the body. Flexible, sturdy flaps of tissue called **valves** control the movement of blood in this direction. Several diseases can affect the heart valves.

valves flaps of tissue that control the flow of blood in the heart

One type of heart valve disease is *mitral valve prolapse*. The mitral valve controls blood flow from the left atrium to the left ventricle and blocks backward blood flow from the ventricle into the atrium. In mitral valve prolapse, however, blood *does* flow backward into the atrium because the valve is defective. In most cases, mitral valve prolapse causes few health issues. In some cases, though, a great deal of reverse blood flow can stress the heart muscle. A valve that functions poorly can be surgically repaired or replaced.

Keep Your Heart Healthy and Active

Plan to get at least
60 minutes
of physical activity each day.
Replace sedentary activities, such as watching TV, with physical activities like dancing, swimming, bicycling, or playing sports.

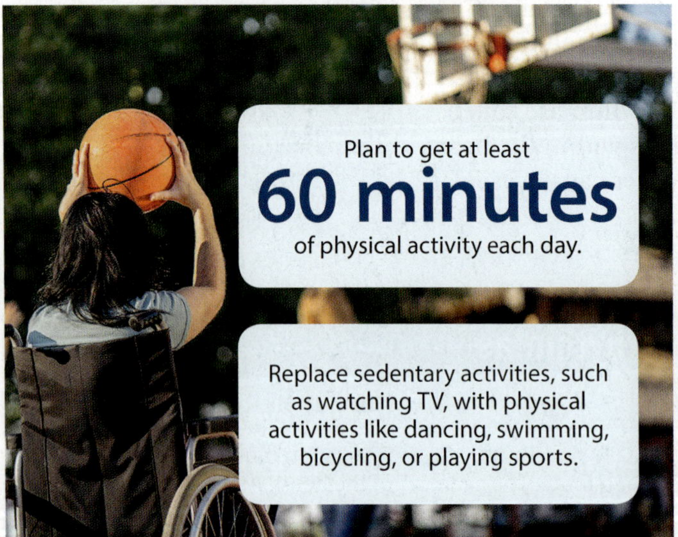

StockPlanets/E+/Getty Images

Figure 20.12 Getting at least 60 minutes of physical activity a day can help strengthen your heart and prevent cardiovascular diseases.

Preventing Cardiovascular Diseases

Preventing cardiovascular diseases involves reducing risk factors and increasing protective factors in your life. Focus on factors you *can* control, such as your habits, lifestyle, and behaviors. Even if you have risk factors you cannot control, reducing your risk in other areas will benefit your health. Some strategies for preventing cardiovascular diseases follow:

- **Be physically active:** Getting enough physical activity will strengthen your heart and help you maintain a healthy blood pressure (**Figure 20.12**). If you have a disability or injury that prevents you from getting some types of physical activity, talk with your doctor about activities you can do or modify.

- **Eat a healthy diet:** Choosing nutritious foods can reduce the amount of cholesterol and fat in your bloodstream. Choose lean protein, such as chicken, fish, or beans, over red meat like beef, pork, and lamb. When cooking, replace animal sources of fat with plant sources such as vegetable oil. Replace fried foods with baked foods.
- **Maintain a healthy body weight:** Reaching and maintaining a healthy weight can reduce strain on your heart.
- **Avoid harmful substances:** Do not use tobacco—by smoking, vaping, or using smokeless tobacco. Nicotine damages the cardiovascular system and is a leading cause of cardiovascular disease. Do not drink alcohol, abuse medications, or use drugs.
- **Manage stress:** Stress makes the heart work harder, which causes strain. Recognize signs of stress, such as irritability, increased heart rate, sweaty palms, and inability to focus. Take breaks or a walk when you feel stressed. Remove yourself from the stressful situation, if possible. Get enough sleep and eat nutritious meals.

Skills for Health and Wellness

Promote Heart Health

Did you know that cardiovascular disease causes one out of every four deaths in the US every year? Fortunately, there are steps you can take now to reduce your lifetime risk of cardiovascular disease. The habits you form as a teen will impact the health of your heart as an adult. You can use the health skills you learned in this textbook to develop and follow healthy habits.

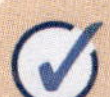

Practice Your Skills

Set Goals

Setting goals can help you make gradual changes in your habits to promote heart health. Both short-term and long-term goals can help you engage in behaviors that reduce your risk for cardiovascular disease.

1. Review the four ways people can change their habits to decrease risk of cardiovascular disease. These methods involve getting physical activity, eating a healthy diet, maintaining a healthy body weight, avoiding harmful substances, and managing stress. You may also identify other ways to promote heart health using reliable, valid resources.
2. Choose three methods for promoting heart health.
3. Assess how successful you are in practicing each method. For example, if you chose to focus on physical activity, you could examine how much physical activity you get. If you focus on a healthy diet, you can keep a food diary to assess your nutritional habits. Consider how you could improve your health behaviors in each area.
4. Create a SMART goal related to each method you chose. Remember that this goal needs to be specific, measurable, achievable, relevant, and timely. Your goal should involve a change in behavior that will promote heart health.
5. Break down each goal into short-term SMART goals, which are the steps you will need to take to achieve the overall goal.
6. Pick a date you plan to have achieved your goals. Record this date on a calendar.
7. Put your goals into action. Follow the steps for each SMART goal for the amount of time you chose. You might want to set reminders to help you remember these steps.
8. Keep track of your progress and take notes about any obstacles you face. Explain how you overcame these obstacles.
9. At the end of the time line you set, evaluate your progress. Reflect on the health benefits you experienced. Discuss goals you can set in the future to keep maintaining the health of your heart.

Methods of Diagnosing Cardiovascular Diseases	
Method	**Description**
Electrocardiogram (ECG)	Detects the electrical rhythm of the heart and determines if blood flow to an area of the heart is disrupted
Stress test	Determines how physical activity affects the heart's function; is an ECG performed while a person walks on a treadmill
Angiogram	Reveals narrow or blocked coronary arteries; dye is injected into a vein and circulates in the coronary vessels
Echocardiography	Visualizes the structure and motion of the heart using sound waves
Cardiac catheterization	Determines how well the heart functions and detects valve disorders; a long, thin, hollow tube called a *catheter* is threaded through blood vessels into the heart to sample the blood in each chamber for oxygen content and pressure

Figure 20.13 Some methods for diagnosing cardiovascular disease are more invasive than others.

stent fine mesh inserted into an artery to crush and push aside plaque, restoring blood flow

Treating Cardiovascular Diseases

To begin treatment for cardiovascular disease, doctors need to determine the exact nature of the disease. **Figure 20.13** lists some methods of diagnosing cardiovascular diseases.

One common treatment for blocked blood vessels involves inserting a stent. A **stent** is a fine mesh shaped like a straw. Doctors insert the stent into a vein and guide it through blood vessels to the blockage. The stent expands to push aside and crush plaque, restoring blood flow. *Bypass surgery* may also repair blocked blood flow. In bypass surgery, a vein from the leg is inserted to route blood around a blocked artery.

Medications can also treat cardiovascular diseases. Blood-thinning medications and aspirin prevent the formation of blood clots. Antihypertensive medications, such as diuretics, lower blood pressure. Some medications decrease the amount of cholesterol in the blood.

Lesson 20.2 Review

Know and Understand

1. Which type of blood vessel supplies the heart with blood and oxygen?
2. Explain the difference between arteriosclerosis and atherosclerosis.
3. What is the healthy range for blood pressure in adults?
4. How are symptoms of a heart attack different between males and females?
5. What causes congestive heart failure?

Think Critically

6. The location of a stroke can determine which brain functions are affected. Research the parts of the brain most often affected by stroke. How does oxygen deprivation affect these areas?
7. Choose one strategy for preventing cardiovascular disease and explain how it benefits the cardiovascular system.

REAL WORLD Health Skills

Practice Health-Enhancing Behaviors Using the information in this lesson, make a list of questions to ask your doctor about cardiovascular diseases. Your questions might be about ways to prevent cardiovascular diseases. They might also relate to responding to a medical emergency like a stroke or heart attack. Keep this list of questions to ask during your next physical exam.

Cancer

Essential Question

How does cancer affect the body?

Lesson **20.3**

Learning Outcomes

After studying this lesson, you will be able to

- explain how cancer develops;
- differentiate between benign and malignant tumors;
- analyze the factors and behaviors that influence cancer risk;
- identify common types of cancer;
- assess strategies for preventing cancer; and
- describe treatment options for cancer.

Key Terms

benign tumors
biopsy
cancer
chemotherapy
colonoscopy
malignant tumors
mammograms
metastasize
tumor

Warm-Up Activity

Cancer: Your Decisions

Make Decisions Your teacher will set a timer for one minute. During that time, list as many decisions that affect a person's risk of cancer as you can. As you read this lesson, add new decisions to your list. Place a check next to decisions you already knew. If any decisions you listed are not discussed in the lesson, research them using reliable and valid resources and note whether they affect risk for cancer. Then write a case study in which a teen uses the decision-making process to make a healthy decision that reduces cancer risk.

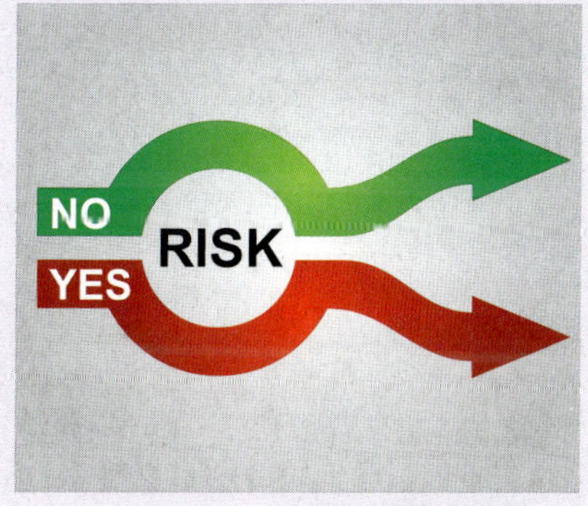

eltoro69/Shutterstock.com

Every year, scientists are learning more and more about cancer. Although scientists do not completely understand this noncommunicable disease, they have worked out many parts of the puzzle. In this lesson, you will learn about the characteristics of cancer, causes of cancer, types of cancer, and methods for prevention and treatment.

What Is Cancer?

Cancer is a complex disease, and different forms of the disease have unique characteristics. All forms of cancer are characterized by an uncontrolled growth of abnormal cells. In a state of health, all cells reproduce, which enables organ growth, tissue repair, and tissue development. These cells control their growth, reproducing only when needed. In contrast, cancerous cells divide rapidly and produce abnormal cells that do not function like normal cells.

cancer complex disease in which abnormal cells reproduce uncontrollably, forming malignant tumors that spread throughout the body

tumor mass of abnormal cells; may be malignant (cancerous) or benign (noncancerous)

benign tumors mass of abnormal cells that is not cancerous; remains in one place and stays small

malignant tumors mass of abnormal, cancerous cells; cells can spread to other areas of the body and invade tissues

metastasize to spread from an original location to other parts of the body

When abnormal cells reproduce, they can form a mass called a **tumor**. Not all tumors are cancerous. **Benign tumors** are masses of noncancerous, abnormal cells. These tumors usually remain in one area of the body, stay small, and do not invade nearby tissues. As a result, they pose few health hazards and may not require treatment. If they do cause health conditions, they are more easily removed than a cancerous tumor.

In contrast, **malignant tumors** are masses of cancerous, abnormal cells. These cells reproduce and invade the tissues around the area they first develop. They can also **metastasize**, or spread to other parts of the body and cause additional tumors to develop. Metastasis is possible because malignant cells can break away from the main tumor and enter blood vessels, which transport the cells throughout the body.

What Causes Cancer?

Interactions between a person's genes, environment, and behavior cause cancer to develop. Factors in all of these areas can increase or decrease a person's likelihood of developing cancer. Diverse forms of cancer often depend on different factors.

Genetics

Genes with *mutations*, or defects, are the basis for cancer. These mutations can change cell function in several ways. For example, they can take away controls over cell growth and division. They can also equip cells to invade neighboring tissues and metastasize.

People can get cancer-causing mutations in a number of ways. Sometimes, people inherit mutations from biological parents. About 5–10 percent of all cancers are caused by these inherited mutations. Other mutations develop during life due to a number of environmental and behavioral factors.

Environmental Influences

Factors in a person's environment also influence cancer risk. One environmental risk factor is exposure to a group of substances called *carcinogens*. Carcinogens cause mutations in genes, leading to cancerous changes in cells. Chemical carcinogens include substances like formaldehyde, asbestos, radon gas, and tobacco smoke. Carcinogens also include some types of radiation, such as ultraviolet (UV) radiation from the sun. In high doses, radiation from X-rays can also cause cancer. Healthcare professionals take care to avoid unnecessarily x-raying patients to limit their lifetime exposure to radiation.

Exposure to pathogens in the environment can also influence cancer risk. Human papillomavirus (HPV), a sexually transmitted infection, is the leading cause of cervical cancer. Both hepatitis B and hepatitis C are capable of causing liver cancer. Infection with human T-lymphotropic virus, Epstein-Barr virus (EBV), and human immunodeficiency virus (HIV) are linked with *lymphoma* (cancer of lymphatic tissue). Additionally, infection with the bacterium *Helicobacter pylori* can cause stomach ulcers and stomach cancer.

Behavior

The decisions people make affect risk for developing cancer. For example, smoking cigarettes is the leading preventable cause of lung cancer. Exposure to secondhand smoke also increases risk for developing lung cancer.

Other known risk factors for cancer include physical inactivity, overweight and obesity, diet, and sun exposure.

Behavioral risk factors have an enormous impact on rates of cancer in a population. For example, the American Cancer Society (ACS) reports that higher rates of some cancers correlate to higher rates of obesity among young adults. Lower rates of smoking have also decreased rates of some smoking-related cancers.

Sun exposure is a modifiable behavioral risk factor for skin cancer, the most common cancer in the US. Most mutations that lead to skin cancer are not inherited from biological parents. Instead, they develop after birth and relate to a person's amount of sun exposure. For skin cancer, behavior is a more significant risk factor than genetics.

Common Cancers

Cancer can affect many different parts of the body. While different cancers can have different signs, **Figure 20.14** lists some common signs and symptoms of all cancers. These symptoms are summarized by the acronym *CAUTION*. Other symptoms include unexplained tiredness, easy bruising, abnormal bleeding, ongoing pain in a part of the body, an unexplained fever or illness that does not go away, frequent headaches, sudden eye or vision changes, and loss of appetite or unplanned weight loss.

Cancers of the skin, lung, breast, and colon are some of the most common types of cancer.

	Signs and Symptoms of Cancer
C	Change in bowel or bladder habits
A	A sore that does not heal
U	Unusual bleeding or discharge
T	Thickening or lump in the breast or any part of the body
I	Indigestion or difficulty swallowing
O	Obvious change in a wart or mole
N	Nagging cough or hoarseness

Figure 20.14 CAUTION summarizes common symptoms of cancer.

Skin Cancer

Skin cancer describes the abnormal growth of cancerous cells in the skin. Skin cancer is caused by exposure to ultraviolet (UV) radiation, which is found in sunlight and in tanning beds and lights. UV radiation directly damages genes and triggers cancerous changes in skin cells.

There are three main types of skin cancer. Two of these types—*basal cell carcinoma* and *squamous cell carcinoma*—are common and curable. *Melanoma* is the most dangerous type of skin cancer because it spreads rapidly throughout the body, sometimes before someone recognizes the initial skin cancer (**Figure 20.15**).

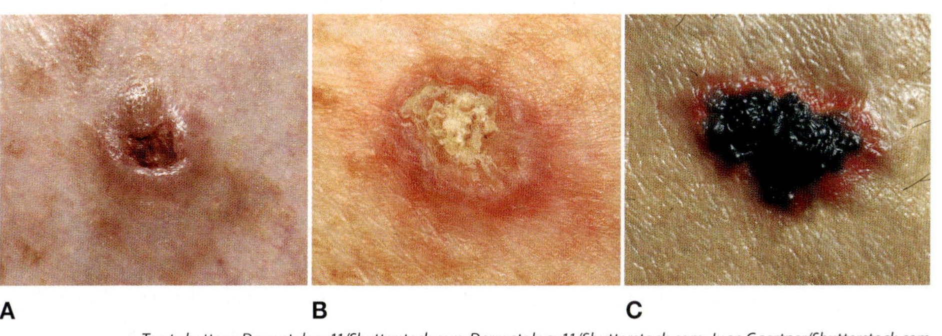

Top to bottom: Dermatology11/Shutterstock.com; Dermatology11/Shutterstock.com; Juan Gaertner/Shutterstock.com

Figure 20.15 Three major types of skin cancer: A) basal cell carcinoma, B) squamous cell carcinoma, C) melanoma. ***Which type of skin cancer is the most dangerous?***

Several unusual changes indicate the development of skin cancer. To recognize these changes, you can use the acronym *ABCDE* to look for the following signs:

- **A** asymmetry (one-half of a mole looks different from the other half)
- **B** border irregularity (the edges of a mole are jagged)
- **C** color, especially uneven color (for example, a purplish center in a black mole)
- **D** diameter (a mole grows bigger in size)
- **E** evolving (a mole changes by becoming bigger, red, itchy, or raised)

Lung Cancer

Abnormal cancerous growth in the lungs is called *lung cancer*. Lung cancer is the leading cause of death from cancer. Most lung cancers begin in the lungs and spread to other organs, including the lymph nodes and brain. A small percentage of lung cancers begins elsewhere in the body and spreads to the lungs.

The chief risk factor for developing lung cancer is smoking cigarettes. In fact, about 80 percent of lung cancers are linked to smoking. This is because cigarette smoke contains many carcinogens. Even breathing secondhand smoke raises the risk for lung cancer, causing up to 7,000 deaths each year. Being exposed to radon gas or asbestos and smoking marijuana can also cause lung cancer.

Signs and symptoms of lung cancer include a cough that gets progressively worse, chest pain, difficulty breathing, and coughing blood. Lung cancer also causes fatigue and weight loss.

Breast Cancer

All people can develop *breast cancer*, or abnormal cancerous growths in breast tissue. Breast cancer affects far more females than males. In the US, breast cancer is the second most common cancer in females, after skin cancer.

Risk factors for breast cancer include genetics, age, and behaviors. Generally, the risk for breast cancer increases with age. Risk factors also include a family history of breast cancer, overweight and obesity, and physical inactivity. About 5–10 percent of all breast cancers are associated with mutations in breast cancer genes 1 and 2, also called *BRCA1* and *BRCA2*.

To detect breast cancer, the ACS recommends yearly **mammograms** (X-rays of the breast) for females 45–49 years of age. Younger females ages 40–44 should discuss with their doctor whether they should get yearly mammograms. A mammogram can detect cancer long before it becomes large enough to notice or feel. If cancer is suspected, a doctor can perform a **biopsy** (removal and testing of a sample of tissue) to confirm or rule out the presence of cancer.

mammograms procedures that use X-rays to image the breast and screen for breast cancer

biopsy procedure in which a sample of tissue is removed and tested for the presence of disease

Colorectal Cancer

Colorectal cancer refers to abnormal cancerous growths in the colon and rectum. The *colon* (also called the *large intestine*) is an organ that carries waste to the *rectum*, which stores feces before elimination. Colorectal cancer can occur in people of all ages, though the majority of cases appear in people 50 years of age or older.

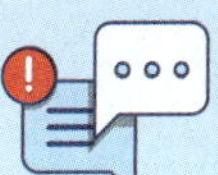

Health in the Media 

Social Media and Disease

Among the many types of media, social media may have the most powerful influence on public and personal health. The Pew Research Center reports about 88 percent of young adults (ages 18–29) in the US use some type of social media. This percentage is closer to 78 percent in adults ages 30–65. Around the world, about three billion people use some form of social media.

The reach of social media can have beneficial or harmful consequences. People who follow health organizations on social media may have access to reliable information about healthcare services, healthy behaviors, and breaking health news. Government agencies and health organizations promote public health by sharing information about healthy lifestyles, effective healthcare products, and preventive care. Social media groups can provide social and psychological support for those living with diseases.

Social media can also have negative consequences. On social media, no one regulates the quality of information. False and harmful information can spread quickly. Corporations can use advertisements with unreliable information to reach millions of customers. Marketing and advertising can promote unhealthy behaviors, such as tobacco or alcohol use, an unhealthy diet, and unsafe sexual activity.

Some skills you can use to find reliable and valid information on social media include the following:

- Limit your exposure to harmful advertising. Use social media settings to screen and block advertising you do not want to see.
- Use skills for evaluating the reliability of health information. You learned these skills in Chapter 2.
- Do not post or share health information you suspect is unreliable.
- Follow only reliable sources of health information.

Practice Your Skills

Access Information

In a small group, browse social media for health content. Find one example of reliable health information shared by a health organization or healthcare facility. Also find one example of an advertisement or article sharing unreliable information. Explain why each example is reliable or unreliable. Also discuss how believing the information shared on social media could impact a teen's health. Then, make a list of reliable sources of health information on social media. Share your list with the class and create a class list to share with your school.

Genetics play a role in colorectal cancer, but inherited genes are linked to only a small number of cases. Other important risk factors include physical inactivity; overweight or obesity; and a diet high in red meat, but low in fruits, vegetables, and fiber.

Early stages of colorectal cancer cause no signs or symptoms. In later stages, symptoms include blood in the feces, stomach pain that does not go away, and unexplained weight loss. Screening is the key to detecting colorectal cancer. A **colonoscopy** is a procedure in which a flexible tube with a camera and small surgical instruments are inserted into the colon. This allows the doctor to see the lining of the rectum and large intestine. The ACS recommends people receive a colonoscopy every 10 years, starting around 45 years of age.

colonoscopy procedure in which a flexible tube with a camera and small surgical instruments are inserted into the colon; a doctor can view the inside of the colon and take samples for testing

Preventing and Treating Cancer

Cancer prevention involves adopting behaviors that reduce the risk of cancer. Often, this means changing habits, including those related to physical activity and diet (**Figure 20.16**).

Reducing Your Risk for Cancer			
Skin cancer	**Lung cancer**	**Breast cancer**	**Colorectal cancer**
• Cover your skin with clothing, a broad-brimmed hat, and sunglasses. • Use broad-spectrum sunscreen with an SPF of 15 or higher every day. • Reapply sunscreen every two hours or immediately after swimming or sweating. • Examine your skin every month. • Avoid tanning and tanning beds. • Get a professional skin exam every year.	• Do not smoke tobacco products, including cigarettes, cigars, and pipes. • Do not smoke marijuana. • Avoid breathing secondhand smoke. • Have your home tested for asbestos and radon. • Get regular physical exams.	• Do not smoke tobacco products. • Limit alcohol consumption. • Maintain a healthy weight. • Get plenty of physical activity. • Avoid radiation and pollution exposure. • Get breast cancer screenings as recommended.	• Do not smoke tobacco products. • Limit alcohol consumption. • Maintain a healthy weight. • Get plenty of physical activity. • Eat vegetables, fruits, and whole grains. • Get colorectal cancer screenings as recommended.

Figure 20.16 Strategies for preventing cancer differ for each type of cancer.

Early detection of cancer allows early treatment and better chances for recovery and survival. Usually, a combination of treatments is more effective than any treatment alone. Surgery is more likely to be effective if the cancer is confined to a small area.

chemotherapy use of medications to kill cancer cells and shrink malignant tumors

Chemotherapy involves the use of medications to kill cancer cells. Chemotherapy can also shrink cancerous tumors to a more manageable size for surgery. Additional treatments include other types of therapy. *Hormone therapy* targets hormones to cut off the conditions cancers need to grow. *Immune therapy* stimulates the body's defenses to attack the cancer. *Radiation therapy* causes damage to cancer cells and triggers their death.

Lesson 20.3 Review

Know and Understand

1. How are cancerous cells different from normal cells?
2. What is the most common cancer in the US?
3. What is the chief risk factor for developing lung cancer?
4. What dietary habits increase risk for colorectal cancer?
5. How does chemotherapy treat cancer?

Think Critically

6. What substances have you heard are carcinogens? Use reliable and valid resources to verify whether or not each substance is a carcinogen.
7. Think of one type of cancer not discussed in this lesson and research its signs and symptoms and ways to prevent it.

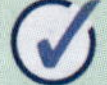

REAL WORLD Health Skills

Communicate with Others Choose one of the methods for preventing cancer discussed in this lesson. Then, create a role-play in which a teen has to make a decision about whether to use one of these methods. For example, a teen could be refusing alcohol or drugs or insisting on bringing sunscreen to the pool. Show effective communication and negotiation skills in your role-play. Share your role-play with a partner and exchange feedback about ways to enhance communication and health.

Other Noncommunicable Diseases

Essential Question?

What other noncommunicable diseases can affect a person's health?

Lesson 20.4

Learning Outcomes

After studying this lesson, you will be able to

- differentiate between type 1 and type 2 diabetes mellitus;
- explain how Alzheimer's disease (AD) affects the brain;
- describe the symptoms of epilepsy;
- identify different types of arthritis;
- describe how osteoporosis affects bone health;
- describe how the body responds in an allergic reaction; and
- explain how asthma impacts breathing.

Key Terms

acidosis
allergy
Alzheimer's disease (AD)
arthritis
autoimmune disease
diabetes mellitus
epilepsy
gout
histamine
hyperglycemia
insulin
osteoarthritis
osteoporosis
rheumatoid arthritis
type 1 diabetes mellitus
type 2 diabetes mellitus

Warm-Up Activity

Your Questions

Access Information So far in this chapter, you have learned about cardiovascular diseases and cancer. These are just two of the many noncommunicable diseases a person can develop. Before reading this lesson, skim the main headings to preview the noncommunicable diseases that will be discussed. With a partner, share your prior knowledge and experience with each noncommunicable disease. Make a list of three questions you have about each disease. After reading the lesson, use the information in the lesson and outside, reliable resources to answer each question. Cite your sources and compare answers with your partner.

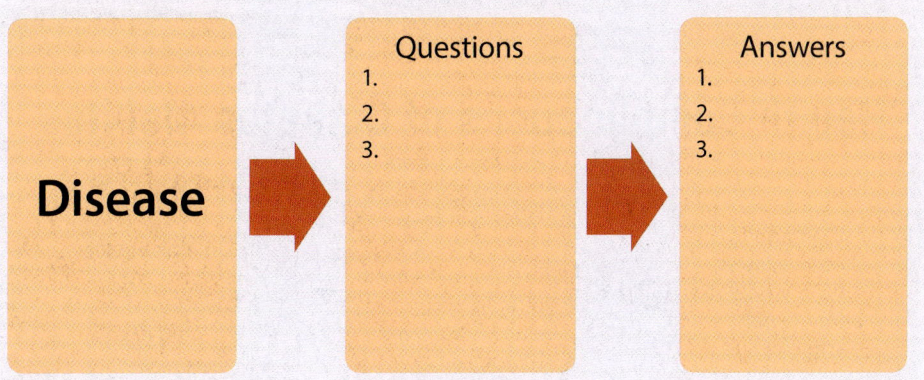

The most common noncommunicable diseases in the US are cardiovascular diseases, cancer, diabetes, and chronic respiratory diseases like asthma. Other common noncommunicable diseases include allergies, arthritis, Alzheimer's disease and other kinds of dementia, epilepsy, and osteoporosis. In this lesson, you will learn about some of these other common noncommunicable diseases.

Diabetes Mellitus

diabetes mellitus disease in which the body is unable to regulate blood sugar

hyperglycemia condition of high blood sugar

Diabetes mellitus, commonly referred to as *diabetes*, is a disease in which the body is unable to regulate glucose in the blood, or *blood sugar*. Diabetes is characterized by **hyperglycemia**, or high blood sugar, which has serious health consequences. Type 1 and type 2 diabetes mellitus have different underlying causes. Both types can lead to health complications if left untreated (**Figure 20.17**).

Type 1 Diabetes Mellitus

type 1 diabetes mellitus autoimmune disease in which the body's immune system destroys insulin-producing cells, decreasing levels of insulin and increasing blood sugar; also called *juvenile-onset diabetes* or *insulin-dependent diabetes*

autoimmune disease type of disease in which the body's immune system attacks its own tissues

insulin hormone that signals cells to move sugar from the blood into surrounding cells; produced by the pancreas

acidosis condition of excess acid in the blood; can lead to coma or death

Type 1 diabetes mellitus is also known as *juvenile-onset diabetes* or *insulin-dependent diabetes*. Type 1 diabetes mellitus can develop at any age, but usually develops between 10 and 14 years of age. Type 1 diabetes mellitus is an **autoimmune disease**, or a disease in which the body's immune system attacks and damages the body's own tissues. It develops because the body's immune system destroys insulin-producing cells in the pancreas. Risk factors include genetics or viral infections.

In type 1 diabetes mellitus, the body becomes unable to make the hormone **insulin**, which the pancreas normally produces. Insulin instructs cells to move sugar from the blood into other cells. Without insulin, sugar remains in the blood, depriving cells of their main source of energy. Starving cells seek their energy from fat and protein. Using fat for energy produces a great deal of acid, which builds to toxic levels in the blood. **Acidosis**, or excess acid in the blood, is dangerous and can lead to coma and death if left untreated.

Common signs and symptoms of type 1 diabetes mellitus include excessive urination, thirst, hunger, and weight loss. As sugar builds up in the blood, the kidneys store extra sugar in the urine. The body loses a large amount of water with the sugar during urination, which triggers thirst.

Treatment for type 1 diabetes mellitus includes insulin, strict diet management, and physical activity. People with this disease must receive insulin through regular injections and monitor their own blood sugar.

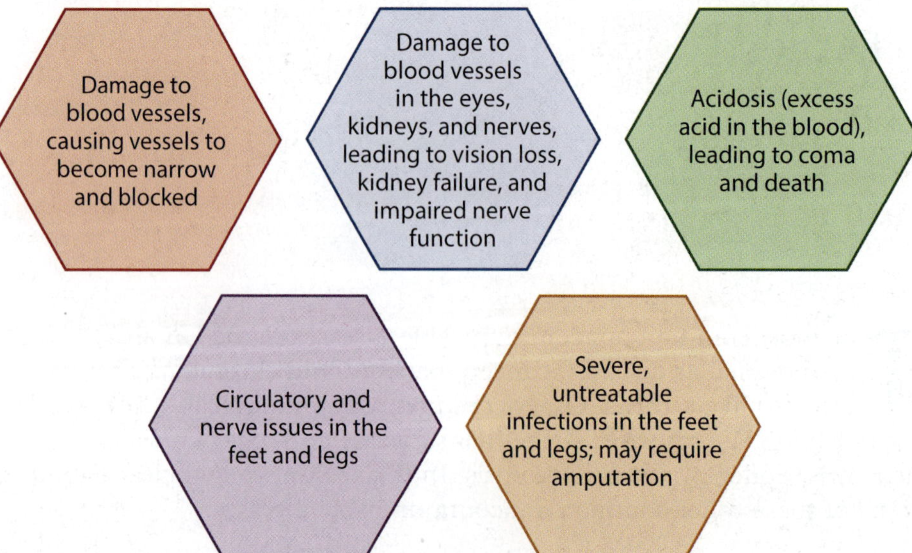

Figure 20.17 Diabetes mellitus can cause many different complications. *What is the term for high blood sugar?*

Some people have an insulin pump implanted in their abdomen that can adjust insulin levels in the bloodstream. They also manage their blood sugar by controlling the amount of food and sugars they eat and getting consistent, moderate physical activity.

Type 2 Diabetes Mellitus

Type 2 diabetes mellitus is also called *adult-onset diabetes* or *insulin-independent diabetes*. Type 2 diabetes mellitus often develops later in life and is associated with obesity. The underlying cause of type 2 diabetes mellitus is *insulin resistance*, meaning the pancreas produces insulin normally, but the body's cells do not respond to insulin. As type 2 diabetes mellitus progresses, the pancreas becomes less able to make insulin, and the liver produces extra sugar. The overall result is high blood sugar, low levels of insulin, and signs and symptoms similar to type 1 diabetes mellitus.

type 2 diabetes mellitus disease in which the body's cells become resistant to insulin, increasing blood sugar; also called *adult-onset diabetes* or *insulin-independent diabetes*

Risk factors for type 2 diabetes mellitus include a family history of the disease, advanced age, obesity, physical inactivity, high blood pressure, and high cholesterol. To help prevent this disease from developing, people can decrease their modifiable risk factors—by being more physically active, for example. Treatment includes modifying diet, managing weight, and taking medications to assist cells with insulin usage. Some people also need insulin injections or other medications if they cannot control the disease with diet and weight management.

Research in Action

Improving Diabetes Treatment

Type 1 and type 2 diabetes mellitus have different causes and some different treatments. Type 1 diabetes mellitus can occur at any age, but is usually first detected in children. Though currently incurable, it can be treated with insulin. In the past, type 2 diabetes mellitus usually affected middle-age adults. Today, type 2 diabetes mellitus is growing more common among teens, young adults, and even younger children. Fortunately, recent research may improve treatments for both type 1 and type 2 diabetes mellitus.

Scientists have found white blood cells known as *T cells* inside the pancreas of people living with type 1 diabetes mellitus. This discovery shows that type 1 diabetes mellitus is an autoimmune disease, in which the immune system attacks the body's organs. In type 1 diabetes mellitus, T cells attack cells in the pancreas that normally make insulin. Scientists have been studying how to control the activities of T cells. One day, it may be possible to treat type 1 diabetes mellitus with medications that turn off destructive T cells.

Type 2 diabetes mellitus is often treated with a combination of diet, lifestyle, physical activity, and medications. A few medications lower the amount of sugar in the blood. Others reduce high blood pressure, and some medications protect cells from the damaging effects of high blood pressure. Recent, promising research aims to develop medications that alter a person's metabolism and the way cells use energy. This approach is not a cure, but may prevent the buildup of sugar in the blood.

Practice Your Skills

Access Information

In a small group, use reliable and valid resources to research the most common noncommunicable diseases among teens. Make a list of these diseases and compare how common they are in teens compared to other age groups. Be sure to evaluate and cite your sources. Present your findings to the class and lead a class discussion about factors that might explain how common these diseases are among teens.

Alzheimer's Disease (AD)

Alzheimer's disease (AD) disease of the brain characterized by dementia, an incurable loss of memory and thinking skills

Alzheimer's disease (AD) is a brain disease characterized by *dementia* (loss of memory and thinking skills). Over time, people living with AD lose memory, thinking, communication, and speaking skills. They also lose control over emotions, especially anger and aggression, and become confused and lost. AD is a *progressive disease*, which means it grows worse over time. Eventually, people lose the ability to eat and care for themselves. It is estimated AD is the third leading cause of death among older adults in the US.

The cause of AD remains unknown. AD causes the brain to shrink and may cause microscopic *plaques* (abnormal clumps of proteins among nerve cells) in the brain. AD is most common in people over 60 years of age, and risk for AD increases with age. Some forms of AD may have a genetic cause. Other risk factors for AD include high blood pressure and cholesterol, brain injury, obesity, smoking, and sleep deprivation.

Medications can ease some of its symptoms, but do not stop AD from progressing. The number of cases of AD is expected to increase steadily as the US population continues to age.

Epilepsy

epilepsy brain disorder characterized by seizures, or interruptions in brain signals; also called *seizure disorder*

Epilepsy, also called *seizure disorder*, is a chronic noncommunicable disease that affects the brain. Epilepsy may be the most common noncommunicable disease of the brain. In fact, the Centers for Disease Control and Prevention (CDC) estimates more than five million people in the US have epilepsy. Often, the cause of epilepsy is unknown, although epilepsy can develop due to other conditions that affect the brain.

Epilepsy causes *seizures*, or interruptions in the usual signaling among brain cells (**Figure 20.18**). Severe epilepsy can interfere with school activities and affect school performance. Epilepsy might also interfere with driving or walking. Often, the seizures associated with epilepsy can be managed with medications.

Arthritis

arthritis disease in which the joints become inflamed, or swollen and painful

Arthritis is a condition characterized by *inflammation*, or pain and swelling, in the joints. Arthritis can cause people to move slowly and stiffly to avoid pain. There are many types of arthritis, each with different causes, treatments, and outcomes.

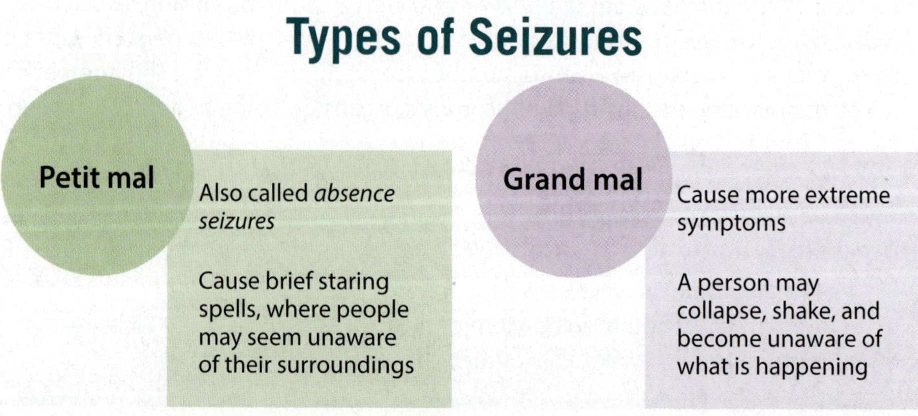

Figure 20.18 Both petit mal and grand mal seizures tend to last from a few seconds to a few minutes.

Osteoarthritis

Osteoarthritis is the most common form of arthritis among adults. It develops as the cartilage that normally pads the surfaces of bones wears down. The bones in joints then come in contact with each other, triggering pain, swelling, and stiffness. Anti-inflammatory medications, pain medications, and mild physical activity can help treat symptoms. Severely damaged joints may require surgery or replacement with an artificial joint.

osteoarthritis disease in which the cartilage normally padding the surfaces of bones wears down, causing swelling and pain

Rheumatoid Arthritis

Rheumatoid arthritis occurs in adults of all ages and is more common in females than males. It affects the joints and usually begins in the hands and feet. It can also affect other parts of the body, including the eyes, heart, lungs, skin, liver, and nervous system. Rheumatoid arthritis is an autoimmune disease of unknown cause. The immune system attacks the joints, causing them to swell painfully. Pain and swelling often come and go, in flare-ups followed by periods of remission. Over time, the damage from this disease can cause crippling changes in the joints. Treatment for rheumatoid arthritis includes anti-inflammatory medications, pain medications, and mild physical activity. Certain medications also target the immune system and block its attack on the joints.

rheumatoid arthritis autoimmune disease in which the body's immune system attacks the joints, causing swelling and pain

Gout

Gout is another type of arthritis that occurs in some aging adults. Gout causes sudden, painful swelling of joints, especially in the feet and big toe. The affected joint may make walking difficult. A family history of gout increases a person's risk of developing the disease. Diets rich in purines (found in red meat, anchovies, and asparagus) and alcoholic beverages can also trigger gout. Medications can significantly reduce pain and swelling.

gout disease characterized by sudden, painful swelling of joints, especially in the feet and big toe

Osteoporosis

Osteoporosis is a disease characterized by weak, brittle bones. During aging, it is normal for healthy bone to lose some strength and thickness. Osteoporosis causes a faster and more severe loss of bone strength. This disease affects both males and females, but most often occurs in females.

osteoporosis disease that makes bones weak, brittle, and prone to fractures

Osteoporosis develops over time and usually causes few symptoms. Most people do not know they have osteoporosis until they experience a bone fracture. In osteoporosis, even minor falls can cause fractures in the wrists, hips, and spine. Other signs and symptoms include losing height as the spine's bones compress and back pain from small spinal fractures and compressed spinal bones.

The risk for osteoporosis is greater in females with smaller bodies, Asian or Caucasian descent, or a family history of the disease. Other risk factors include an inactive lifestyle, tobacco use, alcohol consumption, and a diet low in calcium. Teens and young people can reduce their risk of osteoporosis later in life by decreasing modifiable risk factors—for example, by getting plenty of physical activity. Weight-bearing activities, such as walking, jogging, dancing, and lifting weights, can reduce risk by stimulating bones to grow thick and strong.

The bone changes of osteoporosis cannot be reversed. Medications, lifestyle, and diet can slow the progress of the disease, however. Early prevention, beginning in the teen years, is the key to healthy bones later in life.

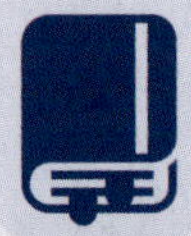

Case Study

Dealing with Illness

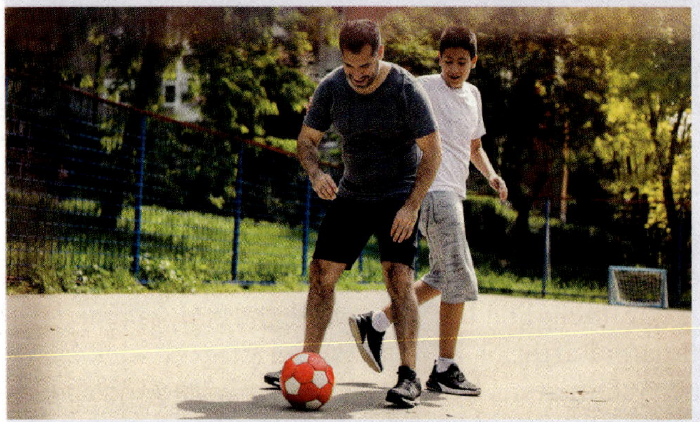

Sladic/E+/Getty Images

Cayden recently witnessed his dad having a heart attack. In the moment, Cayden was terrified and did not know what to do. His mom jumped into action to perform CPR and told Cayden to call 911. They rushed his dad to the hospital. After treatment, the doctor informed Cayden and his family that his dad would be okay. The doctor said his dad would need to monitor his cholesterol levels and get more physical activity. To help his dad adjust to this new lifestyle, Cayden asks his dad to play soccer with him after school. Cayden's family also eats more white meat, fish, and vegetables to lower his dad's cholesterol.

Mr. Perez, the English teacher at Olivia's former middle school, was diagnosed with leukemia a few months ago. Olivia and her friends loved Mr. P as a teacher and were not the only former students who felt this way. When they hosted a 5K fundraiser in Mr. P's honor, it seemed like the entire neighborhood came out to support him. The 5K raised awareness about blood cancers, and the proceeds are helping Mr. P cover the costs of treatment.

Julia was diagnosed with type 1 diabetes mellitus last year. Now, she has to monitor her blood sugar and get physical activity to control her insulin levels. She also has to inject insulin several times per day. Since her diagnosis, Julia has a hard time balancing her health with her social life. When her friends invite her out, she needs to make sure she has enough insulin to make it through the day. She has to be careful not to eat too much sugar. Julia's friends try to be understanding, but are often uncomfortable when Julia injects herself. As Julia adapts to her disease, she has become more comfortable with the way she has to accommodate it to stay healthy.

Practice Your Skills

Advocate for Health

In small groups, choose one of the following noncommunicable diseases: cardiovascular disease, type 2 diabetes mellitus, skin cancer, or lung cancer. Using the information in this chapter and additional resources, research the behavioral risk factors associated with this disease. Together, make a digital poster or animation describing ways to prevent or help treat this disease through changes in behavior. Target teens by making your poster or animation creative, colorful, and engaging. Share your poster or animation with the class.

Allergies

allergy condition in which the body's immune system reacts to a harmless substance like it is a dangerous or disease-causing invader

An **allergy** is a condition in which the body's immune system reacts to a harmless substance like it is a dangerous or disease-causing invader. The substance the immune system reacts to is an *allergen*. Examples of allergens include plant pollen, venom from bee stings, mold, dander, dust, peanuts, or shellfish. An allergen typically enters the body through the mouth, nose, or skin. An *allergic reaction* occurs when the immune system reacts to the allergen. Often, genetics lead to the development of an allergy.

histamine chemical that causes blood vessels to leak fluids into tissues

The effects of an allergic reaction can range from merely annoying to deadly. In an allergic reaction, cells release several chemicals, including **histamine**, which causes blood vessels to leak fluids into tissues. These fluids cause swelling known as *edema*. In the nasal passages, edema causes congestion, irritation, and a runny nose. On the skin, edema causes itchy red spots and bumps called *hives*.

Some allergies are *local*, or restricted to specific organs. For example, the allergy known as *hay fever* mainly affects the respiratory system and eyes. Allergies that affect the entire body are *systemic*. An example of a systemic allergy is the reaction to peanuts. Systemic allergies can cause *anaphylaxis*, a medical emergency in which the lungs fill with fluid and the air passages constrict, blocking breathing and lowering blood pressure to dangerous levels.

People who have severe allergies often carry an emergency supply of epinephrine preloaded in an *EpiPen*®. *Epinephrine* is a chemical that stimulates the heart to beat strongly and restore blood pressure. This reduces the severity of an allergic reaction.

Asthma

Asthma is a respiratory disease in which air passages constrict and fill with mucus, making it difficult to breathe (**Figure 20.19**). Membranes in the airways swell, blocking airflow even more and trapping stale air in the lungs. This triggers wheezing.

Genetics and environment play a role in the development of asthma. People with asthma may also have allergies that can trigger asthma symptoms. Other causes of asthma include anxiety, exertion, infection, and airborne chemicals like those in perfumes. Genetics play a role because asthma often runs in families.

Medications can reduce the number and severity of asthma attacks. In the midst of an asthma attack, people inhale certain medications through *rescue inhalers* to relax the airways quickly. Other asthma medications assist with long-term prevention of asthma attacks.

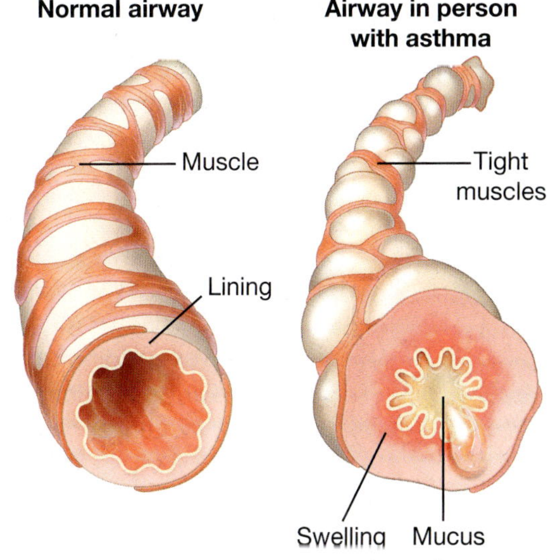

Figure 20.19 During an asthma attack, the muscles surrounding the bronchi tighten, and the bronchial lining swells.

Lesson 20.4 Review

Know and Understand

1. Explain the difference between how type 1 and type 2 diabetes mellitus affect the body.
2. Which form of arthritis is an autoimmune disease?
3. How do people typically find out they have osteoporosis?
4. How does airflow become blocked during an asthma attack?

Think Critically

5. What challenges do you think are unique to Alzheimer's disease, compared to other noncommunicable diseases?
6. What allergens are common in your community? How do these allergens affect people with allergies?

REAL WORLD Health Skills

Practice Health-Enhancing Behaviors Some people have difficulty adjusting to life with a noncommunicable disease. In a small group, brainstorm ways people can stay healthy physically, mentally and emotionally, and socially after being diagnosed with a noncommunicable disease. Include information about community resources for people with noncommunicable diseases. Share the strategies you identify with the class.

Chapter 20 Review and Assessment

Chapter Summary

Noncommunicable diseases develop due to genes, diet, behaviors, and other factors. Unlike communicable diseases, noncommunicable diseases do not spread through contact with living organisms or objects. Treatment for noncommunicable diseases usually involves a combination of methods, including behavioral changes, medications, and therapy. The goals and effects of different treatments vary.

Cardiovascular diseases affect the heart and blood vessels. They include arteriosclerosis and atherosclerosis, hypertension, heart attack, stroke, congestive heart failure, arrhythmias, and mitral valve prolapse. Some strategies for preventing cardiovascular diseases include being physically active, eating a healthy diet, maintaining a healthy body weight, avoiding harmful substances, and managing stress. Treatment methods for cardiovascular disease include insertion of a stent, bypass surgery, and various medications, such as blood thinners and diuretics.

Cancer is a complex disease characterized by an uncontrolled growth of abnormal cells. When these abnormal cells reproduce, they can form a mass called a tumor, and tumors can be malignant or benign. When cancer cells metastasize, they spread to other parts of the body.

Interactions between a person's genes, environment, and behavior cause cancer to develop. Cancer prevention involves adopting behaviors that reduce the risk of cancer. Often, this means changing habits, including those related to physical activity and diet. It also involves avoiding carcinogens and environments that increase the risk of cancer.

Early detection of cancer allows early treatment and better chances for recovery and survival. Cancer treatment methods include surgery and chemotherapy, as well as other types of therapy. Usually, a combination of treatments is more effective than any treatment alone.

While the most common noncommunicable diseases in the US are cardiovascular diseases, cancer, diabetes, and chronic respiratory diseases like asthma, other common noncommunicable diseases include allergies, arthritis, Alzheimer's disease and other kinds of dementia, epilepsy, and osteoporosis.

Vocabulary Activity

Write a brief scene in which 5–10 terms from the chapter are used by medical professionals in a real-life context. Then rewrite the dialogue using simpler sentences and transitions, as though you were describing the same scene to another student. Read both scenes to the class and ask for feedback on whether the two scenes were appropriate for their target audiences.

acidosis	*cancer*	*heart attack*	*relapse*
allergy	*capillaries*	*histamine*	*remission*
Alzheimer's disease (AD)	*cardiovascular diseases*	*homeostasis*	*rheumatoid arthritis*
angina	*chemotherapy*	*hyperglycemia*	*stent*
arrhythmias	*colonoscopy*	*hypertension*	*stroke*
arteries	*complications*	*insulin*	*tumor*
arteriosclerosis	*congestive heart failure*	*malignant tumors*	*type 1 diabetes mellitus*
arthritis	*coronary arteries*	*mammograms*	*type 2 diabetes mellitus*
atherosclerosis	*diabetes mellitus*	*metastasize*	*valves*
autoimmune disease	*epilepsy*	*noncommunicable diseases*	*veins*
benign tumors	*family history*	*osteoarthritis*	
biopsy	*gout*	*osteoporosis*	
blood pressure		*prognosis*	

Review and Recall

Review the information in this chapter by answering the following questions.

1. Which of the following is a period of time without signs and symptoms associated with a disease?
   A. relapse
   B. remission
   C. complication
   D. recurrence
2. What are three methods a doctor may use to diagnose a noncommunicable disease?
3. What is the difference between acute and chronic illness?
4. Which type of blood vessels returns blood from the body's capillaries to the heart?
   A. coronary arteries
   B. aortas
   C. veins
   D. arteries
5. What is the medical term for the chest pain that often accompanies a heart attack?
6. In which disease does blood flow backward into the atrium of the heart because of a defective valve?
7. List three types of therapy that can be used to treat cancer.
8. How do carcinogens cause cancer?
9. Which of the following is a sign or symptom of cancer?
   A. change in bowel or bladder habits
   B. unusual bleeding or discharge
   C. a sore that does not heal
   D. All of the above.
10. Which hormone is needed to instruct cells to take in glucose from the blood?
    A. insulin
    B. cortisol
    C. progesterone
    D. adrenaline
11. Describe the difference between local and systemic allergies.
12. Which chemical causes blood vessels to leak fluids into tissues during an allergic reaction?
13. Why are rescue inhalers used during an asthma attack?

Standardized Test Prep

Reading and Writing Practice

Read the passage below and then answer the following questions.

Cancer is a noncommunicable disease that affects people of all ages. In fact, each year in the US, about 70,000 people ages 15–39 are diagnosed with cancer. Among people 15–24 years of age, the most common cancers are leukemia, lymphoma, testicular cancer, and thyroid cancer.

Because cancer is relatively rare among teens and young adults, finding specialized treatment is important. For some types of cancer, young people may have better outcomes with pediatric treatments, or treatments used for children. Young people with cancer may feel alone with the new diagnosis. Counseling and support groups can help young people cope.

14. Which statement best summarizes this passage?
    A. Cancer is more common in young adults than older adults.
    B. Cancer is harder for younger people.
    C. Cancer can affect young people and pose unique challenges.
    D. Young people have trouble coping with cancer.
15. What are the most common cancers among people 15–24 years of age?
16. What is the meaning of the term *pediatric*?
    A. immature
    B. related to children
    C. childish
    D. specialized

Chapter 20 Skills Assessment

Critical Thinking Skills

Answer the following questions to assess your knowledge of what you learned in this chapter.

1. Think about the behaviors that impact your likelihood of developing a noncommunicable disease. Create a table where one column lists your choices that can help lower your risk of developing a noncommunicable disease, and the other column lists choices that increase your risk of developing a noncommunicable disease.
2. Consider the noncommunicable diseases represented in your family tree. What steps can you take to protect yourself from developing these diseases? What resources are available in your school and community to support early detection of these diseases?
3. Have you ever experienced fear of interacting with someone who has a noncommunicable disease? Explain how this fear is unfounded and how it can be overcome.
4. Explain why arteriosclerosis and atherosclerosis are central to the development of heart diseases.
5. Compare the ways in which fast, slow, and irregular heartbeats can affect the heart. Which do you think would cause the most damage, and why?
6. Create a chart that includes one column for each of the strategies for preventing cardiovascular diseases listed in the chapter. For each strategy, list a specific action you can take to apply the strategy.
7. Compare and contrast the symptoms of a heart attack and stroke. How would you respond differently to each?
8. Are there any health risks associated with benign tumors? Explain your answer.
9. Why is it important to be attentive to even one of the signs or symptoms listed in the *CAUTION* acronym?
10. Select one cancer-related organization to research. What is the history of the organization? What activities is this organization involved in? How could a teen get involved in or contribute to the mission of this organization?
11. Can you think of any communicable diseases that can increase the risk of developing a noncommunicable disease, or vice versa? Discuss your answer with a partner.
12. Which diseases do you think are increasing in frequency, and which ones do you think are decreasing in frequency? Use reliable sources to check your answer. What are some factors that might contribute to what you discovered?
13. Choose one of the noncommunicable diseases discussed in this chapter and use reliable sources to research advancements in treatment of the disease you chose. How do you think treatment of this disease will progress in the future?
14. Choose one of the noncommunicable diseases discussed in this chapter and imagine living with this disease. Create several journal entries describing what life is like living with this disease.

Health and Wellness Skills

Complete the following activities to assess your skills related to health and wellness.

15. **Analyze Influences.** Create a diagram of your family tree that includes your biological siblings, parents, grandparents, and great-grandparents. Then, interview your family members to determine what genetic, environmental, and behavioral risk factors have contributed to disease in your family. Include these risk factors on your family tree diagram. You can also work with a doctor to complete this activity.
16. **Access Information.** Diagnosis of a noncommunicable disease can be scary, no matter the person's age. Using reliable and valid resources, research community and online resources for people adjusting to a new diagnosis and coping with noncommunicable diseases. Include how these resources help and identify any resources that target teens. Share your list of resources with the class.

17. **Communicate with Others.** Making healthy decisions that reduce risk for noncommunicable diseases often requires cooperation from a person's whole family. Identify one lifestyle change you would like to make based on what you learned in this chapter. Then, outline how you could talk about this lifestyle change with your family members to get support and accountability. After outlining your talking points, have this conversation using effective communication and negotiation skills.
18. **Make Decisions.** Imagine that a family friend is over at your home and is acting strangely. He is sweating even though the room is cool, seems short of breath, and complains of pain in his left arm. Use the decision-making process to determine what course of action you should take next.
19. **Set Goals.** Create a plan of action for preventing one noncommunicable disease discussed in this chapter. List the behaviors you already practice to reduce your risk. What additional steps could you take to prevent this disease? Write a specific and detailed plan and schedule for at least one behavior you could engage in to reduce your risk.
20. **Practice Health-Enhancing Behaviors.** A sedentary lifestyle and poor diet contribute to many noncommunicable diseases. For the next week, keep a log of all the physical activity you get and everything you eat or drink. At the end of the week, highlight in green any behaviors that could help reduce your risk for noncommunicable diseases. Highlight in red areas where you could change your behavior to better reduce your risk. Repeat this process for the following week and work toward having more green than red highlights. Write a summary of how you can continue to practice healthy behaviors.
21. **Advocate for Health.** Create a pamphlet explaining the risk factors for cardiovascular disease and ways people can reduce their risk. Include information about a person's diet, physical activity habits, and use of hazardous substances. Include both text and visuals in your pamphlet. Arrange to distribute this pamphlet through a local organization such as a community health center, senior center, or library.

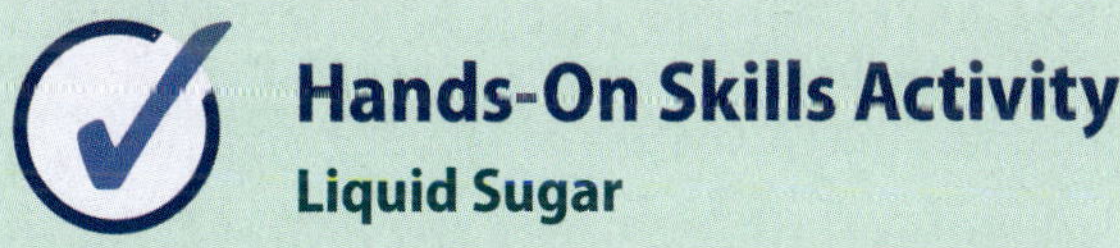

Hands-On Skills Activity

Liquid Sugar

Eating and drinking large amounts of sugar increases a person's risk of developing type 2 diabetes mellitus. This activity will examine just how much sugar is in some popular soft drinks. For this activity, you will need four to six empty drink containers with visible Nutrition Facts labels, small digital scales, bowls, small snack bags, 3 or more pounds of sugar, permanent markers, and poster board.

Steps for This Activity

1. Gather in groups of four to six students. Decide who will bring the required drink containers.
2. The World Health Organization (WHO) recommends that adults obtain less than 5 percent of their daily calories from sugar. This equals about 25 grams of sugar for the average adult. Use a scale to measure out 25 grams of sugar. Then, place the sugar in a snack bag and label it *WHO recommendation for daily sugar intake, 25 g*.
3. In your groups, compare the drink containers you brought. Without looking at the Nutrition Facts labels, predict the grams of sugar in each drink and rank them from least sugary to most sugary.
4. **Access Information.** Next, look at each drink's Nutrition Facts label to determine how many grams of sugar are in each bottle. Multiply the grams of sugar by the number of servings listed, if needed. Measure out the grams of sugar contained in each drink and place the sugar into snack bags with labels for each drink.
5. Compare each drink's sugar content with the WHO-recommended daily sugar intake. Are there any drinks that contain a greater amount of sugar than the WHO recommends for daily consumption?
6. **Practice Health-Enhancing Behaviors.** In your group, discuss how accurate your predictions were. Based on the WHO recommendation for daily sugar intake, which drinks should you avoid?

Unit 8

Human Development and Sexuality

Big Ideas

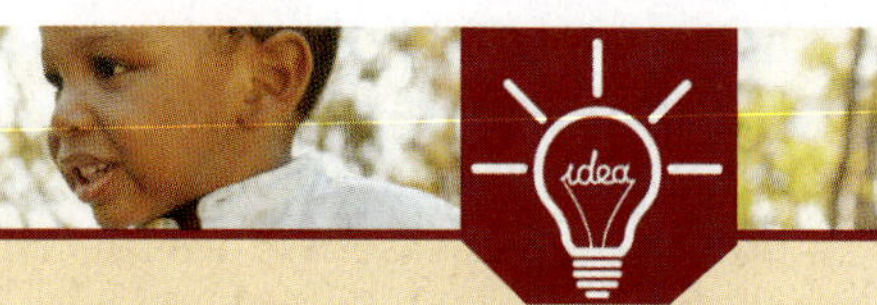

- Sperm are the male sex cells. During sexual intercourse, muscular contractions release sperm from the penis. Organs of the female reproductive system produce hormones and eggs, house a developing baby through pregnancy, and then expel the baby out of the body. Caring for the reproductive systems can help prevent diseases and disorders.
- During sexual intercourse, semen is released into the vagina. If a sperm meets an egg, conception occurs. The fertilized egg implants in the uterus and develops over the course of a pregnancy. Childbirth brings the baby out into the world.
- Teen pregnancy and parenthood affect teen parents, their children and families, and society. To prevent pregnancy, teens can remain sexually abstinent. Several contraceptive methods also reduce the risk of pregnancy.
- Over time, people develop physically, intellectually, emotionally, and socially. While people often reach milestones at certain ages, there are many differences in development.
- Children develop from infancy through the toddler, preschool, and middle-childhood years. In middle childhood, they begin attending school.
- During adolescence, people experience puberty. This time also brings intellectual changes and emotional and social adjustments. People continue to mature through young adulthood, middle adulthood, and older adulthood.
- Sexuality includes a person's biological sex, gender identity and expression, sexual orientation, and sexual experiences and thoughts. While biological sex is assigned at birth, gender identity develops over time. Sexual orientation is a person's enduring pattern of romantic and sexual attraction.
- Sexuality begins developing early in life. Many factors affect a person's sexual behavior, and sexual activity has physical, emotional, and social consequences.
- Contraception helps prevent pregnancy. Methods of contraception include sexual abstinence, barrier methods, hormonal methods, natural methods, and sterilization. These methods work in different ways to prevent the sperm from fertilizing an egg. Emergency contraception helps prevent pregnancy after sexual intercourse occurs.

Monkey Business Images/Shutterstock.com ▶

Health Management Plan ▸ Your Sexual Health and Development

Talking about sexual health and development can be hard and feel awkward. Maybe you feel uncomfortable discussing these topics or do not have much experience communicating about them. These elements of health are a natural and positive part of life, however. Learning to have conversations about them is an essential skill for maintaining your current and future health.

Open your health management plan. Create a new entry called "My Sexual Health and Development." Then, work through these steps to make a plan for promoting health in these areas.

1. Create a table like the one shown. In one column, write everything you think you know about sexual health, sexuality, and development. Also indicate where you received this knowledge—for example, from a doctor or online. In the second column, write the questions you have.

What I Think I Know	My Questions

2. Next, think about your future. List decisions you are making now or that you will need to make in the future regarding your sexual health and development. How will you make these decisions? How could these decisions impact your health?
3. Write down the five most important goals for your life. How will the decisions you make about sexual health and development affect these goals?
4. After reading this unit, come back to your answers. Revise your list of knowledge and questions by correcting any myths you believed and answering your questions. Explain how you will make decisions about sexual health and development now and in the future. Finally, make a plan for defending your goals.

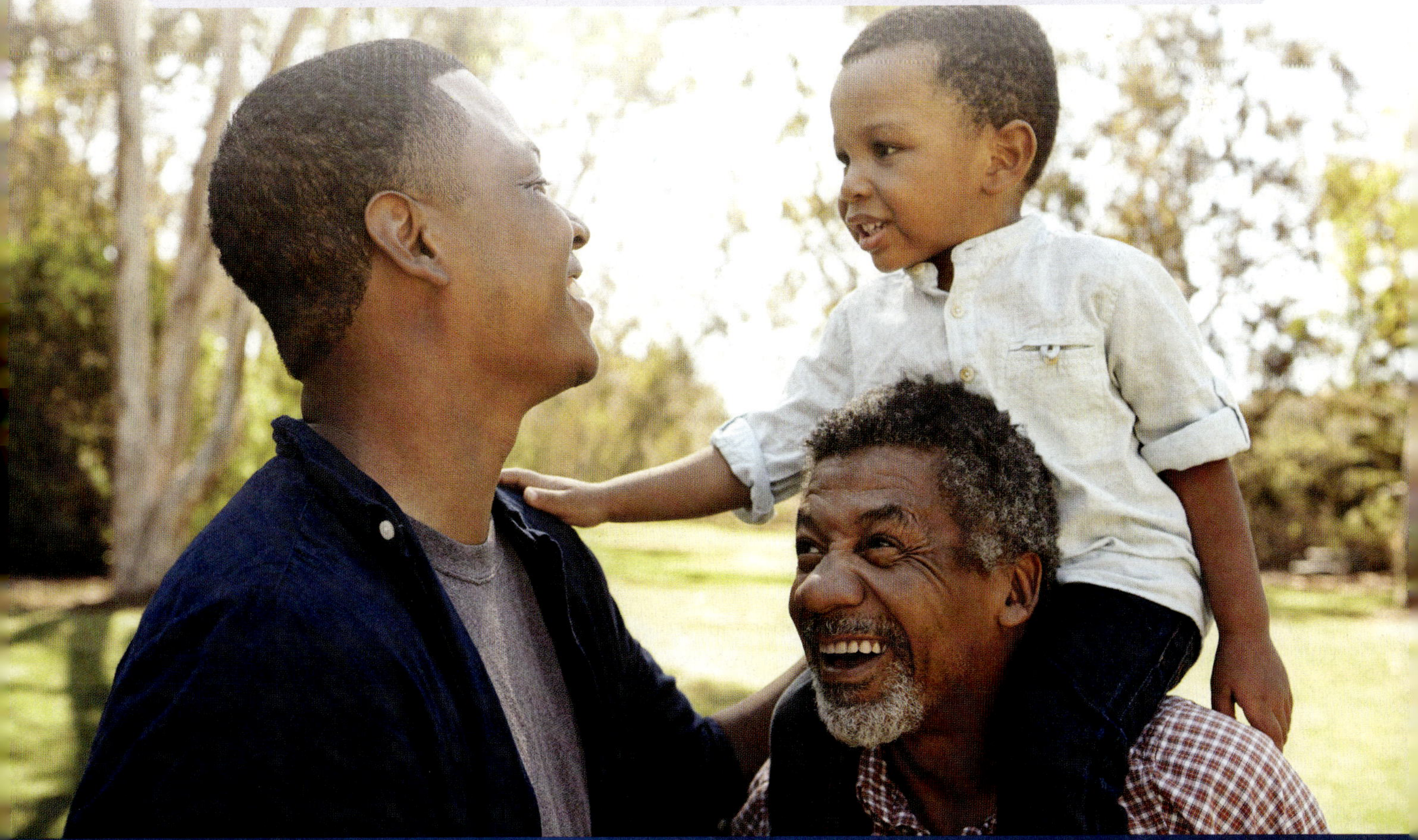

Chapter 21

The Beginning of Life

Look for the skills icon throughout this chapter for opportunities to practice your health skills.

Check Your Health and Wellness Skills

In this chapter, you will learn skills for taking care of your sexual health. To understand the skills you currently use, take the following inventory of your behaviors. Indicate how well you think you use each skill. Use a scale of 1–5, *1* meaning you do not use the skill and *5* meaning you feel completely comfortable using it.

Skill	How Well Do You Use Each Skill?
I can recognize common diseases and disorders of the reproductive system.	
I maintain reproductive hygiene.	
I ask my doctor if I have questions about sexual health.	
I visit the doctor if I notice concerning reproductive symptoms.	
I understand how the male and female reproductive systems work together to create new life.	
I know whom I'd talk to and what I'd say if I had questions about sex or pregnancy.	
I know how to access sexual health resources in my community.	
I show respect and support for teens who are pregnant or parenting.	
I have committed to remain sexually abstinent.	
I know what contraceptive methods help prevent pregnancy.	
	Total:

Add up your responses to each statement. The higher your score, the more comfortable you feel practicing health skills related to sexual health. Which skill do you think is most important for you? Which skill is the most challenging for you? Which skill would you most like to improve? In this chapter, you will learn how to perform these skills better and more often.

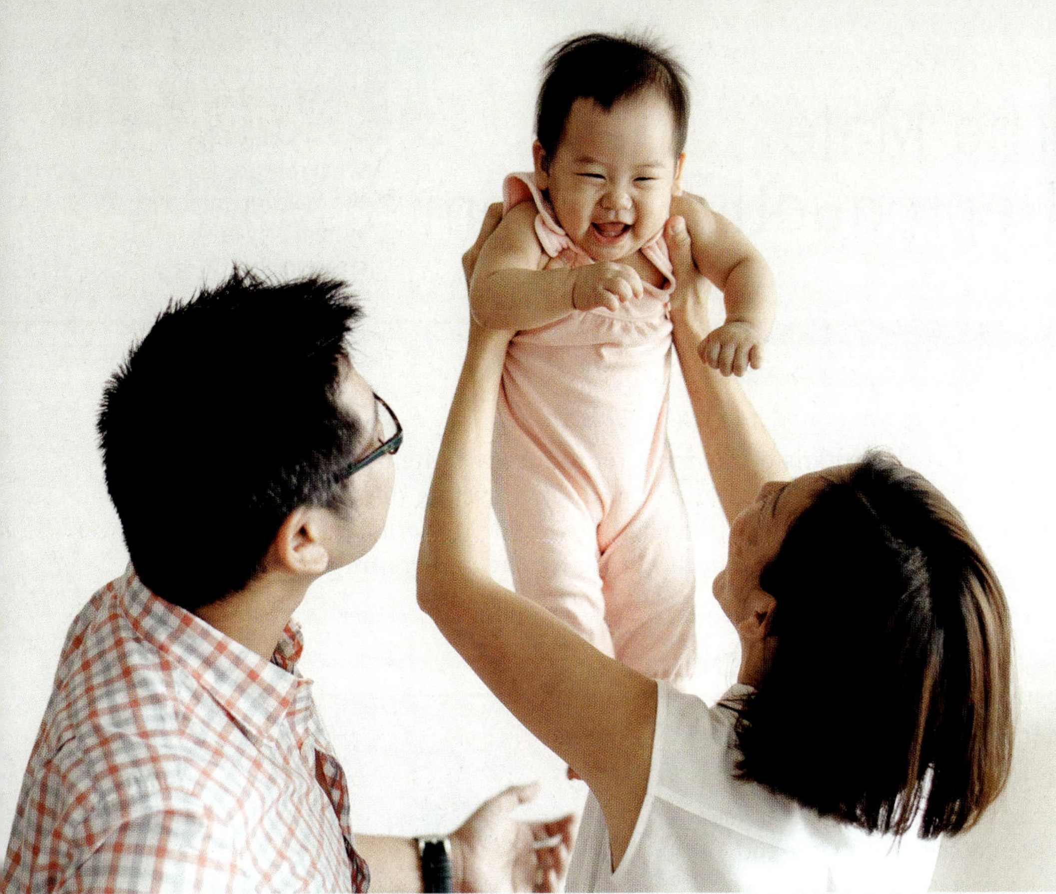

Rawpixel.com/Shutterstock.com

Reading and Notetaking

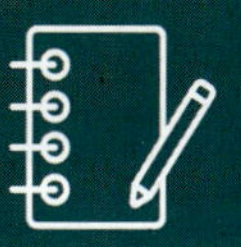

Throughout this chapter, you will read detailed descriptions of the reproductive systems. Specific terminology will help you picture and understand these systems. Before you read the chapter, list the key terms for each lesson and create a list of any key terms with which you are not familiar. Look up these terms in a dictionary or online. Write down the definitions in your own words. As you listen to your teacher present the chapter, revise your definitions as needed. Ask your teacher questions if terms are still unclear to you.

Terms	Definitions	Revised Definitions

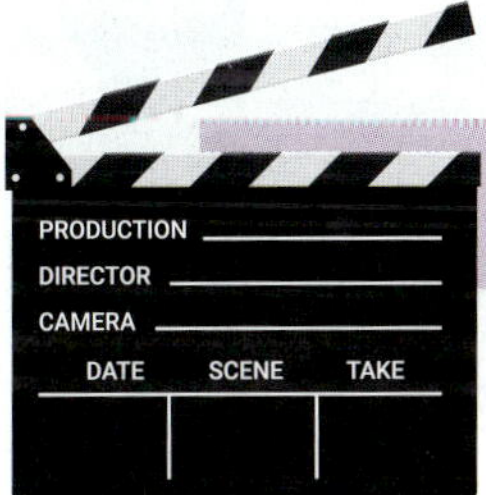

Setting the Scene

Getting to the Facts

This year, some of your friends are getting ready to graduate and go to college. These friends have dated a lot more than you and seem to know a lot about relationships and even sex. Sometimes, you hear your friends saying things about sex you are pretty sure are not true. When you ask questions, your friends say they read their facts online.

To be honest, you have your own questions about sex. You do not know whom to talk to though. You think the conversation would make your parents uncomfortable—or worse, make them worry you were sexually active. You would like to know how to take care of your sexual health. You just are not sure where to start.

Thinking Critically

1. Consider why many teens think conversations about sex will be awkward. How could these conversations be less awkward?
2. In this scenario, whom could you ask questions about your sexual health? Why would you trust this person?
3. What could you say to find out where your friends are getting their facts and help them find reliable information?

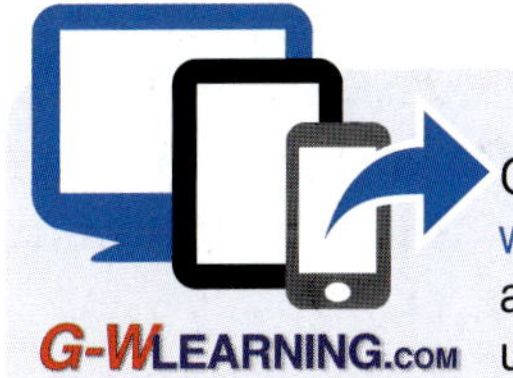

Click on the activity icon or visit www.g-wlearning.com/health/4095 to access online vocabulary activities using key terms from the chapter.

Lesson 21.1

The Male Reproductive System

Essential Question?

What role does the male reproductive system play in creating life?

Learning Outcomes

After studying this lesson, you will be able to

- identify the organs of the male reproductive system;
- analyze the role of the male reproductive system in producing new life;
- describe diseases and disorders of the male reproductive system; and
- explain the steps of properly caring for the male reproductive system.

Key Terms

ejaculation
erection
male reproductive system
penis
prostate
prostate cancer
semen
sexual reproduction
sperm
testes
testicular cancer
testicular self-examination
vas deferens

Warm-Up Activity

Sexual Health

Communicate with Others

Imagine that your little brother recently started puberty, and a lot of physical changes are happening to him. He values your opinion and listens to your advice. He wants to know what he can be doing to maintain his health during this time of change. Before reading this lesson, write down what you think your little brother should know about the male reproductive system. Write a script in which you explain these things using clear, effective communication. After reading, review your script to reflect the new information you learned.

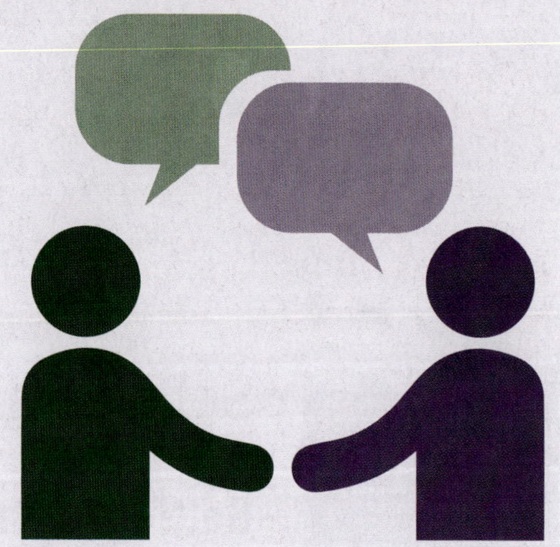

Vaclav Krivsky/Shutterstock.com

Reproduction is a fundamental characteristic of all living creatures. During **sexual reproduction**, the genetic material of two individuals combines to create a new individual.

sexual reproduction process in which the genetic material of two individuals combines to create a new individual

Each type of animal and plant possesses specialized organs for the complex process of reproduction. The human reproductive systems include organs that produce human *sex cells*, or sperm and eggs. In addition, humans have organs for sexual intercourse, which permits a sperm to *fertilize*, or combine with, an egg. The organs of the reproductive systems all play a role in producing new life. The male reproductive system contributes to this end by forming and delivering sperm.

Organs of the Male Reproductive System

The organs of the **male reproductive system** assist with the production and transport of hormones and sperm. These organs include the testes, penis, seminal vesicles, prostate, and vas deferens (**Figure 21.1**). Male sex cells, or **sperm**, are very small, made up of nothing more than a *flagellum* (tail) and a nucleus that contains half of the male's chromosomes.

Males enter *puberty*, or the time period in which reproductive organs mature, in their early teens. Males begin making sperm at puberty and continue to produce sperm throughout their lives.

male reproductive system body system consisting of organs that produce hormones and sperm and enable sexual intercourse; includes the testes, penis, seminal vesicles, prostate, and vas deferens

sperm male sex cells made up of a flagellum and nucleus; contain half of the male's chromosomes

testes organs suspended in the scrotum that produce sperm and testosterone

vas deferens tube that carries sperm from the epididymis to the penis

prostate organ that secretes fluid that mixes with sperm to create semen

semen mixture of fluid and sperm released during ejaculation

Testes and Vas Deferens

An early sign of puberty in males is growth of the **testes**, organs that produce sperm and the hormone testosterone. The two testes are suspended in the *scrotum*, a skin-covered, saclike structure. The testes contain tiny tubes called the *seminiferous tubules*, where sperm develop. When sperm mature, they enter the *epididymis*, a coiled tube along the outer wall of each testis. The epididymis leads into a tube called the **vas deferens**, which carries sperm to the penis.

Seminal Vesicles and Prostate

Located near the base of the urinary bladder, the *seminal vesicles* and **prostate** secrete fluid that mixes with sperm to form **semen**. Semen contains fluid that protects and nurtures sperm. The semen leaves the vas deferens and enters the urethra in the penis. The *urethra* is the tube that carries urine out of the body through the penis. Semen also passes through the urethra. Located beneath the prostate, two *bulbourethral glands* produce mucus to lubricate the urethra.

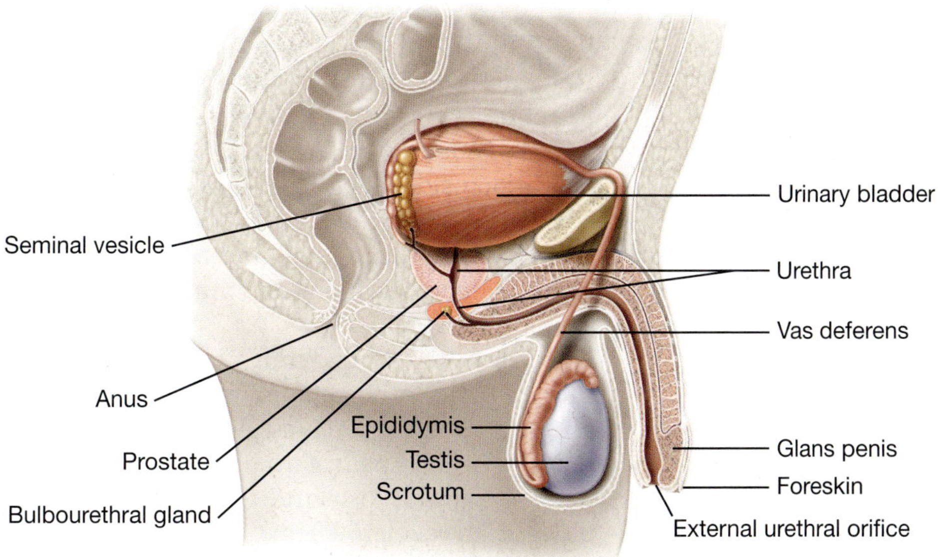

Figure 21.1 Side view of the male reproductive organs. Sperm form in the testes (one testis shown) and are carried to the penis by the vas deferens. The seminal vesicles and prostate secrete fluid to mix with the sperm and form semen. ***What are male sex cells called?***

Penis

penis male organ used in sexual activity; also part of the urinary system

The **penis** is the male organ used for sexual intercourse and is also part of the urinary system. The penis contains *erectile tissue*, or spongy tissue that fills with blood during sexual excitement. The expanded end of the penis is called the *glans penis* and is sensitive to sexual stimulation. A flap of loosely attached skin, called the *foreskin*, covers the glans penis. Sometimes, a procedure called *circumcision* removes this foreskin shortly after birth. This makes the penis easier to wash.

erection lengthening and hardening of the penis due to sexual stimulation; caused by blood flowing into the erectile tissue of the penis

ejaculation series of muscular contractions that forcefully eject semen out of the urethral opening of the penis

In males, sexual stimulation causes blood to flow into the erectile tissue of the penis and results in an **erection**. During vaginal intercourse, the erect penis is inserted into the vagina. Intense sexual stimulation causes contractions in the epididymis and vas deferens, propelling sperm into the urethra. Secretions from the seminal vesicles and prostate mix with the sperm, forming semen. **Ejaculation** occurs when muscular contractions forcefully eject semen out the *external urethral orifice* (opening). *Orgasm* (muscular contractions that cause a pleasurable feeling) usually accompanies ejaculation in males.

Semen contains nutrients for sperm and protects sperm from the acidic environment of the vagina. After ejaculation, sperm remain alive and capable of fertilization for 24–72 hours in the female reproductive tract. In the vagina, sperm swim within seminal fluid and make their way through the cervix, into the uterus, and up the fallopian tubes. The sperm usually meet the egg in the upper third of the fallopian tube.

Diseases and Disorders of the Male Reproductive System

Prostatitis

- Inflammation or infection of the prostate

Epididymitis

- Inflammation of the epididymis

Orchitis

- Inflammation of the testes

Cryptorchidism

- Failure of the testes to descend from the abdominal cavity into the scrotum

Testicular cancer

- Cancer in one or both testes

Prostate cancer

- Cancer in the prostate

Figure 21.2 Inflammation, cancer, and other disorders can disrupt the functions of the male reproductive system and cause serious symptoms.

Diseases and Disorders of the Male Reproductive System

Several diseases and disorders affect the male reproductive system (**Figure 21.2**). Understanding these diseases and disorders can help males recognize abnormal signs and symptoms if they arise.

- **Prostatitis:** Prostatitis is inflammation or infection of the prostate. It is also called *benign prostate hyperplasia (BPH)*. This condition usually begins in middle age. Signs and symptoms include lower back or groin pain, difficulty urinating, and blood in the urine. Pain medications and antibiotics can treat prostatitis.
- **Epididymitis:** Epididymitis is an inflammation of the epididymis. Signs and symptoms include testicular swelling, tenderness, and pain; scrotal pain; painful urination; fever; discharge from the penis; and blood in the semen. Urinary tract infections (UTIs) and a number of sexually transmitted infections (STIs) can cause epididymitis. This condition can be treated with antibiotics.

- **Orchitis:** Orchitis is an inflammation of the testes. The viral infection *mumps,* bacterial infections, or injury can cause orchitis. Signs and symptoms include sudden testicular swelling, pain, and tenderness; nausea and vomiting; fever; discharge from the penis; and prostate enlargement and tenderness. To prevent orchitis, males can receive a vaccination for mumps and use a protective cup during athletic activities.
- **Cryptorchidism:** Cryptorchidism is a failure of the testes to descend from the abdominal cavity into the scrotum. Cryptorchidism can cause infertility and testicular cancer. Treatment includes surgery or hormone therapy.
- **Testicular cancer:** **Testicular cancer** is cancer in one or both testes. Signs and symptoms include testicular swelling, a painless lump on a testicle, and aching in the lower abdomen or scrotum. Males can see a doctor and perform regular self-exams to detect testicular cancer.
- **Prostate cancer:** **Prostate cancer** is cancer in the prostate. The signs and symptoms resemble those of prostatitis. A male's age, 65 years or older, is the single most important risk factor for prostate cancer. Screening for prostate cancer includes a *digital rectal exam* (insertion of a finger into the rectum to feel the prostate) and a *prostate-specific antigen (PSA)* test, which measures the amount of a substance produced by the prostate in the blood.

testicular cancer abnormal cancerous growth in one or both testes

prostate cancer abnormal cancerous growth of the prostate; signs and symptoms resemble those of prostatitis

Caring for the Male Reproductive System

To maintain the health of the reproductive system, males can take several steps to prevent infection and detect any diseases and disorders. Both males and females can reduce risk for STIs by abstaining from sexual activity or using a condom or dental dam.

Practice Hygiene

To maintain hygiene, males should regularly clean the genitals and groin area (between the scrotum and inner thighs). Because this area often remains moist from sweat, bacteria and fungi can grow here. A fungal infection called *jock itch,* a form of *ringworm,* can develop. Males can prevent jock itch by maintaining hygiene, wearing cotton or breathable underwear, and changing underwear regularly.

When cleaning the genitals, males should wash around the head of the penis. Males who have not been circumcised should pull back the penis's foreskin to clean around this area. In practice and competition, males can wear a protective cup that encloses the scrotum and testes to prevent injury.

Perform Testicular Self-Examinations

During the teen years, males should begin to watch for signs of testicular cancer and hernia. Performing a **testicular self-examination** can help males become familiar with the testes' normal shape and size (**Figure 21.3**). With early detection, testicular cancer is treatable and curable. Testicular swelling can also be caused by an infection.

testicular self-examination process of checking the testes for lumps or changes in shape or texture

Steps of a Testicular Self-Examination

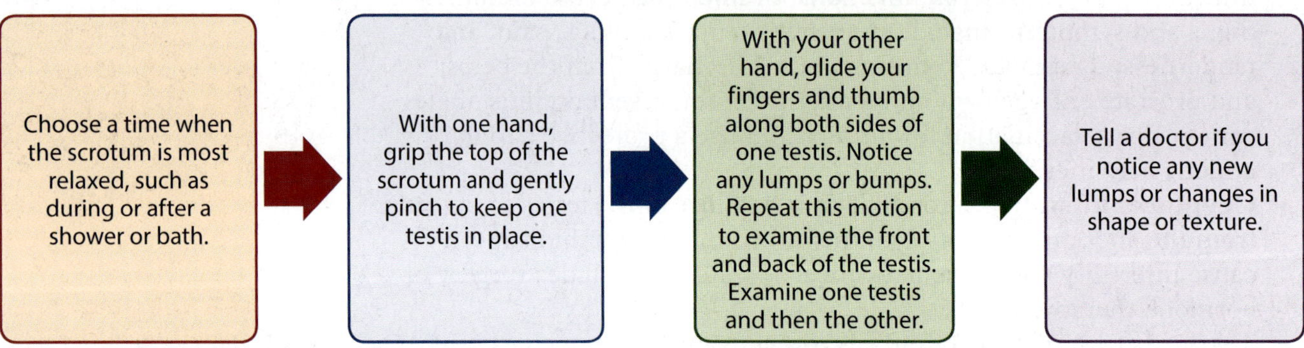

Figure 21.3 A testicular self-examination can help males detect testicular cancer in the early stages, while it is more treatable.

A change in the testes can also be a sign of an inguinal hernia. In an *inguinal hernia*, a portion of the intestine pokes through the abdominal wall into the scrotum. A doctor will need to press on the groin and touch the scrotum to feel for a hernia. If a hernia is detected, surgery can repair it so the intestine does not get injured and cause serious harm.

Visit the Doctor

It is important to visit the doctor regularly to ensure the health of the reproductive system. You should see a doctor right away if you have the following symptoms:

- burning or pain during urination
- blood or pus at the opening of the urethra
- pain or burning in the lower abdomen
- rashes or sores on the penis
- pain, swelling, or new lumps in the testes

Lesson 21.1 Review

Know and Understand

1. Which structures of the male reproductive system produce sperm prior to ejaculation?
2. What happens during an erection?
3. What screenings can help detect testicular and prostate cancer early?
4. What are the steps of a testicular self-examination?

Think Critically

5. What structures does the male reproductive system have in common with the male urinary system?
6. Choose one disease or disorder that affects the male reproductive system and explain how it might impact fertility.

REAL WORLD Health Skills

Access Information Although testicular cancer is rare in teens, it is the most common cancer in males between the ages of 15 and 35. It is important for males to perform a testicular self-examination every month so they can become familiar with the normal size and shape of the testes. Using valid and reliable resources, create a checklist a male could use each month to perform an effective examination. Cite your sources and explain why they are reliable.

The Female Reproductive System

Essential Question

What role does the female reproductive system play in creating life?

Lesson

21.2

Learning Outcomes

After studying this lesson, you will be able to

- explain how the organs of the female reproductive system work together to produce new life;
- describe the menstrual cycle;
- identify diseases and disorders of the female reproductive system; and
- explain the steps in properly caring for the female reproductive system.

Key Terms

breast cancer
breasts
cervix
clitoris
eggs
endometriosis
fallopian tube
female reproductive system
fibroids
labia
menstrual cycle
menstruation
obstetrician/gynecologist (OB/GYN)
ovarian cysts
ovaries
ovulation
premenstrual syndrome (PMS)
toxic shock syndrome (TSS)
uterus
vagina

Warm-Up Activity

Myth or Fact?

Comprehend Concepts Take a few moments to consider the statements about the female reproductive system shown. Your teacher will place a piece of paper with the word *Myth* on one side of the room and a piece of paper with the word *Fact* on the other side of the room. As your teacher reads a statement aloud, move to the *Myth* sign if you believe the statement is false or to the *Fact* sign if you believe the statement is true. Discuss your choice with the other students who made the same choice. Select a spokesperson to explain your decision to the class.

Female reproductive system disorders only affect older adults.	During menstruation, females are easily upset.
Sexually transmitted infections can lead to infertility in females.	Breast cancer is the second leading cause of cancer deaths in females.

The female reproductive system plays a vital role in producing new life. This body system produces female sex cells, called **eggs**, or *ova*, and houses and nurtures a developing baby. During childbirth, the female reproductive system delivers the baby out into the world. The organs of the female reproductive system also help care for a baby after birth.

eggs female sex cells that contain half of the female's chromosomes; stored in the ovaries; also called *ova*

Organs of the Female Reproductive System

female reproductive system body system consisting of organs that produce hormones and eggs, enable sexual intercourse, and nurture a baby; includes the ovaries, fallopian tubes, uterus, vagina, cervix, labia, clitoris, and breasts

The **female reproductive system** includes the ovaries, fallopian tubes, uterus, vagina, cervix, labia, clitoris, and breasts. The female reproductive organs have several functions. The ovaries make hormones. Other organs produce eggs and nurture a fertilized egg as it develops into a baby. Females also have organs for sexual intercourse.

Ovaries

ovaries two small, almond-shaped organs in the lower abdomen that contain thousands of immature eggs

The two **ovaries** are small, almond-shaped organs in the lower abdomen (**Figure 21.4**). Each ovary contains thousands of immature eggs. A single layer of nurturing cells, called a *follicle*, surrounds each egg. Each month, a single egg and its follicle grow toward maturity and are released into the nearby opening of the fallopian tube. Ovaries also make *progesterone* and *estrogen*, the female hormones that control sexual characteristics, the menstrual cycle, and pregnancy.

Fallopian Tubes

fallopian tube tube that leads from each ovary to each side of the uterus

One **fallopian tube** leads from each ovary to each side of the uterus. With the help of finger-like projections called *fimbriae*, the open ends of the fallopian tubes take in an egg as it is released from the ovary. If sperm are in the fallopian tube, fertilization may occur here. The fertilized egg then travels through the fallopian tube to the uterus.

Uterus

uterus hollow, muscular organ that houses the developing baby until it is born

The **uterus** is a hollow, muscular organ. The walls of the uterus contain strong, involuntary muscles and many blood vessels. A fertilized egg implants into the inner lining of the uterus, called the *endometrium*. The uterus then houses the developing baby throughout pregnancy until the baby is born.

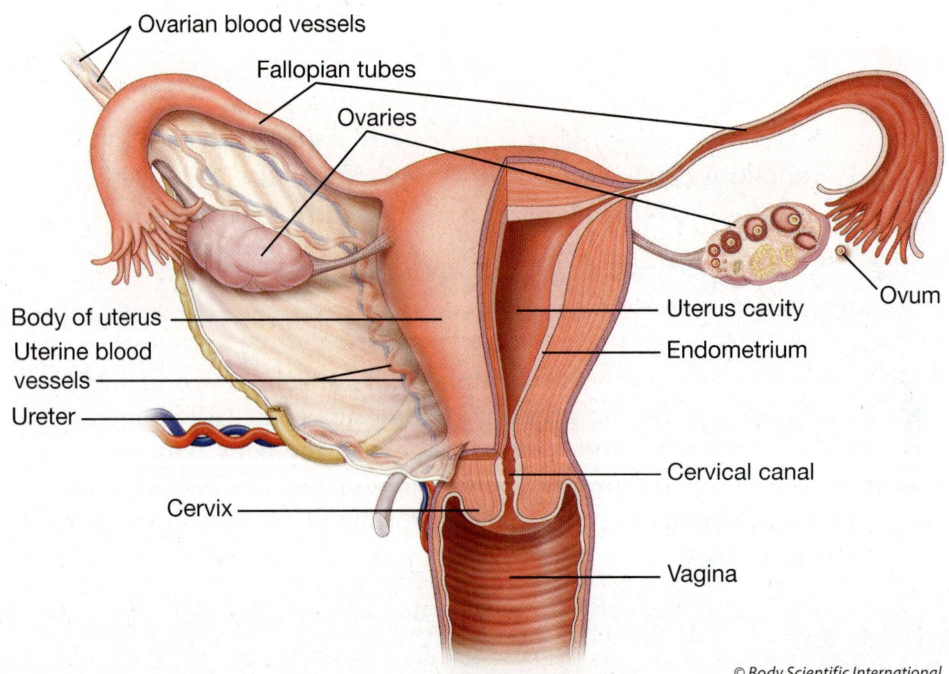

Figure 21.4 In the female reproductive system, eggs (ova) are produced in the ovaries and are then swept into the fallopian tubes. If sperm are deposited in the vagina and swim up to the fallopian tubes, then an egg (ovum) can be fertilized.

Vagina and Cervix

The uterus connects with the vagina through the **cervix**, a narrow passage lined with mucus. This passage *dilates*, or stretches wider, during childbirth.

The **vagina** is a tube-like structure lined with a moist membrane. Its external opening lies between the legs and leads inward and upward to the uterus. Two *greater vestibular glands* on either side of the vaginal opening secrete mucus to aid lubrication. The vagina is the female organ used for sexual intercourse and serves as the *birth canal*, or the passage through which a baby is delivered.

cervix narrow passage that connects the uterus to the vagina

vagina tube-like structure lined with a moist membrane that serves as the birth canal

Labia and Clitoris

On the outside of the female's body, the **labia** protect the vaginal opening (**Figure 21.5**). The labia begin at the *mons pubis*, a pad of fat tissue above the vaginal opening. From the mons pubis, the labia extend downward on each side of the vaginal opening, protecting this area. The outer, larger folds are called *labia majora* (singular *labium majus*), and the inner, smaller folds are the *labia minora* (singular *labium minus*).

Located above the vaginal opening, the **clitoris** contains *erectile tissue*, which is spongy and filled with many small spaces. During sexual arousal, blood flows into these spaces, causing the organ to swell and enlarge. Intense sexual stimulation leads to orgasm. Some females also experience *female ejaculation*, which is an emission of fluid from the urethra.

labia skin folds, including the labia majora and labia minora, that protect the vaginal opening

clitoris mass of erectile tissue that swells and enlarges during sexual arousal

Breasts

The **breasts** contain *mammary glands*, which produce milk after childbirth. Ducts of the milk glands meet and open at the nipple, which is surrounded by a darkly colored area known as the *areola*. Breasts are supported by connective tissue covered with fatty tissue and skin.

breasts structures containing mammary glands that produce milk after childbirth in females

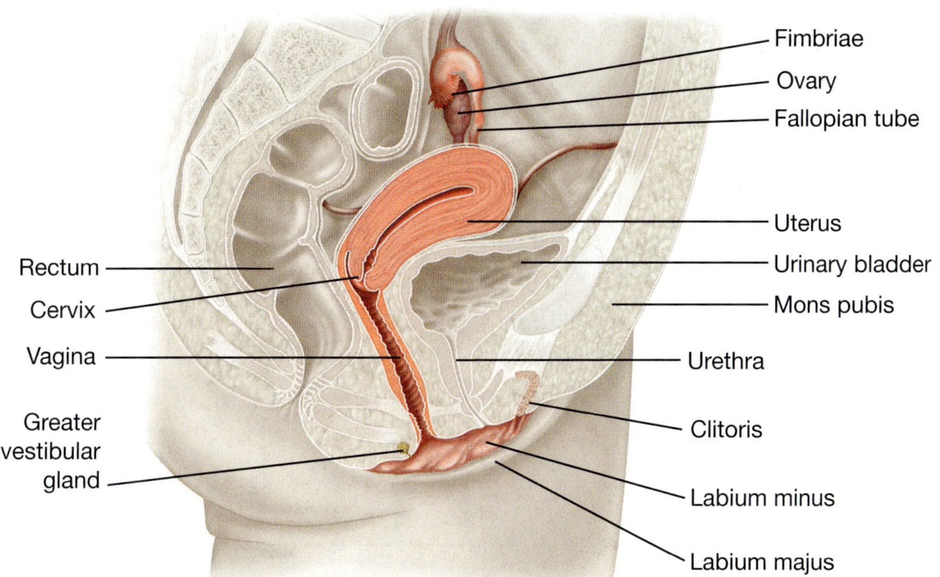

Figure 21.5 The external organs of the female reproductive system include the mons pubis, labia, and clitoris. Internal organs include the cervix, vagina, ovary, fallopian tube, and uterus. ***Which structure of the female reproductive system serves as the birth canal?***

The Menstrual Cycle

menstrual cycle sequence of body changes in females coordinated by the hormones estrogen and progesterone

ovulation release of a mature egg from one of the ovarian follicles

menstruation shedding of the endometrial lining of the uterus; blood and some tissues pass through the vagina

The **menstrual cycle** is a sequence of body changes coordinated by the hormones estrogen and progesterone (**Figure 21.6**). A female's first menstrual cycle, or *menarche*, generally occurs between 10 and 15 years of age. After puberty, females typically experience a menstrual cycle each month.

During the first half of the menstrual cycle, the ovaries secrete the hormone estrogen, which travels in the blood to the uterus. Estrogen stimulates the *endometrium*, or inner lining of the uterus, to thicken and develop more blood vessels. These changes prepare the uterus to deliver nutrients to a developing baby if pregnancy occurs. At the same time, ovarian follicles develop around immature eggs in the ovaries. At the midpoint of the menstrual cycle, ovulation occurs. **Ovulation** is the release of a mature egg from one of the ovarian follicles.

After ovulation, the empty ovarian follicle secretes the hormone progesterone, which stimulates endometrial growth. If pregnancy occurs, the empty follicle continues to make progesterone, which helps maintain the pregnancy. If pregnancy does not occur, progesterone secretion stops, and less estrogen is produced. Declining progesterone and estrogen mark the end of the menstrual cycle. At this point, low hormone levels cause menstruation.

Menstruation is the shedding of the endometrial lining of the uterus. Blood and some tissues from the uterus pass through the vagina out of the body during this time. Menstruation continues throughout a female's life span, except during pregnancy. It usually ends during *menopause*, when the ovaries stop releasing eggs in a female's late 40s or early 50s. Many females use calendars and apps to track their menstrual cycle.

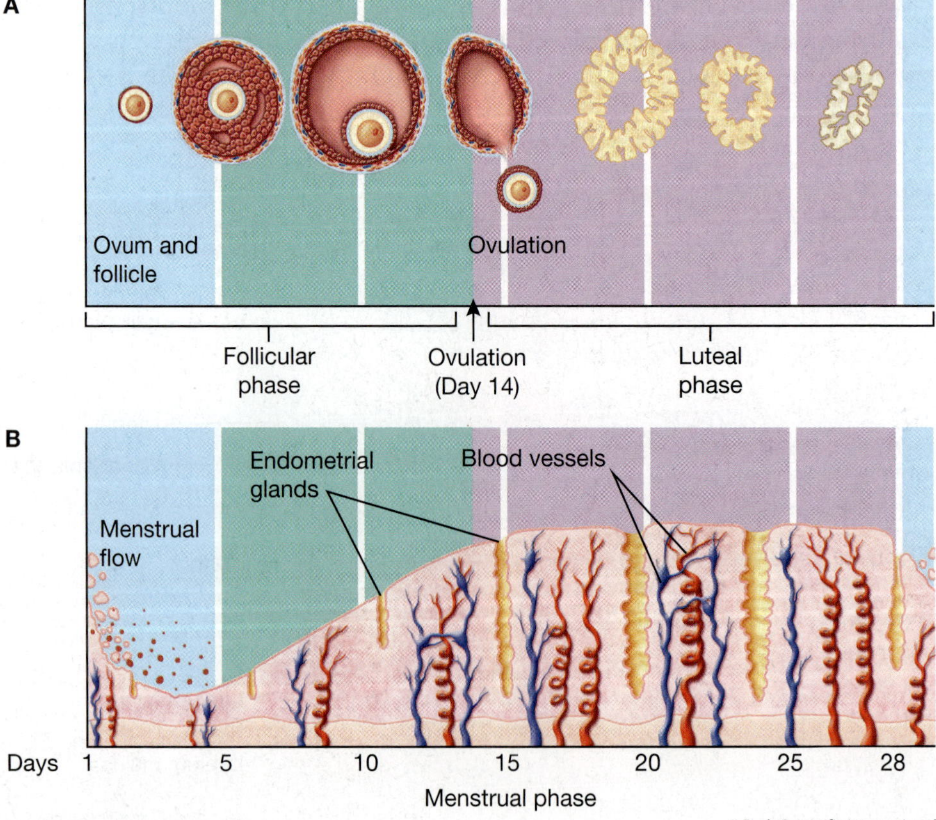

Figure 21.6 During the female menstrual cycle, hormones trigger the release of an egg from the ovaries. The hormone estrogen stimulates the uterus to build endometrial tissue in case of a pregnancy. If no pregnancy occurs, this endometrial tissue is shed.

Diseases and Disorders of the Female Reproductive System

Diseases and disorders of the female reproductive system are common. Most of these disorders affect females during or after puberty.

- **Menstrual disorders:** Though changes in menstrual periods can be normal, some females experience menstrual disorders (**Figure 21.7**). Symptoms of menstrual disorders include lack of menstruation; painful, irregular bleeding; excessive bleeding; and changes in mood, depression, and anxiety.
- **Premenstrual syndrome (PMS):** **Premenstrual syndrome (PMS)** starts one to two weeks before menstruation and stops when menstruation begins. Common symptoms are breast tenderness; acne; bloating; headache and joint pain; food cravings; mood swings, irritability, anxiety, or depression; and fatigue. The cause of PMS is not known, but hormonal changes trigger symptoms. Pain medications and contraceptives may reduce symptoms. Severe PMS that interferes with daily living is called *premenstrual dysphoric disorder (PMDD)*.
- **Endometriosis:** **Endometriosis** is a condition in which endometrial tissue grows outside the uterus. The cause of endometriosis is unknown. Even outside its normal location, endometrial tissue responds to the menstrual cycle by growing and shedding (**Figure 21.8**). Endometriosis can cause pelvic pain, diarrhea or constipation, abdominal bloating, menorrhagia or metrorrhagia, and fatigue. A major complication of endometriosis is *infertility*, or the inability to reproduce. Treatment may include pain medications, hormone therapy, and surgery.

Menstrual Disorders

Disorder	Symptoms	Causes
Amenorrhea	Lack of menstrual period or menstrual periods that stop for several months	Pregnancy, breastfeeding, stress, cancer, hormone imbalance, low body weight, excessive exercise, thyroid disorders, anorexia nervosa, athletic training
Dysmenorrhea	Painful menstruation	Pelvic inflammatory disease, endometriosis, fibroids
Menorrhagia	Excessive menstrual bleeding	Hormonal imbalance, fibroids, pregnancy complications, pelvic inflammatory disease, thyroid disorders, endometriosis, liver or kidney disease; sometimes the cause is unknown
Metrorrhagia	Bleeding between menstrual periods or irregular periods	Fibroids, pelvic inflammatory disease, thyroid disorders, diabetes, blood-clotting disorders

Figure 21.7 Menstrual disorders can include the lack of menstrual periods, painful menstruation, excessive bleeding during menstruation, and irregular menstrual periods.

premenstrual syndrome (PMS) symptoms that start one to two weeks before menstruation and stop when menstruation begins; include breast tenderness, acne, bloating, headaches, mood swings, or fatigue

endometriosis condition in which uterine tissue grows outside the uterus; can cause pain, fatigue, and infertility

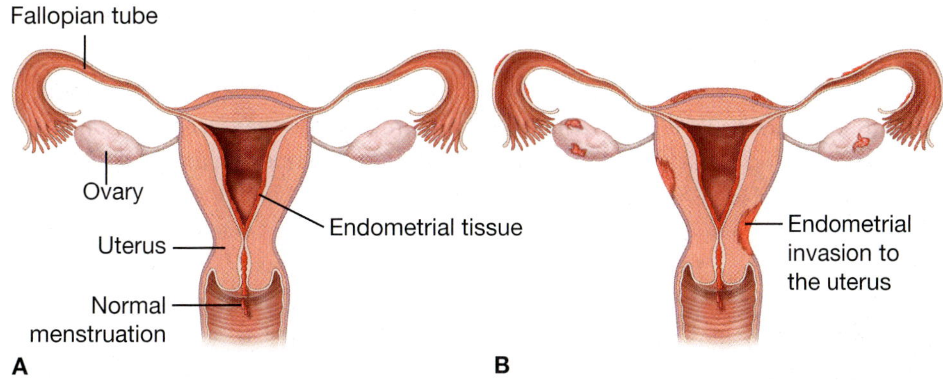

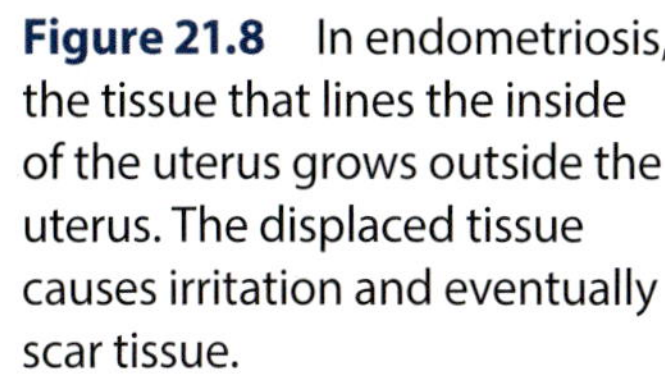
Figure 21.8 In endometriosis, the tissue that lines the inside of the uterus grows outside the uterus. The displaced tissue causes irritation and eventually scar tissue.

© Body Scientific International

- **Pelvic inflammatory disease (PID):** Pelvic inflammatory disease (PID) is a preventable condition often caused by STIs. PID causes inflammation and scarring of the pelvic reproductive organs and can cause chronic pelvic pain, ectopic pregnancy, and infertility.
- **Cervical cancer:** Cervical cancer, or cancer of the cervix, progresses slowly and can be treated effectively with early detection. A *Pap test*, or *Pap smear*, detects abnormal changes in cervical cells before the cells become cancerous. In a Pap test, a doctor swabs the cervix and examines the sample under a microscope to look for abnormal cells. Females should receive Pap tests to screen for cervical cancer every three years between the ages of 21 and 65.
- **Uterine cancer:** Uterine cancer, or cancer of the endometrium, is the most common cancer of the female reproductive organs. The cause is unknown, but estrogen levels appear to be a factor.
- **Fibroid tumors:** Fibroid tumors, also called **fibroids**, are noncancerous tumors of the uterus. They can cause vaginal bleeding, pelvic and abdominal pain, and an enlarged abdomen. Depending on their size and location, they can make pregnancy difficult or impossible.

fibroids noncancerous tumors of the uterus

Local and Global Health

Cervical Cancer Screening

In the US, cervical cancer used to be a leading cause of death among females. In the past 40 years, as Pap tests have helped doctors detect cervical cancer early, the number of deaths from cervical cancer has decreased dramatically. The introduction of the human papillomavirus (HPV) vaccine is also expected to reduce this number. Around the world, access to these technologies influences rates of cervical cancer.

The World Health Organization (WHO) and the United Nations Program on AIDS (UNAIDS) report a growing need to address cervical cancer around the world. This need is most urgent in the world's lowest-income countries.

In these low-income countries, access to Pap tests and the HPV vaccine is limited. Many females have never received the HPV vaccine or a Pap test.

The HPV vaccine and Pap tests could have prevented many of these cancers. Early detection lets doctors remove abnormal cells before the cancer invades other parts of the body. Increasing access to these vaccines and tests could save the lives of females all around the world.

Today, more than 500,000 females around the world are diagnosed with cervical cancer each year.

Worldwide, 300,000 females die from cervical cancer each year.

80% of these females + **90%** of these females live in low-income countries.

Practice Your Skills

Advocate for Health

Rates of cervical cancer vary around the world. They can also vary within a country, state, or community. Since access to vaccines and testing is a critical part of cervical cancer prevention, healthcare access in your community can also influence the number of deaths due to cervical cancer.

To promote cervical cancer testing and vaccination in your community, you need facts about cervical cancer prevention. You also need skills for research and effective communication. In a small group, research rates of cervical cancer in your state or community. Then research facts about preventing cervical cancer and resources to help people get needed testing. Include resources that provide testing for free or at a low cost. Using this information, develop a plan to communicate information for cervical cancer prevention in your community. Design a poster that presents your information and communication plan. Act on your plan and take steps to educate your community.

- **Ovarian cancer:** Ovarian cancer is difficult to detect early, which means it often spreads before symptoms begin. The symptoms of ovarian cancer can be mistaken for a painful menstrual period, except they do not stop after the period.
- **Ovarian cysts:** **Ovarian cysts** are noncancerous tumors on the ovaries. Cysts can be fluid filled or might contain abnormal cells. These cysts are not cancerous, but might need surgical removal if they become large and painful.
- **Tumors of the breast:** Tumors of the breast may be cancerous or noncancerous. **Breast cancer** is the second leading cause of cancer-related death in females. Benign tumors of the breast are common conditions, but are not as serious as breast cancer. Causes of these tumors are not known, but hormones may play a role. Many noncancerous tumors go away without treatment or can be removed surgically. Females can see a doctor and receive regular exams to detect breast cancer.

ovarian cysts noncancerous tumors on the ovaries

breast cancer abnormal cancerous growth of breast cells

Caring for the Female Reproductive System

Females can take several steps to protect the reproductive system and ensure health. To reduce risk for STIs, females, like males, can abstain from sexual activity or use a condom or dental dam. Other steps females can take include practicing hygiene and seeing the doctor.

Maintain Hygiene

Hygiene can help prevent infections of the female reproductive system. To maintain hygiene, females should shower or bathe regularly, wear cotton or breathable underwear, and change underwear daily. After urinating, females should wipe the urethral and vaginal area gently from front to back. This keeps bacteria from the vagina or anus from getting into the urethra, which can cause a urinary tract infection (UTI).

After using the bathroom, females should wash their hands with soap and water. Females should avoid using douches or deodorant sprays to clean the vagina. These products are unnecessary and can irritate the vagina or cause allergic reactions.

Hygiene during a female's menstrual period is especially important. Several different menstrual hygiene products are available to help females manage menstruation. **Figure 21.9** lists these products and steps for using them safely.

Menstrual Hygiene Products

Menstrual Hygiene Product	Description	Use
Pads (sanitary napkins or sanitary pads)	Absorbent material that soaks up blood after it leaves the vagina; are placed in the underwear and come in different sizes, thicknesses, and absorbencies for heavier or lighter periods	To prevent infection, odor, and leakage, check and change every three to four hours or when the pad is soaked. If disposable, place in trash wrapped in toilet paper. Reusable pads need to be cleaned between uses.
Tampons	Cylinders of absorbent material that soak up blood inside the vagina; are inserted into the vagina and come in different sizes and absorbencies	To prevent infection, odor, and leakage, check and change every three to four hours or when the tampon is soaked. If disposable, place in trash wrapped in toilet paper. Reusable tampons need to be cleaned between uses.
Menstrual cup	Flexible, thin cup inserted into the vagina; collects blood before it leaves the vagina and can be washed and reused	To prevent infection, odor, and leakage, remove and empty every few hours or as needed. Wash between uses.

Figure 21.9 Using pads, tampons, and menstrual cups properly can help females maintain hygiene during menstrual periods.

toxic shock syndrome (TSS) medical emergency in which bacteria release toxins that enter the blood

Changing menstrual hygiene products regularly is important. Changing pads infrequently can cause infections of the urethra and vagina. Not changing a tampon or menstrual cup often enough can lead to **toxic shock syndrome (TSS)**, a rare condition in which bacteria in the vagina release toxins that enter the blood. Symptoms of TSS include high fever, vomiting, diarrhea, muscle pain, weakness, dizziness, and a red rash. This condition requires emergency attention.

Practice Breast Awareness

Around the age of 45, females should begin receiving yearly *mammograms* (breast X-rays to detect breast cancer). Some females with a family history of breast cancer or a high risk get mammograms earlier. Breast cancer is extremely rare in teens. Still, teens should become familiar with the structure, look, and feel of their breasts so they can recognize changes.

At one time, the American Cancer Society (ACS) recommended that females perform regular breast self-examinations to detect changes. The ACS no longer recommends this since studies show self-examinations are not effective at distinguishing cancer from normal changes in the breasts. For many females, results caused unnecessary anxiety and follow-up testing.

Skills for Health and Wellness

Skills for Seeking Sexual Healthcare

Sexual healthcare, like any type of healthcare, is a normal part of maintaining your health. For some teens, seeking sexual healthcare or asking questions about sexual health can seem awkward or uncomfortable. Your reproductive system is just like any other body system, however. A doctor can help you care for your body and answer any questions you have.

Talking with a school nurse, doctor, or other trusted adult is a great way of getting answers to your sexual health questions and making any healthcare appointments. In many states, minors can also consent to certain sexual health services. For example, all 50 states allow minors to consent to STI testing and treatment. Twenty-five states allow minors to access contraceptive services.

Practice Your Skills

Access Information

Knowing how to seek sexual healthcare is an important skill. Talking about this topic can make it less awkward and encourage others to get reliable information and seek healthcare for any issues. In this activity, you will get answers to questions about sexual healthcare and share this information with others.

As a class, start by researching answers to the following questions:

- What healthcare facilities offer sexual healthcare in your community? Include doctors' offices, health clinics, any doctors who specialize in sexual health, and free or low-cost options.
- Where in your community could you go to get reliable information about your sexual health?
- In your state, what are minors' rights regarding consent to different sexual healthcare services? What, if any, services require parental notification?
- What symptoms mean a person should seek sexual healthcare? What symptoms indicate a health condition might be an emergency?

Once you have answers to these questions, identify the best way to share your answers with other students. For example, you could create a poster of your findings or post an online FAQ. You could also record a podcast or public service announcement (PSA). Share this information with your fellow students and keep a copy of this information for when you need it.

Each person has different risk factors for breast cancer. Therefore, teens should talk with their doctor about the benefits and risks of various screening methods, including self-examinations. They should also talk with a doctor if they notice any unusual changes, such as

- a hard lump near the armpit;
- dimpled or puckered skin, bulges, or ridges;
- inverted nipples (pointing inward);
- redness, warmth, swelling, or pain;
- itching, scaly skin, sores, or skin rashes; or
- bloody discharge from a nipple.

Symptoms That Need Medical Attention

- Unusual changes in the breasts
- Rashes or sores on the skin or membranes around the vagina
- Burning sensation during urination
- Pain in the pelvic area or lower abdomen
- Fever, red rash, weakness, and pain while using a tampon or menstrual cup
- Unusual discharge, such as pus, from the vagina
- Burning sensation or pain in the vagina or labia

Figure 21.10 Teens should talk to a doctor if they notice any of the symptoms listed. ***What type of doctor specializes in female reproductive health?***

See a Doctor

Seeing a doctor can help teens maintain sexual health. If females have questions about their reproductive system or menstruation, they can talk with a general doctor or with an **obstetrician/gynecologist (OB/GYN)**, a doctor who specializes in female sexual health (**Figure 21.10**).

obstetrician/gynecologist (OB/GYN) doctor who specializes in the health of the female reproductive system; also specializes in pregnancy, labor, and delivery

Lesson 21.2 Review

Know and Understand

1. Which organ transports eggs from the ovaries to the uterus?
2. Why is the vagina sometimes called the birth canal?
3. What change in the body causes menstruation?
4. What is the difference between ovarian cysts and ovarian cancer?
5. Why should females wipe from front to back after urinating?
6. What kind of doctor specializes in female sexual health?

Think Critically

7. How is the clitoris similar to the penis?
8. Choose one disease or disorder that affects the female reproductive system and explain how it might impact fertility.
9. Using reliable resources, research the history of TSS. Has it become more or less common in recent years? Why?

REAL WORLD Health Skills

Communicate with Others Using this lesson, write a question for an advice columnist to answer. Choose a reproductive system disorder, describe the symptoms, and ask the columnist what this condition might be. Be sure not to name the condition in your question. Use as many facts and descriptors as possible. Trade your paper with a partner. Now imagine you are the advice columnist. Using the text, find the symptoms your partner describes. Compose a letter identifying the disorder and explaining your diagnosis. Use effective communication skills in your letter.

Lesson

21.3 Conception, Pregnancy, and Birth

Essential Question?

What happens during pregnancy and birth?

Learning Outcomes

After studying this lesson, you will be able to

- describe how genes from both biological parents influence a person's traits;
- explain what happens during conception;
- outline what happens during the stages of prenatal development;
- explain the importance of prenatal care;
- identify behaviors that help or harm the developing baby; and
- describe what happens during each stage of childbirth.

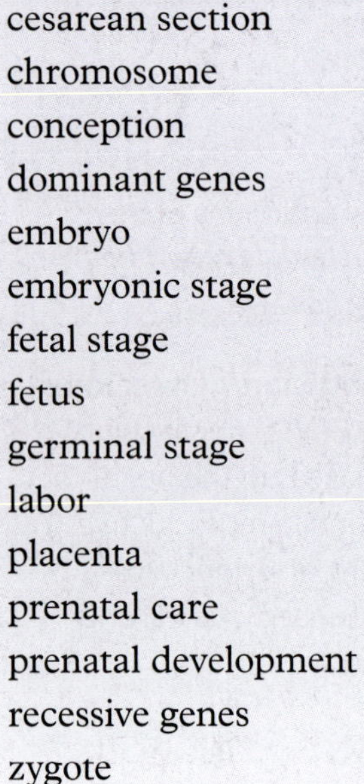

Key Terms

cesarean section
chromosome
conception
dominant genes
embryo
embryonic stage
fetal stage
fetus
germinal stage
labor
placenta
prenatal care
prenatal development
recessive genes
zygote

Warm-Up Activity

Top 10 List

Practice Health-Enhancing Behaviors Suppose you are an obstetrician/gynecologist (OB/GYN). Create a list of the top 10 steps your patients can take to increase their chances of having a healthy pregnancy. This list can include activities pregnant people should and should *not* do. Include explanations of how these activities and behaviors can increase or reduce health risks. Share and compare your list with your classmates' lists.

Top 10
1.
2.
3.
4.
5.
6.
7.
8.
9.
10.

When two people reproduce, their genetic material combines to create a new individual. This new individual has characteristics from both biological parents. This is because the individual has chromosomes from each biological parent. A **chromosome** is a package of genes, which contain the blueprint for the structure and function of your cells. Genes are made of deoxyribonucleic acid (DNA).

chromosome package of genes containing the blueprint for the structure and function of cells

Human cells have 23 pairs of chromosomes, or 46 total chromosomes. Of these, 22 pairs of chromosomes possess similar genetic material. This genetic material influences many of your characteristics, including your eye color, hair color, and risk for certain diseases. Multiple genes influence many of the characteristics you have. Some genes are dominant, and others are recessive.

Dominant genes always cause certain characteristics in a child. **Recessive genes** only cause certain characteristics if the child inherits a recessive gene from each parent.

One pair of chromosomes, called the *sex chromosomes*, differs considerably and determines an individual's biological sex. A female has two X chromosomes in each cell, and a male has one Y chromosome and one X chromosome in each cell. During reproduction, the male and female sex cells (sperm and eggs) each contribute one chromosome to each chromosome pair.

dominant genes DNA segments that always cause certain characteristics in a child

recessive genes DNA segments that only cause certain characteristics if the child has inherited a recessive gene from both parents

Conception

Humans reproduce through sexual intercourse. During intercourse, sperm enter the vagina and swim to the fallopian tube, where the egg is located. There, the sperm and egg combine in a process called *fertilization*. The moment at which the sperm and egg combine is called **conception**.

conception moment at which the sperm and egg combine

At conception, a sperm penetrates an egg. The tip of a sperm can break through the outer layers of an egg. When the first sperm connects with an egg's cell membrane, a chemical reaction sweeps over the surface of the egg, forming a barrier to additional sperm. This ensures that just a single sperm fertilizes the egg.

Research in Action

In Vitro Fertilization (IVF)

Many people experience infertility, the inability to conceive and carry a baby until birth. First used in 1977, *in vitro fertilization (IVF)* is a technology developed by scientists to help couples conceive. During IVF, a female receives hormones that stimulate the ovaries to produce many eggs at once. A doctor removes these eggs and then mixes them with sperm, which fertilize some of them. The doctor then inserts several healthy embryos into the female's uterus for implantation. Inserting multiple embryos increases the chance one will successfully implant.

Since 1978, research has improved the effectiveness and safety of IVF. IVF now makes it possible for thousands of people to have biological children.

IVF can also be used to genetically alter cells that might pass certain diseases to a child. Some people have *mitochondrial diseases*, or incurable genetic diseases in which damaged mitochondria cause lifelong disabilities. A type of IVF called *three-person IVF* can help these people conceive children without passing on this disease. In this procedure, a doctor takes an egg and uses a fine needle to remove its nucleus, which contains mitochondria. The doctor then injects the egg with the nucleus from a female donor's egg. The doctor mixes the egg with sperm and inserts the embryo into the female's uterus. This way, the baby inherits genes from the biological parents without inheriting the mitochondrial disease.

Some people are concerned about the altering of genetic material in eggs and sperm, partially because the baby will pass these genetic changes on during future reproduction. Other genetic alterations, such as those used for gene therapy, do not alter the genes inside sex cells.

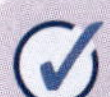

Practice Your Skills

Access Information

Many different factors affect a person's fertility, and fertility treatments such as IVF can help even people with infertility have children. With a partner, research factors that can affect fertility. Use reliable resources and make a list of all the factors for which you find evidence. Write a short blog post identifying steps teens can take now to protect their future fertility. Be sure to explain how these actions affect fertility. Also list fertility treatments that are available or being researched now.

The nucleus of the sperm, which contains its chromosomes, then meets the egg's nucleus. On contact, the nuclei of both cells fuse and combine their chromosomes, forming a nucleus with half of each parent's chromosomes. The fertilized egg is called a **zygote**. The new combination of genes from two parents produces offspring genetically distinct from the two parents.

zygote fertilized egg

Conception usually involves the union of a single sperm with a single egg. In rare cases, however, two different sperm can fertilize two different eggs in the fallopian tubes. If each fertilized egg develops, the result is a pair of *fraternal twins*. Fraternal twins are not genetically identical. They are genetically unique like most siblings. Even rarer are *identical twins*, which develop when a single fertilized egg develops, splits in two, and produces genetically identical babies. Although uncommon, these processes can also result in more than two babies.

Pregnancy

Human *gestation*, or the period of time between conception and birth, is about nine months long. Most babies are born 36–40 weeks after fertilization. Pregnancy can be divided into several stages, and a person's behaviors during pregnancy influence the health of the developing baby.

Stages of Prenatal Development

To become a baby in nine months, a zygote has to change dramatically and rapidly. Development that happens during these nine months is called **prenatal development**.

prenatal development changes that occur when a zygote develops into a baby during the nine months of pregnancy

The Germinal Stage

The **germinal stage** of prenatal development begins at conception and lasts about two weeks. In this phase, the single-celled zygote goes through a process called *cleavage*. During cleavage, a zygote divides itself rapidly into many smaller cells. First, the single cell divides into two. These two cells then each divide, producing four cells. Those cells also divide, and so on. In five days, the zygote divides seven times, forming a ball of 128 cells. This ball of cells, called a *blastocyst*, travels to the uterus (**Figure 21.11**).

germinal stage stage of development that begins at conception and lasts about two weeks; cleavage occurs

After eight to 10 days, the blastocyst implants itself in the endometrium, the inner lining of the uterus. During this process, called *implantation*, the blastocyst burrows into the endometrium, embedding itself within the lining of the uterus. At the site of implantation, the endometrium thickens and develops large, blood-filled spaces called *sinuses*. This implanted mass of cells is called an **embryo**.

embryo implanted, fertilized egg in the uterus

The Embryonic Stage

The **embryonic stage** of prenatal development lasts for about six weeks and is a critical period. During this time, the embryo begins to form the various tissues and organs that make a human. Systems that will help the embryo develop also take shape during this stage. They include the following:

embryonic stage stage of prenatal development that begins at implantation and lasts around six weeks; the embryo begins to form the various tissues, organs, and systems that make a human

- The implanted embryo develops a membrane called the *chorion*. Fingerlike projections called *villi* extend from the chorion into the sinuses of the endometrium. Together, the chorion and another membrane called the *amnion* form the *amniotic sac*, a fluid-filled sac that cushions a developing baby in the uterus.

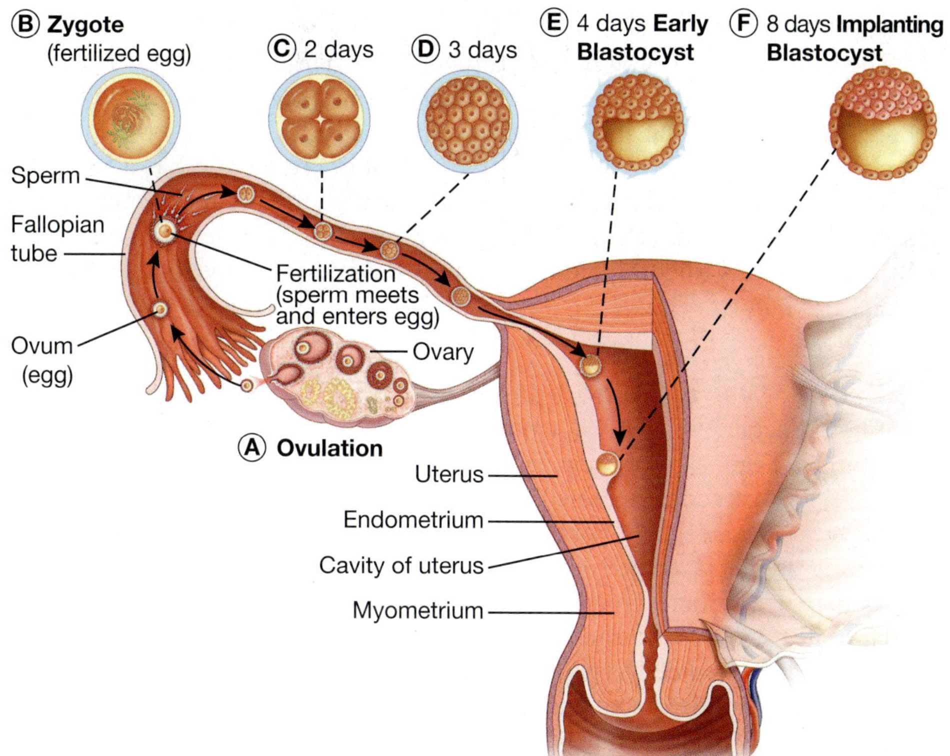

Figure 21.11 During the process of cleavage, a zygote divides until it is a ball of cells called a *blastocyst*. A blastocyst may then implant in the endometrial tissue of the uterus and become an embryo. ***How long does it take for a zygote to grow into a fully developed baby?***

- This merging of embryonic chorion and endometrial tissue creates the **placenta**. Rich in blood vessels, the placenta helps support the embryo (**Figure 21.12**). The placenta secretes the hormone progesterone, which maintains the endometrium in its blood- and nutrient-rich state. The placenta also removes waste and prevents bacteria from reaching the embryo. The placenta blocks some—but not all—harmful substances from reaching the embryo. Chemicals such as alcohol, nicotine, and many drugs can still pass from the pregnant person's body to the embryo. These substances can be very harmful to the developing baby.
- The *umbilical cord* also forms. This tube is full of blood vessels. It connects the placenta to the developing baby at its abdomen. The cord carries nutrients and oxygen from the pregnant person to the embryo.

placenta merged embryonic chorion and endometrial tissue that helps support the developing baby

During the embryonic stage, the embryo begins to form the various tissues and organs of a new individual. This process is called *differentiation*. During differentiation, embryonic cells adopt a variety of specialized structures and functions. As embryonic development proceeds, organogenesis begins. In *organogenesis*, the organs take their familiar forms and locations. Organogenesis continues for several weeks, completing the basic organization of the organs after eight weeks.

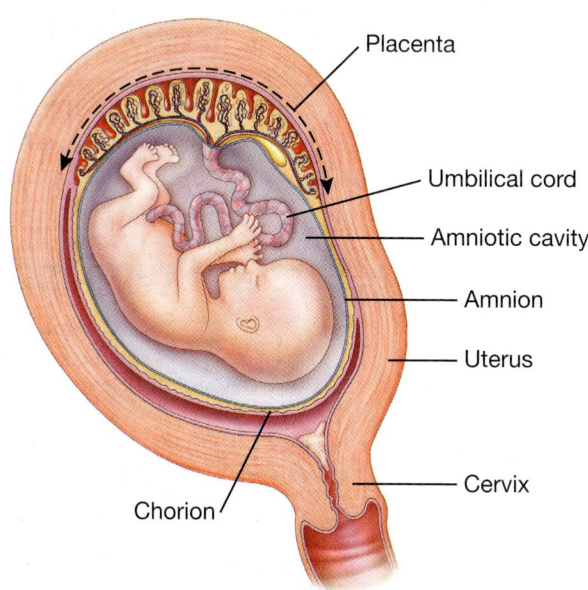

Figure 21.12 The amniotic sac, placenta, and umbilical cord develop to help support an embryo. ***How long does the embryonic stage last?***

The Fetal Stage

fetal stage stage that begins at the ninth week of pregnancy and lasts through birth; the fetus grows considerably

fetus baby during the fetal stage until birth

The ninth week of pregnancy marks the beginning of the **fetal stage**. At this stage, the baby is now called a **fetus**. This stage lasts until the baby is born. During the fetal stage, the fetus grows considerably. By the fourth month, the fetus has grown enough that the pregnant person has a visible bump in the abdomen. After nine months, most of the organs, bones, and muscles of the fetus have completed their development. The lungs and liver are the last organs to complete development. Once they develop, the baby is ready to be born.

Prenatal Care

When pregnancy occurs, hormones stop ovulation and menstruation. Therefore, the first sign of pregnancy is often a missed menstrual period. A pregnancy test can confirm whether a person is pregnant by testing the urine for *chorionic gonadotropin*, a hormone produced by the chorion of the embryo.

prenatal care healthcare for the developing baby and pregnant person before birth

During pregnancy, a person should receive **prenatal care**, or care for the developing baby and pregnant person before birth. This involves making regular visits to an obstetrician/gynecologist (OB/GYN), who specializes in pregnancy, labor, and delivery. On the first visit, the doctor will ask for the date of the person's last menstrual period to estimate the expected birth date, or *due date*. Very few people who are pregnant deliver their babies on the expected date, but this estimate allows the doctor to monitor prenatal development.

Doctors measure pregnancies in weeks and typically divide a pregnancy into three stages called *trimesters* (**Figure 21.13**). During pregnancy, a person typically sees the doctor monthly through the eighth month and weekly during the last month of pregnancy. If a person has pregnancy complications or a health condition, doctor visits will be more frequent.

The first doctor visits might include lab tests for diabetes mellitus and STIs. At follow-up visits, the doctor will perform a routine physical exam to measure the pregnant person's weight, blood pressure, and abdomen. The doctor might prescribe vitamins that are especially needed during pregnancy, such as folic acid to help build the nervous system of the baby.

A person's body changes dramatically during pregnancy. Early in pregnancy, the breasts may grow larger. Skin changes during pregnancy include acne, a blush from increases in blood volume, brown or yellow patches on the face, a dark line running down the abdomen, stretch marks, pronounced moles and freckles, and darker areolas (the area around the nipple). Emotional changes, such as mood swings or sudden tearful outbursts, are also normal.

Some unpleasant side effects of pregnancy include nausea and vomiting (*morning sickness*), leg swelling, varicose veins, hemorrhoids, indigestion and constipation, frequent urination, backache, fatigue, and difficulty sleeping. Knowing what to expect can help a pregnant person note anything out of the ordinary. Visits with a doctor can help people who are pregnant discuss these changes and catch any pregnancy complications (**Figure 21.14**).

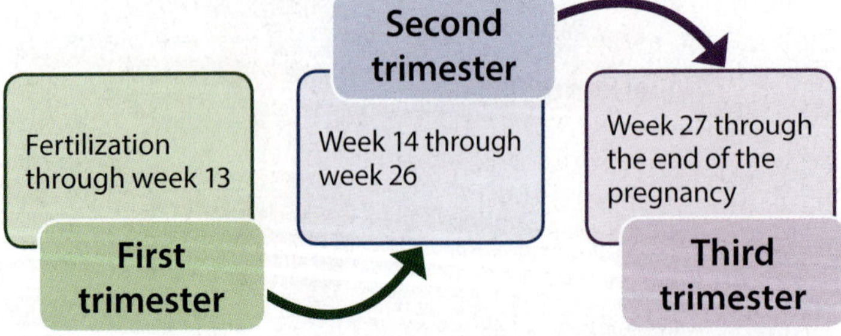

Figure 21.13 A pregnant person will experience different physical developments during each trimester. ***What information is used to estimate a pregnant person's due date?***

Pregnancy Complications	
Complication	**Description**
Ectopic pregnancy	A serious condition in which the embryo attaches and develops inside the fallopian tube where it cannot complete development; rupture of the fallopian tube can cause severe abdominal pain, bleeding, fainting, and shock; often caused by pelvic inflammatory disease (PID) or endometriosis
Miscarriage	A pregnancy that ends before the 20th week; may be caused by genetic abnormalities, injuries, infections, and other diseases
Preeclampsia	High blood pressure during pregnancy; can develop into *eclampsia*, a life-threatening emergency in which a pregnant person's blood pressure rises quickly and seizures occur; risk factors include twins, pregnancy at a young age, history of high blood pressure, diabetes mellitus, and kidney disease
Gestational diabetes mellitus	A condition in which a person cannot make the hormone insulin, which controls the amount of sugar in the blood, during pregnancy; is usually caused by hormone levels associated with pregnancy; risk factors include family history of diabetes mellitus, pregnancy over the age of 35, and smoking
Premature birth	The birth of a baby more than three weeks before the estimated due date; premature babies may have a low birthweight, underdeveloped organs, difficulty getting enough oxygen during birth (which can cause brain damage), more respiratory and digestive diseases, and difficulty feeding, gaining weight, and maintaining body temperature; babies born prematurely may need care in a *neonatal intensive care unit (NICU)*
Stillbirth	The death of a baby after the 20th week of pregnancy, but before birth

Figure 21.14 With prenatal care, a doctor can diagnose pregnancy complications and help treat the pregnant person and the baby.

Healthy Behaviors During Pregnancy

The actions a person takes during pregnancy affect the health of a developing baby. For example, eating well promotes personal health and the health of the baby. Most pregnant people should add about 300 calories to their daily diets. Gaining about 25–35 pounds is normal during pregnancy. Pregnant people also need to drink plenty of water.

Regular physical activity during pregnancy helps maintain circulation, blood pressure, and blood sugar levels. Pregnant people should choose lower-impact activities such as walking and swimming, and should avoid lifting heavy objects during pregnancy.

People who are pregnant should avoid certain substances. These substances include the following:

- **Alcohol:** Alcohol consumption damages a developing baby's brain and can cause serious health conditions called *fetal alcohol spectrum disorders (FASD)*. Because no one knows what amount of alcohol is safe, pregnant people should avoid alcohol completely.
- **Nicotine:** Exposure to nicotine, such as through smoking or vaping, harms fetal brain and lung development. It is not yet clear how other chemicals inhaled during vaping affect a developing baby. Combustible cigarettes produce many additional toxins that harm fetal growth, and smoking is linked to premature birth and stillbirth. Smoking during pregnancy also increases the risk of *sudden unexpected infant death (SUID)*, including *sudden infant death syndrome (SIDS)*, which is the unexplained death of an otherwise healthy baby during sleep.
- **Drugs:** The use of drugs, such as cocaine or marijuana, can cause miscarriage, premature birth, and serious medical conditions, including addiction in the baby. Pregnant people should ask their doctors before taking any medications, herbal supplements, or vitamins. These may be harmful to the baby.

Pregnant people should also avoid certain foods. Foods that contain mercury, such as canned tuna, can damage the fetal brain. Some foods, such as unpasteurized products and raw or undercooked meat, eggs, and fish, can transmit harmful diseases to the baby.

Childbirth

cesarean section surgical procedure to deliver a baby by removing it from the uterus; also called a *C-section*

labor process that pushes a baby out of the uterus and through the vagina

As a baby's due date approaches, hormones prepare the pregnant person's body for childbirth, then trigger and coordinate labor and the delivery of the baby. Making decisions about delivery prior to childbirth can help with the process. For example, the baby may be born in a hospital or birthing center. The doctor may administer *epidural anesthesia* (pain medication injected into the spinal cord of the pregnant person). The baby may be delivered vaginally or through a **cesarean section** (surgery to remove the baby; *C-section*). The doctor may make an incision called an *episiotomy* to help the baby pass through the birth canal.

A process called **labor** pushes a baby out of the pregnant person's body and into the world. Before labor begins, hormones prepare the pregnant person's body for labor and birth. These hormones cause the person's ligaments and joints to soften and relax, permitting the baby to pass through the birth canal. Soon after, labor starts with rhythmic uterine muscle contractions. These contractions cause the cervix to thin, stretch, and open in a process called *dilation*. As labor progresses, the brain releases the hormone *oxytocin*, which causes stronger uterine contractions that push the baby through the cervix and vagina.

There are three stages of labor (**Figure 21.15**):

1. **First stage:** In the first stage of labor, contractions of the uterus cause the cervix to thin (*efface*) and stretch (*dilate*). This opens the cervix and makes room for the baby to pass from the uterus into the vagina.
2. **Second stage:** In this stage, the uterine and abdominal muscles push the baby into the vagina and out of the body.
3. **Third stage:** The placenta is delivered in the final stage of labor.

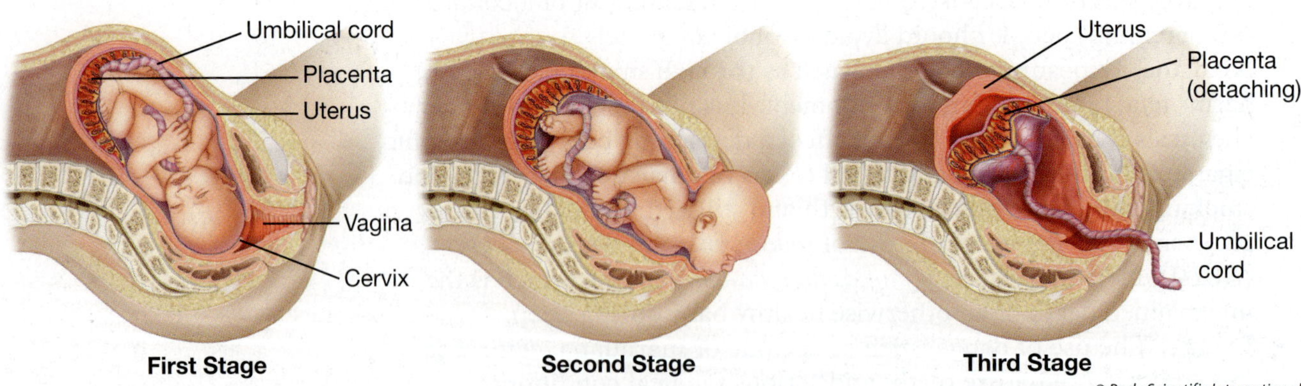

Figure 21.15 In the first stage of labor, the cervix dilates until it is wide enough for the baby to pass through. In the second stage of labor, the baby is pushed out of the body through the vagina. Finally, the placenta detaches and is delivered during the third stage of labor. ***What surgery can be performed to remove the baby from the body?***

Understanding Apgar Scores			
Apgar Condition	**2**	**1**	**0**
Appearance (skin coloration)	Normal color all over (hands and feet are pink)	Normal color (but hands and feet are bluish)	Bluish-gray or pale all over
Pulse (heart rate)	Normal (more than 100 beats per minute)	Fewer than 100 beats per minute	Absent (no pulse)
Grimace (responsiveness)	Pulls away, sneezes, coughs, or cries with stimulation	Facial movement only (grimace) with stimulation	Absent (no response to stimulation)
Activity (muscle tone)	Active, spontaneous movement	Arms and legs flexed with little movement	No movement, "floppy" tone
Respiration (breathing rate and effort)	Normal rate and effort, good cry	Slow or irregular breathing, weak cry	Absent (no breathing)

Figure 21.16 The best possible Apgar score is 10. A score of eight after five minutes means the baby is in good health. Lower scores are common and usually mean the baby needs some attention or more time to adapt. The score after five minutes should be higher than the score at one minute. When a very low score persists, something else may be wrong.

Right after birth, mucus and fluids are suctioned from the baby's mouth and nose to allow the baby to take a first breath. The baby's health, responsiveness, and vital signs are evaluated using the *Apgar test* (**Figure 21.16**). In the hospital, newborns are screened the first day for a variety of diseases and disorders so treatment can begin promptly, if needed.

Lesson 21.3 Review

Know and Understand

1. Explain how the chromosomes of each biological parent determine a baby's biological sex.
2. What event occurs at the end of the germinal stage of prenatal development?
3. How do substances consumed during pregnancy reach the developing baby?
4. Choose one substance pregnant people should not consume and explain why.
5. Which stage of labor pushes the baby into the vagina and out of the body?

Think Critically

6. Why are fraternal twins not genetically identical?
7. What factors do you think determine whether a pregnant person gets adequate prenatal care?

REAL WORLD Health Skills

Advocate for Health Using the top 10 list you created in the *Warm-Up Activity* for this lesson, create a colorful brochure or pamphlet for expecting parents. Elaborate on your list and create a *Pregnancy Wellness* guide that could be given to newly pregnant people at their first prenatal visit. Be sure to identify the target audience for your guide and adapt your language as needed.

Lesson 21.4

Teen Pregnancy and Parenthood

Essential Question?

What are the challenges of pregnancy that occurs during the teen years?

Learning Outcomes

After studying this lesson, you will be able to

- evaluate the benefits of waiting until adulthood to become a parent;
- assess the effectiveness of different methods of preventing pregnancy;
- describe the options available if an unplanned pregnancy occurs;
- analyze risk and protective factors for teen pregnancy;
- explain the physical, social, emotional, and economic challenges of teen pregnancy; and
- identify resources for teens who are pregnant or parenting.

Key Terms

abortion
adoption
child support
custodial parent
custody
legal fatherhood
noncustodial parent
safe haven laws
teen parenthood
teen pregnancy

Warm-Up Activity

Your Goals and Dreams

Set Goals Imagine yourself in 10 years. Consider your goals and dreams for the future. Do you see yourself working in a particular field? Do you want to graduate from college? If you want to live in your own home, describe it. What kind of car will you drive? Do you want to travel and see the world? Are there any other interests you plan to pursue that will cost money? Do you want to be married? How much income will you need?

Now, consider the responsibilities, time, and costs involved in caring for a baby. Using this information as motivation, write a SMART goal for preventing pregnancy until a time you would choose for it to happen. How would having a baby in the next few years affect your ability to pursue your goals and dreams? What would change in your life? Write a letter to yourself describing how pregnancy could affect the plans you have for your present and future.

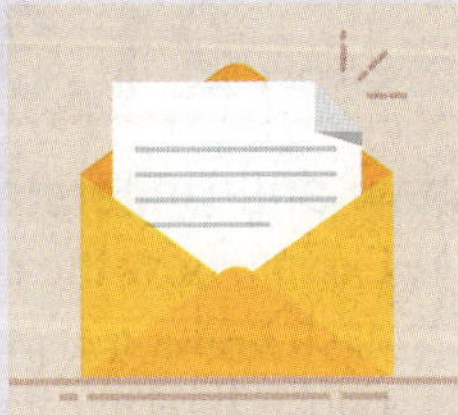

aShatilov/Shutterstock.com

Parenthood has many benefits and rewards for parents, their children, and the community. When teens wait until they are adults to become parents, they are more likely to experience these benefits. In this lesson, you will learn about ways of preventing pregnancy. (You will learn about how to use methods of preventing pregnancy in Chapter 24.) In this lesson, you will also learn about options if pregnancy occurs and the challenges of teen pregnancy and parenthood.

Preventing Pregnancy

The only method that is 100-percent effective in preventing pregnancy is *sexual abstinence*, or the decision to refrain from sexual activity. Many teens choose this method. In addition to preventing pregnancy, abstinence also prevents sexually transmitted infections (STIs) and has social and emotional benefits, such as emotional maturity and more time for personal growth.

Other methods of preventing pregnancy include *contraception*, or the use of certain devices or techniques to stop pregnancy from occurring. Contraceptive methods work by preventing a sperm and egg from meeting, usually by blocking sperm from entering the female reproductive system or inhibiting ovulation (**Figure 21.17**).

Emergency contraception (such as a copper IUD, *ella*®, or *Plan B One-Step*®) can also help prevent pregnancy after sexual activity occurs. The only contraceptive methods that protect against STIs are condoms and dental dams, which you learned about in Chapter 19. You will learn more about contraceptive methods in Chapter 24.

Methods of Contraception		
Contraceptive Method	**Use**	**Number of Pregnancies Expected (per 100 Females)**
Sexual abstinence	Refraining from sexual activity	0
Birth control implant	A small rod implanted into the body by a doctor; releases hormones to prevent ovulation	Less than 1
Intrauterine device (IUD)	A device inserted into the uterus by a doctor; repels sperm; hormonal IUDs also release hormones to thicken cervical mucus and inhibit ovulation	Less than 1
Sterilization	Permanent surgery that alters a male's or female's reproductive system to prevent pregnancy	Less than 1
Birth control shot	An injection of hormones by a doctor every three months; prevents ovulation	6
Birth control patch	A patch placed on the skin every three weeks; releases hormones to prevent ovulation	9
Birth control pill	A pill taken every day; contains hormones that prevent ovulation	9
Vaginal ring	A flexible ring inserted into the vagina; releases hormones to prevent ovulation	9
Diaphragm	A flexible cup inserted into the vagina; blocks sperm from entering the uterus	12
Contraceptive sponge	A sponge inserted into the vagina; contains *spermicide* (a chemical that kills sperm) and prevents sperm from entering the uterus	12–24
Fertility awareness methods (FAM)	Methods that track a female's fertile (unsafe) and infertile (safe) days; include the temperature method, cervical mucus method, and calendar method	12–24
Emergency contraceptive pills	A pill taken within five days of sexual intercourse; contains hormones that prevent ovulation	15 (ella); 11–25 (Plan B)
Cervical cap	A silicone cup inserted into the vagina; prevents sperm from entering the uterus	17–23
External condom	Fits over an erect penis to block sperm from entering the vagina	18
Internal condom	Fits inside the vagina to prevent sperm from entering the uterus	21
Withdrawal	Pulling the penis out of the vagina before ejaculation	22
Spermicide	A substance inserted into the vagina that inactivates sperm	28

Figure 21.17 This chart shows the average effectiveness of various contraceptive methods within the first year of typical use. The effectiveness of these methods depends on whether they are used consistently and perfectly. Forgetting to use a contraceptive method or using a method imperfectly even once significantly reduces effectiveness and increases the chance of pregnancy.

Options if Pregnancy Occurs

If pregnancy occurs, people have several options. Some people choose to give birth to and raise the baby. Others choose to place the child for adoption, or in some cases, end the pregnancy. People benefit from support and counseling from family members, friends, and trusted adults when making these decisions.

Parenting

teen parenthood teen's decision to raise a child independently or with the other parent

When pregnancy occurs, some people choose to become parents and raise the child. **Teen parenthood** involves a teen raising the child independently or with the other parent. In making the decision to parent together, some people choose to marry. Others do not. These decisions require careful consideration. People need to know about the responsibilities of parenting to choose the best course of action.

If people decide to parent their child, they must prepare and learn everything they can about parenthood. From the first day of a child's life, parents have many responsibilities. They must provide for all of the child's physical needs, including nutrition, sleep, hygiene, and healthcare. They should also provide for the child's emotional needs by regularly playing and communicating with the child.

Parents are a child's first teachers. From parents, a child learns language, communication, and social skills. Later, parents should be involved in the child's school education. Perhaps the most important responsibility of parenting is to be dependable and actively present in a child's life. This builds the child's trust, confidence, and self-esteem.

Parents may or may not share the responsibilities of caring for their child. In the US, if parents are married, they both automatically have rights and responsibilities to provide care for their children. If parents do not marry, they can sign a document that assigns legal fatherhood to the male parent. **Legal fatherhood**, or *paternity*, establishes the male parent's right to be involved in the child's life and responsibility to support the child. The female parent has these rights and responsibilities automatically. A parent can also request a paternity test to prove legal fatherhood or get a court order naming the legal father (**Figure 21.18**).

legal fatherhood male parent's right to be involved in the child's life and responsibility to support the child

Benefits of Legal Fatherhood

For Legal Father

- May play a role in making decisions about the child's life
- Has the right to legal visitation with the child
- Has the right to know about the child's health and see the child's medical and school records
- Can be named on the child's birth certificate
- Can seek joint or sole custody if the parents break up or the other parent dies

For Legal Mother

- Can receive help and financial support raising the child
- May receive child support payments
- May have help with childcare
- Might get health insurance for the child through the legal father's employer

For the Child

- Knows the identities of both parents and family origins
- Can receive Social Security, medical, and disability benefits from the legal father
- Can access the legal father's medical history, which can help identify risk factors
- May receive emotional and financial support from both parents
- Can inherit money or property from both parents

Figure 21.18 Establishing legal fatherhood can have benefits for both parents and their child. ***How does the female parent get legal motherhood?***

Unmarried parents have to work out who has **custody** of, or the legal right to care for, the child. In *sole custody*, one parent has this legal right, and the other parent may or may not have *visitation rights* to spend time with the child. In this situation, the baby lives with the **custodial parent**. The other parent is the **noncustodial parent**. Even if the noncustodial parent is not involved with the child, that parent must contribute **child support** for the child's care. Unmarried parents may also choose *joint custody*, in which both parents have legal rights to care for and financially support the child.

In sole custody or joint custody, it is the best for the child if parents can share parenting responsibilities. This type of parenting is only possible if parents have a mature, respectful, and positive relationship, whether they are still romantically involved or not. In shared parenting, people need to

- show respect for each other, the child, and those helping with childcare;
- never involve children in disputes or argue if the child is present;
- communicate with each other and the child respectfully, clearly, and effectively;
- listen to the other parent and be sure to understand what the other parent is saying;
- share information about the child's well-being, health, school, accomplishments, and challenges;
- ask the other parent for help when needed; and
- be reliable by following through on promises and commitments.

custody legal right and responsibility to care for a child and make decisions about care

custodial parent individual who has legal custody of the child; is responsible for the child and has the right to make decisions about the child's care

noncustodial parent individual who is not the primary custody holder of a child, but who has a legal obligation to contribute child support

child support money that one parent gives the other parent to provide financial support for the care of the parents' child

Health in the Media

Teen Pregnancy in the Media

Today, reality TV shows follow the lives of people from many different backgrounds. While these shows may claim to be realistic, they are designed to entertain, like other forms of media.

There are conflicting views about how media depictions of teen pregnancy impact teens. Some people have concerns that media representations of teen pregnancy glamorize it and make teen parents into celebrities. These representations can ignore the negative consequences pregnancy has on a teen's life. Researchers have also found, however, that media representations of teen pregnancy lead teens to do more research about pregnancy and contraceptive methods.

Media can help people understand the lives of others and even encourage viewers to do more research on their own. Still, you cannot rely on media depictions to give a realistic, accurate picture of life. The reality of teen pregnancy is much more complicated than what is on TV.

Practice Your Skills

Analyze Influences

In a small group, reflect on how the media portrays teen pregnancy and parenthood. Following is a list of messages these media representations often communicate. In your group, evaluate each message. Give any examples of shows or movies that communicate this message and assess whether the message is accurate.

- *Teen pregnancy is a common part of high school.*
- *Getting pregnant is a way of getting attention.*
- *Parents can always help the pregnant teen.*
- *Pregnancy and a baby bring teen parents closer.*
- *A teen father does not help the mother.*
- *Teen parents can balance school with childcare.*
- *Teen parents do not work much more than their friends.*

After assessing each message, write a related message that *is* accurate. Share these messages with your class and discuss how each message might impact teens' choices.

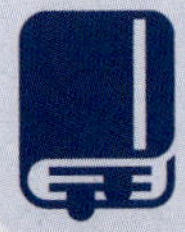

Case Study

Teen Parenthood

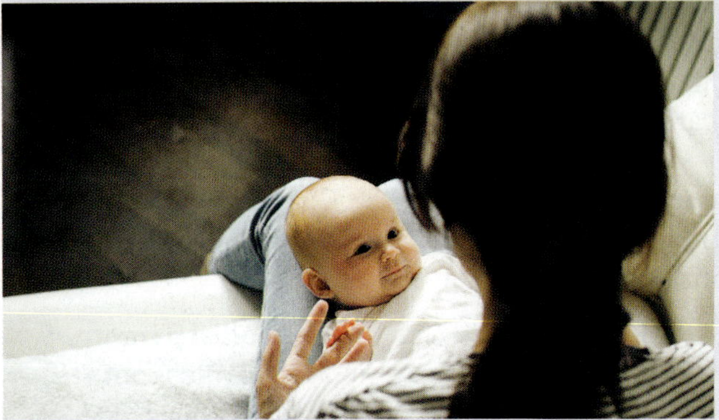

Irina Bg/Shutterstock.com

When 17-year-old Priya had her baby named Tessa last year, she did not realize how isolated and lonely she would feel. While Tessa's father does his best to help raise Tessa, they broke up before Tessa was born. Priya's best friends have all left for college, and she misses them. Priya had to turn down a scholarship to her dream four-year university. She knew she would not be able to raise her daughter and complete school if she moved away from her supportive family. With the limited time she has to socialize, Priya finds most new friendships fizzle once people find out she is a mother.

Sixteen-year-old Deven was not planning on becoming a father until his late 20s, but he and his girlfriend, Chelsea, recently had a son. Deven wants to do everything he can to financially support and take care of Chelsea and the baby. He started a part-time job after school and picks up extra shifts on the weekends. Balancing going to school, working part-time, and helping Chelsea raise their son gets more difficult each day. Deven is thinking about dropping out of school to work full-time.

When Jenny and Karamo found out Jenny was pregnant in high school, they knew they would not have the resources to give their child a happy, stable life. Though they wished they could raise their child, they chose to place the baby for adoption. Sometimes, Jenny and Karamo grieve the loss of this family. Still, adoption has given them the chance to prioritize their goals so they are better prepared to be parents later.

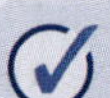

Practice Your Skills

Make Decisions

With a partner, choose one of the scenarios given. Identify the factors that are influencing each person's health positively and negatively. Then, choose three factors the person can change to improve health. Complete the scenario showing how the people involved access supportive resources and use the decision-making process to promote health for themselves and others.

Choosing Adoption

adoption action of legally taking responsibility for and raising another person's biological child

Some people do not feel ready to give birth to and raise a child. In these situations, some people decide to give birth to the child and then place the child for **adoption**. People, and not just teens, make this choice for a variety of emotional, medical, and financial reasons. Parents who choose this route may feel some grief and loss following adoption, but this decision may be best for the child's future and help other couples have children.

Adoption laws vary by state. In some states, the female parent must obtain the consent of the legal father before an adoption can go forward. Pregnant people should also consider the type of adoption. In *open adoptions*, adopted children may have contact with their biological parents. In *closed adoptions*, the biological parents' information is kept private. Adoptive parents must pass criminal background and health screenings. They should have the financial and emotional ability to care for a child in a safe and healthy living environment.

When a pregnancy is unexpected, people can become desperate. Some may consider abandoning a baby after the baby is born. Babies who are abandoned, however, are in great danger. Without regular feedings and a warm place to stay, helpless babies can quickly become sick or die.

Every state has **safe haven laws** (also called *safe surrender laws*) that permit people to leave their babies at certain facilities with no questions asked and with no legal consequences. These laws protect innocent and vulnerable babies from the dangers of abandonment. Each state has age restrictions for a baby who is left at a safe haven. Safe havens include fire stations, police stations, and hospitals. Babies will be well cared for until they can be adopted.

safe haven laws
legislation that permits people to leave their babies at certain facilities with no questions asked; aim to protect babies from abandonment; also called *safe surrender laws*

Ending a Pregnancy

In some cases, people who are not ready to give birth to and raise a child choose to end the pregnancy with a procedure called **abortion**. It is important to realize that abortion is *not* a type of contraception. Contraceptive methods, including emergency contraception, *prevent* pregnancy from happening. Abortion *ends* a pregnancy that has already begun.

abortion procedure that ends a pregnancy

Abortions may be *medical* (use hormones) or *surgical* (use surgery). A person who decides to have an abortion should do so at the earliest possible date. The further along a pregnancy is, the more risks are involved in abortion. In general, abortions performed in the first three months have fewer risks.

You are probably aware that abortion is a controversial topic. Many people strongly oppose abortion. Others believe it is a personal choice. If considering abortion, people can benefit from a strong family support system. Counseling from doctors and advisors can also be helpful.

Understanding Teen Pregnancy and Parenthood

Teen pregnancy refers to a pregnancy that occurs during the adolescent years, when a teen's body is still developing and maturing. Most teen pregnancies are not planned. Once pregnancy occurs, it changes a parent's life forever. A parent's relationships and goals for the future will have to be adjusted.

teen pregnancy
pregnancy that occurs during the adolescent years when a teen's body is still developing and maturing

Several risk and protective factors affect a person's chances of experiencing teen pregnancy. These factors can be either internal or external (**Figure 21.19**).

Risk and Protective Factors of Teen Pregnancy

Risk Factors	Protective Factors
• Limited knowledge of sexual health and contraceptive methods • A parent who had a child before the age of 20 • Unprotected sexual activity • Living in a home with frequent family conflict • Use of alcohol and drugs • Low self-esteem	• Discussions with parents, guardians, and healthcare professionals about contraceptive methods and how to use them properly • Parental or guardian support and a healthy family dynamic • Accurate knowledge of sexual health through healthcare professionals or valid resources • Continuous abstinence, or the commitment to refrain from sexual activity

Figure 21.19 Risk and protective factors affect the chances of teen pregnancy occurring.

Challenges of Teen Pregnancy and Parenthood

Teens who are pregnant or parenting may face various challenges related to physical, emotional, and social health and economic well-being (**Figure 21.20**). The challenges of teen pregnancy and parenthood can be managed in several ways.

Many of the physical challenges of teen pregnancy result from poor prenatal care. Teen parents may neglect prenatal care due to the desire to keep a pregnancy secret, lack of knowledge about proper prenatal care, or other reasons. To ensure the safest possible pregnancy, people should never keep a pregnancy secret. Instead, they should visit a doctor to begin prenatal care as soon as possible. Doctors can advise people who are pregnant about how to care for themselves and their unborn child.

Throughout pregnancy and parenthood, maintaining healthy relationships is important. Healthy relationships can provide teen parents with support and encouragement and satisfy different needs. For example, family members can assist with raising the child with the teen parents and provide emotional support.

Sometimes emotions can become overwhelming for a teen parent. Parents may feel angry, depressed, or stressed because of their new responsibilities. Teen parents can manage these feelings by taking care of their mental and emotional health and getting professional help, if needed.

It is also valuable for teen parents to complete their education. Not completing high school can lead to limited job opportunities, which can result in financial difficulties. On average, only 33 percent of female teen parents complete high school, and only 1.5 percent complete college by the age of 30. For male parents, the likelihood of receiving a high school diploma is 15 percent.

Teens may turn to family for support and childcare. If family members are not available, teen parents can seek out childcare services or look for night classes or online education courses. Receiving at least a high school diploma opens more employment opportunities for teen parents to help financially support their child.

Challenges of Teen Pregnancy and Parenthood	
Parent	**Child**
Physical	
• STIs contracted from sexual intercourse • Anemia • High blood pressure • Complications during childbirth, such as placenta previa (in which the placenta blocks the birth canal), preeclampsia, premature delivery, and prolonged labor	• Low birthweight • Death within the first year of life • Dependence on addictive substances • Slow growth • Infections
Social and Emotional	
• Strained relationships with partner, friends, and family • Anger or depression	• Resentment from parents that harms the child's social and emotional health
Economic	
• Parents' incomplete education and possible difficulty in finding a job	• Financial strain to pay for food, clothing, housing, childcare, and education for the child

Figure 21.20 Many teens need support managing the challenges of teen pregnancy and parenthood.

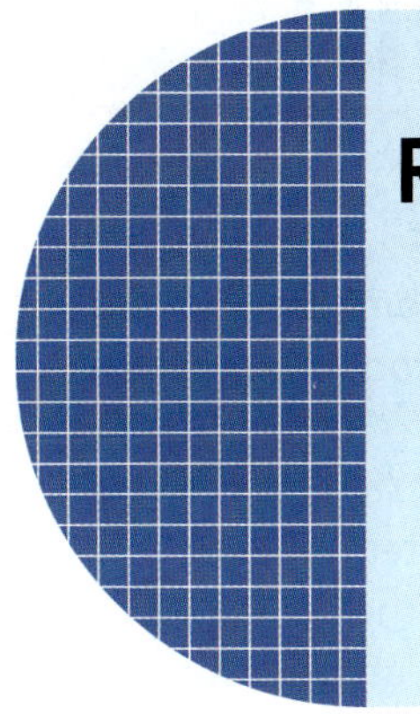

Resources for Teen Parents and Families

- On-site childcare in schools
- Babysitting through school or a community organization after school
- Personal and family counseling
- Career counseling
- Pregnancy and parenting support groups
- Parenting classes that teach the basics of care, feeding, sleeping, diapering, bathing, and child safety
- Online schooling and GED testing services
- Government assistant through Medicaid or the Special Supplemental Nutrition Program for Women, Infants, and Children (WIC)

Figure 21.21 Resources can provide teen parents with financial, emotional, physical, and educational assistance. *What is the term for the legal right to care for a child?*

Resources for Teen Parents

Several resources can help teen parents and their families adjust to the life changes of raising a child (**Figure 21.21**). For example, teen parents can attend local pregnancy and parenting support groups to help them understand and meet the needs of raising a child.

Lesson 21.4 Review

Know and Understand

1. What is the most effective method for preventing pregnancy?
2. How can a teen parent establish legal fatherhood?
3. If a pregnant teen does not want to raise a child, what are that teen's other options?
4. What are the physical health risks of teen pregnancy?
5. Explain why teens who are pregnant should not keep the pregnancy a secret.
6. Why should teen parents make it a priority to finish high school?

Think Critically

7. How do you think adults know when they are ready to become parents?
8. What factors do you think influence how effective a method of contraception is?
9. What misconceptions have you heard about noncustodial parents? How does reality compare to these misconceptions?
10. How would your relationships change if you became pregnant or caused a pregnancy?
11. Research the costs of childcare in your area. If you had a child, how much would you have to spend on childcare to go to school?

REAL WORLD Health Skills

Access Information If parents do not live together, the noncustodial parent typically spends less time with the baby. This parent does, however, still have legal rights and responsibilities regarding the baby. Using this textbook and outside valid and reliable resources, list the rights and responsibilities of a noncustodial parent, according to the laws in your state. Then, design an educational brochure outlining these rights and responsibilities. Include websites and resources a noncustodial parent could view for additional information.

Chapter 21 Review and Assessment

Chapter Summary

During sexual reproduction, the genetic material of two individuals combines to create a new individual. The human reproductive systems include organs that produce human sex cells, or sperm and eggs.

The organs of the male reproductive system include the testes, penis, seminal vesicles, prostate, and vas deferens. To maintain the health of the reproductive system, males can practice hygiene, perform testicular self-examinations, and regularly visit the doctor.

The female reproductive system includes the ovaries, fallopian tubes, uterus, vagina, cervix, labia, clitoris, and breasts. Females can protect the reproductive system and ensure health by practicing hygiene and seeing the doctor regularly.

During vaginal sexual intercourse, sperm enter the vagina. The sperm swim from the vagina to the fallopian tube, where the egg is located. There, the sperm and egg combine in fertilization. The moment at which the sperm and egg combine is called conception.

Pregnancy can be divided into the germinal stage, the embryonic stage, and the fetal stage. During pregnancy, a person should receive prenatal care and be mindful of actions that affect the health of a developing baby.

The only method that is 100-percent effective in preventing pregnancy is sexual abstinence. Other methods of preventing pregnancy include contraception, or the use of certain devices or techniques to stop pregnancy from occurring.

Teen pregnancy and parenthood have many physical, social, emotional, and economic challenges. Teen parents need to know about the responsibilities of parenting to choose the best course of action.

Vocabulary Activity

Working in a small group, discuss what you know about sexual reproduction using basic, everyday language. Review the lesson and your notes and create a digital presentation with visuals summarizing the most important information. In your presentation, use new terms you have learned to describe sexual reproduction. Then, reteach the lesson to your peers using the presentation and at least two activities. Take a few minutes after the presentation to answer any questions.

abortion
adoption
breast cancer
breasts
cervix
cesarean section
child support
chromosome
clitoris
conception
custodial parent
custody
dominant genes
eggs
ejaculation
embryo
embryonic stage
endometriosis
erection
fallopian tube
female reproductive system
fetal stage
fetus
fibroids
germinal stage
labia
labor
legal fatherhood
male reproductive system
menstrual cycle
menstruation
noncustodial parent
obstetrician/gynecologist (OB/GYN)
ovarian cysts
ovaries
ovulation
penis
placenta
premenstrual syndrome (PMS)
prenatal care
prenatal development
prostate
prostate cancer
recessive genes
safe haven laws
semen
sexual reproduction
sperm
teen parenthood
teen pregnancy
testes
testicular cancer
testicular self-examination
toxic shock syndrome (TSS)
uterus
vagina
vas deferens
zygote

Review and Recall

Review the information in this chapter by answering the following questions.

1. What is the role of the vas deferens?
2. Which condition is an inflammation of the testes?
   A. prostatitis
   B. epididymitis
   C. orchitis
   D. cryptorchidism
3. What is menarche?
4. What role does the hormone *progesterone* play in menstruation and pregnancy?
5. At which stage do the ovaries stop releasing ova and the female reproductive years end?
   A. menarche
   B. menstruation
   C. menopause
   D. ovulation
6. Why does the ACS no longer recommend that females perform regular breast self-examinations?
7. How does the conception of fraternal twins differ from that of identical twins?
8. Which test is used to evaluate a newborn baby's health, responsiveness, and vital signs?
9. What happens during organogenesis?
10. Which organ is the last to complete development during the fetal stage?
    A. liver
    B. heart
    C. lungs
    D. A and C.
11. What is the difference between dominant and recessive genes?
12. Explain the difference between an open and a closed adoption.
13. List three expenses related to raising a child.
14. What legal responsibility does the noncustodial parent have?

Standardized Test Prep

Math Practice

Review the following rates of effectiveness for several contraceptive methods. Then, answer the questions that follow.

Contraceptive Method	Number of Pregnancies Expected (per 100 Females)
Sexual abstinence	0
Birth control patch	9
Birth control pill	9
Birth control shot	6
External condom	18
Internal condom	21
Withdrawal	22

15. According to these rates, what percentage of females who use external condoms during sexual intercourse experience pregnancy? What percentage do *not* experience pregnancy?
16. Which of these contraceptive methods is least effective?
    A. withdrawal
    B. birth control patch
    C. internal condom
    D. birth control pill
17. A contraceptive method that is 90 percent effective is more effective than
    A. sexual abstinence
    B. birth control shot
    C. birth control pill
    D. internal condom

Chapter 21 Skills Assessment

Critical Thinking Skills

Answer the following questions to assess your knowledge of what you learned in this chapter.

1. Why does semen contain fluids from the seminal vesicles and prostate?
2. Why do you think some people might choose not to have their child circumcised?
3. List as many characteristics as you can that the male and female reproductive systems have in common.
4. In your own words, summarize the sequence of events in the menstrual cycle.
5. Why is implantation in the endometrium critical for the embryo's survival?
6. Do you think three-person IVF opens the door to manipulation of genes for the unborn? Why or why not? What are some of the ethical issues associated with genetic manipulation and engineering?
7. What factors affect the likelihood that an egg will be fertilized during sexual intercourse?
8. How likely would it be for identical twins to share the same personality traits? Explain your answer.
9. What are some factors that might increase someone's likelihood of becoming a teen parent?
10. Design an educational brochure outlining the benefits of adoption and highlighting the adoption resources available in your community.
11. Make a list of things you most enjoy about being a teen. How would these things change if you were to become a teen parent?
12. What factors might prevent teen parents from receiving the emotional and social support they need?
13. Compare and contrast the financial challenges pregnant teens might face as compared to adults who are pregnant.

Health and Wellness Skills

Complete the following activities to assess your skills related to health and wellness.

14. **Analyze Influences.** Decisions about sexual health are deeply personal for many people. Family members may have strong opinions about whether teens should be sexually active or choose to be parents. Think about your own environment, upbringing, and relationships. What factors influence your thoughts and decisions about sexual health? How? With a partner, discuss how to manage these influences in ways that promote your health and the health of others.
15. **Access Information.** Using reliable and valid resources, research safe haven or safe surrender laws, why these laws exist, and how these laws are defined in your state. Evaluate your sources of information for credibility. Design a poster illustrating where in your community a baby can be left, if there are any age restrictions for the baby, and any other valuable information.
16. **Communicate with Others.** Imagine that your friend Brenda has been sexually active for almost six months. She and her partner have been using condoms, but they have been less than safe a few times when they were out of condoms. Brenda has never been to the gynecologist. Write a persuasive dialogue that highlights the main points why Brenda needs to make an appointment with a gynecologist. In your dialogue, use effective communication skills and show concern for Brenda's health.
17. **Make Decisions.** Lacey and Jeff have been married for two years. Recently, they both graduated from law school and now have entry-level jobs. They are heavily in debt from student loans they took out to attend law school and are trying to save money to buy their own home. Should Lacey and Jeff have a baby at this point in their lives? Use the decision-making process to help Lacey and Jeff make the best decision for their family.
18. **Set Goals.** Review the information in this chapter about caring for the male and female reproductive systems. Then, write a SMART goal for yourself that will help you take care of your reproductive system. Your goal should help you put into action some of the self-care strategies you learned about in this chapter.

19. **Practice Health-Enhancing Behaviors.** Tristan has made a commitment to be sexually abstinent during high school. He is highly motivated, but seems to run into temptations at every turn. Create an advice column for teens who are in this same situation. Include in the column strategies to use during the teen years to maintain sexual abstinence, while still getting to socialize and date.

20. **Advocate for Health.** With a partner or in a small group, research resources for teen parents in your community or state. Examples of resources might include nutrition assistance, educational support, or mental health counseling. Find out what information and support these resources offer. Then, create a social media campaign advertising the resources available to teen parents. Gear your campaign to teen parents who might need to access these resources.

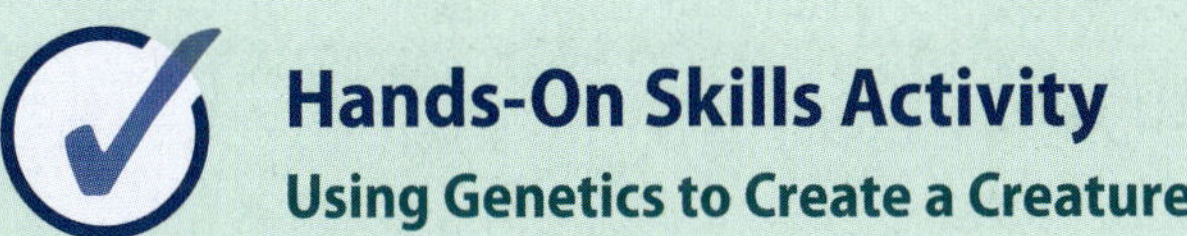

Hands-On Skills Activity

Using Genetics to Create a Creature

You have learned that different patterns of inheritance exist because of the dominant and recessive traits you inherit from biological parents. In this activity, you will create a creature that possesses certain physical traits and learn how a combination of genes works together to create a unique organism. For this activity, you will need water-soluble paint in pink and blue, a small paintbrush, and two coins.

Steps for This Activity

1. Recreate the chart shown. Create a pink coin by painting a thin pink line around the edge. Create a blue coin by painting a thin blue line around the edge.
2. To determine which trait will be expressed, flip both the pink coin and the blue coin. If a coin lands heads-up, check the appropriate "Heads" column. If it lands tails-up, check the appropriate "Tails" column.
3. **Comprehend Concepts.** In the final column of your chart, circle which trait will be expressed in your creature—the dominant trait or the recessive trait. The dominant trait is expressed if either one or both parents passed it on. A recessive trait is only expressed if both parents passed it on.
4. Repeat steps two and three for each trait in your chart.
5. After you have completed the chart, use the traits in the last column to draw your creature. Compare your creature to your classmates' creatures.

	Parent (pink coin)		Parent (blue coin)		Your Creature
Genetic Trait	Dominant (heads)	Recessive (tails)	Dominant (heads)	Recessive (tails)	Creature Trait (circle one) D=Dominant; r=recessive
1. body shape					D= large/round r= small/skinny
2. number of eyes					D= 2 r = 1
3. eye size					D= large r= small
4. eye color					D= blue, green, purple r= red, yellow, orange
5. skin color					D= blue, green, purple r= red, yellow, orange
6. skin texture					D= hairy/furry r = smooth
7. skin design					D= solid color r= polka dots
8. tail length					D= short r= long
9. tail color					D= purple, pink, red r= blue, green, black
10. teeth					D=sharp r= round
11. number of arms					D= 2-4 r= 0-1
12. number of fingers					D= 5-10 r= 2-4
13. claw length					D= long r= short
14. number of claws					D= 5-10 r= 2-4
15. number of legs					D= 2-4 r= 0-1
16. ear size					D= large r= small
17. ear shape					D= round r= pointy or square
18. number of horns					D= 2 r= 1
19. horn shape					D= pointy or jagged r= round or curly
20. horn color					D= orange, yellow, green r= red, pink, purple

Chapter 22

Health Across the Life Span

Lesson 22.1 Understanding Development
Lesson 22.2 Health During the Childhood Years
Lesson 22.3 Adolescence and Puberty
Lesson 22.4 Adulthood and the Nature of Aging

Look for the skills icon throughout this chapter for opportunities to practice your health skills.

Check Your Health and Wellness Skills

In this chapter, you will learn skills for promoting health across the life span. To understand the skills you currently use, take the following inventory of your behaviors. Indicate how well you think you use each skill. Use a scale of 1–5, *1* meaning you do not use the skill and *5* meaning you feel completely comfortable using it.

Skill	How Well Do You Use Each Skill?
I don't stress about developing more quickly or slowly than my peers.	
I value the differences among people and speak up if others make fun of them.	
I know that disabilities don't define a person or make someone incomplete.	
I keep a positive attitude about my unique traits, even when they cause challenges.	
I know whom I'd ask if I had questions about puberty.	
I use a decision-making process to keep myself from being impulsive.	
I seek guidance from people I trust when I face challenging situations.	
I think regularly about my future and how I can set myself up for a healthy one.	
I communicate clearly to build healthy relationships.	
I support those who are grieving.	
	Total:

Add up your responses to each statement. The higher your score, the more comfortable you feel promoting health across the life span. Which skill do you think is most important for you? Which skill is the most challenging for you? Which skill would you most like to improve? In this chapter, you will learn how to perform these skills better and more often.

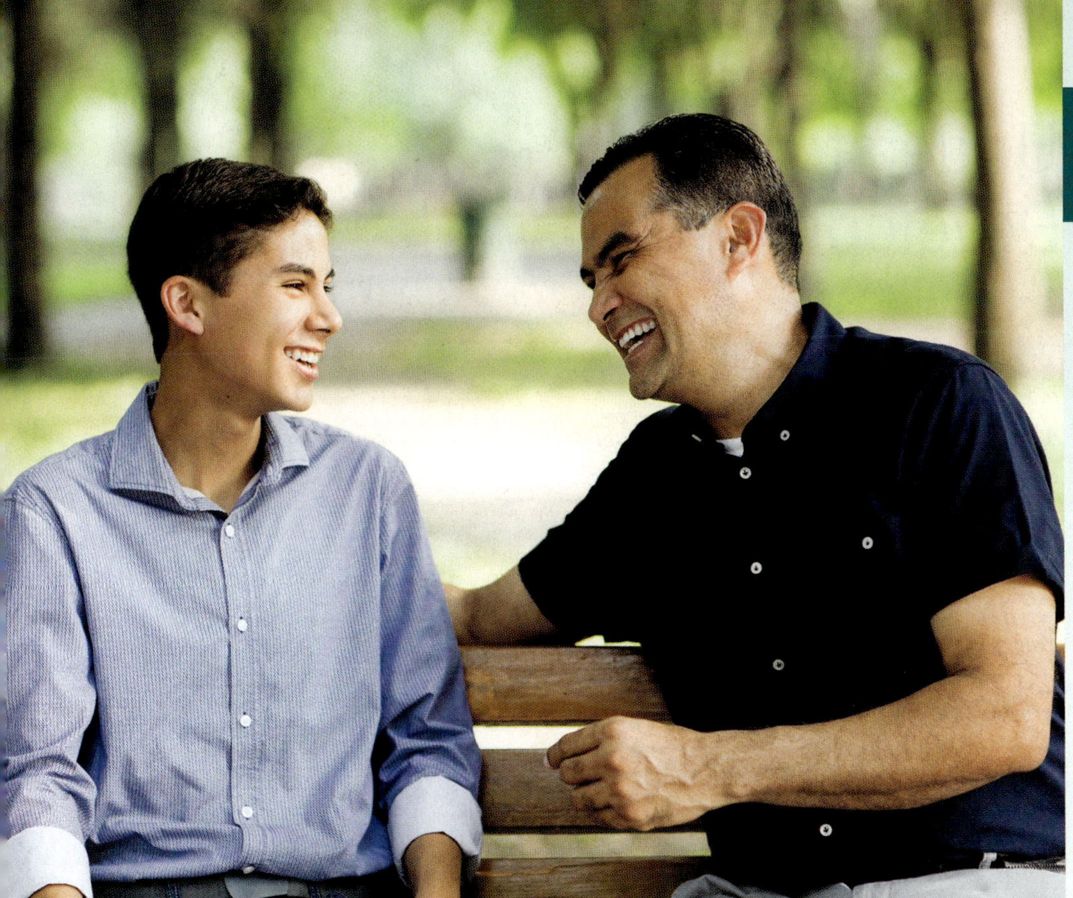
aldomurillo/E+/Getty Images

Reading and Notetaking

Using appropriate vocabulary and maturity, describe how people develop across the life span to a classmate. Start with conception and end with the end of life. As you describe this process, your classmate should listen carefully, take notes on your explanation, and ask questions when something does not make sense or whenever appropriate. After reading this chapter, revise your explanation based on what you learned.

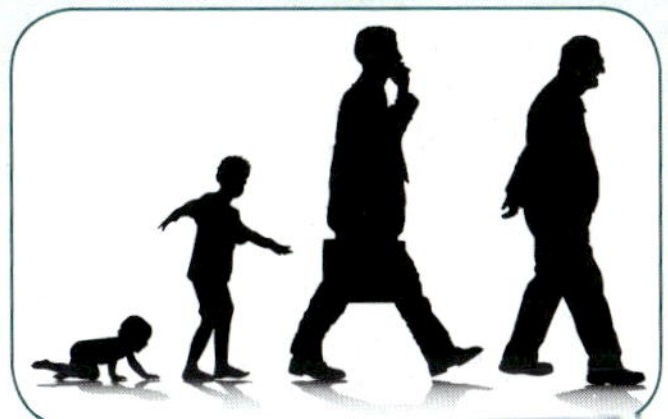
Left to right: grum_l/Shutterstock.com; ducu59us/Shutterstock.com

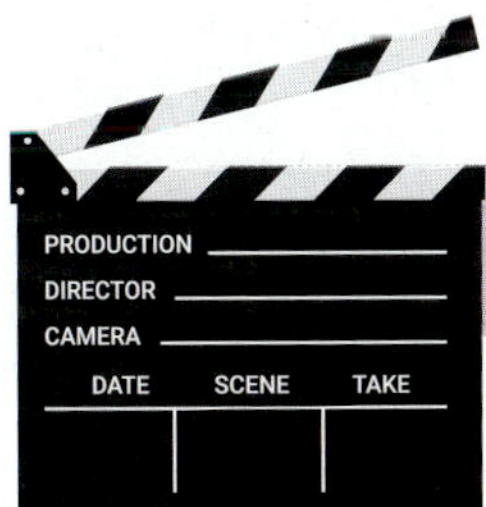

Setting the Scene

Adjustments and Age

This year, you notice you have been experiencing a lot of strong, new emotions. Some days, you feel irritable and emotional, but later you feel excited and silly. Other days, you feel self-conscious and anxious about spending time with your friends.

In the past, you would tell your family about all of these feelings. Lately, though, you get upset when your family asks many questions about your life. You do not understand why you are so easily annoyed. You wonder if this is how it feels to be an adult.

Thinking Critically

1. Are your new emotional experiences in this scenario healthy and normal? How can you learn more about these changes?
2. What are some positive ways you can handle these emotional changes?

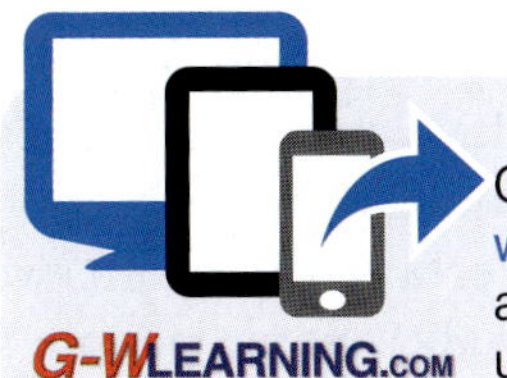

Click on the activity icon or visit www.g-wlearning.com/health/4095 to access online vocabulary activities using key terms from the chapter.

Lesson
22.1

Understanding Development

Essential Question?
How do people develop and change over time?

Key Terms

developmental disabilities
disability
human life cycle
intellectual disabilities
learning disorders
milestones
physical disability

Learning Outcomes

After studying this lesson, you will be able to

- list the stages of development;
- differentiate between types of development;
- analyze internal and external factors that influence development;
- explain how differences in development affect health; and
- describe ways of respecting individual differences in development.

Warm-Up Activity

How Have You Changed?

Comprehend Concepts Before reading this lesson, think about your first memories. How have you changed since you were a child? How do you still hope to change as you enter adulthood? Using a chart like the one shown, consider how you have changed physically, intellectually, emotionally, and socially since your first memories. List as many details as you can. After completing your chart, compare answers with a partner and identify any similarities. Discuss these similarities with the class.

Physical	Intellectual
Emotional	**Social**

Looking at your baby pictures and school photos together would capture how dramatically you have changed since the day you were born. Thanks to continual growth and development, you hardly seem to be the same person. Growth and development are related, but distinct. *Growth* refers to increases in the size of your body and its parts. *Human development* includes growth and the learning of physical, intellectual, mental and emotional, and social skills.

Human Development

Over the course of your life, you will go through several developmental stages. Together, these developmental stages are called the **human life cycle** (**Figure 22.1**). Each developmental stage has certain important events called **milestones** (for example, learning how to walk). Some people reach developmental milestones earlier or later than their peers.

human life cycle series of developmental stages from birth through adulthood and death

milestones events that indicate the development of skills and maturing qualities

Stages of Development

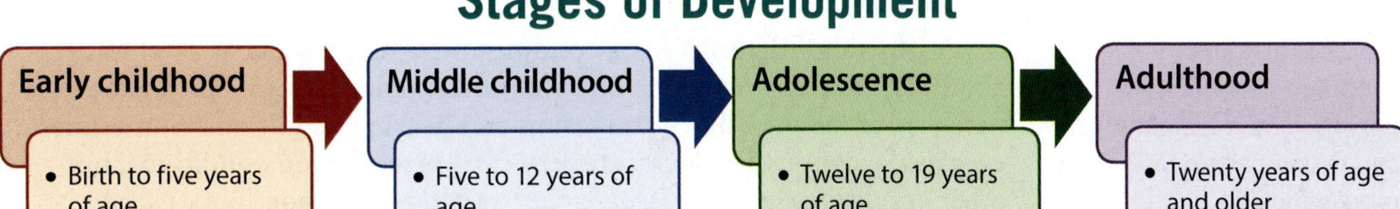

Figure 22.1 Overall, people pass through developmental stages gradually. The most rapid, dramatic changes occur early in life, from early childhood through adolescence. ***What is the term for important events that typically occur during a developmental stage?***

Over time, people develop physically, intellectually, emotionally, and socially. These types of development are related and *interdependent*, meaning they rely on each other:

- **Physical development:** Physical development includes the growth of the body and body parts. Other aspects of human development build on physical development. As the brain develops, a child is better able to process information, learn, and think in sophisticated ways.
- **Intellectual development:** Intellectual development is the maturation of an individual's thinking, information processing, and responsiveness. This includes the development of mature speech and language.
- **Emotional development:** Emotional development refers to the achievement of identity, personality, independence, self-esteem, and other aspects of mental and emotional health. Emotional development normally arises in a healthy and safe environment as the brain matures.
- **Social development:** Social development is the ability to interact in socially acceptable ways. Social and interpersonal skills develop throughout life. Family environment and education strongly influence social development.

Differences in Development

Many factors influence how a person develops. Some are internal, and others are external (**Figure 22.2**). Due to these factors, people develop at different rates. The end results of development can also be different. For example, if someone grows up in a supportive family, that person may develop more social maturity. If someone lives in an environment lacking basic resources, that person may experience malnutrition.

Some differences in development can make it easier or more difficult for a person to perform certain tasks. For example, as you know, mental illnesses can make it more difficult for people to cope with daily life. Noncommunicable diseases can affect the activities a person can do. Another example of a difference is a **disability**, or a condition that impairs a person's ability to perform certain tasks. With treatment and accommodations, people with disabilities can maintain active and rewarding lives.

Factors Affecting Development

Internal Factors	External Factors
Genetic makeup—sets many physical traits, such as hair and eye color; also gives a person certain tendencies, such as likelihood of being tall or short	Relationships—how children are raised impacts their development; behaviors of friends influence personal behaviors
Behavior—impacts relationships and health; getting physical activity influences physical development and aging	Environment—different experiences impact a person's opportunities and development; ability to buy nutritious foods improves physical development

Figure 22.2 People's behaviors, relationships, genetic makeup, and environment all affect their development.

disability condition that impairs a person's ability to perform certain tasks

Physical Disabilities

physical disability
condition that affects a person's physical abilities and makes certain tasks more difficult

A **physical disability** is a condition that affects a person's physical abilities. Some examples include conditions that affect mobility, such as paralysis or loss of a limb, and vision and hearing conditions. Sometimes eyeglasses, contact lenses, or surgery can correct vision conditions, but other conditions, such as *legal blindness* (complete vision loss), cannot be corrected. People with hearing conditions experience hearing loss (called *deafness* in complete hearing loss). Hearing aids and cochlear implants can help restore hearing in some cases.

Physical disabilities change the way people go about daily life and can make certain tasks more difficult. Depending on a person's needs, schools and workplaces can provide adaptations and services to help people with these conditions perform well. For example, people can translate spoken or written words into braille (a system of raised dots) or sign language (a system of gestures) and make buildings accessible to those with limited mobility.

Intellectual Disabilities

intellectual disabilities
conditions that interfere with learning, social behavior, communication, and self-care habits; characterized by an IQ equal to or below 70

Intellectual disabilities are conditions that interfere with learning, social behavior, communication, and self-care habits. Someone with an intellectual disability has an intelligence quotient (IQ) equal to or below 70.

Some factors that can cause intellectual disability include genetic disorders, infections before or after birth, trauma (for example, a brain injury), and environmental factors. For example, two common causes of intellectual disability are the genetic disorders fragile X syndrome and Down syndrome. Usually diagnosed before age two, people living with *fragile X syndrome (FXS)* have mild to moderate intellectual disability and difficulty with social behavior, communication, hyperactivity, and attention. The genetic disorder *Down syndrome* is the most common cause of mild intellectual disability.

Accommodations for intellectual disabilities can include specialized learning strategies and caregiving services. Specific accommodations depend on a person's needs.

learning disorders
conditions that interfere with the brain's ability to process, recall, and apply information

Learning Disorders

Learning disorders interfere with the brain's ability to process, recall, and apply information (**Figure 22.3**). A common learning disorder, *dyslexia*, affects about three million people in the US. Dyslexia does not affect intelligence and does not relate to a person's desire to learn, write, or read. Dyslexia is usually first identified when children begin reading or writing in school.

People can learn adaptive skills that minimize the effects of learning disorders. Accommodations might include specialized learning strategies and accessibility features like changeable fonts.

Common Learning Disorders

Learning Disorder	Causes Difficulty with...
Dyslexia	Reading, writing, identifying words, spelling, forming sentences, and recognizing parts of words
Dyscalculia	Ordering numbers correctly; performing basic math calculations; understanding concepts like time, measurement, or estimation
Processing disorders	Making sense of sensory data (can be visual or auditory)

Figure 22.3 Common learning disorders affect a person's ability to read, write, do math, and process information. ***Which learning disorder affects a person's math abilities?***

Developmental Disabilities

Developmental disabilities are complex, long-term disabilities that affect physical development, intellectual development, or both. These disabilities appear before adulthood. Many physical disabilities and intellectual disabilities may also be developmental disabilities. One developmental disability is attention-deficit hyperactivity disorder (ADHD), which you learned about in Chapter 7. Other examples include the following:

- **Cerebral palsy (CP):** Cerebral palsy (CP) develops in infancy or early childhood and is caused by damage to brain regions that control muscle activity, movement, balance, and posture. Most people with CP have difficulty moving their muscles, and about half can walk on their own. People with CP need different degrees of assistance with daily activities.
- **Autism spectrum disorder (ASD):** Autism spectrum disorder (ASD) is a complex developmental disability that begins in early childhood. ASD causes a range of disabilities with varying levels of severity. People living with ASD typically have difficulty with communication skills and social interactions. They may engage in routine activities or repetitive behaviors that interfere with daily life.
- **Spina bifida (SB):** In spina bifida (SB), the bones that surround the spinal cord do not develop completely. Portions of the spinal cord may bulge between spinal bones, damaging the spinal cord and nerves. Some children with SB may experience paralysis, and some kinds of nerve damage can cause intellectual disabilities.

developmental disabilities complex, long-term disabilities that affect physical development, intellectual development, or both; develop before adulthood

Respecting Developmental Differences

Part of promoting health is respecting individual differences. This means respecting differences in race, nationality, sex, gender identity, sexual orientation, and beliefs. It also means valuing people with conditions like mental illnesses, noncommunicable diseases, and disabilities and reducing stigma. No person is defined by a health condition, and people can achieve positive health even with these conditions.

To show respect for developmental differences, you can treat all people fairly and kindly. If you have stereotypes or negative beliefs about a group of people, challenge these beliefs and keep an open mind. You can promote a culture of respect by treating others well and intervening if you see others showing disrespect.

In the US, several laws protect people with disabilities from discrimination. For example, the *Americans with Disabilities Act (ADA)* gives people with disabilities the same rights as people without disabilities. The ADA also requires public transportation and communication devices like phones to be accessible for use by people with disabilities. The Olmstead Decision, decided by the US Supreme Court, requires states to provide services and support to people with disabilities who prefer living at home. The *Individuals with Disabilities Education Act (IDEA)* protects access to public education for children and teens living with disabilities.

People with disabilities and other differences in development can take steps to improve or maintain their health in each dimension. For example, they can see the doctor regularly, eat a healthy diet, practice hygiene, get enough sleep and physical activity, and receive physical therapy, if needed. They can improve mental and emotional health by managing stress, thinking positively, maintaining healthy relationships, and getting professional help, if needed.

Health in the Media

Disabilities in the Media

Representations of people with disabilities can be hard to find in the media. Until recently, movies and TV shows rarely included any characters with disabilities or other differences in development. As the media begins to include more characters with disabilities, certain patterns have emerged. Often, media representations of characters with disabilities are not realistic. Most of these characters are Caucasian and male and are played by actors without disabilities. Sometimes these characters are insignificant for the story or promote stereotypes. For example, in the media, characters with disabilities commonly

- are portrayed as lacking something or being outside society's expectations;
- show a heroic will to overcome their disabilities;
- face lifelong challenges with superhuman courage; and
- are portrayed as burdens to their families, friends, and communities.

These representations do not portray the diversity among people with disabilities. Unfortunately, they can affect how society understands and behaves toward people with disabilities. These influences can affect the health of people with disabilities and their families and communities.

Practice Your Skills

Analyze Influences

In a small group, choose one movie or TV show that includes a character with a disability. Together, examine how this character is represented. What is the character's race and sex? Is the character played by an actor with a disability? What stereotypes does the character reinforce or contradict? Assess the positive and negative effects this representation could have on someone with a disability and on those without disabilities. Discuss your assessment with the class.

Lesson 22.1 Review

Know and Understand

1. What are the stages of the human life cycle?
2. Explain the difference between an intellectual disability and learning disorder.
3. Give two examples of developmental disabilities.

Think Critically

4. Choose one type of development and identify a time you met a milestone related to that type. Explain why the milestone relates to the type you chose.
5. Choose one factor that affects development (genetics, behavior, relationships, or environment) and review how this factor affects health, as discussed in Chapter 1. Write a reflection about how specifically this factor shapes a person's development and health.
6. With a partner, brainstorm examples of adaptations and services for people with physical disabilities.
7. Write a case study in which a teen demonstrates respect for individual differences in development. Share case studies with a friend and discuss the teens' responses.

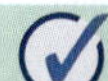

REAL WORLD Health Skills

Make Decisions Think of a time you recently experienced someone showing a lack of respect for differences in development. This could be a time someone made fun of someone with a disability or made an insensitive comment in class, for example. Explain the details of this experience and then go back and imagine what you could have done to promote a more respectful environment. Use the decision-making process to decide how you will respond if you face a similar situation in the future.

Health During the Childhood Years

Essential Question?

What major milestones do people reach during childhood?

Lesson

22.2

Learning Outcomes

After studying this lesson, you will be able to

- describe development during infancy;
- summarize milestones of toddlerhood;
- explain how children change during the preschool years; and
- describe the physical, intellectual, and emotional and social development of school-age children.

Key Terms

attachment
autonomy
early childhood
fine-motor skills
gross-motor skills
middle childhood
temper tantrum

Warm-Up Activity

Growing Like a Weed

Comprehend Concepts

When friends or relatives have not seen a child for a long time, they are often amazed by the child's physical development and may say the child is "growing like a weed." Based on what you already know about child development, what changes do you think children experience? Working with a partner, brainstorm a list of changes, then compare your list with your classmates' lists.

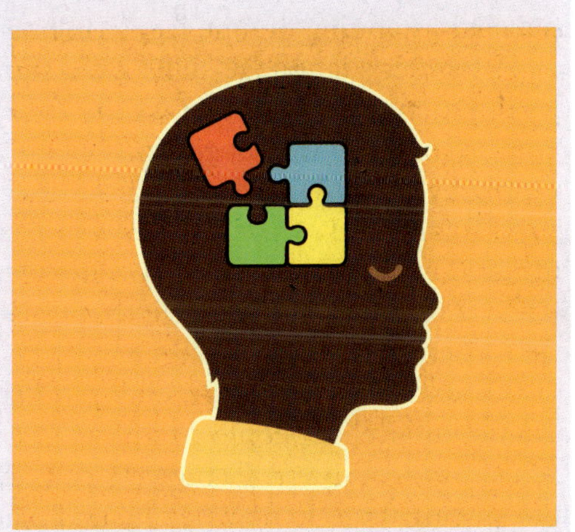

Sudowoodo/Shutterstock.com

The first two stages of the human life cycle are early childhood and middle childhood. Early childhood begins after birth through five years of age, and middle childhood lasts from five years of age until age 12 when adolescence begins. In this lesson, you will learn how children develop physically, intellectually, emotionally, and socially during these years.

Early Childhood

The term **early childhood** describes the time from infancy (birth to one year) through the preschool years (three to five years of age). During this time, infants develop and learn many new skills. They then become toddlers, who are always on the move. Toddlers make great developmental strides as they grow into curious preschoolers. During the preschool years, children immerse themselves in life, soaking up everything they experience and learning and growing faster than ever before.

early childhood
developmental stage from infancy (birth to one year) through the preschool years (three to five years of age)

Infancy

During the first year of life, many infants triple their weight and grow about 12 inches in length. Infants are adapting to life in the outside world after birth. Infants quickly become familiar with the comforting sights, sounds, and smells of their caregivers. They rely completely on their parents or caregivers to meet all of their needs. Responding promptly to an infant's smiling, crying, or other attempts to communicate makes the infant feel safe and loved. As a result, infants form a strong **attachment**, or emotional connection, to their caregivers. As infants grow, they achieve many milestones (**Figure 22.4**).

attachment emotional bond that makes a child feel safe and loved

Toddler Years

Toddlerhood is the period between one and three years of age. Development during toddlerhood is rapid in all areas.

Physically, toddlers begin to lose some of the baby fat—for example, chubby legs and round faces—they had as infants. They develop more teeth, which helps them feed themselves. A major physical milestone for toddlers is taking first steps. Once toddlers learn to walk, they are constantly on the go. Other physical milestones during the toddler years include running, kicking a ball, walking up and down steps alone while holding a railing or wall, sitting in a chair, standing on one leg, stringing beads, and turning pages in a book.

A toddler's language skills are a sign of intellectual growth and development. A child's first words are typically simple ones like *dada* or *mama*. Once children begin to speak, their language skills grow quickly. Simply by listening and talking to others, toddlers absorb many grammar rules. By the end of the toddler years, children can often say several hundred words. In addition, toddlers learn the concept of *object permanence*, which involves understanding that objects and people continue to exist even when they cannot be seen.

Around one year of age, children may become upset, shy, or afraid around unfamiliar people and in new situations. This is a normal milestone called *stranger anxiety*. Caregivers can help children with stranger anxiety by introducing them to new people and places gradually and patiently. Young children may also develop *separation anxiety*, meaning they become upset when away from caregivers. Without an understanding of time, children do not know how long these people will be gone. Separation anxiety is normal and usually stops when a child is between two and three years of age.

During the toddler years, children alternate between displays of **autonomy** (self-directing freedom) and clinging, dependent behavior.

autonomy self-directing freedom

Infant Milestones

- Roll over
- Explore and grasp objects
- Respond to voices
- Learning the concept of *cause and effect* by shaking, pushing, or dropping objects and toys
- Saying first recognizable words or showing signs of understanding words and phrases

Figure 22.4 Some infants may not achieve these milestones in the first year, but should show signs that they soon will. ***What three substages are parts of early childhood?***

Toddlers often react with frustration and anger—including yelling, crying, hitting, biting, or kicking—when they cannot do what they want. This is called a **temper tantrum**. These reactions are normal and a way of testing limits. If caregivers define limits and teach toddlers which behaviors are unacceptable (hitting, for example), toddlers will eventually learn limits.

temper tantrum episode of emotional upset; often includes yelling, crying, hitting, kicking, or biting

As they develop socially, toddlers enjoy watching other children play and like playing near other children. This type of play is called *parallel play* because it is neither cooperative nor interactive. Because toddlers cannot understand empathy yet, they do not understand they can hurt another child's feelings when fighting over toys. While this behavior may seem selfish, it is perfectly normal and common. Toddlers need guidance and occasional intervention from caregivers to learn how to handle conflict with others.

Preschool Years

Preschoolers are children between three and five years of age. During this stage of development, children are usually very active. They show rapid development of the following kinds of motor skills:

- **Gross-motor skills** involve movements that use the large muscles of the body. By the time children enter the preschool years, their upper body and arm strength and greater coordination allow movements to become more refined and efficient (**Figure 22.5**).
- **Fine-motor skills** involve movements that use the body's small muscles. Preschoolers can use the small muscles of their hands to use child-size scissors and hold pencils or crayons to copy simple figures and draw some letters. Preschool children are better able to dress and feed themselves, although they may need occasional help from caregivers.

gross-motor skills movements that use the large muscles of the body

fine-motor skills movements that use the small muscles of the body

Brain development allows preschoolers to observe and develop more ideas about their world. By the preschool years, children develop *classification* skills, which enable them to sort toys and other objects by size, shape, and color. Preschoolers also develop an understanding of time. By five years of age, many children can count and recognize differences in amounts and sizes. They also recognize and assemble patterns using numbers, shapes, colors, and letters. Preschoolers make considerable progress with grammar, vocabulary, and pronunciation. Preschoolers use language to describe objects as being the same or different. They also tell stories and recall the main parts of stories they have heard or read.

During the preschool years, children interact more with adults and seek to please others, especially caregivers, family members, familiar adults, and friends. Preschoolers also begin to develop *empathy*, or a sense of how another person may be feeling. This prepares children to form healthy, close relationships.

When playing with other children, preschoolers move beyond the self-centered behavior of toddlers and engage in *cooperative play*. Because preschoolers realize others have feelings, they cooperate, communicate, trade, and share when playing. Conflicts with other children occur less frequently, and children this age are forming their first friendships.

Preschool Gross-Motor Skills

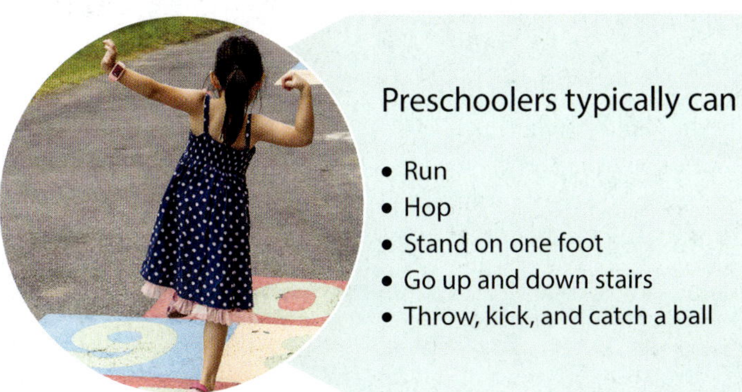

Preschoolers typically can

- Run
- Hop
- Stand on one foot
- Go up and down stairs
- Throw, kick, and catch a ball

supparsorn/Shutterstock.com

Figure 22.5 Physical coordination improves so much between three and five years of age that children can accurately imitate many adult movements by the end of the preschool years.

Preschool children have active imaginations. Many children create imaginary friends at this age. This type of play stimulates preschoolers' emotional growth and development. It is normal for preschoolers to confuse imaginary and real worlds occasionally. They can be confused and frightened by scary stories and movies. By the end of the preschool years, however, children know the difference between fantasy and reality.

Middle Childhood

middle childhood
developmental stage between five and 12 years of age

Middle childhood, or the school-age years, refers to the time between five and 12 years of age. This stage includes another major milestone—children going to school. During these years, important physical, intellectual, emotional, and social growth and development take place.

Physical Development

Children tend to grow at a slow and steady pace during the school-age years. By the end of this period, though, growth may alternate between periods of quick development and slow change. This is why the heights and weights of children who are the same age can be very different (**Figure 22.6**).

Being physically active helps children improve their motor skills. It increases their ease of movement, flexibility, and coordination. Children develop new interests as they engage in physical activities. Many school-age children enjoy playing organized sports, such as baseball or soccer. Children who are active develop muscle strength and coordination faster than children who are less active.

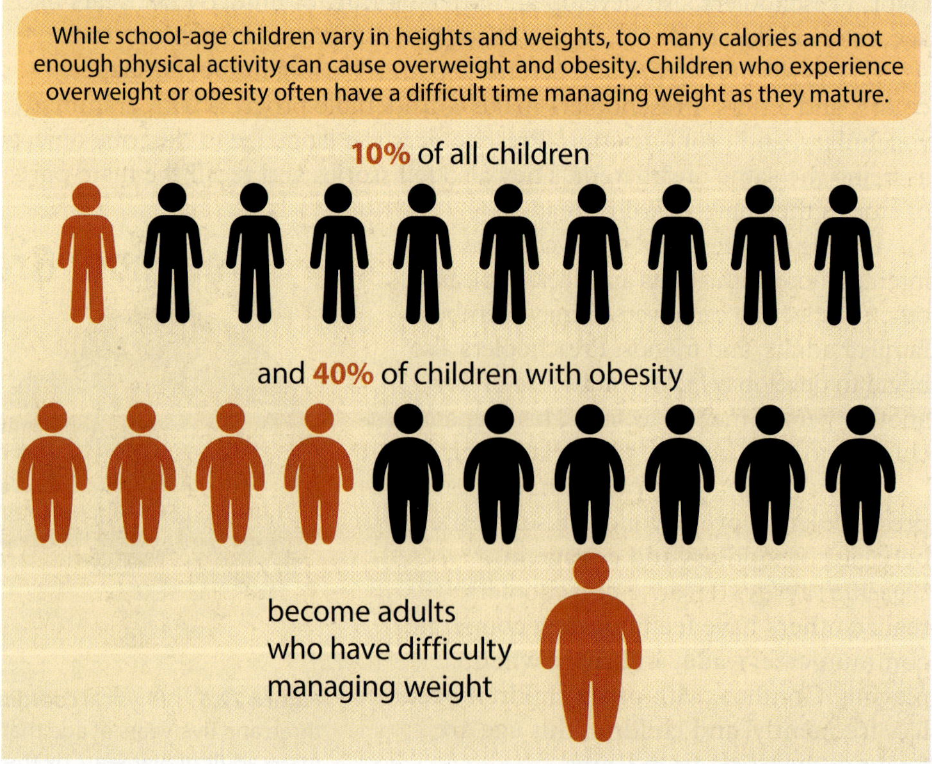

Sudowoodo/Shutterstock.com

Figure 22.6 Establishing healthy habits of eating and physical activity can help children be healthy as they continue to grow and develop. ***Why can school-age children be the same age and varying heights and weights?***

Intellectual Development

Children encounter many new learning opportunities in the school years. Schoolwork increases their language and problem-solving skills. Advances in brain development help school-age children become logical thinkers who learn from previous experiences. Children apply knowledge they have gained in the past to solve current problems.

During the school-age years, children think about their world in a concrete way. This means they think about the present and generally do not think about the future. School-age children often do not link today's actions to future effects. They have not yet developed the skill of planning because they cannot yet think abstractly. School-age children generally think about issues as black or white, right or wrong, and good or bad. They seek answers that are simple and straightforward and do not see the complexity of problems easily.

Emotional and Social Development

School-age children have an expanding social network. These years are characterized by the development of friendships and other relationships outside the family. Children make friends and learn how to be friends. During these years, children spend more time with others after school, on weekends, and during school vacations.

During the school-age years, children also develop *self-esteem*, or sense of worth, purpose, security, and confidence. Healthy self-esteem develops when children have supportive family and friends. It also develops from accomplishments and experience. When children successfully deal with mistakes and accomplish projects at school, they learn to feel confident about their abilities. Handling arguments with friends and adapting to changes at home can also build self-esteem.

Lesson 22.2 Review

Know and Understand

1. What are the three stages of early childhood?
2. Why is it important to respond to an infant's attempts to communicate?
3. Explain why toddlers have temper tantrums.
4. When do children develop empathy?
5. What factors affect the development of self-esteem in school-age children?

Think Critically

6. What factors might affect whether an infant forms an attachment to caregivers? What events might disrupt this process?
7. When did you make your first friends? What skills did you need to make these friends, and how have your skills improved?

REAL WORLD Health Skills

Communicate with Others Most children love to have stories read to them. Reading to children teaches them about language and prepares them to read more on their own. Choose a children's book or a book meant for school-age children and write a few paragraphs explaining why you chose that book, what age group the book is appropriate for, and why the book would fit that age group. Read the book to a small group of classmates and ask them to explain what age group the book is for and why. Take notes and add their comments to your written description.

Lesson

22.3

Adolescence and Puberty

Essential Question?

What changes occur during adolescence and puberty?

Learning Outcomes

After studying this lesson, you will be able to

- explain how sex hormones trigger the physical changes of puberty;
- differentiate between puberty in males and females;
- describe intellectual development during adolescence;
- explain how adolescents develop emotionally;
- analyze how adolescents' social worlds change; and
- assess how to handle common health and wellness issues of adolescence.

Key Terms

adolescence
menarche
nocturnal emissions
primary sexual characteristics
puberty
secondary sexual characteristics

Warm-Up Activity

Adolescent Changes

Access Information Puberty is characterized by developmental changes during adolescence. Using reliable and valid resources, research factors that might influence the age that puberty begins. Has the age that puberty begins changed over the years? How and why? Cite your sources and create a journal entry summarizing what you learned.

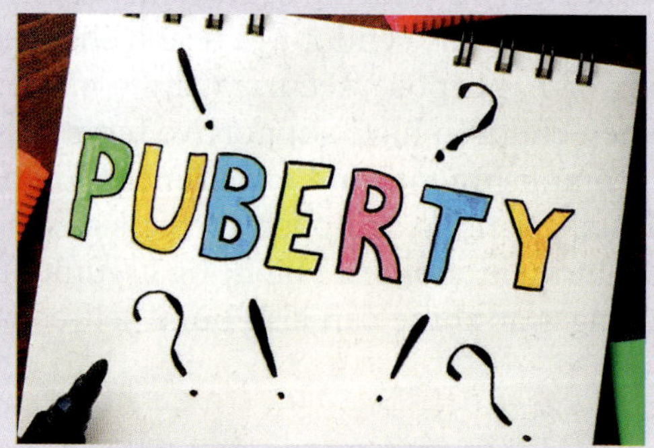

designer491/Shutterstock.com

adolescence developmental stage between 12 and 19 years of age

puberty physical changes that occur as the body's reproductive system matures

During **adolescence**, or the years between the onset of puberty and young adulthood (12–19 years of age), a person's body and mind are transforming. No longer children, but not yet adults, adolescents undergo changes that prepare their minds and bodies for adulthood. During these transitional years, adolescents also gain more responsibility and control over choices regarding their health. On their way to adulthood, adolescents experience many physical, intellectual, emotional, and social changes. These changes begin during **puberty**, when the reproductive system starts to mature.

Physical Development

Significant physical changes are the trademark of adolescence. People complete most of their physical growth during adolescence, achieving their adult height and weight. During adolescence, changes in the levels of sex hormones in the body also trigger the development of sexual characteristics. *Sex hormones* are chemical messengers produced by glands in the body.

They affect specific, targeted areas of the body during adolescence. The types of sex hormones and their target areas are different between males and females (**Figure 22.7**).

Primary sexual characteristics refer to the development of the reproductive organs. The primary sexual characteristics of males are the penis and testes. Female primary sexual characteristics are the ovaries and vagina. **Secondary sexual characteristics** are other features that appear during puberty, such as body hair, a deep voice, or breasts.

primary sexual characteristics
puberty-related physical changes in the reproductive organs (penis, testes, ovaries, and vagina)

secondary sexual characteristics
puberty-related physical changes in parts of the body besides the reproductive organs; for example, growth of hair, deeper voice, or breast development

Physical Development in Males

Puberty usually begins in males between 10 and 16 years of age with the enlargement of the penis and testes. During puberty, males grow taller and gain weight quickly. Their growth rate may double, and males can even grow several inches in one year. By the time puberty ends, a male may have grown 14 inches and gained 40 pounds. Secondary sexual characteristics that appear during puberty in males include pubic, facial, and body hair; a deep voice that may crack as the larynx grows and the body adjusts; broad shoulders; and increased muscle mass.

During puberty, males also experience other changes, such as increased oil production on the skin and scalp. This extra oil can lead to greasy-looking hair and acne on the face, shoulders, and chest. Some males may experience swelling in the breasts, which is normal and usually lessens as adolescence continues. Males also start to experience *erection*, the lengthening and hardening of the penis, in response to sexual excitement or for no reason at all. **Nocturnal emissions**, or ejaculations of semen during the night while sleeping, may occur during puberty. Males may become curious about sex and feel sexually attracted to another person.

nocturnal emissions
release of semen during the night while a male is sleeping

Physical Development in Females

Females begin puberty earlier than males. The first sign of puberty in females is breast development, which typically occurs between 8 and 14 years of age. During puberty, a female's body grows quickly, up to 3 inches per year. By the end of puberty, a female may have grown 10 inches. In females, secondary sexual characteristics include breast development; pubic, leg, and underarm hair; and wide hips. It is also normal for females to gain weight and develop body fat in the hips and buttocks.

Sex Hormones

Puberty begins when the hypothalamus, a gland in the brain, releases gonadotropin-releasing hormone.
- This hormone affects the pituitary gland, which is also located in the brain and controls many other glands in the body.

Gonadotropin-releasing hormone signals the pituitary gland to begin producing *follicle-stimulating hormone* and *luteinizing hormone*.

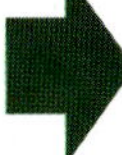

These hormones affect the testes in males and the ovaries in females.
- The testes respond by producing more of the sex hormone *testosterone*.
- The ovaries respond by producing higher amounts of sex hormones called *estrogens*.

Figure 22.7 Male and female bodies release hormones that signal the body to produce more testosterone or estrogen. Testosterone and estrogen are responsible for the development of primary and secondary sexual characteristics. ***What set of physical changes marks the beginning of adolescence?***

It is unhealthy to prevent the development of normal body fat during puberty.

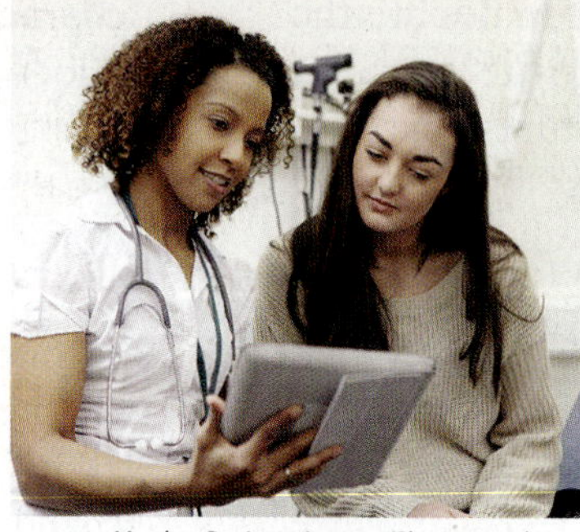

If females have questions about their changing bodies, they should see their doctor for advice about healthy eating habits and healthy, moderate physical activity.

Monkey Business Images/Shutterstock.com

Figure 22.8 Certain amounts of weight and fat gain are necessary developments for females in puberty.

This body fat prepares the body for continued development and the maturation of the female reproductive system (**Figure 22.8**).

The ovaries, vagina, and labia also grow and mature during puberty, and females begin menstruating. As you learned in Chapter 21, during *menstruation*, the inner lining of the female's uterus sheds once a month. A female's **menarche**, or first menstrual period, may be surprising, but parents and guardians or a doctor can help a young female understand what menstruation means and how to prepare for this monthly cycle. Like males, females experience increased oil secretion on the skin and scalp, so they may also develop acne. With these physical changes, females also grow curious about sex and may experience sexual attraction.

menarche female's first menstrual period

Intellectual Development

During adolescence, the brain is still developing, which causes many intellectual changes. As they did during middle childhood, young adolescents think concretely. They view the world in simple terms—in black and white, with few shades of gray—and may not see situations as complex. As adolescents mature, they develop the ability to think more abstractly and see the complexity of issues. An older adolescent is also more likely to think about ways of solving the issue.

Young adolescents may be unable to imagine the future consequences of their actions. As a result, they may act without thinking and take risks. For example, a young adolescent who drinks alcohol at a party might think mainly about the present, the opinions of others, or ways of not being caught. An older adolescent is more likely to think about the short-and long-term consequences of drinking alcohol. The older adolescent may consider alcohol's effects on health and school performance; the risk for accidents, alcohol abuse, and addiction; and consequences of breaking the law.

Advances in intellectual development help adolescents handle more challenging situations, think through complex issues, and understand different points of view. Even older adolescents, however, occasionally fail to predict the consequences of their actions and take risks.

Emotional Development

Adolescents feel the need to establish their independence, be on their own, and rely on their own judgment. School activities, friends, and work offer plenty of opportunities for adolescents to gain independence, which is important for adolescents' emotional growth. Some adolescents emphasize their independence by distancing themselves from their parents or guardians. Adolescents might not be as affectionate as they were in childhood.

During puberty, adolescents experience strong emotions and rapid changes of emotions. Challenging, stressful changes like relationship stress and increased academic pressure can trigger these emotions. Sometimes emotions may also seem to change for no reason. These strong emotions are normal for adolescents, but they are not permanent. These experiences become less intense and frequent in young adulthood.

Research in Action

The Adolescent Brain

Brain activity can be studied using *magnetic resonance imaging (MRI)* and *positron-emission tomography (PET)* scans. These scans reveal the structure of the brain and show which areas are active or inactive under different conditions. Scientists who study how the brain works have found that the adolescent brain is different from the adult brain. Differences in brain development between the adolescent and adult brain may explain why some adolescents are more likely to take risks and act impulsively or emotionally.

Scans of adolescent brains reveal that the brain of an adolescent is not fully developed. The parts of the brain develop at different rates. The *amygdala* is a small structure located deep in the brain and is responsible for emotions; aggressive behavior; and instinctual, emotional reflexes. The amygdala matures fairly early and is well developed in adolescents. At the same time, the *prefrontal cortex*, a region of the brain near the forehead, regulates attention, impulses, and abstract thinking. It helps you plan and predict consequences. This structure, which also regulates the amygdala, may not fully develop until age 24.

Because the amygdala matures earlier than the prefrontal cortex, emotions and impulses strongly influence the adolescent brain. Without oversight from the prefrontal cortex, this can lead to risk taking and impulsive behavior.

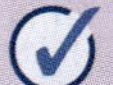

Practice Your Skills

Practice Health-Enhancing Behaviors

Even though brain development makes adolescents more susceptible to impulsive and risky behaviors, adolescents can develop skills to promote their health. With a partner, choose one of the following strategies for promoting health. Then, create a short tutorial teaching other teens how to use this strategy. Include some obstacles teens might face and ways to overcome them.

- Avoid risky situations that increase the chance you will make an unhealthy decision. For example, do not attend unsupervised parties or gatherings where people use drugs or alcohol.
- Decide your views and values regarding risky behaviors like smoking or vaping, using drugs, drinking alcohol, or having unprotected sex. If you experience pressure, you will have thought about these issues beforehand.
- Be prepared to use refusal skills. If you experience pressure, you will be prepared to refuse through your words and actions.
- Use a decision-making process. Do not make fast decisions about things important to you. Avoid making impulsive, risky decisions by slowing down and using a decision-making process.

As they develop, adolescents may feel self-conscious, especially as they compare themselves to their peers. For example, adolescents may compare their families to other families or feel excluded due to differences like disabilities, socioeconomic status, or race. These feelings can cause stress, poor self-image, a sense of not belonging, and sometimes anxiety or depression. Exposure to media can sometimes make these feelings more intense, as adolescents compare themselves to idealized images on social media.

Social Development

During adolescence, a person's social world expands beyond the family and even close friends. The need to feel accepted becomes increasingly important. Adolescents' relationships include new friends, friends of the opposite sex, dating partners, teachers, coaches, and other community members. In these new relationships, adolescents get a taste of what adult life is like.

Adolescents are typically concerned about their peers accepting them. They may seek their peers' approval and try to fit into a peer group to feel like they belong. Peers can be a source of support and fun. Unfortunately, peers can also influence adolescents to engage in risky behaviors they might not otherwise choose. Adolescents need to learn to choose friends wisely and build healthy relationships. They need to learn strategies for saying *no*, setting boundaries in relationships, and communicating and respecting consent.

Another important change in adolescence is the development of identity. Adolescents ask questions like "Who am I?" and "What am I really like?" They may act, talk, and relate to others in different ways over time. These changes are often an attempt to try out different personalities. Adolescents are looking for the one that feels right, when they feel true to themselves. Over time, adolescents come to have a surer sense of who they are. They can base that identity on the values they hold, the goals they have, and the ways of acting that feel most right to them.

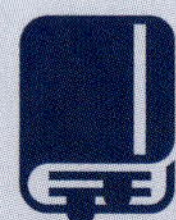

Case Study

Feeling Comfortable with Who I Am

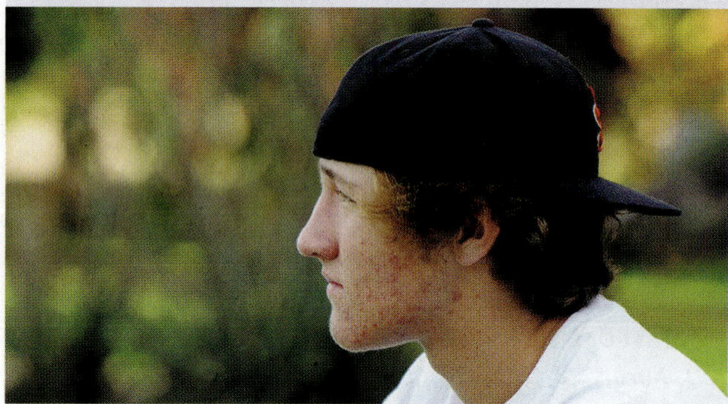

tammykayphoto/Shutterstock.com

At the beginning of his junior year, Emmanuel's face and back suddenly broke out with acne. Emmanuel used to have smooth skin and feels self-conscious at school and his part-time job. He feels like everyone stares at his pimples. Emmanuel talks to his older brother, who also had acne in high school. His brother suggests Emmanuel wash his skin more often to help clean out his pores. Emmanuel takes his brother's advice and washes his face and back in the shower each morning. Over time, Emmanuel's acne begins to fade.

Thomas really enjoyed middle school, but he did not expect high school to be this hard. There is so much to keep track of, from his class schedule to his locker combination to the complicated projects for class. It frustrates Thomas that he struggles more than other kids because he has an autism spectrum disorder. Thomas just wants to fit in and not have to ask for so much help. Thomas' therapist encourages him to focus on things he does well without help, like getting ready in the morning and playing on his baseball team. His therapist reminds him he will need less assistance as he gets used to these new challenges.

Daria has been fighting with her mother a lot since she started high school. She does not understand why her mother is so strict. Last week, Daria had to skip a concert all her friends went to because her mother would not let her stay out late. Daria feels she is old enough to make her own choices about her social life, but her mother still sees her as a child. She needs to prove she is responsible, but is not sure how. She knows her mother wants to keep her safe, but is frustrated by her lack of independence.

Practice Your Skills

Communicate with Others

People go through puberty, develop skills, and build independence at different ages in their lives. Choose an adult you trust—for example, a parent, guardian, older sibling, or other mentor. Using effective communication skills, ask this person about changes that happen throughout high school and into adulthood. When did puberty start for this person? How did this person handle it? When did this person begin to feel fully independent? What advice would this person give to students to guide them through adolescence? Share your favorite story or piece of advice with the rest of the class.

Handling Health and Wellness Issues

Adolescents face some health and wellness issues that are not common in childhood and are not usually associated with adulthood. Some of these issues arise because of newly acquired independence, such as the ability to drive. Other health and wellness issues come with new pressures from peers to engage in risky behaviors. Their developing brain also makes adolescents vulnerable to risk-taking behavior, which can cause health and wellness issues.

Important health and wellness concerns that may affect adolescents include accidents and injuries, overweight and obesity, substance use, sexual health issues, mental illness and suicide, and homicide. You have studied all of these issues throughout this text. To manage these issues, you can use the skills you have learned throughout this text (**Figure 22.9**).

Skills for Handling Health and Wellness Issues

- Learn where to find reliable health information and evaluate health information carefully.
- Understand the physical, intellectual, emotional, and social changes that occur during adolescence.
- Develop methods and refusal skills for handling peer pressure.
- Learn to identify and resist any harmful influences, such as those from social media or advertising.
- Remember the harmful effects of hazardous substances like nicotine, alcohol, and drugs.
- Manage your time so you can balance school, work, physical activity, and fun.
- Maintain sexual health by preventing sexually transmitted infections (STIs) and pregnancy.
- Develop and maintain healthy friendships and relationships with family and community members.
- Practice effective communication and negotiation skills.
- Consult parents or other trusted adults for help with making important decisions.
- Talk with family members or trusted adults to help you solve issues and cope with stress.
- Focus on your strengths, skills, and talents and use positive self-talk.
- Develop and maintain a positive attitude about personal growth, development, and problem solving.
- Set short- and long-term goals and make plans for achieving them.

Figure 22.9 Using skills for time management, refusing peer pressure, or conflict resolution can help teens navigate health and wellness concerns of adolescents.

Lesson 22.3 Review

Know and Understand

1. Which gland releases the hormone that begins puberty?
2. Explain the difference between primary and secondary sexual characteristics.
3. Why do females gain body fat in the hips and buttocks during puberty?

Think Critically

4. What do you think are some common concerns males and females have about puberty? Where can teens get support and information about this process?
5. Give an example of a situation you thought about concretely as a young adolescent that you think about more abstractly now.
6. With a partner, think back to what you have learned in previous chapters and brainstorm strategies teens could use to feel less self-conscious among their peers during adolescence.
7. Why do you think feeling accepted is so important for many teens?
8. What are some examples of health and wellness issues you think teens in your community face more often than adults or children?

REAL WORLD Health Skills

Set Goals The habits you form during adolescence have a huge impact on the kind of adulthood you will lead. Learning skills for maintaining your health now prepares you to lead a healthy adulthood. With a partner, choose one of the skills for handling health and wellness issues in Figure 22.9 Together, brainstorm SMART goals you could set to use this skill. Create one SMART goal each of you will follow and hold each other accountable.

Lesson 22.4

Adulthood and the Nature of Aging

Essential Question

How do people change over the course of life as an adult?

Key Terms

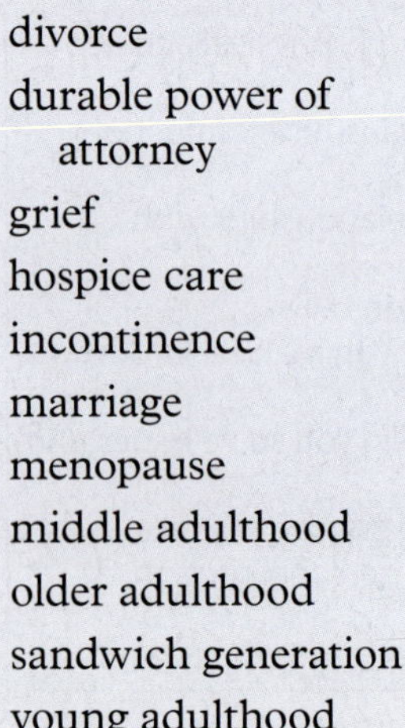

divorce
durable power of attorney
grief
hospice care
incontinence
marriage
menopause
middle adulthood
older adulthood
sandwich generation
young adulthood

Learning Outcomes

After studying this lesson, you will be able to

- compare different definitions of adulthood;
- assess the signs of physical, intellectual, emotional, and social maturity;
- describe the three stages of adulthood;
- identify changes that occur due to aging; and
- explain how people experience and process grief at the end of life.

Warm-Up Activity

Health and Wellness Issues

Access Information With a partner, brainstorm health and wellness issues you think commonly affect adults of different ages. Examine current news stories and scientific studies. Be sure to evaluate whether the information in news stories is reliable and valid. With your partner, make a list of these issues and identify the ages adults usually experience them. Next to each issue, list a skill an adult could use to handle this issue.

Issues	Adults Affected	Skills

How do you know when you have become an adult? Do you become an adult when you reach a certain age—18 or 21, for example? Does a particular event, such as getting a driver's license, graduating from high school or college, or getting married, make you an adult? Do you become an adult when your body is fully developed and capable of reproduction?

In this lesson, you will learn about adulthood and what to expect as you grow older. Some health changes that occur in adulthood are unavoidable, but you can influence other changes by making decisions that enhance health today and throughout life.

Becoming an Adult

Adulthood is defined in various ways. In the US, state and federal governments recognize people as adults when they reach 18 years of age. People who are legal adults have certain privileges and responsibilities. For example, people can vote and marry without a parent's or guardian's permission at 18 years of age. People can purchase alcohol at 21 years of age. A person who is 18 has more legal responsibility for actions and can be treated as an adult in a court of law.

Another definition of adulthood relates to the physical maturity of the body. The young adult's brain and body have reached physical maturity. Young adults have reached their mature height and weight, possess their greatest physical strength and endurance, and enjoy their sharpest cognitive ability.

Many teens have mature reproductive systems and are physically able to create and have children. Teens must mature in many other ways, however, to be considered adults. Perhaps most importantly, teens must still achieve intellectual, emotional, and social maturity. People who are intellectually, emotionally, and socially mature possess the skills they need to

- plan ahead;
- make informed decisions regarding their own welfare;
- consider the impact of decisions on other people and events;
- communicate their feelings; and
- maintain healthy friendships and relationships.

Stages of Adulthood

Adults continue to change and develop physically, emotionally, and socially through various stages of adulthood. **Young adulthood** occurs from 20–40 years of age, **middle adulthood** (*middle age*) occurs from 40–65 years of age, and people in **older adulthood** are 65 years of age and older. Adults in each stage share many experiences, rewards, and challenges.

young adulthood
developmental stage between 20 and 40 years of age

middle adulthood
developmental stage between 40 and 65 years of age

older adulthood
developmental stage from 65 years of age until the end of life

Young Adulthood

Young adulthood is a period of transition and preparation for adulthood. It can be an exciting stage full of possibility and personal growth. Young adults achieve some personal goals or take concrete steps toward some of their life goals.

Local and Global Health

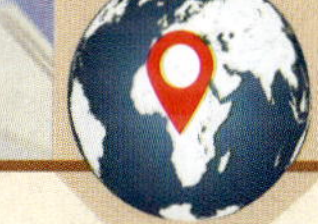

What Does It Mean to Be an Adult?

Many countries and cultures see people as legal adults when they reach a certain age. Some societies also link adulthood to specific life events. For example, many people in North America consider people to be adults when they achieve financial independence, self-responsibility, or independent decision-making. In some societies, adulthood is also associated with taking on certain roles. Adult roles may include completing education and working full-time, being married or in a committed relationship, or becoming a parent.

Over time, the ages at which people are considered adults have steadily risen around the world. Typically, the age of adulthood rises as a society transitions from an agricultural economy, which might depend on early labor, to an information- or computer-based economy.

Practice Your Skills

Analyze Influences

In a small group, consider how people define adulthood in your community. What ages, life events, and roles are associated with being an adult? Do different people in your community hold different views of adulthood? Then, use reliable and valid resources to research how adulthood is defined in another culture. Learn about the events and ages that define adulthood and what roles adults are expected to hold. In your group, analyze what factors you think describe the differences between your chosen culture and your community. How do both definitions of adulthood affect health for teens?

People achieve full physical maturity during young adulthood. Young adults also mature emotionally. With years of experience behind them, they become better at managing emotions and stress. In addition, the brain completes development in the early years of young adulthood. This helps young adults plan and regulate their behavior.

In the US, many young adults become fully responsible for their lives, which can mean having an income and living independently or with people they choose. There is no "typical" young adult in the US, however. Young adults may be single, married, or divorced, and not all young adults have children. Some live alone or with their parents or guardians, and some live with other young adults.

marriage legal union between two partners in a couple

During adulthood, many people make decisions about entering a committed relationship or marriage. **Marriage** is a formal, committed relationship with a defined, legal status. Married couples share resources and legal responsibility for any children they have. In some states, couples who live together for an extended period of time may be considered married even if they do not marry formally.

In a marriage or committed relationship, partners benefit from developing a plan for sharing responsibilities and roles. For example, they decide how to share work inside and outside the home. They may divide or take turns with various tasks and responsibilities related to the home or children.

divorce legal end of a marriage due to the desire of one or both partners

Leaving a marriage is more complicated than leaving a dating relationship, since it involves a legal union. To end a marriage, partners must seek a legal **divorce**.

Marriage and divorce are major, life-changing events. In the US, the age of marriage has risen steadily. Today, many adults are not married, and adults who do marry often wait until they are older and more mature. Statistics show that men typically wait to marry until they are 29 years of age, while many women wait until they are 27 years of age.

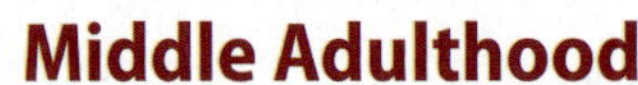

Middle Adulthood

In the US, adults who are 40–65 years of age tend to be fairly healthy and active. In fact, today's adults are not only living longer, but also have more healthy and productive days over their lifetime. After years of experience, adults may make some of their greatest achievements during this time. Compared with younger adults, middle-age adults tend to be more flexible and adapt well to changing circumstances. They have learned to reconsider their priorities and goals when necessary.

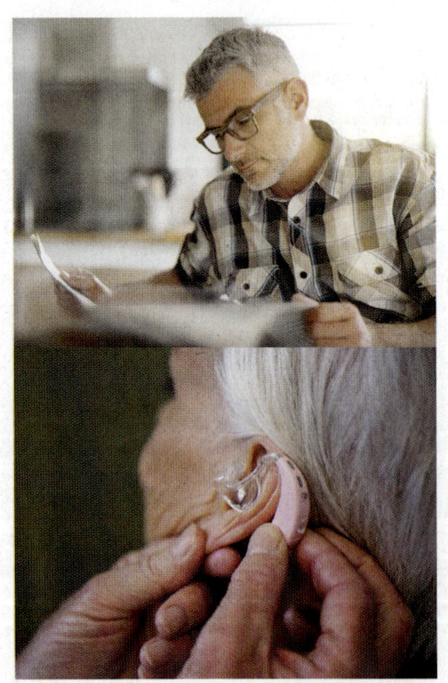

Top to bottom: goodluz/Shutterstock.com; wavebreakmedia/Shutterstock.com

Figure 22.10 Adults can adjust to vision or hearing loss by adapting their behavior or using reading glasses or hearing aids.

Health changes during middle adulthood are gradual, and most middle-age adults adapt well to their changing bodies. Though physical strength, coordination, and endurance begin to gradually decline, adults' thinking skills and memory usually remain strong. Some loss of hearing and vision may occur during middle adulthood (**Figure 22.10**). For example, normal changes to the eyes' lenses can make it difficult to read small print or see details of small objects. Adults can adjust by adapting their behavior or using reading glasses or hearing aids.

Middle-age and older adults may have adolescent or adult children. As these children grow up and leave home, adults adjust to new relationships with their children. In addition, adults may experience new relationships with grandchildren. Adults also often have increased work responsibilities.

Some adults care for aging parents or family members who need medical and financial help. This can be difficult for adults, especially those who also have children. Adults who care for their parents as well as their own children are called the **sandwich generation**. Fortunately, many communities have resources to help adults care for children and aging relatives. These include healthcare professionals who provide services for aging adults; after-school activities and care for children; and counseling to help adults balance personal and professional responsibilities.

sandwich generation
adults who are caring for aging parents or family members and their own children

Older Adulthood

Advancing age brings rewards and new challenges. Many older adults show self-confidence, knowledge, and judgment and maintain cognitive skills. They have experience coping with life's hardships and are better able to manage emotions, make compromises, and understand other viewpoints. These qualities lead many to consider older adults wise.

When older adults retire from work, they find time to pursue new opportunities, such as new jobs, hobbies, and other interests. These activities often lead to new friendships. Older adults must also adjust to a reduced income during retirement.

Naturally, older adults may also experience declining health and independence and loss of some friends and family. After retirement, older adults find ways to maintain a social life, feel productive, and remain active. Some ways retired adults can fulfill these needs include working part-time jobs; volunteering at schools, hospitals, or museums; or taking courses at local community colleges.

The Aging Process

What can you expect to experience as your body ages? Aging happens to everyone, regardless of health status. It is normal for many body functions to change as the body grows older.

Physical Changes Associated with Aging

The changes associated with aging are sometimes easy to notice. For example, you can see wrinkles or graying hair. Aging also affects other organs and areas of the body in ways that people do not see. Over time, aging affects the following body systems.

Muscular and Skeletal Systems

Muscles normally lose mass and strength with age, though physical activity helps maintain strength, flexibility, and endurance. Changes in aging muscles may cause older adults to become tired more quickly. Additionally, bones lose strength, mass, and density. As bones become more fragile, older adults may experience more fractures. Over time, the cartilage that covers the ends of bones also wears down. This can lead to *arthritis*, or inflammation of the joints (**Figure 22.11**). Moderate physical activity maintains bone health and slows age-related changes.

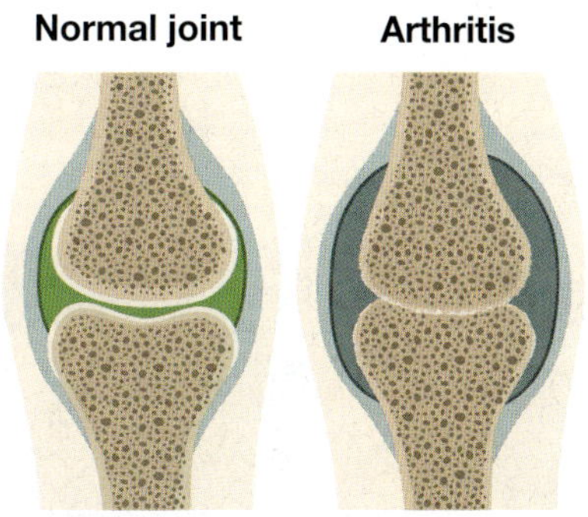

Normal joint

Arthritis

Olga Bolbot/Shutterstock.com

Figure 22.11 As cartilage wears down in the joints over time, older adults have an increased risk of health conditions such as arthritis.

Cardiovascular System

Blood vessels stiffen and narrow with age, which can cause high blood pressure. Avoiding tobacco products, eating low-fat diets, and staying active can slow these age-related changes in blood vessels and the heart.

Physical activity and a healthy lifestyle can maintain heart strength and efficiency and reduce the risk for cardiovascular disease in aging adults.

Respiratory System

The respiratory system works with the cardiovascular system to obtain oxygen and deliver it to the blood. At rest, most people get enough oxygen, but physical activity requires people to breathe faster and more deeply. This becomes more difficult as the chest and rib muscles become less flexible and the lungs become less elastic. As a result, older adults often get tired more easily and run out of breath sooner compared to younger adults.

The membrane that lines the respiratory system also thins with age. The respiratory membrane produces less mucus and does not protect as well against pathogens. This is why older adults have an increased risk for respiratory diseases, such as influenza and pneumonia. Fortunately, vaccines can reduce the risk for influenza and bacterial pneumonia in older adults.

Nervous System

The most noticeable nervous system changes occur in the brain and spinal cord. Memory may falter more often with age, but usually remains intact unless a person develops *dementia*, or a condition of declining cognitive function. Reflex and reaction time slow as people get older, reflecting an aging spinal cord and nerves. Major changes in personality or language are signs of a nervous system disorder.

Sensory System

The skin shows the first outward, obvious signs of aging. People may develop wrinkles, age spots (flat, brown spots), and skin tags (small, raised growths).

Other changes in the sensory organs occur gradually. In middle age, vision-related changes make it more difficult for people to focus on close objects or read small print. Declining hearing is also common as adults get older. Older adults may have difficulty hearing the TV or radio and may not hear a doorbell ring. Certain medications can alter a person's ability to taste and smell food (**Figure 22.12**).

Changes to the senses of taste and smell cause people to lose their appetites, which can cause weight loss and malnutrition.

Older adults can improve the flavor and appeal of food in healthy ways, such as by adding pepper, seasoning, spices, or herbs.

Rawpixel.com/Shutterstock.com

Figure 22.12 Sometimes, older people lose their appetites due to loss of taste and smell. Learning to season food well can bring their appetites back.

The Digestive System

Aging affects all parts of the digestive system, from the mouth to the large intestine. As people age, they produce less saliva, which causes dry mouth. This means bacteria can remain in the mouth. As a result, older adults have more risk for developing cavities and inflammation of the gums, known as *gingivitis*.

The lining of the intestines thins as people grow older, slowing digestion and absorption. The muscles in the intestinal walls act more slowly, causing waste to remain in the intestine longer. This makes it difficult to pass waste, a condition called *constipation*.

Liver function also declines with age. As a result, older adults with declining livers are more sensitive to medications and more likely to experience side effects.

Doctors and pharmacists can advise older adults about using medications safely. The liver also makes clotting factors to control blood loss. Since clotting factors may not be as abundant, older adults bruise easily and can lose more blood from minor injuries.

Urinary System

With age, the kidneys become less efficient and excrete more water from the body. Loss of extra water puts older adults at risk for dehydration. The muscles controlling urination also weaken with age. This can cause **incontinence**, or the inability to prevent urination when urine collects in the bladder. In addition, the urinary bladder weakens, so the bladder does not completely empty anymore. Urine does not thoroughly wash bacteria from the bladder and urethra, which can lead to urinary tract infections. Regular urinary habits can prevent infections by washing bacteria out of the urinary system.

incontinence inability to prevent urination when urine collects in the bladder

Reproductive System

Females typically begin **menopause** in their late 40s to middle 50s. During menopause, egg production and menstruation stop because estrogen levels drop. Rapidly dropping levels can cause irregular menstruation, dry skin, thinning hair, sudden swings in body temperature (called *hot flashes*), and chills. Emotional changes and stress can make it difficult to sleep. Lifestyle changes or medications can help manage these symptoms.

menopause period during which egg production stops and estrogen levels drop in females; usually occurs in late 40s to middle 50s

Hormones decline in males, too, but not as rapidly as estrogen in females. Males often remain fertile, but make fewer sperm. Males typically lose muscle mass and strength and experience thinning hair and dry, thin skin. Sometimes, the prostate enlarges in middle age. An enlarged prostate may block urine flow, making it difficult to urinate and increasing risk for urinary tract infections (UTIs).

Adaptations to Aging

By adapting to physical changes, most aging adults can maintain an active, healthy life. Adaptations include technologies that compensate for reduced abilities. Hearing aids and telephone amplification devices assist older adults with hearing loss. Eyeglasses with lenses that have two parts, called *bifocals*, improve reading. Large print books and larger fonts on digital devices make reading easier for older adults.

Some older adults have more difficulty than others with mobility, strength, and balance. These adults may use canes, wheelchairs, and other assistive devices to remain active and mobile. At home, ramps can replace steps, which may be difficult to climb. Adults with physical disabilities can share rides with friends and family members or use public transportation. The home can be modified to minimize falls, and housing options for older adults can help reduce the risk of an accident or health condition (**Figure 22.13**).

Adults can continue to be physically active by adapting activities as they age. Instead of running, older adults can walk, bike, or swim to reduce impact on joints and bones. If endurance becomes difficult, older adults can be active more frequently, but for shorter periods of time. Older adults should see their doctors regularly to help prevent diseases. Doctors can identify and treat any health conditions before they become worse.

Reducing the Risk of Falls in Older Adults

- Manage health conditions and medications that may cause dizziness, dehydration, or blurry vision
- Make sure to have and use eyeglasses with a current prescription from an eye doctor
- Increase lighting throughout the home, especially near the top and bottom of stairs
- Install secure rails on all stairs
- Install grab bars or a shower chair and handheld showerhead in the bathtub or shower
- Get physical activity to improve strength, balance, coordination, and flexibility
- Wear properly fitting, sturdy shoes with nonslip soles
- Secure or remove loose rugs
- Make sure to keep cords and objects out of walkways

Figure 22.13 Older adults and their loved ones can make certain adaptations to prevent injuries from falls. ***What are eyeglasses with lenses that have two parts called?***

Loss and Grief

durable power of attorney individual who is legally assigned to make healthcare decisions for a person in the event the person becomes incapable of deciding

hospice care healthcare that provides comfort at the end of a person's life

grief complex emotion characterized by a sense of loss

The human life cycle ends in death. Death can occur at any time and can be sudden or expected. Sometimes, people can prepare for death. People can assign others to make health and financial decisions for them if they become unable. A **durable power of attorney** is a person legally designated to make healthcare decisions for someone who cannot. People can also prepare for death by creating a *living will*, which outlines how money and property will be divided after a person's death. Before death, people often receive **hospice care**, which provides comfort when a person is not expected to live longer than six months.

When death occurs, it is usually accompanied by a complex emotion called *grief*. **Grief** is a profound sense of loss and sadness. A person who is grieving experiences many feelings following the death of a family member, partner, or friend. People who are grieving need love and support from family and friends. Some people may also need professional help to cope with loss. If people do not get the help they need, they could be at risk for developing depression, anxiety, or other mental health conditions and illnesses.

Skills for Health and Wellness

Working Through Grief

Grief is a profound sense of loss and sadness, often in response to the death of a close family member or friend. Grieving may be a new emotional experience for some teens. Familiar or not, grieving is a complex process and unique to each person. When grieving, teens can use healthy coping skills, express their feelings, and care for their emotional, social, and physical health.

Strategies for Coping

- Talk with friends, family members, and other trusted adults about your feelings.
- Get physical activity to reduce stress.
- Take part in calming, soothing activities, like listening to music, walking, or reading.
- Spend time doing enjoyable activities with people who care about you.
- Experience and express your feelings by taking time to cry or journaling about your loss. You might write a letter expressing your thoughts and feelings.
- Take part in creative activities, such as drawing, playing music, and making art.
- Talk with others who may have shared your loss and learn how they express grief.
- Maintain social activities and relationships with friends and family.
- Reach out to community resources for support and get professional help from a therapist or counselor, if needed.

Practice Your Skills

Communicate with Others

Knowing how to cope with grief and help someone who is grieving are two important skills. In this activity, you and a partner will play the roles of a teen and the teen's grieving friend. The grieving friend will express thoughts and feelings about a recent loss. The other teen will listen, show empathy and support, and make suggestions for handling the grief. In your role-play, use effective communication skills. After role-playing this scenario, discuss what you learned. What are the most challenging aspects of grief? What strategies worked in your scenario? What strategies did not work? What resources or professionals can help people grieving in your school and community?

All people experience grief, loss, the death of a loved one, and eventually their own death. These emotional experiences are personal and unique. Even so, people generally pass through certain stages when they are grieving their own death or the loss of someone else. You learned about these stages in Chapter 7.

Grieving is a normal and healthy process (**Figure 22.14**). People might need to mark the loss with a ritual, such as a funeral. While people who are grieving might need time alone, sharing their feelings with someone—family members, friends, an advisor, or a professional counselor—can also help them heal.

People who are grieving should avoid making difficult decisions. They should also avoid life changes that bring additional stress, such as moving, changing jobs, or making large purchases. If such decisions are necessary, they can consult with close family members who can help them think through the decision carefully. Grief causes great physical and emotional stress. A person who is grieving may need help with self-care during this difficult time. Nutrition, physical activity, and adequate sleep help the body and mind face the challenges of grieving.

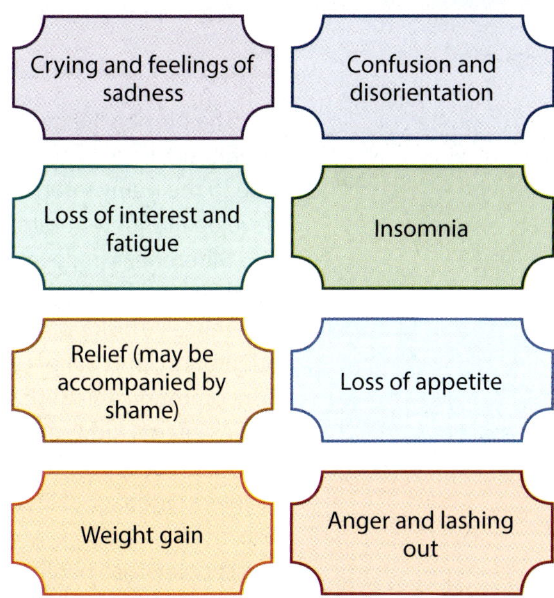

Figure 22.14 Each person may grieve in a different way.

Lesson 22.4 Review

Know and Understand

1. In the US, when can a person vote and marry without permission from a parent or guardian?
2. List three signs of intellectual, emotional, and social maturity.
3. How is marriage different from a dating relationship?
4. Why do older adults have an increased risk for influenza and pneumonia?

Think Critically

5. What is your family's definition of adulthood? Talk with your parents or guardians if you are unsure and share your answer with a partner.
6. What might be the challenges of caring for a child while also caring for an aging parent or other family member?
7. Choose one change associated with aging and explain how an adult could adapt to this change to maintain health.
8. Think of a time you experienced grief or talk with a family member who has experienced grief. Make a list of strategies for handling grief and coping well.

REAL WORLD Health Skills

Advocate for Health People of a certain life stage or generation typically share certain characteristics because of their similar experiences and events in the world around them. This can lead to different views, experiences, and behaviors. As with any other difference, it is important to respect differences between people of various life stages and generations. In a small group, identify one issue in your community that shows a lack of respect for differences due to generation and life stage. In your group, create a social media campaign to promote respect for these differences. Adapt your language for your target audience: your community. Put your campaign into action.

Chapter 22 Review and Assessment

Chapter Summary

The human life cycle is made up of early childhood, middle childhood, adolescence, and adulthood. Over time, people develop physically, intellectually, emotionally, and socially. Due to the many internal and external factors that influence how a person develops, people develop at different rates.

Differences in development include physical disabilities, intellectual disabilities, learning disorders, and developmental disabilities. Part of promoting health is respecting individual differences. This means respecting differences in race, nationality, sex, gender identity, sexual orientation, and beliefs. It also means valuing people with conditions like mental illnesses, noncommunicable diseases, and disabilities and reducing stigma.

As infants grow, they achieve many milestones. Development during toddlerhood is rapid in all areas of development, and a major physical milestone for toddlers is taking first steps. A toddler's language skills are a sign of intellectual growth and development. During preschool age, children are usually very active and show rapid development of gross- and fine-motor skills. Preschoolers also begin to develop empathy and engage in cooperative and imaginative play. Middle childhood includes another major milestone—children going to school. During these years, important physical, intellectual, emotional, and social growth and development take place.

On their way to adulthood, adolescents experience many physical, intellectual, emotional, and social changes. These changes begin during puberty, when the reproductive system starts to mature. During adolescence, changes in the levels of sex hormones in the body trigger the development of sexual characteristics, which vary between males and females. Important health and wellness concerns that may affect adolescents include accidents and injuries, overweight and obesity, substance use, sexual health issues, mental illness and suicide, and homicide.

Adulthood is defined in various ways. In the US, state and federal governments recognize people as adults when they reach 18 years of age. Adults continue to change and develop physically, emotionally, and socially through young adulthood, middle adulthood, and older adulthood. Adults in each stage share many experiences, rewards, and challenges. Over time, aging affects the cardiovascular, respiratory, nervous, sensory, digestive, urinary, and reproductive systems.

The human life cycle ends in death, which is usually accompanied by a complex emotion called grief. Grief is a profound sense of loss and sadness and causes great physical and emotional stress. Nutrition, physical activity, and adequate sleep help the body and mind face the challenges of grieving.

Vocabulary Activity

In teams, create categories for the terms below. Then, classify as many of the terms as possible within the categories your team selected. Share your ideas with another team and discuss your categories.

adolescence	*hospice care*	*nocturnal emissions*
attachment	*human life cycle*	*older adulthood*
autonomy	*incontinence*	*physical disability*
developmental disabilities	*intellectual disabilities*	*primary sexual characteristics*
disability	*learning disorders*	*puberty*
divorce	*marriage*	*sandwich generation*
durable power of attorney	*menarche*	*secondary sexual characteristics*
early childhood	*menopause*	*temper tantrum*
fine-motor skills	*middle adulthood*	*young adulthood*
grief	*middle childhood*	
gross-motor skills	*milestones*	

Review and Recall

Review the information in this chapter by answering the following questions.

1. The achievement of individual identity is a part of which type of development?
   A. social
   B. emotional
   C. physical
   D. intellectual
2. Which developmental disability is caused by damage to brain regions that control muscle activity, movement, balance, and posture?
3. Which law protects access to public education for children and teens living with disabilities?
4. At which stage of early childhood do children form their first friendships?
5. Explain the difference between gross- and fine-motor skills.
6. What is the difference between parallel play and cooperative play?
7. What is the understanding that objects and people continue to exist even when they cannot be seen?
   A. attachment
   B. cause and effect
   C. classification
   D. object permanence
8. What is the first sign of puberty in males?
   A. a deeper voice that cracks occasionally
   B. hair growth on the face and under the arms
   C. enlargement of the penis and testes
   D. nocturnal emissions
9. Why do females gain weight and develop body fat in the hips and buttocks during puberty?
10. What is the difference between concrete and abstract thinking?
11. List three health and wellness concerns that may affect adolescents.
12. What are the three stages of adulthood? Include each stage's age range in your answer.
13. What is meant by the term *sandwich generation*?
14. Which part of the body shows the first outward, obvious signs of aging?
    A. skin
    B. lungs
    C. muscles
    D. heart

Standardized Test Prep

Math Practice

The following results are from a survey of children who have disabilities. Review the results of this survey and answer the questions that follow.

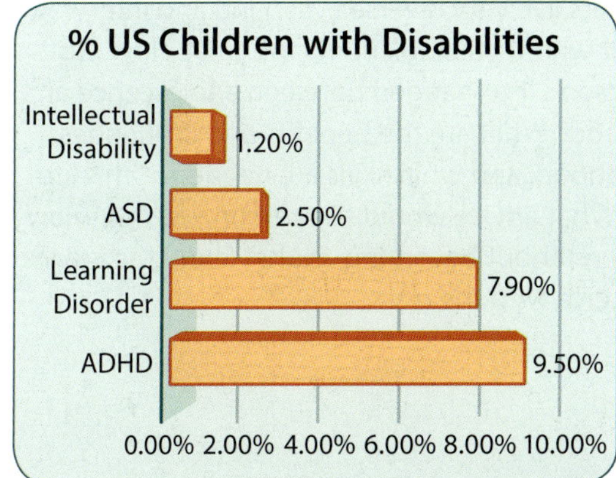

Zablotsky, Benjamin, et al. "Prevalence and Trends of Developmental Disabilities among Children in the United States: 2009–2017." American Academy of Pediatrics.

15. What was the most common disability among children in this survey?
16. Approximately how many children in this survey had ASD?
    A. one out of 30
    B. one out of 100
    C. one out of 50
    D. one out of 10
17. Which disability had a prevalence closest to 8 percent?

Chapter 22 Skills Assessment

Critical Thinking Skills

Answer the following questions to assess your knowledge of what you learned in this chapter.

1. Give one example of each of the four types of human development. How do these areas relate to and depend on one another?
2. Assess your school's level of accessibility for individuals with disabilities. What are some ways your school does a good job of accommodating the needs of individuals with disabilities? What are some ways accessibility could be improved?
3. What steps could you take to better respect differences in development?
4. Interview someone living with one of the disabilities discussed in this chapter. Write several journal entries describing what you learned.
5. Why is the development of empathy important?
6. Describe several ways toddlers begin to display their autonomy and independence.
7. How important is it that people read to infants, toddlers, and preschoolers? What impact does this have on the development of their language skills?
8. With a partner, brainstorm as many strategies as you can for dealing with emotions in a healthy manner during adolescence.
9. Explain how personal relationships with friends and family might change during adolescence.
10. Many of the health and wellness concerns that affect adolescents can be prevented with effective decision-making. What are some strategies you can use to avoid these concerns and keep yourself healthy?
11. Why is the age at which US state and federal governments recognize people as adults different from the age at which people can legally purchase alcohol?
12. How are older adults cared for in your family? How does this reflect the ways in which your family views aging and older adulthood?
13. Choose two online or print articles about coping with grief and the loss of a loved one. Analyze the articles and identify effective ways of coping with grief.
14. How do people in different stages of development interact with and relate to one another? How might people benefit from interacting with others who are in different stages of development?

Health and Wellness Skills

Complete the following activities to assess your skills related to health and wellness.

15. **Analyze Influences.** In a small group, discuss what factors you think influence whether a society or community is accepting of differences among people, including people with disabilities. How do attitudes in a society or community influence the health of people with disabilities? Do these attitudes translate into media representations? How much power do you think teens have to change attitudes about people with disabilities?
16. **Access Information.** Adulthood is always changing, and adults live very diverse lives. Find and interview an adult whom you look up to and trust. How has this person's life changed between adolescence and adulthood? What are the benefits and challenges of adulthood, and what skills are needed in this life stage? What advice would the person you interview give teens about becoming adults? Share the advice you receive with the class.

17. **Communicate with Others.** Many older adults enjoy conversations with younger people, and younger people can benefit from the wisdom older adults have to offer. In small groups, find a senior center or assisted living facility in your community that would welcome visitors. Plan some activities for your visit, such as talking to older adults, serving a meal, singing holiday carols, or leading a game. Set up a time at the facility and then visit. Afterward, share your experience with the rest of the class. Discuss how the visit benefited your health and the health of the older adults there.
18. **Make Decisions.** As a teen and soon-to-be young adult, you are getting ready to establish your own independence. At the same time, you are still developing intellectually, emotionally, and socially and benefit from guidance at this stage in life. Make a list of decisions you feel you can make on your own. Also make a list of decisions you would want guidance on or would want to make collaboratively. Next to each decision, explain your reasoning.
19. **Set Goals.** Right now, it may be difficult to look ahead 20, 30, or even 40 years. Try to imagine yourself as a middle or older adult. Think about how your goals and dreams may change as time passes. Standing in the shoes of an older version of yourself, write three SMART goals you think you might make at that time in your life. How do these goals differ from the goals you have now?
20. **Practice Health-Enhancing Behaviors.** You have probably experienced the grieving process, either firsthand or through someone you know. Think of a time you experienced loss or witnessed a friend or family member go through the stages of grief. Write a poem, letter, reflection, or song about the experience. Include how the loss felt, how grief was processed, and how the experience changed you or the other person.
21. **Advocate for Health.** Community resources can benefit people at all stages of life. In a small group, research resources in your school and community. Indicate the populations and ages these resources serve. Make a guide for yourself listing the community resources that might be helpful to you now and during each stage of life. Then, as a class, create one guide for the students at your school. Make your guide engaging and creative and keep your target audience in mind.

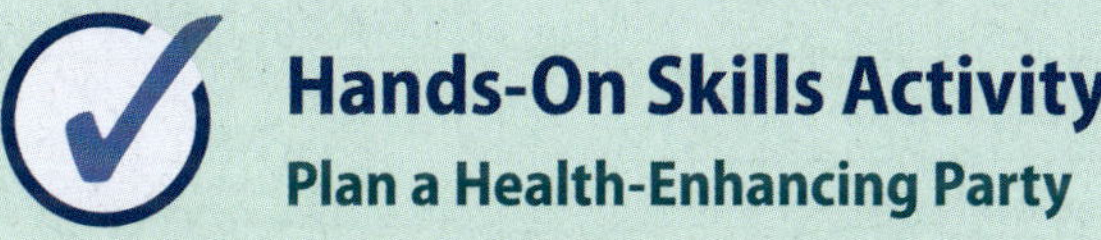

Hands-On Skills Activity

Plan a Health-Enhancing Party

In this activity, your class will be divided into small groups. Each group will plan a party for someone in a particular age group. Each group will then host a Party Day during class to present their ideas.

Steps for This Activity

1. Decide whose party you will be planning. If possible, choose a real or fictional person who does not belong to your age group. Your teacher may assign the age group. Choose a health-enhancing party theme that is appropriate for the guest and follows school rules.
2. Design an invitation to the party. Consider what is appropriate for the guest when choosing the party date, time, and location.
3. **Make Decisions.** As a group, decide on two age-appropriate activities or games for the party, keeping in mind what might be healthy activities for the guest. Be prepared to have someone in your group play or lead one of these activities on Party Day.
4. **Practice Health-Enhancing Behaviors.** Plan a party menu of two to three nutritious party foods. Use your knowledge of healthy food and snack choices for the guest's age group.
5. **Analyze Influences.** Choose two to three presents for the guest. Research presents that will have a positive influence on the guest's health and development, and be able to explain why you chose the presents.
6. On your group's Party Day, present a description of your guest, a sample invitation, the activities, the menu, a picture or sample of the party food, and the presents. Explain your group's choices in each category.

Chapter 23 Understanding Sexuality

Lesson 23.1 Aspects of Sexuality

Lesson 23.2 Sexual Feelings and Behavior

Look for the skills icon throughout this chapter for opportunities to practice your health skills.

Check Your Health and Wellness Skills

In this chapter, you will learn skills for making healthy decisions about sexuality. To understand the skills you currently use, take the following inventory of your behaviors. Indicate how well you think you use each skill. Use a scale of 1–5, *1* meaning you do not use the skill and *5* meaning you feel completely comfortable using it.

Skill	How Well Do You Use Each Skill?
I understand that sexuality is a normal part of development.	
I show respect for people of different sexes, gender identities, and sexual orientations.	
I feel confident in who I am, whether I fit gender stereotypes or not.	
I speak up if I witness other people showing homophobia.	
I know that portrayals of sex in the media aren't usually realistic.	
I understand my own values and beliefs about sexual activity.	
I know how the consequences of a sexual relationship could change my future.	
I discuss my expectations, consent, and boundaries about sexual activity with a partner.	
I respect others' consent and boundaries about sexual activity.	
I use the decision-making process to make healthy decisions about sexual activity.	
	Total:

Add up your responses to each statement. The higher your score, the more comfortable you feel making healthy decisions about sexuality. Which skill do you think is most important for you? Which skill is the most challenging for you? Which skill would you most like to improve? In this chapter, you will learn how to perform these skills better and more often.

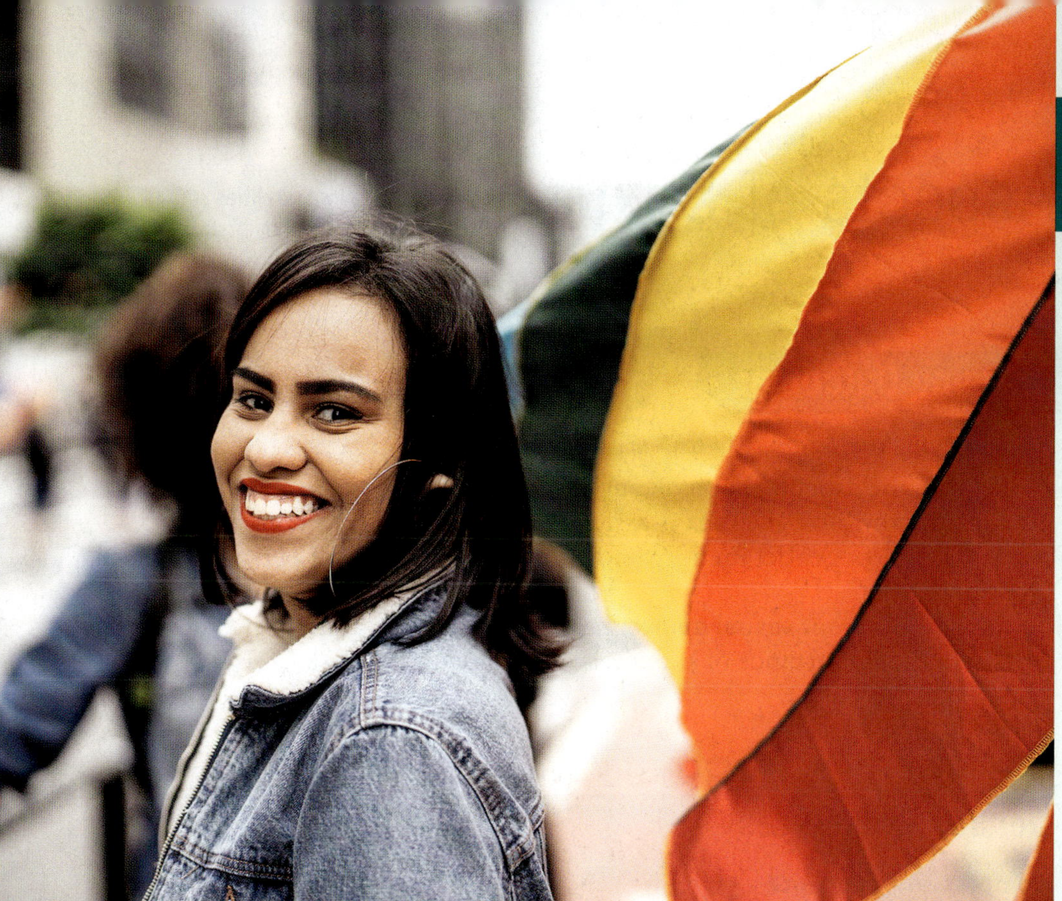

FG Trade/E+/Getty Images

Reading and Notetaking

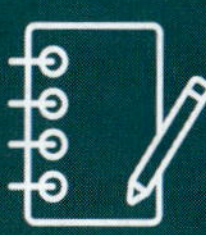

Before you hear about the content in this chapter, think about how you would answer the following questions:

- What is sexuality?
- Are sexual orientation and gender identity the same thing?
- What are the consequences of sexual relationships?

As you listen to your teacher present this lesson, take notes about these topics using a graphic organizer like the one shown. Use the text to add any additional notes you may have missed.

What is sexuality?	
Are sexual orientation and gender identity the same thing?	
What are the consequences of sexual relationships?	

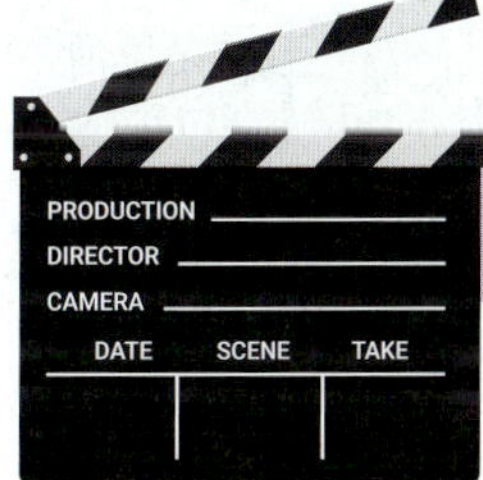

Setting the Scene

Views of Sexuality

After you attended a very small middle school, life at your new high school is full of exciting opportunities and challenges. One of these challenges is adjusting to the culture at your new school. In your middle school, most students had similar views about sexuality. At your new high school, people have many different attitudes about sex, sexuality, and how people of the same or opposite sex should interact.

You know you are not the only one going through this adjustment. Some of your classmates from middle school make fun of students who have different views. You know this approach is wrong, however. You do not have to compromise your own values and decisions to respect others. You want to learn more about the different attitudes of your classmates, but sometimes it feels awkward or scary to ask.

Thinking Critically

1. What factors have influenced your views on sex and sexuality?
2. How are your views on sex and sexuality different from the views of your peers? How are your views similar?
3. Why is it important to respect other people's views about sex and sexuality? What questions could you ask to learn more about a person's views?

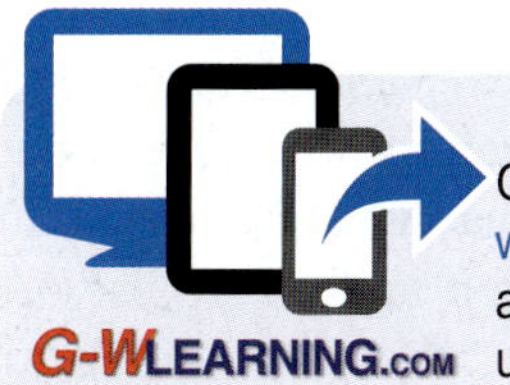

G-WLEARNING.com

Click on the activity icon or visit www.g-wlearning.com/health/4095 to access online vocabulary activities using key terms from the chapter.

Lesson

23.1 Aspects of Sexuality

Essential Question?

What qualities and behaviors make up a person's sexuality?

Learning Outcomes

After studying this lesson, you will be able to

- identify the aspects that make up a person's sexuality;
- explain how biological sex is assigned;
- describe how gender identity and expression influence a person's sexuality;
- analyze different sexual and romantic orientations; and
- assess the importance of support for individuals who are LGBT+.

Key Terms

cisgender
disorder of sex development (DSD)
gender binary
gender nonconforming
homophobia
LGBT+
nonbinary
same-sex marriage
sexuality
sexual orientation
transgender

Warm-Up Activity

Gender Stereotypes

Comprehend Concepts

Gender stereotypes are assumptions made about an individual based on gender. Before reading this lesson, think of a trait commonly associated with a gender stereotype you have encountered. For example, your trait might be "being good at math" or "being sensitive." Take turns reading each trait to the class. If you relate to the trait described in a statement, stand up. Once all statements have been read, discuss observations as a class. Did the pattern of who stood up or stayed seated fit feminine or masculine stereotypes? Why or why not? Then, discuss how gender stereotypes can be harmful.

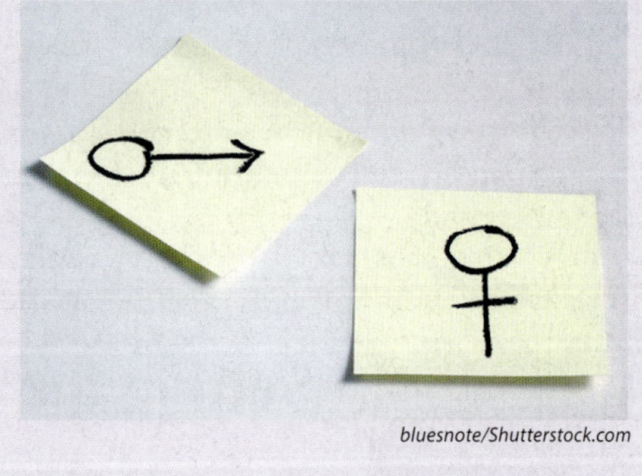

bluesnote/Shutterstock.com

When you hear the word *sexuality*, what do you think of? Maybe you think about your decision to abstain from sexual activity or your sexual orientation. Sexuality includes these factors, but it also includes other aspects of your identity. You do not have to be sexually active to explore and understand your sexuality.

sexuality element of identity that includes a person's biological sex, gender identity and expression, sexual orientation, and sexual experiences and thoughts

Sexuality is an important part of identity and is the expression of gender and sexual feelings. It includes how you look, feel, think, and behave (**Figure 23.1**). It also affects how other people perceive and treat you and the roles you play in your family and in society.

You learned about some of these aspects in Lesson 4.2: *Embracing Your Identity*. You will learn more about each aspect of sexuality in this lesson.

Biological Sex

As you learned in Lesson 4.2, *biological sex* refers to whether you are genetically and physically male or female. The sex chromosomes you inherited from your biological parents determine your biological sex. Eggs and sperm contain these sex chromosomes. If both the egg and the sperm contribute X chromosomes, a person will be female. If the sperm contributes a Y chromosome, a person will have one X chromosome and one Y chromosome and be male. Sex chromosomes direct the development and growth of the reproductive organs and other sexual characteristics. Much of this growth and development occurred before you were born.

Aspects of Your Sexuality

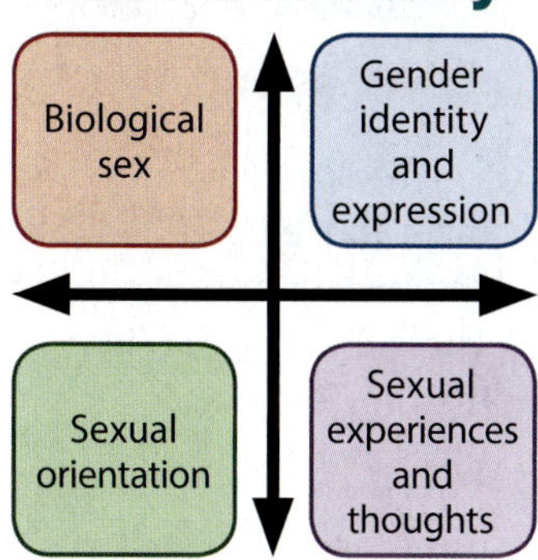

Figure 23.1 Your sexuality involves more than just your sexual orientation or sexual behaviors.

How Biological Sex Is Assigned

Though biological sex is usually assigned at birth, doctors can often detect a person's biological sex even before birth. At about the seventh week of prenatal development, a doctor can use a blood test to determine a baby's biological sex. After the 18th week of development, an ultrasound can help visualize a baby's reproductive organs. Typically, a doctor can determine a baby's biological sex at birth by observing the external reproductive organs. According to this observation, the baby is assigned a biological sex. For this reason, biological sex is sometimes called *assigned sex*.

Disorders of Sex Development (DSDs)

Most babies can be identified at birth as either male or female. Some babies, however, are born with or develop an ambiguous, or unclear, biological sex. This condition is called a **disorder of sex development (DSD)**, though some people prefer to call it a *difference of sex development (DSD)* or *intersex*. DSDs are relatively common, occurring in as many as 1–2 percent of live births. Babies with DSDs have external reproductive organs that are not obviously male or female.

disorder of sex development (DSD) condition of being born with or developing an ambiguous biological sex; also called a *difference of sex development (DSD)* or *intersex*

In most cases, DSDs occur because reproductive organs have not developed fully and cannot be identified. For example, male organs may appear small or resemble female organs. In other cases, external reproductive organs do not match a baby's chromosomal sex. That is, some babies with XY chromosomes are born with female characteristics, and some babies with XX chromosomes develop male characteristics. When this occurs, doctors may order blood tests to identify the baby's sex chromosomes and the type of DSD. These tests and the baby's anatomy help parents understand the baby's sexual development. Parents may assign a sex to the baby and choose to raise the baby as male or female. These babies may or may not grow up comfortable with their assigned sex.

Some sex chromosome combinations cause ambiguous sexual development later in life. For example, babies with *Turner Syndrome* have one X chromosome from one parent and no sex chromosome from the other. *Klinefelter Syndrome* describes the presence of two X chromosomes and one Y chromosome. Babies with Turner Syndrome or Klinefelter Syndrome do not show signs of ambiguity at birth. Instead, their sexually ambiguous traits appear during puberty. These observations indicate that being male or female is more complicated than possessing certain sexual anatomy or sex chromosomes.

Local and Global Health

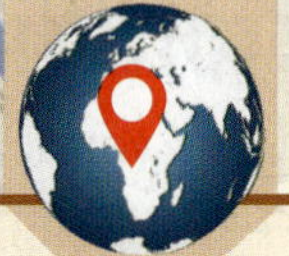

The Evolving View of Biological Sex

The United States officially recognizes two sexes: male and female. Medical professionals have long known that a small percentage of children have DSDs. These children may face challenges as they grow and mature if their assigned biological sex conflicts with their own gender identity.

In the US, a number of states are adapting to science's improved understanding of gender and sex. For example, some states allow people to identify as *male*, *female*, or *X* on their driver's licenses. This is more inclusive of people who are nonbinary. Many US businesses and other organizations also give people the option to select a third sex for documents such as airline tickets and college applications.

This evolving view of gender and sex is also evident around the world. In 2013, Germany became the first European country to allow parents to assign a third sex to a child born with an ambiguous biological sex. Norway recognizes that adults may want to change their assigned sex. Adults in Norway can do this by submitting paperwork to the government and do not need a doctor's recommendation or surgery. Australia recently enacted a law to protect people with DSDs from discrimination.

Practice Your Skills

Advocate for Health

People who have DSDs may or may not be comfortable with the biological sex they are assigned at birth. With a partner, search online or read an article or book about a person with a DSD. Read about this person's experience, feelings, and challenges. Then, with your partner, discuss what steps you could take to increase awareness and acceptance for people with DSDs in your community. What small changes could your community make to help people with DSDs feel more accepted? What information do you think people in your community need to know about DSDs? Then, create a communication campaign to spread these messages in your community. Adapt the information for your audience and share this information on social media, through flyers, or in a public service announcement (PSA).

Negative Effects of Gender Stereotypes

- Mental and emotional strain
- Lack of support
- Discomfort in social situations
- Distorted expectations
- Pressure to exhibit extreme gender traits
- Low self-esteem
- Increased conflict and violence
- Barriers to success and achievement

Figure 23.2 Because gender stereotypes do not reflect reality, they can cause internal and interpersonal conflict. ***What are the behaviors considered "appropriate" for a particular gender?***

Gender

Gender describes the characteristics a society associates with a biological sex. These expectations vary among societies and cultures and change over time. For example, some people believe in strict *gender roles*, or behaviors considered "appropriate" for each gender. Some people also have *gender stereotypes*, or assumptions based on gender. These traits, roles, and stereotypes influence how people think and behave (**Figure 23.2**).

The Gender Binary

Movies, advertisements, and other media often present unrealistic, exaggerated images of the traits associated with *masculinity* (being male) and *femininity* (being female). In some cases, the media implies that extreme masculinity and femininity are normal and desirable. These influences, along with other cultural and societal influences, can lead to extremely opposite perceptions of what it means to be male or female.

These perceptions are an example of the **gender binary**, or the idea that the genders of man and woman are entirely opposite. Seeing gender this way is unrealistic. No person exhibits traits associated with each gender to the extreme, and no one can attain them to the degree portrayed by the media (**Figure 23.3**).

gender binary view that the genders of man and woman are entirely opposite; ignores gender expressions that fall between these opposites

For these reasons, the expression of masculinity and femininity can be a source of insecurity. People may feel insecure about the way others perceive them. They think they are supposed to be entirely "masculine" or "feminine," not realizing these are just descriptions, or stereotypes, and not something that exists in real individuals.

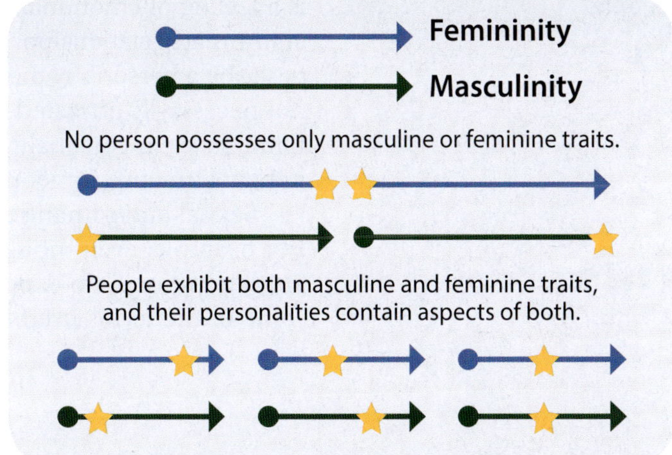

Figure 23.3 Most people's behavior lies somewhere between the extremes of completely feminine and completely masculine. ***What is the name of the idea that the genders of man and woman are opposites?***

Gender Identity and Expression

Gender identity describes a person's internal, deeply held thoughts and feelings about gender. Gender identity influences a person's *gender expression*, or outward display of gender. Gender expression includes the way a person dresses, acts, and talks. It also includes how a person wants to be treated by others.

A child's sense of gender becomes well-established around five years of age. During childhood, most boys will play with other boys, and girls will play with other girls. This may be a way for children to solidify and support their own sense of gender identity. It is normal, however, for some children to role-play as the opposite sex or prefer to play with children of the opposite sex.

Most people identify with the gender associated with their biological sex. These people are called **cisgender**. Some people realize they are not comfortable with the gender associated with their biological sex. This happens for many reasons. People who identify with a gender that does not match their biological sex are called **gender nonconforming**.

cisgender identifying with the gender associated with one's biological sex

gender nonconforming identifying with a gender that is not associated with one's biological sex

For example, a person with female reproductive organs may be raised as a girl, but later in life feel like a boy, regardless of anatomy or chromosomes. This person may choose to identify as a man and assume the associated role and behaviors. This person is considered to be **transgender**. People who are transgender identify with the gender opposite their biological sex. A woman who is transgender is born with male sexual anatomy, but identifies as a woman. A man who is transgender is born with female sexual anatomy, but identifies as a man. Some people who are transgender choose to change their appearance, clothing, and name to match the gender with which they identify.

transgender identifying with the gender opposite the one that is associated with one's biological sex

Other people who are gender nonconforming may be **nonbinary**. This means they have a gender identity that falls outside the categories of man or woman. These people may identify with neither gender (*agender*) or both genders (*bigender*). Some people may have a *fluid*, or changing, gender identity.

nonbinary identifying with a gender that falls outside the categories of man or woman

Sexual Orientation

sexual orientation
enduring pattern of a person's romantic and/or sexual attraction to other people

A person's sexual orientation is separate from gender identity. People of all gender identities can have any orientation. **Sexual orientation** describes the enduring pattern of a person's romantic and/or sexual attraction to other people. *Sexual attraction* involves interest in a person's physical qualities and desire for sexual activity with that person. *Romantic attraction* is a feeling of emotional connection to another person and the desire for an intimate relationship. Some people use the word *romantic orientation* to describe a person's romantic attraction. People of various orientations are not necessarily attracted or unattracted to all people of a particular gender. Differences in personality, appearance, and gender expression all play a role in how attractive someone finds a person.

Sexual and romantic orientation correlate for many, but not all, people. For example, even though people who are asexual do not experience sexual attraction, some do experience romantic attraction. **Figure 23.4** contains some of the terms used to describe sexual and romantic orientation.

Sexual and Romantic Orientations	
Sexual Orientations	
Sexual Orientation	**Description**
Heterosexual	Having sexual attraction for people of the opposite gender; also called *straight*
Homosexual	Having sexual attraction for people of the same gender; sometimes called *gay* or *lesbian*
Androsexual	Having sexual attraction for masculinity
Gynesexual	Having sexual attraction for femininity
Bisexual	Having sexual attraction for both men and women
Polysexual	Having sexual attraction for multiple genders (including nonbinary genders)
Skoliosexual	Having sexual attraction for people who are nonbinary
Pansexual	Having sexual attraction for all genders (including nonbinary genders)
Demisexual	Developing sexual attraction only with a deep emotional bond
Asexual	Not having any sexual attraction for other people
Romantic Orientations	
Romantic Orientation	**Description**
Heteroromantic	Having romantic attraction for people of the opposite gender
Homoromantic	Having romantic attraction for people of the same gender
Androromantic	Having romantic attraction for masculinity
Gyneromantic	Having romantic attraction for femininity
Biromantic	Having romantic attraction for both men and women
Polyromantic	Having romantic attraction for multiple genders (including nonbinary genders)
Skolioromantic	Having romantic attraction for people who are nonbinary
Panromantic	Having romantic attraction for all genders (including nonbinary genders)
Demiromantic	Developing romantic attraction only with a deep emotional bond
Aromantic	Not having any romantic attraction for other people

Figure 23.4 Everyone has both a sexual orientation and a romantic orientation. ***Can a person's romantic orientation be different from sexual orientation? Give an example.***

People of all orientations can be found in all races, ethnicities, cultures, countries, and social and economic backgrounds. People who are unsure about their orientation are often called *questioning*. Many factors, some unknown, influence the development of a person's sexual orientation. Known factors include a person's genes, environment, and experiences.

It is not unusual for some teens to be unsure of or confused about their sexual orientation. At times, some teens who are heterosexual feel romantic or sexual attraction to people of the same gender. This does not necessarily mean they are nonheterosexual. For example, a girl might develop a "crush" on another girl in her school or on a female celebrity. This type of sexual curiosity is fairly common while adolescents are maturing and is due in part to increased hormone levels. In time, most teens sort out their feelings and understand their sexual orientation (**Figure 23.5**).

Support for LGBT+ Youth

During adolescence, teens are exploring their sexuality. Regardless of their gender identity and sexual orientation, teens think about and want to discuss their feelings and dating experiences. Teens who are gender nonconforming, nonbinary, and nonheterosexual often feel, however, that they must hide this part of themselves from others. Hiding this part of identity is sometimes called being *closeted* or *in the closet*.

LGBT+ is a common acronym used to identify people of these sexual orientations and gender identities. It stands for *lesbian*, *gay*, *bisexual*, and *transgender*. The plus sign indicates the inclusion of other sexual orientations and gender identities as well. For example, the acronym *LGBT* is sometimes expanded to include *Q* (queer or questioning), *I* (intersex), and *A* (asexual). Some people argue that, despite efforts to be inclusive, this acronym does not represent every sexual orientation or gender identity. Additionally, not everyone wants to be defined by this acronym. As the LGBT+ community evolves, so will the terminology used to describe it.

LGBT+ acronym used to identify people who are nonheterosexual and/or gender nonconforming

LGBT+ Discrimination

Generally, people who are LGBT+ are accepted more widely today than in the past. Still, these individuals experience varying degrees of prejudice, rejection, bullying, sexual harassment, and violence.

Questions About Sexual Orientation

Do not put pressure on yourself. Many people need time to explore their identities throughout their teen years, and even during their whole lives.

You do not have to decide on one label, and even if you do, this may change in later years.

Ask yourself some questions and reflect honestly about how you feel. If you feel confused or upset about your gender identity or sexual orientation, trusted adults and professionals can listen and help.

Remember that dreams or fantasies may not indicate anything about your sexual orientation. They can, however, help you explore your feelings safely and privately without acting on them.

Figure 23.5 Throughout your teen years, you may find yourself developing sexual feelings toward a particular gender or biological sex. As you do, reflecting on these feelings can help you explore this aspect of your identity.

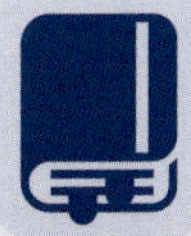

Case Study

The LGBT+ Community

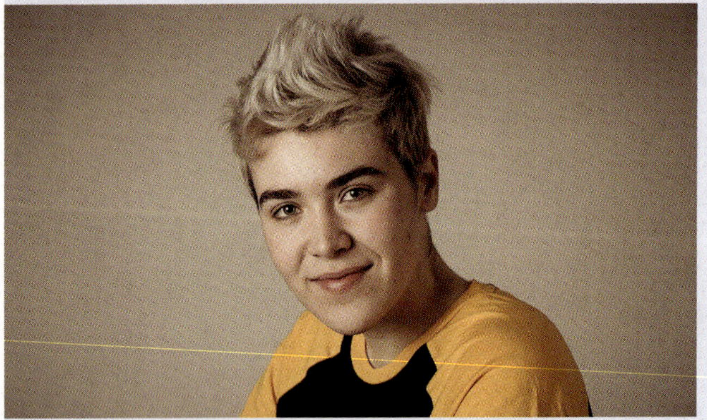

sam thomas/iStock / Getty Images Plus/Getty Images

Bailey took a big risk coming out to family members as gender nonbinary. Bailey's family had not talked much about LGBT+ people, so Bailey was not sure what to expect. Bailey was relieved when the family expressed support and understanding. Bailey's family members do occasionally forget to use Bailey's they/them pronouns, but Bailey can tell they are trying. A gentle reminder is all it takes for Bailey's family to remember the correct way to address them.

Growing up, Leesa was confused by her sexual orientation. When all her friends started to have crushes on boys or male celebrities, Leesa did not. She did not have crushes on girls either. For a while, Leesa feared something was wrong with her. When she read an article from an LGBT+ website about asexuality, she felt relieved and no longer felt alone. She recently joined a group on social media for people who are asexual and has made a few friends who share her experiences.

Dominick was walking out of school with his friend when he noticed Leah, a girl from his history class, being taunted by two other classmates. The two classmates were calling Leah degrading names, mocking her for being a lesbian, and blocking her path as she tried to walk away. Dominick turned to his friend and told him to find a teacher, while Dominick stepped in front of Leah. He told the two classmates to walk away and asked Leah if she was all right.

Practice Your Skills

Communicate with Others

Conversations about sexuality can be difficult to navigate, but are important to maintaining personal health and healthy relationships. In small groups, create a script scenario in which Bailey, Leesa, Dominick, or Leah has a conversation about sexuality. This conversation can be with a family member, friend, or trusted adult. Write the script using effective communication skills. Turn in your script to your teacher to share with the class.

Compared with their peers, teens who are LGBT+ have a greater risk of developing depression or anxiety, dropping out of school, running away from home, or attempting suicide. To avoid harassment, many people who are LGBT+ hide their sexual orientation or gender identity, although it can be difficult and painful to deny this basic part of who they are.

homophobia hostility, anger, exclusion, and violence directed at people who are LGBT+

The term **homophobia** was first used in 1969 to describe an irrational fear of homosexuality. Today, it refers to hostility, anger, exclusion, and violence directed at people who are LGBT+. Teens who are LGBT+ may face the negative attitudes and actions associated with homophobia occasionally or on a daily basis.

Despite the discrimination that is still present, many teens who are LGBT+, especially those who have strong support systems, do feel comfortable with themselves. Many go through the process of "coming out" and tell trusted family members, friends, and others about their sexual orientation or gender identity. It is important for teens who are LGBT+ to have a supportive and accepting group of people around them. Many schools have student organizations for students who are LGBT+ and their *allies*, or students who support them. An example is a *gay straight alliance* or *GSA*.

Laws Protecting LGBT+ Individuals

Governments have passed laws to protect people who are LGBT+ from discrimination. Federal laws, including the Civil Service Reform Act of 1978 and the Civil Rights Act of 1991, prohibit workplace discrimination against employees because of their sexual orientation or gender identity.

You read briefly about hate crimes in Chapter 15. *Hate crimes* are criminal acts motivated by the offender's bias against a person's actual or perceived race, religion, disability, ethnicity, gender identity, or sexual orientation. People who are LGBT+ are frequent targets of these crimes.

The Matthew Shepard and James Byrd, Jr., Hate Crimes Prevention Act protects people from crimes that target people because of their sexual orientation, gender identity, disability, and race. Matthew Shepard was a young man who was murdered because he was gay. James Byrd, Jr., was killed by a white supremacist because he was African-American.

On June 26, 2015, the US Supreme Court legalized **same-sex marriage**, or the legal marriage between two people of the same sex. This established that same-sex couples have the right to marry. Therefore, all states must issue marriage licenses to same-sex couples, and states must recognize same-sex marriages legally performed in other states. The court's decision was based on the Fourteenth Amendment of the US Constitution, which guarantees all US citizens have the same rights.

same-sex marriage legal marriage between two people of the same biological sex

Research in Action

Children of Same-Sex Parents

The US Census Bureau estimates about 105,000 children live in families with same-sex parents. Today, many of these same-sex parents are legally married.

The American Academy of Pediatrics (AAP), the leading organization for the scientific study of children's health in the US, reviewed more than 30 years of research about the well-being of children who have same-sex parents. The AAP concluded that having same-sex parents had no effect on children's emotional or physical health. Also, children fared as well having two male parents as they did having two female parents.

A recent study confirmed that family stability is the most important factor affecting children's health. This study found that the well-being of children was better if children's parents were legally married. This applied whether children had same-sex or opposite-sex parents.

Practice Your Skills

Advocate for Health

Conduct research on new findings about same-sex parents. What new scientific evidence expands on the health effects of being raised by same-sex parents? Summarize your findings in small groups and explain why your resources are valid and reliable sources of health information.

In these same groups, assess how well your school promotes acceptance and tolerance among people of all sexual orientations and gender identities. Do people of all sexual orientations and gender identities feel accepted at your school? Are all family structures treated with respect? Examine what your school community does well and what it could do better. Together, brainstorm strategies your school community can use to foster an environment that promotes respect for other people.

Select a specific target audience for your information and choose the most effective method of communicating these strategies. Incorporate information from your research and provide resources for people who want more information.

Safe Zones

As teens who are LGBT+ learn more about their gender identity and sexual orientation, they may feel out of place and need support. Programs called *safe zones* are designed to help people in the LGBT+ community feel welcome. These programs are important for students who are LGBT+, since they are more likely to experience bullying and exclusion. High schools with these programs designate specific parts of the school as spaces where people will be accepted for who they are. This space could be a room, a particular staff member or teacher, or an entire school. A specific logo or symbol identifies this space. In a safe zone, students know they will be accepted and can discuss LGBT+ issues openly.

Providing safe zones increases inclusiveness and support in a school. One study conducted in a high school found that safe zones led to greater feelings of safety, tolerance, and respect for students who are LGBT+. Even subtle reminders of safe zones can lead to more positive feelings about school climate. Another study, conducted at the State University of New York, compared how students felt after seeing a syllabus that did or did not include a safe zone symbol. Students who saw the safe zone symbol said their college campus had a more positive climate for students who are LGBT+. These findings suggest that safe zone programs lead to an overall more positive school climate.

Lesson 23.1 Review

Know and Understand

1. Why is biological sex sometimes called *assigned sex*?
2. Why is the gender binary an unrealistic view?
3. Explain the difference between being cisgender, gender nonconforming, and nonbinary.
4. How is romantic attraction different from sexual attraction?
5. Give an example of what homophobia looks like today.

Think Critically

6. What factors do you think influence whether a person with a DSD grows up comfortable with the sex assigned at birth?
7. What are some examples of traits associated with the genders man and woman? How realistic are these traits, and how would believing them influence a person's health and decisions?
8. Why do you think people who are LGBT+ sometimes face discrimination? What steps can people take to help them feel welcome and accepted?

REAL WORLD Health Skills

Practice Health-Enhancing Behaviors Individually or in small groups, brainstorm the different factors that you have observed influence gender stereotypes. Together, identify some ways teens at your school could combat or challenge these factors and change these stereotypes. Turn these influences and strategies into a social media campaign or PSA to share with your peers.

Sexual Feelings and Behavior

Essential Question?
What skills can you use to make healthy decisions about your sexuality?

Lesson 23.2

Learning Outcomes

After studying this lesson, you will be able to

- describe early sexual feelings in children and adolescents;
- list the phases of the human sexual response cycle;
- analyze factors that affect a person's sexual behavior;
- explain the physical, emotional, and social impacts of sexual relationships; and
- make responsible decisions about sexual activity.

Key Terms

human sexual response cycle
masturbation
orgasm
sexual history

Warm-Up Activity

You Want to Talk About Sex?

Set Goals Being curious about sex is a normal part of a teen's development. Understanding positive sexual health and practices is important, not only for your adolescent years, but also for your lifetime. Why is it important to talk about this subject? Why do you think some people have a hard time talking about sex? Whom might you need to talk to about sex? If you have a hard time discussing this subject, what might make it easier? Think about answers to these questions and then share your thoughts with a classmate. Then, set three SMART goals for identifying a trusted adult who can answer your questions about sex, developing a healthy relationship, and reaching out when you need to talk.

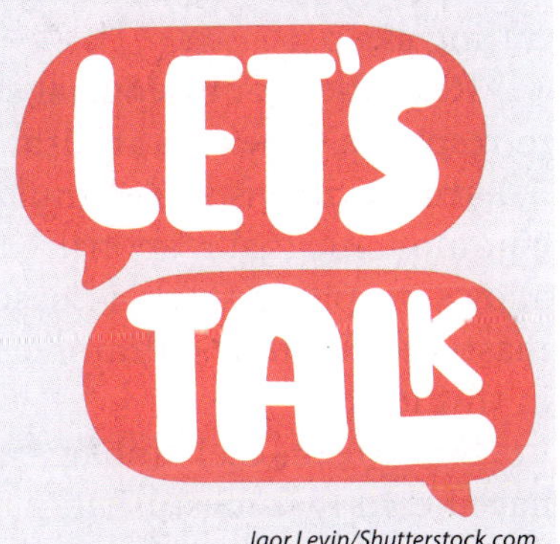

Igor Levin/Shutterstock.com

Sexuality is a natural and important part of human biology and behavior. During puberty, sexual development speeds up. As a result, adolescents experience physical changes and unfamiliar, intense drives and emotions.

It is normal for adolescents to become curious about sex, sexual development, and romantic relationships at this point in their lives. These new thoughts and emotions can be confusing. You probably have questions, which is only natural. Your thoughts, questions, and emotions are the result of human biology unfolding during puberty.

For a happy and healthy transition to adulthood, you need to have reliable information and develop effective skills for dealing with sex, sexuality, and relationships. This lesson should answer some of your questions and help you develop the skills you need to address these important topics.

Early Sexual Feelings

Sexuality is a part of your identity that begins developing long before puberty. In fact, even children experience feelings related to their sexuality and engage in sexual behaviors. From an early age, children are curious about their bodies. Even at a very young age, children may show their genitals to others, touch their genitals for comfort or pleasure, try to look at naked people, or play "doctor" with other children. These actions would be considered inappropriate in older people, but are normal during the development of children.

During the teen years, sexual feelings increase, and people start to become curious about sex. It is normal to feel sexual excitement, or *arousal*, which can be caused by sexual thoughts, daydreams, or images. Teens may find themselves thinking about sex often or having sexual dreams and fantasies about celebrities or people they know. Males may also experience erections and *wet dreams*, or ejaculation that occurs during sleep.

Regardless of biological sex, teens might begin masturbating in response to sexual arousal caused by dreams and fantasies. **Masturbation** is self-stimulation of the reproductive organs and is a common, normal response to sexual excitement. The act of masturbation allows people to safely release sexual tension. During adolescence, masturbation may culminate in orgasm, which you will read about later in this lesson.

masturbation self-stimulation of the reproductive organs in response to sexual excitement

Some teens feel embarrassed or guilty about masturbating. They may have heard that masturbation can cause acne, blindness, or other issues. These beliefs are myths. Masturbation does not cause these issues and is a normal, exploratory behavior. Teens who are uncertain about how to respond to sexual excitement can talk about masturbation with a doctor, nurse, parent or guardian, or other trusted adult.

Human Sexual Response Cycle

During adolescence, many teens experience feelings of sexual attraction. The reproductive organs and brain produce hormones that influence sexual development and these feelings. The combination of romantic and sexual attraction is new, complicated, and intense, but is a normal part of human biology and development.

Sexual attraction often leads to sexual arousal. When a person becomes sexually aroused, physical changes occur in the body. These physical changes progress through four phases: excitement, plateau, orgasm, and resolution. Together, these phases make up the **human sexual response cycle** (**Figure 23.6**).

human sexual response cycle physical changes that occur in the body in response to sexual arousal and activity

Excitement Phase

The excitement phase of sexual response begins with increased blood flow to the sensitive reproductive organs. In females, the clitoris responds by growing longer and swelling. The labia swell, flush with color, and separate. In males, the penis responds by lengthening and hardening.

Sexual stimulation in females causes increased vaginal secretions, which lubricate and prepare the vagina for sexual intercourse. Blood flow increases to the vagina, labia, and clitoris, causing a warm sensation. The breasts swell and become sensitive.

Sexual stimulation in males causes blood to flow into the penis' erectile tissue and results in an erection. The erect penis becomes hard, elongated, and capable of being inserted for sexual intercourse. Heart rate and blood pressure increase in both males and females.

Plateau Phase

During the plateau phase, heart rate and blood pressure continue to rise. In females, blood flow increases to the vaginal wall, the labia continue to swell and flush with color, and the clitoris withdraws under tissue called a *hood*. In males, the penis becomes fully erect, and the testes swell.

Orgasmic Phase

After the plateau phase, sexual excitement may increase and proceed to the orgasmic phase. **Orgasm** is the climax of sexual excitement, characterized by pleasurable sensations in the genital area. This phase is marked by rhythmic muscular contractions in the reproductive organs and throughout the body.

In males, orgasm usually accompanies ejaculation. During ejaculation, muscular contractions forcefully eject semen out of the urethral opening of the penis. Orgasm in females occurs as rhythmic vaginal contractions. Females may also ejaculate fluid from their urethra. During orgasm, males and females experience an intense sense of pleasure and release.

Resolution Phase

During the resolution phase, blood pressure lowers, and heart rate slows down. Less blood flows to the reproductive organs. In females, the labia and clitoris reduce in size and return to their unexcited state. Males lose their erections, and the testes return to their unexcited size and position.

Factors Affecting Sexual Behavior

Many factors influence people's values, views, beliefs, and decisions about sexual behavior. Understanding these factors can help people examine their attitudes about sexual behavior and make healthy decisions.

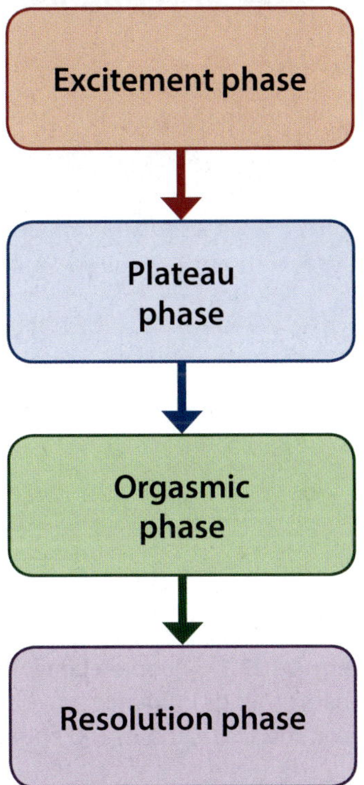

Figure 23.6 The phases of the human sexual response cycle are accompanied by different physical changes.

orgasm climax of sexual excitement characterized by pleasurable muscular contractions in the reproductive organs and throughout the body

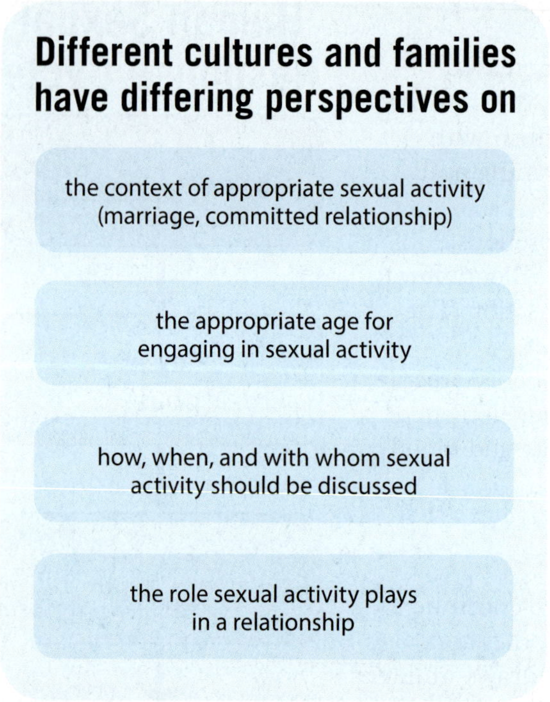

Different cultures and families have differing perspectives on

the context of appropriate sexual activity (marriage, committed relationship)

the appropriate age for engaging in sexual activity

how, when, and with whom sexual activity should be discussed

the role sexual activity plays in a relationship

Figure 23.7 People's family and cultural backgrounds influence how they value, communicate about, and engage in sexual activity.

Cultural and Family Background

Different cultures and families have different attitudes regarding sexual behavior and activity (**Figure 23.7**). For example, some cultures see sexual activity as only acceptable in the context of marriage. Other cultures are accepting of sexual activity in committed relationships. Cultures also have varying ideas about what age is appropriate for sexual activity and how openly sexual activity should be discussed. In this way, a person's culture and society shapes opinions and norms regarding sexual activity.

A person's family may also influence attitudes and beliefs. Family members may teach children about the role of sexual activity in a relationship. Through their discussions, they also model for children how sexual activity should be discussed. If sexual activity is treated like a normal part of development, children are more likely to be prepared for handling sexual feelings. If it is not, teens may feel negatively about their sexual feelings and drives.

Many families also have strong beliefs about when sexual activity should begin. These beliefs also influence a person's decisions. For example, teens are more likely to be sexually abstinent if their family members have an unfavorable view of teen sexual activity.

Family and Peer Relationships

Teens' relationships have a significant influence on the decisions they make about sexual activity. One important influence is the quality of these relationships. Teens with positive, stable family relationships are less likely to be sexually active. This is also the case for teens with positive, healthy peer relationships. Lower-quality relationships increase the chance a teen will choose to be sexually active.

Relationships also influence what teens perceive as norms surrounding sexual activity. If teens think their peers are sexually active, they are more likely to be sexually active themselves. In reality, however, most teens are not sexually active.

Media

Between social media, music, online videos, and TV, teens use media as many as nine hours per day. This exposure to media can shape a person's values, expectations, attitudes, and behavior. As a result, media with sexual content has an enormous influence on teen sexual activity.

In the US, about 80 percent of TV programs show sexual content, and up to 85 percent of music videos contain sexual or sexually suggestive content. Sexual content in the media often portrays unrealistic and casual attitudes toward sex. Rarely, if ever, do couples in the media discuss their decision to have sex, contraception, or the consequences of sex. These depictions do not reflect the reality of sexual relationships. Sexually explicit media can sometimes show sexual relationships without consent and respect.

Unrealistic or harmful attitudes and expectations can influence people to make unhealthy, uninformed decisions about sexual activity. Fortunately, people can protect themselves from this influence using skills for analyzing and interpreting media messages (**Figure 23.8**). Instead of accepting that media depictions represent reality, teens can question sexual content they see and remember that sexual activity has consequences and many teens are not sexually active.

Questions to Ask About Media

Who created this?	Was it a company? an individual? Was it an anonymous source?
Why did they make this?	To inform? to change your mind or behavior? to get you to buy something?
Who is the target audience?	Kids, teens, or adults? boys or girls? students? athletes?
What makes this source credible?	Does it have information from a content expert? Does it provide data from a scientific study?
Were there details left out? If so, why?	Does it only present one side? Do you need more information to fully understand?

Figure 23.8 Teens can ask specific questions to analyze and interpret media. ***What percentage of US TV programs shows sexual content?***

Goals and Values

Teens who set and work toward clear goals are more likely to avoid risky behaviors, including sexual activity. Clear goals bring into focus the importance of making responsible decisions each day. Each daily, weekly, and monthly decision can impact whether people achieve their goals. For example, having clear goals for the future can make teens less likely to risk the short- and long-term consequences of teen pregnancy or a sexually transmittted infection (STI).

A person's *values*, or what a person considers important, also influence decisions about sexual activity. Values often come from a person's family, culture, society, or education. They guide decisions and behaviors throughout life. Teens who understand their own values are better able to make healthy decisions and are less likely to be pressured into risky behaviors.

Consequences of Sexual Relationships

Sexual activity has many effects on each person in a romantic relationship. The consequences of sexual activity are physical, emotional, and social and can last for a person's lifetime.

Physical Consequences

Sexual activity can have many long-lasting physical consequences. These consequences can alter a person's goals and future decisions and opportunities. Having vaginal sex even once, and even for the first time, can lead to pregnancy and the birth of a baby. As you have learned, becoming a teen parent changes a person's life dramatically and can lead to health conditions for the pregnant person and baby.

Sexual activity of any kind puts people at risk for STIs. Because some STIs are asymptomatic, some people do not know they have an STI. Even so, STIs can lead to infertility and other health conditions. While some are easily treated, others stay for the rest of a person's life.

Emotional Consequences

Just as hormones direct the development of the reproductive system during puberty, they also influence emotions and behavior during and after sexual activity. The hormone *oxytocin* is released by the brain during several different situations, including in-person conversations, holding hands, hugging, sexual activity and orgasm, labor and childbirth, and breastfeeding.

Health in the Media

Portrayal of Sex in the Media

TV shows, movies, music videos, and music use sexual images to get their audience interested and keep them watching. The aim of these images is to entertain, not to educate. As a result, portrayals of sex in the media are often fiction. These portrayals do not show the communication that is part of healthy sexual relationships.

Sometimes, the media can even spread potentially destructive messages about sex. For example, some media portrayals treat people as objects for sexual activity. Others associate sexual activity with aggressive behavior or violence. Media portrayals can also reinforce gender stereotypes and normalize teen sexual activity.

All of these factors can have negative influences on how teens view sexual activity. Media portrayals that normalize unhealthy behaviors can harm health, and teens may develop unrealistic expectations about sexual relationships. Controlling media exposure and analyzing media messages can help teens manage this influence and make healthy decisions.

Practice Your Skills

Analyze Influences

View a music video or popular TV show that features young adults or teens. Evaluate the video or show according to the following statements. Use a chart like the one shown to decide whether each statement about sexual behavior is *true* of the video or *false* of the video. Then answer the questions that follow.

After evaluating the music video or TV show, create a blog post or video in which you answer the following questions:

- What were the results of your evaluation? Based on these results, does the video or show you chose have a *realistic* or *unrealistic* portrayal of sex? Why?
- Think about the sexual or romantic situations in the music video or TV show. How do these differ from your real-life experiences?
- Is there anything wrong with portraying people as sexual objects? How do these portrayals affect people's behavior? Explain.
- Do you think the images and messages in the video or show you chose influence teens' views about sex? If so, how? Explain your answer.

Statement	True?	False?
People are portrayed as objects for sexual activity.		
People often wear revealing clothes.		
People's physical appearances seem more important than other personal qualities.		
Kissing and sexual activity are important parts of the story or plot.		
Most of the dialogue focuses on discussions about sexual relationships or sexual activity.		
Most scenes that portray romantic relationships show or imply sexual activity.		
People assume (do not actively seek) consent for sexual activity.		
Abstinence or contraceptive use is not shown, implied, or discussed.		

Skills for Health and Wellness

Use the Decision-Making Process: Sexual Activity

Decisions about sexual activity can be difficult to make, especially if you feel pressured or feel like everyone around you is having sex. In hard decisions like this one, it is especially important to use decision-making skills and follow the decision-making process. You learned about the six steps of the decision-making process in Chapter 2. Following is an example of how you could apply it to a situation where someone is asking you to have sex.

Using the Decision-Making Process: Sexual Activity	
Step 1: Define the decision or problem.	You know you do not want to have sex, but your partner keeps asking you. In the past, you have just ignored your partner's question and changed the subject. You need to make a decision about how you will remain abstinent in this situation.
Step 2: Explore alternatives and options.	With a friend, you brainstorm ways of handling the situation. You think of the following alternatives: • Wait until your partner gives up on asking you. • Change your mind about waiting to have sex. • Use your refusal skills the next time your partner asks you. • Start a conversation with your partner about your views on sex. • End the dating relationship.
Step 3: Consider the consequences.	You work on identifying the potential consequences of each alternative. Waiting until your partner stops asking might ruin your relationship, and ending the relationship will mean not dating your partner anymore. Changing your mind will compromise your values. Using refusal skills will work, but it might be easier to start the conversation ahead of time instead of waiting until your partner next wants to have sex.
Step 4: Identify the best alternative.	You choose to start a conversation with your partner. It is time to discuss both of your views about sex.
Step 5: Decide and act.	You put your decision into action by telling your partner you want to meet up and talk about something. You practice what you want to say ahead of time with your friend.
Step 6: Evaluate and revise.	After talking with your partner, your partner seems surprised, but will respect your decision. You decide to use refusal skills if your partner asks again. If your partner tries to pressure you, you will end the dating relationship.

Practice Your Skills

Make Decisions

What tough decisions do teens in your school have to make about sex? Think about this question and then write a realistic case study about a teen facing a difficult decision related to sex. For example, the teen in your story could be debating whether to be sexually abstinent or trying to get real answers to questions about sex. After writing your case study, place it in a pile with the case studies of your classmates. Choose another classmate's case study at random and read it.

Now, use the decision-making process to help the teen in the case study you chose make the decision or solve the problem. Go through each step of the decision-making process and explain how the teen makes the decision. Complete the case study with the outcome of the decision and then return the case study to the person who wrote it. Assess the decision made in the case study you wrote. Would you have made a different decision? Explain.

Oxytocin, often called the *cuddling hormone*, also affects the brain by causing sensations of bonding, closeness, and nurturing. Sometimes, these sensations can be very intense. Most teens are not ready to handle the intense emotions associated with a sexual relationship like jealousy or vulnerability. Many teens may feel overwhelmed by these new emotions. Teens may also have to cope with the stress of a possible pregnancy or STI. After forming an intimate bond, a couple will have a harder time after a breakup.

Social Consequences

Teens who have a sexual relationship may face unexpected social consequences. Sometimes peers view sexually active teens negatively. Sexual activity can also cause conflict in family relationships if family members disapprove of teens' decisions.

When teen couples become sexually active, they often spend more time together and less time with other friends. This can harm friendships and other relationships. Friends who disapprove of teen sexual relationships may avoid the couple, leaving them isolated.

Making Decisions About Sex

According to experts, the most responsible decision teens can make related to sexual activity is *sexual abstinence*. Sexual abstinence involves refraining from sexual activity. Its benefits, which you learned about in Lesson 14.5, include protection from pregnancy and STIs, emotional maturity, time for personal growth and relationships, and greater enjoyment of nonsexual activities. Abstinence can be hard to practice, but will help you protect your health, relationships, and future dreams and goals.

When making decisions about sex, couples should be able to discuss sex openly (**Figure 23.9**). Both partners should carefully consider their values, their goals for the future, and the risks associated with sex. During this conversation, couples should do the following:

- *Discuss* their views on sex and ways to handle STIs or an unplanned pregnancy. This discussion should occur early in the relationship, before people become sexually involved or aroused. Both partners should be able to give their views openly and honestly, knowing their partner will listen and understand. If a person is undecided about sex, that person should make a decision before beginning a romantic relationship. It takes maturity to share, communicate honestly, and trust.
- *Respect* the other person's decision about sex. Partners must respect each other's commitment to sexual abstinence. Before having sex, each partner must consent to sex. One person cannot make the decision for the other person or assume the other person will go along.
- *Agree* on the methods for carrying out the decision. If the couple decides to be sexually abstinent, they should discuss how they will stick to that decision. Couples who are sexually active should agree on methods for preventing pregnancy and STIs. You will learn more about methods for preventing pregnancy in Chapter 24.
- *Share* information about their **sexual history**, or past sexual activity and partners. If either partner has an STI, the couple must discuss this and take steps to prevent transmission.

sexual history
information about a person's past sexual activity and partners

Openly and honestly discuss views on sex

You should know your views on sex before engaging in a sexual relationship.

Respect each other's decisions about sex

Each person should respect their partner's decision to practice sexual abstinence and only engage in sex if both people consent.

Agree on the methods for carrying out the decision

Methods for maintaining abstinence or preventing pregnancies and STIs should be decided together.

Share information about sexual history

Talk to each other about past sexual activity and partners, including any history of STIs.

Figure 23.9 If teens do not know their views on sex and cannot talk openly and honestly with their partner about sex, they are not be ready to have a sexual relationship.

Lesson 23.2 Review

Know and Understand

1. What happens during orgasm in males and females?
2. How does family background influence a teen's decisions about sexual activity?
3. Why are sexual relationships more emotionally intense than relationships without sexual activity?
4. What is the most responsible decision teens can make related to sexual activity?

Think Critically

5. Why is masturbation a safer release of sexual tension than teen sexual activity?
6. Why do you think high-quality relationships make teens less likely to engage in sexual activity?
7. What unrealistic expectations about sexual activity have you seen media depictions set?
8. Why is it important for couples to share their sexual histories before becoming sexually active?

REAL WORLD Health Skills

Access Information When it comes to sex, people sometimes say that "everyone is doing it." The media may support this belief by portraying teens and young adults involved in casual sexual relationships with no responsibilities attached. Using reliable and valid resources, research the latest statistics on teens and sexual activity. How many teens are actually sexually active? Are these sexual relationships truly casual, with no responsibilities attached? Record a short video, podcast episode, or PSA discussing the phrase "everyone is doing it."

Chapter 23 Review and Assessment

Chapter Summary

Sexuality is a part of identity that includes your biological sex, gender identity and expression, sexual orientation, and sexual experiences and thoughts. Biological sex describes whether you are genetically and physically male or female. Biological sex is often assigned at birth, but can be ambiguous. In contrast, gender describes the characteristics society associates with a biological sex.

Society often assumes particular gender roles and stereotypes. Gender stereotypes can harm self-esteem and a person's relationships, especially since people do not exhibit only masculine or feminine traits. Gender identity refers to a person's deeply held, internal thoughts and feelings about gender. People who are gender nonconforming have a gender identity that does not match their biological sex. People who are nonbinary have a gender that falls outside the categories of man or woman.

Sexual orientation is a person's enduring pattern of romantic and/or sexual attraction to others. People use many different words to describe sexual and romantic orientation. Often, people who are gender nonconforming or have a nonheterosexual orientation identify as LGBT+. People who are LGBT+ may face discrimination. Being an upstander and advocating for safe zones can help these people feel accepted.

Sexual feelings increase during the teen years, and people start to become curious about sex. Some teens may feel sexual excitement, or arousal. Some may have sexual fantasies or wet dreams. Teens might masturbate in response to this arousal. Physical changes in the body during sexual arousal are called the human sexual response cycle and include the following phases: excitement, plateau, orgasm, and resolution.

Sexuality develops over a person's lifetime, starting in childhood. Many factors affect sexual behavior, including cultural and family background, relationships, media, and goals and values. Sexual relationships have lasting physical, emotional, and social consequences. Therefore, it is important to make responsible decisions about sex and discuss this decision with a partner. Making wise decisions about sex is part of promoting personal health.

Vocabulary Activity

Imagine you want to have a conversation with a trusted adult about one of the topics in this chapter. Write a script in which you have this conversation, using the key terms shown appropriately. Express your thoughts and feelings, as well as what you believe the trusted adult's thoughts and feelings would be. After writing the script, reflect on what you have written. Why is it important to use these key terms accurately? How could you educate people who do not know them about their meanings?

cisgender	*human sexual response cycle*	*same-sex marriage*
disorder of sex development (DSD)	*LGBT+*	*sexual history*
gender binary	*masturbation*	*sexual orientation*
gender nonconforming	*nonbinary*	*sexuality*
homophobia	*orgasm*	*transgender*

Review and Recall

Review the information in this chapter by answering the following questions.

1. What is the difference between gender identity and sexual orientation?
2. Which chromosome combination results in a biological male? biological female?

3. What does it mean to be born with a disorder of sex development (DSD)?
4. Which of the following is *not* an aspect of sexuality?
   A. sexual orientation
   B. hormonal balance
   C. biological sex
   D. sexual experiences
5. When do sexually ambiguous traits begin to appear in children with Turner Syndrome or Klinefelter Syndrome?
6. Which term describes people who identify with the gender opposite their biological, anatomical sex?
   A. bisexual
   B. heterosexual
   C. homosexual
   D. transgender
7. What defines expectations for masculinity and femininity?
   A. society
   B. nature
   C. birth
   D. biological sex
8. Which hormone is often called the *cuddling hormone* and affects the brain by causing sensations of bonding, closeness, and nurturing?
9. What are the four phases in the human sexual response cycle?
10. During which phase of the human sexual response cycle do heart rate and blood pressure continue to rise?
    A. excitement
    B. plateau
    C. orgasm
    D. resolution
11. What is the climax of sexual excitement?
    A. orgasm
    B. masturbation
    C. arousal
    D. plateau
12. What is one thing couples should discuss when making decisions about sex?
13. What is another term for sexual excitement?
    A. wet dream
    B. masturbation
    C. arousal
    D. orgasm

Standardized Test Prep

Reading and Writing Practice

Read the passage below and then answer the following questions.

The phrase "coming out" is short for "coming out of the closet." When people who are LGBT+ come out, they are telling their family members, friends, and others about this part of their identity.

Coming out can be scary, especially if family members or friends do not seem accepting. Coming out, however, can be empowering and help people embrace their identities and develop closer, more honest relationships. It can also help a person connect with the larger LGBT+ community and be a role model for others. This can help debunk stereotypes and myths and educate others.

Generally, the process of coming out begins with coming out to one's self. Then it involves coming out to others.

14. Which statement best describes the main point of this passage?
    A. People who are LGBT+ should always come out.
    B. Coming out is scary for many people.
    C. People need to be educated about LGBT+ issues.
    D. Coming out has many benefits for people who are LGBT+ and others.
15. What is the first stage in coming out?
16. The phrase "coming out" is short for what other phrase?

Chapter 23 Skills Assessment

Critical Thinking Skills

Answer the following questions to assess your knowledge of what you learned in this chapter.

1. What is the advantage of allowing individuals with DSDs to select their gender when they grow up? Do you think a person should be required to select a gender?
2. Is developing a "crush" on a member of the same sex always an expression of homosexuality in an adolescent? Why or why not?
3. Does your school have an LGBT+ support group? If not, do you think one is needed? With a partner, brainstorm some steps you could take to start one.
4. What can be done to help teens who are unsure about their gender identities or sexual orientations?
5. Do you think the term LGBT+ is an adequate and accurate term? Why or why not? Can you think of a better term? Explain your answer.
6. What does the term homophobia mean to you? In what ways have you seen it displayed?
7. How can you respect other people's views on sexuality, even if they differ from your own?
8. Is gender identity chosen or assigned? Explain your answer.
9. With a partner, discuss several examples of inaccurate depictions of sex in the media. What are some ways you can protect yourself from unrealistic views of sexual activity presented in the media?
10. How might a sexually active relationship affect other relationships?
11. What might prevent romantic partners from discussing their views on sex?
12. What are some examples of situations that might make sexual abstinence difficult?
13. Make a list of questions you have about sex. Then, create an action plan to help you consult reliable sources and trusted adults for the answers to your questions.

Health and Wellness Skills

Complete the following activities to assess your skills related to health and wellness.

14. **Analyze Influences.** Think about all of the factors that influence your sexual behaviors and decisions. What factors do you think have had a positive influence on your sexual behaviors and decisions? Describe examples. What factors have had a negative influence? Describe these as well. What strategies could you use to avoid the negative factors and increase the positive?
15. **Access Information.** Learning about sex from unreliable sources can lead teens to believe myths and misconceptions about sex. Research places you could go to get credible, reliable, and valid information about topics related to sex. These places may be online or in your community. Create an infographic or one-page handout listing the resources you found and describing what makes them credible, reliable, and valid.
16. **Make Decisions.** Making the decision to remain sexually abstinent can be difficult, but can prevent many health risks. Write down five factors you should consider before making this decision. Are these factors strong enough for you to stick with your decision to remain sexually abstinent? Are there some considerations you could focus on that would help you remain abstinent? Underline the strong considerations and cross out the weak ones. Add any additional considerations that are strong considerations.
17. **Set Goals.** Gender roles and stereotypes can cause confusion and strain for people and their relationships. With a partner, discuss how gender roles and stereotypes influence you. Then, create three SMART goals to help you navigate gender roles and stereotypes and promote an environment that is respectful of gender diversity. Act on one of these goals and evaluate how it influences you personally and those around you.

18. **Communicate with Others.** Imagine your school has an anonymous hotline where students can call in for advice about different situations. You are a member of the student group trained to answer these calls and provide advice. You answer a call from a student who is questioning personal gender identity and sexual orientation. What would you say to this student to encourage healthy thoughts and help the person open a line of communication with a trusted adult?
19. **Practice Health-Enhancing Behaviors.** Although sexual abstinence is the most responsible decision for teens, some teens make the decision to become sexually active. If teens decide to be sexually active, what are some factors these teens should talk about with each other to try and reduce the associated risks? Create a journal entry that discusses these factors. Consider how these factors could also affect a future sexual relationship during adulthood.
20. **Advocate for Health.** Research and define the term *homophobia*. What views does homophobia include? Do these views exist in your community? in your school? In small groups, list some examples of homophobia, including physical, mental, emotional, sexual, and verbal abuse or bullying and cyberbullying. Next, discuss actions you could take to help someone experiencing these types of bullying. As a group, come up with a positive message that could take the place of the homophobic message. Share your work with the class.

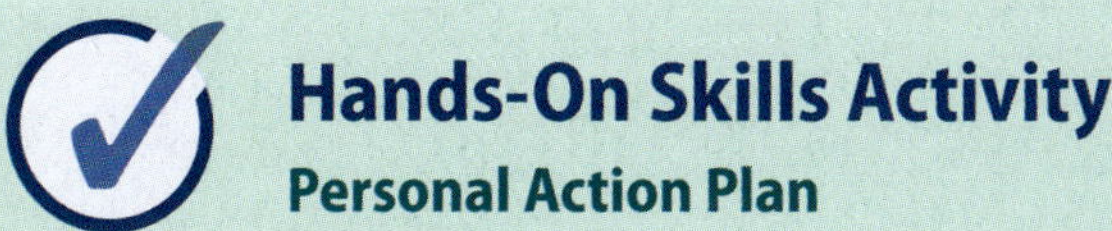

Hands-On Skills Activity

Personal Action Plan

In this chapter, and in other chapters, you have learned about healthy teen relationships, the risks of being sexually active as a teen, and the benefits of remaining sexually abstinent. In this activity, you will formulate a *Personal Action Plan* you can use when faced with challenges to your own sexual values and decisions.

Steps for This Activity

1. On a separate sheet of paper or electronically, create a chart as described in the following steps.
2. **Set Goals.** Consider your current goals and dreams. In a box labeled *Now*, list your short-term goals. Where do you hope to be in one year? What are your current dreams and hobbies? What do you enjoy about your life? In a box labeled *Later*, list your long-term goals and dreams. Where do you hope to be in 10 years? What do you want your life to look like? What do you want to achieve?
3. Explore your own personal values. What beliefs are important to you and why? Could you defend these values and beliefs, if challenged? How do these values and beliefs fit into your present and future goals and dreams? How do your values and beliefs affect your sexual behavior and your reaction to challenges of a sexual nature? At the bottom of your chart, list your most important values and beliefs and how they relate to challenges of a sexual nature.
4. **Practice Health-Enhancing Behaviors.** In boxes between *Now* and *Later*, formulate pledges or promises to yourself that will help you reach your *Later* goals. These pledges are personal oaths or statements you can use when faced with sexual challenges. The pledges could range from not drinking alcohol or using drugs, to only kissing, to communicating your consent, boundaries, and wishes to your partner. As you formulate these pledges, think about the different challenging situations you might face. How far would you be willing to go sexually if someone asked you? How might alcohol, drugs, or being in a bedroom affect your decisions?
5. When complete, keep your *Personal Action Plan* in a place where you can reference it or change it, if needed.

Chapter
24 Pregnancy Prevention

Look for the skills icon throughout this chapter for opportunities to practice your health skills.

Check Your Health and Wellness Skills

In this chapter, you will learn skills for preventing pregnancy. To understand the skills you currently use, take the following inventory of your behaviors. Indicate how well you think you use each skill. Use a scale of 1–5, *1* meaning you do not use the skill and *5* meaning you feel completely comfortable using it.

Skill	How Well Do You Use Each Skill?
I know where to get reliable information about contraception.	
I verify the things I hear people saying about contraception before I believe them.	
I feel comfortable discussing my boundaries and consent about contraception with a dating partner.	
I enforce my boundaries and know how to say *no* if someone asks me to cross them.	
I follow the directions on devices and medications exactly.	
I think of and ask questions if I don't understand how to use a device or medication.	
I compare the effectiveness, pros, and cons of devices and medications before purchasing them.	
I have people to go to for advice if I decide to use contraception.	
I understand the importance of using contraception correctly every time.	
I can differentiate between contraceptive methods that are effective or ineffective.	
	Total:

Add up your responses to each statement. The higher your score, the more comfortable you feel preventing pregnancy. Which skill do you think is most important for you? Which skill is the most challenging for you? Which skill would you most like to improve? In this chapter, you will learn how to perform these skills better and more often.

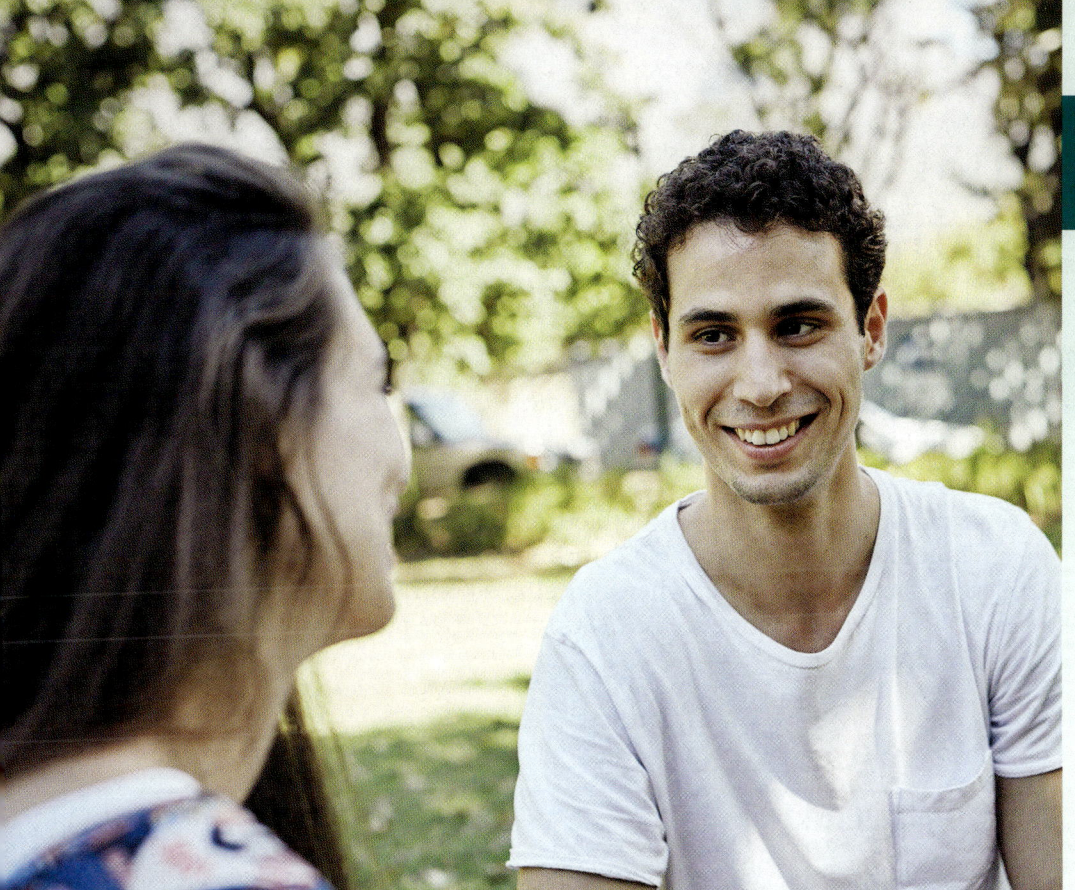

RapidEye/E+/Getty Images

Reading and Notetaking

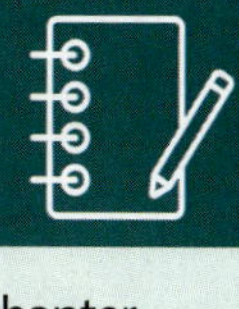

Before reading this chapter, write 12 statements describing what you already know about pregnancy prevention and contraceptive methods. List these statements in a graphic organizer like the one shown. As you read this chapter, decide whether each statement is accurate or not. Add key information from the chapter to your organizer, writing notes as statements. After reading, read your statements aloud with a partner. Check each other's statements for correct spelling, grammar, and pronunciation and revise as needed.

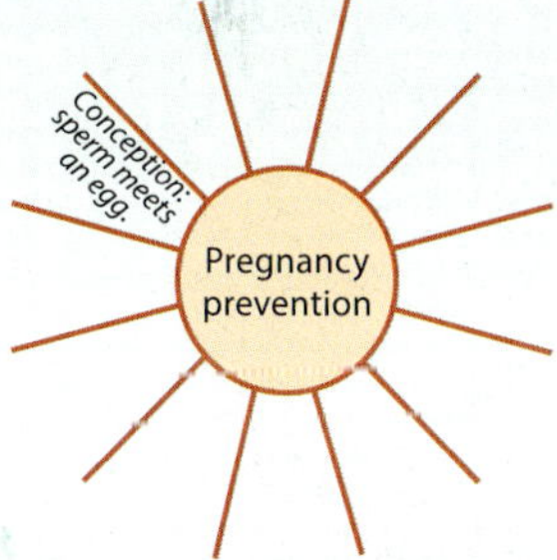

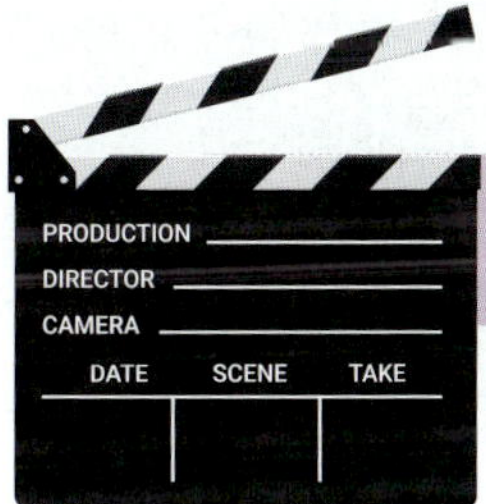

Setting the Scene

Any Risk Is Too Big

You have been dating your partner for nine months. You love your partner and hope you will stay together after high school. Sometimes, you dream about marrying your partner. You often think you have found "the one."

So far in your relationship, you and your partner have decided to be sexually abstinent. Sticking to this decision has been getting harder recently. The other day, your partner said maybe it was time to reconsider the decision. "Contraceptives prevent pregnancy, and some even prevent STIs," your partner said. You love and want to feel close to your partner, but are also nervous. You have a lot of big, long-term goals for your life. You want absolutely no risk for pregnancy.

Thinking Critically

1. Should teens worry about pregnancy, even if they are using contraceptives? Why or why not?
2. What do you think is the most effective way for teens to prevent pregnancy?
3. In this scenario, how could you explain your feelings to your partner clearly and respectfully? What reliable resources could you use to get facts about the effectiveness of contraception?

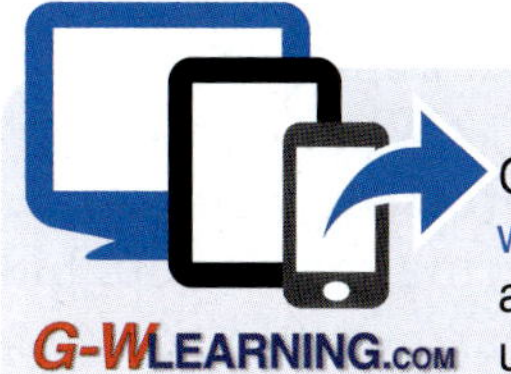

Click on the activity icon or visit www.g-wlearning.com/health/4095 to access online vocabulary activities using key terms from the chapter.

Lesson

24.1 What Is Contraception?

Essential Question

What is the purpose of contraception, and what is the most effective method?

Learning Outcomes

After studying this lesson, you will be able to

- define *contraception*;
- recognize pregnancy prevention facts and myths;
- explain how to identify reliable information about sexual health;
- identify factors to consider when choosing a contraceptive method; and
- assess why sexual abstinence is the most effective method of contraception.

Key Terms

barrier methods
contraception
hormonal methods
natural methods
sterilization

Warm-Up Activity

What Do You Know?

Comprehend Concepts You may have heard the term *contraception* in the media or in your own family. What does the term mean to you? What specifically comes to mind when you hear the term *contraception*? What does *sexual abstinence* mean to you? What do you think are some possible benefits of remaining sexually abstinent? Write a paragraph containing your answers to these questions.

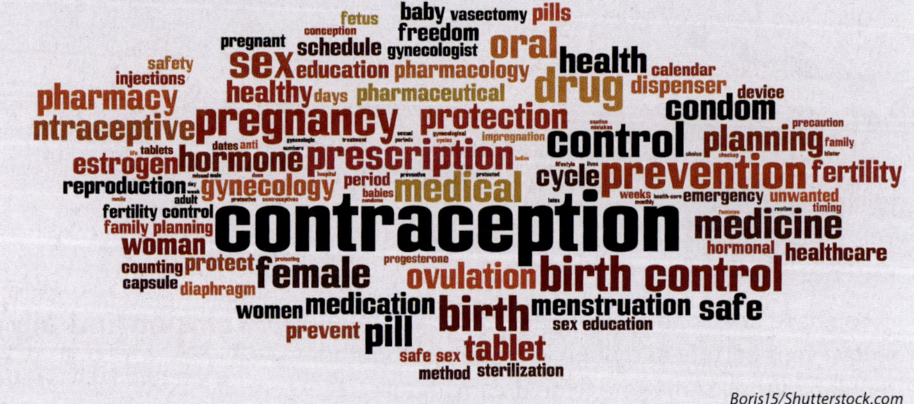

Boris15/Shutterstock.com

Many young people dream of someday having their own families. Parents know, however, that pregnancy and family life demand attention, money, time, and emotional maturity. For people who want to delay having children or do not want children, **contraception** helps prevent pregnancy. It also allows people to remain childless if they choose.

contraception any method that reduces the risk of pregnancy resulting from sexual activity

What would you say if a friend asked you how to prevent pregnancy? if you heard someone say pregnancy could be prevented by urinating or douching after sex? How would you react if your dating partner told you pregnancy was not possible the first time you had sex?

As your peers talk about sexuality and sex, you have probably heard many misconceptions or myths. Unfortunately, false information about pregnancy prevention can have serious consequences. Not knowing the facts about contraception can lead to an unplanned pregnancy, now during adolescence or in your adult future. In this chapter, you will learn the facts about contraception, including common types and how to use them.

Health in the Media

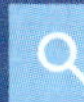

Media Messages About Contraception

Some teens spend fewer hours in school than they do using some form of media, including TV shows, online videos, music, and social media. Most media content is entertainment and is not trying to share reliable information. As a result, teens consume a lot of media containing mixed messages, unrealistic situations, and untrue information.

Because sexual activity is common in media portrayals, teens are exposed to a lot of unrealistic information about sex and contraception. For example, most movies with sexual content do not show or discuss the consequences of sexual activity, such as pregnancy and STIs. Most movies also have no information about contraception and show people engaging in sexual activity without even discussing pregnancy prevention.

Movies also commonly depict sexual activity involving people who do not discuss the decision to have sex, consent, contraception, or the potential consequences of sex. In fact, it is unusual for movies to show *any* serious consequences of sex.

As a result of these representations, teens may not realize discussing contraception and STI prevention is an essential part of having a healthy sexual relationship. Teens may think talking about contraception is unromantic or interrupts the mood. In reality, discussing contraception is a way of showing care and respect and protecting both partners from the potentially negative consequences of sex.

Practice Your Skills

Advocate for Health

Think about the movies, books, TV shows, online videos, and music you have seen, read, or listened to in the past six months. Which of these forms of media contained sexual content? List all the media that contained sexual content and then assess each one using the following criteria. Tally how often the statements were true or false of the media you consumed. Then, in a group, discuss how often the statements were true or false. How do you think these messages affect teens? Create an alternative, realistic, health-enhancing message for each statement. Make sure your statements appeal to your target audience: teens. Share these messages with your peers.

Media Message	True	False	Alternative Realistic Message
Having sex once can't cause pregnancy.			
Adults are not worried about becoming pregnant.			
Having sex has no negative consequences.			
People don't talk about using contraception before having sex.			
Having casual sex has no negative consequences.			
You don't have to worry about STIs when you have sex.			

Myths and Facts About Pregnancy Prevention

Many myths exist about how pregnancy occurs and can be prevented. Believing these myths can have life-changing consequences. The best way to guard against myths is to learn the facts about contraception and pregnancy and evaluate sources carefully (**Figure 24.1**). Following are some common myths and facts about pregnancy prevention:

Myth #1: A female who urinates after sex will not get pregnant.
Fact: Urinating after sex does *not* prevent pregnancy.

Myth #2: Douching, or cleaning the inside of the vagina, after sex prevents pregnancy.
Fact: Douching after sex does *not* prevent pregnancy. In fact, douching can increase the likelihood of pregnancy by pushing semen deeper into the vagina. Douching also does not prevent the transmission of STIs and HIV.

Myth #3: Pregnancy cannot occur the first time people have sex.
Fact: Someone *can* become pregnant the first time people have sex. Having sex or using contraception that is not 100 percent effective can lead to pregnancy and STI transmission any time people have sex, including the first time.

Myth #4: A female cannot become pregnant while menstruating.
Fact: Females *can* become pregnant during menstruation. It is unlikely, but possible. Females with regular menstrual cycles of 28–32 days will typically not become pregnant during menstruation. Many females, however, have irregular periods. Some have shorter cycles (24 days, for example), and some ovulate earlier than the 14th day. These people can become pregnant during menstruation.

Myth #5: Pregnancy cannot occur if the male withdraws, or "pulls out," before ejaculating.
Fact: Someone *can* become pregnant even if a male withdraws before ejaculation. Often, the penis releases some fluid containing sperm before ejaculation. *Withdrawal*, covered later in this chapter, is the least effective method of contraception.

Myth #6: Pregnancy will not occur if someone stands up during or after sex.
Fact: People *can* become pregnant no matter the position during and after sex. Standing up during or after sex will not prevent pregnancy.

Myth #7: A female younger than 18 years of age cannot become pregnant.
Fact: Females younger than 18 years of age can and do become pregnant. Someone who has begun menstruating can become pregnant regardless of age.

Evaluating Information About Sexual Health

Ask Yourself	Why?
Does the source have medical expertise?	Because contraception is based on anatomy and physiology, sources should have medical and scientific expertise. For example, a reliable source might be a medical organization, such as the Mayo Clinic, a hospital and research facility. The Mayo Clinic employs doctors with MD degrees and expert researchers with PhD or MS degrees.
What is the mission or objective of the source?	An organization's website should list its mission, or purpose and goals. A reliable source is dedicated to promoting physical and mental health. Employees should have medical and scientific expertise.
Does the source describe alternatives?	Contraception is complicated. Some methods may not be right for certain people. Therefore, a source should offer several options, and their advantages and disadvantages. This allows people to make a responsible decision.
Is the source a profit-making organization?	Some organizations are businesses with the goal of making money. The information these organizations present may be biased. For example, a company that makes a certain type of contraception may present incomplete or misleading information about abstinence or other contraceptive methods.

Figure 24.1 Asking yourself specific questions can help you verify sources will contain accurate and relevant information for your health.

Myth #8: People will not contract an STI or HIV as long as they use a condom during sexual activity.
Fact: If used properly and consistently, latex, polyurethane, and polyisoprene condoms can reduce—but not eliminate—the risk of contracting an STI or HIV.

Myth #9: Pregnancy is not that common after sex.
Fact: In a given year, 85 out of 100 females who have sex without contraception will become pregnant. If you have sex without contraception, you only have a 15 percent chance of *not* getting pregnant.

Myth #10: Pregnancy will not occur if people use contraception during sex.
Fact: Using contraception reduces, but does not eliminate, the risk of pregnancy. The chance of becoming pregnant depends on the contraceptive method used. Some methods are more effective than others. The risk of pregnancy also depends on whether people use contraception consistently and correctly. Abstinence is the *only* way to avoid pregnancy completely.

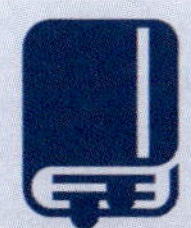

Case Study

Is That Really True?

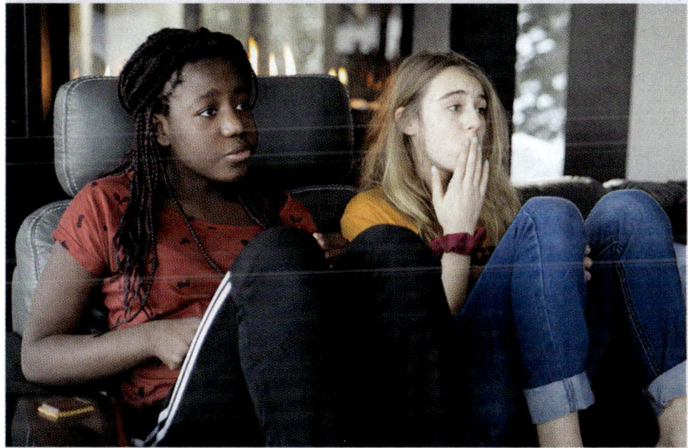

marieclaudelemay/iStock / Getty Images Plus/Getty Images

Raegan was scrolling through social media when she came across an article claiming she cannot become pregnant while on her period. Raegan knows you cannot believe everything you see online and she does not think this sounds right. Raegan also recognizes this article is not a credible source of health information. She is not completely sure, however. Raegan wants to find reliable information about this claim, but does not know where to look.

Sitting at home, Jayden overhears his older brother's conversation on the phone. His older brother says, "Condoms and birth control are such a hassle. Why doesn't he just pull out? Problem solved." Jayden knows his brother is wrong. Pulling out is not that effective and does not protect against STIs. He does not know if it is his place to correct his brother. At the same time, he worries his brother will spread this misinformation if he says nothing.

One night, Sonja was watching her favorite show with her best friend. During the show, two characters had sex, and the female character was worried about becoming pregnant since they did not use a condom. The male character told her, "Don't worry. It was only one time. You won't get pregnant." Sonja's friend scoffed at this, and Sonja was confused. Was the male character wrong?

Practice Your Skills

Make Decisions

In these scenarios, each teen has a decision to make about how to get reliable information or share that information with others. Using the decision-making process, complete one scenario to show how the teen gets factual information or corrects a myth. Explain how the teen completes each step of the decision-making process. Have the teen go back and revise the decision if it does not work. Then, share the factual information the teen found with the class and cite your sources.

barrier methods contraceptive methods that prevent sperm from traveling through the female reproductive system and fertilizing an egg

hormonal methods contraceptive methods that alter a person's hormone levels to thicken cervical mucus and inhibit ovulation (the release of an egg)

natural methods contraceptive methods that time sexual activity with a female's menstrual cycle and the sexual response cycle to prevent the sperm and egg from meeting

sterilization contraceptive method that permanently prevents pregnancy by altering the reproductive system, often through surgery

Types of Contraception

There are many contraceptive methods, and people must choose the method that works best for them. People can consult a healthcare professional if they have questions about selecting a method. A healthcare professional and the manufacturer's instructions for the product or device provide information about how to use contraceptives. The main categories of contraceptive methods are

- *sexual abstinence*—is the only 100-percent effective method of preventing pregnancy;
- **barrier methods**—prevent sperm from traveling through the female reproductive system and fertilizing an egg;
- **hormonal methods**—alter a person's hormone levels to thicken cervical mucus and inhibit ovulation;
- **natural methods**—time sexual activity with a female's menstrual cycle and the sexual response cycle; and
- **sterilization**—permanently prevents pregnancy by altering the reproductive system, often through surgery.

You will learn more about each of these methods later in this chapter.

Contraceptive methods are only effective if they are used correctly every single a time a person has sexual intercourse. Not using contraception correctly just one time can lead to pregnancy. If a person forgets to use contraception during sexual intercourse or notices a contraceptive method fails (for example, if a condom breaks), *emergency contraception* can help prevent pregnancy. Emergency contraception does *not* end a pregnancy that has already begun. Instead, it uses hormones to prevent pregnancy from occurring.

Even with contraception, sexual activity is risky, especially during adolescence. Though condoms and dental dams help protect people against STIs and HIV, other contraceptive methods do not. Only sexual abstinence is 100 percent effective in preventing pregnancy and STIs.

Questions to Consider When Selecting Contraception

How effective is it in preventing pregnancies?

Does it also protect against STIs and HIV?

How easy is it to use? Can you forget to use it or use it incorrectly? Can it break?

How much does this method cost? What are the up-front costs, and how much will it cost over time?

Do I need a doctor's prescription for this method?

Is this method reversible?

Figure 24.2 Different methods of contraception vary in effectiveness, cost, ease of use, and availability. To determine the right method for you, reflect on these questions. ***Which category of contraception permanently prevents pregnancy?***

Factors to Consider When Selecting Contraception

Each contraceptive method has advantages and disadvantages (**Figure 24.2**). People should consider their goals, sexual history, and any STIs when selecting a method. Is the goal to prevent pregnancy and have protection from STIs and HIV? Certain methods, such as condoms, can reduce the risk of pregnancy, STIs, and HIV. Other methods, such as hormonal contraception, reduce the risk of pregnancy, but do not protect from STIs and HIV.

People should also consider the cost and availability of contraception. Some methods, such as a condom or spermicide, are inexpensive and can be obtained without a doctor's prescription. Other methods, such as the intrauterine device (IUD), require a doctor's visit. A person using the birth control shot must visit the doctor regularly.

Some people want to use a *reversible* method of contraception so they can choose to have children in the future. Others would prefer a method that is permanent. Sterilization is permanent and practically irreversible. You will learn about sterilization in Lesson 24.4.

Ease of use is another important factor. Each method of contraception is effective only when used correctly every time, which may not always be convenient or possible. Some people cannot use certain types of contraception, such as hormonal methods, because of health conditions or activities like smoking.

Skills for Health and Wellness

Answering Questions About Your Sexual Health

Many teens have questions about their sexual health and contraception. Turning to unreliable sources for answers or believing myths can have negative consequences and lead to pregnancy. It is best to get answers using reliable resources, such as credible websites, books, or magazines; healthcare professionals; or other trusted adults. Different people prefer to use different resources, depending on their level of comfort and relationships. Learning how to answer these important questions will help you protect your health now and into adulthood.

Practice Your Skills

Access Information

What is one question you have related to sexual health or contraception? Be specific about what you want to know. Then get a factual answer by accessing reliable information. For this activity, try to find your answer online. Use the following steps:

1. Start by searching for online resources that answer your question. Use search terms that clearly relate to your question.
2. Visit websites with reliable information. If possible, navigate directly to a website you know is reliable. For example, you could visit the website of a professional health organization like the ones that follow and search for an answer there.

Sources for Information About Adolescent Sexual Health	
American Academy of Pediatrics	www.aap.org
American Sexual Health Association	www.ashasexualhealth.org
Center for Young Women's Health	www.youngwomenshealth.org
Centers for Disease Control and Prevention	www.cdc.gov
Mayo Clinic	www.mayoclinic.org
US Department of Health and Human Services	www.healthfinder.gov
Young Men's Health	www.youngmenshealthsite.org

3. To evaluate whether a website is reliable, ask the following questions:
   - What is the URL stem? Websites ending with .org, .gov, or .edu are most reliable. Websites ending with .com are usually business or commercial and may be making money related to the information they provide.
   - Does the website advertise products or belong to a business that sells products? You cannot trust websites that are trying to sell products or services.
   - Who is the author or sponsor of the website? Do not rely on opinion articles, editorials, or blogs. Use websites and articles authored by someone with medical expertise from the professional healthcare or health science field.
   - Does the website cite specific scientific studies to support its information?
   - Is the source current? Progress in science and technology can make information out of date.
4. Check the information you find against other sources. You should be able to find the same facts from other reliable sources, such as professional health organization or hospital websites. You could also check your information with a doctor or other healthcare professional.

After getting an answer to your question, create a social media post, blog post, or journal entry explaining the answer. Be sure to cite your sources.

Sometimes, people have strong preferences and views about contraception. Fortunately, the least expensive method of preventing pregnancy is also the most effective: sexual abstinence.

Abstinence: The Most Effective Method of Contraception

There is only one 100 percent effective method of preventing pregnancy, and that is sexual abstinence. Abstinence is also 100 percent effective at protecting against STIs. In addition, abstinence has other social and emotional benefits, which you learned about previously. These benefits include emotional maturity, time for personal growth and relationships, enjoyment of nonsexual activities, and the freedom to pursue one's goals without worrying about pregnancy or STIs.

Abstinence does not involve purchasing devices such as condoms, visiting the doctor for a shot, or taking a pill at the same time every day. Because of this, abstinence costs nothing. It is not expensive like some methods of contraception.

For some people, practicing abstinence can be difficult. People may feel pressured to have sex or get caught up in sexual attraction. By remembering their goals, avoiding risky situations, and using refusal skills, people can face these challenges and stay committed to abstinence. This commitment will help them pursue their goals, build healthy relationships, and prepare for a healthy adulthood.

Lesson 24.1 Review

Know and Understand

1. What is the purpose of contraception?
2. Why is it important to get reliable, factual information about contraception?
3. How are barrier methods different from hormonal methods of contraception?
4. Why is ease of use an important factor when choosing contraception?
5. What advantages does sexual abstinence have over other methods of contraception?

Think Critically

6. List one myth you have heard about contraception. What is the fact that debunks the myth?
7. Why are contraceptive methods only effective if they are used correctly every single time a person has sexual intercourse?

REAL WORLD Health Skills

Set Goals Create a dream board of you and your ideal life in 10 years. Note whether you have a romantic partner or are single. Draw or find pictures of the kind of home, belongings and experiences, and job you want. Where would you like to live? Do you have kids at this point in your life? Now, imagine you are in your senior year and contract an incurable STI or are due to have a child the month you graduate. How would this picture change? Would accomplishing this picture be possible? Would it be harder? Would it take longer? How would being sexually active affect your goals? What short-term goals could you set to make sure you reach your long-term goals?

Barrier Methods

Essential Question?

How do barrier methods help prevent pregnancy?

Lesson 24.2

Learning Outcomes

After studying this lesson, you will be able to

- explain how barrier methods reduce the risk of pregnancy;
- list the steps in applying and removing an external condom;
- describe how to apply and remove an internal condom;
- discuss how the contraceptive sponge helps prevent pregnancy;
- understand how to use a diaphragm for contraception; and
- analyze how people use the cervical cap to avoid pregnancy.

Key Terms

cervical cap
contraceptive sponge
diaphragm
spermicide

Warm-Up Activity

Talk About Condoms

Analyze Influences Barrier methods are some of the most common methods of contraception used. As a class, discuss the following question: *What have you heard about condoms?* Share what you have heard about condoms from advertisements, conversations, and media portrayals. List these messages in a chart like the one that follows. Then assess whether you think each message is accurate or not. How do these messages influence teens?

Message	Is It Accurate?	Influence on Teens

Barrier methods are a common type of contraception. These methods physically reduce the risk of fertilization and pregnancy by preventing sperm from reaching the egg inside the female reproductive system. Each barrier method has advantages and disadvantages. For example, condoms protect against STIs and HIV, while other methods do not.

No barrier method is 100 percent effective in preventing pregnancy or STI transmission. For example, even if a person with genital herpes or human papillomavirus (HPV) does not have visible sores, the virus may be present on skin not covered by a condom. The virus can then spread to the person's partner during sexual activity.

Some barrier methods are easier to use than others. Barrier methods of contraception include external condoms, internal condoms, the diaphragm, the cervical cap, and the contraceptive sponge (**Figure 24.3**).

Figure 24.3 To be effective, each method must be used correctly every time a person has sexual intercourse.

Barrier Methods

Method	Use	Requires a Doctor's Visit	Estimated Cost	Number of Pregnancies Expected (per 100 Females)
Diaphragm	A flexible cup inserted into the vagina; blocks sperm from entering the uterus	Yes	\$0–\$250 (including doctor's visit) depending on insurance	12
Contraceptive sponge	A sponge inserted into the vagina; contains *spermicide* (a chemical that kills sperm) and prevents sperm from entering the uterus	No	\$15 for three	12–24
Cervical cap	A silicone cup inserted into the vagina; prevents sperm from entering the uterus	Yes	\$0–\$275 (including doctor's visit) depending on insurance	14–29
External condom	Fits over an erect penis to block sperm from entering the vagina	No	\$2–\$6	15
Internal condom	Fits inside the vagina to prevent sperm from entering the uterus	No	\$2–\$3 each	21
Spermicide	A substance inserted into the vagina that inactivates sperm	No	\$8–\$15 per kit	28

External Condoms

The *external condom*, sometimes called the *male condom*, is designed to fit over the erect penis during sexual activity. There are several types of external condoms:

- *latex condoms*—made from a form of natural rubber derived from the sap of rubber trees
- *polyurethane condoms*—made from various forms of plastic
- *polyisoprene condoms*—made from synthetic, latex-free rubber
- *natural condoms*—made from the walls of animal intestines; these condoms contain small pores through which pathogens can pass, so they do *not* prevent STIs and HIV

External condoms help prevent pregnancy by catching the semen released during ejaculation and preventing sperm from reaching the egg. In addition, external condoms can be coated with **spermicide**, a substance that inactivates sperm (**Figure 24.4**). An external condom must be applied after an erection and before the penis touches a partner's genitals. This is important because the penis can release fluids containing sperm and possibly pathogens that cause STIs prior to ejaculation. External condoms cannot be reused; a new condom must be used each time intercourse occurs.

spermicide substance that inactivates sperm

Using external condoms has no health-related side effects unless one partner has a latex allergy, which can trigger an allergic reaction if latex condoms are used. People who have a latex allergy should use a different type of condom or a different method of contraception.

External condoms become dry, brittle, and ineffective over time. It is important to check the expiration date and discard expired condoms. People should not store condoms in hot or cold places (like cars) or in wallets, where they can be damaged or punctured. Petroleum-based lotions or lubricants such as Vaseline should not be used with a latex condom. These substances will break down the latex barrier.

Using an external condom is easy, but people should take care to prevent spilling semen. It is a good idea to practice applying and removing a condom before engaging in sexual activity. People can practice by applying an external condom over an object shaped like a penis (**Figure 24.5**).

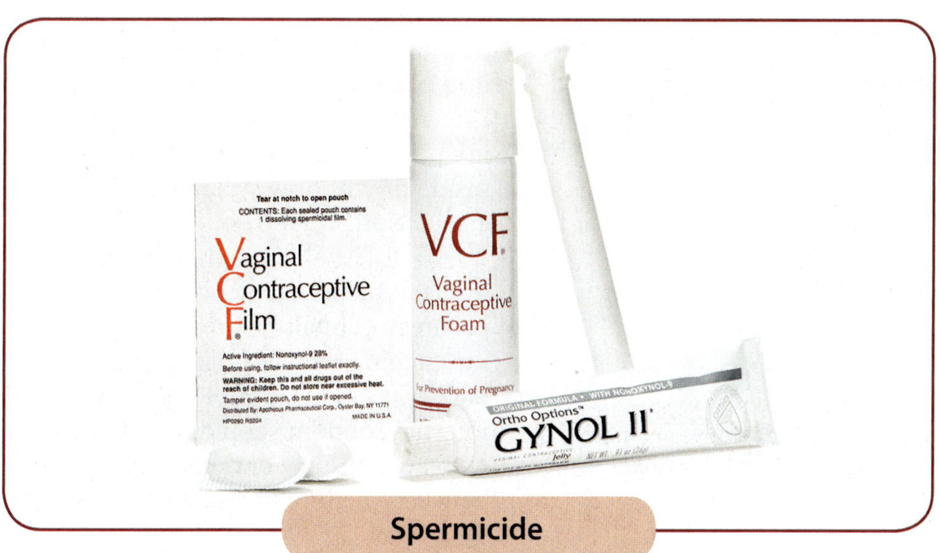

© Planned Parenthood Federation of America

Figure 24.4 Spermicide can also be inserted into the vagina on its own to inactivate sperm or be used with other barrier methods like diaphragms and cervical caps. ***Which type of condom does not prevent the transmission of STIs and HIV?***

Using an External Condom

Applying an External Condom

1. Gently tear open the condom package at its edge. Do not use teeth or scissors to do this. If the package is wet or sticky, discard it. Each condom is rolled into a ring within its package.
2. Determine which way the condom unrolls using a finger.
3. Pinch the condom tip to remove air. This will prevent breakage when the condom fills with semen. Leave a small amount of space at the tip to collect semen.
4. Place the condom at the tip of the erect penis.
5. The condom will not roll if it is placed incorrectly. Once the condom is positioned correctly, roll it to the base of the penis.
6. Apply some water-based lubricant if the condom is not lubricated. Never use petroleum-based lotions or lubricants such as Vaseline with a latex condom.

Removing an External Condom

1. Remove the penis from the partner's genitals before it softens. Otherwise, the condom can fall off and spill semen.
2. Hold the base of the condom at its ring while withdrawing to keep the condom from coming off the penis.
3. Pull off the condom and dispose of it in the trash. Wash your hands.
4. Never reuse a condom. Use a new condom for each erection.

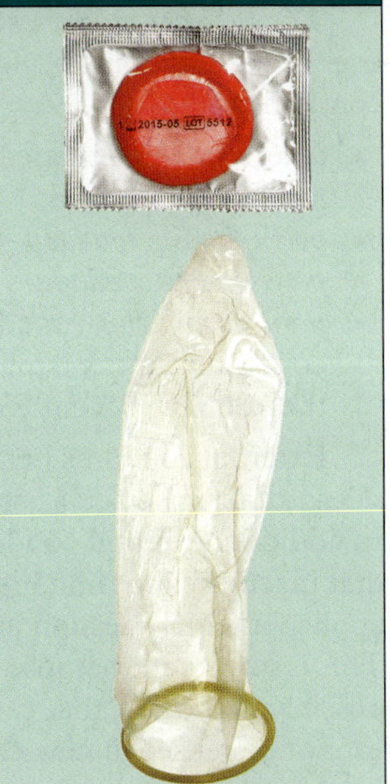

Top to bottom: kaarsten/Shutterstock.com; Dragan Milovanovic/Shutterstock.com

Figure 24.5 To effectively prevent pregnancy, a person must know when and how to apply and remove an external condom. ***Why should people not use external condoms past their expiration date?***

Using an Internal Condom

Applying an Internal Condom

1. Apply spermicide to the inside of the inner ring of the condom.
2. Squeeze the inner ring at the closed end of the condom and push it into the vagina or rectum as deep as it will go. The outer ring should rest just outside the vagina or rectum.
3. Hold the outer ring against the vaginal or rectal opening while the penis is inserted. The penis should not slide outside the condom.

Removing an Internal Condom

1. Hold the outer ring and twist the end of the condom to trap semen inside and prevent spillage.
2. Pull the condom out and discard it in the trash. An internal condom can only be used once. A new condom must be used each time a person has sexual intercourse.

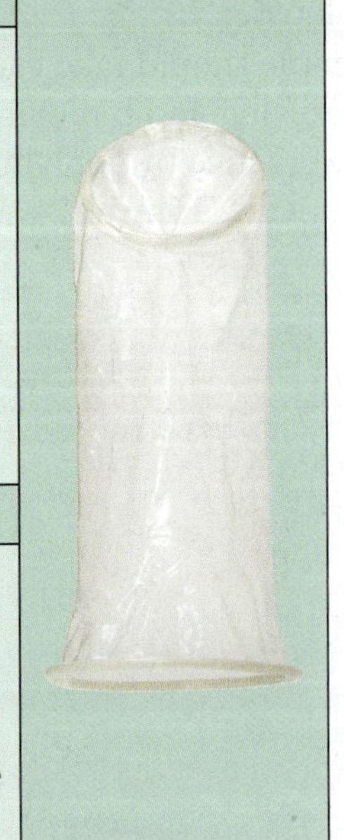

© Planned Parenthood Federation of America

Figure 24.6 People should take care to insert and remove an internal condom properly to prevent semen from spilling. ***What can make internal condoms more effective?***

Internal Condoms

An *internal condom*, sometimes called a *female condom*, is a device similar to a pouch, which is placed inside the vagina or rectum. Internal condoms are made of plastic, so they do not cause allergic reactions in people allergic to latex. Each end of the condom has a flexible ring to help a person insert the condom and to hold it in place while the penis is inserted. Internal condoms are more effective if a person adds spermicide to the inside or withdraws the penis before ejaculation.

An internal condom must be inserted before the penis touches a partner's genitals. It prevents pregnancy by catching semen. It also forms a barrier to STIs (**Figure 24.6**). An internal condom should not be worn with an external condom, since friction between them reduces effectiveness.

Contraceptive Sponge

The **contraceptive sponge** is a barrier method that helps block sperm from entering the uterus (**Figure 24.7**). The contraceptive sponge is inserted into the vagina and positioned to cover the cervix. A person can insert it several hours (at least 10 minutes) before sexual intercourse and leave it in place for 30 hours.

contraceptive sponge contraceptive device made of plastic foam; covers the cervix to prevent sperm from entering the uterus and contains spermicide

Unlike condoms, the contraceptive sponge does not have to be replaced each time people have sexual intercourse. The same sponge can be used more than once during a 30-hour period. A small loop makes it easier to pull out of the vagina.

The contraceptive sponge does not protect against STIs and HIV, so the female's partner should still wear a condom. Contraceptive sponges are less effective in preventing pregnancy than external and internal condoms. They are more effective at preventing pregnancy for people who have never given birth, as compared to people who have given birth.

Diaphragm

diaphragm cup-shaped contraceptive device made of silicone; covers the cervix to prevent sperm from entering the uterus and is bigger than the cervical cap

The **diaphragm** is a flexible, cup-shaped disk that is inserted into the vagina. It covers the cervix and helps block sperm from entering the uterus (**Figure 24.8**). Unlike with condoms and contraceptive sponges, getting a diaphragm requires an exam and prescription. During the exam, the healthcare professional checks the health of the cervix and uterus and prescribes the correctly sized diaphragm. A person can then purchase a diaphragm with a prescription at drugstores.

The diaphragm's package contains directions for correct insertion, removal, and care. A person must use it each time intercourse occurs and cover it with spermicide before insertion. Spermicide causes the sperm to stop moving and prevents them from entering the uterus.

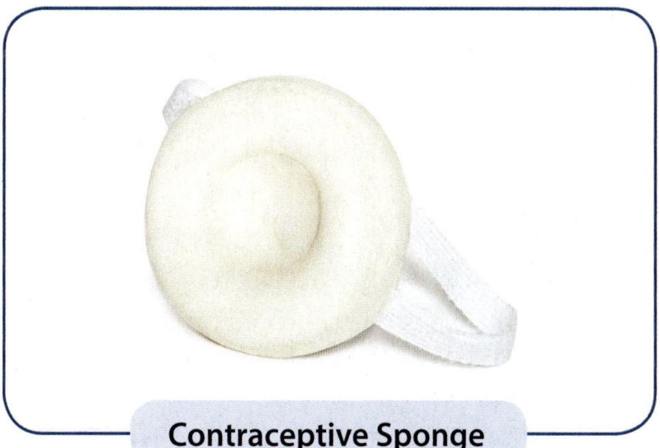

© Planned Parenthood Federation of America

Figure 24.7 A contraceptive sponge is made of plastic foam, is about 2 inches in diameter, and contains spermicide.

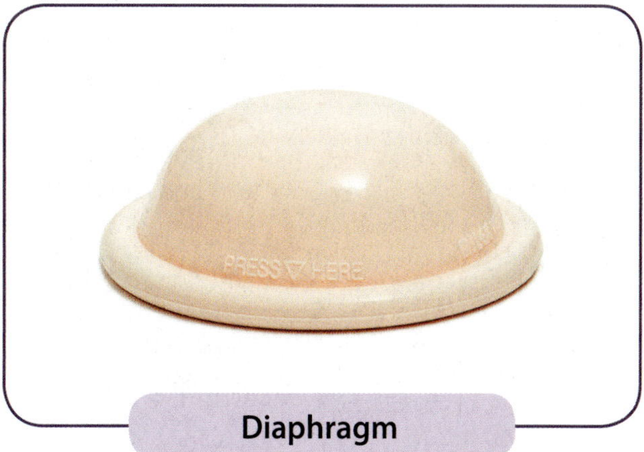

© Planned Parenthood Federation of America

Figure 24.8 Diaphragms are made of silicone, a material that usually does not cause discomfort. ***What part of the body does a diaphragm cover?***

cervical cap cup-shaped contraceptive device made of silicone; covers the cervix to prevent sperm from entering the uterus and is smaller than the diaphragm

A diaphragm costs more than a condom or contraceptive sponge, but a person can use it multiple times and for much longer than other barrier methods. While initial costs are relatively high, the diaphragm is inexpensive for long-term contraception.

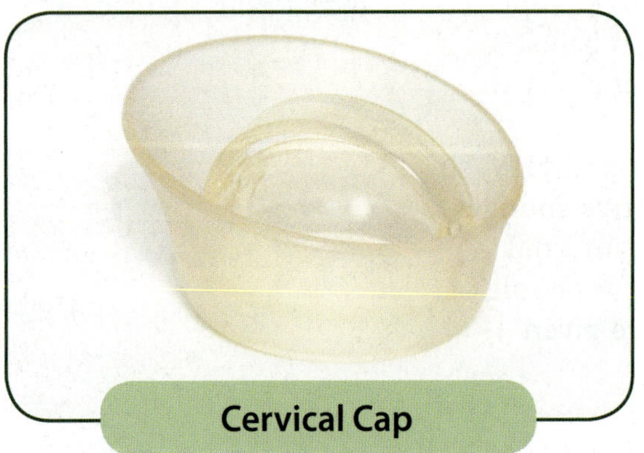

© Planned Parenthood Federation of America

Figure 24.9 The cervical cap is smaller than a diaphragm and may be more difficult to position correctly.

Cervical Cap

The **cervical cap** is a flexible cup that covers the cervix and helps block sperm from entering the uterus (**Figure 24.9**). Like the diaphragm, the cervical cap is made of silicone. A person must see a doctor or other healthcare professional to obtain a prescription for a cervical cap. During the exam, a doctor checks the health of the cervix and uterus and prescribes the correct size. The cervical cap works best for people who have never given birth.

The cervical cap's package contains directions for correct insertion, removal, and care. A person must cover the cap with spermicide and insert it before intercourse. Like the diaphragm, the cervical cap is expensive at first, but can be used for a long time.

Lesson 24.2 Review

Know and Understand

1. Which barrier methods are worn by females to prevent pregnancy? by males?
2. Which type of condom does *not* also protect against STIs?
3. When during sexual activity should an external or internal condom be applied?
4. What are the similarities and differences between the contraceptive sponge, diaphragm, and cervical cap?

Think Critically

5. What factors might make external and internal condoms difficult to use correctly?
6. Choose two barrier methods and compare them in terms of effectiveness, ease of use, and cost. What factors might affect which method people choose?

REAL WORLD Health Skills

Practice Health-Enhancing Behaviors To be effective, contraceptive methods need to be used correctly every time. On a piece of paper, brainstorm factors that might get in the way of people using barrier methods and abstinence effectively to prevent pregnancy and STIs. Then, list several strategies people could use to make sure they use these methods correctly. Create a journal entry reflecting on what strategies might work best for you now and in the future.

Hormonal Methods

Essential Question?

How do hormonal methods work to prevent pregnancy?

Lesson 24.3

Learning Outcomes

After studying this lesson, you will be able to

- understand how hormonal methods prevent pregnancy;
- distinguish between different types of oral contraceptives;
- explain the use of the birth control patch;
- describe the function of the vaginal ring;
- identify what a person must do to get the birth control shot;
- analyze the effectiveness of the birth control implant;
- contrast the two types of intrauterine devices (IUDs); and
- explain how emergency contraception helps prevent pregnancy after sexual intercourse.

Key Terms

birth control implant
birth control patch
birth control shot
emergency contraception
intrauterine device (IUD)
oral contraceptives
vaginal ring

Warm-Up Activity

What Are the Facts?

Access Information What do you already know about hormonal contraceptive methods? For each hormonal method listed, indicate whether you have never heard of it, have heard of it, or know how it works. Share what you know with a partner and then use a reliable resource to verify two facts you and your partner think you know. Were your facts correct? Verify the other facts you shared as you read this lesson.

Method	Never Heard of It	Heard of It	Know How It Works
Birth control implant			
Birth control patch			
Birth control pill			
Birth control shot			
Emergency contraceptive pill			
Intrauterine device (IUD)			
Vaginal ring			

Hormonal methods of contraception prevent pregnancy by using *hormones*, or chemical substances that control many body functions, including reproduction. Hormonal methods of contraception use the hormones estrogen and *progestin* (synthetic progesterone) to thicken cervical mucus, thin the endometrial lining of the uterus, and inhibit *ovulation*, which is the release of an egg. Because hormonal methods work in this way, they also help control the menstrual cycle to treat severe menstrual pain, endometriosis, and other reproductive disorders.

Hormonal Methods				
Method	**Use**	**Requires a Doctor's Visit**	**Estimated Cost**	**Number of Pregnancies Expected (per 100 Females)**
Birth control implant	A small rod implanted into the body by a doctor; releases hormones to prevent ovulation and must be replaced after five years	Yes	$0–$1,300 (including doctor's visit), depending on insurance	Fewer than 1
Intrauterine device (IUD)	A device inserted into the uterus by a doctor; repels sperm; hormonal IUDs also release hormones to thicken cervical mucus and inhibit ovulation; is effective for 3–12 years	Yes	$0–$1,300 (including doctor's visit), depending on insurance	Fewer than 1
Birth control shot	An injection of hormones by a doctor every three months; prevents ovulation	Yes	$0–$250 (including doctor's visit), depending on insurance	6
Birth control patch	A patch placed on the skin every week for three weeks; releases hormones to prevent ovulation	Yes	$0–$150 per month, depending on insurance	9
Birth control pill	A pill taken every day; contains hormones that prevent ovulation	Yes	$0–$50 per month, depending on insurance	9
Vaginal ring	A flexible ring inserted into the vagina; releases hormones to prevent ovulation and must be replaced monthly	Yes	$0–$200 per month, depending on insurance	9
Emergency contraceptive pill	A pill taken within five days of sexual intercourse; contains hormones that prevent ovulation	Yes (ella®); No (Plan B One-Step®)	$50–$67 (ella®); $40–$50 (Plan B One-Step®)	15 (ella®); 11–25 (Plan B One-Step®)

Figure 24.10 Most hormonal methods require a doctor's visit, but each type will vary in cost, effectiveness, and how long it will last. ***Which two hormones are used in hormonal methods of contraception?***

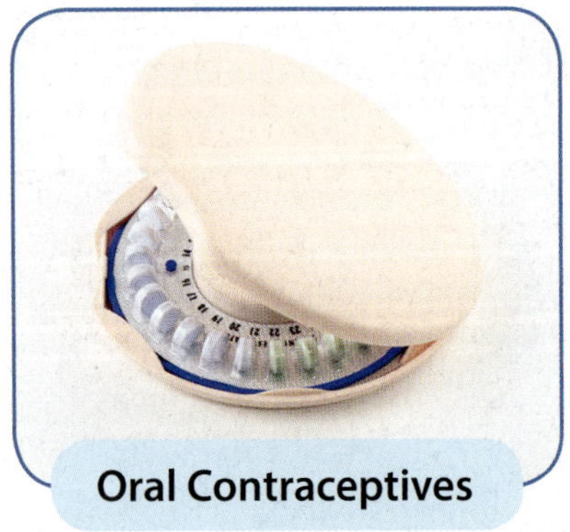

Oral Contraceptives

Jacob Kearns/Shutterstock.com

Figure 24.11 Oral contraceptives are usually called the *birth control pill* or just *the pill*.

oral contraceptives
medications containing hormones that stop ovulation; are taken every day

In this lesson, you will learn about several types of hormonal methods (**Figure 24.10**). All of these methods use hormones to influence the female reproductive system. No hormonal methods currently exist for males, but several different options are being researched and developed.

Oral Contraceptives

Oral contraceptives are medications containing hormones that reduce the likelihood of pregnancy. These medications are taken *orally* (by mouth) at the same time each day (**Figure 24.11**). The hormones in birth control pills help prevent pregnancy by preventing ovulation, or the release of an egg, and thickening cervical mucus to slow sperm down. If ovulation does not occur, there is no egg for a sperm to fertilize. Birth control pills do not prevent STIs or HIV. In fact, some research suggests people who use birth control pills have an increased risk of STIs.

People need to visit a doctor or other healthcare professional and get a prescription to begin taking birth control pills. During the exam, a doctor will make sure no health conditions will make taking the pill dangerous. The pill is very effective at preventing pregnancy if taken *exactly as prescribed.* Skipping even one pill increases the chance of becoming pregnant.

Local and Global Health

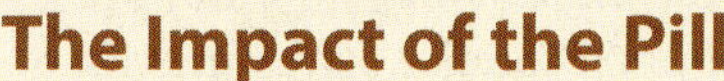

The Impact of the Pill

The birth control pill, introduced in 1960, was a breakthrough in contraception. In the US today, about 16 percent of females ages 15–49 take the birth control pill. Around the world, this number is closer to 9 percent.

When it was introduced, the pill gave females an effective way to plan and space pregnancies. This and other factors contributed to social change. Since 1960, the number of females in the workplace has tripled, and females have more financial independence. Before 1960, only 6 percent of females in the US completed a college education. This number rose to 37 percent in the decades after.

Apart from contraception, the birth control pill also has other health benefits. Taking the birth control pill reduces menstrual cramping, symptoms of endometriosis, premenstrual syndrome (PMS), and the risks of an ectopic pregnancy and ovarian and uterine cancer. Females have lighter periods using the pill, which helps prevent iron deficiency and anemia.

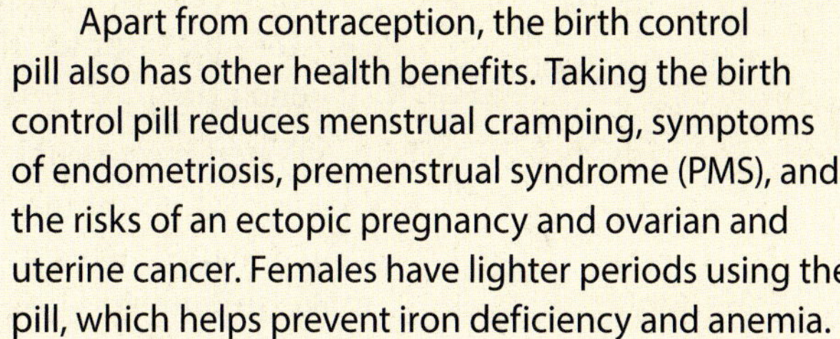

The birth control pill has also benefited females globally, though some countries have not seen as much social change. Fewer females with low incomes bear the economic burden of raising more children, and fewer females fear the health risks of pregnancy and childbirth.

Practice Your Skills

Access Information

Since the birth control pill was introduced, it has evolved and become a safer and more reliable method of contraception. In a small group, use reliable resources to research answers to the following questions about the birth control pill and its evolution:

- What were the first birth control pills like? How have these pills changed over the years?
- What are the potential side effects of taking birth control pills? Have these effects changed over time? What precautions help protect females from these side effects?
- How exactly do birth control pills prevent pregnancy? How effective are they?
- Where can females go to learn more about or get birth control pills?

Many people use apps or alarms to help them remember to take the pill (**Figure 24.12**). The birth control pill comes in two basic forms: the combination pill and the progestin-only pill.

Combination Pill

Most people who take birth control pills take the *combination pill*, which contains the hormones estrogen and progestin. The combination pill comes in a pack of 21, 28, 91, or 365 pills. All of these packs have *active pills*, which contain hormones. Packs of 28 and 91 also have *inactive pills*, which do not contain hormones and help a person stay in the habit of taking a pill every day. Packs of 91 or 365 pills are sometimes called *continuous* or *extended-cycle birth control*. Following is a summary of these options:

- **21-pill pack:** Someone using the 21-pill pack takes an active pill every day for three weeks and then no pills for one week. After that week, the person starts a new 21-pill pack.

Some apps can
- send reminders to take the pill
- provide advice if you skip a pill
- track symptoms to spot any side effects of the pill
- record and analyze how your menstrual cycle changes over time
- predict when you will begin menstruating or ovulating

bsd/Shutterstock.com

Figure 24.12 Any information an app provides about a female's menstrual cycle should come from a reliable source.

- **28-pill pack:** Someone using the 28-pill pack takes one active pill each day for three weeks, then one inactive pill every day for one week. The last seven pills have no effect on the female reproductive system, but help with keeping the daily habit of taking the pill.
- **91-pill pack:** Someone using the 91-pill pack takes active pills for 12 weeks and inactive pills for one week.
- **365-pill pack:** These packs contain 365 active pills that are taken each day.

When using packs of 21, 28, or 91 pills, females experience *withdrawal bleeding* while taking the inactive pills. This bleeding is not the same as menstruation (the shedding of the uterus's thickened lining). Active pills make the uterine lining shed during withdrawal bleeding much thinner.

Progestin-Only Pill

birth control patch plastic contraceptive device applied to the skin as a patch; releases hormones to stop ovulation

Some people take a form of the birth control pill that contains only progestin. This *progestin-only pill*, also called the *minipill*, contains no estrogen. The progestin-only pill comes in a 28-pill pack, and all of the pills contain active hormones. People who take the progestin-only pill tend to experience fewer side effects.

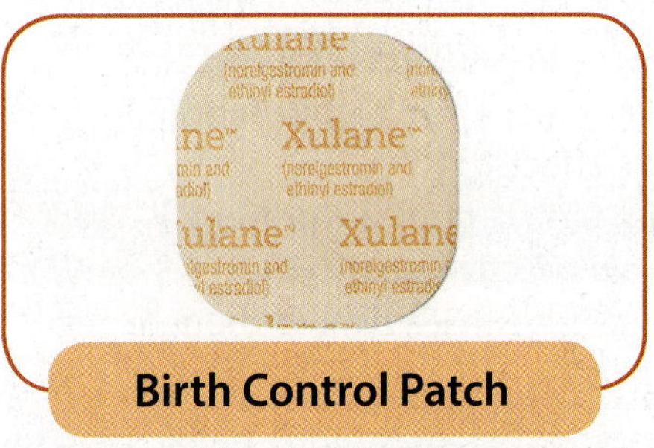

© Planned Parenthood Federation of America

Figure 24.13 Like the birth control pill, the patch contains the hormones estrogen and progestin.

Birth Control Patch

The **birth control patch** (often called the *patch*) is a thin, 2- to 3-inch, plastic patch applied to the skin like a bandage (**Figure 24.13**). The patch works like the birth control pill, except that hormones are absorbed in a *transdermal* way (from the patch through the skin into the blood). The birth control patch prevents ovulation and thickens cervical mucus, slowing down sperm.

Females who use this method apply one patch to the skin for one week and then remove it. They replace the old patch with a new patch for the second week. After removing the second patch, they wear a third patch for the third week. No patch is worn during the fourth week (during withdrawal bleeding).

The patch's package contains directions for applying and removing birth control patches. The patch must be worn in specific locations. The directions should state what people should do if a patch falls off or they forget to replace one.

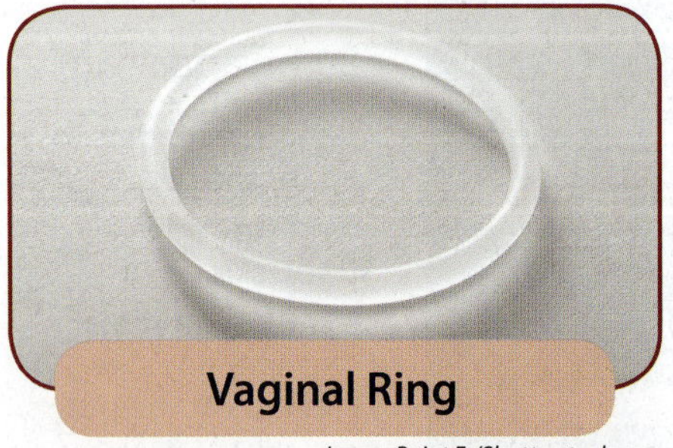

Image Point Fr/Shutterstock.com

Figure 24.14 People should follow the package's directions for proper storage, insertion, and removal of the vaginal ring. ***For how long is a vaginal ring used?***

Vaginal Ring

The **vaginal ring** is a small, flexible ring that contains the hormones estrogen and progestin (**Figure 24.14**). The ring works by releasing hormones that prevent ovulation and thicken cervical mucus to slow sperm movement.

The vaginal ring is inserted into the vagina for three consecutive weeks. Exactly three weeks after insertion, a person should remove the ring, ideally at the same time it was inserted, and discard it. No ring is used during the fourth week (during withdrawal bleeding).

vaginal ring flexible, ring-shaped contraceptive device inserted into the vagina; releases hormones to stop ovulation

Birth Control Shot

The **birth control shot**, often called *Depo-Provera*, is an injection of the hormone progestin. The progestin in the shot helps prevent pregnancy by preventing ovulation and thickening cervical mucus. A female who uses this method must see a healthcare professional to receive the shot every three months. Depending on the type of shot, it can be given in the arm or buttocks. The birth control shot is highly effective in preventing pregnancy if a person receives injections according to schedule.

birth control shot
contraceptive method in which a female receives an injection of progestin every three months to stop ovulation

birth control implant
flexible, toothpick-sized contraceptive device inserted under the skin of the upper arm; releases progestin to stop ovulation

Birth Control Implant

The **birth control implant** is a flexible, toothpick-sized rod containing the hormone progestin (**Figure 24.15**). The implant releases progestin, which prevents ovulation and thickens cervical mucus. The implant can be left in place for three or four years, during which time it gradually releases doses of progestin.

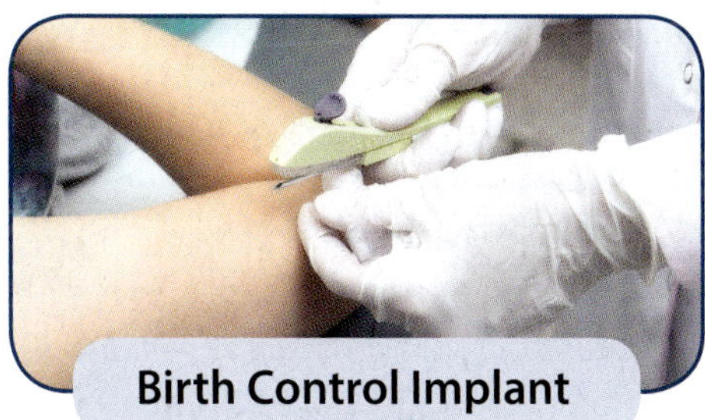

PAKULA PIOTR/Shutterstock.com

Figure 24.15 A doctor inserts the birth control implant under the skin of a female's upper arm, where the implant releases progestin.

Intrauterine Device (IUD)

An **intrauterine device (IUD)** is a small, T-shaped device a doctor inserts into the uterus. IUDs can also be removed by a doctor, making IUDs a reversible method of contraception. Two types of IUDs exist: copper IUDs (*ParaGard®*) and hormonal IUDs (*Mirena®*, *Liletta®*, *Skyla®*, or *Kyleena®*) (**Figure 24.16**). These IUDs work in different ways to prevent pregnancy:

- **Copper IUD:** The copper ParaGard® IUD is thought to interfere with sperm movement, fertilization, and implantation. The advantage of the ParaGard® IUD is it can be left in place for 12 years and does not affect a person's hormone levels. The ParaGard® IUD can also be used as a form of emergency contraception.
- **Hormonal IUDs:** Hormonal IUDs release hormones that inhibit ovulation and cause mucus in the cervix to thicken, making it difficult for sperm to reach the uterus. Hormonal IUDs last for years and can reduce menstrual cramps and significantly lighten or even stop menstruation.

Both copper and hormonal IUDs can be removed if a female wants to become pregnant.

intrauterine device (IUD)
small, T-shaped contraceptive device inserted into the uterus; copper IUDs interfere with sperm movement, and hormonal IUDs release hormones to thicken cervical mucus and inhibit ovulation

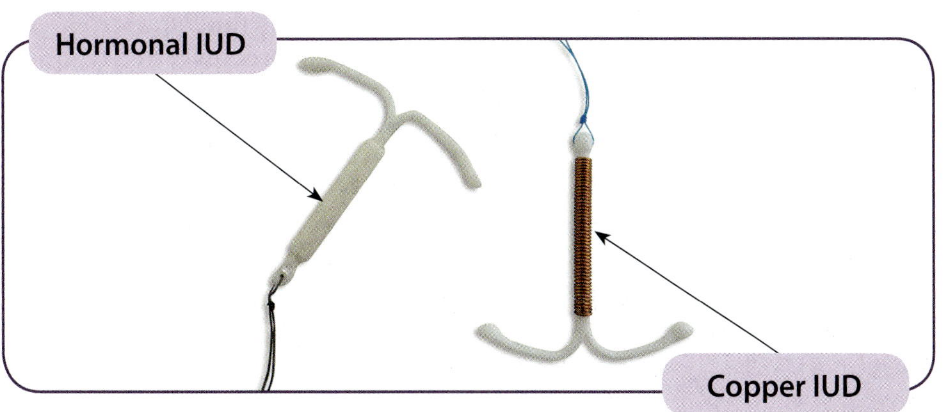

iStock.com/Lalocracio

Figure 24.16 Both copper and hormonal IUDs must be inserted and removed by a doctor. ***Into what female reproductive organ is an IUD inserted?***

Research in Action

Hormonal Contraceptives for Males

Since the introduction of the birth control pill, females have had access to long-term, reversible hormonal contraception. These contraceptive methods include oral contraceptives; the birth control shot, patch, or implant; the vaginal ring; and IUDs. Each method reduces the risk of pregnancy.

In recent years, scientists have also been testing the safety and effectiveness of hormonal contraceptives for males. Two oral contraceptives have been tested in small groups of males. One is called *dimethandrolone undecanoate*, and the other is called *11-beta-MNTDC*. Both oral contraceptives contain a combination of hormones that lower testosterone production in males. Since testosterone is needed for sperm production, a drop in testosterone means the testes stop making sperm. These oral contraceptives are taken once daily and affect sperm production after two to three months. Sperm production begins again a few days after a male stops taking the pills.

Practice Your Skills

Comprehend Concepts

With a partner, discuss why it is important to have hormonal contraceptive methods available for both males and females. What advantages would hormonal contraceptives have over other forms of contraception for males? During your discussion, complete the table that follows comparing the advantages and disadvantages of different methods of male contraception. Research any method with which you are not familiar. If a male hormonal contraceptive was approved, do you think males would use it? Why or why not?

Male Contraceptive Methods	Advantages	Disadvantages
Sexual abstinence		
External condom		
Sterilization		
Withdrawal		
Male hormonal contraceptive pill		

Emergency Contraception

Even when partners agree to use contraception and try to use it correctly, mistakes can happen. For example, an external condom can break, leak, or slip off. An internal condom might leak or slip out of position. A person might forget to insert a diaphragm or take the birth control pill.

emergency contraception contraceptive method used to prevent pregnancy when normal contraception has failed; includes the copper ParaGard® IUD and emergency contraceptive pills containing hormones

In these cases, **emergency contraception** can help prevent pregnancy. Emergency contraception can also help prevent pregnancy in the case of sexual assault. One type of emergency contraception is the ParaGard® copper IUD. If inserted within five days of sexual intercourse, this IUD is the most effective method of emergency contraception.

Several types of emergency contraceptive pills can also prevent pregnancy. These pills, such as *ella*® and *Plan B One-Step*®, contain hormones that prevent ovulation and thicken cervical mucus. Emergency contraception is similar to other hormonal methods, but contains a greater amount of the same hormones. Emergency contraception prevents fertilization. It does *not* stop or interrupt a pregnancy that has already occurred. It also does not reduce the risk of STIs and HIV.

Most emergency contraceptive pills are available at drugstores without a prescription, and anyone can buy them, regardless of age. The emergency contraceptive pill ella® requires a doctor's prescription and is the most effective emergency contraceptive pill. Emergency contraceptive pills can reduce the chance of pregnancy by up to 89 percent when used within five days of sexual intercourse. The earlier emergency contraception is taken, the more effective it will be.

While effective as a backup method, emergency contraception is less effective than standard birth control pills and several other contraceptive methods. Emergency contraception is not intended for regular use and should not be used as regular birth control for several reasons. Long-term use can cause irregular and unpredictable menstruation. Other forms of contraception are much less expensive and much more effective.

Lesson 24.3 Review

Know and Understand

1. What hormones are used in hormonal contraceptives to inhibit ovulation in females?
2. Explain the difference between active and inactive pills in oral contraceptives.
3. How is the vaginal ring different from the diaphragm or cervical cap?
4. Describe the difference between the birth control patch, shot, and implant.
5. Which type of IUD does not affect a female's hormone levels?

Think Critically

6. What factors do you think influence whether a female chooses to take oral contraceptives or use another hormonal method?
7. How is emergency contraception different from other hormonal methods of contraception? How is it different from the decision to end a pregnancy?

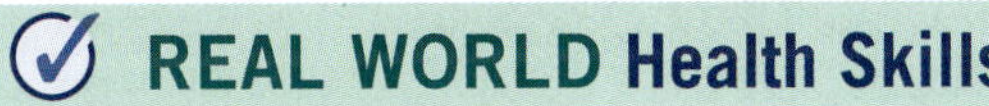

Communicate with Others As a class, identify a person in your community who is an expert on hormonal contraceptives. This person could be a gynecologist, doctor, or therapist or counselor who specializes in sexual health. As a class, schedule an interview with this person or contact the person electronically to ask about hormonal contraceptive options. Get answers to the following questions about each hormonal contraceptive method:

- How effective is this method, and what factors influence effectiveness?
- What are the short-term side effects?
- What are the long-term side effects?
- Are teens more likely to have side effects compared to adults?
- How much does it cost?
- What are the advantages and disadvantages of using this method?
- How old do you have to be to purchase this contraceptive?

Lesson

24.4

Natural Methods and Sterilization

Essential Question

How do natural methods and sterilization help reduce the risk of pregnancy?

Learning Outcomes

After studying this lesson, you will be able to

- explain how fertility awareness methods (FAM) reduce the risk of pregnancy;
- analyze why the withdrawal method is ineffective;
- describe the process of male sterilization; and
- explain how female sterilization is performed.

Key Terms 

fertility awareness method (FAM)
tubal ligation
vasectomy
withdrawal

Warm-Up Activity

Thoughts and Decisions

Analyze Influences Read the statements that follow and write what thoughts come to mind when you read each one. Have you ever thought something similar to these statements? How have these thoughts influenced your decisions? As you read this lesson, refer back to these statements and note how your thoughts about them change. How might your thoughts about them influence your decisions in the future?

I know my body. We won't get pregnant if we have sex today.

I've been watching the calendar for a month. I can't get pregnant, so there's no need for a condom.

If I just withdraw, nothing will get inside.

In this lesson, you will learn about natural methods of contraception and sterilization. Natural methods are methods that do not use barriers, devices, or hormones. Instead, these methods prevent pregnancy by tracking a female's cycle of fertility and taking actions such as withdrawal during sexual intercourse. Sterilization involves physically altering the reproductive system, usually permanently (**Figure 24.17**).

Natural Methods

Some people prefer natural methods of contraception because they do not use devices or medications. This preference might be a result of a person's values and beliefs or medical reasons. Additionally, the cost of contraceptive devices or medications may mean some people want to use natural methods, which do not cost money. Although they are less expensive, natural methods are harder to use correctly, which means they are less effective at preventing pregnancy for most people.

Natural Methods and Sterilization				
Method	**Use**	**Requires a Doctor's Visit**	**Estimated Cost**	**Number of Pregnancies Expected (per 100 Females)**
Tubal ligation (female sterilization)	Surgery to cut or block the fallopian tubes	Yes	$0–$6,000 (including doctor's visit), depending on insurance	Fewer than 1
Vasectomy (male sterilization)	Surgery to cut or block the vas deferens, which transport sperm from the testes to the penis	Yes	$0–$1,000 (including doctor's visit), depending on insurance	Fewer than 1
Fertility awareness methods (FAM)	Methods that track a female's fertile (unsafe) and infertile (safe) days; include the temperature method, cervical mucus method, and calendar method	No (but recommended)	$0–$20	12–24
Withdrawal	Pulling the penis out of the vagina before ejaculation	No	$0	22

Figure 24.17 Natural methods do not require a doctor's visit and are usually free. Sterilization can be expensive, depending on insurance, and requires a doctor's visit. ***How many pregnancies are expected when using tubal ligation?***

Fertility Awareness Methods (FAM)

A **fertility awareness method (FAM)** is a contraceptive method that takes advantage of the natural rhythm of a female's fertility. People who use FAM track when ovulation occurs and which days an egg is capable of being fertilized. As you know, the menstrual cycle typically lasts 28 days. In general, sexual intercourse on seven of those days can result in an egg being fertilized. This is because an egg lives for about one day, while sperm can live for three to five days. This means pregnancy is possible three to five days before ovulation, on the day of ovulation, and on the first and possibly second day after ovulation.

fertility awareness method (FAM)
contraceptive method that tracks a female's cycle of fertility and avoids sexual activity on days an egg can be fertilized

FAM is extremely useful for planning a pregnancy, but is only somewhat helpful for preventing pregnancy. There are several types of FAM:

- **Temperature method:** A person can track ovulation by measuring *basal body temperature* (resting temperature) first thing every morning. Body temperature rises slightly after ovulation and stays higher than normal for most of the remainder of that menstrual cycle. Temperature drops back to normal near the end of the cycle, when menstruation begins. To prevent pregnancy, someone should only have sex three days after body temperature rises until temperature declines (about the time of menstruation). During ovulation, body temperature rises just tenths of a degree. Because the change is so small, people should use a special basal temperature thermometer and record daily temperatures on a chart or app.

A female's body temperature might change at any time due to alcohol consumption, sleep, stress, or other factors. For this reason, people should record several months of temperature readings so they can recognize natural variations.

- **Cervical mucus method:** *Mucus* is a thick, watery secretion present in many parts of the body, including the cervix. The consistency of cervical mucus changes during the menstrual cycle (**Figure 24.18**). According to this method, pregnancy can occur two or three days before slippery mucus begins, for about three days after slippery mucus reaches its greatest amount, and possibly at the end of menstruation. Pregnancy is less likely when slippery mucus begins to decline, when mucus becomes sticky or cloudy, and during the dry days that follow this decline. Females examine cervical mucus by placing their fingers inside their vagina or examining mucus discharged on their underwear. Many extraneous factors can affect a female's cervical mucus.
- **Calendar-based methods:** People using a calendar-based method mark the day a female begins menstruating and then mark days pregnancy is likely or unlikely to occur. Generally, pregnancy will not occur during the six days following the beginning of menstruation and during days 19–32 after menstruation begins. People may use calendars, apps, or cycle beads to keep track of days. Calendar-based methods are not precise. A female's cycle can change at any time due to illness or stress. This method is especially unreliable for people with irregular cycles.

FAM has several drawbacks. FAM requires attention and record keeping and is subject to many mistakes. This is why many people use several methods of FAM together. Still, many people who use FAM do not use the methods regularly and correctly. As a result, about 25 out of 100 people become pregnant, which is a very high rate of pregnancy compared to other contraceptive methods. Furthermore, FAM does not prevent STIs. FAM is best for people who are in a position to raise and support a child. For these reasons, FAM is not recommended for teens.

Figure 24.18 A female can determine likelihood of a pregnancy occurring based on the consistency of cervical mucus.

Cervical Mucus During the Menstrual Cycle

Stage	Cervical Mucus
Menstruation	Blood flow prevents observation of mucus.
Post-menstruation	Little or no mucus is present (*dry days*).
Pre-ovulation	Mucus increases and is yellow or cloudy and sticky. Just before ovulation, mucus becomes clear and slippery for four days (*slippery days*).
Ovulation	Mucus is very wet, thick, and sticky.
Post-ovulation	Mucus reduces and becomes cloudy.
Pre-menstruation	Little or no mucus is present, especially one to two days before menstruation.

Withdrawal

Withdrawal, or *pulling out*, is one of the least effective contraceptive methods. When people use withdrawal, a male pulls the penis out of the female's vagina before ejaculating. This may keep sperm out of the vagina and reduce the risk of pregnancy.

withdrawal contraceptive method that involves pulling the penis out of the vagina before ejaculation

Withdrawal is *not* an effective method of preventing pregnancy for several reasons. Withdrawal is difficult to time correctly and requires self-control. It is not always easy for a male to withdraw during intense sexual excitement. In addition, before ejaculation, *pre-ejaculate fluid* containing sperm can leak from the penis and cause pregnancy. Withdrawal results in many pregnancies and does not protect people from STIs (**Figure 24.19**).

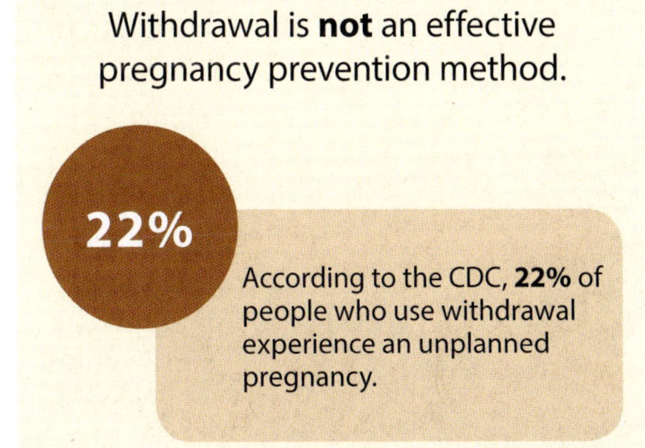

Figure 24.19 When used alone, withdrawal is one of the most ineffective methods of contraception. ***How can a person become pregnant even if a penis is withdrawn before ejaculation?***

Sterilization

Sterilization prevents pregnancy by permanently altering the male or female reproductive system. These alterations work by preventing the sperm and egg from uniting. They do not protect against STIs and HIV.

Sterilization may be the best choice for adults who know they do not want children or any more children. Sterilization is not appropriate for everyone, however. Reversing sterilization is difficult and often unsuccessful. Therefore, people considering sterilization must be sure they do not ever want children (**Figure 24.20**).

Choosing Sterilization

Reasons to Choose Sterilization	Reasons Not to Choose Sterilization
• Adults know they do not want to have more children. • Adults find other contraceptive methods unacceptable. Hormonal methods may be dangerous for some people, or pregnancy may carry serious risks. • Adults have a genetic disease or disorder they do not want to pass on to children. • Adults know they are and will never be emotionally or financially able to raise a family.	• Adults might want children, but do not want them now. If there is *any* chance adults might someday want children, they should not select sterilization. • Adults feel pressured to be sterilized. Adults should make their own decisions since they will live with the effects. • Adults have other personal issues, such as financial or personal stress or relationship conflict. These problems might go away; sterilization will not.

Figure 24.20 There are many reasons to choose sterilization, but adults should be aware that sterilization is often irreversible.

Male Sterilization

vasectomy surgical procedure that cuts or blocks the vas deferens, permanently preventing pregnancy

Male sterilization involves a surgery called a **vasectomy**, which a doctor performs. During a vasectomy, the *vas deferens* (two tubes that carry sperm from the testes to the penis) are cut or blocked. This prevents sperm from leaving the testes and entering semen. Vasectomy is nearly 100 percent effective.

A doctor usually performs a vasectomy in a doctor's office or hospital. The surgery involves making a small incision or puncture in each side of the scrotum. The doctor then cuts or blocks the vas deferens through this incision (**Figure 24.21**).

Most males who have a vasectomy return home the same day and recover quickly with no side effects. Some males experience bruising, swelling, and discomfort after the procedure. After a vasectomy, the prostate and seminal vesicles continue to function. Males still ejaculate normally and continue to produce semen. The testes keep making testosterone, so males can get erections and have sex just as they did prior to the surgery. Vasectomies are much less expensive than female sterilization.

After three months, a doctor will use an X-ray to confirm the vas deferens were successfully blocked. People should use an alternative form of contraception until that time.

Female Sterilization

Female sterilization works by blocking the fallopian tubes, which prevents sperm from reaching an egg released from an ovary. It does not affect the function of the ovaries. A female continues to make female hormones and ovulate after this procedure. Sterilization does not affect a female's sexual characteristics, sexual arousal, ability to have sex, or onset of menopause.

tubal ligation surgical procedure that cuts or blocks the fallopian tubes, permanently preventing pregnancy

The surgical procedure for female sterilization is **tubal ligation** (**Figure 24.22**). This surgery makes it impossible for sperm to reach an egg, which means that tubal ligation is nearly 100 percent effective in preventing pregnancy.

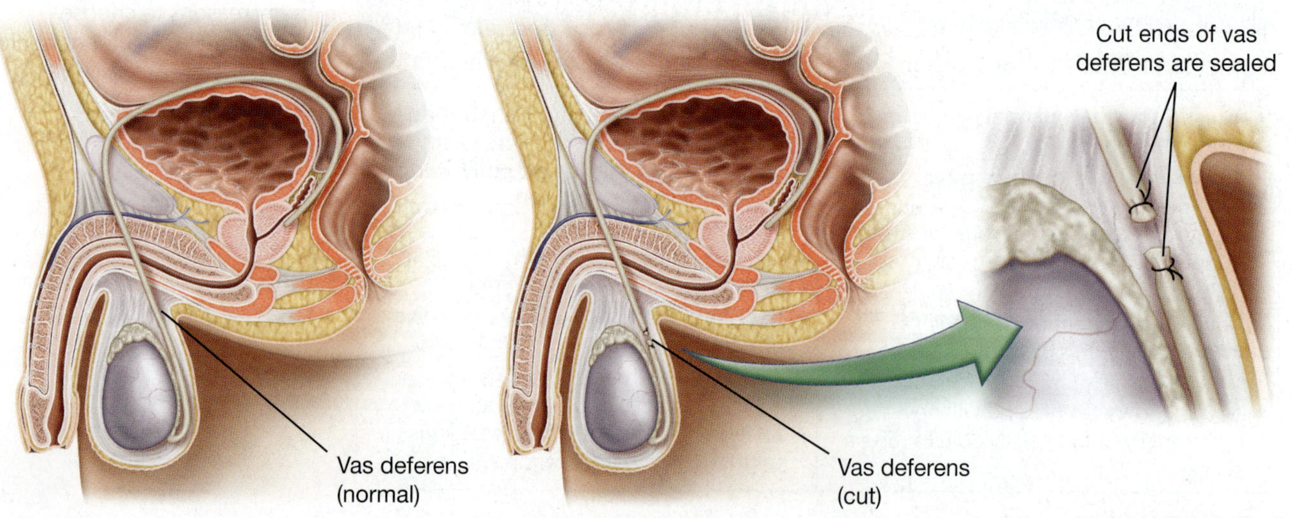

Figure 24.21 In a vasectomy, the vas deferens are cut or blocked and then sealed to stop the release of sperm.

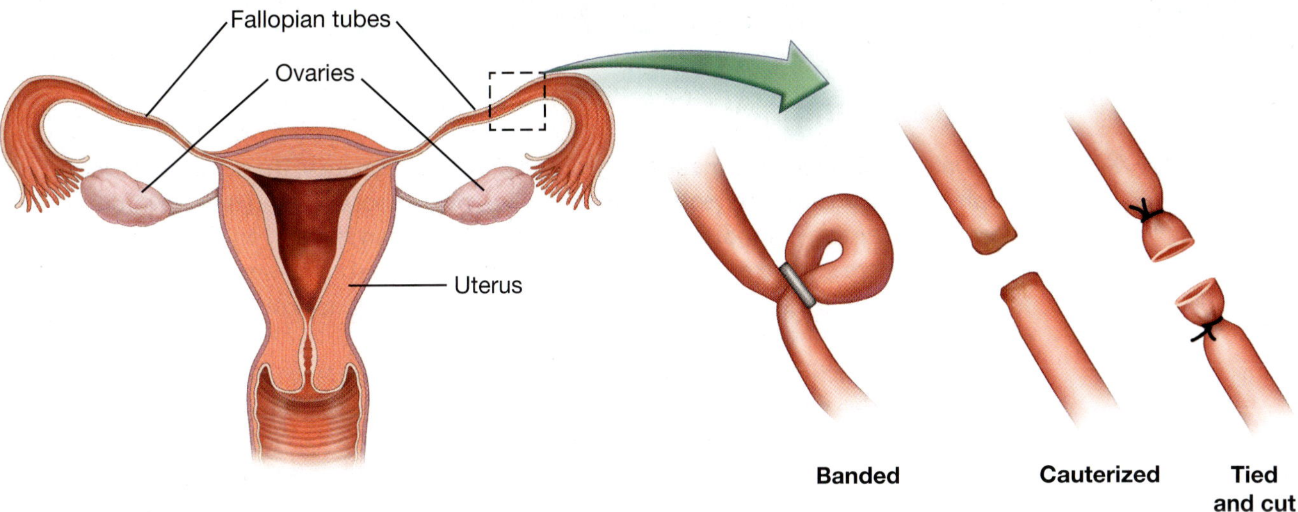

Figure 24.22 In tubal ligation, a doctor cuts or blocks the fallopian tubes. ***How does tubal ligation affect the function of the ovaries?***

Many tubal ligations are done in a hospital, while others are done in an outpatient surgery clinic. Depending on the type of surgery, some females return home the same day, while others recover in the hospital. Three months after surgery, doctors view an X-ray to confirm the tubes were successfully blocked. During those first three months, people should use an alternative form of contraception.

Lesson 24.4 Review

Know and Understand

1. Why is FAM not recommended for teens?
2. Explain why withdrawal is not an effective method of contraception.
3. Why should people be sure they never want children before choosing sterilization?

Think Critically

4. What factors make it difficult to track a female's cycle of fertility?
5. What are the similarities and differences between a vasectomy and tubal ligation?

REAL WORLD Health Skills

Analyze Influences With a partner, discuss why people might choose natural methods of contraception over other methods. Why are these methods described as *natural*? What beliefs, ideas, and viewpoints might influence people to prefer these methods? Brainstorm with your partner to analyze these influences. Then, write a paragraph about situations that are appropriate for using natural methods. Create a podcast where you discuss the following question with your partner: *What factors affect people's decisions about contraception? How do these factors change over time?*

Chapter 24 Review and Assessment

Chapter Summary

Contraception includes methods meant to prevent pregnancy. These methods help people plan pregnancy and remain childless when they choose. Having reliable information about contraception is important. Unreliable information can result in an unplanned pregnancy. There are five major types of contraception: sexual abstinence, barrier methods, hormonal methods, natural methods, and sterilization. Emergency contraception can help prevent pregnancy if these methods fail.

The most effective method of contraception is sexual abstinence. Abstinence is also the most effective method of preventing STI and HIV transmission. It has many social and emotional benefits and costs less than other methods.

Barrier methods work by physically blocking sperm from traveling through the female reproductive system and fertilizing an egg. Internal and external condoms are examples of barrier methods that also reduce the risk of STI and HIV transmission. Other barrier methods include the contraceptive sponge, diaphragm, and cervical cap.

Hormonal methods contain hormones that influence the female reproductive system. These methods help prevent pregnancy by thickening cervical mucus, thinning the lining of the uterus, and inhibiting ovulation (the release of an egg). Oral contraceptives are hormone-containing pills a female takes every day. Other methods include the birth control patch, vaginal ring, birth control shot, birth control implant, and intrauterine devices (IUDs). Emergency contraception is a hormonal method that helps prevent pregnancy within five days of sexual intercourse. It does not end a pregnancy that has already begun.

Natural methods of contraception include fertility awareness methods (FAM) and withdrawal. FAM tracks a female's menstrual cycle to time sexual intercourse when there is no egg for sperm to fertilize. Withdrawal involves pulling the penis out of the vagina before ejaculation and is not effective when used alone. Sterilization is a permanent method of birth control that involves surgically altering the reproductive system.

Vocabulary Activity

Write a short dialogue that narrates a discussion between two people about sexual health decisions. In your dialogue, the two people might talk about choosing abstinence or about factors that affect the decision to use a certain type of contraception. They should use effective communication and negotiation skills. Use and define at least five terms from this chapter in your dialogue.

barrier methods	*diaphragm*	*oral contraceptives*
birth control implant	*emergency contraception*	*spermicide*
birth control patch	*fertility awareness method (FAM)*	*sterilization*
birth control shot		*tubal ligation*
cervical cap	*hormonal methods*	*vaginal ring*
contraception	*intrauterine device (IUD)*	*vasectomy*
contraceptive sponge	*natural methods*	*withdrawal*

Review and Recall

Review the information in this chapter by answering the following questions.

1. Is it possible for someone to become pregnant while menstruating? Explain.
2. Which type of contraception permanently alters the reproductive system?

3. Which contraceptive method protects against STIs and HIV?
   A. condom
   B. birth control pills
   C. sterilization
   D. withdrawal
4. How is emergency contraception different from other forms of contraception?
5. What factors should people consider when choosing a method of contraception?
6. Which method of contraception is most effective at preventing pregnancy and STIs?
7. How do barrier methods work to prevent pregnancy?
8. Explain why a condom should be applied before the penis touches a partner's genitals.
9. Why should an external and internal condom not be worn together?
10. Which of the following does *not* protect against STIs?
    A. dental dam
    B. spermicide
    C. external condom
    D. internal condom
11. Explain how the hormones in birth control pills help prevent pregnancy.
12. Which hormonal method delivers hormones into the blood in a transdermal way?
    A. birth control implant
    B. IUD
    C. birth control patch
    D. birth control implant
13. How often should the birth control shot be given to prevent pregnancy?
14. How does the copper IUD help prevent pregnancy?
15. What are the different forms of emergency contraception?
16. List two factors, besides ovulation, that can change a female's resting body temperature.
17. Which contraceptive method is also called "pulling out"?
18. What are the two surgeries used for male and female sterilization?
19. How long should people use an alternative form of contraception after sterilization?

Standardized Test Prep

Math Practice

Incorrect or inconsistent use decreases the effectiveness of contraception. Read the information below and then answer the following questions.

Effectiveness Rates of Contraception, By Method

Contraceptive Method	Perfect Use	Typical Use
Contraceptive pill	99%	91%
Vaginal ring	99%	91%
Diaphragm	94%	88%
Contraceptive sponge	80–91%	76–88%
External condom	98%	85%
Internal condom	95%	79%
Withdrawal	96%	78%
Spermicide	82%	72%

20. If 5,000 high school students use withdrawal as their primary method of contraception this year, how many will experience a pregnancy?
21. For typical use, what percentage of teens using external condoms will experience a pregnancy?
22. How much more effective is the contraceptive pill than spermicide for perfect use? for typical use?

Chapter 24 Skills Assessment

Critical Thinking Skills

Answer the following questions to assess your knowledge of what you learned in this chapter.

1. What sources of information about sexual health have you accessed? Were these sources reliable? Why or why not?
2. How do people's goals, sexual histories, and any STIs affect decisions about contraception? Explain.
3. What benefits does sexual abstinence have over other forms of contraception? What, if any, weaknesses does it have compared to other forms of contraception?
4. Which barrier methods do you think would be easiest to use? hardest to use? Why?
5. Correct use is an essential part of effectively using barrier methods. Where could you go to get more reliable information about using barrier methods effectively? How would you know the information is reliable?
6. What factors do you think explain why some barrier methods require a doctor's prescription, while others do not?
7. Why do almost all forms of hormonal contraception require a doctor's visit? How does this protect the health of people who use these methods?
8. What resources can people use to learn more about hormonal methods and use them effectively? What apps are available? How do these help with correct use?
9. Which hormonal method do you think would be easiest for someone to use? Why? Explain your reasoning.
10. Do you think most teens understand how emergency contraception works? What misconceptions might teens have? Correct these misconceptions and share with a partner.
11. Why do you think some people prefer natural methods of contraception?
12. Why do many people who use FAM use it to plan a pregnancy and become pregnant?
13. Using reliable resources, research your state's laws about minors' rights to consent to contraceptive services, including sterilization. Discuss these laws in a small group.

Health and Wellness Skills

Complete the following activities to assess your skills related to health and wellness.

14. **Analyze Influences.** Cultural background and beliefs have a significant influence on people's attitudes about teen sexual activity. Consider what beliefs and cultural expectations have shaped your attitude toward teen sexual activity. To do this, you might need to research the different cultures and beliefs in your family. Make a video about your findings and reflect on how these attitudes have influenced your personal opinions about teen sexual activity.
15. **Access Information.** Using reliable resources, research the sterilization options available for males and females. For each sterilization procedure, list what the procedure does, how and where the procedure is performed, how much the procedure costs, advantages and disadvantages of the procedure, and how effective it is. Are there any barriers that might get in the way of people choosing this procedure? After gathering your information, create an informative pamphlet or brochure with this information. Present your final product to the class.
16. **Communicate with Others.** As a class, contact a person you know, in-person or online, who had a baby early in life (preferably before or during college). Think of several questions you would like answered and then interview this person about the experience. After the interview, write an essay describing what you learned.
17. **Make Decisions.** A crucial step in accomplishing your goals is getting the right support. To get this support, choose one trustworthy adult with whom you can have open conversations, even about sensitive topics. Once you have chosen this adult, write a brief statement addressed to the adult and explain your choice. In this statement, be sure to include your short- and long-terms goals and the topics you plan to discuss openly and honestly.

Describe what support you need from the adult and ask if the adult is comfortable with this role in your life. If you both agree, sign the statement. Keep it in a safe place so you can use it as a conversation starter when difficult topics arise.

18. **Set Goals.** Create a time line for your life. What are your goals for the next five years? the next 10 years? Do you want children? Remember that to reach your goals, you also need to set restrictions that will defend your goals and help you achieve them. Identify events or pressures that might deter you from living the life you have planned. Include events related to sexual activity and pregnancy. Then describe how you might avoid these obstacles.
19. **Practice Health-Enhancing Behaviors.** Knowing about contraception can not only protect your health, but can also help you promote the health of others. For each scenario given, write exactly what advice you would give to the friend asking you. Use what you learned in this chapter to help.
    - A. Your friend, who is not dating anyone, is approached by an acquaintance at an event. This acquaintance clearly likes your friend and suggests going somewhere alone. Your friend asks to talk to you for a minute. What advice do you give?
    - B. Two of your friends have been in a relationship for a year. They are two years apart, and the older partner has been sexually active in the past. Each friend comes to you separately looking for advice, since the couple is disagreeing about whether to be sexually active. What advice do you give each friend?
20. **Advocate for Health.** Create a social media campaign to outline the potential outcomes of unprotected sexual activity during the teen years. In your campaign, be sure to include risks related to pregnancy and STI transmission. Explain why sexual abstinence is a positive choice and also compare options for avoiding STI transmission and pregnancy.

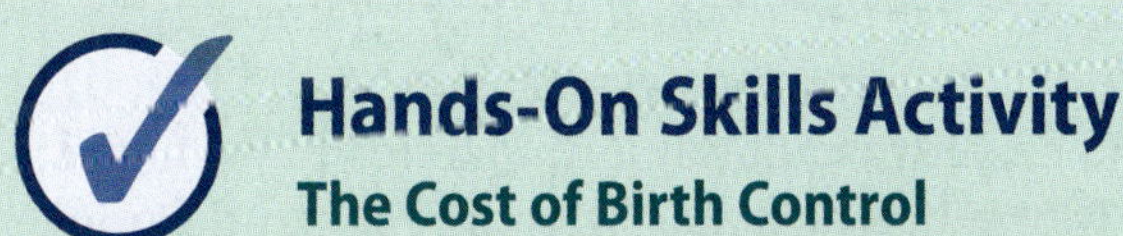

Hands-On Skills Activity

The Cost of Birth Control

Contraception can seem expensive to those who are buying it often or considering buying it. The costs of purchasing contraception are minimal, however, compared to the costs of giving birth to and caring for a baby or treating an incurable STI. In this activity, you will do research or visit local stores to compare the costs of purchasing contraception for one year versus the cost of having and caring for a baby for one year.

Steps for This Activity

1. Choose two contraceptive products discussed in this chapter. The products you choose should be available at a store or pharmacy. Research or estimate how often a person might need to purchase these products if the person was sexually active.
2. **Access Information.** Develop a comprehensive list that includes all the products a person would need to purchase to care for a newborn baby. Include cribs, carriers, baby clothes, and repeat purchases such as diapers, wipes, and food. Calculate the costs of the items on your list. Check prices online or go to local stores. Also research and record the cost of giving birth to a baby at your local hospital and getting testing and treatment for an incurable STI.
3. Multiply the cost of the contraceptive products you chose by the number of times a person would purchase them in one year of being sexually active. This is the cost of using contraception for one year. Then, add up the prices of the items a person would need to care for a newborn baby for one year. Make sure to multiply the costs of repeat purchases, such as diapers. Finally, add the cost of giving birth to a baby. Separately, add up the costs of testing and treatment for an incurable STI.
4. Compare the three total costs. How big is the difference between the cost of using contraception for one year and the cost of having and caring for a baby or getting testing and treatment for an STI? On a poster, write these numbers and attach pictures of all the items a person would purchase in each situation. Present your poster to the class.

Background Lesson 1 The Body Systems

Background Lesson 1.1 Organization of the Body

Understanding the organization and structures of the body is an important part of understanding health. The human body is organized into cells, tissues, organs, and body systems. *Cells* are the basic unit of all living things, including humans.

A *tissue* is an organized group of similar cells. Each type of tissue plays a different role in the body (**Figure BL1.1**). Some tissues form glands. *Glands* release substances into the body. For example, the salivary glands release saliva, a liquid that softens and helps break down food, into the mouth.

An *organ* is made of different tissues. Each organ performs a specific job. For example, the stomach is made of muscle, nervous, and connective tissue and glands that work together to store and digest food.

A group of organs that works together is a *body system*. For example, the stomach works with other organs of the digestive system. Different body systems work closely together. For example, the respiratory system transfers oxygen to the blood, and the cardiovascular system carries oxygenated blood to the body's cells. Many organs and body systems are located within body cavities.

In this background lesson, you will learn about major body systems of the human body. You learned about the male and female reproductive systems in Chapter 21: *The Beginning of Life*. This lesson will review the other major body systems.

Types of Tissues	
Type	**Description**
Connective tissue	• Supports and protects the body • Found in bone, cartilage, fat (adipose), and the dermis
Epithelium	• Protects the surfaces of most organs, forms glands, and absorbs nutrients and water • Found in the skin and internal and external surfaces of the digestive organs, blood vessels, and other organs
Muscle	• Moves bones and other parts of the body • Found in the muscles, heart, intestines, and stomach wall
Nervous tissue	• Controls muscles and glands and interprets and responds to information from the senses • Found in the brain, spinal cord, nerves, and sensory organs

Figure BL1.1 Tissues are groups of similar cells.

Background Lesson 1.2 Integumentary System

The *integumentary system* covers and protects the entire body. This system includes the skin, hair, and nails.

Skin

The *skin* protects the body and does a surprising number of important jobs. If spread flat, it would cover 17–20 square feet, about the size of a bedsheet. Skin thickness ranges from 0.5 millimeters on the eyelids to 4 millimeters on the soles of the feet.

The skin has three layers: the epidermis, dermis, and hypodermis (**Figure BL1.2**).

1. The *epidermis* is the outermost layer. Most cells in the epidermis contain *keratin*, a tough protein that protects the skin from infections and injuries. The epidermis grows continually from its base. New cells push up older cells, which die, fall off, and are replaced. The epidermis contains *keratinocytes*, which make keratin and vitamin D, and *melanocytes*, which make *melanin* (skin pigment).
2. The *dermis* lies below the epidermis and firmly anchors skin to the body. This layer contains oil glands and sweat glands. Oil glands, called *sebaceous glands*, produce oil that keeps skin moist and prevents hair from becoming brittle. Sweat glands produce sweat, which helps cool the body. The dermis also contains nerve fibers and *dermal ridges*, which make up fingerprint patterns.
3. The *hypodermis* lies under the dermis. It contains fat (adipose), which insulates the body and stores energy, and blood vessels.

Hair and Nails

Hair and nails, like the skin, protect the body. For example, eyelashes and eyebrows protect the eyes. Head hair shields the scalp from the sun, and hairs protect the nose from foreign objects.

The hair and nails are made of keratin. Hair grows from *hair follicles* and lengthens as new cells push up older cells. All skin surfaces grow hair, except the palms, soles, lips, nipples, and some genital areas. Genes determine hair color and texture.

Nails protect the ends of the fingers and toes. Nails grow from cells in *nail beds* on the upper sides of the fingers and toes near the ends. Nails lengthen as new nail pushes out older nail.

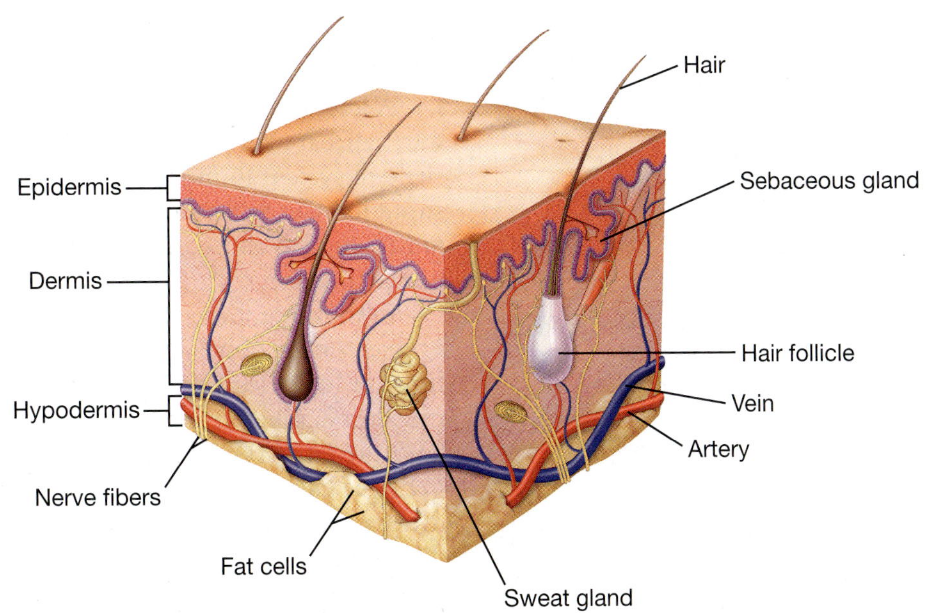

Figure BL1.2 The epidermis, dermis, and hypodermis make up the skin.

Background Lesson 1.3 Skeletal System

The *skeletal system* is made of 206 bones, which protect organs, give the body structure, and enable movement (**Figure BL1.3**).

Bone Tissue

Bones are made of minerals, proteins, and living cells. Bone hardness comes from the minerals *calcium* and *phosphate*, which the blood delivers to bone tissue. Bone strength and flexibility comes from the protein *collagen*. Living bone cells make collagen.

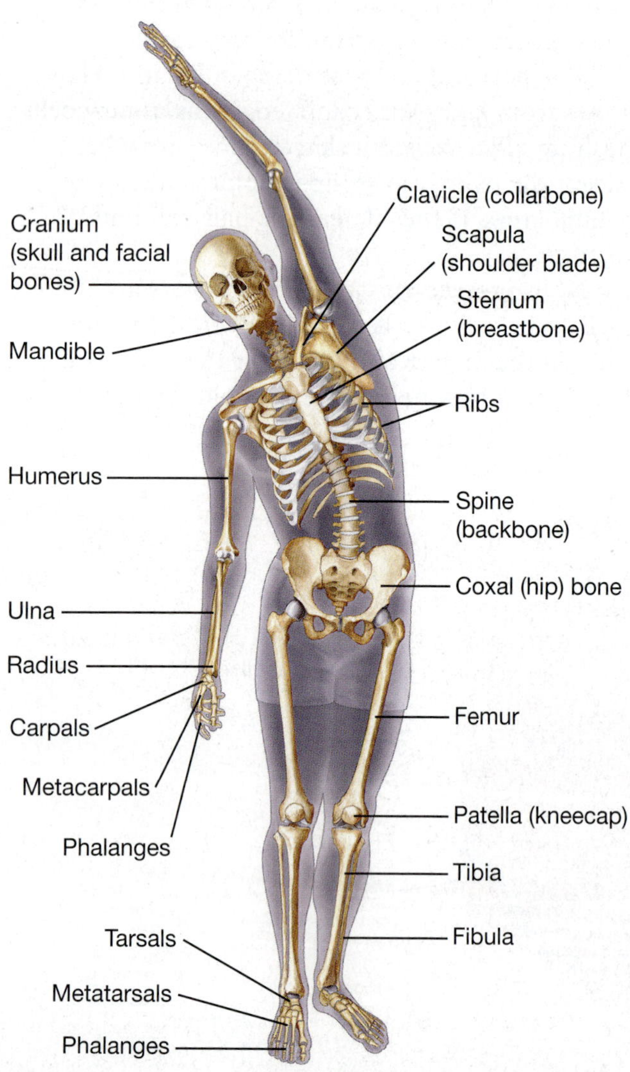

Figure BL1.3 Bones make up the skeletal system. Shown here are some major bones of the body.

Bones develop, grow, heal, and adapt throughout a person's life. Bone cells called *osteoblasts* use collagen and minerals to make new bone tissue. *Osteoclasts* break down and dissolve bone tissue. Weight-bearing activities like running and lifting weights put stress on bones. This stress pushes osteoblasts to make dense, strong bone tissue.

Bone Structure

Bones come in many shapes and sizes. For example, bones of the fingers, arms, and legs are long and cylindrical. Bones of the skull, hip, and backbone are flat or have an irregular shape. A layer of dense, strong bone tissue covers most bones. Under that dense bone is spongy bone tissue that contains *bone marrow*. The bone marrow makes most of the body's blood cells. Bone tissue also contains arteries and veins.

When people are born, the ends of many bones are made of *cartilage*, which is not as hard as bone. This cartilage slowly turns into bone tissue, causing growth. After this cartilage is used up, bone growth stops. Bone growth stops in some people when they reach their mid-teens. In other people, bones continue growing into the mid-twenties.

Joints

A *joint* is a location where two or more bones meet and are held together. Joints enable the skeletal system to move. Some joints, such as the shoulder, can move in several directions. Other joints, such as those in the skull, do not allow bones to move.

In movable joints, strong bands of tissue called *ligaments* hold bones together. For example, the tibia, or lower leg bone, and the femur, or large thighbone, meet at the knee joint. Ligaments hold the femur and tibia together and limit how the knee can move. Ligaments can be injured if the knee is forced to move or twist in different directions. A special fluid inside movable joints reduces the amount of friction between bones. In movable joints, cartilage protects bones and absorbs shock where bones meet.

Background Lesson 1.4 Muscular System

The *muscular system* contains muscles that help parts of the body move (**Figure BL1.4**). When muscle tissue shortens, or *contracts*, it can make attached bones move. A bone can move when a muscle stretches too. Nerves stimulate muscles to contract or stretch.

Muscles are connected to bones by bands of tissue called *tendons*. Tendons can shorten or lengthen when muscles pull them. Muscles, bones, and tendons work closely together.

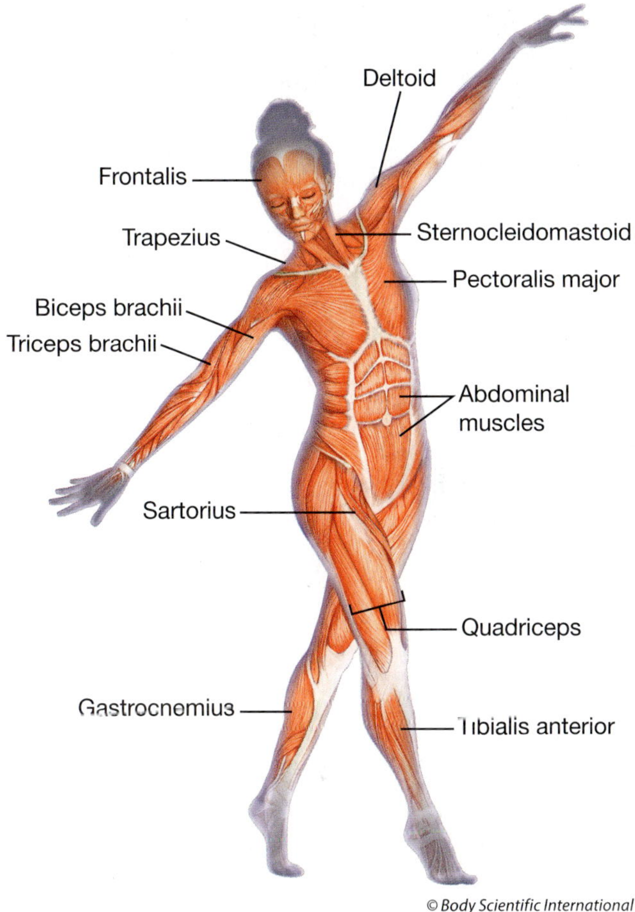

Figure BL1.4 Shown here are some major muscles of the muscular system.

Muscle Tissue

Muscles are built from muscle cells. There are three types of muscle:

- *Skeletal muscles* attach to bones. They are *voluntary*, which means you can control them. For example, you can move your leg muscles to walk or use your hand muscles to type.
- *Smooth muscles* are *involuntary*, which means they cannot be controlled. These muscles work without you realizing it. For example, smooth muscles in your stomach mix and digest food without your control.
- *Cardiac muscle* is involuntary muscle found in the heart. Without conscious effort, cardiac muscle pumps blood throughout the body.

Muscle Pairs

Throughout the body, most skeletal muscles work in pairs to move certain body parts. For example, the biceps brachii contract to bend the arms at the elbows. The triceps brachii contract to straighten the arms at the elbows.

Some muscles stabilize joints. For example, muscles hold the shoulder joint firmly in place when you bend and extend your arm at the elbow. Other muscles of the neck, back, and trunk maintain posture when you are standing, sitting, and walking.

Background Lesson 1.5 Cardiovascular System

The *cardiovascular system* provides the body with a continuous supply of blood containing oxygen and nutrients. It includes the heart, blood vessels, and blood (**Figure BL1.5**).

Heart

The *heart* is a hollow, muscular organ located in the center of the chest. The heart pumps blood through blood vessels around the body.

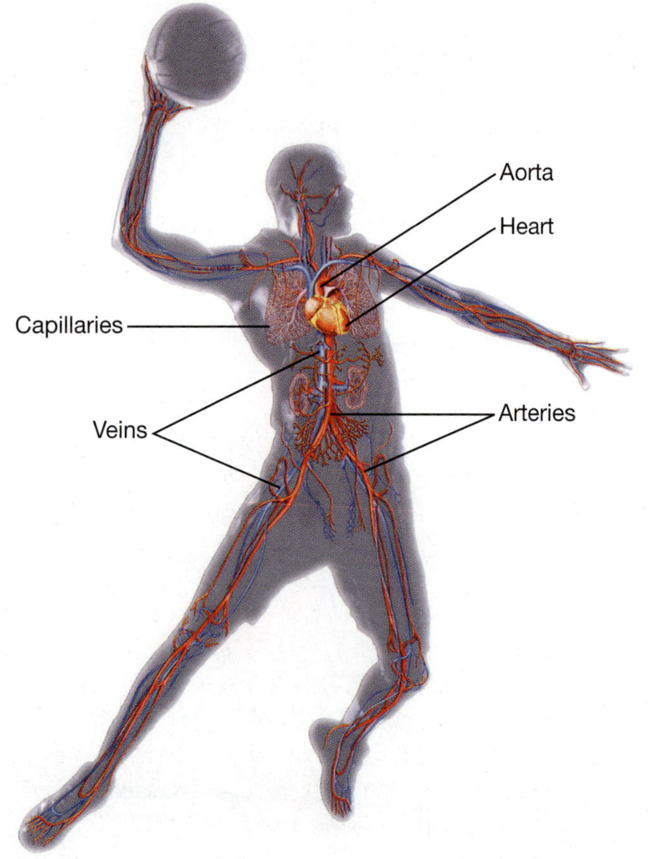

© Body Scientific International

Figure BL1.5 The cardiovascular system is made up of the heart, blood vessels (arteries, veins, and capillaries), and blood.

At 70 beats per minute, the heart pumps about 2,000 gallons of blood each day.

The heart contains four chambers. The top two chambers are the *atria*. The atria receive blood and pass it to the lower two chambers, called *ventricles*. The muscular ventricles pump blood out of the heart into blood vessels. Structures called *valves* open and close to permit one-way blood flow from the atria to the ventricles and from the ventricles into blood vessels (**Figure BL1.6**).

The heart has a natural *pacemaker*, composed of specialized cardiac tissue in the wall of the right atrium. The pacemaker sends regular signals to the atria and ventricles, causing them to contract. Stress, physical activity, hormone levels, and other factors can change the rate of pacemaker signaling, which changes heart rate.

Blood Vessels

Blood vessels carry blood between the heart and the rest of the body. *Arteries* carry blood from the heart to the rest of the body. The *aorta* is an artery and the largest blood vessel in the body. *Capillaries* are the smallest blood vessels. They deliver oxygen and nutrients to cells and pick up cells' waste. *Veins* carry blood from the rest of the body to the heart.

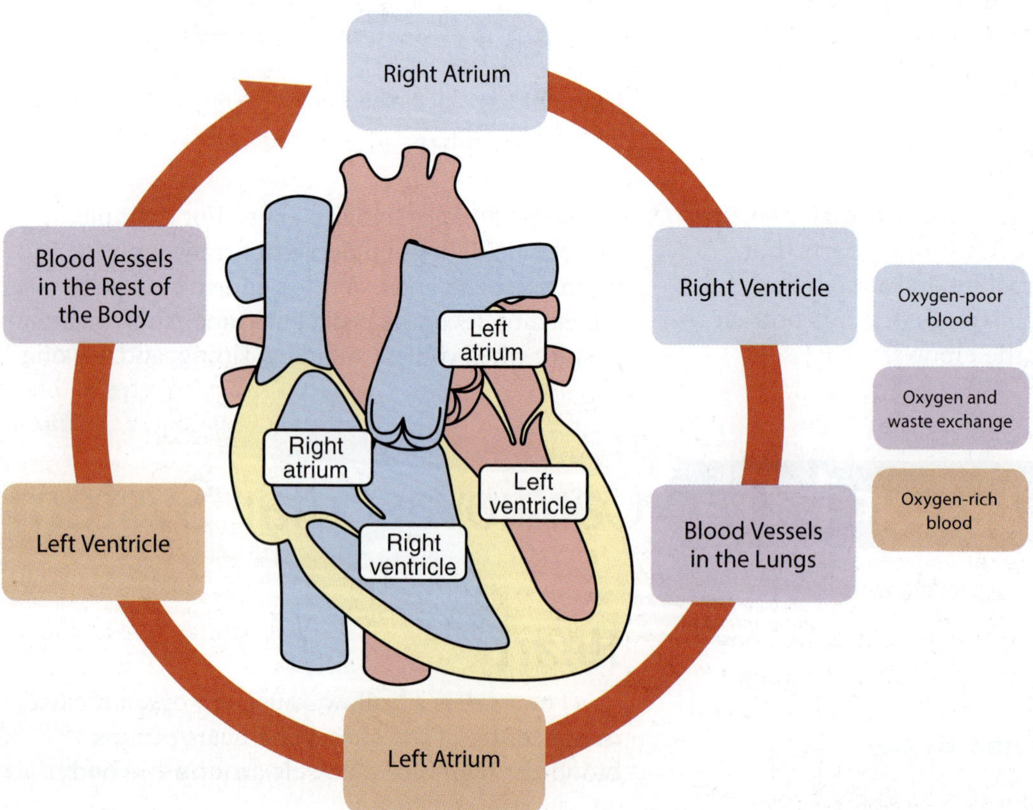

Figure BL1.6 Blood flows from the right atrium into the right ventricle. The right ventricle then pumps blood into the lungs, where the blood receives oxygen. Blood returns into the left atrium of the heart and then passes into the left ventricle. The left ventricle pumps oxygen-rich blood into the rest of the body. Once oxygen passes from the blood into the body's various tissues, oxygen-poor blood returns to the right atrium of the heart, and the process begins again.

Goodheart-Willcox Publisher

Blood

The adult body holds 5–6 liters of blood. Blood is mostly water. The watery portion of blood, called *plasma*, transports all the substances carried by blood. Blood also contains the following blood cells:

- *Red blood cells* are the most numerous blood cell. They contain a substance called *hemoglobin*, which enables them to carry and release oxygen. Red blood cells also have certain sugars on their surfaces that determine a person's blood type.
- *White blood cells* help defend the body against infections. Many white blood cells live in lymphatic organs of the body.
- *Platelets* are responsible for blood clotting. Clotting stops blood from flowing outside the wall of an injured blood vessel.

Background Lesson 1.6 Respiratory System

The *respiratory system* draws air into the lungs and delivers oxygen to the blood. It also takes carbon dioxide—another gas—out of the blood and sends it outside the body (**Figure BL1.7**). The process of inhaling and exhaling air is *external respiration*. The exchange of oxygen and carbon dioxide in the lower respiratory system is *internal respiration*.

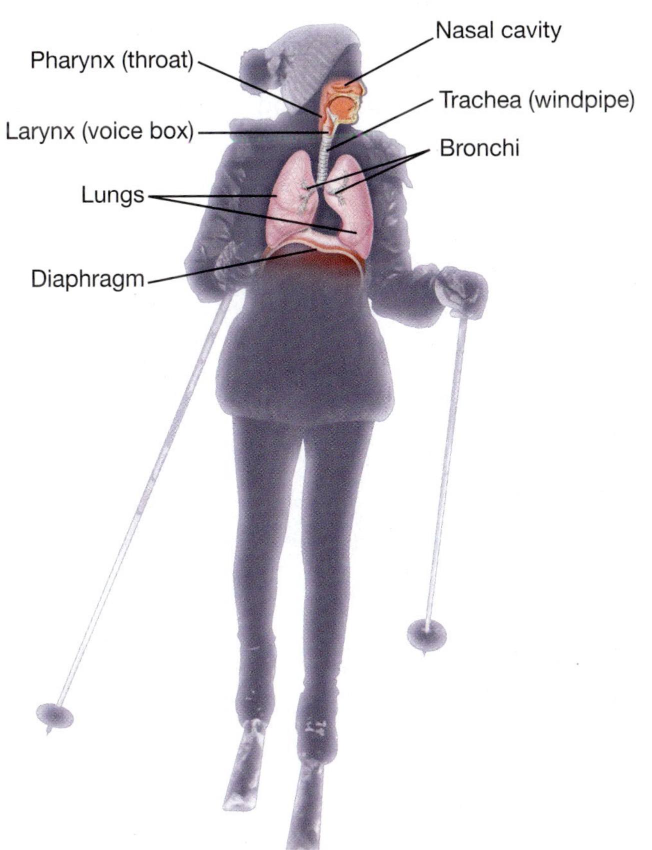

Figure BL1.7 Organs of the upper and lower respiratory systems make up the respiratory system.

Upper Respiratory System

The upper respiratory system brings air containing oxygen into the body. Air enters the nose and mouth and passes down through the *pharynx* (throat) to the *larynx* (voice box) and then through the *trachea* (windpipe) to the lungs. You can feel the larynx as a bump in the front of your throat. It vibrates when you speak, as air passes across the vocal cords. A structure called the *epiglottis* covers the larynx when you swallow and prevents food from entering the trachea.

The inner walls of the respiratory passages make a moist, sticky substance called *mucus*. Mucus traps bacteria and dust particles so they cannot enter the lungs. The passage behind the nose is also lined with mucus and blood vessels that warm and moisten air.

Lower Respiratory System

The trachea branches into two *bronchi*, or air passages that lead to each *lung*. The bronchi divide into smaller passages, called *bronchioles*, inside the lungs. These airways end as thin-walled sacs called *alveoli*. When you inhale, air fills the alveoli. Oxygen moves from air in the alveoli into the blood through capillaries. Carbon dioxide also moves out of the blood into air that is then exhaled.

The chief muscle that enables inhalation is the *diaphragm*, located beneath the lungs and above the abdomen. As the diaphragm moves down, the chest expands. Other chest muscles also help the chest expand. Exhalation happens when these muscles relax. The chest collapses and squeezes air out the mouth and nose.

Background Lesson 1.7 Lymphatic and Immune Systems

The *lymphatic system* is responsible for removing foreign substances from the body. This body system also includes organs and tissues of the *immune system* that help fight infections. The main organs of the lymphatic and immune systems include lymphatic vessels, lymph nodes, tonsils, the spleen, the thymus, and white blood cells.

Lymphatic Vessels and Lymph Nodes

The *lymphatic vessels* are similar to blood vessels, but they do not carry blood. Instead, they carry extra fluid that builds up in tissues of the body. This fluid becomes *lymph* when it enters the lymphatic capillaries and flows into other lymphatic vessels. Lymphatic vessels collect and transport lymph to veins in the chest. There, lymph rejoins the blood.

Lymph is filtered by *lymph nodes* before it reenters the blood. Inside the lymph nodes, white blood cells remove bacteria and viruses from the fluid.

Tonsils are small masses of tissue that guard the throat from infection. They are located on the sides and top of the back of the throat. The tonsils also contain white blood cells. When the throat is infected, tonsils enlarge and become red.

Spleen and Thymus

The *spleen* is an organ filled with white blood cells and filters blood. It also removes dead red blood cells from the blood. The spleen is located to the left of the stomach and is shaped like a flattened bean. The *thymus* is a lymphatic organ located in front of the large blood vessels in the upper chest. In the thymus, certain kinds of white blood cells learn how to recognize and attack bacteria and viruses.

White Blood Cells

White blood cells are part of the lymphatic system. Some take in and destroy bacteria. Others specialize in controlling viruses. Some white blood cells make *antibodies*, or proteins that stick to bacteria and viruses and help destroy these invaders. All these white blood cells are a vital part of the body's immune system.

Background Lesson 1.8 Nervous System

The *nervous system* allows people to think, use the senses, move, and maintain important body processes. The nervous system is organized into two parts. The *central nervous system (CNS)* includes the brain and spinal cord. The *peripheral nervous system (PNS)* includes all other nerves (**Figure BL1.8**).

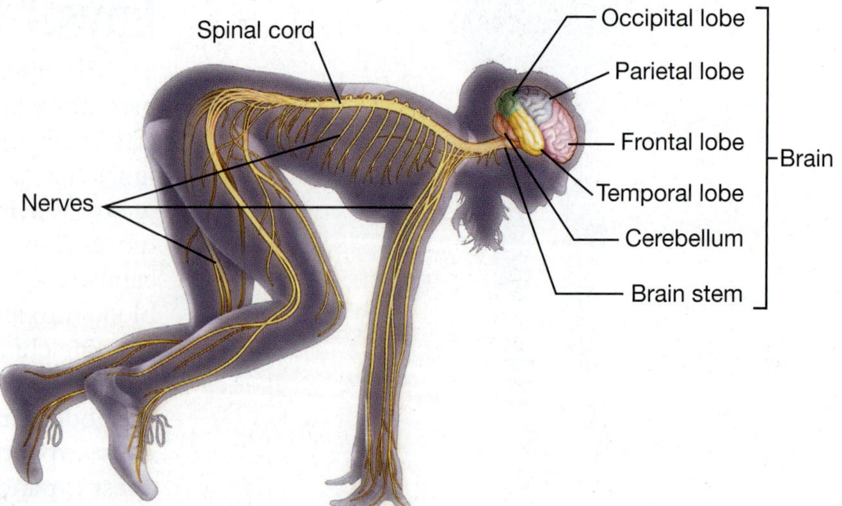

Figure BL1.8 The nervous system contains the brain, spinal cord, and nerves.

Neurons

Neurons, or cells specialized to receive and send signals, are the building blocks of the nervous system.

Neurons make up the brain, spinal cord, and nerves. *Sensory neurons* carry signals from the body to the CNS. *Motor neurons* carry information from the CNS to muscles and glands of the body.

Brain

The *brain* controls nearly all body functions. It is responsible for learning, memory, and interpreting information from the sensory organs.

The bones of the skull protect the brain. The brain is also protected by three layers of membrane called *meninges*. *Cerebrospinal fluid (CSF)* circulates over the brain and cushions and protects it.

The largest part of the brain is the *cerebrum*, which interprets sensory information, controls muscles, and is responsible for intelligence, learning, memory, and personality. The cerebrum is divided into two nearly equal halves—the left and right hemispheres. The halves are connected by nerves so they can communicate.

Different parts of the cerebrum have different functions:

- The *frontal lobes* control muscles, including speech muscles. They also control personality, judgment, and memory.
- The *temporal lobes* are responsible for hearing, taste, and smell. The left temporal lobe helps understand spoken language.
- The *parietal lobes* interpret signals from the senses and muscles from the opposite side of the body.
- The *occipital lobes* interpret information from the eyes.

Beneath the occipital lobe lies the *cerebellum*, which coordinates muscle activity. The *brain stem* connects the base of the brain to the spinal cord and controls heartbeat and breathing.

Spinal Cord

The *spinal cord* carries nerve signals between the brain and the body. It is protected by meninges, CSF, and bones of the spine called *vertebrae*. Nerves in the spinal cord branch to all areas of the body. The spinal cord also controls some *reflexes*, or automatic responses to a sensation.

Background Lesson 1.9 Sensory Organs

You are probably familiar with the senses of sight, sound, hearing, taste, and touch. Other senses include balance, pressure, pain, and temperature. Senses are made possible by nerve endings and structures specialized for detecting certain kinds of information.

Eyes

The eyes and brain work together to make vision possible. Nerve endings in the eyes detect light. Nerves then carry this information to the occipital lobe of the brain, which forms images from the information it receives. Numerous structures help the eye capture light and send signals to the brain (**Figure BL1.9**).

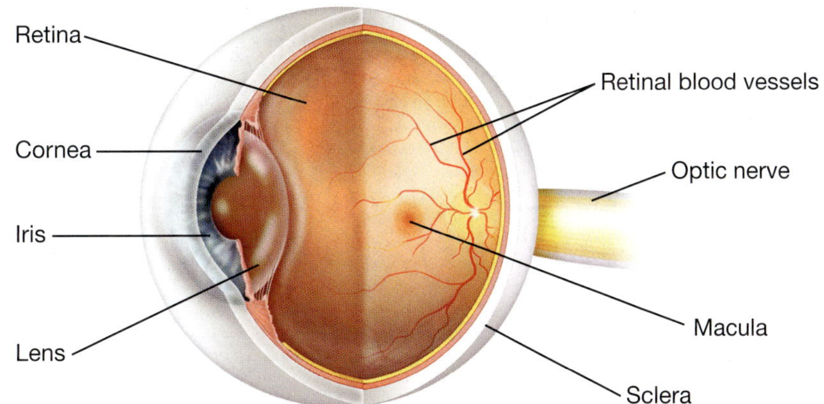

Figure BL1.9 The structures of the eye bring in light and then send information to the brain to interpret the images.

The *sclera* is a strong tissue that gives the eye its shape. You can see the front of the sclera where it forms the white of your eye. The inner, back layer of the eyeball is the *retina*. The retina is made of nerve endings that respond to light. In the center of the retina is the *macula*, an area rich in nerve endings. This area is responsible for forming sharp images.

The front of the eyeball is protected by a clear layer called the *cornea*. Light passes through the cornea to the *lens*, which focuses light on the retina. The *iris*, the colored part of the eye, lies between the lens and cornea. The black, circular opening in the iris is the *pupil*, which allows light into the eyeball. The iris can change the pupil's size and adjust the amount of light entering the eye.

The *eyelids* can close and protect the eye. Tear glands produce tears that lubricate and clean the eye's outer surface.

Ears

The ear is responsible for the senses of hearing and balance. The ear has three regions: the outer ear, middle ear, and inner ear (**Figure BL1.10**). The *outer ear* begins with the visible, external ear and a tube called the *auditory canal*. Sound travels through the auditory canal to the *eardrum*, a thin wall of connective tissue. The middle ear begins at the eardrum and includes three tiny bones called the *malleus*, *incus*, and *stapes*.

The *inner ear* begins with the *cochlea*, a snail-shaped organ connected to sensory nerves from the brain. The inner ear also contains balance organs. These detect the head's position and movement.

The visible, external ear helps direct sound to the auditory canal. Sound traveling through the auditory canal causes the eardrum to vibrate against the middle ear bones. These vibrate against the cochlea, which sends information about sound to the brain via the *vestibulocochlear nerve*.

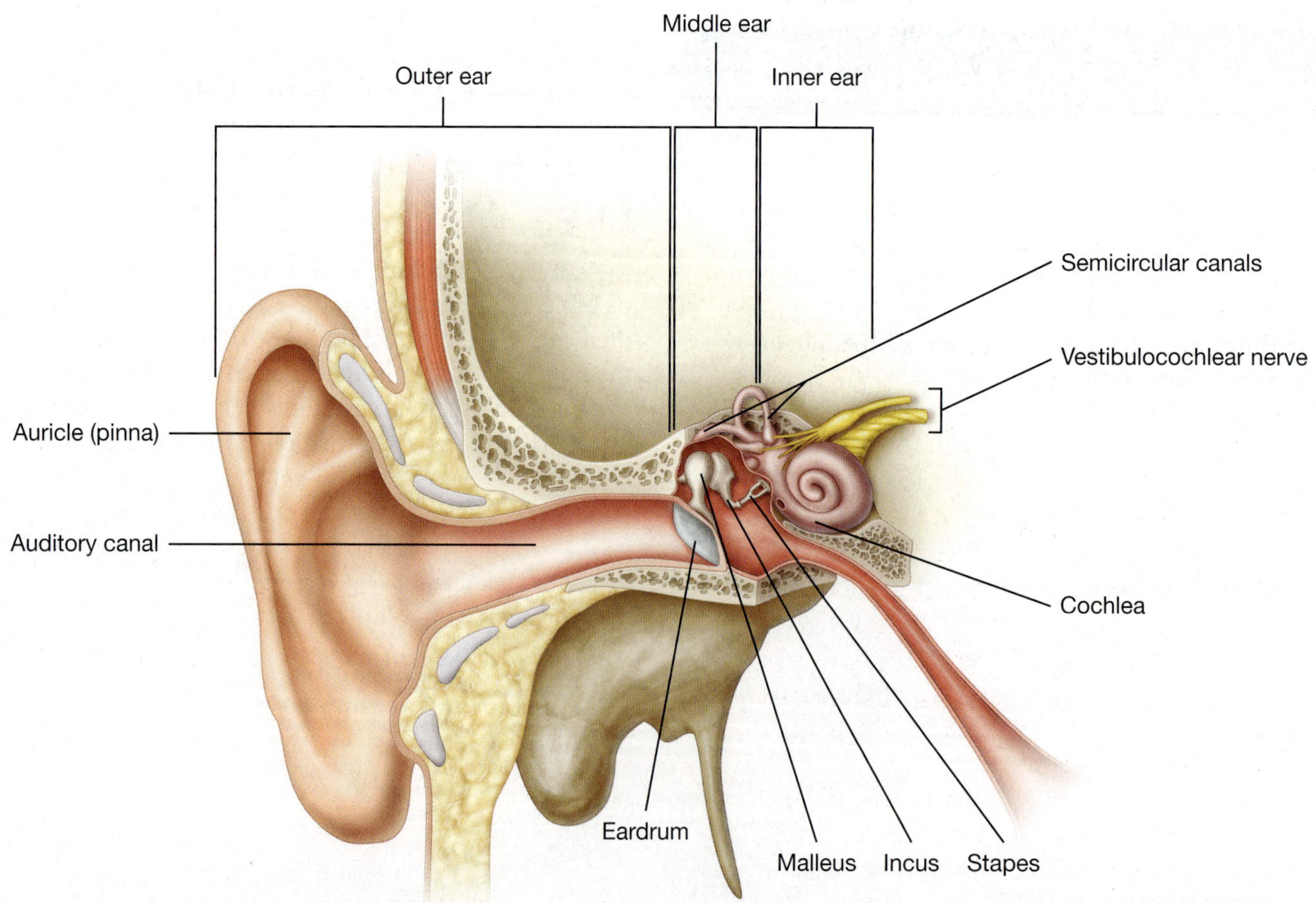

Figure BL1.10 The structures of the ear bring in sound and convert it into vibrations that are sent to the brain.

Background Lesson 1.10 Endocrine System

The *endocrine system* controls the body using hormones. Organs of the endocrine system make and release hormones into the bloodstream, which carries hormones around the body (**Figure BL1.11**).

Pituitary Gland

The *pituitary gland*, often called the *master gland*, is located beneath the hypothalamus in the brain. Pituitary hormones control endocrine glands and affect other organs and tissues, directing processes like growth, birth, and puberty. The pituitary gland itself is controlled by the hypothalamus.

Thyroid

The *thyroid* is a gland located on the front of the neck, just below the larynx. It makes *thyroid hormone*, which increases the rate at which the body uses energy. This hormone also controls the body's temperature.

Parathyroid Glands

The *parathyroid glands* are four tiny glands located on the back of the thyroid gland. These glands make *parathyroid hormone (PTH)*. PTH controls blood levels of calcium and phosphate, which are minerals important for bone and cell growth.

Adrenal Glands and Pancreas

One *adrenal gland* is located on top of each kidney. These glands produce hormones that control blood levels of minerals and salts. Adrenal hormones control how the body uses energy sources such as carbohydrates.

The adrenal glands also make *adrenaline*, which prepares the body to cope with stress by increasing heart and breathing rate. Adrenaline also increases blood flow to the muscles, heart, lungs, and brain.

The *pancreas* is an endocrine organ and also part of the digestive system. As part of the endocrine system, the pancreas makes the hormone *insulin*, which lowers blood sugar.

Ovaries and Testes

The *ovaries* and *testes* are part of the endocrine system and also part of the reproductive system. As you read in Chapter 21, the ovaries produce the hormones estrogen and progesterone. These hormones regulate the sexual development of females and the menstrual cycle. The testes produce testosterone, which controls the sexual development of males.

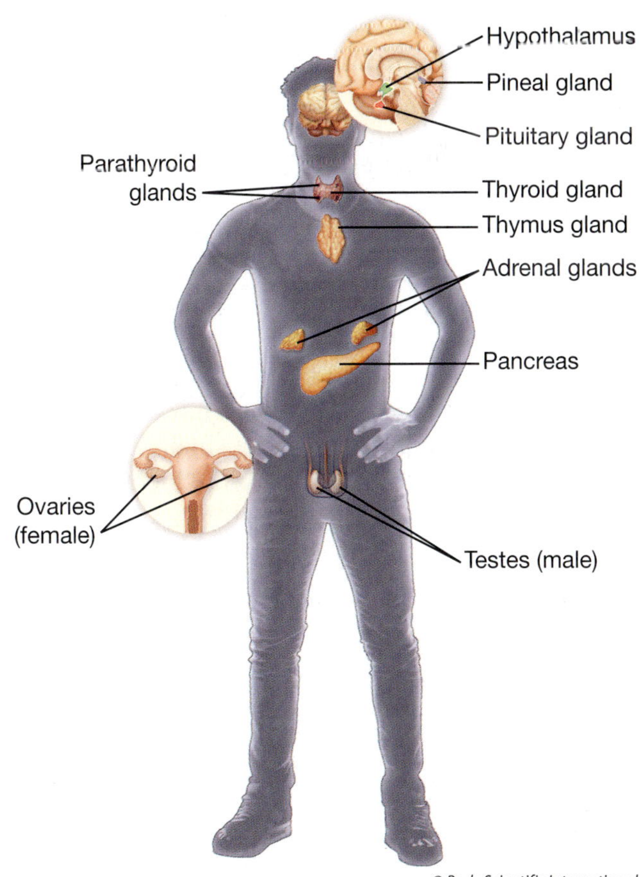

Figure BL1.11 The organs of the endocrine system release hormones that guide body processes.

Background Lesson 1.11 Digestive System

The *digestive system* brings food into the body, breaks it down (called *digestion*), and absorbs nutrients into the blood. It also removes solid waste from the body (**Figure BL1.12**).

Mouth and Teeth

Digestion begins in the mouth. Here, teeth break down food into a soft mass. *Salivary glands* around the mouth release saliva, which moistens food. The muscular tongue pushes chewed food into the *pharynx* (throat). Swallowed food passes from the pharynx into the esophagus.

Esophagus

The *esophagus* is a muscular tube that transports chewed, moistened food to the stomach. A small, donut-shaped muscle called a *sphincter* opens to let food pass into the stomach and closes to prevent backflow into the esophagus.

Stomach and Small Intestine

The *stomach* is a muscular organ that mixes food with acid and enzymes to break it down further. Food passes from the stomach into the *small intestine*. Muscles in the small intestine's walls push food through the small intestine, where enzymes continue digestion. The small intestine absorbs nutrients and water into the bloodstream, so blood can transport them to other cells.

Pancreas, Liver, and Gallbladder

The pancreas, liver, and gallbladder aid in this stage of digestion. The *pancreas* releases digestive enzymes into the small intestine. The *liver* makes *bile*, which helps breaks down fat. The *gallbladder* stores bile and releases it into the small intestine.

Large Intestine

From the small intestine, undigested food passes into the *large intestine*, also called the *colon*. The large intestine prepares solid food waste for removal from the body.

The large intestine absorbs any water left in undigested food. The remaining solid waste is eliminated as *feces*. Feces are stored in a part of the large intestine called the *rectum*. Muscles of the large intestine eliminate feces through an opening called the *anus* at the end of the large intestine.

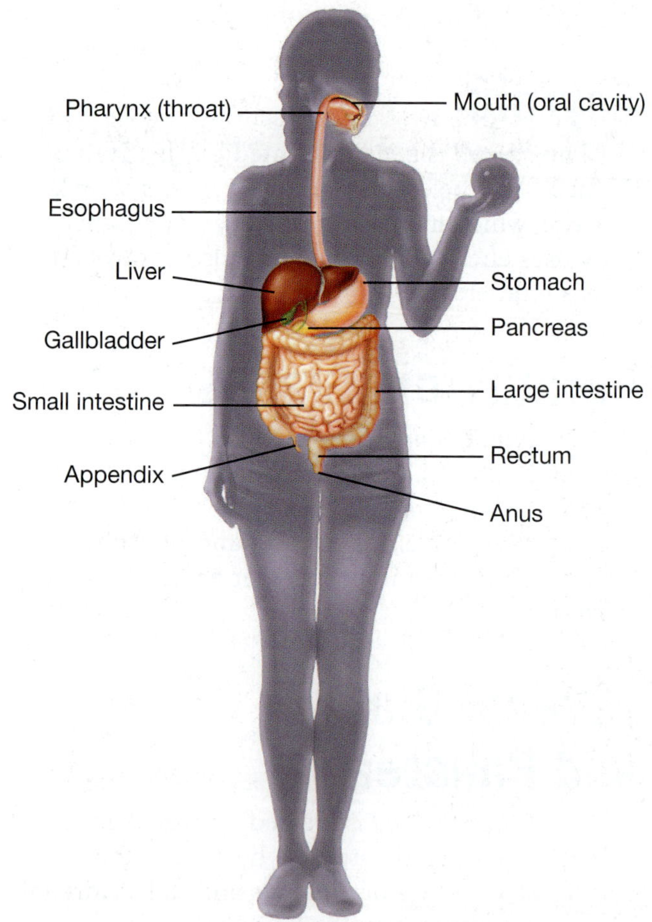

Figure BL1.12 The organs of the digestive system facilitate the digestion, absorption, and elimination of substances you consume.

Background Lesson 1.12 Urinary System

The *urinary system* removes liquid waste from the body. The urinary system includes two kidneys and ureters, the bladder, and the urethra (**Figure BL1.13**).

Kidneys

Two bean-shaped *kidneys* begin the process of urine production by filtering blood and removing waste. Kidneys also control the amounts of water, minerals, and acid in blood. As blood moves through the kidneys, the liquid waste that is filtered out becomes *urine*. Urine exits each kidney through a ureter. Cleansed and filtered blood returns to the cardiovascular system.

Kidneys must continually filter waste from blood and form urine. You would not live long if your kidneys stopped working. Waste would build up in the blood quickly and poison every organ, including the brain.

Ureters, Bladder, and Urethra

The *ureters* are tubes that carry urine from each kidney to the bladder. Each ureter enters the top of the bladder.

The *urinary bladder* is a muscular organ that stores urine. When the bladder is full, the bladder muscle squeezes urine into the urethra. Two sphincters join the urethra to the bladder. The outermost sphincter gives you some control over urination.

The *urethra* is a small tube that transports urine out of the body. The urethra exits males at the tip of the penis. The urethra is shorter in females and exits above the vagina.

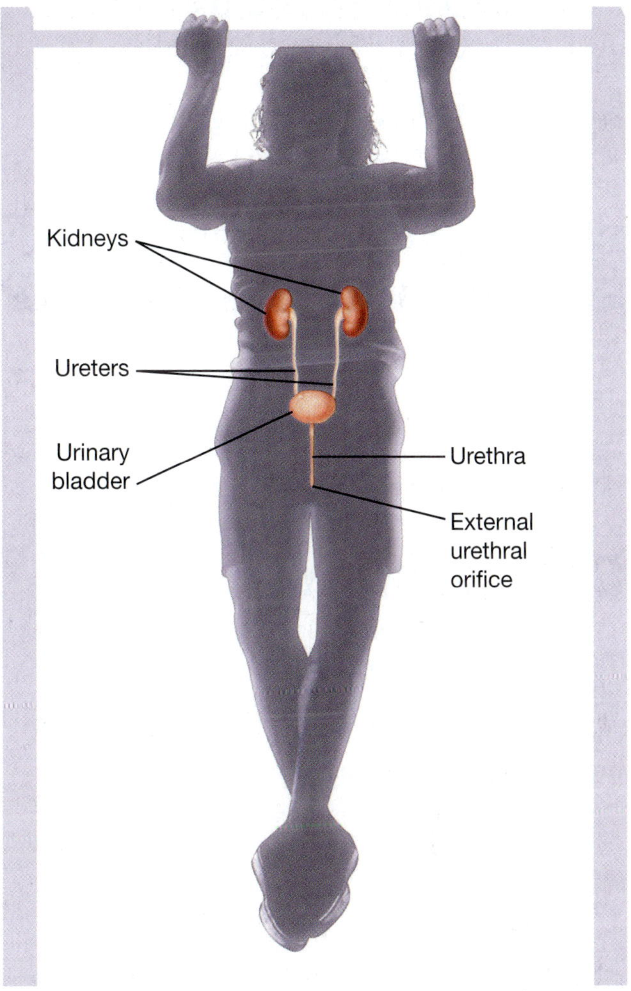

Figure BL1.13 The organs of the urinary system filter blood and remove liquid waste from the body.

Background Lesson 2 Personal Hygiene

Background Lesson 2.1 Caring for Your Skin

The skin plays a very important role in keeping you healthy. You learned about the anatomy of the skin in Background Lesson 1.2. Caring for the skin is an important part of maintaining health.

Basic Skin Care

Keeping your skin healthy requires daily care. Taking a bath or shower every day will keep your skin clean and prevent body odor. When bathing or showering, use a mild soap and warm water. After bathing, applying a lotion or moisturizer can keep skin from becoming too dry. Applying a deodorant or antiperspirant will prevent body odor. A *deodorant* covers up the odor of sweat. An *antiperspirant* dries up sweat and helps reduce sweating.

Caring for your skin also involves healthy lifestyle choices. Eating nutritious foods, such as fruits and vegetables, and drinking lots of water can keep your skin looking its best. Getting enough sleep each night, managing stress, and avoiding substance use can also keep your skin looking healthy.

Managing Common Skin Conditions

Caring for your skin can help you manage common skin conditions that affect teens and people of all ages.

Sun Damage

Spending time in the sun can damage your skin and increase risk for skin cancer. To prevent this, find a shady spot when you are outside and wear clothing that protects any exposed skin. Wear a hat with a large brim to protect your face, head, ears, and neck.

Even in social situations, it is important to use sun protection. You may need to use refusal skills if people discourage you from being safe. *Sunscreens* protect the skin by absorbing, reflecting, or scattering ultraviolet (UV) light from the sun. A sunscreen's *sun protection factor (SPF)* describes its effectiveness at blocking UV rays. The higher the SPF of a product, the greater the protection it provides. You should use sunscreen with an SPF of at least 15. For the best protection, apply sunscreen 30 minutes before going outdoors and reapply sunscreen every two hours, or more often if you sweat or swim.

Finally, avoid tanning beds, tanning booths, and sunlamps. The UV rays produced by these machines are just as dangerous as those from the sun.

Acne

At some point, most teens experience *acne*, a skin condition that causes pimples. Acne is partly caused by elevated levels of hormones during puberty, which increase oil production in the body. Pimples form when *pores*, or hair follicles under the skin, become clogged with oil. As the outer layer of skin sheds, dead skin cells can become stuck together inside a pore. This creates a blockage.

Over time, oil and bacteria leak into the skin surrounding a pore, causing infection and inflammation. A *whitehead* is a pimple characterized by whitish pus. A *blackhead* is a yellow or blackish bump inside a clogged pore and is more open to the air.

Strategies you can use to prevent acne breakouts and help them clear up quickly include the following:

- Wash your face gently twice a day. After washing your face, rinse so that the soap does not stay on your skin.
- Do not squeeze or pick at pimples. This can lead to permanent acne scars.

- Avoid touching your face with your fingers. This can spread bacteria and cause inflammation and irritation.
- Keep clean anything that touches your face, including eyeglasses, headbands, and hats. Keep your hair clean and pulled away from your face.
- If you wear makeup, buy brands that are oil-free and *noncomedogenic* or *nonacnegenic*. Throw away old makeup, which can contain bacteria. Be sure to wash all makeup off your skin before you go to sleep.
- Be careful when shaving your face. Try to shave lightly, and not too frequently, to avoid accidentally cutting a skin blemish.

If acne persists, you can see a dermatologist, who can share useful information about caring for your skin type. *Cystic acne* is a particularly severe type of acne that does not clear up without medication.

Eczema

Eczema, or *dermatitis*, is a condition that causes swollen, red, dry, and itchy patches of skin. When these patches are scratched, they can become infected. Eczema is a chronic condition, which means it continues over time. Some people are more likely to develop this condition than others. Eczema is not contagious. You cannot catch it from someone else.

Eczema flare-ups can be triggered by colds or other minor illnesses, as well as irritating substances. Stress is also associated with eczema flare-ups. If you have eczema, do not scratch the affected area of skin. To relieve dryness and itching, apply a lotion or cream when the skin is damp. This locks in moisture and can help reduce itching. Symptoms of eczema can also be treated using over-the-counter (OTC) products.

Tattoos and Piercings

Tattoos are designs created by inserting colored ink under the skin with a needle. *Body piercing* involves making a hole in the skin where jewelry can be inserted.

Although getting a tattoo or a body piercing may seem harmless, health conditions can develop whenever needles are inserted into the body. If they are not sterilized, needles used for piercings and tattoos can spread bloodborne diseases like hepatitis or human immunodeficiency virus (HIV). Some people can also experience an allergic reaction, typically to jewelry worn in the pierced area or to tattoo ink.

To reduce the risk of these complications, you should only have tattoos and piercings done at clean, safe, and well-regarded facilities by licensed professionals. If you get a piercing or tattoo, it is important to follow instructions to care for it and decrease the possibility of infection. Keep in mind that having a tattoo removed is often an expensive, time-intensive process that may leave scarring.

Background Lesson 2.2 Caring for Your Hair

You lose about 50 to 100 hairs every day through normal activities such as washing, brushing, or combing your hair. These hairs are replaced by new hairs, which grow from the same follicle.

Teens and adults can experience several common hair conditions. A common issue for teens is having oily hair. This is often due to sebaceous glands producing too much oil during puberty. Some teens may also have *dandruff*, or white flakes of dead skin in the hair and on the shoulders. Dandruff can be caused by dry skin; infrequent shampooing, which allows oil and skin cells to build up; and excessive shampooing, which can irritate the scalp.

Another hair condition is caused by *lice*, or tiny insects that attach to hair and feed on human blood. Lice spread easily from one person to another through direct head-to-head contact or through sharing combs, brushes, or hats. Although lice do not cause any major health conditions, they are very itchy and can be uncomfortable.

Some strategies you can use to keep your hair healthy and prevent these conditions follow:

- Wash your hair regularly to keep it clean.
- Eat a nutritious diet. Some hair conditions are partly caused by a lack of certain vitamins and fats.
- If you have dandruff, try a medicated shampoo. If dandruff continues, see your doctor or a dermatologist.
- Avoid sharing items that have touched your hair with other people.
- If you have lice, use a medicated shampoo to kill the lice and their eggs (called *nits*). Wash all bedding, towels, and other items that have touched your hair in hot water.

Background Lesson 2.3 Caring for Your Nails

Fingernails and toenails are made up of layers of *keratin*, a hard protein. Nails protect the sensitive tissues on the tips of your toes and fingers and grow from the area at the base of the nail.

Healthy nails are smooth, free from spots or discoloration, and consistent in color. Some nail irregularities, such as white spots or vertical ridges, are normal. Nail discoloration, curled nails, or redness and swelling around the nail can sometimes indicate health conditions.

To take care of your nails, keep them dry and clean. This prevents bacteria and other organisms from growing under your fingernails. If you must soak your hands or use harsh chemicals, wear gloves. Trim your nails regularly using clippers, manicure scissors, or a nail file. Also be sure to moisturize your hands regularly, including your fingernails and cuticles. Do not bite your fingernails, pick at your cuticles, or pull off hangnails. Doing so can cause infections.

Before visiting a nail salon, make sure the salon and nail technician are licensed. All tools should be properly sterilized between customers to avoid spreading infections.

Background Lesson 2.4 Caring for Your Teeth

Each tooth consists of three distinct parts (**Figure BL2.1**). The *crown* is the visible portion of the tooth. It is protected by *enamel*, a hard, white substance made of calcium. The *neck* connects the crown to the root of the tooth at the gum line. The *root* contains blood vessels and nerve endings that connect the tooth to the jaw. The adult mouth typically contains 32 teeth. Different types of teeth have different shapes, locations in the jaw, and functions.

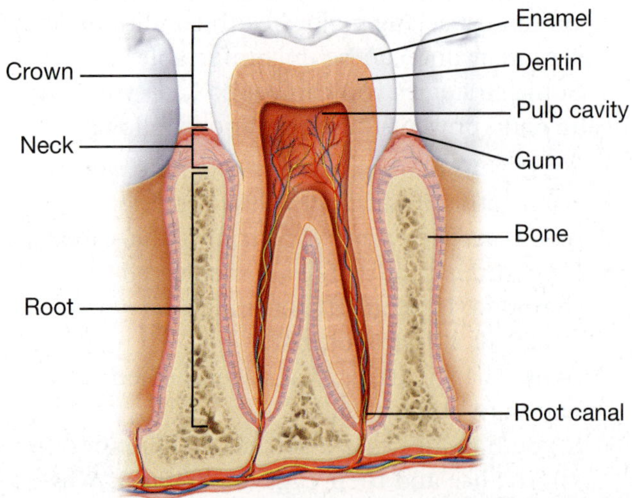

Figure BL2.1 The crown, neck, and root make up the tooth.

Common Conditions of the Mouth and Teeth

When you eat or drink something, your saliva helps breaks down food particles and sugars so they can be digested. This process turns everything you eat or drink into a type of acid. This acid then combines with bacteria in your mouth, as well as saliva and small food particles, to form plaque. *Plaque* is a sticky, colorless film that coats the teeth and dissolves their protective enamel. If plaque is not removed, it mixes with minerals to become *tartar*, a harder substance that requires professional cleaning to be removed.

If you do not brush and floss your teeth daily, food particles remain in your mouth and promote bacterial growth. This results in tooth decay. Over time, tooth decay causes *cavities* (also known as *dental caries*), or holes in the teeth that occur when plaque eats into a tooth's enamel. As decay continues, the hole gets deeper and eventually reaches the nerve layer known as *dentin* under the enamel. This causes painful nerve damage and can lead to *death of the tooth* if the decay reaches the deepest layer of the tooth (the *pulp cavity*).

A buildup of plaque and tartar causes toxins to form in the mouth, which irritates the gums. Over time, this irritation can lead to *gingivitis*, an inflammation of the gums. It can also lead to *periodontitis*, or *periodontal disease*, which is an infection caused by bacteria getting under the gums and destroying gums and bone. Early signs of gingivitis and periodontitis include swelling and bleeding of the gums.

Other common conditions of the mouth and teeth are listed in **Figure BL2.2**.

Preventing Mouth and Teeth Conditions

Sometimes you can treat mouth and teeth conditions at home. For example, a person with bruxism can wear a mouth guard. For other conditions, people need to see a medical professional for treatment. For example, tooth sensitivity may indicate a cavity, which requires treatment from a *dentist*. Many teens wear braces, which need to be applied by an *orthodontist*.

Strategies you can use to prevent and manage common mouth and teeth conditions include the following:

- Brush your teeth, including your tongue, at least twice a day. Use a soft-bristle brush and toothpaste that contains fluoride.
- Get a new toothbrush when the bristles wear out, which is usually about every three months.
- Floss your teeth every day to help remove food particles that are stuck between your teeth and cannot be reached by brushing.
- Avoid using any type of tobacco product, including cigarettes, vaping devices, and chewing tobacco.
- Eat nutritious foods, including fruits and fiber-rich vegetables. Avoid eating sticky foods that are high in sugar and starch, such as candy, cakes, and soda. If you eat these types of foods, brush your teeth as soon as possible afterward.

Mouth and Teeth Conditions

Condition	Description
Bruxism	Teeth grinding; may be caused by stress, anxiety, or sleep disorders; can damage the teeth and jaw over time
Cold sores (also called *fever blisters*)	Small, red, swollen blisters on the lips and inside the mouth; caused by a virus spread through saliva and can last several days to two weeks
Halitosis	Bad breath caused by poor dental hygiene, gum disease, certain foods, or other health conditions
Impacted wisdom teeth	Condition in which wisdom teeth become stuck under the gum tissue or may only be able to partially come through the gums; impacted wisdom teeth need to be removed
Overbite	Condition in which the upper teeth protrude significantly past the lower teeth
Underbite	Condition in which the lower teeth protrude significantly past the upper teeth

Figure BL2.2 Dental professionals, such as dentists and orthodontists, can help diagnose and treat conditions of the mouth.

- If you have bad breath, use an antiseptic mouth rinse, which reduces the bacteria that cause bad breath.
- See your dentist twice a year. Your dentist will catch conditions early on, when they can be more easily treated.
- Wear a mouth guard during activities that can result in broken teeth, such as football or ice hockey.
- If cold sores are painful, treat them using a skin cream or ointment to speed up healing and ease the pain.

Background Lesson 2.5 Caring for Your Eyes

Keeping your eyes healthy is important. Fortunately, there are several simple strategies you can use to keep your eyes as healthy as possible throughout your lifetime. For example, you should wear protective eyewear when playing some contact sports. Also use protective gear during activities that can create flying debris that could hit the eyes, such as mowing the lawn, sawing wood, or sanding.

When spending time outdoors, wear sunglasses to block harmful UV rays. Look for sunglasses that claim to block at least 99 percent of UVB and UVA rays or that provide UV 400 protection. One of the most important steps for protecting eye health is to get regular eye exams from a medical professional who specializes in eye health (for example, an *ophthalmologist* or *optometrist*).

Many people have vision conditions that require them to wear eyeglasses or contact lenses. Examples of these conditions are shown in **Figure BL2.3**. Some of these vision conditions can also be corrected by surgery. If you wear contact lenses as a result of one of these conditions, care for your lenses properly to avoid infection. This includes washing your hands with soap and water before putting in contact lenses, cleansing them with a sterile solution, and removing them before swimming or showering.

Common Vision Conditions	
Condition	**Description**
Astigmatism	Condition in which the eye does not focus light evenly onto the retina, causing objects to appear blurry and stretched out
Farsightedness (also called *hyperopia*)	Condition in which distant objects are seen more clearly than nearby objects; light focuses behind the retina instead of on the retina
Glaucoma	Condition in which the optic nerve becomes damaged, leading to vision loss; often caused by fluid buildup, which creates pressure in the eye
Nearsightedness (also called *myopia*)	Condition in which objects close to the eye appear clear, while objects farther away appear blurry; light focuses in front of the retina instead of on the retina
Presbyopia	Condition that affects aging adults; the lens of the eye loses its elasticity, making it harder to see close objects clearly

Figure BL2.3 An ophthalmologist or optometrist can screen for and help someone decide on the right treatment for these vision conditions.

Background Lesson 2.6 Caring for Your Ears

The sense of hearing allows you to listen to music, talk with friends, and be aware of approaching cars and other dangers. Taking care of your ears can help you protect this sense.

Some people are born without the sense of hearing. For others, hearing loss develops over time, often due to damage to the inner ear. Repeated exposure to loud sounds (louder than 85 decibels) causes this damage, and louder sounds cause more damage. In fact, 12.5 percent of children and teens (6–19 years of age) experience hearing loss from using headphones or earbuds at too high a volume.

Hearing loss can also develop more suddenly from a ruptured eardrum. Loud blasts of noise, sudden changes in pressure, the insertion of an object into the ear, or an infection can rupture the eardrum. In fact, just one exposure to a very loud sound, blast, or impulse (at or above 120 decibels) can cause hearing loss.

Many people do not notice gradual hearing loss. Early signs of this loss include difficulty hearing relatively soft sounds, such as doorbells; difficulty understanding speech during telephone conversations or in noisy environments; and *tinnitus* (pain or ringing in the ears) after exposure to excessively loud sounds.

Once hearing is lost, it cannot be completely brought back. It is important, therefore, to protect your ears. You can do this by avoiding exposure to very high levels of noise, such as at rock concerts, dances, or construction sites. Wearing earplugs in these settings can also protect hearing. Avoid listening to music at high volume levels (above 85 decibels), especially when using headphones or earbuds. Do not insert anything into the ear, even to clean it. Inserting an object into the ear can cause injury that leads to hearing loss.

Sleep

Background Lesson 3

Background Lesson 3.1 Understanding Sleep

While you are sleeping, your body and brain are performing healing tasks essential to your health. For these activities to occur, mechanisms in the body must cause sleep or wakefulness by affecting when you feel drowsy or awake.

Circadian rhythms are naturally occurring physical, behavioral, and mental changes in the body that typically follow the 24-hour cycle of the sun. Most circadian rhythms are controlled by the body's master biological "clock," called the *suprachiasmatic nucleus* or *SCN*.

The SCN works in two ways to regulate sleep. First, it monitors light in the environment, so the body is more active when there is more light. In the late evening, the SCN also causes the pineal gland to release the hormone *melatonin*, which increases feelings of relaxation and sleepiness. Compared with adults, melatonin in teens is typically released later in the evening and remains at high levels until later in the morning. This explains why teens have trouble falling asleep earlier in the evening and waking up early the next morning.

When the body's natural circadian rhythm is disrupted, the biological clock needs time to readjust. Working night shifts, adjusting to daylight savings, or simply being exposed to *blue light* (light that produces large amounts of energy) at night can trick your body into an unnatural circadian rhythm.

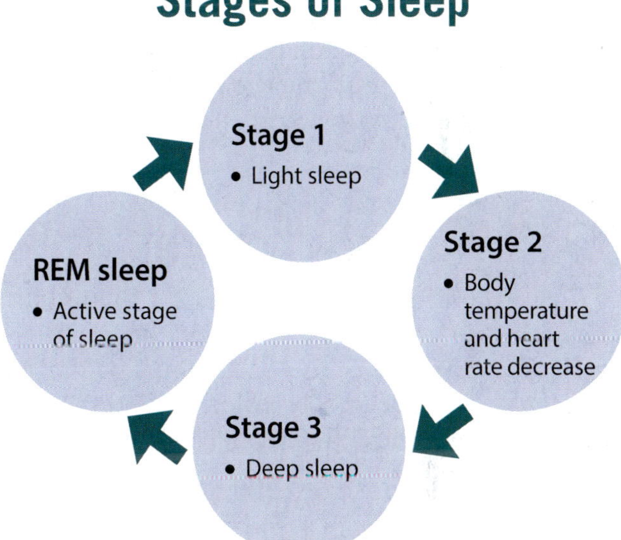

Figure BL3.1 The first period of REM sleep usually occurs 70–90 minutes after you fall asleep. The first sleep cycles of your night's rest contain relatively short REM periods and long periods of deep sleep (stage 3). REM sleep periods get longer, while deep sleep periods get shorter in each successive sleep cycle.

Stages of Sleep

Each night, you usually pass through several stages of sleep (**Figure BL3.1**). A complete sleep cycle—from stage 1 through REM sleep—lasts about 90–110 minutes. During stage 1, you sleep lightly. In stage 2, body temperature and heart rate decrease. Stage 3 includes deep sleep and progresses into *REM sleep*, which has many important functions. The brain regions used for learning are stimulated during REM sleep, and the production of proteins that help your body build and maintain tissues and fight off infections increases.

Sleep Needs

The amount of sleep that people need varies at different ages. Teens ages 13–17 need eight to 10 hours of sleep each night. Because of the role sleep plays, *sleep deprivation*, or a pattern of not getting enough sleep, can have serious effects on physical, mental, and emotional health. Some effects of sleep deprivation include health conditions such as diabetes mellitus and cardiovascular disease, obesity, difficulty paying attention and concentrating, and impairments that can lead to serious injuries.

Background Lesson 3.2 Getting Enough Sleep

Getting enough sleep is an essential part of staying healthy. It can be hard to get enough sleep and also do your homework, participate in extracurricular activities, talk with friends, and get to school on time. Using healthy sleep strategies, however, can help you get the sleep you need.

Set and Follow a Schedule

Following a consistent schedule means going to bed at approximately the same time each night and getting up at approximately the same time each morning. It is important to use the same schedule throughout the week—not just Monday through Friday.

Be Physically Active

Being physically active for even 20–30 minutes a day can help you fall and stay asleep. Try to be physically active at least five or six hours before you plan to go to sleep. Physical activity in the evening can make it difficult to fall asleep.

Understand Substances That Affect Sleep

Avoiding substances that make it harder to sleep can help you fall asleep more quickly and sleep more deeply. One example is *stimulants*, or substances that increase energy, alertness, and attention. Caffeine is one type of stimulant. Avoiding drinks, foods, and medications that contain caffeine (for example, coffee, chocolate, energy drinks, soft drinks, nonherbal teas, and diet pills) can help you sleep better.

Relax Before Bedtime

When people try to fall asleep at the end of the day, they sometimes find themselves focusing on stressful experiences or worrying about upcoming events. If you are worrying about what you need to remember the next day, write a quick note to yourself. If you cannot sleep, or if you wake up and cannot get back to sleep, get out of bed and do a relaxing activity.

Control Exposure to Light

If you spend the evening exposed to blue light from a TV, phone, or computer screen, your body may produce less melatonin, making it harder to feel sleepy. This exposure to blue light can disrupt your circadian rhythm. Strategies for regulating exposure to light and your body's production of melatonin are shown in **Figure BL3.2**.

Strategies for Controlling Light Exposure	
During the Day (AM / PM)	**At Night** (AM / PM)
• When you wake up, open the blinds or curtains and turn on bright lights to jump-start your biological clock and help you feel more awake and alert. • Talk to your teachers about keeping curtains and blinds open in the classroom to increase the amount of natural light you get during the day. • Spend time outside during the day whenever possible. Before or after school are great times for a quick walk or socializing outside with friends.	• Use an app to reduce the amount of blue light your phone, tablet, television, or computer produces at night. • Set a "turn-off time" for all digital devices at least one or two hours before you want to go to bed. • If possible, keep all digital devices outside the bedroom. If you sleep near your phone, move it away from your bed so you are not tempted to check it. Turn your phone to silent so notifications do not disturb you. • Use a night-light in the bathroom to avoid turning on a bright light in the middle of the night.

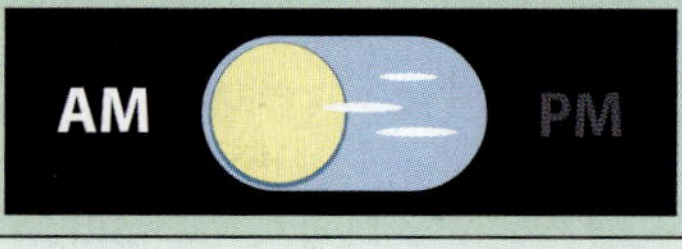

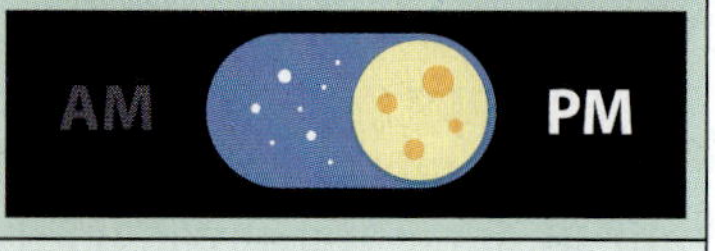

BadBrother/Shutterstock.com

Figure BL3.2 Making a few small changes can help control your exposure to light. For example, if you like to read before bed, avoid reading from your computer or phone. Instead, read from a physical book or e-reader that does not produce blue light.

Glossary/Glosario

English

A

"all-or-nothing" mind-set: way of thinking that classifies behaviors as either total successes or total failures.

abortion: procedure that ends a pregnancy.

abuse: violent behaviors that cause physical, emotional, sexual, or financial harm to another person.

acid reflux disorder: condition in which a mixture of digested food and acid moves from the stomach to the lower esophagus, resulting in heartburn.

acidosis: condition of excess acid in the blood; can lead to coma or death.

acquaintances: people in a person's social circle who may not be close enough to be friends.

acquired immunodeficiency syndrome (AIDS): health condition in which the body can no longer fight infections and disease; caused by the progression of human immunodeficiency virus (HIV).

active listening: act of concentrating on the person talking and acknowledging what one has heard.

added sugars: sugars that do not occur naturally in foods.

addictive disorders: mental illnesses in which people develop a psychological dependence on certain processes or behaviors.

adolescence: developmental stage between 12 and 19 years of age.

adoption: action of legally taking responsibility for and raising another person's biological child.

advocate: to take actions that show support.

aerobic: using oxygen to break down energy for use in the muscles.

aerosol: suspension of fine particles or droplets in the air.

affirmations: statements that acknowledge a person's value and strengths.

affirmative consent: direct, verbal, freely given agreement that occurs when someone clearly says *yes*.

age of consent: age at which a person can legally agree to engage in sexual activity.

aggressive: making demands of and insulting others; an ineffective communication style.

agility: ability to rapidly change the body's momentum and direction.

Air Quality Index (AQI): tool for reporting daily air quality and how air quality impacts different health concerns.

Español

mentalidad de "todo o nada": forma de pensar que clasifica los comportamientos como éxitos totales o fracasos totales.

aborto: procedimiento que pone fin a un embarazo.

abuso: comportementos violentos que causan daño físico, emocional, sexual o financiero hacia otra persona.

trastorno de reflujo ácido: afección en la que una mezcla de alimentos digeridos y ácido se mueve desde el estómago hasta el esófago inferior, lo que provoca acidez estomacal.

acidosis: condición de exceso de ácido en la sangre; puede conducir a un estado de coma o la muerte.

conocidos: personas dentro del círculo social de una persona que no son lo suficientemente cercanas como para ser consideradas amigas.

síndrome de inmunodeficiencia adquirida (SIDA): afección de salud en la que el cuerpo ya no puede combatir infecciones y enfermedades; causado por la progresión del virus de inmunodeficiencia humana (VIH).

escucha activa: acción de concentrarse en la persona que habla y reconocer lo que se ha escuchado.

azúcares añadidos: azúcares que no se encuentran naturalmente en los alimentos.

trastornos adictivos: enfermedades mentales en las cuales las personas desarrollan una dependencia psicológica de ciertos procesos o comportamientos.

adolescencia: período de desarrollo entre los 12 y 19 años de edad.

adopción: acción de asumir legalmente la responsabilidad y criar al hijo biológico de otra persona.

abogar: realizar acciones que muestren apoyo.

aeróbico: uso del oxígeno para descomponer la energía para su uso en los músculos.

aerosol: suspensión de partículas finas o microgotas en el aire.

afirmaciones: declaraciones que reconocen el valor y las virtudes de una persona.

consentimiento expreso: acuerdo verbal, directo y voluntario que ocurre cuando alguien dice que *sí* con claridad.

edad para dar consentimiento: edad a la que una persona puede aceptar legalmente participar en actividades sexuales.

agresivo: hacer demandas e insultar a otros; un estilo de comunicación inefectivo.

agilidad: capacidad para cambiar rápidamente la dirección y el impulso del cuerpo.

Índice de calidad del aire (Air Quality Index, AQI): herramienta para informar la calidad diaria del aire y cómo esta impacta sobre diferentes cuestiones de salud.

English

airbrushing: digitally altering an image to eliminate blemishes, cellulite, bulges, or wrinkles.

alcohol: addictive depressant with the active ingredient ethanol; alters brain function.

alcohol poisoning: medical emergency in which a person consumes more alcohol than the body can break down; alcohol suppresses the nervous system and vital body functions to dangerous levels; also called *alcohol overdose*.

alcohol use disorder (AUD): substance use disorder in which a person has an addiction to alcohol and continues to consume it despite negative health effects.

Alcoholics Anonymous (AA): support group and program for people with an alcohol use disorder (AUD); outlines 12 steps for overcoming alcohol addiction.

allergy: condition in which the body's immune system reacts to a harmless substance like it is a dangerous or disease-causing invader.

alternatives: courses of action one can take.

Alzheimer's disease (AD): disease of the brain characterized by dementia, an incurable loss of memory and thinking skills.

amenorrhea: abnormal absence of menstrual period.

anaerobic: powering the body without the use of oxygen.

analgesics: medications that relieve pain.

anaphylaxis: severe allergic response in which fluid fills the lungs and air passages narrow, restricting breathing.

angina: pain in the chest that often accompanies a heart attack; may feel like pressure or squeezing or a dull or sharp pain.

anonymity: notion that others do not know who a person is online.

antibiotic-resistant bacteria: bacteria that do not respond to treatment with certain antibiotics.

antibiotics: medications that target and kill disease-causing bacteria.

antibodies: chemicals that attach to pathogens and label them as foreign bodies to be destroyed.

antiretroviral therapy (ART): treatment for human immunodeficiency virus (HIV)/acquired immunodeficiency syndrome (AIDS) that includes a mixture of three medications, each of which interferes with the reproduction of HIV inside the body.

anxiety disorder: mental illness in which feelings of worry and dread interfere with daily life.

arrhythmias: abnormal heart rhythms; include fast, slow, and uncoordinated heartbeats.

Español

aerografía: alterar digitalmente una imagen para eliminar manchas, celulitis, protuberancias o arrugas.

alcohol: depresivo adictivo con el ingrediente activo etanol; altera la función cerebral.

intoxicación por alcohol: emergencia médica en la que una persona consume más alcohol del que el cuerpo puede descomponer; el alcohol suprime el sistema nervioso y las funciones vitales del cuerpo a niveles peligrosos; también se llama *sobredosis de alcohol.*

trastorno por consumo de alcohol (alcohol use disorder, AUD): trastorno por consumo de sustancias en el que una persona tiene una adicción al alcohol y continúa consumiéndolo a pesar de los efectos negativos para la salud.

Alcohólicos Anónimos (AA): grupo y programa de apoyo para personas con un trastorno por consumo de alcohol (AUD); describe 12 pasos para superar la adicción al alcohol.

alergia: afección en la que el sistema inmunológico del cuerpo reacciona a una sustancia inofensiva como si fuera un invasor peligroso o que causa enfermedades.

alternativas: medidas que uno puede tomar.

enfermedad de Alzheimer (Alzheimer's disease, AD): enfermedad del cerebro caracterizada por demencia, una pérdida incurable de memoria y habilidades de pensamiento.

amenorrea: ausencia anormal del período menstrual.

anaeróbico: energizar el cuerpo sin el uso de oxígeno.

analgésicos: medicamentos que alivian el dolor.

anafilaxia: respuesta alérgica grave en la que los pulmones se llenan de líquido y las vías respiratorias se estrechan, lo que restringe la respiración.

angina: dolor en el pecho que a menudo acompaña a un ataque cardíaco; puede sentirse presión u opresión, o un dolor sordo o agudo.

anonimato: noción de que otros no saben quién es una persona en línea.

bacteria resistente a los antibióticos: bacteria que no responde al tratamiento con ciertos antibióticos.

antibióticos: medicamentos que atacan y matan las bacterias que causan enfermedades.

anticuerpos: sustancias químicas que se adhieren a los patógenos y los identifican como cuerpos extraños para ser destruidos.

terapia antirretroviral (TARV): tratamiento para el virus de inmunodeficiencia humana (VIH)/síndrome de inmunodeficiencia adquirida (SIDA) que incluye una mezcla de tres medicamentos, cada uno de los cuales interfiere con la reproducción del VIH dentro del cuerpo.

trastorno de ansiedad: enfermedad mental en la cual los sentimientos de preocupación y temor interfieren con la vida diaria.

arritmias: ritmos cardíacos anormales; incluyen latidos cardíacos rápidos, lentos y descoordinados.

English

arsenic: element normally found in soils and rocks; is poisonous and carcinogenic at high levels.

arteries: large, muscular blood vessels that deliver blood from the heart to the rest of the body.

arteriosclerosis: disease in which the walls of the arteries thicken, harden, and become inflexible.

arthritis: disease in which the joints become inflamed, or swollen and painful.

asbestos: natural mineral in soils; was formerly used for insulation and fire protection, but can cause cancer when inhaled.

assertive: clearly stating needs, wants, and feelings; most effective communication style.

asthma: chronic condition in which airways constrict and fill with mucus; blocks airflow to and from the lungs.

asymptomatic: showing few or no signs of infection or disease.

atherosclerosis: disease in which fatty deposits collect in the walls of arteries, restricting blood flow.

athlete's foot: fungal infection of the skin between the toes or in the groin; causes an itchy, burning rash.

attachment: emotional bond that makes a child feel safe and loved.

attitude: pattern of viewing and reacting to events in a certain way.

attraction: physical and emotional connection, or chemistry, that draws people together.

autoimmune disease: type of disease in which the body's immune system attacks its own tissues.

automated external defibrillator (AED): device that delivers a controlled, precise shock to the heart to restore a person's heartbeat.

autonomy: self-directing freedom.

B

bacteria: single-celled microorganisms with no nucleus; are mostly beneficial, but can cause disease.

barrier methods: contraceptive methods that prevent sperm from traveling through the female reproductive system and fertilizing an egg.

bath salts: synthetic drugs that contain the stimulant methylenedioxypyrovalerone (MDPV); are often marketed as household products.

behavioral factors: choices and behaviors that affect a person's chance of developing a disease, unhealthy condition, or injury.

Español

arsénico: elemento que normalmente se encuentra en suelos y rocas; en altas concentraciones es venenoso y cancerígeno.

arterias: vasos sanguíneos grandes y musculares que conducen la sangre desde el corazón hacia el resto del cuerpo.

arteriosclerosis: enfermedad en la que las paredes de las arterias se ensanchan, se endurecen y se vuelven inflexibles.

artritis: enfermedad en la que las articulaciones se inflaman o hinchan, lo que causa dolor.

asbesto: mineral natural en suelos; anteriormente se usaba para aislamiento y protección contra incendios, pero puede causar cáncer cuando se inhala.

asertivo: claramente indicando necesidades, deseos y sentimientos; estilo de comunicación más efectivo.

asma: condición crónica en la cual las vías respiratorias se contraen y se llenan de mucosidad; bloquea el flujo de aire hacia y desde los pulmones.

asintomático: evidencia pocos o ningún signo de infección o enfermedad.

ateroesclerosis: enfermedad en la cual los depósitos grasos se acumulan en las paredes de las arterias, restringiendo el flujo sanguíneo.

pie de atleta: infección micótica de la piel entre los dedos del pie o en la ingle; causa una erupción cutánea con picazón y ardor.

apego: vínculo emocional que hace que un niño se sienta seguro y amado.

actitud: patrón de ver y reaccionar a los eventos de cierta manera.

atracción: conexión física y emocional, o química, que une a las personas.

enfermedad autoinmune: tipo de enfermedad en la cual el sistema inmunológico del cuerpo ataca sus propios tejidos.

desfibrilador externo automático (DEA): dispositivo que administra un choque controlado y preciso al corazón para restablecer los latidos cardíacos de una persona.

autonomía: libertad autodirigida.

bacteria: microorganismos unicelulares sin núcleo; son principalmente beneficiosos, pero pueden causar enfermedades.

métodos de barrera: métodos anticonceptivos que evitan que los espermatozoides viajen a través del sistema reproductor femenino y fertilicen un óvulo.

sales de baño: drogas sintéticas que contienen el estimulante metilendioxipirovalerona (MDPV); a menudo se comercializan como productos para el hogar.

factores de conducta: elecciones y comportamientos que afectan las posibilidades de una persona de desarrollar una enfermedad, una afección poco saludable o de sufrir una lesión.

English

benign tumors: mass of abnormal cells that is not cancerous; remains in one place and stays small.

biological sex: label assigned at birth based on physical factors such as hormones, chromosomes, and genitalia.

biopsy: procedure in which a sample of tissue is removed and tested for the presence of disease.

bipolar disorder: mood disorder characterized by extreme highs (mania) and lows (depression).

birth control implant: flexible, toothpick-sized contraceptive device inserted under the skin of the upper arm; releases progestin to stop ovulation.

birth control patch: plastic contraceptive device applied to the skin as a patch; releases hormones to stop ovulation.

birth control shot: contraceptive method in which a female receives an injection of progestin every three months to stop ovulation.

bisphenol A (BPA): chemical used to make some plastics; may be harmful to humans.

blood alcohol concentration (BAC): percentage of alcohol in a person's blood.

blood pressure: force that blood exerts on the arterial walls; measured in millimeters of mercury (mmHg).

body compassion: feelings of acceptance, care, and kindness toward one's body.

body composition: ratio of the various components—fat, bone, and muscle—that make up the body; influenced by genetics, eating patterns, and physical activity.

body-fat distribution: locations of fat deposits on a person's body.

body image: subjective mental image of one's own body; established based on self-observation and the reactions of others.

body mass index (BMI): tool used to determine whether a person's weight is healthy for that person's height; BMI = weight (lbs.)/height (in.)^2 × 703.

body neutrality: focus on what the body can do, rather than how it looks.

body positivity: appreciation of body-type diversity; involves valuing the body and understanding it will change.

body scan: relaxation technique that involves paying careful attention to the body, scanning it for signs of tension, and then releasing that tension.

boundaries: rules about what behaviors are acceptable or unacceptable.

Español

tumores benignos: masa de células anormales no cancerosa; permanece en un lugar y su tamaño es pequeño.

sexo biológico: denominación asignada al nacer basada en factores físicos como hormonas, cromosomas y genitales.

biopsia: procedimiento en el que se extrae una muestra de tejido y se analiza la presencia de una enfermedad.

trastorno bipolar: trastorno del estado de ánimo caracterizado por altibajos extremos (manía) y bajos (depresión).

implante anticonceptivo: dispositivo anticonceptivo flexible del tamaño de un mondadientes que se inserta debajo de la piel en la parte superior del brazo; libera progestina para detener la ovulación.

parche anticonceptivo: dispositivo anticonceptivo de plástico aplicado a la piel como parche; libera hormonas para detener la ovulación.

vacuna anticonceptiva: método anticonceptivo en el que la hembra recibe una inyección de progestina cada tres meses para detener la ovulación.

bisfenol A (bisphenol A, BPA): químico utilizado para fabricar algunos plásticos; puede ser perjudicial para los humanos.

concentración de alcohol en la sangre (blood alcohol concentration, BAC): porcentaje de alcohol en la sangre de una persona.

presión sanguínea: fuerza que ejerce la sangre sobre las paredes arteriales; medido en milímetros de mercurio (mmHg).

compasión corporal: sentimientos de aceptación, cuidado y bondad hacia el cuerpo.

composición corporal: proporción de los diversos componentes (grasa, hueso y músculo) que conforman el cuerpo; influenciada por la genética, los patrones de alimentación y la actividad física.

distribución de grasa corporal: lugares de depósitos de grasa en el cuerpo de una persona.

imagen corporal: imagen mental subjetiva del propio cuerpo; establecida en base a la auto observación y las reacciones de los demás.

índice de masa corporal (IMC): herramienta utilizada para determinar si el peso de una persona es saludable para su altura; IMC = peso (lb)/altura (pulg.)^2 × 703.

neutralidad corporal: foco en lo que el cuerpo puede hacer, en lugar de en cómo se ve.

positividad corporal: apreciación de la diversidad de tipo corporal; implica valorar el cuerpo y comprender que cambiará.

exploración del cuerpo: técnica de relajación que implica prestar especial atención al cuerpo, escanearlo en busca de signos de tensión y luego liberar esa tensión.

límites: reglas sobre qué comportamientos son aceptables o inaceptables.

English

breakup: end of a romantic relationship.
breast cancer: abnormal cancerous growth of breast cells.

breasts: structures containing mammary glands that produce milk after childbirth in females.
bullying: aggressive behavior toward someone that causes the person injury or discomfort; can be physical or psychological; also called *peer abuse.*

burnout: state of emotional, physical, and mental exhaustion; occurs due to prolonged stress.
bystander effect: situation in which a bystander is less likely to intervene and stop violent, harmful, or unsafe behavior because the person thinks someone else will.

bystanders: people who are present at a situation, but do not participate or intervene.

C

calories: units of energy in food.
cancer: complex disease in which abnormal cells reproduce uncontrollably, forming malignant tumors that spread throughout the body.

capillaries: tiny blood vessels with thin walls through which oxygen, nutrients, and waste can pass.

carbohydrates: nutrients that are the major source of energy for the body; can be found in fruits, vegetables, grains, and dairy products.

carbon monoxide: poisonous gas that interferes with the ability of red blood cells to carry oxygen throughout the body.
carcinogens: cancer-causing substances.
cardiopulmonary resuscitation (CPR): emergency procedure that uses chest compressions and sometimes rescue breathing to restore heartbeat.

cardiorespiratory fitness: ability of the cardiovascular and respiratory systems to deliver oxygen and nutrients to muscles and cells.
cardiovascular diseases: health conditions that harm and hinder the function of the heart and blood vessels.

cardiovascular system: body system that transports blood throughout the body; consists of the heart and blood vessels.
catfishing: luring someone into a relationship online by creating a fake profile.
cervical cancer: abnormal cancerous growth of the cervix; often caused by the human papillomavirus (HPV).

Español

ruptura: final de una relación romántica.
cáncer de mama: crecimiento canceroso anormal de las células mamarias.
senos: estructuras que contienen glándulas mamarias que producen leche después del parto en las hembras.
intimidación (bullying): comportamiento agresivo hacia alguien que causa lesiones o malestar a la persona; puede ser físico o psicológico; también se denomina *abuso entre pares.*
agotamiento: estado de agotamiento emocional, físico y mental; ocurre debido al estrés prolongado.
efecto espectador: situación en la que un espectador tiene menos probabilidades de intervenir y detener un comportamiento violento, dañino o inseguro porque cree que alguien más lo hará.
espectadores: personas que están presentes en una situación, pero que no participan ni intervienen.

calorías: unidades de energía en los alimentos.
cáncer: enfermedad compleja en la cual las células anormales se reproducen sin control, formando tumores malignos que se extienden por todo el cuerpo.
capilares: pequeños vasos sanguíneos con paredes delgadas a través de las cuales pasan oxígeno, nutrientes y desechos.
carbohidratos o hidratos de carbono: nutrientes que son una fuente importante de energía para el cuerpo; se encuentran en frutas, verduras, granos y productos lácteos.
monóxido de carbono: gas venenoso que interfiere con la capacidad de los glóbulos rojos para transportar oxígeno por todo el cuerpo.
carcinógenos: sustancias que provocan cáncer.
reanimación cardiopulmonar (RCP): procedimiento de emergencia que utiliza compresiones torácicas y, a veces, rescata la respiración para restablecer los latidos del corazón.
aptitud cardiorrespiratoria: capacidad de los sistemas cardiovascular y respiratorio para suministrar oxígeno y nutrientes a los músculos y las células.
enfermedades cardiovasculares: afecciones de salud que dañan y dificultan la función del corazón y los vasos sanguíneos.
sistema cardiovascular: sistema corporal que transporta sangre por todo el cuerpo; consiste en el corazón y los vasos sanguíneos.
catfishing: atraer a alguien a una relación en línea creando un perfil falso.
cáncer de cuello uterino: crecimiento canceroso anormal del cuello uterino; a menudo causada por el virus del papiloma humano (VPH).

English

cervical cap: cup-shaped contraceptive device made of silicone; covers the cervix to prevent sperm from entering the uterus and is smaller than the diaphragm.

cervix: narrow passage that connects the uterus to the vagina.

cesarean section: surgical procedure to deliver a baby by removing it from the uterus; also called a *C-section.*

chemotherapy: use of medications to kill cancer cells and shrink malignant tumors.

child abuse: any intentional physical, emotional, or sexual act committed by an adult that harms or threatens to harm a child.

child support: money that one parent gives the other parent to provide financial support for the care of the parents' child.

chlamydia: bacterial sexually transmitted infection (STI) with few or no symptoms; can cause pelvic inflammatory disease (PID) and infertility in the female reproductive system.

chromosome: package of genes containing the blueprint for the structure and function of cells.

chronic bronchitis: condition in which the bronchial tubes become swollen and irritated, narrowing the pathway to the lungs.

chronic obstructive pulmonary disease (COPD): group of conditions that make breathing more difficult; includes chronic bronchitis, emphysema, and asthma.

cirrhosis: buildup of scar tissue in the liver.

cisgender: identifying with the gender associated with one's biological sex.

Clean Air Act: federal law that regulates air pollution levels to protect people's health.

clique: small group of friends who deliberately exclude other people from joining or being a part of their group.

clitoris: mass of erectile tissue that swells and enlarges during sexual arousal.

cocaine: highly addictive stimulant that comes from the leaves of a coca plant.

cognition: ability to think, reason, and remember.

cognitive distortions: unhealthy patterns of thinking that are often not grounded in reality.

cognitive empathy: ability to see the world from another person's perspective.

collaborative decision-making: process of working with others to make a decision.

colonoscopy: procedure in which a flexible tube with a camera and small surgical instruments are inserted into the colon; a doctor can view the inside of the colon and take samples for testing.

Español

capuchón cervical: dispositivo anticonceptivo en forma de copa de silicona; cubre el cuello uterino para evitar que el esperma ingrese al útero y es más pequeño que el diafragma.

cuello uterino: paso estrecho que conecta el útero con la vagina.

cesárea: procedimiento quirúrgico para dar a luz a un bebé retirándolo del útero.

quimioterapia: uso de medicamentos para matar las células cancerosas y reducir los tumores malignos.

abuso infantil: cualquier acto físico, emocional o sexual intencional cometido por un adulto que daña o amenaza con dañar a un niño.

manutención de los hijos: dinero que uno de los padres le da al otro para proporcionar ayuda financiera para el cuidado del hijo de ambos.

clamidia: infección de transmisión sexual (ITS) bacteriana con pocos o ningún síntoma; puede causar enfermedad inflamatoria pélvica e infertilidad en el sistema reproductor femenino.

cromosoma: paquete de genes que contiene el modelo para la estructura y función de las células.

bronquitis crónica: afección en la cual los bronquios se hinchan e irritan, estrechando la vía hacia los pulmones.

enfermedad pulmonar obstructiva crónica (EPOC): grupo de afecciones que dificultan la respiración; incluye bronquitis crónica, enfisema y asma.

cirrosis: acumulación de tejido cicatricial en el hígado.

cisgénero: identificarse con el género asociado con el sexo biológico.

Ley del Aire Limpio: ley federal que regula los niveles de contaminación del aire para proteger la salud de las personas.

camarilla: pequeño grupo de amigos que deliberadamente excluyen a otras personas de unirse o formar parte de su grupo.

clítoris: masa de tejido eréctil que se hincha y se agranda durante la excitación sexual.

cocaína: estimulante altamente adictivo que proviene de las hojas de una planta de coca.

cognición: capacidad de pensar, razonar y recordar.

distorsiones cognitivas: patrones de pensamiento poco saludables que a menudo no se basan en la realidad.

empatía cognitiva: capacidad de ver el mundo desde la perspectiva de otra persona.

toma de decisiones colaborativa: proceso de trabajar con otros para tomar una decisión.

colonoscopia: procedimiento en el cual se inserta un tubo flexible con una cámara y pequeños instrumentos quirúrgicos en el colon; un médico puede ver el interior del colon y tomar muestras para analizarlas.

English

common cold: viral disease usually caused by the rhinovirus; spreads through droplets in the air and primarily affects the nose and throat.

communicable diseases: diseases caused by pathogens that spread through contact among living organisms and objects; also called *infectious diseases.*

communication: exchange of spoken or unspoken messages between people.

communication process: series of actions people use to exchange ideas, thoughts, feelings, and information.

community health: overall health of a group of people who live in the same area and interact with one another.

community resources: organizations and programs that help the environment and people within a community.

community service: actions that promote the environment and health of a community.

complications: health conditions that develop as a result of another disease.

compost: mixture of food scraps and other organic matter that breaks down in the environment; can be used to fertilize gardens.

compromise: agreement in which two sides come together and each side gives in a little.

conception: moment at which the sperm and egg combine.

concussion: brain injury that results from a blow or jolt to the head or upper body.

condom: device that acts as a barrier against pathogens during sexual activity; also acts as a barrier method of contraception.

conflict: disagreement or argument that occurs due to misunderstandings or differing priorities, values, goals, or needs.

conflict-resolution skills: strategies for working through a disagreement or argument in positive, productive ways.

congestive heart failure: condition in which the heart becomes too weak to circulate blood effectively through the body.

constipation: infrequent or delayed hard, dry bowel movements.

consumer: anyone who purchases goods and services.

contraception: any method that reduces the risk of pregnancy resulting from sexual activity.

contraceptive sponge: contraceptive device made of plastic foam; covers the cervix to prevent sperm from entering the uterus and contains spermicide.

Español

resfriado común: enfermedad viral generalmente causada por el rinovirus; se propaga a través de microgotas en el aire y afecta principalmente la nariz y la garganta.

enfermedades transmisibles: enfermedades causadas por agentes patógenos que se propagan a través del contacto entre organismos y objetos vivos; también denominadas *enfermedades infecciosas.*

comunicación: intercambio de mensajes hablados o no hablados entre personas.

proceso de comunicación: serie de acciones que las personas usan para intercambiar ideas, pensamientos, sentimientos e información.

salud comunitaria: salud general de un grupo de personas que vive en la misma área e interactúa entre sí.

recursos comunitarios: organizaciones y programas que ayudan al medio ambiente y a las personas dentro de una comunidad.

servicio comunitario: acciones que promueven el medio ambiente y la salud de una comunidad.

complicaciones: afecciones de salud que se desarrollan como resultado de otra enfermedad.

compost (abono): mezcla de restos de comida y otra materia orgánica que se descompone en el medio ambiente; se puede utilizar para fertilizar jardines.

compromiso: acuerdo en el que dos partes se unen y cada una cede algo.

concepción: momento en el que se combinan el esperma y el óvulo.

contusión cerebral: lesión cerebral producto de un golpe o impacto en la cabeza o la parte superior del cuerpo.

condón: dispositivo que actúa como barrera contra los patógenos durante la actividad sexual; también actúa como un método anticonceptivo de barrera.

conflicto: desacuerdo o argumento que ocurre debido a malentendidos o prioridades, valores, metas o necesidades diferentes.

habilidades de resolución de conflictos: estrategias para resolver un desacuerdo o argumento de manera positiva y productiva.

insuficiencia cardíaca congestiva: afección en la cual el corazón se vuelve demasiado débil para hacer circular la sangre de manera efectiva a través del cuerpo.

estreñimiento: movimientos intestinales secos, duros y poco frecuentes o retardados.

consumidor: cualquier persona que compra bienes y servicios.

anticoncepción: cualquier método que reduzca el riesgo de embarazo como resultado de la actividad sexual.

esponja anticonceptiva: dispositivo anticonceptivo hecho de espuma plástica; cubre el cuello uterino para evitar que el esperma ingrese al útero y contiene espermicida.

English

co-occurring disorders: two conditions that affect health at the same time; for example, substance use disorders and other mental illnesses.

cooldown: activity that helps the body wind down after physical activity; helps heart rate return to normal level.

copyright: right of a creator to exclusively own original material and use it in any way.

core values: part of identity that describes what a person believes and finds important; guide personal behaviors and choices.

coronary arteries: blood vessels that supply the heart muscle with blood containing oxygen and nutrients.

coworkers: people who work for the same employer or do the same kind of work.

cross training: act of participating in various types of physical activity to help improve skill in another type.

crystal meth: form of methamphetamine that consists of clear crystal chunks.

culture: beliefs, values, customs, and arts of a particular group or society.

custodial parent: individual who has legal custody of the child; is responsible for the child and has the right to make decisions about the child's care.

custody: legal right and responsibility to care for a child and make decisions about care.

cyberbullying: use of the internet or electronic communication to mistreat or frighten someone.

cyberstalking: following and repeatedly contacting someone using electronic communication or the internet; causes the person to feel scared, nervous, or threatened.

cycle of abuse: four stages of abuse (tension building, incident, reconciliation, and calm) that repeat as long as the abuse continues.

D

Daily Values: recommended daily intake amounts for specific nutrients based on a 2,000-calorie eating plan.

dating: regularly spending time or communicating with someone whom a person is interested in romantically.

decision-making process: steps for making a healthy decision; include identifying the decision, brainstorming alternatives, evaluating alternatives, making the decision, carrying out the decision, and evaluating the decision.

defense mechanisms: mental processes used to avoid conscious conflict, feelings, or thoughts.

Español

trastornos concurrentes: dos condiciones que afectan la salud al mismo tiempo; por ejemplo, trastornos por uso de sustancias y otras enfermedades mentales.

enfriamiento: actividad que ayuda al cuerpo a relajarse después de la actividad física; ayuda a que la frecuencia cardíaca vuelva al nivel normal.

derechos de autor: derecho de un creador a poseer exclusivamente material original y utilizarlo de cualquier manera.

valores centrales: parte de la identidad que describe lo que una persona cree y encuentra importante; guia las conductas y elecciones personales.

arterias coronarias: vasos sanguíneos que suministran al músculo cardíaco sangre que contiene oxígeno y nutrientes.

compañeros de trabajo: personas que trabajan para el mismo empleador o hacen el mismo tipo de trabajo.

entrenamiento cruzado: acto de participar en varios tipos de actividad física para ayudar a mejorar la habilidad de otro tipo.

metanfetamina cristalina: forma de metanfetamina que consiste en trozos de cristal transparente.

cultura: creencias, valores, costumbres y arte de un grupo o sociedad particular.

padre con custodia: individuo que tiene la custodia legal del menor; es responsable del niño y tiene derecho a tomar decisiones sobre su cuidado.

custodia: derecho legal y responsabilidad de cuidar a un niño y tomar decisiones sobre su cuidado.

ciberacoso: uso de internet o comunicación electrónica para ejercer maltrato o atemorizar a alguien.

acecho cibernético: seguimiento y contacto reiterado con alguien mediante comunicación electrónica o internet; hace que la persona se sienta atemorizada, nerviosa o amenazada.

ciclo del abuso: cuatro etapas de abuso (desarrollo de tensión, incidente, reconciliación y calma) que se repiten mientras el abuso continúa.

valores diarios: cantidades recomendadas de ingesta diaria de nutrientes específicos según un plan de alimentación de 2,000 calorías.

salir en citas: pasar tiempo regularmente o comunicarse con alguien con quien una persona tiene un interés romántico.

proceso de toma de decisiones: pasos para tomar una decisión saludable; incluyen la identificación de la decisión, la lluvia de ideas sobre las alternativas, la evaluación de alternativas, la toma de la decisión, la ejecución de la decisión y la evaluación de la decisión.

mecanismos de defensa: procesos mentales utilizados para evitar conflictos conscientes, sentimientos o pensamientos.

English

deforestation: condition in which forests are removed faster than they can grow.

dehydration: condition in which the body does not have enough fluid to perform basic functions.

dental dam: condom-like sheet that fits between one person's mouth and another's reproductive organs; helps prevent the transmission of sexually transmitted infections (STIs).

deoxyribonucleic acid (DNA): chemical that carries genetic information, which determines many traits; found in chromosomes.

depressant: substance that slows down the central nervous system, including the brain.

detoxification: process that allows the body to clear itself of all alcohol or drugs.

developmental disabilities: complex, long-term disabilities that affect physical development, intellectual development, or both; develop before adulthood.

dextromethorphan (DXM or DM): type of opioid-like medication that suppresses coughing; found in many over-the-counter cough and cold medications.

diabetes mellitus: disease in which the body is unable to regulate blood sugar.

diaphragm: cup-shaped contraceptive device made of silicone; covers the cervix to prevent sperm from entering the uterus and is bigger than the cervical cap.

diet pills: medications that claim to help reduce a person's weight.

dietary fiber: complex carbohydrate found only in plant-based foods; cannot be completely digested, but has many health benefits.

Dietary Guidelines for Americans: guidelines published by the US Department of Agriculture (USDA) and US Department of Health and Human Services (HHS) that provide recommendations for establishing eating patterns to promote health.

digestive system: body system consisting of organs that take in foods, pass nutrients from these sources into the bloodstream, and then expel waste out of the body.

digital citizenship: practice of taking responsible, healthy actions as part of the digital community.

digital footprint: all of the content people share, access, or have shared about them online.

dignity: recognition that all people have the right to be valued and respected for who they are.

Español

deforestación: condición por la que los bosques se eliminan más rápido de lo que pueden crecer.

deshidratación: condición por la cual el cuerpo no tiene suficiente líquido para realizar funciones básicas.

barrera bucal: película similar a un condón que se ajusta entre la boca de una persona y los órganos reproductivos de otra; ayuda a prevenir la propagación de infecciones de transmisión sexual (ITS).

ácido desoxirribonucleico (ADN): químico que transporta información genética y que determina muchos rasgos; se encuentra en los cromosomas.

depresivo: sustancia que ralentiza el sistema nervioso central, incluido el cerebro.

desintoxicación: proceso que le permite al cuerpo eliminar todo el alcohol o las drogas.

discapacidades del desarrollo: discapacidades complejas a largo plazo que afectan el desarrollo físico, intelectual o ambos; se manifiestan antes de la edad adulta.

dextrometorfano (DXM o DM): tipo de medicamento similar a los opioides que suprime la tos; se encuentra en muchos medicamentos de venta libre para la tos y el resfriado.

diabetes mellitus: enfermedad en la que el cuerpo no puede regular su nivel de azúcar en sangre.

diafragma: dispositivo anticonceptivo en forma de copa de silicona; cubre el cuello uterino para evitar que el esperma ingrese al útero y es más grande que el capuchón cervical.

pastillas para adelgazar: medicamentos que dicen ayudar a reducir el peso de una persona.

fibra dietética: carbohidrato complejo que se encuentra solo en alimentos de origen vegetal; no se puede digerir por completo, pero tiene muchos beneficios para la salud.

Pautas Alimentarias para Estadounidenses: pautas publicadas por el Departamento de Agricultura de los EEUU (US Department of Agriculture, USDA) y el Departamento de Salud y Servicios Humanos de los EEUU (US Department of Health and Human Services, HHS) que proporcionan recomendaciones para establecer patrones de alimentación para promover la salud.

sistema digestivo: sistema del cuerpo que consiste en órganos que toman los alimentos, pasan nutrientes de estas fuentes al torrente sanguíneo y luego expulsan los desechos del cuerpo.

ciudadanía digital: práctica de realizar acciones responsables y saludables como parte de la comunidad digital.

huella digital: todo el contenido que las personas comparten, acceden o han compartido sobre ellas en línea.

dignidad: reconocimiento de que todas las personas tienen derecho a ser valoradas y respetadas por quienes son.

English

direct transmission: method of disease transmission in which infectious material and pathogens travel from their origin to an individual.

disability: condition that impairs a person's ability to perform certain tasks.

disaster: large-scale event that causes harm to people or property.

dislocation: condition in which bones move out of their normal positions.

disordered eating: range of irregular eating behaviors; may or may not lead to diagnosis of a specific eating disorder.

disorder of sex development (DSD): condition of being born with or developing an ambiguous biological sex; also called a *difference of sex development (DSD)* or *intersex*.

distress: stress that causes negative feelings and harmful health effects.

diuretics: substances that help the body eliminate sodium and water, mostly through increased urination; can cause a drop in weight and dangerous side effects; also called *water pills*.

diversity: differences in many areas, such as a person's race, ethnicity, sex, gender identity, sexual orientation, or spiritual beliefs.

divorce: legal end of a marriage due to the desire of one or both partners.

dominant genes: deoxyribonucleic acid (DNA) segments that always cause certain characteristics in a child.

dopamine: chemical in the brain that causes feelings of pleasure; motivates behaviors like eating and drinking.

driving under the influence (DUI): operating a motor vehicle with a blood alcohol concentration at or over 0.08% for adults; for teens, this level is lower and varies by state; also known as *driving while intoxicated (DWI)* or *drunk driving*.

drought: extended period with no rainfall.

drug abuse: act of consuming addictive, illegal substances.

drug allergy: immune response in which the body treats a particular substance as if it is harmful to the body; causes an allergic reaction if the person consumes the substance.

drugs: substances that cause physical or psychological changes in the body; may have medical or nonmedical purposes.

drug sensitivity: increased likelihood of developing negative side effects in response to a particular substance.

durable power of attorney: individual who is legally assigned to make healthcare decisions for a person in the event the person becomes incapable of deciding.

Español

transmisión directa: método de transmisión de enfermedades en el que el material infeccioso y los patógenos viajan desde su origen a un individuo.

discapacidad: condición que afecta la capacidad de una persona para realizar ciertas tareas.

desastre: evento a gran escala que causa daños a personas o bienes.

dislocación: afección en la cual los huesos se salen de su posición normal.

alimentación desordenada: rango de conductas alimentarias irregulares; puede o no conducir al diagnóstico de un trastorno alimentario específico.

trastorno del desarrollo sexual (disorder of sex development, DSD): condición de nacer o desarrollar un sexo biológico ambiguo; también se denomina *diferencia de desarrollo sexual (DSD)* o *intersexual*.

angustia: estrés que provoca sentimientos negativos y efectos nocivos para la salud.

diuréticos: sustancias que ayudan al cuerpo a eliminar el sodio y el agua, principalmente a través del aumento de la micción; puede causar una disminución del peso y efectos secundarios peligrosos; también se denominan *píldoras de agua*.

diversidad: diferencias en muchas áreas, como la raza, etnia, sexo, identidad de género, orientación sexual o creencias espirituales de una persona.

divorcio: fin legal de un matrimonio debido al deseo de uno o ambos cónyuges.

genes dominantes: segmentos de ácido desoxirribonucleico (ADN) que siempre causan ciertas características en un niño.

dopamina: químico en el cerebro que causa sensaciones de placer; motiva comportamientos como comer y beber.

conducir intoxicado (driving under the influence, DUI): operar un vehículo motorizado con una concentración de alcohol en sangre igual o superior a 0.08% para adultos; para los adolescentes, este nivel es más bajo y varía según el estado; también denominado *conducir en estado de ebriedad (driving while intoxicated, DWI)* o *conducir ebrio*.

sequía: período extendido sin precipitaciones.

abuso de drogas: acción de consumir sustancias adictivas e ilegales.

alergia a los medicamentos: respuesta inmune en la cual el cuerpo trata una sustancia particular como si fuera perjudicial para el cuerpo; provoca una reacción alérgica si la persona consume dicha sustancia.

drogas: sustancias que causan cambios físicos o psicológicos en el cuerpo; pueden tener o no fines médicos.

sensibilidad a los medicamentos: mayor probabilidad de desarrollar efectos secundarios negativos en respuesta a una sustancia en particular.

poder notarial duradero: persona que ha sido legalmente asignada para tomar decisiones de atención médica por otra persona si esta se vuelva incapaz de decidir.

English

E

early childhood: developmental stage from infancy (birth to one year) through the preschool years (three to five years of age).

eating disorder: mental illness characterized by abnormal eating or disturbances in eating habits.

ecosystems: natural systems made of interrelated biotic and abiotic parts.

edible: food mixed with a drug or a drug's active ingredients.

eggs: female sex cells that contain half of the female's chromosomes; stored in the ovaries; also called *ova*

ejaculation: series of muscular contractions that forcefully eject semen out of the urethral opening of the penis.

elder abuse: behaviors or neglect that cause harm to someone 60 years of age or older.

e-liquid: substance made of nicotine or another drug and other chemicals; is heated during vaping.

embryo: implanted, fertilized egg in the uterus.

embryonic stage: stage of prenatal development that begins at implantation and lasts around six weeks; the embryo begins to form the various tissues, organs, and systems that make a human.

emergency contraception: contraceptive method used to prevent pregnancy when normal contraception has failed; includes the copper ParaGard® intrauterine device (IUD) and emergency contraceptive pills containing hormones.

emergency healthcare: medical care that treats life-threatening health conditions.

emergency preparedness: steps one takes to ensure safety before, during, and after an emergency or natural disaster.

emerging infectious diseases: communicable diseases that are new or increasing unexpectedly.

emotional abuse: attitudes, controlling behaviors, or words that harm a person's mental and emotional health; also called *mental*, *verbal*, or *psychological abuse*.

emotional empathy: ability to experience the emotions another person is feeling.

emotional health: dimension of health that refers to the expression of thoughts and feelings, including emotions, moods, feelings about one's self, and views about the world.

emotional intelligence (EI): skill in perceiving, understanding, and managing emotions and feelings.

emotions: strong feelings experienced based on one's circumstances, relationships, or moods.

Español

primera infancia: etapa del desarrollo desde la infancia (nacimiento hasta un año) hasta la edad preescolar (tres a cinco años de edad).

trastorno alimentario: enfermedad mental caracterizada por una alimentación anormal o alteraciones en los hábitos alimenticios.

ecosistemas: sistemas naturales hechos de partes bióticas y abióticas interrelacionadas.

comestible: alimentos mezclados con una droga o los ingredientes activos de una droga.

óvulos: células sexuales femeninas que contienen la mitad de los cromosomas femeninos; se forman en los ovarios.

eyaculación: contracciones musculares que expulsan enérgicamente el semen de la abertura uretral del pene.

maltrato de ancianos: comportamientos o abandono que causan daño a alguien mayor de 60 años de edad.

e-líquido: sustancia hecha de nicotina u otra droga y otras sustancias químicas; se calienta durante el vapeo.

embrión: óvulo implantado y fecundado en el útero.

etapa embrionaria: etapa de desarrollo prenatal que comienza con la implantación y dura alrededor de seis semanas; el embrión comienza a formar los diversos tejidos, órganos y sistemas que forman un ser humano.

anticoncepción de emergencia: método anticonceptivo utilizado para prevenir el embarazo cuando la anticoncepción normal ha fallado; incluye el dispositivo intrauterino (DIU) ParaGard® de cobre y las píldoras anticonceptivas de emergencia que contienen hormonas.

atención médica de emergencia: atención médica que trata afecciones de salud potencialmente mortales.

preparación para emergencias: pasos que se toman para garantizar la seguridad antes, durante y después de una emergencia o desastre natural.

enfermedades infecciosas emergentes: enfermedades transmisibles nuevas o que presentan un aumento inesperado.

abuso emocional: actitudes, comportamientos de control o palabras que dañan la salud mental y emocional de una persona; también se denomina *abuso mental*, *verbal* o *psicológico*.

empatía emocional: capacidad para experimentar las emociones que siente otra persona.

salud emocional: dimensión de la salud que se refiere a la expresión de pensamientos y sentimientos, incluyendo emociones, estados de ánimo, sentimientos sobre uno mismo y puntos de vista sobre el mundo.

inteligencia emocional (emotional intelligence, EI): habilidad para percibir, comprender y manejar las emociones y los sentimientos.

emociones: sentimientos fuertes experimentados según las circunstancias, relaciones o estados de ánimo.

English

empathy: ability to understand and share the feelings of another person.

emphysema: condition that causes the lungs to lose elasticity; permanently enlarges airways and destroys the alveoli in lung tissue.

empty calories: units of energy that supply few or no nutrients to the body.

enabling: protecting a person from the negative consequences of chosen behaviors.

endemic: disease that naturally occurs at low levels in a particular area.

endocrine system: body system that consists of glands, which secrete hormones to regulate body processes.

endometriosis: condition in which uterine tissue grows outside the uterus; can cause pain, fatigue, and infertility.

endorphins: brain chemicals that improve mood; released during physical activity.

endurance: ability to continue performing a physical activity over time.

environment: circumstances, objects, or conditions that surround a person in everyday life.

environmental health: field of health that focuses on interactions between different natural systems.

environmental justice: aspect of community and world health concerned with populations exposed to harmful environmental and societal factors through no fault of their own.

Environmental Protection Agency (EPA): US government agency that sets and enforces laws related to protecting the environment and human health.

environmental protection hierarchy: graphic created by the Environmental Protection Agency (EPA) that shows four different ways of protecting the environment: disposal or release, treatment, recycling, and source reduction.

epidemic: disease that occurs in unexpectedly large numbers over a particular area.

epilepsy: brain disorder characterized by seizures, or interruptions in brain signals; also called *seizure disorder*.

erection: lengthening and hardening of the penis due to sexual stimulation; caused by blood flowing into the erectile tissue of the penis.

ergonomics: practices that ensure health and safety during the performance of a task.

escape plan: document that outlines safe routes and procedures for leaving an area or building during an emergency.

ethnicity: one's connection to a particular social group that shares similar cultural or national ties.

Español

empatía: capacidad para comprender y compartir los sentimientos de otra persona.

enfisema: afección que hace que los pulmones pierdan elasticidad; agranda permanentemente las vías respiratorias y destruye los alvéolos en el tejido pulmonar.

calorías vacías: unidades de energía que suministran pocos o ningún nutriente al cuerpo.

posibilitar: proteger a una persona de las consecuencias negativas de los comportamientos elegidos.

endémica: enfermedad que ocurre naturalmente en niveles bajos en un área particular.

sistema endocrino: sistema corporal que consiste en glándulas que secretan hormonas para regular los procesos corporales.

endometriosis: afección en la cual el tejido uterino crece fuera del útero; puede causar dolor, fatiga e infertilidad.

endorfinas: sustancias químicas del cerebro que mejoran el estado de ánimo; se liberan durante la actividad física.

resistencia: capacidad de continuar realizando una actividad física a lo largo del tiempo.

entorno: circunstancias, objetos o condiciones que rodean a una persona en su vida diaria.

salud ambiental: campo de la salud que se centra en las interacciones entre diferentes sistemas naturales.

justicia ambiental: aspecto de la salud comunitaria y mundial relacionado con las poblaciones expuestas a factores ambientales y sociales nocivos sin culpa propia.

Agencia de Protección Ambiental (Environmental Protection Agency, EPA): agencia del gobierno de los Estados Unidos que establece y hace cumplir las leyes relacionadas con la protección del medio ambiente y la salud humana.

estructura de protección ambiental: gráfico creado por la EPA que muestra cuatro formas diferentes de proteger el medio ambiente: eliminación o liberación, tratamiento, reciclaje y reducción de fuentes.

epidemia: enfermedad que se produce en cantidades inesperadamente grandes en un área particular.

epilepsia: trastorno cerebral caracterizado por convulsiones o interrupciones en los impulsos cerebrales; también se denomina *trastorno convulsivo*.

erección: alargamiento y endurecimiento del pene debido a la estimulación sexual; causado por la sangre que fluye hacia el tejido eréctil del pene.

ergonomía: prácticas que garantizan la salud y la seguridad durante la realización de una tarea.

plan de evacuación: documento que describe rutas y procedimientos seguros para abandonar un área o edificio durante una emergencia.

etnicidad: conexión de uno con un grupo social particular que comparte vínculos culturales o nacionales similares.

English

euphoria: intense pleasurable feeling.

eustress: positive stress that encourages growth and motivation.

exclusive: romantically involved only with a dating partner.

exercise: physical activity that is structured, planned, and has the purpose of increasing physical fitness.

extended family: distant relatives, including aunts, uncles, cousins, and grandparents.

external condom: device that fits over an erect penis to prevent semen from coming in contact with other organs; helps prevent many sexually transmitted infections (STIs) and can reduce the chance of pregnancy occurring during sexual intercourse; also called the *male condom*.

F

fad diets: stylish weight-loss plans that promise significant weight loss in short periods of time, often through cutting out food groups or buying premade meals.

fallopian tube: tube that leads from each ovary to each side of the uterus.

family history: record of diseases among close biological relatives.

family therapy: treatment method in which family members meet together with a therapist to build positive, functional relationships and strengthen interactions.

famine: widespread hunger and starvation caused by lack of food.

fats: nutrients, largely made up of fatty acids, that provide a valuable source of energy for muscles and help in the absorption and transport of vitamins and nutrients.

fat-soluble vitamins: type of vitamin that dissolves in the body's fats and can be stored for later use.

feedback: constructive response to a message.

female athlete triad: three health conditions related to intense physical activity in females; disordered eating, amenorrhea, and osteoporosis.

female reproductive system: body system consisting of organs that produce hormones and eggs, enable sexual intercourse, and nurture a baby; includes the ovaries, fallopian tubes, uterus, vagina, cervix, labia, clitoris, and breasts.

fentanyl: prescription opioid 50 to 100 times more powerful than morphine; prescribed for pain other opioids cannot control.

Español

euforia: sensación intensa y placentera.

eustrés: estrés positivo que fomenta el crecimiento y la motivación.

exclusivo: involucrado románticamente solo con una pareja de citas.

ejercicio: actividad física estructurada y planificada que tiene el propósito de aumentar la condición física.

familia extensa: parientes lejanos, incluidos tíos, primos y abuelos.

condón externo: dispositivo que se ajusta sobre un pene erecto para evitar que el semen entre en contacto con otros órganos; ayuda a prevenir muchas infecciones de transmisión sexual (ITS) y puede reducir la posibilidad de que ocurra un embarazo durante las relaciones sexuales; también se denomina *condón masculino*.

dietas de moda: planes modernos para perder peso que prometen una pérdida de peso significativa en cortos períodos de tiempo, a menudo mediante la eliminación de grupos de alimentos o la compra de comidas preparadas.

trompa de Falopio: conducto que conecta cada ovario con cada lado del útero.

antecedentes familiares: registro de enfermedades entre parientes biológicos cercanos.

terapia familiar: método de tratamiento en el que los miembros de la familia se reúnen con un terapeuta para forjar relaciones positivas y funcionales y fortalecer las interacciones.

hambruna: hambre generalizada causada por la falta de alimentos.

grasas: nutrientes, compuestos principalmente de ácidos grasos, que proporcionan una valiosa fuente de energía para los músculos y ayudan a la absorción y transporte de vitaminas y nutrientes.

vitaminas solubles en grasa: tipo de vitamina que se disuelve en las grasas del cuerpo y puede almacenarse para su uso posterior.

retroalimentación: respuesta constructiva a un mensaje.

tríada de la atleta femenina: tres condiciones de salud relacionadas con la actividad física intensa femenina; alimentación desordenada, amenorrea y osteoporosis.

sistema reproductivo femenino: sistema corporal que consiste en órganos que producen hormonas y óvulos, permiten las relaciones sexuales y nutren a un bebé; incluye los ovarios, las trompas de Falopio, el útero, la vagina, el cuello uterino, los labios vaginales, el clítoris y los senos.

fentanilo: opioide recetado 50 a 100 veces más potente que la morfina; recetado para el dolor que otros opioides no pueden controlar.

English

fertility awareness method (FAM): contraceptive method that tracks a female's cycle of fertility and avoids sexual activity on days an egg can be fertilized.

fertilizers: chemicals applied to farmland, gardens, and lawns to promote growth.

fetal alcohol spectrum disorders (FASD): set of health conditions that affect the baby born to a person who has consumed alcohol during the pregnancy.

fetal stage: stage that begins at the ninth week of pregnancy and lasts through birth; the fetus grows considerably.

fetus: baby during the fetal stage until birth.

fever: body temperature over 98°F (37°C); body temperature rises as part of the immune response.

fibroids: noncancerous tumors of the uterus.

fight-or-flight response: physiological stress reaction in which the body mobilizes its resources to fight off or escape from a perceived threat; also called the *stress response*.

financial abuse: behaviors that involve using money to exert power in a relationship; may include controlling finances and using money to make others act in certain ways.

fine-motor skills: movements that use the small muscles of the body.

fire triangle: representation of the three elements (fuel, heat, and oxygen) needed to start a fire.

first aid: treatment given in the first moments after an accident or injury, usually before medical professionals arrive.

first-aid kit: collection of necessary items to treat minor injuries.

five-and-five method: procedure of responding to choking that involves a series of back blows alternating with abdominal thrusts.

fixed mind-set: belief that a person's most basic abilities and feelings are permanent and cannot be changed.

flaming: writing mean and hateful comments with the intention of hurting others.

flexibility: ability to fully and easily move the joints.

food additives: substances added to food products to cause desired changes to flavor, shelf life, or other reasons.

food allergy: condition in which the body's immune system reacts to a food as if the food is harmful; sudden symptoms can be caused by tiny amounts of the food.

Español

método de conciencia de fertilidad (fertility awareness method, FAM): método anticonceptivo que controla el ciclo de fertilidad femenino y evita la actividad sexual en los días en que un óvulo puede ser fertilizado.

fertilizantes: químicos aplicados a tierras de cultivo, jardines y céspedes para promover el crecimiento.

trastornos del espectro alcohólico fetal (fetal alcohol spectrum disorders, FASD): conjunto de afecciones de salud que afectan al bebé nacido de una persona que ha consumido alcohol durante el embarazo.

etapa fetal: etapa que comienza en la novena semana de embarazo y dura hasta el nacimiento; el feto crece considerablemente.

feto: bebé durante la etapa fetal hasta el nacimiento.

fiebre: temperatura corporal superior a 98°F (37°C); la temperatura corporal aumenta como parte de la respuesta inmune.

fibromas: tumores no cancerosos del útero.

respuesta de lucha o huida: reacción de estrés fisiológico en la que el cuerpo moviliza sus recursos para luchar o escapar de una amenaza percibida; también se denomina *respuesta al estrés*.

abuso financiero: comportamientos que implican usar dinero para ejercer poder en una relación; podría incluir el control de las finanzas y el uso del dinero para hacer que otros actúen de ciertas maneras.

habilidades de motricidad fina: movimientos que utilizan los músculos pequeños del cuerpo.

triángulo de fuego: representación de los tres elementos (combustible, calor y oxígeno) necesarios para iniciar un incendio.

primeros auxilios: tratamiento dado en los primeros momentos después de producido un accidente o lesión, generalmente antes de que los profesionales médicos lleguen a la escena.

botiquín de primeros auxilios: colección de artículos necesarios para tratar lesiones menores.

método de cinco y cinco: procedimiento de respuesta a la asfixia que implica una serie de golpes en la espalda que se alternan con empujes abdominales.

mentalidad fija: creencia de que las capacidades y sentimientos más básicos de una persona son permanentes y no se pueden cambiar.

mensaje hostil: escribir comentarios malos y llenos de odio con la intención de lastimar a otros.

flexibilidad: capacidad de mover completa y fácilmente las articulaciones.

aditivos alimentarios: sustancias agregadas a los productos alimenticios para causar los cambios deseados en el sabor, la vida útil u otras razones.

alergia alimentaria: condición en la cual el sistema inmunológico del cuerpo reacciona a un alimento como si fuera perjudicial; los síntomas repentinos pueden ser causados por pequeñas cantidades del alimento.

English	Español
Food and Drug Administration (FDA): federal organization that regulates and ensures the safety of food, health products, and medications.	**Administración de Alimentos y Medicamentos (Food and Drug Administration, FDA)**: organización federal que regula y garantiza la seguridad de los alimentos, productos para la salud y medicamentos.
foodborne illnesses: illnesses that are transmitted by food; also called *food poisoning*.	**enfermedades transmitidas por los alimentos**: enfermedades que se transmiten a través de los alimentos; también se denomina *intoxicación alimentaria*.
foodborne infection: foodborne illness that occurs when food is handled or prepared improperly; is caused by bacteria, viruses, or parasites.	**infección transmitida por los alimentos**: enfermedad transmitida por los alimentos que ocurre cuando se manipulan o preparan de manera inadecuada; es causada por bacterias, virus o parásitos.
foodborne intoxication: foodborne illness caused by toxins, which are produced by organisms present in a food.	**intoxicación transmitida por los alimentos**: enfermedad transmitida por los alimentos causada por toxinas que son producidas por organismos presentes en un alimento.
food desert: area without nearby full-service grocery stores.	**desierto alimentario**: área sin tiendas de comestibles de servicio completo.
food diary: daily record of what a person eats; used to track eating patterns and calorie intake.	**diario de alimentos**: registro diario de lo que come una persona; se utiliza para controlar los patrones de alimentación y el consumo de calorías.
food intolerances: conditions in which a person's body cannot properly digest particular types of food; can develop gradually as a person eats large quantities of a certain food frequently.	**intolerancias alimentarias**: condiciones en las que el cuerpo de una persona no puede digerir adecuadamente determinados tipos de alimentos; puede desarrollarse gradualmente a medida que una persona come grandes cantidades de ciertos alimentos con frecuencia.
food preferences: opinions about different types of food; influenced by genetics, age, feelings and thoughts, cultural background, and social environment.	**preferencias de alimentos**: opiniones sobre diferentes tipos de alimentos; influenciadas por la genética, edad, sentimientos y pensamientos, antecedentes culturales y entorno social.
fossil fuels: natural gas, coal, and oil; are burned to produce energy.	**combustibles fósiles**: gas natural, carbón y petróleo; se queman para producir energía.
fracture: break in a bone.	**fractura**: quebradura de un hueso.
friendship: relationship between two or more people who share common interests, values, and goals and support each other.	**amistad**: relación entre dos o más personas que comparten intereses, valores y metas comunes y se apoyan mutuamente.
frostbite: condition in which the skin and the body tissues beneath it freeze.	**congelación**: condición en la cual la piel y los tejidos del cuerpo debajo de ella se congelan.
fungi: multicellular organisms that produce spores; are mostly beneficial, but can cause disease.	**hongos**: organismos multicelulares que producen esporas; son principalmente beneficiosos, pero pueden causar enfermedades.

G

English	Español
gangs: groups of people who engage in violent and illegal activities.	**pandillas**: grupos de personas que participan en actividades violentas e ilegales.
gender: behavioral, cultural, or psychological traits and roles society associates with a biological sex.	**género**: rasgos y roles conductuales, culturales o psicológicos que la sociedad asocia con un sexo biológico.
gender binary: view that the genders of man and woman are entirely opposite; ignores gender expressions that fall between these opposites.	**binarismo de género**: razón que los géneros de hombre y mujer son completamente opuestos; ignora las expresiones de género que se encuentran entre estos opuestos.
gender identity: component of identity that describes internal, deeply held thoughts and feelings about one's gender.	**identidad de género**: componente de identidad que describe pensamientos y sentimientos internos y muy arraigados sobre su propio género.

English

gender nonconforming: identifying with a gender that is not associated with one's biological sex.

gender roles: societal or cultural expectations about how people of a certain gender should behave, dress, speak, and act.

gender stereotypes: preconceived ideas, roles, and characteristics people associate with a certain gender.

generally recognized as safe (GRAS): proven by the Food and Drug Administration (FDA) to be safe for consumption.

genes: deoxyribonucleic acid (DNA) segments that contain the blueprint for the structure and function of a person's cells; affect development, personality, and health.

genetically modified organism (GMO): living thing with genetic material that has been altered through genetic engineering.

genetic disorders: health conditions that develop due to a person's genes; do not require the presence of other risk factors.

genetic predisposition: increased likelihood of developing a health condition due to genes inherited from biological parents.

genital herpes: herpes simplex virus (HSV) infection of the reproductive organs.

genital warts: abnormal growths on the skin and membranes around the reproductive organs and anus; caused by some forms of human papillomavirus (HPV).

geography: land features and any bodies of water present in an area.

germinal stage: stage of development that begins at conception and lasts about two weeks; cleavage occurs.

germ theory: scientific theory that specific pathogens cause specific diseases.

glucose: simple carbohydrate and the preferred source of energy for the brain and central nervous system.

goal: specific endpoint that signifies a condition one hopes to reach.

gonorrhea: bacterial sexually transmitted infection (STI) with mild or no symptoms; primarily affects the rectum, throat, and reproductive tract.

gossip: hurtful rumors about a person that may or may not be true.

gout: disease characterized by sudden, painful swelling of joints, especially in the feet and big toe.

gratitude: appreciation for what one has.

greenhouse gases: gases in Earth's atmosphere that trap heat, acting like the glass walls and roof of a greenhouse.

Español

no conformidad de género: identificarse con un género que no está asociado con el sexo biológico de uno.

roles de género: expectativas sociales o culturales sobre cómo las personas de cierto género deben comportarse, vestirse, hablar y actuar.

estereotipos de género: ideas preconcebidas, roles y características que las personas asocian con un determinado género.

generalmente reconocido como seguro (generally recognized as safe, GRAS): verificado por la Administración de Alimentos y Medicamentos (Food and Drug Administration, FDA) como seguro para el consumo.

genes: segmentos de ácido desoxirribonucleico (ADN) que contienen el código para la estructura y función de las células de una persona; afectan el desarrollo, la personalidad y la salud.

organismo genéticamente modificado (OGM): ser vivo con material genético que ha sido modificado a través de la ingeniería genética.

trastornos genéticos: afecciones de salud que se desarrollan debido a los genes de una persona; no requieren la presencia de otros factores de riesgo.

predisposición genética: mayor probabilidad de desarrollar una afección de salud debido a genes heredados de padres biológicos.

herpes genital: infección por el virus del herpes simple (VHS) de los órganos reproductivos.

verrugas genitales: crecimientos anormales en la piel y las membranas alrededor de los órganos reproductivos y el ano; causado por algunas formas de virus del papiloma humano (VPH).

geografía: características de la tierra y cualquier cuerpo de agua presente en un área.

etapa germinal: etapa de desarrollo que comienza en la concepción y dura aproximadamente dos semanas; se produce la segmentación.

teoría de los gérmenes: teoría científica de que patógenos específicos causan enfermedades específicas.

glucosa: carbohidrato simple y la fuente de energía preferida del cerebro y el sistema nervioso central.

meta: punto final específico que significa una condición que uno espera alcanzar.

gonorrea: infección de transmisión sexual (ITS) bacteriana con síntomas leves o asintomática; afecta principalmente el recto, la garganta y el tracto reproductivo.

chismes: rumores hirientes sobre una persona que pueden ser ciertos o no.

gota: enfermedad caracterizada por hinchazón repentina y dolorosa de las articulaciones, en especial en los pies y el dedo gordo.

gratitud: aprecio por lo que uno tiene.

gases de efecto invernadero: gases en la atmósfera de la Tierra que atrapan el calor, actuando como las paredes de vidrio y el techo de un invernadero.

English

green products: items that have a less harmful impact on the environment than some traditional (nongreen) items.

grief: complex emotion characterized by a sense of loss.

gross-motor skills: movements that use the large muscles of the body.

group dating: spending time in a group that includes someone a person is interested in romantically.

growth mind-set: belief that a person's most basic abilities and feelings can be changed through hard work and dedication.

H

hacking: cybercrime that uses computer code to open and read files on computers, websites, or other digital locations.

hallucinogens: drugs that change a person's perception of reality; can cause hallucinations, affect mood, and alter a person's sense of time.

hand washing: practice of using soap and water to clean the hands.

hangover: negative symptoms caused by excessive alcohol use; for example, nausea, fatigue, and headaches.

happiness: positive emotion linked to well-being and contentment with life.

harassment: aggressive behavior that targets and hurts another person because of a particular part of the person's identity, such as race, religious beliefs, sex, gender identity, or sexual orientation.

hate crime: any kind of violence or threat of violence that targets people because of their race, ethnicity, disability, sexual orientation, gender identity, or religion.

hazing: type of bullying that uses group pressure to make someone do an embarrassing or dangerous activity to be accepted in a group.

health: state of complete physical, mental and emotional, and social well-being.

healthcare: medical care that seeks to prevent and treat health conditions.

health fraud: illegal activity related to health products and services; for example, deceptive labeling or advertising.

health literacy: ability to locate, evaluate, apply, and communicate information pertaining to health.

health promotion: process of advocating for the health of families and communities by sharing health information.

Español

productos ecológicos: productos que tienen un impacto menos dañino sobre el medio ambiente que los productos tradicionales (no ecológicos).

duelo: emoción compleja caracterizada por una sensación de pérdida.

habilidades de motricidad gruesa: movimientos que utilizan los músculos grandes del cuerpo.

citas grupales: pasar tiempo en un grupo que incluye a alguien con quien una persona está interesada románticamente.

mentalidad de crecimiento: la creencia de que las capacidades y sentimientos más básicos de una persona se pueden cambiar a través del trabajo duro y la dedicación.

piratería: ciberdelito que usa códigos informáticos para abrir y leer archivos en computadoras, sitios web u otros sitios digitales.

alucinógenos: drogas que cambian la percepción de la realidad de una persona; pueden causar alucinaciones, afectar el estado de ánimo y alterar el sentido del tiempo de una persona.

lavado de manos: práctica de usar agua y jabón para limpiar las manos.

resaca: síntomas negativos causados por el consumo excesivo de alcohol; por ejemplo, náuseas, fatiga y dolores de cabeza.

felicidad: emoción positiva vinculada a la plenitud y satisfacción con la vida.

acoso: comportamiento agresivo que es dirigido hacia y lastima otra persona debido a una particularidad de su identidad, como raza, creencias religiosas, sexo, identidad de género u orientación sexual.

crimen de odio: cualquier tipo de violencia o amenaza de violencia dirigida a personas debido a su raza, origen étnico, discapacidad, orientación sexual, identidad de género o religión.

novatadas: tipo de intimidación que utiliza la presión grupal para hacer que alguien realice una actividad vergonzosa o peligrosa para ser aceptado en un grupo.

salud: estado de completa plenitud física, mental, emocional y social.

cuidado de la salud: atención médica que busca prevenir y tratar afecciones de salud.

fraude a la salud: actividad ilegal relacionada con productos y servicios de salud; por ejemplo, información o publicidad engañosas.

educación sobre: capacidad de localizar, evaluar, aplicar y comunicar información relacionada con la salud.

promoción de la salud: proceso de abogar por la salud de las familias y las comunidades mediante el intercambio de información sobre la salud.

English

health-related fitness: body's ability to perform daily activities with ease and energy.

heart attack: medical emergency in which the coronary arteries that supply blood to the heart become narrow or blocked, disrupting blood flow to the heart.

heat cramps: painful muscle spasms caused by overheating of the body.

heat exhaustion: health condition caused by overheating of the body; characterized by nausea, dizziness, weakness, headache, weak pulse, disorientation, and fainting.

heatstroke: medical emergency caused by overheating of the body; can lead to shock, coma, and even death.

hepatitis: inflammation of the liver; caused by the hepatitis A, B, or C virus.

herbicides: chemicals used to kill unwanted plants, such as weeds.

heroin: naturally occurring, illegal opioid; comes as a white powder often mixed with other substances.

histamine: chemical that causes blood vessels to leak fluids into tissues; released during an allergic reaction.

homelessness: state of being without regular, consistent housing.

homeostasis: body's internal, steady state of balance; the body maintains homeostasis by regulating body temperature, the amount of sugar in the blood, blood pressure, and oxygen level in tissues.

homicide: act of killing a person.

homophobia: hostility, anger, exclusion, and violence directed at people who are LGBT+.

honesty: truthfulness about one's actions, desires, and feelings.

hormonal methods: contraceptive methods that alter a person's hormone levels to thicken cervical mucus and inhibit ovulation (the release of an egg).

hospice care: healthcare that provides comfort at the end of a person's life.

human immunodeficiency virus (HIV): bloodborne virus that infects and kills the body's cells, weakening the immune system.

human life cycle: series of developmental stages from birth through adulthood and death.

human papillomavirus (HPV): common sexually transmitted infection (STI) that infects cells in the skin and membranes, causing them to grow abnormally.

human sexual response cycle: physical changes that occur in the body in response to sexual arousal and activity.

Español

estado físico relacionado con la salud: la capacidad del cuerpo para realizar actividades diarias con facilidad y energía.

ataque cardíaco: emergencia médica en la cual las arterias coronarias que suministran sangre al corazón se estrechan o bloquean, interrumpiendo el flujo sanguíneo al corazón.

calambres por calor: espasmos musculares dolorosos causados por el sobrecalentamiento del cuerpo.

agotamiento por calor: afecciones de salud causadas por el sobrecalentamiento del cuerpo; caracterizado por náuseas, mareos, debilidad, dolor de cabeza, pulso débil, desorientación y desmayos.

golpe de calor: emergencia médica causada por sobrecalentamiento del cuerpo; puede provocar conmoción, coma e incluso la muerte.

hepatitis: inflamación del hígado; causado por el virus de la hepatitis A, B o C.

herbicidas: productos químicos utilizados para matar plantas no deseadas, como las malas hierbas.

heroína: opioide ilegal de origen natural; viene como un polvo blanco a menudo mezclado con otras sustancias.

histamina: sustancia química que hace que los vasos sanguíneos derramen líquidos en los tejidos; liberada durante una reacción alérgica.

sin hogar: estado de estar sin vivienda regular y constante.

homeostasis: estado de equilibrio interno y estable del cuerpo; el cuerpo mantiene la homeostasis al regular la temperatura corporal, la cantidad de azúcar en la sangre, la presión arterial y el nivel de oxígeno en los tejidos.

homicidio: acto de matar a otra persona.

homofobia: hostilidad, ira, exclusión y violencia dirigida a personas que están LGBT+.

honestidad: veracidad sobre las propias acciones, deseos y sentimientos.

métodos hormonales: métodos anticonceptivos que alteran los niveles hormonales de una persona para ensanchar mucosidad cervical y inhibir la ovulación (la liberación de un óvulo).

cuidado de enfermos terminales: atención médica que brinda comodidad al final de la vida de una persona.

virus de inmunodeficiencia humana (VIH): virus transmitido por la sangre que infecta y mata las células del cuerpo, debilitando el sistema inmunológico.

ciclo de vida humana: serie de etapas de desarrollo desde el nacimiento hasta la edad adulta y la muerte.

virus del papiloma humano (VPH): infección de transmisión sexual (ITS) común que infecta las células de la piel y las membranas, haciendo que crezcan de manera anormal.

ciclo de respuesta sexual humana: cambios físicos que ocurren en el cuerpo en respuesta a la excitación y actividad sexual.

English	Español
human trafficking: form of modern slavery in which people are forced or pressured to perform labor or sexual acts against their will.	**trata de personas**: forma de esclavitud moderna en la que las personas son forzadas o presionadas a realizar actos laborales o sexuales en contra de su voluntad.
hyperglycemia: condition of high blood sugar.	**hiperglucemia**: afección de azúcar alta en la sangre.
hypertension: disease characterized by high blood pressure.	**hipertensión**: enfermedad caracterizada por presión arterial alta.
hypothermia: medical emergency in which body temperature is too low; can lead to shock, coma, and death.	**hipotermia**: emergencia médica en la que la temperatura corporal es demasiado baja; puede provocar conmoción, coma y la muerte.
hypoxia: condition in which the body does not receive the oxygen it needs, resulting in widespread cell damage.	**hipoxia**: condición en la cual el cuerpo no recibe el oxígeno que necesita, lo que resulta en un daño celular generalizado.

I

English	Español
identity: characteristics and qualities that distinguish who a person is.	**identidad**: características y cualidades que distinguen quién es una persona.
identity formation: process of discovering and establishing one's identity through physical, cognitive, and social changes.	**formación de identidad**: proceso de descubrir y establecer la identidad a través de cambios físicos, cognitivos y sociales.
identity theft: act of using people's personal information to pretend to be them.	**robo de identidad**: acto de usar la información personal de las personas para pretender ser ellas.
illness: poor overall state of health in which a person cannot function normally; caused by factors such as disease, risky behaviors, hazardous substances, and concerns with mental or emotional health.	**padecimiento**: mal estado de salud general en el que una persona no puede funcionar normalmente; causada por factores como condiciones, conductas de riesgo, sustancias peligrosas y preocupaciones con la salud mental o emocional.
immediate family: close relatives, including parents or guardians, children, and siblings.	**familia inmediata**: parientes cercanos, incluidos padres o tutores, hijos y hermanos.
immune system: body system consisting of organs, tissues, and cells that defend against infection.	**sistema inmunológico**: sistema del cuerpo que consiste en órganos, tejidos y células que defienden contra la infección.
impersonation: act of pretending to be another person online.	**suplantación de identidad**: acto de pretender ser otra persona en internet.
incontinence: inability to prevent urination when urine collects in the bladder.	**incontinencia**: incapacidad para evitar orinar cuando la orina se acumula en la vejiga.
indirect transmission: method of disease transmission in which infectious material and pathogens pass to a person from a source that acts solely as a carrier.	**transmisión indirecta**: método de transmisión de enfermedades en el que el material infeccioso y los agentes patógenos pasan a una persona desde una fuente que actúa únicamente como portador.
infatuation: intense romantic feelings for another person that develop suddenly and are usually based on physical attraction.	**enamoramiento**: sentimientos románticos intensos por otra persona que se desarrollan de forma repentina y generalmente se basan en la atracción física.
inflammation: immune response characterized by redness, heat, swelling, and pain.	**inflamación**: respuesta inmune caracterizada por enrojecimiento, calor, hinchazón y dolor.
influenza: disease caused by the influenza virus; causes respiratory symptoms and body aches; also called the *flu*.	**influenza**: enfermedad causada por el virus de la influenza; causa síntomas respiratorios y dolores corporales; también se denomina *gripe*.
inhalants: chemicals that people breathe to experience some type of high; often take the form of household substances.	**inhalantes**: sustancias químicas que las personas aspiran para experimentar algún tipo de sensación de euforia; a menudo toman la forma de sustancias domésticas.
inhibition: psychological restraint that keeps people from acting in dangerous ways.	**inhibición**: restricción psicológica que impide que las personas actúen de manera peligrosa.
inpatient facilities: healthcare facilities in which patients reside for the duration of treatment.	**instalaciones para pacientes hospitalizados**: instalaciones de atención médica en las que los pacientes residen durante el tratamiento.

English	Español
insulin: hormone that signals cells to move sugar from the blood into surrounding cells; produced by the pancreas.	**insulina**: hormona que indica a las células que muevan el azúcar de la sangre a las células circundantes; es producida por el páncreas.
intellectual disabilities: conditions that interfere with learning, social behavior, communication, and self-care habits; characterized by an intelligence quotient (IQ) equal to or below 70.	**discapacidades intelectuales**: condiciones que interfieren con el aprendizaje, el comportamiento social, la comunicación y los hábitos de autocuidado; caracterizadas por un coeficiente intelectual (CI) igual o inferior a 70.
intensity: amount of energy the body uses per minute during an activity.	**intensidad**: cantidad de energía que el cuerpo usa por minuto durante una actividad.
internal condom: device that fits inside the vagina or rectum to prevent semen from entering; is less effective than an external condom at preventing some sexually transmitted infections (STIs); also reduces the chance of pregnancy occurring during sexual intercourse; also called the *female condom.*	**condón interno**: dispositivo que se ajusta dentro de la vagina o el recto para evitar la entrada de semen; es menos efectivo que un condón externo para prevenir algunas infecciones de transmisión sexual (ITS); también reduce la posibilidad de que ocurra un embarazo durante las relaciones sexuales; se denomina también *condón femenino.*
internet predators: people who use personal information to find and harm people or violate their privacy.	**depredadores de internet**: personas que usan información personal para encontrar y dañar a personas o violar su privacidad.
intimate partner violence: violent behaviors between two people who are or were married, dating, or in a romantic relationship.	**violencia de pareja**: comportamientos violentos entre dos personas que están o estuvieron casadas, saliendo o en una relación romántica.
intrauterine device (IUD): small, T-shaped contraceptive device inserted into the uterus; copper IUDs interfere with sperm movement, and hormonal IUDs release hormones to thicken cervical mucus and inhibit ovulation.	**dispositivo intrauterino (DIU)**: pequeño dispositivo anticonceptivo en forma de T que se inserta en el útero; los DIU de cobre interfieren con el movimiento de los espermatozoides y los DIU hormonales liberan hormonas para ensanchar mucosidad cervical y inhibir la ovulación.
I-statements: words that explain how the speaker feels without judging the receiver.	**mensajes "yo"**: palabras que explican cómo se siente el hablante sin juzgar al receptor.

J

English	Español
jealousy: emotion characterized by wanting or being unhappy about another person's positive experiences or circumstances.	**celos**: emoción caracterizada por querer o ser infeliz por las experiencias o circunstancias positivas de otra persona.

L

English	Español
labia: skin folds, including the labia majora and labia minora, that protect the vaginal opening.	**labios**: pliegues de la piel, incluidos los labios mayores y los labios menores, que protegen la abertura vaginal.
labor: process that pushes a baby out of the uterus and through the vagina.	**trabajo de parto**: proceso que empuja a un bebé fuera del útero y a través de la vagina.
landfills: locations where waste is buried between layers of soil.	**vertederos**: lugares donde los desechos están enterrados entre capas de suelo.
lanugo: fine hair that grows all over the body as a result of starvation due to anorexia nervosa.	**lanugo**: cabello fino que crece en todo el cuerpo como resultado del hambre debido a la anorexia nerviosa.
laryngectomy: surgical procedure that removes the larynx, requiring a person to breathe through an opening in the neck.	**laringectomía**: procedimiento quirúrgico que elimina la laringe y requiere que la persona respire a través de una abertura en el cuello.
law enforcement: community workers who make sure laws are followed.	**agentes de aplicación de la ley**: trabajadores comunitarios que se aseguran de que se cumplan las leyes.
lead: soft gray metal mined from the ground; was used in some products and then banned due to its toxicity.	**plomo**: metal gris suave extraído del suelo; fue utilizado en algunos productos y luego prohibido debido a su toxicidad.

English

learning disorders: conditions that interfere with the brain's ability to process, recall, and apply information.

legal fatherhood: male parent's right to be involved in the child's life and responsibility to support the child.

leukoplakia: condition characterized by thickened, white, leathery spots inside the mouth; can develop into oral cancer.

LGBT+: acronym used to identify people who are nonheterosexual and/or gender nonconforming.

life expectancy: length of time a person is expected to live.

lifelong learning: practice of always seeking to gather new information and learn new skills.

life span: actual number of years a person lives.

long-term non-progressors: people living with human immunodeficiency virus (HIV) who progress very slowly through the latency stage of HIV.

love: intense affection for and attachment to another person.

M

major depressive disorder: mood disorder characterized by feelings of intense sadness, worthlessness, and hopelessness; also called *clinical depression*.

male reproductive system: body system consisting of organs that produce hormones and sperm and enable sexual intercourse; includes the testes, penis, seminal vesicles, prostate, and vas deferens.

malignant tumors: mass of abnormal, cancerous cells; cells can spread to other areas of the body and invade tissues.

malnutrition: form of poor nutrition in which a person does not get or properly absorb the recommended amounts of essential nutrients.

mammograms: procedures that use X-rays to image the breast and screen for breast cancer.

mandated reporters: individuals required by law to report signs of abuse.

marijuana: mind-altering, addictive drug made up of dried parts of the cannabis plant.

marriage: legal union between two partners in a couple.

Maslow's hierarchy of human needs: model of human needs, in which basic needs are met before higher-level needs.

masturbation: self-stimulation of the reproductive organs in response to sexual excitement.

Español

trastornos del aprendizaje: condiciones que interfieren con la capacidad del cerebro para procesar, recordar y aplicar información.

paternidad legal: el derecho del padre varón a participar en la vida del niño y la responsabilidad de mantenerlo.

leucoplasia: afección caracterizada por manchas gruesas, blancas y coriáceas dentro de la boca; puede convertirse en cáncer oral.

LGBT+: acrónimo utilizado para identificar personas no heterosexuales y/o sin conformidad de género.

esperanza de vida: tiempo que se espera que viva una persona.

aprendizaje permanente: práctica de buscar siempre recopilar nueva información y aprender nuevas habilidades.

período de vida: cantidad real de años que vive una persona.

progresores lentos: personas que viven con el virus de inmunodeficiencia humana (VIH) que progresan muy lentamente a través de la etapa de latencia del VIH.

amor: afecto intenso y apego por otra persona.

trastorno depresivo mayor: trastorno del estado de ánimo caracterizado por sentimientos de tristeza intensa, inutilidad y desesperanza; también se denomina *depresión clínica.*

sistema reproductivo masculino: sistema del cuerpo que consiste en órganos que producen hormonas y esperma y permiten las relaciones sexuales; incluye los testículos, el pene, las vesículas seminales, la próstata y el conducto deferente.

tumores malignos: masa de células cancerosas anormales; las células pueden extenderse a otras áreas del cuerpo e invadir los tejidos.

malnutrición: forma de mala nutrición en la que una persona no obtiene o absorbe adecuadamente las cantidades recomendadas de nutrientes esenciales.

mamografías: procedimientos que usan rayos X para obtener imágenes de la mamay detectar el cáncer de mamas.

denunciantes obligatorios: personas que están obligadas por ley a denunciar signos de abuso.

marihuana: droga adictiva y que altera la mente compuesta de partes secas de la planta de cannabis.

matrimonio: unión legal entre dos personas en una pareja.

jerarquía de las necesidades humanas de Maslow: modelo de necesidades humanas en el que las necesidades básicas se satisfacen antes que las necesidades de nivel superior.

masturbación: autoestimulación de los órganos reproductivos como respuesta a la excitación sexual.

English

maximum heart rate: number of heartbeats per minute when the heart is working its hardest.

MDMA: synthetic club drug that increases the activity of dopamine, norepinephrine, and serotonin in the brain; also called *ecstasy* or *Molly*.

media: in-person and online communication channels, such as books, TV shows, movies, social media, and advertisements.

mediation: strategy for resolving difficult conflicts through a neutral third party.

mediator: neutral third party who attempts to help people involved in a conflict reach an agreement.

medical emergency: urgent, life-threatening situation.

medication: substance that treats disease or relieves symptoms.

medication abuse: use of a medication in an unintended or harmful way; includes using medications for unintended purposes, sharing or selling medications, taking too much of a medication, or combining medications without a doctor's approval.

medication-assisted treatment (MAT): strategy for treating substance use disorders that involves using medications and teaching a person how to handle cravings and avoid abusing the substance again.

medication misuse: act of unintentionally not following the instructions for taking a medication.

menarche: female's first menstrual period.

meningitis: inflammation of the membranes around the brain and spinal cord; can cause brain and nerve damage, disability, and death if untreated.

menopause: period during which egg production stops and estrogen levels drop in females; usually occurs in late 40s to middle 50s.

menstrual cycle: sequence of body changes in females coordinated by the hormones estrogen and progesterone.

menstruation: shedding of the endometrial lining of the uterus; blood and some tissues pass through the vagina.

mental distress: short-term mental and emotional state in which negative thoughts and feelings impair relationships, daily tasks, and enjoyment of life.

mental health: dimension of health that describes how a person observes and interprets information to make decisions, solve problems, and examine situations.

mental health conditions: patterns of thinking and feeling that decrease mental and emotional health; can be everyday worries or serious mental illnesses.

Español

frecuencia cardíaca máxima: cantidad de latidos por minuto cuando el corazón funciona al máximo.

MDMA: droga sintética que aumenta la actividad de la dopamina, la noradrenalina y la serotonina en el cerebro; también se denomina *éxtasis* o *Molly*.

medios: canales de comunicación en persona y en internet, como libros, programas de televisión, películas, redes sociales y anuncios publicitarios.

mediación: estrategia para resolver conflictos difíciles a través de un tercero neutral.

mediador: tercero neutral que intenta ayudar a las personas involucradas en un conflicto a llegar a un acuerdo.

emergencia médica: situación urgente y potencialmente mortal.

medicamento: sustancia que trata la enfermedad o alivia los síntomas.

abuso de medicamentos: uso de un medicamento de manera no intencional o perjudicial; incluye el uso de medicamentos para fines no deseados, compartir o vender medicamentos, tomar demasiados medicamentos o combinar medicamentos sin la aprobación de un médico.

tratamiento asistido con medicamentos (medication-assisted treatment, MAT): estrategia para tratar los trastornos por consumo de sustancias que implica utilizar medicamentos y enseñar a una persona a manejar los antojos y evitar volver a abusar de la sustancia.

uso indebido de medicamentos: acto deliberado de no seguir las instrucciones para tomar un medicamento.

menarquia: primer período menstrual femenino.

meningitis: inflamación de las membranas alrededor del cerebro y la médula espinal; puede causar daño cerebral y nervioso, discapacidad y muerte si no se trata.

menopausia: período durante el cual la producción de óvulos se detiene y los niveles de estrógeno disminuyen en las hembras; por lo general, ocurre entre finales de los 40 y mediados de los 50.

ciclo menstrual: secuencia de cambios corporales femeninos coordinados por las hormonas estrógeno y progesterona.

menstruación: desprendimiento del revestimiento endometrial del útero; la sangre y algunos tejidos pasan a través de la vagina.

angustia mental: estado mental y emocional a corto plazo en el que los pensamientos y sentimientos negativos perjudican las relaciones, las tareas diarias y el goce de la vida.

salud mental: dimensión de la salud que describe cómo una persona observa e interpreta la información para tomar decisiones, resolver problemas y examinar situaciones.

afecciones de salud mental: patrones de pensamiento y sentimiento que disminuyen la salud mental y emocional; pueden ser preocupaciones cotidianas o enfermedades mentales graves.

English

mental health medications: substances that cause changes in the brain to reduce the symptoms of a mental illness.

mental illness: health condition in which negative or unhelpful feelings or thoughts become so severe they interfere with daily life.

mentors: people who guide others in positive ways.

mercury: silver metal that is liquid at room temperature; is naturally found in coal, oil, and other fuels.

metabolism: rate at which the body uses energy to carry out basic physiological processes.

metastasize: to spread from an original location to other parts of the body.

methamphetamine: extremely addictive, synthetic stimulant; is powerful enough a person can develop an addiction on first use.

methicillin-resistant Staphylococcus aureus (MRSA): dangerous disease caused by antibiotic-resistant *Staphylococcus aureus*; can infect the skin, bone, lungs, and bloodstream.

middle adulthood: developmental stage between 40 and 65 years of age.

middle childhood: developmental stage between five and 12 years of age.

milestones: events that indicate the development of skills and maturing qualities.

mindfulness: state of concentrated, judgment-free awareness of what is happening in the present moment.

mindfulness-based stress reduction (MBSR): act of using relaxation techniques, such as deep breathing, visualization, focused attention, and guided movements, while focusing intensely on the present.

mind-set: person's thought pattern, attitude, and mood.

minerals: inorganic nutrients absorbed from plants, water, and animal food sources.

minors: people under the age of 18.

misunderstandings: failures in communication that lead to conflict.

mold: fungus that grows in moist areas.

mononucleosis: disease caused by the Epstein-Barr virus (EBV); causes fever, sore throat, fatigue, swollen lymph nodes, and a swollen spleen; also called *mono* or *kissing disease*.

mood swings: sudden shifts in emotion.

muscle dysmorphia: disorder characterized by extreme concern with becoming more muscular.

Español

medicamentos para la salud mental: sustancias que causan cambios en el cerebro para reducir los síntomas de una enfermedad mental.

enfermedad mental: condición de salud en la cual los sentimientos o pensamientos negativos o inútiles se vuelven tan severos que interfieren con la vida diaria.

mentores: personas que guían a otros de maneras positivas.

mercurio: metal plateado que es líquido a temperatura ambiente; se encuentra naturalmente en el carbón, el petróleo y otros combustibles.

metabolismo: ritmo al cual el cuerpo usa energía para llevar a cabo procesos fisiológicos básicos.

metástasis: extender desde un lugar de origen a otras partes del cuerpo.

metanfetamina: estimulante sintético extremadamente adictivo; es lo suficientemente poderoso como para que una persona pueda desarrollar una adicción al primer uso.

Staphylococcus aureus resistente a la meticilina (SARM): enfermedad peligrosa causada por el *Staphylococcus aureus* resistente a antibióticos; puede infectar la piel, los huesos, los pulmones y el torrente sanguíneo.

edad adulta media: etapa de desarrollo entre los 40 y 65 años de edad.

infancia media: etapa de desarrollo entre los cinco y 12 años de edad.

hitos: eventos que indican el desarrollo de habilidades y cualidades de maduración.

atención plena: estado de conciencia concentrada y libre de juicio de lo que está sucediendo en el momento actual.

reducción del estrés basada en la atención plena (REBAP): acto de usar técnicas de relajación, como respiración profunda, visualización, atención enfocada y movimientos guiados, con un enfoque intenso en el presente.

mentalidad: patrón de pensamiento, actitud y estado de ánimo de la persona.

minerales: nutrientes inorgánicos absorbidos de plantas, agua y fuentes de alimentos para animales.

menores: personas menores de 18 años.

malentendidos: fallas en la comunicación que conducen al conflicto.

moho: hongo que crece en zonas húmedas.

mononucleosis: enfermedad causada por el Virus de Epstein-Barr (VEB); provoca fiebre, dolor de garganta, fatiga, ganglios linfáticos inflamados e inflamación del bazo; también se la llama *enfermedad del beso*.

cambios de humor: cambios repentinos en la emoción.

dismorfia muscular: trastorno que se caracteriza por una necesidad extrema de volverse más musculoso.

English

MyPlate: food guidance system created by the US Department of Agriculture (USDA); reminds people about the proportions of the five different food groups they should eat at a meal.

Español

MyPlate: sistema de orientación alimentaria creado por el Departamento de Agricultura de los EEUU (US Department of Agriculture, USDA); recuerda a las personas las proporciones de los cinco grupos de alimentos diferentes que se deben ingerir en una comida.

N

natural disasters: emergencies caused by naturally occurring events, such as floods, earthquakes, wildfires, or hurricanes; cause great damage or loss of life.

desastres naturales: emergencias provocadas por eventos naturales, como inundaciones, terremotos, incendios forestales o huracanes; causan grandes daños o pérdidas de vidas.

natural methods: contraceptive methods that time sexual activity with a female's menstrual cycle and the sexual response cycle to prevent the sperm and egg from meeting.

métodos naturales: métodos anticonceptivos que regulan la actividad sexual en función del ciclo menstrual femenino y el ciclo de respuesta sexual para evitar que el esperma y el óvulo se encuentren.

natural resources: materials in the natural environment that people can use, such as water, oil, timber, and soil.

recursos naturales: materiales en el entorno natural que las personas pueden usar, como agua, petróleo, madera y tierra.

negative peer pressure: social pressure among people of the same age or status that encourages unhealthy behaviors or is not respectful.

presión negativa de pares: presión social entre personas de la misma edad o estatus que fomenta comportamientos poco saludables o no es respetuosa.

neglect: form of child abuse that occurs when an adult intentionally or unintentionally does not meet a child's basic physical, emotional, medical, or educational needs.

negligencia: forma de abuso infantil que ocurre cuando un adulto, con o sin intención, no satisface las necesidades físicas, emocionales, médicas o educativas básicas de un niño.

negotiation: process of working together to resolve conflict and find acceptable solutions; involves identifying the cause, asking for solutions from both parties, agreeing on and carrying out a solution, and evaluating the solution and renegotiating, if necessary.

negociación: proceso de trabajar juntos para resolver conflictos y encontrar soluciones aceptables; implica identificar la causa, pedir soluciones a ambas partes, acordar y llevar a cabo una solución, y evaluar la solución y renegociar, si es necesario.

nervous system: body system that consists of the brain, spinal cord, and nerves that trade information throughout the body.

sistema nervioso: sistema corporal que consiste en el cerebro, la médula espinal y los nervios que intercambian información en todo el cuerpo.

nicotine: toxic substance that gives tobacco products their addictive quality.

nicotina: sustancia tóxica que le da a los productos de tabaco su cualidad adictiva.

nicotine replacement: treatment for nicotine addiction that continues to put some nicotine into the body; lessens withdrawal symptoms and cravings, making it easier to quit.

reemplazo de nicotina: tratamiento para la adicción a la nicotina que continúa introduciendo algo de nicotina en el cuerpo; disminuye los síntomas de abstinencia y los antojos, facilitándole a la persona que deje de fumar.

nocturnal emissions: release of semen during the night while a male is sleeping.

emisiones nocturnas: liberación de semen durante la noche mientras un varón duerme.

noise pollution: exposure to unnatural, harmful noise.

contaminación acústica: exposición a ruidos no naturales y nocivos.

noise-related hearing loss: condition in which hearing worsens due to exposure to loud or long-lasting sounds.

pérdida auditiva relacionada con el ruido: condición en la que la audición empeora debido a la exposición a sonidos fuertes o duraderos.

nonbinary: identifying with a gender that falls outside the categories of man or woman.

no binario: identificarse con un género que queda fuera de las categorías de hombre o mujer.

noncommunicable diseases: health conditions that develop over time as a result of genes, environment, and behaviors; do not spread between living organisms and objects.

enfermedades no transmisibles: condiciones de salud que se desarrollan con el tiempo como resultado de genes, medio ambiente y comportamientos; no se propaga entre organismos vivos y objetos.

English

noncustodial parent: individual who is not the primary custody holder of a child, but who has a legal obligation to contribute child support.

nonverbal communication: use of body language, tone and volume of voice, and other wordless signals to send a message.

nutrient-dense foods: foods that provide vitamins, minerals, and other substances that either contribute to adequate nutrition intake or have positive health effects; contain little or no saturated fats, added sugars, refined starches, and sodium.

nutrients: chemical substances that provide the nutrition essential for growth, energy, and function.

nutrition: process of choosing and consuming food necessary for health and growth.

Nutrition Facts label: Food and Drug Administration (FDA)-required label on all packaged foods; contains information about serving size, number of servings, number of calories, amounts of different nutrients, and daily values for nutrients.

O

obesity: condition of excess body fat or excessive overweight.

obstetrician/gynecologist (OB/GYN): doctor who specializes in the health of the female reproductive system; also specializes in pregnancy, labor, and delivery.

older adulthood: developmental stage from 65 years of age until the end of life.

online etiquette: positive behaviors and effective communication techniques that are expected online.

opioids: prescription medications that relieve severe or long-lasting pain.

opportunistic infections: diseases that develop by taking advantage of a weakened immune system.

optimal health: state of excellent health and wellness, including physical, mental and emotional, and social health.

optimistic: expecting good outcomes for actions and feeling or showing hope for the future.

oral contraceptives: medications containing hormones that stop ovulation; are taken every day.

organ donation: act of allowing your organs to be donated and transplanted into another person, typically upon your death.

organic: produced without the use of chemical fertilizers, pesticides, or other artificial chemicals.

Español

padre sin custodia: individuo que no es el titular principal de la custodia de un menor, pero que tiene la obligación legal de contribuir con la manutención de los hijos.

comunicación no verbal: uso del lenguaje corporal, tono y volumen de voz y otras señales sin palabras para enviar un mensaje.

alimentos ricos en nutrientes: alimentos que proporcionan vitaminas, minerales y otras sustancias que contribuyen a una ingesta nutricional adecuada o tienen efectos positivos para la salud; contienen poca o ninguna grasa saturada, azúcares agregados, almidones refinados y sodio.

nutrientes: sustancias químicas que proporcionan la nutrición esencial para el crecimiento, la energía y la función.

nutrición: proceso de elección y consumo de alimentos necesarios para la salud y el crecimiento.

etiqueta de información nutricional: etiqueta requerida por la Administración de Alimentos y Medicamentos (Food and Drug Administration, FDA) en todos los alimentos envasados; contiene información sobre el tamaño de la porción, cantidad de porciones, cantidad de calorías, cantidades de diferentes nutrientes y los valores diarios de nutrientes.

obesidad: condición de exceso de grasa corporal o sobrepeso excesivo.

obstetra / ginecólogo (OB/GYN): médico que se especializa en la salud del sistema reproductivo femenino; también se especializa en embarazo, trabajo de parto y parto.

edad adulta mayor: etapa de desarrollo desde los 65 años hasta el final de la vida.

etiqueta en línea: comportamientos positivos y técnicas efectivas de comunicación que se esperan en línea.

opioides: medicamentos con receta que alivian el dolor intenso o prolongado.

infecciones oportunistas: enfermedades que se desarrollan aprovechando un sistema inmunológico debilitado.

salud óptima: estado de salud y bienestar excelente, que incluye la salud física, mental, emocional y social.

optimista: esperar buenos resultados para las acciones y sentir o mostrar esperanza para el futuro.

anticonceptivos orales: medicamentos que contienen hormonas que detienen la ovulación; se toman todos los días.

donación de órganos: acto de permitir que tus órganos sean donados y trasplantados a otra persona, generalmente después de tu muerte.

orgánico: producido sin el uso de fertilizantes químicos, pesticidas u otros productos químicos artificiales.

English

orgasm: climax of sexual excitement characterized by pleasurable muscular contractions in the reproductive organs and throughout the body.

oropharyngeal cancer: abnormal cancerous growths on the back of the throat, base of the tongue, and tonsils; often caused by the human papillomavirus (HPV).

orthorexia: disordered eating pattern characterized by an obsession with healthy eating; leads to negative consequences.

osteoarthritis: disease in which the cartilage normally padding the surfaces of bones wears down, causing swelling and pain.

osteoporosis: disease that makes bones weak, brittle, and prone to fractures.

outlook: way of thinking or feeling about a situation.

outpatient facilities: healthcare facilities that patients visit for treatment and then leave.

ovarian cysts: noncancerous tumors on the ovaries.

ovaries: two small, almond-shaped organs in the lower abdomen that contain thousands of immature eggs.

overdose: act of taking more of a substance than the body can break down at one time; can lead to serious health consequences and death.

overnutrition: form of malnutrition caused by consuming too many of some nutrients.

over-the-counter (OTC) medications: substances that can legally be sold without permission from a healthcare professional in a particular country.

overweight: condition of excess body weight from fat, bone, muscle, water, or a combination of these factors.

ovulation: release of a mature egg from one of the ovarian follicles.

oxytocin: hormone released during sexual activity that promotes bonding and connection.

P

pandemic: disease that spreads to much of the world.

panic attacks: episodes of intense fear characterized by fast heartbeat, dizziness, shaking, trouble breathing, and chest pain.

parasites: microorganisms that live on or inside other organisms (*hosts*).

particulates: tiny particles suspended in the air.

passion: typically short-lived attraction, based on physical attraction rather than a deeper, longer-lasting emotional connection.

passive: hiding or not clearly stating needs, wants, and feelings.

Español

orgasmo: clímax de excitación sexual caracterizado por contracciones musculares placenteras en los órganos reproductivos y en todo el cuerpo.

cáncer orofaríngeo: crecimientos cancerosos anormales en la parte posterior de la garganta, la base de la lengua y las amígdalas; a menudo causada por el virus del papiloma humano (VPH).

ortorexia: patrón de alimentación desordenado que se caracteriza por una obsesión con una alimentación saludable; conduce a consecuencias negativas.

osteoartritis: enfermedad en la cual el cartílago que normalmente recubre las superficies de los huesos se desgasta, causando hinchazón y dolor.

osteoporosis: enfermedad que debilita los huesos, los hace quebradizos y propensos a fracturas.

perspectiva: forma de pensar o sentir acerca de una situación.

instalaciones para pacientes ambulatorios: instalaciones de atención médica que visitan los pacientes para recibir tratamiento y luego se van.

quistes ováricos: tumores no cancerosos en los ovarios.

ovarios: dos órganos pequeños con forma de almendra en la parte inferior del abdomen que contienen miles de óvulos inmaduros.

sobredosis: acto de tomar más sustancia de la que el cuerpo puede descomponer a la vez; puede conducir a graves consecuencias para la salud e incluso la muerte.

sobrenutrición: forma de malnutrición causada por el consumo de demasiados nutrientes.

medicamentos de venta libre (over-the-counter, OTC): sustancias que se pueden vender legalmente sin permiso de un profesional de la salud en un país en particular.

sobrepeso: condición de exceso de peso corporal por grasa, hueso, músculo, agua o una combinación de estos factores.

ovulación: liberación de un óvulo maduro de uno de los folículos ováricos.

oxitocina: hormona liberada durante la actividad sexual que promueve la unión y la conexión.

pandemia: enfermedad que se propaga a gran parte del mundo.

ataques de pánico: episodios de miedo intenso caracterizados por latidos cardíacos rápidos, mareos, temblores, dificultad para respirar y dolor en el pecho.

parásitos: microorganismos que viven encima o dentro de otros organismos (*huéspedes*).

partículas: pequeñas partículas suspendidas en el aire.

pasión: atracción de corta duración, por lo general, la cual se basa en la atracción física en lugar de una conexión emocional más profunda y duradera.

pasivo: esconder o no indicar claramente las necesidades, deseos y sentimientos.

English

passive-aggressive: using techniques that do not clearly state needs, wants, and feelings to make demands of and insult others.

pathogens: disease-causing microorganisms.

pedestrians: people on foot or using methods of transportation with small wheels (for example, bicycles, skateboards, or wheelchairs).

peer mediation: process in which specially trained students work with other students to resolve conflicts.

peer pressure: social pressure among people of the same age or status; can make people feel like they need to do and like the same things to be liked or respected.

pelvic inflammatory disease (PID): infection of the fallopian tubes and pelvic cavity that sometimes leads to infertility.

penis: male organ used in sexual activity; also part of the urinary system.

Per- and Polyfluoroalkyl Substances (PFAS): chemicals used to make some nonstick coatings on cookware and water- and stain-resistant fabrics.

perfectionism: personal standard or attitude that rejects anything less than ideal performance.

performance-enhancing drugs (PEDs): medications that people abuse in hopes of improving strength, speed, and stamina.

personality: combination of thoughts, feelings, and behaviors that make a person unique.

personality disorders: mental illnesses characterized by consistent patterns of inappropriate behavior.

pessimistic: expecting only bad outcomes for actions and feeling unhopeful for the future.

pesticides: chemicals used to destroy insects or other organisms that harm plants or animals.

phagocyte: white blood cell that specializes in engulfing and destroying pathogens, especially bacteria.

phishing: pretending to represent companies or government agencies and asking for personal information.

phobia: extreme, unrealistic fear of an object or situation.

physical abuse: behaviors that cause bodily harm to another person.

physical activity: any action in which the body uses energy.

Español

pasivo-agresivo: uso de técnicas que no establecen claramente las necesidades, deseos y sentimientos para exigir e insultar a los demás.

patógenos: microorganismos causantes de enfermedades.

peatones: personas a pie o que utilizan medios de transporte con ruedas pequeñas (por ejemplo: bicicletas, patinetas o sillas de ruedas).

mediación entre pares: proceso en el que estudiantes especialmente capacitados trabajan con otros estudiantes para resolver conflictos.

presión de los compañeros: presión social entre personas de la misma edad o estatus; puede hacer que las personas sientan que deben hacer y que les deben gustar las mismas cosas para que sean aceptados o respetados.

enfermedad inflamatoria pélvica (pelvic inflammatory disease, PID): infección de las trompas de Falopio y la cavidad pélvica que algunas veces conduce a la infertilidad.

pene: órgano masculino utilizado en la actividad sexual; también forma parte del sistema urinario.

sustancias per- y polifluroalquiladas (PFAS): productos químicos utilizados para hacer algunos recubrimientos antiadherentes en utensilios de cocina como así también telas resistentes al agua y a las manchas.

perfeccionismo: estándar o actitud personal que rechaza cualquier cosa menos que el rendimiento ideal.

medicamentos para mejorar el rendimiento (performance-enhancing drugs, PED): medicamentos que las personas abusan con la esperanza de mejorar la fuerza, la velocidad y la resistencia.

personalidad: combinación de pensamientos, sentimientos y comportamientos que hacen que una persona sea única.

trastornos de la personalidad: enfermedades mentales caracterizadas por patrones constantes de comportamiento inapropiado.

pesimista: que espera solo malos resultados para las acciones y se siente desafortunado para el futuro.

pesticidas: productos químicos utilizados para destruir insectos u otros organismos que dañan las plantas o los animales.

fagocito: glóbulo blanco que se especializa en envolver y destruir patógenos, especialmente bacterias.

phishing: pretender representar a empresas o agencias gubernamentales y solicitar información personal.

fobia: miedo extremo, poco realista a un objeto o situación.

abuso físico: comportamientos que causan daño corporal a otra persona.

actividad física: cualquier acción en la cual el cuerpo usa energía.

English

Physical Activity Guidelines for Americans: recommendations published by the US Department of Health and Human Services about how much physical activity children, teens, and adults should get.

physical disability: condition that affects a person's physical abilities and makes certain tasks more difficult.

physical fitness: body's ability to perform daily activities and meet unexpected demands with energy to spare.

physical health: dimension of health that refers to how well the body functions.

pinkeye: infection of the surface of the eye; causes itchy, red, watery eyes and dry crust on the eyelids.

placenta: merged embryonic chorion and endometrial tissue that helps support the developing baby.

pneumonia: infection in which tiny air sacs in the lungs swell, making breathing difficult.

poisonous: capable of causing illness or death on entering the body.

pollen: dry, dusty powder made by flowers.

pollution: presence of waste in the environment.

popcorn lung: condition that damages the lungs' smallest airways; leads to coughing and shortness of breath.

positive peer pressure: social pressure among people of the same age or status that contributes to good health and can be beneficial.

positive reappraisal: act of thinking about the good aspects of stressful events.

post-exposure prophylaxis (PEP): emergency course of antiretroviral therapy (ART) that a person can take within 72 hours of potential exposure to human immunodeficiency virus (HIV).

post-traumatic stress disorder (PTSD): stress-related disorder characterized by flashbacks, feelings of numbness, and difficulty sleeping after an extremely stressful event.

pre-exposure prophylaxis (PrEP): combination of two medications in one pill taken daily to prevent human immunodeficiency virus (HIV) transmission.

premenstrual syndrome (PMS): symptoms that start one to two weeks before menstruation and stop when menstruation begins; include breast tenderness, acne, bloating, headaches, mood swings, or fatigue.

Español

Pautas de Actividad Física para Estadounidenses: recomendaciones publicadas por el Departamento de Salud y Servicios Humanos de EE.UU. sobre la cantidad de actividad física que deben realizar los niños, adolescentes y adultos.

discapacidad física: condición que afecta las capacidades físicas de una persona y hace que ciertas tareas sean más difíciles.

aptitud física: la capacidad del cuerpo para realizar actividades diarias y satisfacer demandas inesperadas con energía de sobra.

salud física: aspecto de la salud que hace referencia a cómo funciona el cuerpo.

conjuntivitis: infección de la superficie del ojo; provoca picazón, lagrimeo y enrojecimiento de los ojos y costra seca en los párpados.

placenta: corion embrionario y tejido endometrial fusionados que ayuda a apoyar al bebé en desarrollo.

neumonía: infección en la que se hinchan pequeños sacos de aire en los pulmones, lo que dificulta la respiración.

venenoso: capaz de causar una enfermedad o la muerte al ingresar al cuerpo.

polen: polvillo seco hecho de flores.

contaminación: presencia de residuos en el medio ambiente.

pulmón de palomitas de maíz: afección que daña las vías respiratorias más pequeñas de los pulmones; provoca tos y falta de aliento.

presión positiva de pares: presión social entre personas de la misma edad o estatus que contribuye a la buena salud y puede ser beneficiosa.

reevaluación positiva: acto de pensar sobre los buenos aspectos de los eventos estresantes.

profilaxis posterior a la exposición (post-exposure prophylaxis, PEP): curso de emergencia de la terapia antirretroviral (TAR) que una persona puede tomar dentro de las 72 horas después a una posible exposición al virus de la inmunodeficiencia humana (VIH).

trastorno de estrés postraumático (post-traumatic stress disorder, PTSD): trastorno relacionado con el estrés caracterizado por recuerdos retrospectivos, sensación de entumecimiento y dificultad para dormir después de un evento extremadamente estresante.

profilaxis previa a la exposición (pre-exposure prophylaxis, PrEP): combinación de dos medicamentos en una píldora tomada diariamente para prevenir la transmisión del virus de inmunodeficiencia humana (VIH).

síndrome premenstrual (premenstrual syndrome, PMS): síntomas que comienzan una o dos semanas antes de la menstruación y se detienen cuando comienza la menstruación; incluyen sensibilidad en sénoslas mamas, acné, hinchazón, dolores de cabeza, cambios de humor o fatiga.

English

prenatal care: healthcare for the developing baby and pregnant person before birth.

prenatal development: changes that occur when a zygote develops into a baby during the nine months of pregnancy.

prescription medications: substances that can legally be sold only with permission from a doctor or other qualified healthcare professional.

pressure: motivation to do an activity or take on certain qualities; can be internal or external.

preventive healthcare: medical care that seeks to prevent health conditions from developing; includes annual physical or wellness exams, checkups, vaccinations, and screenings.

primary care physician (PCP): healthcare professional who provides routine checkups, screenings, treatments, prescriptions, and preventive services.

primary sexual characteristics: puberty-related physical changes in the reproductive organs (penis, testes, ovaries, and vagina).

privacy settings: features for controlling who can see personal information online.

professional communication: process of sending and receiving messages in a formal environment, such as a workplace or school.

prognosis: statement about the likely outcome of a disease; made by a medical professional.

progressive muscle relaxation: relaxation technique that involves tensing and then relaxing each part of the body until the whole body feels relaxed.

prostate cancer: abnormal cancerous growth of the prostate; signs and symptoms resemble those of prostatitis.

prostate: organ that secretes fluid that mixes with sperm to create semen.

protective factors: aspects of people's lives that reduce risk and increase the likelihood of optimal health.

protein: nutrient the body uses to build and maintain cells and tissues and provide energy; may also act as hormones or enzymes.

pseudoscience: theories and health claims that are described as science-based when they are not.

puberty: physical changes that occur as the body's reproductive system matures.

public health: science-based approach to protecting and improving the health of populations as a whole.

public service announcements (PSAs): media messages that support public health.

purging: attempts to rid the body of food.

Español

atención prenatal: atención médica para el bebé en desarrollo y para la persona embarazada antes del nacimiento.

desarrollo prenatal: cambios que ocurren cuando un cigoto se convierte en un bebé durante los nueve meses de embarazo.

medicamentos con receta: sustancias que pueden venderse legalmente solo con el permiso de un médico u otro profesional de la atención médica calificado.

presión: motivación para realizar una actividad o adquirir ciertas cualidades; puede ser interno o externo.

atención médica preventiva: atención médica que busca prevenir el desarrollo de condiciones de salud; incluye exámenes anuales físicos o de bienestar, chequeos, vacunas y exámenes de detección.

médico de atención primaria (primary care physician, PCP): profesional de la salud que brinda chequeos de rutina, exámenes, tratamientos, recetas y servicios preventivos.

características sexuales primarias: cambios físicos relacionados con la pubertad en los órganos reproductivos (pene, testículos, ovarios y vagina).

configuración de privacidad: funciones para controlar quién puede ver información personal en línea.

comunicación profesional: proceso de envío y recepción de mensajes en un entorno formal, como un lugar de trabajo o una escuela.

pronóstico: declaración sobre el resultado probable de una enfermedad; hecho de un profesional de la salud.

relajación muscular progresiva: técnica de relajación que implica tensar y luego relajar cada parte del cuerpo hasta que todo el cuerpo se sienta relajado.

cáncer de próstata: crecimiento canceroso anormal de la próstata; las señales y los síntomas se parecen a los de la prostatitis.

próstata: órgano que secreta líquido que se mezcla con esperma para crear semen.

factores protectores: aspectos de la vida de las personas que reducen el riesgo y aumentan la probabilidad de una salud óptima.

proteína: nutriente que el cuerpo usa para construir y mantener células y tejidos y proporcionar energía; también puede actuar como hormonas o enzimas.

pseudociencia: teorías y declaraciones de salud que se describen como basadas en la ciencia cuando no lo están.

pubertad: cambios físicos que ocurren a medida que madura el sistema reproductivo del cuerpo.

salud pública: enfoque basado en la ciencia para proteger y mejorar la salud de las poblaciones en su conjunto.

anuncios de servicio público (public service announcements, PSA): mensajes de medios que apoyan la salud pública.

purga: intentos de limpiar al cuerpo de alimentos.

English

purpose: stable and generalized intention to accomplish something that is both meaningful to the self and consequential for the world beyond the self.

Q

quality of life: extent to which a person experiences a healthy, happy, and fulfilling life.

R

radon: colorless, odorless, tasteless gas produced naturally from soil and rocks that contain uranium.

rape: sexual intercourse that occurs without consent.

recessive genes: deoxyribonucleic acid (DNA) segments that only cause certain characteristics if the child has inherited a recessive gene from both parents.

reciprocal: shared or exhibited by both sides.

recycling: treating or processing used or waste products to make them suitable for reuse.

refusal skills: set of skills designed to help someone avoid participating in unhealthy behaviors.

rehabilitation program: treatment for a substance use disorder in which a healthcare professional oversees recovery; may involve a combination of medicinal and behavioral treatment.

reinfection: recurrence of a communicable disease.

relapse: (1) act of taking a substance again after deciding to stop; (2) recurrence of a disease, in which signs and symptoms return after a period of remission.

relationships: connections that people form and maintain with others.

relaxation response: physiological reaction in which the body returns to its resting state after a stressful event.

remission: period of time without signs and symptoms associated with a disease.

renewable energy: energy that comes from the Earth's natural resources, such as wind, water, and sunlight; cannot be used up.

reproductive system: body system consisting of organs that work together to create new human life; is different between males and females.

resilience: ability to recover from traumatic and stressful events.

Resource Conservation and Recovery Act: federal law that provides rules and regulations about the management of hazardous wastes.

Español

propósito: intención estable y generalizada de lograr algo que sea significativo para el ser y consecuente para el mundo más allá del ser.

calidad de vida: medida en que una persona experimenta una vida sana, feliz y satisfactoria.

radón: gas incoloro, inodoro e insípido producido naturalmente a partir del suelo y rocas que contienen uranio.

violación: relaciones sexuales que ocurren sin consentimiento.

genes recesivos: segmentos de ácido desoxirribonucleico (ADN) que solo causan ciertas características si el niño ha heredado un gen recesivo de ambos padres.

recíproco: compartido o exhibido por ambas partes.

reciclaje: tratamiento o procesamiento de productos usados o de desecho para hacerlos adecuados para su reutilización.

habilidades de rechazo: conjunto de habilidades diseñadas para ayudar a alguien a evitar participar en comportamientos poco saludables.

programa de rehabilitación: tratamiento para un trastorno por uso de sustancias en el que un profesional de la salud supervisa la recuperación; podría implicar una combinación de tratamiento medicinal y conductual.

reinfección: recurrencia de una enfermedad contagiosa.

recaída: (1) acto de tomar una sustancia nuevamente después de decidir parar; (2) recurrencia de una enfermedad, en la cual las señales y los síntomas regresan después de un período de remisión.

relaciones: conexiones que las personas forman y mantienen con los demás.

respuesta de relajación: reacción fisiológica en la que el cuerpo vuelve a su estado de reposo después de un evento estresante.

remisión: período de tiempo sin señales ni síntomas asociados con una enfermedad.

energía renovable: energía que proviene de los recursos naturales de la Tierra, como el viento, el agua y la luz solar; no se puede agotar.

sistema reproductivo: sistema del cuerpo que consiste en órganos que trabajan juntos para crear una nueva vida humana; es diferente entre el varón y la hembra.

resiliencia: capacidad para recuperarse de eventos traumáticos y estresantes.

Ley de Conservación y Recuperación de Recursos: ley federal que proporciona reglas y regulaciones sobre el manejo de desechos peligrosos.

English

respect: acknowledgment that each person has worth and deserves to have needs met; is shown through kindness and considerate behavior.

respiratory etiquette: behaviors that prevent the spread of disease through droplets.

response substitution: treatment for nicotine addiction where people practice responding to difficult feelings and situations using stress management, relaxation, and coping skills instead of tobacco use.

rheumatoid arthritis: autoimmune disease in which the body's immune system attacks the joints, causing swelling and pain.

risk factors: aspects of people's lives that increase the chances they will develop a disease or disorder or experience an injury or decline in health.

roofies: club drug made of Rohypnol® that makes a person unable to move or respond to events.

rumination: act of thinking deeply or obsessively about negative feelings or situations.

S

Safe Drinking Water Act: federal law that requires drinking water be tested for more than 90 different pollutants.

safe haven laws: legislation that permits people to leave their babies at certain facilities with no questions asked; aim to protect babies from abandonment; also called *safe surrender laws.*

safe zones: spaces where students can go to feel safe and supported, no matter what.

same-sex marriage: legal marriage between two people of the same biological sex.

sandwich generation: adults who are caring for aging parents or family members and their own children.

saturated fats: type of fat found primarily in animal-based foods; are typically solid at room temperature.

schizophrenia spectrum disorders: mental illnesses characterized by irregular thoughts, delusions, and hallucinations.

school violence: any violent behavior that occurs on school property, at school-sponsored events, or on the way to or from school or school events.

science: body of knowledge based on observation and experimentation; answers questions about the natural world.

Español

respeto: reconocimiento de que cada persona tiene valor y merece que se satisfagan sus necesidades; se muestra a través de la amabilidad y el comportamiento considerado.

etiqueta respiratoria: conductas que evitan la propagación de la enfermedad a través de microgotas.

sustitución de la respuesta: tratamiento para la adicción a la nicotina en el que las personas practican responder a sentimientos y situaciones difíciles utilizando el manejo del estrés, la relajación y las habilidades para superar las situaciones en lugar del consumo de tabaco.

artritis reumatoide: enfermedad autoinmune en la cual el sistema inmunológico del cuerpo ataca las articulaciones, causando hinchazón y dolor.

factores de riesgo: aspectos de las vidas de las personas que aumentan sus posibilidades de desarrollar una enfermedad o un trastorno, o de experimentar una lesión o deterioro de la salud.

roofies: droga de club hecha de Rohypnol® que hace que una persona no pueda moverse o responder a los eventos.

rumiación: acto de pensar profunda u obsesivamente sobre sentimientos o situaciones negativas

Ley de Agua Potable Segura: la ley federal que exige que el agua potable se analice en más de 90 contaminantes diferentes.

leyes de refugio seguro: legislación que permite a las personas dejar a sus bebés en ciertas instalaciones sin hacer preguntas; su objetivo es proteger a los bebés del abandono; también denominadas *leyes de entrega segura.*

zonas seguras: espacios donde los estudiantes pueden ir para sentirse seguros y apoyados, independientemente de lo que ocurra.

matrimonio del mismo sexo: matrimonio legal entre dos personas del mismo sexo biológico.

generación sándwich: adultos que cuidan a sus padres o miembros de la familia que están envejeciendo y a sus propios hijos.

grasa saturada: tipo de grasa que se encuentra principalmente en alimentos de origen animal; por lo general es sólida a temperatura ambiente.

trastornos del espectro esquizofrénico: enfermedades mentales caracterizadas por pensamientos irregulares, delirios y alucinaciones.

violencia escolar: cualquier comportamiento violento que ocurre en la propiedad escolar, en eventos patrocinados por la escuela o en el recorrido hacia o desde la escuela o en eventos escolares.

ciencia: cuerpo de conocimiento basado en observación y experimentación; responde preguntas sobre el mundo natural.

English

secondary sexual characteristics: puberty-related physical changes in parts of the body besides the reproductive organs; for example, growth of hair, deeper voice, or breast development.

secondhand aerosol: suspension of fine particles that people inhale involuntarily when someone nearby is vaping.

secondhand smoke: smoke that people inhale involuntarily when someone nearby is smoking.

sedentary behaviors: activities that consist of sitting or lying down and using very little energy.

self-actualization: feeling of reaching one's full potential through creativity, independence, spontaneity, and a grasp of the real world.

self-care: process of actively taking care of one's own well-being and health, especially during periods of stress.

self-compassion: attitude of kindness and understanding toward one's self, even when experiencing setbacks and disappointments.

self-esteem: confidence in one's own worth and abilities.

self-image: mental picture of one's abilities, appearance, and personality based on experiences and interactions with others.

self-medicate: to abuse medications or drugs to cope with symptoms of a health condition.

self-respect: pride and confidence in one's self.

self-talk: one's thoughts about one's self throughout the day.

semen: mixture of fluid and sperm released during ejaculation.

sexting: sending sexual content in the form of digital text, pictures, or videos.

sexual abstinence: decision to refrain from sexual activity for physical, social, or emotional reasons.

sexual abuse: behaviors that involve sexual activity to which one person does not or cannot consent.

sexual activity: actions that involve contact with a person's reproductive organs; can include sexual intercourse and other activities.

sexual assault: act of threatening, pressuring, or forcing someone into sexual activity.

sexual harassment: verbal or nonverbal sexual attention that occurs without consent.

sexual history: information about a person's past sexual activity and partners.

Español

características sexuales secundarias: cambios físicos relacionados con la pubertad en partes del cuerpo además de los órganos reproductivos; por ejemplo, crecimiento de vellos, voz más profunda o desarrollo de los senos.

aerosol de segunda mano: pequeñas partículas en suspensión que inhalan las personas involuntariamente cuando alguien está vapeando cerca.

humo de segunda mano: humo que inhalan involuntariamente las personas cuando alguien está fumando cerca.

comportamientos sedentarios: actividades que consisten en sentarse o acostarse y consumen muy poca energía.

autorrealización: sentimiento de alcanzar el máximo potencial propio a través de la creatividad, la independencia, la espontaneidad y la comprensión del mundo real.

autocuidado: proceso de cuidar activamente la propia plenitud y salud, especialmente durante los períodos de estrés.

autocompasión: actitud de amabilidad y comprensión hacia uno mismo, incluso cuando se experimentan contratiempos y decepciones.

autoestima: confianza en el valor y las capacidades de uno mismo.

autoimagen: imagen mental de las capacidades, apariencia y personalidad de uno mismo basado en experiencias e interacciones con los demás.

automedicarse: abusar de medicamentos o drogas para superar los síntomas de una afección de salud.

autoestima: orgullo y confianza en uno mismo.

diálogo interno: los pensamientos sobre uno mismo durante el día.

semen: mezcla de líquido y esperma liberado durante la eyaculación.

sexting: envío de contenido sexual en forma de texto digital, imágenes o vídeos.

abstinencia sexual: decisión de abstenerse de la actividad sexual por razones físicas, sociales o emocionales.

abuso sexual: comportamientos que implican actividad sexual para la cual una persona no da su consentimiento o no puede dar su consentimiento.

actividad sexual: acciones que implican contacto con los órganos reproductivos de una persona; puede incluir relaciones sexuales y otras actividades.

agresión sexual: acto de amenazar, presionar u obligar a alguien a tener actividad sexual.

acoso sexual: atención sexual verbal o no verbal que ocurre sin consentimiento.

historia sexual: información sobre la actividad sexual pasada de una persona y sus parejas.

English

sexual intercourse: sexual activity that involves penetration, or insertion of a body part or object into another body part.

sexual orientation: enduring pattern of a person's romantic and/or sexual attraction to other people.

sexual reproduction: process in which the genetic material of two individuals combines to create a new individual.

sexual violence: sexual behaviors that occur without consent.

sexuality: element of identity that includes a person's biological sex, gender identity and expression, sexual orientation, and sexual experiences and thoughts.

sexually transmitted infections (STIs): communicable diseases that spread from one person to another during sexual activity; also called *sexually transmitted diseases (STDs).*

shock: life-threatening condition in which the vital organs do not receive enough blood and oxygen.

sibling abuse: chronic physical, emotional, or sexual mistreatment of one sibling by another.

sibling rivalry: competitive feelings between siblings; siblings may compete for material or nonmaterial items.

side effects: unintended changes that develop in response to a medication.

skill-related fitness: ability to perform successfully in a particular sport or leisure activity.

SMART goal: endpoint that is specific, measurable, achievable, relevant, and timely.

smokeless tobacco: tobacco product that is chewed or snuffed rather than smoked.

social health: dimension of health that refers to how well a person gets along with others.

socialize: to teach to behave in ways society accepts.

specialists: healthcare professionals who have additional training in treating certain types of diseases and disorders.

sperm: male sex cells made up of a flagellum and nucleus; contain half of the male's chromosomes.

spermicide: substance that inactivates sperm.

sprain: injury to a ligament.

stalking: following and repeatedly contacting someone in a way that causes the person to feel scared, nervous, or threatened.

Español

relaciones sexuales: actividad sexual que implica penetración o inserción de una parte del cuerpo u objeto en otra parte del cuerpo.

orientación sexual: patrón duradero de la atracción romántica y/o sexual de una persona hacia otras personas.

reproducción sexual: proceso en el cual el material genético de dos individuos se combina para crear un nuevo individuo.

violencia sexual: conductas sexuales que ocurren sin consentimiento.

sexualidad: elemento de identidad que incluye el sexo biológico, identidad y expresión de género, orientación sexual y experiencias y pensamientos sexuales de una persona.

infecciones de transmisión sexual (ITS): enfermedades transmisibles que se transmiten de una persona a otra durante la actividad sexual; también llamadas *enfermedades de transmisión sexual (ETS).*

choque: condición potencialmente mortal en la que los órganos vitales no reciben suficiente sangre y oxígeno.

abuso de hermanos: abuso crónico físico, emocional o sexual de un hermano por otro.

rivalidad entre hermanos: sentimientos competitivos entre hermanos; los hermanos pueden competir por temas materiales o no materiales.

efectos secundarios: cambios no deseados que se desarrollan en respuesta a un medicamento.

estado físico relacionado con la habilidad: capacidad para desempeñarse de forma exitosa en un deporte en particular o actividad de ocio.

meta SMART: punto final que es específico (specific), mensurable (measurable), alcanzable (achievable), relevante (relevant) y oportuno (timely).

tabaco sin humo: producto de tabaco que se mastica o se inhala en lugar de fumarlo.

salud social: aspecto de la salud que hace referencia a qué tan bien se relaciona una persona con los demás.

socializar: enseñar a comportarse de una manera aceptada por la sociedad.

especialistas: profesionales de la salud que tienen capacitación adicional en el tratamiento de ciertos tipos de enfermedades y trastornos.

esperma: células sexuales masculinas formadas por un flagelo y un núcleo; contienen la mitad de los cromosomas masculinos.

espermicida: sustancia que inactiva el esperma.

esguince: lesión de un ligamento.

acecho: seguimiento y contacto reiterado con alguien a través de maneras que provocan que la persona se sienta atemorizada, nerviosa o amenazada.

English

standard precautions: infection control practices to prevent the spread of disease during first aid.

statutory rape: sexual intercourse between an adult and anyone under the age of consent.

stent: fine mesh inserted into an artery to crush and push aside plaque, restoring blood flow.

sterilization: contraceptive method that permanently prevents pregnancy by altering the reproductive system, often through surgery.

stigma: negative, false, unfair beliefs associated with a circumstance, quality, or person.

stimulants: substances that cause the brain to release adrenaline, increasing energy, alertness, and attention.

stimulus control: treatment for nicotine addiction that involves avoiding tempting situations and managing feelings that lead to nicotine use.

stomach flu: infection of the intestines (*gastroenteritis*) caused by the norovirus; characterized by vomiting, diarrhea, fever, and stomach cramps.

strep throat: disease caused by the *Streptococcus* bacterium; characterized by a painful sore throat and swollen, tender tonsils.

stress: body's physical and psychological reactions to situations people perceive as threats.

stress hormones: chemicals that coordinate the fight-or-flight response; include epinephrine, norepinephrine, and cortisol.

stress management: process of using strategies to reduce the impact of the stress response and handle threatening situations in positive ways.

stressors: factors that lead to stress.

stress-related disorder: mental illness that develops as a result of stressful events; examples include acute stress disorder and post-traumatic stress disorder (PTSD).

stroke: medical emergency in which blood vessels in the brain become narrow or blocked or burst, disrupting blood flow to a part of the brain.

substance use disorder: mental illness in which a person continues using a substance despite negative effects on health and life.

suicide: intentional act of ending one's own life.

suicide clusters: series of suicides in a particular community that occur in a relatively short period of time.

suicide contagion: copying of suicide attempts after exposure to another person's suicide.

Español

precauciones estándar: prácticas de control de infecciones para prevenir la propagación de la enfermedad durante los primeros auxilios.

estupro: relaciones sexuales entre un adulto y cualquier persona menor de edad.

stent: malla fina insertada en una arteria para aplastar y apartar la placa, restaurando el flujo sanguíneo.

esterilización: método anticonceptivo que previene de forma permanente el embarazo al alterar el sistema reproductivo, a menudo mediante cirugía.

estigma: creencias negativas, falsas e injustas asociadas con una circunstancia, calidad o persona.

estimulantes: sustancias que hacen que el cerebro libere adrenalina, aumentando la energía, el estado de alerta y la atención.

control de estímulos: tratamiento para la adicción a la nicotina que consiste en evitar las situaciones tentadoras y manejar los sentimientos que conducen al consumo de la nicotina.

gripe estomacal: infección de los intestinos (*gastroenteritis*) causada por el norovirus; caracterizado por vómitos, diarrea, fiebre y dolores estomacales.

faringitis estreptocócica: enfermedad causada por la bacteria *estreptococo*; caracterizada por dolor de garganta doloroso e inflamación y sensibilidad de las amígdalas.

estrés: reacciones físicas y psicológicas del cuerpo ante situaciones que las personas perciben como amenazas.

hormonas del estrés: sustancias químicas que coordinan la respuesta de lucha o huida; incluyen epinefrina, noradrenalina y cortisol.

manejo del estrés: proceso de usar estrategias para reducir el impacto de la respuesta al estrés y manejar situaciones amenazantes de manera positiva.

estresores: factores que conducen al estrés.

trastorno relacionado con el estrés: enfermedad mental que se desarrolla como resultado de eventos estresantes; los ejemplos incluyen trastorno de estrés agudo y trastorno de estrés postraumático (PTSD).

accidente cerebrovascular: emergencia médica en la cual los vasos sanguíneos en el cerebro se estrechan, bloquean o explotan, interrumpiendo el flujo sanguíneo a una parte del cerebro.

trastorno por consumo de sustancias: enfermedad mental en la cual una persona continúa usando una sustancia a pesar de los efectos negativos sobre la salud y la vida.

suicidio: acción intencional de quitarse la vida uno mismo.

grupos de suicidios: series de suicidios en una comunidad en particular que ocurren en un periodo relativamente corto.

contagio de suicidio: copia de intentos de suicidio después de haber estado expuesto al suicidio de otra persona.

English

supervisor: person who oversees one's work in an organization.

support group: treatment method in which people who have faced or are facing similar challenges meet together to discuss obstacles and ways of overcoming them.

survivors: people who have lost someone to suicide.

sustainability: actions that help maintain the natural resources in the environment.

syphilis: bacterial sexually transmitted infection (STI) that is fatal if untreated and has four stages: primary syphilis, secondary syphilis, latent syphilis, and late-stage syphilis.

T

tar: residue consisting of small, thick, sticky particles; builds up in the lungs as a result of smoking.

target heart rate: number of heartbeats per minute that is safe and effective for a given intensity.

technostress: type of stress caused by the constant presence of technology.

teen parenthood: teen's decision to raise a child independently or with the other parent.

teen pregnancy: pregnancy that occurs during the adolescent years when a teen's body is still developing and maturing.

temper tantrum: episode of emotional upset; often includes yelling, crying, hitting, kicking, or biting.

terrorism: ideologically motivated use of violence and threats to frighten and control groups of people.

testes: organs suspended in the scrotum that produce sperm and testosterone.

testicular cancer: abnormal cancerous growth in one or both testes.

testicular self-examination: process of checking the testes for lumps or changes in shape or texture.

tetanus: disease caused by a toxin that leads to painful muscle contractions that can interfere with breathing.

therapist: healthcare professional who diagnoses mental illnesses and delivers therapy.

therapy: treatment method that changes the way a person thinks, interprets information, behaves, and experiences and expresses emotions; involves communicating with a therapist.

thirdhand smoke: particles and gases left over after someone smokes a cigarette; remains on surfaces nearby.

Español

supervisor: persona que supervisa el trabajo en una organización.

grupo de apoyo: método de tratamiento en el que las personas que se han enfrentado o se enfrentan a desafíos similares se reúnen para discutir los obstáculos y las formas de superarlos.

sobrevivientes: personas que han perdido a alguien por suicidio.

sostenibilidad: acciones que mantienen los recursos naturales del medio ambiente.

sífilis: infección de transmisión sexual (ITS) bacteriana que es mortal si no se trata y tiene cuatro etapas: sífilis primaria, sífilis secundaria, sífilis latente y sífilis en etapa tardía.

alquitrán: residuo que consiste en partículas pequeñas, gruesas y pegajosas; se acumula en los pulmones como resultado de fumar.

frecuencia cardíaca objetivo: número de latidos por minuto que es seguro y efectivo para una intensidad dada.

tecnostress: tipo de estrés causado por la presencia constante de tecnología.

paternidad adolescente: decisión del adolescente de criar a un niño independientemente o con el otro padre.

embarazo adolescente: embarazo que ocurre durante los años de la adolescencia cuando el cuerpo de un adolescente aún se está desarrollando y madurando.

rabieta: episodio de malestar emocional a menudo incluye gritar, llorar, golpear, patear o incluso morder.

terrorismo: uso de violencia y amenazas, motivado ideológicamente con el fin de asustar y controlar a grupos de personas.

testículos: órganos suspendidos en el escroto que producen esperma y testosterona.

cáncer testicular: crecimiento canceroso anormal en uno o ambos testículos.

autoexamen testicular: proceso de verificación de los testículos en busca de bultos o cambios en la forma o textura.

tétanos: enfermedad causada por una toxina que provoca contracciones musculares dolorosas que pueden interferir con la respiración.

terapeuta: profesional de la salud que diagnostica enfermedades mentales y brinda terapia.

terapia: método de tratamiento que cambia la forma en que una persona piensa, interpreta información, se comporta y experimenta y expresa emociones; implica comunicarse con un terapeuta.

humo de tercera mano: partículas y gases que quedan después de que alguien fuma un cigarrillo; permanece en superficies cercanas.

English

time management: practice of devoting the appropriate amount of time to each task, only committing to tasks you have time for, and prioritizing tasks; helps people reach goals and reduce stress.

tobacco: plant with leaves that contain the chemical nicotine.

tolerance: body's need for an increased amount of a substance to experience the effects once felt with smaller amounts.

toxic shock syndrome (TSS): medical emergency in which bacteria release toxins that enter the blood.

toxic stress: stress caused by repeated, long-lasting exposure to severe stressors, such as neglect and abuse, violence, or loss of a loved one.

traditions: patterns of behavior passed down in a culture.

***trans* fat**: type of fat historically found in many processed foods; can also occur naturally in animal-based foods.

transgender: identifying with the gender opposite the one that is associated with one's biological sex.

trauma: extreme stress due to deeply disturbing events, such as disasters, sexual assault, or violence.

trichomoniasis: common sexually transmitted infection (STI) caused by a protozoan; is easily treated once diagnosed.

trolling: drawing others into arguments and disrupting discussions.

trust: belief in another person's reliability and good intentions.

tubal ligation: surgical procedure that cuts or blocks the fallopian tubes, permanently preventing pregnancy.

tumor: mass of abnormal cells; may be malignant (cancerous) or benign (noncancerous).

type 1 diabetes mellitus: autoimmune disease in which the body's immune system destroys insulin-producing cells, decreasing levels of insulin and increasing blood sugar; also called *juvenile-onset diabetes* or *insulin-dependent diabetes.*

type 2 diabetes mellitus: disease in which the body's cells become resistant to insulin, increasing blood sugar; also called *adult-onset diabetes* or *insulin-independent diabetes.*

U

undernutrition: form of malnutrition caused by the body not receiving or absorbing needed nutrients.

Español

gestión del tiempo: práctica de dedicar la cantidad de tiempo adecuada a cada tarea, solo comprometiéndose con las tareas para las que tienes tiempo y priorizando las tareas; ayuda a las personas a alcanzar metas y a reducir el estrés.

tabaco: planta con hojas que contienen el químico nicotina.

tolerancia: la necesidad del cuerpo de una cantidad mayor de una sustancia para experimentar los efectos que alguna vez se sintieron con cantidades más pequeñas.

síndrome de choque tóxico (toxic shock syndrome, TSS): emergencia médica en la cual las bacterias liberan toxinas que ingresan a la sangre.

estrés tóxico: estrés causado por la exposición repetida y duradera a estresores severos, como negligencia y abuso, violencia o pérdida de un ser querido.

tradiciones: patrones de comportamiento que se transmiten en una cultura.

grasas *trans*: tipo de grasa históricamente encontrada en muchos alimentos procesados; también puede ocurrir naturalmente en alimentos de origen animal.

transgénero: identificarse con el género opuesto al que está asociado con el sexo biológico de uno.

trauma: estrés extremo debido a eventos profundamente perturbadores, como desastres, agresión sexual o violencia.

tricomoniasis: infección de transmisión sexual (ITS) común causada por un protozoo; se trata fácilmente una vez diagnosticada.

trolling: conducir a otros a enfrentamientos y discusiones perturbadoras.

confianza: creencia en la confiabilidad y buenas intenciones de otra persona.

ligadura de trompas: procedimiento quirúrgico que corta o bloquea las trompas de Falopio, evitando permanentemente el embarazo.

tumor: masa de células anormales; puede ser maligno (canceroso) o benigno (no canceroso).

diabetes mellitus tipo 1: enfermedad autoinmune en la cual el sistema inmunológico del cuerpo destruye las células productoras de insulina, disminuyendo los niveles de insulina y aumentando el azúcar en la sangre; también denominada *diabetes de inicio juvenil* o *diabetes insulinodependiente.*

diabetes mellitus tipo 2: enfermedad en la cual las células del cuerpo se vuelven resistentes a la insulina, aumentando el azúcar en la sangre; también denominada *diabetes de inicio en adultos* o *diabetes no insulinodependiente.*

desnutrición: forma de malnutrición causada por el cuerpo que no recibe o absorbe los nutrientes necesarios.

English

underweight: condition of a body weight that is too low compared with others of the same sex and age.

unsaturated fats: type of fat found in plant-based foods; are liquid at room temperature.

upstander: person who recognizes when a behavior is wrong, takes steps to intervene and stop the behavior, and promotes positive change; also called an *ally*.

uterus: hollow, muscular organ that houses the developing baby until it is born.

V

vaccination: process of introducing a dead pathogen or nontoxic part of a pathogen into the body to provoke an immune response that prevents a certain disease; also called *immunization*.

vaccine: substance containing a dead pathogen or nontoxic part of a pathogen; introduced into the body to provoke an immune response.

vagina: tube-like structure lined with a moist membrane that serves as the birth canal.

vaginal ring: flexible, ring-shaped contraceptive device inserted into the vagina; releases hormones to stop ovulation.

values: qualities or priorities one considers important.

valves: flaps of tissue that control the flow of blood in the heart.

vandalism: deliberate destruction of or damage to someone else's property.

vaping devices: tobacco products that heat tobacco or synthetic nicotine without burning it, producing an aerosol.

vas deferens: tube that carries sperm from the epididymis to the penis.

vasectomy: surgical procedure that cuts or blocks the vas deferens, permanently preventing pregnancy.

veins: blood vessels that deliver blood from the rest of the body back to the heart.

verbal communication: use of words, spoken or written, to send a message.

violent behavior: intentional use of actions or words that cause or threaten to cause harm to a person or object.

viral load: amount of human immunodeficiency virus (HIV) in the blood.

virus: piece of computer code that changes the way a digital device works to disrupt functions or steal personal information.

Español

bajo peso: condición de un peso corporal demasiado bajo en comparación con otras personas del mismo sexo y edad.

grasa no saturada: tipo de grasa que se encuentra en alimentos de origen vegetal; es líquida a temperatura ambiente.

espectador activo: persona que reconoce cuando un comportamiento es incorrecto, toma medidas para intervenir y detener el comportamiento, y promueve un cambio positivo; también denominado un *aliado*.

útero: órgano muscular hueco que alberga al bebé en desarrollo hasta que nace.

vacunación: proceso de introducir un patógeno muerto o una parte no tóxica de un patógeno en el cuerpo para provocar una respuesta inmune la cual previene una determinada enfermedad; también denominada *inmunización*.

vacuna: sustancia que contiene un patógeno muerto o una parte no tóxica de un patógeno; introducido en el cuerpo para provocar una respuesta inmune.

vagina: estructura en forma de tubo forrada con una membrana húmeda que sirve como canal de parto.

anillo vaginal: dispositivo anticonceptivo flexible con forma de anillo insertado en la vagina; libera hormonas para detener la ovulación.

valores: cualidades o prioridades que uno considera importantes.

válvulas: colgajos de tejido que controlan el flujo de sangre en el corazón.

vandalismo: destrucción deliberada o daño a la propiedad de otra persona.

dispositivos de vapeo: productos de tabaco que calientan tabaco o nicotina sintética sin quemarlo, produciendo un aerosol.

conducto deferente: tubo que transporta esperma desde el epidídimo hasta el pene.

vasectomía: procedimiento quirúrgico que corta o bloquea los conductos deferentes, evitando permanentemente el embarazo.

venas: vasos sanguíneos que llevan sangre del resto del cuerpo de regreso al corazón.

comunicación verbal: uso de palabras, habladas o escritas, para enviar un mensaje.

comportamiento violento: uso intencional de acciones o palabras que causan o amenazan causar daño a una persona u objeto.

carga viral: cantidad de virus de inmunodeficiencia humana (VIH) en la sangre.

virus: fragmento de código informático que cambia la forma en que funciona un dispositivo digital para interrumpir funciones o robar información personal.

English

viruses: pathogens that invade cells and direct them to create more viruses.

visualization: relaxation technique that involves imagining one's self in a pleasant environment.

vitamins: organic nutrients that promote growth and development, help regulate body processes, maintain healthy skin, and help the body release energy.

volatile organic compounds (VOCs): chemicals found in paint, varnish, cleaning supplies, and other sources; evaporate in the air.

W

warm-up: activity that prepares the body for physical activity; gets blood pumping to the muscles and stretches muscles.

water-soluble vitamins: type of vitamin that dissolves in water; are used immediately by the body or removed during urination.

weapon: any object used to cause damage to an object or person.

weight stigma: flawed belief that having a thinner body or lower weight is always better.

well-being: person's ability to function positively and overall satisfaction that life's present conditions are good.

wellness: process of identifying one's state of health and taking steps to improve it.

withdrawal: (1) negative symptoms that develop when a person with a physical dependence stops using a substance; (2) contraceptive method that involves pulling the penis out of the vagina before ejaculation.

world health: health of human populations around the world.

Y

young adulthood: developmental stage between 20 and 40 years of age.

Z

zygote: fertilized egg.

Español

virus: patógenos que invaden las células y las dirigen para crear más virus.

visualización: técnica de relajación que implica imaginarse a uno mismo en un ambiente agradable.

vitaminas: nutrientes orgánicos que promueven el crecimiento y el desarrollo, ayudan a regular los procesos corporales, mantienen una piel sana y ayudan al cuerpo a liberar energía.

compuestos orgánicos volátiles (volatile organic compounds, VOC): químicos encontrados en pintura, barniz, productos de limpieza y otras fuentes; se evaporan en el aire.

calentamiento: actividad que prepara al cuerpo para la actividad física; hace que se bombee sangre a los músculos y estira los músculos.

vitaminas solubles en agua: tipos de vitaminas que se disuelven en el agua; el cuerpo las utiliza de inmediato o se eliminan con la orina.

arma: cualquier objeto usado para causar daño a un objeto o persona.

estigma de peso: creencia errónea de que tener un cuerpo más delgado o un peso más bajo siempre es mejor.

plenitud: capacidad de una persona para funcionar de forma positiva y satisfacción general de que las condiciones actuales de la vida son buenas.

bienestar: proceso de identificar el estado de salud y tomar medidas para mejorarlo.

abstinencia/retiro: (1) síntomas negativos que se desarrollan cuando una persona con una dependencia física deja de usar una sustancia; (2) método anticonceptivo que consiste en sacar el pene de la vagina antes de la eyaculación

salud mundial: salud de las poblaciones humanas en todo el mundo.

adulto joven: etapa de desarrollo entre 20 y 40 años.

cigoto: óvulo fertilizado.

Index

Note: Page numbers followed by *f* indicate figures.

B

C

D

E

F

G

H

M

N

O

P

Q

R

S

T

U

V

W

Y

Z